Natural Healing *for* Bipolar Disorder

A Compendium of Nutritional Approaches

Eva Edelman

Borage Books
Eugene, Oregon, USA

NATURAL HEALING FOR BIPOLAR DISORDER: A COMPENDIUM OF NUTRITIONAL APPROACHES
by Eva Edelman

First edition, March, 2009
Published by BORAGE BOOKS

For information contact:
BORAGE BOOKS, 3003 WEST 11TH AVE, #144, EUGENE, OR 97402, USA
tel: (541) 683-8720
email: msgs@boragebooks.com
web: www.boragebooks.com

Foreword by Abram Hoffer, MD, PhD

Illustrated by Eva Edelman

PUBLISHER'S CATALOGING IN PUBLICATION DATA
Edelman, Eva
Natural healing for bipolar disorder: A compendium of nutritional approaches / Eva Edelman — 1st ed.
x, 382p. : ill. ; 28cm. ;
Includes bibliographical references, glossary and index.
ISBN 978-0-9650976-0-4 pbk.
1. Manic-depressive illness — Treatment. 2. Manic-depressive illness — Nutritional aspects. 3. Affective disorders — Treatment. 4. Mental illness — Nutritional aspects. 5. Orthomolecular therapy. 6. Alternative medicine. 7. Vitamin therapy.
RC516
616.895--dc22

The author welcomes any comments, additions, critiques, or relevant experiences sent c/o BORAGE BOOKS.

For ordering information, see page 378.

Printed and bound in the United States of America
Printed on recycled, acid-free paper

Acknowledgments

Warmest thanks to the following individuals for their generous gifts of time and information: Abram Hoffer, MD, PhD, William J Walsh, PhD, Michael Lesser, MD, Hyla Cass, MD, Joan Matthews Larson, PhD, Bradford S Weeks, MD, Maggie McClure, DC, and Andrew Cutler, PhD. And to all researchers, physicians, and natural health practitioners devoted to the development and perpetuation of effective and humane therapies for the mentally ill.

Warmest thanks also to Dan Stradford, Gayle Brown, Katya Blissenbach, Dev Rana, PhD, Barbara Eisenhardt, Steve DeLang, David Moyer, LCSW, Tom Lane, Alan Darman, Nancy Raymond, MS, Chris Foulke, Michelangelo Markus, Maureen, Valerie, Mary McCollough, RN, Ellen Klowden, Roberta Aronson, MSW, and everyone else who has offered insights, inspiration, support, warmth, or encouragement over these past seven years.

And from the bottom of my heart, thank you to my children, Eartha and Enoch, my brother, Martin, and my good friend, David, for their love.

This book is written
in loving memory
of my mother
Louise Edelman

Disclaimer

As in most human endeavors, particularly in the field of medicine, information held to be fact today often later proves inaccurate or incomplete. Research into the brain's functioning, and its effect on mood, along with the role played by nutrition, is ongoing, and new perspectives are constantly evolving. Thus the material in this book should be considered subject to revision, as new information is uncovered. And, although every effort has been made to insure accuracy, please do not assume this material, nor the author's presentation, for that matter, is entirely free of error or omission.

Since each individual is biochemically unique, no book can rightly take the place of informed medical diagnosis and treatment. This book provides general information and should in no way be construed as specific clinical advice. None of the material herein is to be taken as diagnosis or prescription for any mental or physical illness, as a directive concerning any particular form of treatment, or as an endorsement of any particular product or service. It is presented solely for educational purposes and does not constitute treatment recommendations for the nonclinician.

Neither the author, editor, publisher, distributor, nor any related party can take responsibility for the results of any experimentation with the therapies described. Not do they make make any claims or recommendations concerning them. For the origin of any claims, check the references.

There is always a risk in treating any medical condition. Bipolar disorder is frought with life-endangering risk, whatever the treatment, or lack of it, for that matter. This book is not to be construed as advice on whether to take, or alter intake, of psychiatric (or any other) medications. If you have an affective disorder, or any other medical or psychiatric condition, please seek the services of a knowledgeable physician. In some cases, this will be an orthomolecular, naturopathic, or other nutritionally-oriented physician. Any questions or concerns should be brought to your physician.

How to use this book

This book describes nutrients and other natural approaches sometimes used in bipolar therapy or explored in the research. It is generally structured, as follows:

Contents overview

Part I: Nutrients
— Mania & Stabilization
— Mania & Depression
— Depression

Part II: Biotypes
— Pyrrole Disorder
— Methylation imbalances

Part III: Toxins
— Metals
— Other toxins

Part IV: Health

Part V: Lifestyle

Part VI: Related disorders

Page content

General overview:

☐ **THE LARGE INTERIOR COLUMNS** — describe influences of nutrients, biotype, and health status on mood and mental health.

☐ **THE CALLOUT** — contains quotes, anecdotes, interesting tidbits, and some relevant studies.

Technical information:

☐ **"CONSIDERATIONS" BOX** — contains information on nutrient functions and sources, symptoms, susceptible populations, lab tests, contraindications, etc.

☐ **OTHER BOXES** — contain such information as:
— the role of nutrients in brain biochemistry
— some related health issues
— limited comparisons to pharmaceuticals

Study this material

This material distills the essence from years of work by many individuals, who have devoted their lives to the search for effective and nontoxic treatments for mental illness. It is necessarily dense, and needs to be studied thoroughly to be absorbed. The reader may want to approach this as a reference, and start with sections of greatest personal interest.

Table of Contents

Continued on next page

Table of Contents *Continued*

Foreword

Orthomolecular psychiatry

I have been practicing psychiatry since 1950. I started out as an orthodox psychiatrist. We were more or less left on our own in Saskatchewan, and depended on observations made by previous psychiatrists. Patients diagnosed schizophrenic or manic depressive (now called bipolar) rarely recovered. We had palliative treatment only.

In the 1950's, as antipsychotics started to take hold in North America, we were developing the adrenochrome hypothesis. This logically led to the use of large doses of vitamins B3 and C for treating schizophrenia. We introduced the first double blind placebo-controlled trials to psychiatry. These showed that adequately large doses of B3 doubled the two year-recovery rate. Our research expanded with the help of Linus Pauling, Roger Williams, and other esteemed colleagues, into what is now called orthomolecular psychiatry.

Our present recovery rate is eighty to ninety percent, except for very chronic and abused patients immobilized by the drugs they have been given. My definition of recovery includes paying income tax, often along with practicing excellent medicine, writing magnificent poetry, or otherwise reaching toward one's potential.

Edelman's book

Since the early days of our research, the rapidly developing field of orthomolecular medicine has uncovered intricate and profound connections between nutrients and brain function. Thus specific conditions respond best to a complex of nutrients, while nutrients have numerous clinical properties and are therapeutic for multiple conditions (e.g., the niacin used for schizophrenia, may concurrently improve arthritis, hypercholesterolemia, etc.).

Books which gather, digest, and make understandable this now massive body of research are essential. This compendium by Edelman is just such a book, chock full of useful information for patient and physician alike.

Edelman's book is directed at bipolar psychoses but, in my opinion, applies to all psychiatric disorders, as most are expressions of underlying biochemical/ nutritional factors. It serves as one of the major references on the role of nutrients in mental health.

It reminds me of the compendiums released each year by Big Pharma, with the critical difference being that this compendium describes the value of a large number of nutrients, essential to health, and comprises the subject matter of orthomolecular medicine, while Pharma's compendiums are all about the toxicity and danger of drugs. The tragedy is that the drug compendiums are widely distributed and the negative information therein often ignored. It would be a major gift to humanity if this excellent compendium were distributed as widely, and attended to.

Current choices

Around 1954, the antipsychotic drugs discovered in France reached North America. These drugs were very effective in controlling undesirable behavior. Control was misinterpreted as recovery, leading to massive discharge of patients from inadequate mental hospitals, reputedly "cured."

The drugs defined the new psychiatry, which has been stuck in the same paradigm ever since. Billions of dollars and many physician lifetimes have been consumed in research comparing the original drugs with the latest incarnations, only to show that the new drugs are neither appreciably better nor more effective than the old ones (though sometimes more toxic). But they are more expensive, and have made the drug companies rich beyond measure.

Everyone has benefitted except the patients, their families, and society, which has the burden of looking after millions of people trapped in their illness. Dr Bernard Rimland dubbed this "toximolecular" psychiatry — a term seconded by Linus Pauling.

A case in point: Antipsychotic drugs are prescribed to vast numbers of unfortunate patients worldwide, including many bipolars. They have the following side effects: tardive dyskinesia and other neurological disease, deterioration of brain function, permanent social incapacity, tranquilizer psychosis, metabolic syndrome (diabetes, high blood cholesterol, high triglycerides, morbid obesity), and cardiovascular complications. They play a substantial role in untold broken marriages and homes, addictions to street drugs and alcohol, homelessness, welfare dependence, suicides, homicides, and imprisonments. And the recovery rate is less than ten percent, as tranquilizers complicate the natural psychosis by superimposing on it the psychosis induced by the drug.

Why would any intelligent society preferentially mandate such drugs when nontoxic alternatives are available that are safe and effective?

Consider the following anecdote, as written by my patient, Miss LH, and printed with her permission:

Recovery from Bipolar Psychosis, by Miss LH

I was diagnosed with bipolar disorder nine years ago, when I was seventeen years old. I always knew I was "different." As a child, I had severe night terrors, unexplained stomachaches, irritable rages that would appear out of nowhere and be gone just as suddenly, a constant restlessness prevalent hyperactivity — there were days that I don't think I ever sat still for more than five minutes. I remember staying up all night reading with a flashlight from the time I was five years old, sleeping maybe two hours at most, but never feeling tired. And then there were days when I couldn't seem to wake up, and would sleep twenty hours or more. At school I was always a good student, but would finish my work quickly, then become easily bored and somewhat disruptive.

I have always experienced extremes of emotion. I could go from laughter to tears in a second… smiling and happy to irritable and raging in the blink of an eye… completely agitated and unable to sit still, then catatonic ten minutes later.

My mood swings typically involved major fluctuations in energy levels, and increased sensitivity. Normal lights would seem too bright and I would quite often wear sunglasses indoors. The radio, the TV, people talking or shuffling papers, the hum of the refrigerator or the fluorescent lights would be too loud, and might drive me to the edge of insanity.

When in a crowd, I'd hear little pieces of every single conversation going on around me all at once, all overlapping together. When manic (or mixed), and running on high speed, I could listen to five conversations simultaneously without losing focus. I'd sometimes listen to the radio, watch TV, talk on the phone and read or write — all at once! And if I didn't stay busy enough, I couldn't keep my mind under control and it would escape without me into another reality. This can all be very tiring, with every day feeling like three.

When depressed, I had no motivation or physical energy to do anything. I'd become completely nonfunctional, and could barely take care of myself. Doing laundry or washing dishes could reduce me in seconds to a puddle of tears on the floor. Then I'd feel guilty, and the negative voices in my mind would start to take over, telling me that I'm a horrible, worthless person who can't do anything right.

I suffered agoraphobia — especially when I needed to go out by myself. I was scared of being alone in a crowd in case it became too much for me to handle and I was unable to get out of a potentially awkward and embarrassing social situation. Grocery shopping, or crossing the road became very difficult; taking the bus, impossible. Running simple & necessary errands became overwhelming.

On top of that, the instability of my moods was challenging for me and others to deal with. I became very socially isolated. And I couldn't concentrate, consistently attend classes, hold a job, or even eat or sleep regularly.

The prognosis for severe bipolar I with psychosis is generally not very good — I often felt I had little to look forward to in life; I was constantly trying to survive the chronic symptoms of depression & mania, mixed states & psychosis and, at times, rapid cycling through all these moods.

I was doing the best I could to function, and constantly trying to become more independent and strive for stability to improve the basic quality of my life. But the rapid and extreme mood swings were becoming unmanageable, and all too easily sent me into a state of crisis; and they were getting progressively worse. When I became severely suicidal and started having hallucinations, I was forced to seek help.

Unfortunately, I would not find the stability I wanted and desperately needed for eight long years.

I was eventually prescribed almost every major drug that can be used for a mood disorder. Sometimes I would improve slightly for a few weeks, only to plateau and then end up worse off than before. Other times, the drugs wouldn't even make a difference — or they aggravated my mood swings and caused more severe episodes, which they were supposed to prevent. And the physical side effects — the dizziness, grogginess, nausea, clumsiness, poor balance, etc. — made me very sick, made life even more difficult, and caused a lot of stress and anxiety.

For a while, the medications were allegedly "working" — at least, my doctors told me that I finally seemed normal to them. However, I was sluggish and depressed; I could barely stay awake eight hours a day. My white blood cell count was always abnormally elevated and I had week-long flu symptoms every month — yet my doctors were unable to find any infection or other explanation. Although they could see my overall health deteriorating rapidly, they were primarily concerned with treating my mood disorder, despite the fact that their meds were making me physically sicker every day.

My doctors had tried many of the prescription drugs several times in the course of my treatment, in every combination imaginable, yet nothing seemed to work the way they thought it would, so they started to give up on me. The only solution they could offer was heavy tranquilizers/antipsychotics. The antipsychotics seemed to make my doctors feel more comfortable, since I was too groggy to show any sign of emotion. But they were torture for me — it's like being buried alive: your mind is still racing but you can barely lift your head, let alone communicate the ideas that are flying by. You are doing some of the basic things you need to do in life, but trapped in a shell of a body, looking out at the outside world, not able to truly live.

I'd always been told to weigh the benefits and risks of taking the medications compared to those of living with this disorder. The message I got from the majority of the medical community was that ANYTHING was better than living with a mental illness. I wasn't expected to "compromise," I was expected to sacrifice my basic quality of life!

The compounded side effects of the drugs became more and more severe over time, while any helpful results have always quickly disappeared. I am still suffering some toxic effects — even from some I stopped taking years ago. However my doctors continued to insist that this was the best course of treatment.

My mood was never stabilized longer than a few weeks. And I worried that eventually the meds would have left me too sedated to live independently and I would require full-time care. I wondered how these drugs could be "helping" me to have a better life.

Finally the psychiatrists ran out of ideas. Several specialists refused to see me since I did not respond to medications the way they thought I should. And I was so sick I couldn't stand to be alive. But I wasn't ready to die — so I started to look for alternatives. I kept telling myself there had to be another way.

That's when I started seeing Dr. Hoffer and taking the large doses of vitamins and supplements he prescribed. I had already been taking some vitamins, but he was able to provide proper guidance for a treatment plan personalized for my bipolar symptoms. I still remember the first time I met him. He respectfully listened to everything I had to say and proceeded to tell me with confidence that he thought he could help, though he warned me, there are no "quick fixes" in this world; it would take time to get me well.

After all these years of trying to find a way to survive and manage my illness I was done looking for "easy" solutions, because they had only served to make my life much harder. I had been told the medications would help within a month but, instead, every month for the past eight years, my severe episodes had only been getting progressively more severe.

But now, my routine of therapeutic doses of vitamins, a reduced stress lifestyle, acupuncture, & other coping skills are allowing me to finally live virtually symptom-free. The extremes of mood have been eliminated, although I still have some minor episodes. My life overall is becoming more manageable. For the first time, I feel an overwhelming sense of hope & acceptance for who I am. For the first time in a long time I don't feel "crazy" and out-of-control. And it's a really nice feeling.

Until this past year, I had to choose between severe agitation & psychosis, or major sedation leaving me unable to pour a glass of water. To me, that is not an acceptable "choice" to be forced to make about your life — it's not a way to live.

Now, it's like waking up out of a coma, after eight years... Even though I was walking around, going through the motions of life — I wasn't living.

I have never felt this alive before — the colors in the world are all brighter somehow... the trees are shades of green that I don't remember seeing before... I can laugh again, and smile... and actually feel happy. I don't remember the last time I really felt happy — certainly it was before I was on any medication.

These changes started within a few months of beginning the holistic treatment of vitamins, etc. and steadily lowering my medications. So far I have had no major episodes and have been able to function much better than when I was heavily medicated.

I also haven't felt this physically healthy in years. My white blood cell count is finally within normal, and I've hardly been sick at all. I hadn't realized how sick I had been until my body started to recover and regain strength — what it would be like to not feel nauseous every day, or to live without the constant fog over my brain that didn't allow me to think or see the world clearly, or to walk without constantly stumbling and falling.

The past year has been one of the best I can remember — although I'm not completely "better" because recovery is a slow process — I am definitely well on my way to a happier & healthier life!

I am on the least amount of medication I have taken since first beginning treatment, yet I have made such great progress that many of my doctors are dumbfounded.

I think I have changed more than anyone could have ever imagined or even hoped for. And everyone around me is so relieved.

I am closer to having a real life than I have ever been. The stability that has constantly eluded me, despite heavy medications, is now within reach. I can FEEL emotions, instead of being completely numb and dead to the world like I used to be when I was taking the drugs.

The proof for me that Dr. Hoffer's advice & expertise have been significantly beneficial to me lies in the fact that I was finally able to finish my University degree, and am starting to slowly get back into the work force. This time, last year, my doctors were struggling (unsuccessfully) to keep me out of the hospital and alive.

I wish this information had been available to me when I was younger and first went for treatment, because it's what has saved me. I have no doubt that without this routine of vitamins and supportive therapies, I would be struggling to find stability for an indefinite amount of time, if not my entire life…

Now, I finally feel like my life is worth living — and I wonder how I managed to make it this far without that feeling. I have learnt that everything can change…

Without the medication side effects, and without a constantly unstable mood, it's as though a great weight has been lifted from my shoulders

I think stability is not a lack of chaos — rather, it is an inner peace that is found within the midst of natural chaos. I try to treasure the balance that is making its way into my life, and I am slowly finding my peace.

Thank you, Dr. Hoffer, for helping me to get my life back — the way I was meant to live: happy & stable.

Comment

This is the sort of feedback I would like every therapist to experience. This excellent compendium will help make this possible. I endorse this book for the good it will do for patients. I think that every patient who values his or her own health and the health of others should educate themselves with the information gathered into this useful volume. This knowledge may save their lives.

Orthomolecular treatment of patients is also beneficial to the physicians who treat them. Practicing medicine is a very stressful occupation. The degree of stress depends to a large degree on the recovery rates of patients being treated. Several doctors who had planned to retire because they found the stress so severe learned orthomolecular medicine. When they began to see the results they immediately gave up any plan do so and were much more cheerful. There is nothing as satisfying to a healer as seeing what was considered a hopelessly ill patient recover.

And usually doctors who see the beneficial effects of the nutrients start taking them. They too will feel better and live longer.

— Abram Hoffer MD PhD FRCP (C) RNCP
October, 2008

Introduction

Causes & old paradigms

"Any psychiatrist using nutrients is forced to accept that they are involved in the causes."

Abram Hoffer MD, PhD

"I give my critics full credit for having delayed the introduction of orthomolecular medicines into the medical world, and for having denied life, health and happiness for innumerable patients. Supporters of old paradigms never realize how much damage they do by... [rigid] adherence to old theories."

Abram Hoffer MD, PhD
Father of orthomolecular medicine

"Why nutrition is the way forward"

"Drugs are foreign to the body's natural biochemistry and thus produce side effects. Nutrients are part of us, so side effects are minimal, rarely lethal... Vitamins, amino acids, and trace elements existed ever since cells began to congregate to form tissues, and tissues organize to form skin, glands, muscles, bones, and nerves. Nutrients were in beneficial biochemical action before mind ever formed thought or tongues touched teeth to speak... "

Carl C Pfeiffer, PhD, MD

The future

"The present medical focus on drug therapy may not pass the test of time. It is entirely possible that future progress in molecular biology may elucidate the basic mechanisms and causes of most diseases. It seems likely that the next century's treatments will implement natural body chemicals that restore the patient to a normal condition, rather than drugs that result in an abnormal condition."

William J Walsh, PhD

1. Why nutrients

"[I was grateful for] *the calming, soothing effect of the vitamins. They seemed to go to the root of the problem, to the fibre of my mind and body...*

"[Vitamins create a] *physical feeling of solidity at one's very core — so different from the hollowness, the vacuum experienced during the illness."*

Patient recovering under orthomolecular treatment

"[With vitamins] your body says, in essence, 'Thanks for enabling me to make the enzyme which will get me out of trouble.' [To the drug, it says]... 'You've blocked my ability to make that enzyme and... I need that enzyme so what can I do now?'"

Robert Atkins, MD

"When in doubt, try nutrition first."

Roger J Williams, PhD

"What if some psychiatric patients could be treated with inexpensive vitamins and minerals rather than expensive patented pharmaceuticals? Or what if some doses of psychiatric drugs could be reduced by the concurrent use of nutrients?"

Charles W Popper, MD, 2001

Natural therapies

More than half a century of medical research and clinical practice have created a flood of information on the role of nutrients in psychiatric function, and have been accompanied by recovery or great improvement in tens of thousands of patients.

Bipolar research to-date suggests significant, cumulative long-term benefit, markedly more sustainable than with pharmaceuticals alone. Such work merits careful consideration. This book is offered as a compendium and guide to these emerging approaches, in the hope of educating the public, facilitating physician access to the material, and stimulating further medical investigations.

The brain depends on nutrition

Since brain cells are made of nutrients, and run on nutrients, the potency of nutrients in bipolar therapy should not be suprising. After all, nutrients directly influence how our genetics manifests.

Supplying depleted nutrients, and eliminating substances, stresses, and disorders which interfere with function, gives the brain the raw materials of healing. Thus, Patrick Quillin, PhD, (1987) notes that the brain needs amino acids, vitamin and mineral cofactors, EFAs, and phospholipids to construct neurotransmitters (which communicate messages from one nerve cell to another), receptors (gatekeepers to the cell), and second messengers (which carry transmitter information into the cell); also, appropriately balanced electrolytes (minerals) to accurately convey messages along the neural axon. Moreover, the brain depends on nutrients in the body which metabolize food into glucose, and then demands 25% of that glucose, along with those nutrients which turn it into energy, and which maintain cellular energetics. The brain also usurps at least 20% of the oxygen available to the body, plus nutrients which support its transport and use. Nutrients are also crucial in protecting the brain from free radicals, heavy metals, allergens, toxins and microbes; and in maintaining healthy function in other body systems serving the brain. Hence, a reasonable therapeutic goal might be an optimal diet, plus optimal relevant supplementation, and elimination of that which is harmful.

Sustainability of nutrients (LARSON 2001, WALSH 2006, KIDD 2004, PFEIFFER 1987, 88)

Factors promoting the sustainability of an accurately-tailored nutritive approach (or nutrients augmenting meds):

□ Nutrients nourish brain and body, and are, *by definition*, required for viability and healthy function.

□ Nutrients usually work synergistically (consider, the multi-nutrient combos in healthy food).

□ Most (but not all*) nutrients produce a *gradual* improvement, reducing the risk of triggering a new episode.

□ Once requirements are established, therapy is usually furthered by continued intake. If "tolerance" to a nutrient seems to occur,** response can readily be reestablished.***

□ Over time, appropriate nutrients often enable lower doses of concurrent meds, and may, as well, afford protection from some of the side effects, thereby decreasing damage due to chronic drug treatment, and increasing therapeutic efficacy.

* Exceptions usually involve the more acutely potent nutrients, e.g., SAMe, phenylalanine, etc., especially high doses, or if not indicated.

** As when ongoing high doses reduce absorption or effectiveness.

*** E.g., by stopping that nutrient for a day or so, while temporarily substituting a nutrient with similar benefits. (Note: Not appropriate before episodes tend to start, if rapid cycling, or with other mood instability.)

Bipolar outcome

Some preliminary indications of nutritional outcome

Critical single nutrients

A number of small controlled or double blind studies *restricted to single critical nutrients* (e.g., omega 3, various aminos, magnesium, vitamin C, etc.) have suggested considerable improvement, often comparable to pharmaceuticals short-term, and with a better profile long-term. Not all isolated nutrients will be as effective. Studies are referred to throughout Part I of this book. (See, for instance: Kay 1984, Heiden 1999, Stoll 1999, Poldinger 1991)

Outcome with multiple nutrients

Clinical results suggest *multiple nutrients,* accurately tailored to individual biochemical requirements, *can compound the benefit significantly.* Thus, data on affectives who fit certain "biotypes" suggest remarkable success:

□ In a depression* outcome study by Dr. William J Walsh, PhD, President, Walsh Research Institute, 60% of 200 depressives experienced major improvement (contrast this to the 25% or less reported with pharmaceuticals); another 32%, partial improvement. Overall, two-thirds improved to the extent that they were able to discontinue or reduce meds. (WALSH 1997, 2006) (Of course, unipolar results are not always applicable to bipolars. (COMPTON 2001))

□ From accumulated data on over 1800 bipolars, given at least 90 lab assays each, Walsh reports that of the approximately 80% of bipolars with biotype imbalances, 70% of those who stuck with the nutrient program (always an issue with bipolars) improved significantly; and 50% of those treated recovered to the extent that they no longer required medication.* Results were best when biotype treatment was begun early. This may represent the best well-substantiated bipolar outcome thus far, whatever the treatment, either nutritionally or pharmaceutically-based.(WALSH 2007, 08)

* Important: Reductions in medication are *not even considered til after at least 3-4 months of biotype therapy.* Subsequently, if indicated, reductions are prescribed in *gradual steps, tied to nutritive healing.* See: *If dose reduction is indicated,* p. 289).

□ Dr Michael Lesser, MD, one of the early orthomolecular pioneers, similarly finds nutrient treatment addressing biotype, other nutrient imbalances, blood sugar, allergies, immune status, etc, is successful in up to 85% of bipolars, "as long as the patient is dedicated to following treatment, and the family, supportive." He states: "If they really cooperate, a tremendous amount can be done. Most can eventually go off medication. Others need minimal maintenance, but can work, go to school and do fine. Even if patients become frustrated, stop therapy, and go downhill, the overall outcome is still better than if they hadn't tried at all, because they have had the experience of the temporary gains." (LESSER 2008)

On the degree of improvement

"Patients get well to a degree not seen by [mainstream] therapists, [many of whom] believe that orthomolecular therapists are prone to exaggeration. Those [who actually see] the results are astonished."

Abram Hoffer, MD, PhD

Dual diagnosis outcome (LARSON 2008)

Joan Larson, PhD, is the founder of Health Recovery Center in Minnesota, which mainly serves clients with alcohol or substance abuse (ubiquitous in bipolars). HRC results with dual diagnosis bipolars (usually primary alcoholism/addictions, secondary mood disorder) suggest attention biotype, hypoglycemia,* etc., plus nutrients to counter addictions (often IV), along with psychosocial support, improves virtually all accompanying mood symptoms. Larson states, "Once you find the nutrients which address the patient's unique genetics,** symptoms just seem to melt away." She finds that bipolars almost always improve and, in the course of the six weeks of therapy, are usually able to wean from psych meds.*** She says, "It never fails to astound me how fast it works." The earlier treatment can be instituted, the better the results.****

For a summary of Larson's protocol for bipolars, see p. 18.

* Which is highly prevalent, especially with very rapid cycling.

** Suggested by symptom and response history for individual and family members, confirmed with labs.

*** Often through IV therapies (e.g., for benzo withdrawal, IV taurine-C-glutathione, perhaps B, etc.; plus oral GABA and other nutrients, *as relevant*).

**** But note: Bipolar disorder secondary to alcoholism may be milder, and respond more readily (if alcoholism can be resolved) than primary bipolar disorder. (See *How alcoholism manifests,* p. 186.)

Drugs & nutrients are not mutually exclusive

"To me a bipolar patient who becomes "well" with greatly-reduced medication requirements has achieved complete success. I don't believe that medication doses need to go to zero, as long as side effects are absent and long-term effects are minimal or absent." — William J Walsh, PhD, 2006

"Management of bipolar disorder is at a turning point. The pathophysiology, risk factors, and treatment modalities are now sufficiently well clarified to enable a broader integrative approach… Because [it] remains such a challenging condition to treat, dogmatic adherence to either a purely pharmaceutical approach or a purely "alternative" approach is not tenable. Patients… are so vulnerable to setbacks from environmental risk factors that effective management demands lifestyle and dietary reform and stress reduction. Pharmaceuticals still have an important role… but preferably in conjunction with comprehensive dietary supplementation. Nutrients [provide] their own benefits [and] can also facilitate effective drug activity at lower dosages and help guard against the adverse effects associated with these potent pharmaceuticals." — Paris M Kidd, PhD, 2004

Importance of preventing early episodes

"It doesn't matter how you get manic, it's that the brain has seen mania." — Terrence Ketter, MD, 2000

Once mania first occurs, *whatever the cause,* 90-95% of people go on to further mood episodes. That's why bipolar I is identified by a single manic episode. (WINOKUR 1969, TOHEN 1990).

Cumulative episodes increase deterioration. Each mania increases the risk of more episodes, closer together, and progressively more severe. *Thus, preventing early episodes improves outcome.* (MASTERS 1996, GOLDBERG 1999B)

Functional outcome (mainstream)

During an episode, job loss is at least 80%. (WINOKUR 1969) After, especially after mania, (HARROW 1990) work and schooling often suffer. (CORYELL 1993) Three to five years later, 15-73% are unemployed, or working at reduced status. (CORYELL 1989, 90, 93, TOHEN 1990A, 2000AB, KLERMAN 1992, CARLSON 1974, DION 1988)

Subclinical symptoms continue in many, (GITLIN 1995, KELLER 1992, TOHEN 1990) creating chronic psychosocial difficulties (BELLACK 1989, LARSON) (e.g., social withdrawal, discontent, family discord) in one to two-thirds; (MACQUEEN 2001, O'CONNELL 1991, HASTINGS 1958, CARLSON 1974, BRATFOS HAUG 1968, CORYELL 1989, 99, TOHEN 2000AB) 90% of marriages end in divorce. (MARANO, 2005)

RECOMMENDED READING:
Cass Hyla, MD, *Supplement Your Prescription,* 2007

Warning: This material is in no way intended as a directive on the use of pharmaceuticals. Such decisions often entail life-or-death repercussions. With any concerns, speak with your physician.

Outcome with pharmaceuticals alone

Orthodox treatment offers an estimated additional ten years of effective activity at work, school, and family life, nine years of normal health, after which function diminishes. (GELENBERG 1993)

Over the past 60 years, bipolar incidence has steadily increased, (GERSHON 1987, KLERMAN 1992) and symptoms have become more severe, (WOLPERT 1990) and more drug-resistant. (KIDD 2004) The median number of lifetime episodes used to be ten, (GOLD 1987) but has increased considerably. Bipolars can now spend up to one-fifth of their lives in mood episodes, (ANGST 2000) generally more depressed than manic. (HADDAD 2002, BRIGHAM 2001) Rapid cycling and very rapid cycling have become prevalent, as have mixed episodes. (Thus, in one study of 570 affectives, very rapid mood cycling did not occur in 1960, became apparent in 1975, and prevalent in 1985. (WOLPERT 1990)) Psychotic mania is also increasing. Such changes usually represent an exacerbation of the illness, making it more difficult to treat. (Also see, *Functional outcome,* at left.)

Certainly, the modern proliferation of junk food, substance abuse, and environmental pollution contribute to the deteriorating statistics. (KIDD 2004) Nonetheless, pharmaceuticals cannot be presumed without blame. Thus, though antidepressants do pull many bipolars back from the brink of death, at some point, they trigger mania in an estimated 30-50%, may also increase depression, and significantly increase the risk of rapid cycling. (KETTER 2001, FRYE, KETTER 2001, POST 2003, BRIGHAM 2001) Medications for hyperactivity (which pervades childhood histories of bipolars) pose similar risk. (BRIGHAM 2001, FRYE 2000) Some researchers also question the repercussions of significant use of antipsychotics (even atypicals). (WHYBROW 1997, BRIGHAM 2001) Moreover, bipolars who withdraw from such meds, may be beset with a particularly persistent rebound, further destabilizing mood, and often resulting in unending prescriptions. (GOLD 1987, RICHMAN 1992)

Mood stabilizers, on the other hand, seem to afford most bipolars years to decades of relative respite. Unfortunately, with enough time, potency tends to wane; or cycling may be pushed toward depression or mania. Higher doses and drug cocktails may then be instituted, but also, for many patients, eventually lose potency, while adverse effects increase, perhaps including intense manias which break through the tranquilization and further destabilize mood. (FRYE, KETTER 2001, MOLLER 2003, TRIMBLE 1996, KUKOPULOS 1995, MAJ 1989, POST 1990, 93AB, 95, 99, WERRY 1991, GILLBERG 1993, SWANN 1997, DENICOFF 1997, GELENBERG 1989, O'CONNELL 1991, SARANTIDIS 1981, WEISS 1995) Many patients thus become unresponsive to medication, and much more difficult to treat by any method. (KETTER, FRYE 2001) (See p. 285-86.)

Hence, an increased interest in therapeutic use (often adjunctive) of omega 3, thyroid hormone, B complex, and other natural brain biochemicals.

Nutritional Research

A definitive cure for bipolar disorder remains elusive, whatever the treatment. Nonetheless, though further work is needed, nutritional research (noted throughout this book) is promising. Investigations have included:

Nutritional studies

□ Double blinds and other controlled studies — Mainstream and orthomolecular studies of key nutrients, taken alone,* or adjunctive to pharmaceuticals.

□ Outcome studies, usually for multiple nutrients, tailored to individual biotype requirements — these often involve extensive biochemical and nutritive data on blood, urine, and hair, correlated with psychiatric rating scales and clinical results. In a number of cases, nutrient treatment is discontinued,** and then resumed, providing an ABA (on, off, on) experimental design, in which patients serve as their own controls.

□ Other clinical data.

* Not necessarily reflecting optimal benefits, as the influence of each nutrient can be subtle, as compared to the results of a comprehensive nutrient protocol.

** Usually not deliberately depriving the patient, but due, for example, to the patient's economic constraints, or decisions to stop taking nutrients because they feel like they've recovered.

Research on related disorders, with implications for bipolars

□ Biotype research for related psychiatric conditions.

□ Other nutritional/herbal research on associated psychiatric conditions (e.g., GABA's effects on anxiety; valerian's benefit to insomnia, etc.).

□ Research on nutritional, herbal, and medical therapies for confounding physical conditions (thyroid disorder, allergy, Candida, sugar imbalance, neurotoxicity, etc.)

Supportive material

□ Anecdotal reports — obviously not proofs, but traditionally an inspiration for the development of numerous medications and other medical treatments.

□ Extrapolations from pharmaceutical studies to corresponding nutrients, suggesting therapeutic approaches for further investigation (thus, SSRI studies suggest looking at serotonin precursors (tryptophan or 5HTP); studies of benzodiazepines (which act on GABA receptors) focus attention on GABA; studies of CCBs, on magnesium (a natural CCB); etc.).

Limits to all bipolar research (both pharmaceutical & nutrient) (BAUER 1996, FRYE, KETTER 2001, BRIGHAM 2001)

Unfortunately, the very nature of bipolar illness poses problems in experimental design. Both pharmaceutical and nutritional studies are rarely definitive, because:

The cyclical nature of the illness obscures therapeutic effects (e.g., "improvements" may merely reflect a shift in the cycling pattern, etc.).

Manics may not cooperate, or even stay in the study. Moreover, patients often fail to report hypomania or mania so episodes may pass unnoted.

Bipolar vulnerability to stress (even mild stressors, or the study itself) may distort results.

Intricate interactions of treatment with individual biochemistry and health are difficult to control for.

Responsive subgroups are not readily distinguished. (What heals one patient may hurt another.)

Paucity of data on long-term outcome. Most studies are short, and so do not adequately account for the effects of cycling, of time lags before therapeutic benefit or rebound reactions emerge, etc.

Data on adverse effects is often lost due to the high drop-out rate common in pharmaceutical studies.*(HORROBIN 2002)

The effects of drugs, polypharmacy, (COMPTON 2001) and drug discontinuation (especially when abrupt) are not easily separated from effects of illness.**

The high cost of large double blinds largely shapes what is convincingly studied to proposals for which large pharmaceuticals companies and other wealthy concerns are willing to pay.*** (ABRAMSON 2004)

Moral considerations may restrict research, e.g., whether the proposed treatment (or lack of it in controls) might trigger a new episode, promote rapid cycling, or otherwise increase severity, or fatality). (COMPTON 2001)

In part to avoid such dilemnas, mainstream studies often compare a proposed medication to one already in use. This makes conclusions about the new drug dependent on the lack of flaws in studies of the original drug.

* Horrobin points out that 40-60% of subjects typically drop out of six-to-eight-week studies of psychiatric medications, mostly to avoid side effects; in one-year studies, 60-90%. Benefits are thus validated for only a small percentage of patients.

** For example, medication withdrawal in the course of a study, especially if abrupt, can produce rebounds easily mistaken for bipolar exacerbations. (Lithium, for instance, in many of the early studies, was abruptly withdrawn from controls (a practice now known to promote mania), thus distorting results. (Ketter 2001, Bauer, Gold 1987)

*** Abramson (2004) claims that studies financed by drug companies are five times more likely to find in favor of the company's drug of choice.

Evolving experimental designs (BAUER 1996, COMPTON 2001 FRYE 2001)

Because of such factors, (BAUER 1996) really well-controlled double blinds studying bipolar disorder are uncommon. (COMPTON 2001) (So, for instance, despite prior "controlled" double-blind research, decades passed before recognizing that significant antidepressant intake often fosters rapid cycling, or may otherwise worsen long-term outcome.) (POST 2003, KETTER, FRYE 2001)

Consequently, some mainstream researchers now recommend open, naturalistic, longitudinal studies. This type of design particularly lends itself to exploring how bipolars fare, long term, with multiple nutrients, tailored to health, diet, medication, evolving biochemistry, cycling pattern, etc.

Individualizing nutritional therapy

"Defective enzymes can be forced to function at normal levels with an increase of cofactors (vitamins) and activators (trace metals)."

Antonio J DeLiz, MD, PhD, 1979

"Individual patients will differ greatly in their treatment preferences and capacities, history of response to previous treatments, family history of treatment response, and tolerance for different side effects. Therefore, the experts first-line recommendations certainly will not be appropriate in all circumstances."

Peter M Whybrow, MD, 1997

Nutritional requirements vary widely from one person to another. Average requirements will not address everyone's needs, even assuming that the average has been correctly determined. Similarly, multivitamins are not universally helpful, and specific supplements which work for some, or even, most individuals, may not work for others.* The key is to discover exactly which nutrients and what doses each person uniquely requires.

Attention to the individual's unique biochemical profile is important, in identifying unique nutrient requirements and contraindications. For example, supplemental folic acid, DMAE, phenylalanine, copper, iron, methionine, SAMe, 5HTP, choline, inositol, glutamine, or certain other nutrients may reduce or increase symptoms, depending on whether they're actually needed or contraindicated. (PFEIFFER 1987, WALSH 2006)

Also see: *Fine tailoring therapy,* p. 290.

Biochemical individuality (WILLIAMS 1956)

Dr. Roger Williams, PhD, the pioneer of biochemical individuality research, points out that body parts sport a great variety of shapes, sizes, functions and strengths: lungs can have three lobes instead of two; hearts can be located in different parts of the chest; tolerance for sugar or protein can vary widely.

Nutritional individuality (WILLIAMS 1956)

Williams found the inherent need for specific vitamins often varies by a factor of 20, in some cases, 40. Mineral requirements are less varied, but need for calcium, for instance, can vary fourfold. Similarly, with food: one person can thrive on goat milk, another need to avoid all dairy; one may do well as a meat-eater, another as a vegetarian. Herbs affect people differently: valerian helps most people sleep, but stimulates others; kava sedates most, irritates some, etc.

Enzyme individuality

Enzymes mediate the biochemical reactions of the body. Enzymes are formed from nutrients. The quantity of enzymes available to different people can vary markedly, to the extent that some people do not have any appreciable quantity of a particular critical enzyme.* For example, people born with phenylketonuria (PKU) lack enzymes which change phenylalanine into tyrosine. (HOFFER 1973)

* Low levels can be due to: lack of nutritive components; metabolic error in its chemistry; interference with synthesis by toxins; inefficient transport; maladaptive response to the enzyme, etc. (Pfeiffer 1987)

Nutrient dependencies (HOFFER 1973, 74, 83, PFEIFFER, 1987)

Nutrient dependencies are chronic needs for large doses of particular nutrients. Orthomolecular physicians find people often recover from genetic disorders involving a lack of enzymes, when given optimal doses of corresponding nutrients, usually lifelong. Hoffer gives the following example: Genetic deficiency of enzymes which convert vitamin B3 to NAD,* can lead to depression, anxiety, or psychosis; while optimal doses of NAD's precursor (B3) and supportive nutrients (e.g., B6) encourage NAD formation, and symptom improvement.

Dependencies are not always genetic. Hoffer reports on the creation of dependencies for megadoses of B1 and B3 in soldiers subjected to severe malnutrition and stress as World War II POW's; dependency for B1, in many alcoholics; B6, in some who chronically eat too much milk and protein.

Most nutrient assays (and MDRs) are calibrated to average required levels and do not take possible dependencies into account. Assays of key enzymes which use that nutrient** can increase diagnostic sensitivity. (PFEIFFER 1987)

* A crucial enzyme in brain metabolism and respiration.
** Especially those which give some indication of being subfunctional.

Therapeutic implications

Thus, even if a finite number of biotype or other protocols roughly address most cases, treatment works best when fine-tuned to individual chemistry.

RECOMMENDED READING

Williams, Roger, PhD, *Biochemical Individuality,* 1956.

Reminder: This information in this book is presented for educational purposes only, and not to be construed as medical advice. If you need treatment for affective disorder, or any other medical condition, please seek the services of a knowledgeable physician.

Caveats for the patient

Juggling our health

Envision the grand health experiment in which each of us courageously engages. We start off with certain vulnerabilities and strengths. We find fullfillment as we can, confront what stresses we will. Risk surrounds us, especially in an age replete with junk food, pesticides, street drugs, and industrial pollution. Even when aware of contraindications (e.g., too much caffeine and sugar, too little sleep, too much stress, etc.), we sometimes make the wrong choice anyway.

Mental health is manipulated by our choices: what we eat; what nutrients we take, and when; the quality of light and air to which we are exposed; whether and how we exercise, conduct friendship, let go of resentments, interact with nature, and relate to the Divine.

The optimal balance of such factors is uniquely defined for each individual, and modifies how genetics manifests. Discovering that balance is an art. As we pay attention to how our choices affect us, as we learn what helps us and what hinders, and as we adjust our goals through life, we become more able to consciously move toward what keeps us well.

Commitment and perseverance required

☐ ***REMEMBER THAT NATURAL HEALING TAKES TIME.*** It can take anywhere from a few weeks to a year or more to become apparent.

☐ ***PAY ATTENTION TO SUBTLE IMPROVEMENTS.*** Symptomatic improvement is often slow, daily changes subtle, leading some to attribute recovery to other influences (e.g., relaxation, friends, getting a job, etc.). If nutrients are then discontinued, deterioration is likely, though again, often gradual. Unfortunately, some people are not convinced til they have struggled through a number of such cycles.

☐ ***MAINTAIN NUTRITIVE INTAKE.*** Nutrients usually must be increased when under stress, or when a mood episode threatens. Stopping mood-modulating nutrients, even when feeling recovered, usually leads to relapse. Former levels of improvement may then become more elusive, take longer to attain, and require higher nutrient doses. (Hoffer 1983A)

☐ ***TAKE NUTRIENTS ON SCHEDULE.*** Missed doses, especially of the more acutely effective nutrients, may worsen, perhaps trigger, an episode. The risk increases, the longer the lapse.

☐ ***BE MODERATE.*** Attune your lifestyle to natural biorhythms (regular meals, exercise, and bedtime; sufficient sleep, etc.). Avoid undue stress, sugar, junk food, caffeine, alcohol, street drugs, tobacco, etc.

Interact with your doctor

☐ ***LEARN ALL YOU CAN*** about bipolar disorder and nutrition, and what works for you. This is a lifelong process.

☐ ***CHOOSE A KNOWLEDGEABLE PHYSICIAN*** to whom you can relate, and actively participate in treatment decisions.

☐ ***BE PATIENT.*** Determining the precise nutrients which fit your unique biochemical profile may involve a number of trials. And as your chemistry changes, further trials may be needed.

☐ ***TRACK SYMPTOMS.*** Track symptoms (including reactions to treatment and to stressors) and express any concerns to your doctor.

☐ ***BE PREVENTIVE.*** Learn what triggers you, what helps, and which symptoms precede episodes. Work with your doctor on preventive measures.

"Your importance in healing"

"In my opinion the ONLY person who can cure bipolar is the bipolar person in question (his or her self). An alternative doctor may help us to get well by partially educating us in what we need to know... and/or steering us in the right directions, but we need to do most of what needs to be done (diet correction, Candida control, supplementation, etc.) to get well and/or stay well on our own."

Alan Darman

Handfuls of pills

Some people object to taking "handfuls" of pills. Some suggestions:

Clinics or compounding pharmacies may formulate supplements to suit requirements.

Commercial supplements may contain a number of nutrients you need (e.g., a Candida or pyrrole formulation).

You may be able to combine some liquid, or powdered nutrients.

Sublingual nutrients may be easier to take (and absorb).

Otherwise, just pretend the caps or tabs are little pieces of your favorite food, think about what they can do for your body and mind, and send them to work.

By the way, pills should be swallowed one at a time; with water, juice, or herb tea; sequentially — not by the handful.

Keep a mood/treatment diary (Brigham 2001)

Mapping nutrients, meds, diet, stressors, reactions and symptoms, helps clarify risks, cycling patterns, and relapse cues.

Attend to relapse cues & seek therapy

Cues vary. Possibilities include:

For mania: Increasing insomnia, irritability, unusual thought, expansiveness, increased risk taking, etc. (Altman 1992)

For depression: Conceptual disorganization, stress, difficulty with daily life, etc. (Altman 1992)

For suicide: Renewed energy before depression resolves,(Stoll 1999) hopelessness, irritability, discontent, fall from prior achievements, isolation, rigid thinking, etc. (Beck 1999, Ellis 1996) (See p. 267.)

History: A brief overview of the beginnings of nutrient-based (orthomolecular) psychiatry

"Nutrients are gentle, slow, and effective in the long term. They do not blunt the patient's vitality in a few weeks or cause the serious side effects and toxicity now associated with tranquilizers. You do not get tardive dyskinesia from vitamins." — Abram Hoffer, MD, PhD

Earlier nutrient cures (Joliffe 1940, Spies 1938, Kaufman 1939, Checkley 1939, Green 1971, Kahan 1977, Hoffer 2005, Murray 1991, Stone 1974)

Scurvy and pellagra, with their often prominent affective components, offered early examples of mood syndromes cureable by individual nutrients. In 1742, James Lind proposed a nutritional etiology for scurvy; in 1928, Joseph Goldberger did the same for pellagra. The effectiveness of vitamins C and B3, respectively, inspired further research into the role of nutrients in mental health. Such investigations came to a virtual halt during World War II.

The founding of Megavitamin & Orthomolecular therapy

In the early fifties, Doctors Abram Hoffer, MD, PhD, and Humphrey Osmond, MRCS, DPM, introduced use of high-dose vitamins B3 and C for schizophrenia with the first double blinds in the history of psychiatry. Thus began "Megavitamin Therapy." (Hoffer 1957, 62, 72, 73, 83, 2005, Dhalla 1989, Mathews 1985)

In 1968, Dr. Linus Pauling, two-time Nobel laureate, in a classic article in *Science,* renamed it "Orthomolecular Psychiatry," based on the concept that the brain could heal if provided with the right (*ortho*) molecular environment, i.e., by optimizing concentrations of substances naturally present in the brain, and removing that which is toxic.

As therapy evolved, other nutrients were studied. Guided by each patient's unique biochemical requirements, physicians supplied minimal to mega doses (in some cases, ten to over a hundred times the orthodox RDA) of relevant vitamins, and more modest doses of minerals, EFAs, and amino acids (with considerable variation between patients). (Hawkins 1973, Cott 1977, Williams 1979, Hoffer 1987, 2005, Pfeiffer 1987, 88, Kahan 1977)

Biotypes (Hoffer 2005, Pfeiffer 1987, 88)

Starting in the late 1960s, Dr. Hoffer, Carl C Pfeiffer, MD, PhD, and others found that nutrients addressing histamine imbalance and/or pyroluria produced improvement, in most patients; often great improvement or recovery when the illness was caught early. (See pp. 145-68.)

Applicability to bipolar disorder

At the time, the trend was to diagnose many bipolars as schizophrenic. So the earlier "schizophrenia" treatments were used on, and perhaps benefitted, some bipolars. Researchers have since successfully applied nutrient and biotype approaches to bipolar disorder, depression, autism, behavior disorder, and a number of other severe psychiatric conditions. (Walsh 2006, 07)

Evolving approaches (Cott 1977, Hoffer 2005, Pfeiffer 1987, 88, Kahan 1977)

Doctors Theron Randolph, Arthur Coca, Walter Alvarez, and Herbert Rinkel laid the groundwork for clinical ecology, and for a view of allergic response which includes mental symptoms. Doctors Elizabeth Rees, Marshall Mandell, and William Philpott introduced orthomolecular therapists to the role of allergies in mental disorders.

Hoffer has emphasized the importance of a varied, natural, whole foods diet, eliminating junk and processed food; Dr. Michael Lesser, the usefulness of organic food, if possible. Alan Cott, MD, and Jack Ward, MD, drew attention to the influence of blood sugar; David Horrobin, MD, PhD, and Donald Rudin, MD, to the role of essential fatty acids; William Crook, MD, and Orion Truss, MD, to the role of yeast infestation.

Others emphasized the role of additional co-occuring medical conditions, such as, hormone imbalances, convulsive disorders, toxic overload, etc.

William Walsh, PhD, has pointed out the relevance of methylation and metal metabolism status to histamine biotypes. Biotype work is also continued by Patrick Holford, Michael Lesser, MD, Joan Matthews Larson, PhD, and numerous others.

Mainstream studies

A 1999 multicenter study led by Andrew Stoll, MD, of Harvard, spotlighted the use of omega 3 in bipolar depression and marked a turning point in mainstream attention to natural substances for the treatment of bipolar disorder. Numerous mainstream studies are listed herein.

Current status

Ongoing worldwide research continues to reveal intricate connections of brain function with nutrition and health, i.e. how what we feel, think, and do, is interwoven with how well we nourish and protect our cells.

The Future: A nutrients & mental health wishlist

(1) Comprehensive education of the general population, before completing high school, as to the uses of nutrients to maintain mental and physical health.

(2) Increasingly widespread availability of information on nutritional approaches.

(3) Unrestricted public access to quality nutrient supplements.

(4) Extensive training of physicians as to the profound influence of nutrients on biochemistry and health.

(5) The development of protocols which consider nutrients as first-line treatment, wherever medically possible, with treatment tailored to each individual's unique biochemical requirements.

(6) Hospitals equipped to provide state-of-the-art nutritional analysis and treatment (including IV and IM therapies, *as relevant*), and which use nutritional approaches preferentially (*where indicated*).

(7) Inclusion of the patient as a partner in healthcare decisions.

(8) Generous funding for nutritional research. An emphasis on naturalistic, longitudinal studies.

2. Some Definitions

At this stage of medical understanding, any biochemical definition of bipolar disorder would probably involve an intricate web of factors, perhaps somewhat like those presented in this book. Until more direct mechanisms are determined, the DSM IV definition roughly serves as a common denominator and, just as with a "diagnosis of "fever," helps alert patient and physician to the need for further attention. Note: Most of the following definitions are taken from DSM IV.

Episodes

A mood episode is a mania, depression or mixed state. Episodes can be isolated, switch continually, or be separated by relatively nonsymptomatic intervals. Bipolar disorder is characterized by prolonged, often extreme and debilitating episodes, difficult to dislodge, even when circumstances improve.

Manic episode

DSM IV generally defines a manic episode as:

An abnormally elevated, expansive or irritable mood lasting at least a week, and consisting of three or more of the following symptoms (four if only irritable):

- □ Grandiosity, inflated self-esteem.
- □ Less need for sleep.
- □ More talkative than usual, or pressure of speech.
- □ Flight of ideas, racing thoughts.
- □ Distractibility.
- □ Increased goal-directed activity or psychomotor agitation.
- □ Indulgence in pleasurable activities with little regard for risk (e.g., spending sprees, gambling, sexual liasons, unwise business ventures).*

Also: Symptoms impair social relationships or function at work, include psychotic features (e.g., delusions, hallucinations),* or lead to hospitalization due to risk of harm to self or others.

And: Not a mixed episode. Not directly due to a medical condition, or reactions to antidepressants or other medication, or street drugs.

* See *Bipolar delusions & psychosis,* p. 268.

Hypomanic episode (BRIGHAM 2001)

Hypomanias are defined by the occurence of some of the above symptoms over at least four days, without impairing social or occupational function, without psychotic features, and not requiring hospitalization.

Hyperthymic (overactive) temperament* (BRIGHAM 2001)

Hyperthymia is defined as two persistent symptoms of hypomania, with no mania for at least the first two years, and lack of manic or organic etiology.

Hyperthymics tend to be optimistic, active, perhaps great achievers. Brigham (2001) suggests 30% of severe melancholics, especially males, may be intolerant of depression, and so instead appear hyperthymic.

* Temperaments may be primary or secondary to psychiatric or medical disorders, and can co-occur with affective illness.

"[Delerious mania] begins very suddenly, only sleeplessness, restlessness, or anxious moodiness may already be conspicuous one or two days beforehand. Consciousness rapidly becomes clouded and the patient becomes confused and bewildered, completely losing orientation to time and place... Numerous hallucinations appear and the mood changes rapidly from being timid and lacrimous...to unrestrainedly merry, erotic or ecstatic."

Emil Kraepelin, MD, 1921

Irritable manias

"Most manias were euphoric a generation ago, but now two-thirds are accompanied by irritability, anger, and/or depression."

HE Marano, 2005

"[Manics typically develop] indiscriminate enthusiasm for interpersonal, sexual, or occupational interactions, with abusive, violent, or other antisocial behavior, common."

Paris Kidd, PhD, 2004

"[Many manics have] irritable or paranoid reactions to anyone who stands in the way of their achievements."

Priscilla Slagle, PhD, 2006

"What is reality
to this synthetic doll
who should smile, who should shift gear,
should spring the doors open in a wholesome disorder,
and have no evidence of ruin or fears?"

Anne Sexton, from "Self," June 1958

"[There are] two kinds of spleen, one mocking, active passionate, malignant; the other morose and wholly passive, when one's only wish is for silence and solitude and the oblivion of sleep. For anyone possesed by this latter kind, nothing has meaning, the destruction of a world would hardly move him. At such times I could wish the earth were a shell filled with gunpower, to which I would put a match for my diversion."

Hector Berlioz, from "Memoirs"

"From my rotting body flowers shall grow and I am in them and that is eternity."

Edvard Munsch

"It was the season of Light, it was the season of Darkness, it was the spring of hope, it was the winter of despair, we had everything before us, we had nothing before us..."

Charles Dickens, from *Tale of Two Cities*, 1859

"The fires of a supreme zest for living and the most gnawing desire for death alternate in my heart, sometimes in the course of a single hour. I know only one thing: I cannot go on like this."

Gustav Mahler, at nineteen

Major depressive episode (WEISSMAN 1991, LARSON, www.mental-health-today...)

DSM IV generally defines a major depressive episode as:

Mood disturbance or loss of interest in almost all usual activities for most of the day, most days, for at least two weeks, with five or more of the following symptoms, including either depressed mood or loss of interest (*the first two listings, below*):

- ☐ Depressed mood (e.g., sadness, emptiness, pessimism, uncontrollable crying).
- ☐ Marked loss of interest or pleasure in usual activities (e.g, social withdrawal, or loss of interest in sex).
- ☐ Significant alteration in weight or appetite.
- ☐ Insomnia or too much sleep.
- ☐ Psychomotor agitation (e.g., irritability, impatience, hostility) or retardation (e.g., slowed speech, movement, response).
- ☐ Fatigue, lethargy, loss of energy or motivation.
- ☐ Feelings of worthlessness, helplessness, or unmerited guilt.
- ☐ Difficulty thinking, concentrating, or making decisions.
- ☐ Recurrent thoughts of death, self-destructive behavior, suicidality.
- ☐ Certain physical complaints (e.g., head or back aches, gastrointestinal symptoms, blurred vision).

Also: Symptoms significantly impair social, educational, or occupational function, or mandate hospitalization due to risk to self or others.*

And: Not a mixed episode. Symptoms are not directly due to medication, street drugs or medical condition and are not better accounted for by bereavement.

Note: The Diagnostic Guidelines Task Force of the International Society for Bipolar Disorder, (GHAEMI 2008) suggests symptoms of *bipolar* depression commonly include *atypical symptoms* such as psychotic features, pathological guilt, or leaden paralysis.

Dysthymic temperament (impaired moods)

Dysthymia is defined by two persistent symptoms of depressive disorder plus tearfulness and hopelessness, absence of major depression during the first two years, and lack of depressive or organic etiology.

Dysthymics tend to be introverted and withdrawn, and consider life a struggle, though stimulation may enable them to be conscientious, self-disciplined, and cheerful. Many chronic dysthymics will eventually experience at least one major depression. (BRIGHAM, 2001)

Mixed episode or dysphoric mania

Mixed states are more common than pure mania or hypomania. Thus, during mania, the majority score high on depression scales, and suicide rates are significant. (BRIGHAM, 2001)

DSM IV generally defines a mixed state as:

Criteria for both mania and major depression are met nearly every day for at least one week, along with marked impairment in occupational or social function, hospitalization to prevent harm to self or others, or presence of psychotic features.

And: Symptoms are not directly due to a medical condition, medication, street drugs, or antidepressant treatment.

Subclinical mixed states can also occur.

Bipolar I

DSM IV generally defines bipolar I as:

A history or presence of at least one manic or mixed episode, regardless of whether major depression has occurred.*

Bipolar II

DSM IV generally defines bipolar II as:

A history or presence of at least one major depressive and at least one hypomanic episode, but no manic or mixed episodes.*

Rapid cycling

DSM IV generally defines rapid cycling as:

At least four episodes in the previous year that meet criteria for major depressive, manic, mixed, or hypomanic episodes, with some remission between states, or a switch to the opposite polarity episode.

Also: Symptoms cause significant clinical distress or significantly impair social, occupational, or other functioning.*

A very rapid alternation of manic and depressive symptoms (over days) is often diagnosed Bipolar Disorder not otherwise specified.

* And: Symptoms are not better accounted for by schizoaffective disorder; not superimposed on schizophrenia, delusional disorder, or psychotic disorder NOS and not directly due to medical conditions, medication, street drugs, or antidepressant treatment.

Cyclothymic temperament (circular moods)

Cyclothymia is generally defined by numerous hypomanic and mild depressive episodes over at least two years (one year in children) with no symptom-free intervals lasting more than two months, and no full-blown affective episodes.

Note: 15-50% may subsequently develop bipolar I or II. (BRIGHAM 2001)

Bipolar spectrum

Many physicians now view bipolar disorder as a continuum, with some patients not fitting criteria for mixed state, rapid cycling, or bipolar I or II, though symptoms, family history and difficulty with antidepressants suggest an evolving mood disorder, within a bipolar spectrum.(BRIGHAM 2001, AKISKAL 2005)

"There is a particular kind of pain, elation, loneliness and terror involved in this kind of madness... The ideas and feelings are fast and frequent like shooting stars.. But, somewhere, this changes. The fast ideas are far too fast, and there are far too many; overwhelming confusion replaces clarity. Everything previously moving with the grain is now against - you are irritable, angry, frightened, uncontrollable... It will never end, for madness carves its own reality."

Kay Redfield Jamison, PhD, 1995

Brief definitions

Bipolar I: 1+ manias

Bipolar II: 1+ hypomanias & 1+ major depressions

Rapid cycling: 4+ episodes per year

Mixed states: manic and depressive states more or less co-occur.

"'Bipolar disorder' is a behavioral, not a true medical diagnosis. It is a wastebasket term that doesn't get to the molecular basis. You're still left to figure out the underlying disorder."

Michael Lesser, MD, 2008

Initial presentation & typical course

Bipolars usually report good family life and adjustment to work before the illness. (BRATFOS 1968) In one study, 92% had finished high school, 60% had further education. (PLUMLEE 1986)

Initial diagnosis is most often mid to late teens, but occurs at moderate frequency through the twenties and thirties. (RUSH 2003, MARANO 2005, CABF 2002, GOODWIN 2007)

Males have a greater tendency to mania in their first episode, are more prone to mania in general, and tend to experience more extreme manias. Bipolar I females are more prone to depression. (MACQUEEN)

The typical untreated mania lasts a couple of months; (FRYE 2001) depression, two to thirteen, (GOODWIN 1990, HADDAD 2002, KETTER 2001) Episodes tend to become more severe over time, and psychosis may emerge or increase. (KETTER, FRYE, 2001, BOWDEN 1999, TRIMBLE 1996)

Concurrent disorders (HUDSON 1999)

Concurrent psychiatric disorders are prevalent, (STRAKOWSKI 1992, AMADEO 1992, PESELOW 1995, O'CONNELL 1991) and may mask bipolar illness, or increase cycling and mixed states. (BAUER 1993, 94AB, MCELROY 1992) They can include: anxiety and panic disorders, substance abuse, borderline, agorophobia and other phobias, PTSD,(FREEMAN 2002) ADD, hyperactivity, autism, Tourette's, OCD, (KAPLAN 2000) pathological gambling, eating disorders, body dysmorphic disorder, kleptomania, pyromania, trichotillomania, intermittent explosive disorder, prolonged anger, child or spousal abuse, criminal activity or incarceration.

See *Related conditions* pp. 263-76.

3. Gifts & Trials

"I am often amazed at the intellectual & creative abilities of my patients with apparent mental disturbances."

Walter Lemmo, ND

"And if we musicians live so often, as you know we do, on sunny heights, the sadness of reality cuts all the deeper when it lies naked before our eyes."

Robert Schumann, 1849

"Though my dark side is dormant right now, it continues to play a big role in whatever capacity I have to be creative — that's the well I'm able to tap into where all the anguish, rage and sadness are stored."

Jessica Lange, 1995

"There is a fine and at times invisible line between mania and creativity... Mild elation or hypomania can give the needed extra boost to creative people... Creativity is probably a delicate special balance of talent, discipline and inherited chemical energy... Manic elation... in small doses [helps sustain] the great effort that is usually required to perfect something really innovative."

Ronald Fieve, MD, 1976

"The drive to express their inner creativity is heightened in many gifted individuals, and when [blocked] it implodes into numbness, rage, depression, and hopelessness."

Annemarie Roeper, 1996

Mood & expressive styles (Jamison 1980, 92, 93, Zimmerman 1942, Reitman 1950, Dax 1953, Enachescu 1971, Wadeson 1976, Goodwin 1990)

Manics talk more, more rapidly, and more powerfully. Their words are more vivid and they use more action verbs. (Anderson 1976)

Similarly, manic art tends to be created rapidly; seems more imaginative, active, and sexual; and often has a swirling, agitated quality. Colors are brighter, more intense, and highlighted with more use of contrast.

Art of the depressed tends to be created more slowly, and often focuses on death and decay. It generally seems more barren and cold, with darker colors, and less motion.

In some ancient tribes, the mentally ill were revered as spiritual teachers and healers. Those respectful attitudes are echoed today in the accolades and wide girth given moody writers and artists, brilliantly eccentric political and military leaders, and certain lone and insightful individuals on a spiritual quest. In fact, a disproportionate number of bipolars (and their families) exhibit heightened creativity, leadership, or spirituality.

In the depths of illness, such gifts can taunt, rather than inspire. Nonetheless, many use them as a ladder out of those depths, torturous though that ascent might be. And the insights revealed often offer a glimmer of light to both the bipolar, and society in general.

Creativity

Note to bipolars who think they are "not creative"

In the author's opinion, creativity is not elitist. Although many have been discouraged from doing so, all people benefit by pursuing creative expression if, for nothing else, then as a means of exploring ourselves and our place in the universe. It doesn't matter whether you think you are "talented" or not, so long as you focus on discovering what is true for you, on what you really feel and choose; and you keep engaging in your art. (*Note: It can take two weeks or more to develop a habit.*)

Intersection with mood

Mood disorder seems to be over-represented among individuals classically recognized as creative (Janza 2004) and may, to some extent, help drive the aspiring poet, playwright, or musician. (Fieve 1976)

Chemically, it may be that mania, with its increased fronto-limbic stimulation, and correspondingly enhanced cognition, feeling, awareness, and motivation, fuels creativity; or becomes the inspiration for work that is created later, during euthymia or even depression.

In an extensive review of historical observations, biographies, scientific surveys, and psychiatric evaluations, Janza (2004) found bipolar symptoms more frequent in the "creative." Moreover, during intense creative expression, artists and writers frequently report hypomanic-type symptoms (Janza 2004), and most seem to experience a mood/creativity interaction. (Andreason 1987, Fieve 1976)

In a survey of 47 British writers and artists, Kay Jamison, PhD, (1989) found the greatest psychiatric problems in poets, then writers. Half the poets, two-thirds of the playwrights, 20% of biographers, 13% of painters had been treated for depression. 17% of poets had been treated for mania. All poets, novelists, and artists, 88% of playwrights, and 20% of biographers experienced intense creative episodes characterized by enthusiasm, euphoria, high energy, confidence, fast mental associations, and fluid thought. 63% of playwrights had been treated for mood disorder. 38% of the entire group had received treatment for affective illness (a rate six time that of the general population); one third of the group had severe mood swings; one fourth, intense elated mood states, 50% had taken psychiatric medications, 20% had been previously hospitalized, and 90% reported creative highs lasting an average of two weeks (a typical span for manic elation). (Jamison 1989)

Similarly, Andreason (1987) found substantially greater affective illness, particularly bipolar disorder, among 30 writers (teachers at the University of Iowa creative writing workshop) studied over 15 years. 80% of had experienced a mood episode (compared to 30% in controls); 37%, major depression (17% in controls); 30%, alcoholism (7%, controls). Most wrote during normal mood. First degree relatives also showed greater affective disorder and creativity.

In Arnold M Ludwig's biographical survey of 1005 famous persons in the 20th century, rates of psychosis, suicide attempts, mood disorder, drug and alcohol use was two-to three fold greater in writers and artists than in people successful in business, science or public life. Mania and suicide occured most in poets. Writers and relatives had very high rates of bipolar psychosis.

Commonalities

Temperament, cognitive style, and mood, are notably similar in "creative" individuals and bipolars (particularly bipolar IIs). The bipolar syndrome, for example, involves such creative characteristics as manic love of words, sexual seduction via the arts (poetry, music art, food, fashion, etc.), hypersensitivity to others, etc. (JANZA 2004, AKISKAL 2005, FIEVE 1976, NETTLE 2002, KUBIE 1961)

Conversely, creatives often experience such bipolar traits as:

- ☐ Creative surges and blocks similar to mood swings. (KUBIE 1961, FIEVE 1976)
- ☐ Sudden change of mood immediately preceding creative periods (in perhaps 50%). (JAMISON 1989)
- ☐ Affective temperaments. Cylcothymia. (NOWAKOWSKA 2005)
- ☐ Tendency to emotional problems and vulnerability. (FIEVE 1976)
- ☐ Emotional flooding; confusing, conflicting passions and ideas; unconventional or restless behavior. (ANDREASON 1987)
- ☐ Overinclusive thinking, rich associations, or hypomania. (JANZA 2004)
- ☐ Reduced sleep, or sudden early waking prior to creative episodes. (JAMISON 1989)
- ☐ Unique, unconventional, eccentric, erratic perceptions. (ANDREASON 1987, FIEVE 1976)
- ☐ Ornamental, flamboyant (red and bright colors). (AKISKAL 2005)
- ☐ Tolerance for ambiguity. (ROTTENBERG 2001)
- ☐ Curiosity, risk taking, adventuresome. (ANDREASON 1987, ROTTENBERG 2001)
- ☐ Creativity, novelty-seeking (NOWAKOWSKA 2005), impulsivity. (AKISKAL 2005)
- ☐ Eminence, creative achievement, professional instability. (AKISKAL 2005)
- ☐ High energy and activity. (ROTTENBERG 2001)
- ☐ Excess sociability, frequent moving, different jobs. (ANDREASON 1987, FIEVE 1976)
- ☐ Multiple marriages. (AKISKAL 2005)
- ☐ Multiple substance abuse, addiction (ANDREASON, AKISKAL 2005)
- ☐ Comorbidity, irritability, anxiety, neuroticism. (NOWAKOWSKA 2005)

Virginia Woolf

"[Virginia Woolf's imagination] .. flew rapidly ahead, parting company with reality... magnifying simple words and experiences. One would hand her a bit of information, as dull as a lump of lead, and she would hand it back glittering with diamonds... Virginia was a life enhancer."

Nigel Nicolson, 1992

On writing & mood

"The truth is people scarcely care for each other... never become attached to anything outside themselves." (June 4, 1923)

"[To write] one must get out of life... become externalized; very, very concentrated, all at one point." (August 22, 1922)

"[I am possessed by] some inner loneliness... And no one knows how I suffer, walking up this street, engaged with my anguish." (October 11, 1929)

"Writing is effort: writing is despair." (May 31, 1933)

"Few people can be so tortured by writing as I am." (June 23, 1936)

"I pitched into my great lake of melancholy...The only way I keep afloat is by working... Directly I stop working I feel that I am sinking down, down... I feel that if I sink further I shall reach the truth... That is the only mitigation... I shall make myself face the fact that there is nothing — nothing for any of us." (June 23, 1929)

"The only exciting life is the imaginary one." (April 21, 1928)

"There is a luxury in being quiet in the heart of chaos." (June 23, 1927)

"The creative power at once brings the whole universe to order." (July 27, 1934)

"The poetry of existence... overcomes me." (June 13, 1923)

Moods (our world.compuserve.com.... bipolar.about.com...)

Adeline Virginia Stephen was born in 1882 to a family of intellectuals, writers, and affectives. Her sister was a painter; her father, a writer.

Virginia did not go to school, but devoured the extensive family library.

Her first "nervous breakdown" occurred in 1895, at age 13, after her mother died; another, in 1904 after her father's death. In 1912, she married Leonard Woolf; then had a severe breakdown after her first novel, a year later.

She couldn't write when ill, but came up with most book ideas when manic. Heightened productivity may have followed life-threatening moods from 1912-15.

*"Forward forward let us range,
Let the great world spin forever down
the ringing grooves of change."*

Alfred Lord Tennyson
from *Locksley Hall*, 1837-38 1842

*"...heroic hearts,
Made weak by time and fate, but strong
in will
To strive, to seek, to find, and not to
yield."*

Alfred Lord Tennyson, *Ulysses*, 1833-42

"Let us have faith that might makes right; and in that faith let us to the end, dare to do our duty as we understand it."

President Abraham Lincoln

"Power always thinks it has a great soul and vast views beyond the comprehension of the weak."

President John Adams

Mania & leadership

"[Many] intelligent manic leaders can persuade others to do almost anything... [and are] able to perceive the defects in others most rapidly... People... are attracted by [their] vitality. [They think] big and are generally able to seduce others into relinquishing their... scruples."

Ronald R. Fieve, MD, 1976

Fieve (1976) believes hyperthymia or mild bipolar II may have given some politicians the drive to produce exceptional leadership. He suggests that such leaders often attract a devoted following, as long as they're not crossed, and don't become paranoid or irrational.

Qualities that can be common to leadership & hypomania (Fieve 1976, Akiskal 2005)

- ☐ Exploration, territoriality, mating dominance.
- ☐ Manic charm, likeability, vitality, enthusiasm.
- ☐ Ability to work all night, get by on little sleep.
- ☐ Extraordinary focus and concentration.
- ☐ Penetrating assessment of defects in other people.
- ☐ Ability to attract a following, convince others, impose one's will.
- ☐ Thrive on legal battles.

Spirituality

Increased spiritual preoccupation is considered a "symptom" of bipolar disorder (and epilepsy and schizophrenia), is subject to the delusions created by the illness, and may be fostered by the overactive nervous system. Nonetheless, especially if delusions can be weeded out, the heightened spiritual focus can be a gift, bringing with it deep devotion, study, and spiritual connection.

Theodore Roosevelt: Perhaps hyperthymic or mild bipolar II (Fieve 1976)

"I wish to preach, not the doctrine of ignoble ease, but the doctrine of the strenuous life; the life of toil and effort; of labor and strife; to preach that highest form of success which comes, not to the man who desires a more easy peace, but to the man who does not shrink from danger, from hardship or from bitter toil, and who out of these wins the splendid ultimate triumph..."

"No man has had a happier life than I did, a happier life in every way."

President Theodore Roosevelt

Fieve suggests Theodore Roosevelt was mostly hypomanic, and may have been bipolar II or hyperthymic.

He had been a talkative, active, and precocious child, fascinated with nature. As a student at Harvard, he was nervous and enthusiastic, always running, occasionally depressed, and relatively outcast.

He nonetheless went on to a workaholic and highly successful political career. He was involved in violent disputes at the US Civil Service Commission, and the New York City police board (to which he was elected chair in 1895), but rose rapidly to become a member of the NY State Assembly and then, by 1899, governor of New York.

Roosevelt's enthusiasm for war helped spur US participation in the Spanish-American War, where he led his "Rough Riders" (who idolized him) in the infamous and dangerous, but pivotal charge up San Juan Hill.

As US president, he was at his desk by 7:30 in the morning, in constant interaction with the public, legistlators, and foreign dignatories, surrounded by fascinating people and endless projects.* Before dinner, he would walk, ride horses, or box. At night he'd devour volumes of specialized literature. He slept little.

He said he liked "to be working the levers of the great machine." He was colorful, active, joyous, and undiplomatic. He'd rage, distort facts, contradict himself. Reactionaries pronounced him criminal; the righteous, insane. Mark Hanna, Republican chair, called him a "madman." The public loved him. The "teddy" bear was named after him.

* He wrote over 100,000 letters between governorship and presidency. And he expanded the National Forest System, busted trusts, pushed through the Meat Inspection and the Pure Food and Drug Acts, mediated labor disputes and the Russo-Japanese war, manipulated Panamanian politics to insure construction of the Panama canal, etc.

Churchill's moods (Moran 1966, Storr 1969, 90, Rowse 1956, Pearson 1991, Mather 2006)

"When I was young, for two or three years, the light faded out, I did my work barely, sat in the House of Commons, but black depression settled on me... I don't like standing near the edge of a platform when an express train is passing through. I like it wider between me and the train... I don't want to go out in the world... at such moments."

Prime Minister, Winston Churchill

"Do not let us speak of darker days; let us rather speak of sterner days. These are not dark days: these are great days — the greatest days our country has ever lived; and we must all thank God that we have been allowed to play a part in making these days memorable in [history]."

Winston Churchill, Harrow School, Oct 29 1941

"[He was] forceful, driving, tireless, and in need of very little sleep, ...able to achieve whatever he wished, to conquer any impossible situation, to succeed brilliantly as a writer, politician, warrior or Prime Minister."

Randolph Churchill

"[Churchill's] prolific... ideas, explod[ed] in different directions like machine-gun bullets."

Lord Beaverton

"Had he been a stable and equable man, he could never have inspired the nation. In 1940, when all the odds were against Britain, a leader of sober judgment might well have concluded we were finished."

Anthony Storr, 1969

Famous persons believed to have suffered mood disorders THE MOODYNEWS. COM..., MENTALJOKES.COM..., BIPOLARSURVIVOR.COM...

People who have stated so publicly, or who have been "diagnosed" retroactively.

Poets: Lord Byron, Alfred Lord Tennyson, Walt Whitman, William Blake, Edna St Vincent Millay, Robert Frost, Sylvia Plath, Robert Lowell, Anne Sexton, TS Eliot.

Writers: Plato, Hans Christian Andersen, Victor Hugo, Honore de Balzac, F. Scott Fitzgerald, Leo Tolstoy, Mark Twain, Charles Dickens, Edgar Allen Poe, Robert Louis Stevenson, Jack London, Agatha Christie, Ernest Hemingway, Tennessee Williams, Theodore Roethke, Kate Millett.

Musicians: Ludwig von Beethoven, Amadeus Mozart, Hector Berlioz, Gustav Mahler, Cole Porter, Rosemary Clooney, Connie Francis, Charley Pride, Brian Wilson, Axl Rose, Tony Orlando, Alvin Alley (dancer).

Actors: Marilyn Monroe, Jim Carrey, Carrie Fisher, Patty Duke, Robert Downey Jr., Margot Kidder.

Stage or film directors: Tim Burton (& artist), Francis Ford Coppola, Rod Steiger (& writer), Joshua Logan (& writer), Moss Hart (& playwright).

Artists: Francesco Goya, Vincent Van Gogh, Paul Gauguin, Edvard Munsch, Jackson Pollack, Georgia O'Keefe.

Psychiatrists, psychologists, physicians: Clifford Beers, Sigmund Freud, Mark Vonnegut, Kay Redfield Jamison.

Scientists: Isaac Newton, Nicola Tessler.

Politicians, military: John Adams, Robert E. Lee, Abraham Lincoln, John Brown, Napoleon Bonaparte, George S. Patton, Theodore Roosevelt, Winston Churchill.

Enterpreneurs: Ted Turner, JC Penney, Larry Flynt.

Summary

Although mild bipolar disorder may, in some, accentuate creative, spiritual, or leadership attributes, the cost of the illness can, nonetheless, be overwhelming, accompanied, as it can be, by feelings of worthlessness, inexorable psychic pain, escalating anger, an often constant threat of death, and other such gems. What's needed is greater power over mood, so that moods serve instead of control — to make brain response more flexible, and to counteract paranoia, confusion, psychosis, and despair. Nutrients such as omega 3, magnesium, zinc, niacin, B complex, vitamin C, taurine and GABA target just such attributes. (*Therapy, of course, must be tailored by the physician to each patient's unique biochemical profile.*) Read on...

"Sickness insanity and death were the angels that surrounded my cradle and they have followed me throughout my life."

Edvard Munsch

Genetics & epidemiology

Risk to family members (Gold 1987)

Inheritance of bipolar disorder is fairly well-established. However, not everyone with genetic susceptibility becomes bipolar. Environmental factors influence whether NIMH and how the genetics manifests, e.g., nutrition, toxic exposures, health, psychosocial stressors, etc. (Gold 1987)

An identical twin, whether raised with, or apart from, a bipolar co-twin, incurs an estimated 57-80% risk of developing the disorder.*(Bertlesen 1977, Walsh 2006) or more, (Whybrow 1993, Gurling 1995, Rush 2003b) perhaps up to 93%. (Kallman) (In major depression concordance is estimated at 40-70%.)

For children of a bipolar parent, the risk of becoming bipolar may be at least 15%. (van Gent, Gold 1987) perhaps 10-30%. (CABF 2002) One sibling or fraternal twin bipolar poses a risk of about 20-32% for other siblings. With one child and one parent bipolar, the risk to other children is estimated at 25% or more; with both parents bipolar, 70%. (CABF 2002, Walsh 2006)

The risk of developing bipolar I has been variously estimated at 4-24% in immediate relatives of the bipolar; the risk of developing bipolar II, at 1-5%. (mental-health-today.com...)

The rate of illness is greater in relatives of early-onset bipolars. (Strober 1992) Later onset suggests lower genetic load; thus, less affective illness in family members. (Post 2001) Late onset may be secondary to other illness, drug use, or other factors. (Young 1992)

Common genetics with unipolar depression & schizophrenia

70%-90% of bipolars have a close relative who is also bipolar. (Moore 1998, Kluger 2002) A somewhat smaller percentage have a relative with another affective illness. (Gershon 1982, Maier, 1999, Moore 1998) Unipolars, on the other hand, tend to have mainly unipolar relatives. (Gold 1987) Consistent biological distinctions between bipolar and unipolar disorders are not obvious, (Yatham1997) while overlap can be substantial. (Rush 2003) From this, Gold (1987) hypothesizes bipolar illness could be a severe form of unipolar. The risk of switching from major depression to bipolar disorder is considerable, and has been estimated [perhaps conservatively] to be at least 10%. (Goodwin 2007)

Schizophrenia, and unipolar and bipolar disorders may also share some genetics.* Over several generations, many family lines contain members with all three disorders. Patients, themselves, can show features of all three. (Moller 2003, Horrobin 2003, Kidd 2004)

* Commonalities can include neural membrane dysfunction, serotinergic abnormalities, etc.

Multiple genes

Bipolar inheritance may be through a number of genes, such as those that control calcium and sodium ion channels, (Sklar 2008) PLA2 activity, (Horrobin 2000) methylation, pyrrole production, metal metabolism, (Walsh 2007) anterior cingulate function, B vitamin absorption and use, hormonal balances, tendency to limbic seizures, suceptibility to allergies or environmental illness, sensitivity to seasonal change, etc.

Populations

Clinical studies find bipolar disorder more common in professionals and people with greater than average educational and social achievements.*(Welner 1979, Winokur 1969, 82, Woodruff 1971) Type II bipolars, especially, are often highly successful or creative, and found in higher socioeconomic strata. (Coryell 1989, Lenzi 1993) Bipolar families also tend to be more prosperous. (Goodwin 1990) Otherwise, no major distinctions have been found across cultures, age or gender, (Bauer 1994ab) except that women may be at greater risk for rapid cycling.

Consistent demographic data is sparce and can be distorted. (Strakowski 1992) A study by Woods (1993), for instance, found US psychiatrists more likely to diagnose African Americans as schizophrenic, rather than bipolar. Youth are also more subject to misdiagnosis. Cultural knowledge and sensitivity are critical.

* Gold (1987) suggests that mild bipolar genetics (or more severe susceptibility moderated by a calm balanced life and/or optimal nutrition) may promote increased energy, goal directedness, and optimism, while a greater genetic load, unopposed, may predispose to psychosis.

Lifetime risk

Recently, researchers have suggested that 1% of the US population is severely bipolar, with milder illness in another 5%. (Marano 2005) Lifetime risk of bipolar I has been estimated at 0.8 to 1.6%; (Kessler 1994) with bipolar II, at 0.5-0.8%.*(Weissman 1991, 96, Bauer 1994ab) However rates are difficult to assess, as many bipolars are never treated.

Other countries show similar rates, though criteria can vary. Taiwan reports 0.3%; New Zealand, 1.5%; (Weisman 1996) In general, worldwide lifetime prevalence varies from 1.0 to 3.7% for the whole bipolar spectrum. (Hirschfeld 2003, Rush 2003)

Rates in the young for both depression (Weissman 1991, Gershon 1987) and mania (Gershon 1987, Lasch 1990) have increased markedly over the past 50 (Gershon 1987) to 80 years. (Lasch 1990, CABF 2002) Onset is also earlier. (McInnis 1993, CABF 2002)

In 2007, the 21st European Neuropsychopharmacological Congress in Barcelona, Spain, bringing together European and US surveys, has suggested 2% of the population will be bipolar at some time in their lives, with another 6% part of a bipolar spectrum. (Goodwin 2007)

* Major depression, on the other hand, affects at least 5% of Americans; (Weissman 1991) 7-8%, if confounding illnesses are not teased out, (Tsuang 1984, Robbins 1984, Winokur 1982, 1987); 10% of females. (Gold 1987) Average onset is ten years later than bipolar disorder. Rates vary from 1.5% in Taiwan to 19% in Beirut. (Weissman 1996, Robins 1984)

4. Survey of nutritional approaches

Some key approaches are listed below (*and integrated into Frameworks 1-3, pp.22-3, 84-5*). Contraindications, studies, references, and other details are given throughout this book. *Beware! The illness, the various therapies and meds, or the lack of them, all involve potentially life-or-death choices. Persons needing treatment for mood disorders should consult a knowledgeable physician who will tailor treatment to individual biochemistry.*

Biotype protocol (Walsh 1997, 2000, 03, 06, 07, Pfeiffer 1987, 88)

From work with over 1800 bipolars (see pp. 3, 145), Dr. William J. Walsh, PhD, of Walsh Research Institute, has found the following biotypes most common:

□ Pyrrole disorder, primary in an estimated 18-20% of bipolars, and characterized by a continual depletion of zinc and B6, compromising serotonin formation and ability to handle stress.

□ Undermethylation/high folate (histadelia), primary in approximately 35%. Undermethylated patients do not readily activate antidepressant neurotransmitters, and certain other brain and body biochemicals, and so are often subject to severe suicidal depressions.

□ Overmethylation/low folate (histapenia), primary in about 25%, and often, especially in more severe cases, associated with metal metabolism dysfunction and high copper. Grandiosity and hypomania are common, due to overactivated stimulating neurotransmitters.

Note: In some cases, biotypes 2 & 3 switch with mood.

□ Other considerations: metal metabolism disorders, autoimmune and allergy issues (especially, gluten), low lithium, oxidative stress, thyroid and other endocrine imbalance, convulsive disorders, malabsorption, Candida, toxicity, blood sugar issues, immune illness, etc.

Therapy is individualized to each patient's unique biochemical requirements, taking into account biotype, further nutrient and health needs, and lifestyle factors.

Essential fatty acids & phospholipids

A 1999 study by Dr. Andrew Stoll, MD, of Harvard, drew mainstream attention to the effectiveness of omega 3, especially in bipolar depression. Omega 3 (particularly EPA) supports flexible receptor and second messenger response to brain stimulation, opposes inflammatory immune chemicals implicated in depression, (Maes 1998), counters Candida, alters stress chemistry, (Horrobin 1999) and balances histamine levels.

On the other hand,with pyroluria, especially when severe, GLA is often preferable. (Bibus 2003) (*See page 92*)

Supportive nutrients include B vitamins, and therapies which reduce oxidative stress (plentiful antioxidants, avoiding excitotoxins, redress of any metal metabolism dysfunction, etc.). Also, phospholipids, which house neural membrane EFAs. Phosphatidyl choline is often useful for manic and overmethylated persons; phosphatidyl inositol, for many who are depressed and undermethylated. (Walsh 2006) (See pp. 47-52, 86-98.)

Note: Optimal EFA and phospholipid intake is part of many of the approaches described on these pages.

Hoffer's general approach

Dr. Abram Hoffer, PhD, MD, has developed the following general protocol, which he modifies to address individual biochemical requirements. (Hoffer 2008)

□ Vitamin B3 — Hoffer's research and clinical work has, for decades, highlighted the importance of high-dose B3 in reversing voices, dysperceptions, paranoia, and psychosis. B3 has powerful antianxiety benefits (and like benzodiazepines, stimulates GABA receptors). (Mohler) Moreover, it promotes formation of acetylcholine and COMT (which moderate stimulation), and of serotonin (which does so for some bipolars). And it's a critical component of the brain enzyme, NADH, which is antidepressant and critical to brain metabolism. B3 also helps regulate dopamine and form histamine, making it particularly useful for low histamine and metal metabolism disordered patients, and often for pyrolurics. (Histadelics, especially with psychosis, anxiety, agitation, or insomnia, may also benefit, though usually at more moderate doses. (Walsh 2006))

□ Vitamin C — supports formation of antidepressant transmitters (norepinephrine and serotonin), and counters vanadium toxicity. Hoffer (2005) reports profound benefit to psychosis. It can also be antimanic. (Tolbert points out that it targets the same receptors as tranquilizers and antipsychotics, and at high doses, is as potent as strong neuroleptics.) C also helps redress histamine imbalances, supports metal metabolism, improves pyroluria and cerebral allergies, and protects neurotransmitter systems from oxidative stress.

□ B complex— often depleted in bipolars; supports neurological function and prevents deficiencies during high intake of B3 or other individual B vitamins.

□ Vitamin B6 — required in forming most mood-modulating neurotransmitters.

□ Folic acid — antidepressant; supports formation of dopamine, norepinephrine, serotonin. *Restrict if histadelic.*

□ Zinc (citrate)— Moderates mood, anxiety, hyperactivity, paranoia, and psychosis.

□ Vitamin D — antidepressant; supports sleep cycle.

□ EFAs — especially with depression. Usually omega 3. *Pyrolurics often preferentially need GLA.*

□ Antioxidants — protect the brain and EFAs from oxidative stress (selenium (which is also antiviral; check blood to assess need); E (also antianxiety); etc.)

□ Redress any nutrient depletion or dependency. Treat food sensitivities, blood sugar and endocrine imbalances, toxicity, etc. Support sleep, minimize stress, address trauma. Consider effects of antidepressants, etc.

Antiseizure-based approaches (SLAGLE 2001, ROSS 2001)

Anticonvulsive vitamins and minerals (magnesium, zinc, B3, B6, C, etc.), alone, or combined with inhibitory, anticonvulsive, aminos (taurine, GABA, glycine). With depression, add precursors and cofactors for producing dopamine, norepinephrine, and/or serotonin, *as relevant.**

* These precursors are usually not appropriate for histapenics.

Larson's approach

Dr. Joan Matthews Larson, PhD, of Health Recovery Center, in Minnesota which primarily treats alcoholism and substance abuse, has developed this protocol to address bipolar disorder in her dual diagnosis patients.

□ B100 — [3x/day (2x if taking lithium), with food]

□ Ester C — [1300 mg, 2 to 3x/day, with food.]

□ Lithium orotate — [20 mg, 3x/day with food]

□ EFAs

□ Taurine — a major anticonvulsive/inhibitory transmitter. Larson finds it comparable to lithium in stabilizing mood. [500 mg, 3x/day, on an empty stomach] *Note: If instead, taking prescription lithium:* skip the taurine; take B, C, EFAs, *as above*; add CalMag [50/150 mg, 3x/day, w. food]. *Check for low thyroid, folate, C.*

□ Biotype treatment. Larson finds histadelia prevalent in bipolars.

□ Balance blood sugar. Hypoglycemia is ubiquitous in very rapid cyclers.

□ Oral GABA, zinc, B3, other vitamins and minerals, perhaps multis, antidepressant nutrients *as relevant*, etc., *as per individual genetics/biochemistry/response.*

□ IVs *when indicated*, e.g., high-dose C, or taurine-C-glutathione, perhaps B complex, *as relevant.*

Focus on neural energetics, plasticity, stress

Nutrients that support: receptor & second messenger flexibility (EFAs, phospholipids, etc); balanced mitochondrial energy production (carnitine, pyruvate, NADH, CoQ10, B2, magnesium, etc.); appropriate glucocorticoid signalling; protection from free radicals and excitotoxins (antioxidants, zinc, magnesium, correction of any metal metabolism dysfunction, etc.). (MCGINNIS 2004, QUIROZ 2004)

General approach (CASS 2008, PFEIFFER 1987, WALSH 2008, LESSER 2008)

Orthomolecular treatment of the individual patient is generally guided by ongoing signs, symptoms, histories, clinical response, and relevant labs which, taken together, point to specific nutritional and health imbalances, and toxicity issues.

Additional considerations

Allergies, Sugar, Digestive issues, Malnutrition, Low lithium (LESSER 2008, TRUSS 1980, 81, 83, 84, TROWBRIDGE 1986, PHILPOTT 1978AB, 82, 87, ROGERS 1997)

Allergies and sensitivities. Environmental illness. Blood sugar dysregulation. Malabsorption, Candida, other parasites. Acidity. Low enzymes, bile, hydrochloric acid. Malnutrition. Low environmental or dietary lithium.

Neuroendocrine balance (SEE REFERENCES IN CORRESPONDING CHAPTERS)

Especially thyroid, pancreas and adrenal function, and dysregulation of the hypothalamus/pituitary/endocrine axis. *Note: Activity tends to change with mood or stress.*

Confounding illness & toxicity (SEE REFERENCES IN CORRESPONDING CHAPTERS)

□ Autoimmune, immune and chronic illness.

□ Neurotoxicity — metal metabolism disorder, oxidative stress, excitoxicity, substance abuse, drug side effects, pollutants. (KAPCZINSKI 2004)

Lifestyle moderation (SEE REFERENCES IN CORRESPONDING CHAPTERS)

Regular sleep, meals, exercise, etc., in tune with natural biorhythms. Optimize diet.

Reduce exposure and susceptibility to stressors.

Psychological support for cases of abuse/trauma.

When depressed: Sunlight and exercise, especially in the morning. Social support. Creativity. Work.

When manic: Minimize stimulation.

Diet. Multiples, only if indicated. (WALSH 2006, COUSENS 2001, HOFFER 1987)

Bipolars often have poor diets, low in minerals, aminos, EFAs, B vitamins, and antioxidants, and high in junk food; perhaps confounded by substance abuse. And nutrient absorption is often poor.

A good diet, tailored to individual needs, is always helpful. *Some* also respond to relatively low-to-moderate doses of high-quality (perhaps restricted*) multiples, to complement therapeutic nutrients and to redress overall depletion.

However, many bipolars (e.g., with methylation, metal metabolism, pyrrole, convulsive, or toxicity issues) are already overloaded with certain nutrients, or reactive to them, and do *NOT* do well with most multiples. Thus, *depending on chemistry,* supplemental copper, iron, folic acid, methionine, SAMe, manganese, choline, inositol, *will variously promote healing, or cause deterioration.* *(WALSH 2002)

Moreover, multi-minerals, or multi-aminos (free-form or otherwise) may compete with minerals or aminos that are particularly needed, impeding absorption and use.

* E.g., copper-and-amino-free multivitamin/mineral for some histapenics and pyrolurics; hypoallergenic multis for patients with primary food sensitivities.

Pfeiffer's checklist (PFEIFFER 1987, 88)

□ Daily cycling: Look for allergies, hypoglycemia, Candida, abuse of caffeine, alcohol, cocaine, etc.

□ Weekly: Test for pyroluria, and B6 and zinc deficiency. Check for weekly sources of stress.

□ Monthly: Check for PMS, excess copper stimulation with low zinc, and seasonal allergies.

Some interesting anecdotal approaches

Warning: These approaches have been used by only a small number of bipolars, and are cited for illustative-educational purposes only. Individuals can react adversely to specific components or require others that are lacking. Inappropriate choices can cause harm. Persons needing treatment for mood disorders should consult a knowledgeable physician who will tailor treatment to individual biochemistry.

Margot Kidder (2008)

Margot Kidder recovered from severe bipolar I with psychotic features, using this protocol.

Morning: One hour sunlight. Choline/inositol combo (500 mg). Multi with generous B vitamins.
Tyrosine (1000 mg) (*not if rapid cycling or manic*)
L-glutamine (500 mg) (*only if stimulation is needed*)
Phenylalanine (500 mg) (*only if needed for depression*)

Evening: Taurine (500-1000 mg); GABA (500-2000 mg) Tryptophan (1000 mg) (*do not take with SSRIs*). Multi.

Alan Darman (2000, 07, 08)

*Darman (2000) recovered from years of severe rapid cycling bipolar I with this approach, which he developed based on the work of Drs S Rogers, P Slagle, J Balch, and others.**

Address malabsorption (bentonite & fiber, and glutamine, separated by several hours); allergies, Candida. (*See p. 199, and Rogers 1997*)

Ongoing, inhibitory, anti-manic, mood-stabilizing, sleep-promoting nutrients (focusing on aminos).

At the first hint of mania (less sleep, irritability, increased drive, excitement, etc.) increase antimanic nutrients (taurine, GABA, glycine, choline, etc.)* *and stop exclusively antidepressant nutrients* (if used).

At the first hint of depression, antidepressant nutrients, especially aminos (e.g., tyrosine, tryptophan, phenylalanine) *with care not to overdo them,* added to ongoing stabilizing nutrients. (*See Slagle 2001.*)

* After a number of years on this protocol, Darman (2007, 08) finds he now responds to a full range of free form amino acids, plus full spectrum vitamins and minerals (*see Balch 2000*), with additional EFAs, choline, carnitine, certain other nutrients; and continued attention to malabsorption issues.

George Eby (2006)

Magnesium glycinate (typically, 200 mg, 4x/day) plus other supportive nutrients.

Patty E Fleener, MSW (2005)

Omega 3 (2-3x/day)
B (100 mg, 3x/day); P5P (50 mg, *divided over the day*)
Vitamin B12 (2x/day, *on an empty stomach*)
Vitamin C (3-6 gm, *divided over the day*)
Zinc (50 mg; *keep total over all supplements below 100 mg*)
Magnesium-citrate or -glycinate (350-750 mg, *divided over the day. Alert your physician if you have kidney disease.*)
Calcium (up to1500 mg if you don't eat dairy regularly; *divided over the day; do not use calcium carbonate*)
Taurine (500 mg, 3x/day, *on an empty stomach)*
Multi-vitamin/mineral with high B, no iron. (2-3x/day)
Free-form aminos. (2x/day, *on an empty stomach*)

For mania prevention: Mild calming tea. Limit stress, noise. Dim lights. Close eyes. Breathe slowly and deeply. Use guided imagery (*to a safe, beautiful, relaxing place*).

Generally antidepressant:
L-tyrosine (500 mg) + B6 (50 mg) + C (100 mg). (2x/day, *on an empty stomach; don't take with milk*)
St Johns Wort, with mild depression (takes 6-8 weeks); or 5HTP or SAMe for more rapid reponse. *Avoid if trying to get pregnant or prone to breast cancer.*
Medication as prescribed. Work with your doctor.

The True Hope approach

The multiple, formulated by David Hardy, an animal nutritionist, provides high-dose minerals, substantial antioxidants; and support for oxygenation (ginkgo, germanium) and gut integrity (glutamine). It is augmented by suggestions for dietary improvements, limiting coffee and sugar, avoiding alcohol and street drugs, addressing Candida, getting enough sleep and relaxation, and reducing stress. Added omega 3 is especially advised with depression; phosphatidyl choline, with mania; inositol, with anxiety. An amino acid supplement is also provided, where indicated.

In two small preliminary trials, improvement was reported in about 60% of bipolars who stayed in the studies. (Kaplan 2001, Simmons 2003) Anecdotal reports seem to be about evenly divided; some claim to do very well with this approach, others deteriorate.* A large double blind is now underway.

The formula may be particularly relevant for some whose primary imbalance involves malnutrition, malabsorption, allergies, addictions, blood sugar fluctuations, certain EFA problems, etc., and for some who tend more toward depression. However, the vanadium content can be problematic. And, of the major biotypes, the formula would seem to best address undermethylation (histadelia) — except for the high doses of folate, especially at the outset — while the high copper and other factors, would probably make it counterproductive for histapenia and pyroluria.**

Undeniably, this approach offers significant quantities of a variety of good nutrients, which may address underlying imbalances in a considerable number of bipolars. And it is relatively convenient. On the other hand, as Lesser says, "one formula can't work for the whole world." Thus, Walsh points out, for any given patient, the dose for certain required nutrients can be much too low, while harmful choices may be oversupplied. (Walsh 2008) So the issue becomes how well the formula matches the patient's needs.

* And in some cases, it serves as a starting point, after which further progress occurs with a more individualized approach.

** If histapenic, the methionine, phenylalanine and high copper can be disastrous, inositol will not necessarily be helpful, while B3 and B6 doses appear inadequate. If pyroluric, the copper is again a major problem; B6 is low; the eventual reductions in zinc and manganese may cause flareups; and, with moderate-to-severe pyroluria, the added omega 3 may be counterproductive (with GLA, preferable).

A note on addressing symptoms vs. underlying causes (WALSH 2006, 07)

Symptomatic attention is often life-saving, and may be necessary thoughout therapy. On the other hand, attention to underlying causes becomes critical to long-term stability.

While many natural anti-manic or anti-depressant choices discussed in Part I may also address causes, others (especially *certain* herbs, aminos, and other acutely potent nutrients) may mainly improve symptoms.

Attention to methylation imbalances, pyrrole disorder, oxidative stress, hormonal issues, neurological problems, metal metabolism dysfunction, allergies, toxicity, etc. (all discussed later in this book) — as well as, nutrient dependencies, depletion or overload — may get closer to the root of the bipolar illness, creating a more sustainable solution.

The overall balance of such factors is dictated by each patient's unique requirements.

Theories of bipolar etiology & some potentially corresponding nutrients (SCHERK 2004, YURGELUN-TODD 2000. SEE RELEVANT CHAPTERS FOR FURTHER REFERENCES)

Some proposed etiologies (described further throughout this book) are mentioned here [*with several potentially relevant nutrients italicized and in brackets*].

□ Altered receptor density and sensitivity, intracellular signalling and gene expression. (DILSAVER 1986, MCENANY 1990, STOLL 1996, KAPCZINSKI 2004) [*Omega 3, phospholipids, magnesium, etc.*]

□ Interruptions in mood-regulating limbic, prefrontal, striatum, etc., circuits. Limbic subconvulsive seizures. Kindling. (KAPCZINSKI 2004) [*GABA, taurine, magnesium, zinc, manganese, B6.*] Laterality issues. [*Copper/zinc, cognitive exercises* (PFEIFFER 1987, 88)]

□ Methylation/folate imbalances, pyroluria, metal metabolism dysfunction, etc. [*See Biotypes,* pp. 145-68.]

□ Electrolyte dysfunction/imbalance. (DILSAVER 1986) [*Magnesium, zinc, potassium foods, C, perhaps calcium, restrict vanadium*]

□ Reduced cell plasticity and resilience [*EFAs, phopholipids, antioxidants*], maladaptive stress reponse [*C, B5, relevant minerals, GABA, taurine*] (including problems with neurotrophic regulation, glucocorticoid signaling, phosphodiesterase activity, glutamate throughput; mitochondrial function [*Carnitine, pyruvate, CoQ10, tyrosine, etc.*]). (STORK 2005, QUIROZ 2004).

□ Imbalances between stimulating and inhibitory systems (BOULLIN 1979, DILSAVER 1984, MCENANY 1990 KAPCZINSKI 2004). [*Inositol, tyrosine, phenylalanine; versus choline, taurine, GABA, perhaps tryptophan*]

A pharmaceutical approach & some potentially corresponding nutrients (NUTRIENT REFERENCES CAN BE FOUND IN RELEVANT CHAPTERS)

Pfeiffer's Law: *"If there's a drug that can alter the brain's biochemistry, there's usually a combination of nutrients that can achieve the same thing without side effects."*

Below is a hypothetical glimpse of how a pharmaceutical approach (derived from Sachs (2000) and Ketter (2001)) might start to be translated into a protocol for nutrients and herbs [*with some nutrients which may address the same issues in italics and brackets*].

IMPORTANT: WHAT FOLLOWS IS AN INCOMPLETE AND GENERALIZED OUTLINE OF THIS PHARMACEUTICAL APPROACH, AND DOES NOT CONSTITUTE TREATMENT SUGGESTIONS.

□ Mood stabilizers, on an ongoing basis, usually life-long. They are the base to which mood-specific treatments are added. [*Anticonvulsive/inhibitory nutrients, e.g., GABA, taurine, magnesium glycinate, B, B1, B3, B6, zinc, manganese, perhaps melatonin, nutritional doses of lithium, lecithin, etc.*]

□ For mania: optimize mood stabilizers [*above nutrients*]. If insufficient, consider antianxiety meds [*B3, B complex, C, E, zinc, GABA, etc.*], CCBs [*magnesium*], or omega 3. With unresponsive psychotic features or severe mania, consider atypical antipsychotics. [*B3, C, zinc, B6, etc.; biotype therapy.*]

□ For bipolar depression: stabilizers. If necessary, an antidepressant least likely to trigger mania [*omega 3 (GLA if pyroluric), calcium, C, B3 or NADH, B6, B12, carnitine, folate (if histapenic), inositol (if histadelic), etc.*], often, an SSRI [*5HTP, tryptophan, St. Johnswort*], in some cases, meds targeting catecholamines [*tyrosine or phenylalanine plus B6, C, etc.*].

Note: Before starting nutrients interactions of meds, especially with amino acids, or herbs, should be ruled out by the physician. Taking nutrients does not mean one can suddenly stop taking meds (this can entail life-or-death risk), though, as the patient improves, physicians frequently find careful, gradual reductions in medication are indicated. *See p. 289.*

I: Nutrient survey

a: Mania & Stabilization

"Bring me my Bow of burning gold!
Bring me my Arrows of desire!
Bring me my Spear; O clouds unfold!
Bring me my Chariot of fire!"

William Blake
"And did those feet in ancient time," 1804-10

"[As a celebrity,] it was easy for me to check into hotels with nothing. I had nothing. I certainly never had any cash. There were also times when I didnt have credit cards or checkbooks or anything. Still the door opened. The piper had to pay later on, but it was certainly a manic's dream."

Patty Duke, *A Brilliant Madness,* 1992

"Here is the liberation of the caged wild animals of the earth."

Sarah Clemmens
Mark Twain's daughter, on her father's anger

See also:
Mania & Depression, pp. 57-83.

The following two frameworks roughly bring together some of the nutritional approaches described throughout this book. Although definitive cures do not exist, the physician or researcher may find these frameworks helpful in evaluating therapeutic options. For the general public, the material in this book is presented for strictly educational purposes, to facilitate understanding, and should not be construed as treatment suggestions.

Framework 1: Nutrition & mood stabilization

(REFERENCES CAN BE FOUND IN RELEVANT CHAPTERS)

The key is determining, for each individual, the precise therapeutic equation potent enough to stabilize mood, prevent breakthrough episodes, and bring down intractable manias, without moving cycling toward depression, or discouraging participation in treatment, i.e., the least suppressive therapy which works.

Biotypes

Treatment of biotype imbalances (pyroluria, over or under-methylation) may be the overriding consideration in most bipolars.

See Part II, pp. 145-68.

Potentially therapeutic nutrients

Dose, timing, and choice of nutrients should be tailored to biotype and unique biochemical requirements. Take into account ongoing response, including variations in symptom intensity over the day.

□ **MAGNESIUM** — a calcium channel blocker; may be especially useful for stabilization, mania, rapid cycling.

□ **ZINC, NUTRITIONAL LITHIUM, PERHAPS CHROMIUM, SELENIUM** — and other minerals, *as relevant*.

□ **VITAMIN C** — a natural tranquilizer; counters anxiety, mania, depression, psychosis, vanadium toxicity; benefits pyroluria, methylation, and metal metabolism disorders.

□ **B VITAMINS** — support brain communication, maintenance, and mood stability. Bipolar levels are often low. Specific vitamins (e.g., B3, B1, B6) are often needed.

□ **TAURINE, GABA, GLYCINE**— anticonvulsive, sleep-promoting, and mood-stabilizing; inhibitory neurotransmitters. *Individuals may respond best to only one, or some specific combination.*

□ **TRYPTOPHAN OR 5HTP** — helps moderate mood and maintain some patients (*but fosters mania in others*).

□ **PHOSPHATIDYL CHOLINE** — decreases mania, helps moderate mood, particularly in histapenics. (*Be cautious, as bipolars can be particularly sensitive to choline, excess of which can trigger depression, perhaps especially in histadelics.)*

□ **APPROPRIATE EFAS** — critical to mood and to receptor function. Take with B vitamins and antioxidants.

□ **ANTIOXIDANTS & OTHER NEUROPROTECTIVE NUTRIENTS** — protect brain neurotransmitter systems, neural membrane fatty acids, and overall brain health.

□ **OTHER NUTRIENT NEEDS** – may reflect depletion, dependency, malnourishment, or genetic issues.

See Part I, pp. 21-144.

Attention to confounding health conditions

□ Metal metabolism disorders and metal toxicity.

□ Allergies, sensitivities.

□ Malabsorption. Candida. Malnutrition.

□ Sugar metabolism imbalances.

□ Thyroid, adrenal and other endocrine imbalance.

□ Seizures and other neurological conditions.

□ Chronic oxidative stress, excitotoxicity, substance abuse, toxic reactions to medication, other toxicity.

□ Physical illness. Autoimmune, or immune issues.

See Parts III and IV, pp. 169-250.

Diet

□ Fresh whole foods, freshly prepared, with an emphasis on vegetables, sufficient protein (especially fish and legumes; perhaps, high-quality meat, poultry, and/or dairy), and antioxidant-rich foods. Moderate portions of seeds, nuts, whole grains (preferably sprouted), fresh low-glycemic fruit.

□ Tailor diet to address biotype, blood sugar, allergies, Candida, etc.

□ Calming herb teas, and foods (e.g., nutritional yeast, lecithin (*especially if histapenic*), etc.), *as relevant.*

□ Avoid allergens, sugar, white flour, altered or fried fat, processed food, MSG, aspartame,® street drugs, alcohol. Limit caffeine, salt, vanadium sources (soy, etc.).

See Part V, pp. 254-56.

Lifestyle factors

□ Be alert for signs of a mood episode.

□ Adjust daily activities to natural biorhythms (e.g, sleep at night, regular meals, etc.).

□ Avoid triggers. Reduce stress.

□ Breathwork. Physical exercise (at moderate levels).

□ Psychosocial support, cognitive exercises, creative outlets, meditation, prayer.

See Part V, pp. 251-62.

Increase support during seasonal change, illness, injury, emotional or other stressors.
Medication as prescribed. Consult with your physician.

Framework II: Nutritive approaches for mania

(REFERENCES CAN BE FOUND IN RELEVANT CHAPTERS)

Prevention of mania is critical. Mania not only begets more manic and depressive episodes, and general deterioration, but the potent treatment sometimes required may also worsen the illness. Prevention entails:

- □ Optimizing ongoing nutritive and other support for mood stabilization and brain flexibility.
- □ Adjusting dose, frequency, and timing of nutrient intake to address times of the day when symptoms tend to become worse (e.g., morning depression, nightly insomnia, whatever).
- □ Attention to triggers and signs of mania; immediate increases in nutritive support.
- □ A commitment by the patient to do what it takes to avoid or mitigate mania (e.g., reduce external stimulation, avoid triggers, take additional stabilizing nutrients, consider feedback from trusted persons, etc.).

Optimize biotype support

Pyroluria, and/or methylation imbalances, perhaps confounded by metal metabolism dysfunction, may often be the overriding consideration.

See Part II, pp. 145-68.

Potentially therapeutic nutrients

Dose, timing, and choice of nutrients should be tailored to biotype and unique biochemical requirements. Take into account ongoing response, including variations in symptom intensity over the day.

□ Continue relevant mood-stabilizing therapies, and adjust, *as relevant.*

□ Increase the more potent stabilizers to reduce symptoms, e.g., GABA, taurine, magnesium glycinate, phosphatidyl choline (*especially for histapenia*), time-release melatonin, etc.; perhaps, B1, B3, B, C, zinc, etc.; *as relevant*.

□ Consider, *as relevant*, kava, valerian, skullcap, ladies slipper, wood betony, etc., perhaps mixed with some of the milder herbs, such as, hops, chamomile, passion flower, Bach Rescue Remedy.

□ Stop the stronger antidepressant supplements (e.g., SAMe, 5HTP, phenylalanine, rubidium, rhodiola, Korean ginseng, etc.),* if used. Also, *if contributing to mania,* reduce or eliminate, *as appropriate,*** glutamine, carnitine, tryptophan, cesium, iron, ginkgo, tyrosine, methionine, inositol, germanium, multiples, Siberian or American ginseng, noni, goji berries, etc. Similarly, *if indicated,*** reduce calcium, manganese, chromium, vitamin D, GLA, omega 3 (or switch the focus to DHA rather than EPA), etc.

See Part I, pp. 21-144.

* The physician will probably also reduce antidepressant meds.

** Taking into account overall mental and physical health needs.

Physical health & lifestyle

Treat allergies, Candida, malabsorption, blood sugar and hormonal imbalances, neurological illness, oxidative stress, excitotoxicity, other toxins and confounding health conditions.

See Parts III , IV, and V, pp. 169-262.

Address triggers

Address diet and lifestyle factors. Avoid allergens, coffee, alcohol, drugs, sugar, foods which promote Candida, fried food, excitotoxins, stimulating foods or nutrients.

Reduce exposure and sensitivity to stressors and stimulants, including stimulating social interactions, overpursuit of goals, etc.. Darkness, quiet, and rest are helpful (e.g., retreat to a quiet room; dim the lights; relax).

See Part V, 251-62.

Treat early

Treat at the first hints of emerging mania (less sleep, irritability; increased drive, excitement, etc.).

Natural therapies for acute or nonresponsive mania may involve nutrient IVs; or, with psychotic mania, a short-term, high-meat diet. (See *Acute therapies,* p. 56; and *Psychotic mania,* p. 268.)

Monitor & adjust

Carefully monitor reactions and adjust therapy accordingly. If therapy overshoots, producing signs of depression, cautiously add antidepressant nutrients to the mood-stabilizing regimen, and consider reducing the stronger antimanics. And *vice versa.* Averting episodes becomes easier as experience with the individual's response to specific nutrients and herbs accumulates. Patient education and participation in this process enhances outcome.

Medication as prescribed. Consult with your physician.

Cautions & reminders

Individual biochemical requirements are not identical, and supplements helpful for one patient can be detrimental for another. Fullcontraindications, interactions with med, dosage information, etc. are not included.

Persons needing treatment for affective disorder, or other medical conditions, should seek the services of a knowledgeable physician, who will tailor treatment to individual biochemical requirements.

Inappropriate dose reduction or withdrawal from affective drugs can be life-threatening. Amino acids, herbs, and some other nutrients may interact with drugs.

I. Minerals

Minerals regulate neural messages. They support creation and use of neurotransmitters, mediate release into the synapse, guide receptor activity, and convey messages along the neural axon. They are the cofactors that make brain enzymes work, and are critical in brain cell communication, metabolism and immune defense.

" Minerals ....[are] required by any and all body functions from the basic subcellular molecular biological 'metallic fingers' of RNA and DNA to electrochemical, catalytic, structural, reproduction, maintenance, repair and a plethora of miscellaneous functions."

"A potentially apocalyptic mixture of mining, deforestation, farming, irrigation and acid rain has shifted, eroded, or leached [the earth's] mineral rich land."

Joel D Wallach, ND, 1994

Unfortunately, our food no longer provides enough of the minerals we need, as soil depletion has vastly accelerated over the past century.* Minerals are also leached from our bones during stress. Except for communities clustered around the few regions on earth endowed with rich veins of minerals, most people are mineral-deficient, and suffer mental and physical repercussions. (WALLACH 1994)

* Due to deforestation, flooding, irrigation, deep plowing, monocropping, lack of fallow periods, use of fertilizers with limited minerals (rather than ash, compost or manure), and general overuse. (Wallach 1994)

Bipolars generally require more of certain minerals, and do poorly with certain others. In some cases, the appropriate minerals (or minerals, vitamins, and EFAs), may be sufficient to reverse mania and maintain stability; in others, aminos may be central to therapy.

Mineral requirements vary over individuals. Lab assessments, and careful evaluation of signs, symptoms and response help map need. Some of the more important minerals for manics may include:

- ☐ Magnesium — may often be important in moderating mood, even severe mania or rapid cycling.
- ☐ Zinc — shows benefit to mania and some depressions. It's sedative at very high doses, a potent antioxidant, and critical in treating pyroluria and metal metabolism dysfunction.
- ☐ Lithium — lithium-containing soils and water sources have long been reputed to calm behavior. Physiologic amounts (a small fraction of the psychiatric dose) have benefitted mood.
- ☐ Selenium — antioxidant; helps protect brain function. (See p. 78.)
- ☐ Chromium — especially with blood sugar imbalance. (pp. 127-28.) *though it's not necessarily indicated, as it may overstimulate some manics.*

Magnesium (Mg)

Moderating mood & mania (Pfeiffer 1975, 88, Werbach 1991, Jaffe 1992, Eby 2001)

Research suggests magnesium can, in many cases, moderate mood, (Weston 1921) even rapid cycling, (Chouinard 1990) and drug-resistant mania. (Giannini 2000, Heiden 1999, Blabicher 1997) (See box, below.)

Some of the research

Weston, 1921 — IV magnesium sulfate produced relaxation, sleep, and sedation in 50 patients with mania, agitation or agitated depression.

Blabicher 1997 — IV magnesium sulfate was effective as an adjunct for severe mania.

Heiden 1999 — in an open study, seven of ten severely agitated treatment-resistant manics improved markedly on up to 23 days of IV magnesium sulfate, added to medication. Neuroleptic and benzo doses were able to be significantly reduced.

Giannini 2000 — magnesium oxide augmentation of verapamil was significantly more effective for mania as compared to controls on the drug alone.

Chouinard 1990 — in a small, open-label trial, response in at least 50% of severe, treatment-resistant, rapid cyclers was equivalent to, or better than, that to lithium.

Deficiency has been associated with mania, hypomania, and such related symptoms as emotional stress, restlessness, excessive talking, irritability, agitation, hyperactivity, anxiety, panic attacks, insomnia, hyperemotionality, moodiness, anger, rage, tantrums, fear, paranoia, belligerance, aggression, violence, obsessions, compulsions, odd behavior, and heightened sensitivity to light and sound. (Hall 1973, Slagle 1995, Mason, Durlach 1995, Eby 2001, 06, Beitman 1991, Standley 1994, 95, Pfeiffer 1975, 88, Werbach 1991, Jaffe 1992) *Consider its effects on the following conditions:*

- □ Anxiety — Magnesium is sedative in itself, and also enhances benzodiazepine anti-anxiety activity. (Slagle 1995)
- □ Sleep disturbance — Magnesium promotes sleep. (Penland 1988) Deficiency has been associated with fatigue, insomnia, and fitful sleep. (Pfeiffer 1975) Chronic insomnia decreases magnesium further; as can sleeping pills or antihistamines. (Eby 2001, 06, Cousens 2001)
- □ Psychosis & paranoia — Magnesium can be low in some schizophrenias and, especially when severely low, can produce personality change, paranoia, hallucinations, or delirium. (Slagle 1995, Pfeiffer 1975, 87, 88)
- □ Depression — Magnesium can be antidepressant. (See p. 126.)
- □ SAD — Up to 70% of SAD patients are magnesium-deficient. Aside from light therapy, magnesium and D3 can be useful in treatment. (Eby 2001, 06)
- □ Intellectual dysfunction — Studies suggest magnesium supports memory, concentration, intelligence, and learning ability. (Larson 2001, Slagle 1995, NIH)
- □ Hyperactivity — Magnesium can be low in children with hyperactivity (prevalent in bipolar histories), (Mousain-Bosc 2004, 06, Starabrat-Hermelin 1997) concentration problems, or neuroses. (Nizankowska-Blaz 1993) In one study, magnesium was deficient in 95% of 116 hyperactive children. When no coexisting disorders were present, hyperactivity improved as magnesium increased (as compared to controls on pharmaceuticals alone). (Starabrat-Hermelin 1998)
- □ Other — autism, PTSD, OCD, isolation, seizures, bedwetting, PMS. (Pfeiffer 1975, Marlowe 1984, Standley 1994, 95, Walsh 2007)

Biotype considerations (Pfeiffer 1975, 87, 88, Walsh 2007)

Magnesium benefits all biotypes. It helps counter histadelia (by decreasing mast cell histamine secretion, and helping metabolize methionine to SAMe). It is also often indicated in pyroluria, especially with agitation, and can help moderate histapenic anxiety. (See pp. 145-68.)

Effects on the brain which influence mood

- Helps prevent adrenalin buildup.
- Modulates the influence of stimulating neurotransmitters.
- Blocks calcium and sodium uptake into the nerve cell.
- Influences second messengers and certain receptors.
- Helps block excitotoxicity.
- Supports neural membrane stability. Anticonvulsive.

See *Neurochemistry,* next page.

Physical functions which can influence mood

(Slagle 1995, Pfeiffer 1975, Garrison 1985, Balch 1990, Page 1992, Quillin 1987, Lieberman 1990, Murray 1996)

- Helps prevent insulin resistance, and support sugar metabolism and storage.
- Supports secretion of, and response to, parathyroid hormone, which regulates calcium.
- Improves female hormone balance.
- Benefits hyperthyroid, & aldosteronism.
- Supports cell energy production.
- Supports creation of antibodies, resistance to infection, chelation and elimination of heavy metals, protection by the liver from toxic chemicals.
- Supports appetite, aids digestion. Helps maintain acid/alkaline balance.

"Magnesium permits one to support adversity with more serenity."

ML Robinet, 1934, who also found (1921) sparsity of soil magnesium strikingly related to suicides

Brain & neurological symptoms of magnesium depletion

Chronic headaches or migraines. (SLAGLE 1995)

Noise & light sensitivity. (SLAGLE 1995)

Tingling, prickling, or creeping sensation. (SLAGLE 1995)

Incoordination, bizarre movement. Pronounced startle, muscle twitching, tremors, spasms, shakiness, tetany, seizures, convulsions. (DURLACH 1995, PFEIFFER 1975, LARSON 2001, SLAGLE 1995, STANDLEY 1994, 95)

Cold hands and feet. (DURLACH 1995)

Increased tendency to mini-strokes, dementias, retardation.* (HALL 1973, KIROV 1990, 94, SLAGLE 1995, PFEIFFER 1975)

* One study in JAMA reports 70% lower incidence of mental retardation, and 90% lower incidence of cerebral palsy in children whose mothers were supplemented with magnesium in pregnancy.

Neurochemistry (SLAGLE 1995, EBY 2001, 06)

Magnesium regulates neural communication, particularly at the synapse and receptors. Deficiency leaves the nervous system overreactive. (SIMONTACCHI 2000)

Neurotransmission effects (PFEIFFER 1975, 87, 88, COLODNY 1998, SLAGLE 1995)

- ☐ Calms overstimulation from dopamine, serotonin, norepinephrine, and acetylcholine, and reduces receptor oversensitivity.
- ☐ Helps create tyrosine, serotonin, SAMe, COMT. May interfere with adrenal catecholamine release. (FRIEDMAN 96)
- ☐ Helps regulate NMDA and 5-HT3 receptors, countering pain and sleep deprivation.

Neural membrane

- ☐ Helps optimize neural membrane fatty acids. (SLAGLE 1995) With B1, supports fat metabolism. (RAYSSIGUIER 1981)
- ☐ Supports creation of DHA and conversion of EFAs to prostaglandins. (COUSENS 2001)
- ☐ Supports membrane permeability and enzyme transport across the neural membrane. (PFEIFFER 1975, COLODNY 1998)

Calcium channel blocking

- ☐ Controls calcium pumps and blocks calcium uptake to the nerve cell, reducing stimulation. (ABRAHAM1982, ALTURA 1985, HOSCHL 1991, PFEIFFER, COLODNY 1998, WESTON 1921, ISERI 1984)

Second messenger activity

- ☐ Influences* neural creation of inositol. (COLODNY 1998)
- ☐ Important in G protein/cAMP signals (which are blunted in depression). (FRIEDMAN 1996)

* The magnesium enzyme, IMPase, hydrolyzes inositol monophosphate into inositol. (See p. 96.)

Sodium/potassium activity

- ☐ Helps maintain cellular electrical potential. (PFEIFFER 1975)
- ☐ Deficiency can damage the sodium pump causing cellular water retention and swelling, (PFEIFFER 1975) with accompanying irritability and depression. (CACH 1988, ROGERS 1997)

Neuroprotective effects

- ☐ Anticonvulsive. (STANDLEY 1994, 95, EBY 2001)
- ☐ Helps block excitotoxic reactions. (BLAYLOCK 1995) (pp.191-3)
- ☐ May reduce cerebral aluminum accumulation (especially as magnesium malate, which readily crosses the blood brain barrier and binds to aluminum). (PFEIFFER 1975)

Hippocampus

- ☐ Magnesium is important in the hippocampus, which mediates emotional memory. (RAJKOWSKA 2000)

Role in stress chemistry (EBY 2001, 06, BARNETT, SLAGLE 1995, BAUMEL 1995, PFEIFFER 1975, 88, MCGUIRE 1984, HENROTTE 1986)

- ☐ Modulates stress, but gets used up interacting with calcium, adrenalin, and stress transmitters; and compensating for low oxygen (which acidifies the blood).*
- ☐ Depletion then reduces calcium channel blocking, increases liver sugar release, promotes adrenalin buildup, accelerates heartbeat, and may alter pituitary function; all of which worsen stress and further destabilize mood.

CCBs, magnesium, & mood (CURRIER 1998, DUBOVSKY 1995, POST 1999)

Calcium channel blockers (CCBs) inactivate calcium channels, reducing calcium entrance into the cell and increasing levels without (e.g., serum), generally increasing inhibition. (BRUNET 1990, CURRIER 1998, DUBOVSKY 1983, 86, HOSCHL 1991)

Effects on mood

Trials suggest CCBs support mood stabilization in some bipolars, (POST 1996, 99, DUNN 1998) particularly rapid, (POST 1990, GOODNICK1995) and ultra rapid cyclers. (PAZZAGLIA 1993) CCBs may be most effective in mania,*(MASTERS 1996. HOSCHL 1989, 91, DUBOVSKY 1982, 86, 95, GARZO-TREVINO 1992, DOSE 1986, GIANNINI 1984, 85, DINAN 1988, BROTMAN 1986, BRUNET 1990, CAILLARD 1985, GOODNICK 1996, BARTON 1987) and, with lithium, may be preventive. (MCDERMUT 1995, MANNA 1991, AUBY 1992, POST 1999) They may help some bipolar depressions, (MASTERS 1996) and have been used to counter panic and agitation. (GOLDSTEIN 1985, POLLACK 1987)

Magnesium, a nutritional CCB, seems to convey similar effects on mood. (ISERI 1984)

Calcium blocking by the major mood stabilizers

The three primary mood stabilizers also block calcium entry into the neuron,*(POST 1999) thereby moderating signalling. (STOLL 1996)

* Carbamazepine, via NMDA receptors; valproate via T-type calcium receptors, and lithium via the phosphinositide system.

Antionvulsant effects

As with the major mood stabilizers, animal and clinical data suggest some anticonvulsant activity, (DE FALCO 1992) and blocking of dopamine stimulation. *(PANI 1990, POST 1996)

* CCBs are also known to reduce spasms (so have been used in certain cardiovascular conditions, esophageal spasm, asthma, premature labor, migraines, Tourettes, cerebrovasopasm, etc.) (Eby 2001, 06)

Considerations (PFEIFFER 1975, 88, WERBACH 1991, JAFFE 1992, BALCH 1990, GARRISON 1985, PAGE 1992, QUILLIN 1987, LIEBERMAN 1990, MURRAY 1996, SLAGLE 1995)

Need may be suggested by

Mood instability, insomnia, hyperactivity, anxiety, irritability, paranoia, overreactive to stress, marked startle response, heightened hearing.

Depression, SAD. Light-headedness, dizzy. Confusion, poor memory, dementia. (DURLACH 1992)

Weakness, lethargy, fatigue, chronic fatigue.* (WESSELEY 1991, COX 1991, CLAGUE 1992, DURLACH 1992)

Carbohydrate or chocolate craving, sugar imbalance.

Pale, puffy face. Swollen gums. Small artery and skin lesions. Dry mouth and eyes. Slow tissue repair.**

Numbness, tingling, tremors. Spasmatic conditions (asthma, migraines, difficulty swallowing or breathing, hypertension, premature labor, (MULLER 1971) bedwetting, seizures, etc. (DURLACH 1995, SLAGLE 1995)

Weak adrenals (crave salt, low sexual vitality, etc.). (SLAGLE)

Muscle tension, tightness, aches, cramps (especially if low relative to calcium). With severe deficit, prolonged contractions, e.g., chronic lower back or fibromyalgic pain.***(DURLACH 1995, COUSENS 2001)

Malabsorption, constipation, nausea, anorexia, ulcerative colitis, irritable bowel, leaky gut syndrome, etc.

Heart/arterial spasms. Rapid or irregular heart-beat, weak sensitive heart, chest pain, high cholesterol and triglycerides, high blood pressure, clots, vessel degeneration, arteriosclerosis. Prone to mitral valve prolapse, stroke, heart attack.**** (SLAGLE 1995, DURLACH 1995, COUSENS 2001, WORSE)

Temperature dysregulation.

Female hormonal problems.*****

Some thyroid issues. (DISHASHI 1996, NEGUIB 1963)

Kidney hypofunction, kidney or gallstones.******

Symptoms of elevated calcium.

Growth or genetic defects.*******

Sensitivity to toxins. Prone to infection.

Possibly, noise-induced hearing loss, glaucoma, SIDS.

* Supports energy production and transfer, formation of cAMP in the Kreb's cycle, mitochondrial ATP reactions, oxidative phosphorylation. (Slagle)
** Works with C to build collagen and connective tissue.
*** Deficiency dysregulates NMDA and 5-HT3 receptors, increasing pain and insomnia. Lack of sleep causes further depletion. (Worse, Eby 2001, 06)
**** Magnesium strengthens the heart; improves flexibility, contractibility and oxygen access; acts as a CCB; dilates, relaxes, supports blood vessels; enhances circulation, lowers cholesterol; balances blood clotting mechanisms. Depletion increase thromboxane B2, fostering coronary arterial spasms and clots. (Slagle 1995, Larson 2001, Pfeiffer 1975, Worse)
***** PMS, menstrual cramps or bloating, excess lactation, pregnancy or postpartum complications, premature infants. Natural estrogen helps move magnesium into the cells. (Eby 2001, 06)
****** Low magnesium allows calcium to crystalize, forming stones. Magnesium helps dissolve calcium phosphate kidney stones, and may prevent formation of calcium oxalate stones.
******* Helps create protein, DNA and other genetic materal. Binding agent for RNA. May help create growth hormone.

Populations

Deficiency is common in industrialized countries (perhaps 15 to 70%) (DURLACH 1992, 95) and in psychiatric patients. Cousens (2001) finds up to 80% of his patents deficient.

Conditions promoting deficiency (SLAGLE 1995, LARSON 2001, PFEIFFER 1975, 87, 88, EBY 2001, 06)

Malnutrition, long fasts, dieting. Malabsorption, gastrointestinal disorders, molds, parasites. Too much sugar or fat, diabetes,* imbalanced protein, too much or too little calcium or D. Alcoholism (60-80%). Celiac disease. Kidney or liver damage. Chronic fluid loss, e.g., extensive vomiting, diarrhea, perspiration, diuretics, etc.. Acid/alkaline imbalances. Radiation, surgery, shock. Aging. Stress, mood disorder, insomnia, other severe psychiatric conditions. Pyroluria, porphyria. Female. (GEORGE 1994, HERZBERG 1972). Extended intake of synthetic estrogens, antibiotics, (SLAGLE 1995) lithium,** CCBs, (EBEL) neuroleptics.

* Insulin helps return magnesium to the cells.
** Lithium (which has similar chemical properties) competes for binding sites (Layden 2000, Srinivasan 1999) and displaces magnesium, (Amari 1999, Dunner 1975, Herzberg 1977, Ananth 1979, Pavlinac 1979) increasing blood levels and, perhaps, diarrhea. Eventually bone magnesium can become depleted. (Plenge 1982)

Nutrient interactions (SLAGLE 1995, PFEIFFER 1975)

Enhances B1 activity and supports use of other B vitamins, C and E.

Low magnesium decreases serum potassium, calcium, and phosphorus, which may not improve til it increases.

Magnesium enhances the effectiveness of zinc and potassium, supports calcium metabolism and uptake, and potassium uptake.

Supports amino acid and carbohydrate metabolism.

Lab

Blood tests are insensitive (99% is within the cell), even in severe depletion (e.g., fatal heart conditions). (EBY 2001, 06, ROGERS 1997) Imbalance in either direction can heighten manic or depressive reactions.*(KIROV 1990, 94) RBC is slightly more accurate than serum. (SLAGLE 1995, RAJKOWSKA 2000) 24-hr urine reflects loss, not necessarily cell levels. (JAFFE 1992) Loading may give better results. (COLODNY 1998)

Consider diet and medical history, (SLAGLE 1995), and relationsip to calcium and other stimulating nutrients. (LEVINE 1999)

A trial of magnesium is often helpful. (ROGERS 1997)

* Lab results may not reflect functional status or requirements. (Lesser, Smith, Ananth 1979, Pavlinac 1979) Confounding variables include: disordered metabolism, depressed pumps (Kirov 1994), preferential absorption due to greater need (e.g, in mania), (Young1996) increased loss (common in affectives) via sweat, urine, feces), increased extracellular with reduced neural levels due to stress. (Levine 1999) Also, lithium increases blood magnesium, but moves it out of cells.

Sources (COUSENS 2001, LARSON 2001, SLAGLE 1995, BALCH 1990, NUTRICIRCLES® 1996)

Chlorophyl sources: dark leafy greens (beet greens, spinach, chard, collard greens, parsley, dandelion). Spirulina, chlorella, other algae. Kelp, dulse, other seaweeds. Avocado, artichokes, garlic, squash, beets, broccoli, cauliflower, carrots, celery, asparagus, legumes; sprouts (sunflower, buckwheat, lentils, etc.); other vegetables. Blackstrap molasses. Bananas, figs, apricots, dates, apples, grapefruit, watermelon, blackberries. Wheat germ and bran, brewer's yeast. Salmon, halibut, shrimp, tuna, crab, other fish/seafood, eggs, liver. Almonds, cashews, brazil nuts, filberts, pecans, walnuts, coconut; pumpkin, sesame and sunflower seeds, etc. Whole grains (if phytates are disabled).*

* Low in refined grain, meat, boiled vegetables, food from poor soil.

Considerations *continued*

Supportive nutrients

Manganese, lecithin, and omega 3 support use. (ROGERS 1997, EBY 2001, 06, SLAGLE 1995) Magnesium also works with B6, C, D, CoQ10, potassium, calcium, phosphorus, protein, and boron. (SLAGLE 1995) B6, medium chain triglycerides, and thyroid enhance absorption. (ROGERS 1997) Walking supports absorption into cells.

Competing nutrients, foods, etc

Refined carbohydrates overcooked or processed foods, oxidized fats, too little or too much protein; and too much alcohol, caffeine, or salt deplete magnesium. Oxalic (e.g in spinach and sorrel) and phytic acids (in uncooked grains) decrease availability. (PFEIFFER 1975, 88, COUSENS 2001, EBY 2001, 06, SLAGLE 1995, LARSON 2001)

Though magnesium is rich in fatty foods, it binds with animal and saturated fats (including dairy), creating insoluble salts, which interfere with absorption (EBY 2001, 06, SLAGLE 95)

Excessive sodium, phosphorus, iron, zinc, potassium, D; very high calcium; and aluminum, fluoride, and phosphate decrease absorption, and cause urinary loss. (SLAGLE 1995, PFEIFFER 1975, EBY 2001, 06)

Very high B, B6, B2, and perhaps folic acid may increase use of and need for magnesium. (SLAGLE 1995)

Adrenalin, stress, insomnia (EBY 2001, 06), and synthetic estrogen (SLAGLE 1995) use up magnesium.

Supplements (SLAGLE 1995, JAFFE 1992, EBY 2006)

Magnesium taurate — particularly useful for bipolars. (MCCARTY 1996, EBY 2006)

Magnesium glycinate — particularly useful for bipolars, well absorbed, supports REM. (EBY 2001, 06) *Start with coated tablets, or with milk to avoid the metallic taste.*

Magnesium chloride — cheaper and easy to absorb. Taurine or glycine can be taken separately.

Magnesium malate (found in apples) — used in fibromyalgia, well-absorbed, creates a rapid response.

Magnesium citrate, gluconate, orotate or slow-release lactate — also readily absorbed. (COLODNY 1998)

Time-release — helps minimize laxative effect.

AVOID: Magnesium-aspartate or -glutamate, which may be hidden in "amino acid chelates," and can foster oxidative stress and worsen depression. Also, magnesium sufate (epsom salt) and -hydroxide (milk of magnesia), which are laxative and not absorbed well in any case. Magnesium oxide is also poorly absorbed. (EBY 2001, 06)

Dose

Eby suggests starting with coated magnesium glycinate at 200-400 mg, 2-3x/day and adjusting up or down to what works. Slagle (1995) suggests a total of 400-2000 mg, if necessary, depending on symptoms & response.* Divide doses over the day to prevent rebound. If intake stops, symptoms re-emerge, but subside on resumption. (EBY 2001, 06)

Conditions promoting excess

Excess is rare with normal doses, but may occur with insufficient urinary excretion, over-absorption, certain bone tumors, female cancers, IM or IV injections (e.g., for convulsions or high blood pressure); high oral intake for cathartic or antacid effects. (PFEIFFER 1975, COUSENS 2001, EBY 2001, 06)

Calcium/magnesium balance

Inadequate magnesium compromises calcium absorption. Skye Weintraub, ND, points out that the commonly recommended 2:1 calcium/magnesium ratio doesn't work for everyone. Some do better with equal or more magnesium than calcium. Bipolars often need more magnesium. (EBY 2001, 06)

Along with labs, watch for symptoms of deficiency of either, and adjust accordingly. Diarrhea may suggest a need for more calcium or for probiotics.

Effects of excess, contraindications (LARSON 01, SLAGLE 95, PFEIFFER 75, GOLD 87)

Early morning waking. (500 mg calcium, PM, may help.)

Skin flushing, thirst, nausea, diarrhea, vomiting.

Light headed, uncoordinated, dizzy, blurred vision (if due to high dose Mg-glycinate, -citrate or -chloride may help)

Lethargy, fatigue, weakness, drowsiness, stupor.

Epsom salt (magnesium sulfate) baths, especially if taking sedatives, risk oversedation and drowning.

Moderate toxicity is associated with depression, and perceptual, personality, and intellectual changes.

Too much can cause CNS suppression, loss of reflexes, low blood pressure, slow heart beat and respiration.

High doses can inhibit insulin release from the pancreas or decrease thyroid function.

Contraindicated in myasthenia gravis, Addisons disease; adrenal, liver or kidney failure.*

Extreme excess contributes to a rare bone softness & deformity (osteomalacia), and can cause anesthesia, heart failure, coma or death.

* Mild kidney disorders compromise reabsorption, depleting magnesium. Medically supervised supplementation can prevent severe deficit. (Slagle)

Preventing diarrhea (EBY 2001, 06)

At mood-modulating doses, magnesium can be antibiotic (depleting intestinal bacteria), reduce other nutrients and, if poorly absorbed, attract too much water to the large intestines, thus becoming laxative. Therapeutic possibilities:

Calcium and/or omega 3 — counterbalances magnesium, but do not overdo, as excess may overstimulate.

Generous beneficial intestinal bacteria. Eby (2001, 06) suggests several billion live (refrigerated) microorganisms, 3-5x/day. Take separately from magnesium.

Time-release magnesium may help.

Use absorbable forms of magnesium.

Eat oats, grits, other soluble fiber. Also bananas, rice, apples, tea, toast.

Potassium rich foods to help eliminate the water.

Avoid nonsoluble fiber, greasy food, sugars. Limit dairy, *as appropriate.*

Treat leaky gut syndrome.

If necessary, metamucil or psyllium with fluids.

If necessary, reduce magnesium and substitute mood-moderating nutrients (zinc, amino inhibitors, etc.).

Zinc (Zn)

Interaction with mood

Clinical results suggests zinc is frequently an important influence on mood, and may be particularly useful in moderating mania and overstimulation, and improving mood in pyroluria and other zinc-depleted conditions. (Pfeiffer 1975, 88, Walsh 1996, 2000)

Low zinc has been reported in some manias, and with such manic symptoms as agitation, irritability, (Prasad 1978) anxiety; (Gold 1987) and such related conditions as hyperactivity, (Torren 1996) behavior disorders, (Walsh, 1996) paranoia, epilepsy, and psychosis.* (Irvine 1969, Prasad 1978, Hoffer 1983ab, Pfeiffer 1987) Deficiency can also be associated with depression, seasonal affective disorder, confusion, apathy, rigid/irritable personality, panic, eating and behavior disorders, learning disabilities, memory impairment, and excitotoxicity. (Little 1989.Moynahan 1976, Pfeiffer 1972, 74, 83, 88, Prasad 1978, Jaffe 1992, Kimura 1965, Murray 1996, Gold 1987, Werbach 1991, Hoffer 1983, Walsh 1996, 2000, Caldwell, Prasad 1978, Wallwork 1981)

* Supplementation has been shown to reduce need for major tranquilizers in many psychotic patients. (Pfeiffer 1975, 87, 88)

Interaction with stress

Zinc is crucial in handling stress, and is used up thereby, allowing catecholamines to rise even more, further compromising resistance to stress, anxiety, and other mood symptoms. (Wallwork 1981, Slagle 1992, McLardy 1973, Garbarg 1974, Harrison 1991ab)

Biotype & allergy connections (Walsh 1991, 96, 2000, Jaffe 1992, Pfeiffer 1975, 87, 88ab)

Zinc has, for decades, been shown to benefit the major biotypes (see pp. 145-68), which can play a critical role in mood :

- □ Pyroluria — a condition commonly associated with mood disturbance, hyperexcitability, suicidal depression, behavior disorder, anxiety, and irritability; and occuring in perhaps 18% of bipolars. Numerous studies find zinc crucial in treating pyroluria.
- □ Histadelia (undermethylation/high folate) — which typically manifests as constant severe depression, obsessions, and compulsions; and occurs in an estimated 35% of bipolars. Zinc supports methylation (helps convert homocysteine to cysteine or methionine).
- □ Histapenia (overmethylation/low folate) — can be associated with overstimulation, anxiety, hypomania, depression and psychosis, and occurs in an estimated 25% of bipolars. Zinc is important to treatment. It counters catecholamine elevation, regulates histamine levels, and facilitates normal histamine storage in basophils.
- □ Metal metabolism disorder — often complicates histapenia, fostering psychosis and paranoia. Zinc is critical in reducing the high copper, and in supporting MT function.
- □ Allergy to dairy or glutenous grains — Zinc is used in small intestine enzymes which metabolize casein and gluten. Thus, intake, especially if previously depleted, often improve dairy and wheat allergies. (Walsh 2006)

See *Biotypes*, pp. 145-68.

Zinc's sedative effects

A case report, (Murphy 1970) pointed out by Pfeiffer, illustrates the sedative potency of large quantities of zinc. A 16-year-old boy in Tehran, hearing that zinc was good for him, but unaware of appropriate dose, consumed the equivalent of 12,000 mg. elemental zinc* in a peanut butter sandwich. (Supplements commonly contain 10-30 mg. Though pyrolurics may be prescribed 100-150 mg, this mainly replaces the zinc they continuously disable and excrete, and would otherwise be a very high dose. The boy consumed 120 times that.)

The peanut butter slowed zinc release and symptom onset. The boy became dizzy, and staggered, and his writing became relatively illegible. He slept most of the time, and was increasingly difficult to waken over five to six days. As the zinc left his body, he completely recovered.

Uses of zinc in the brain

- □ Helps prevent dopamine and norepinephrine elevation, thereby moderating stimulation and reducing susceptibility to mania or psychosis (especially in histapenia). (Pfeiffer 1975, 87, McLardy 1973, Garbarg 1974, Harrison 1971ab, Wallwork 1981)
- □ Helps form, metabolize and regulate GABA. Deficiency decreases GABA. (Walsh 2008)
- □ Critical if taking taurine. (See *Low zinc concerns,* p. 38.)
- □ Helps counter excitotoxins. With P5P, it's required in forming GAD, which helps block excitotoxicity. (Blaylock 1995)
- □ Important in membrane transport, EFA and prostaglandin synthesis. (Ferbabdez-Madrif 1973)
- □ With histamine, may help integrate thought memory and emotion in the hippocampus. (Harrison 1971ab, Ibata 1969, McLardy 1973, Kimura 1965)
- □ Potent antioxidant activity; protects sulfhydryls and lipids, and helps maintain A, glutathione, E, glutathione peroxidase, and superoxide dismutase, all antioxidant. (McGinnis 2004)
- □ Induces metallothionein, an antioxidant enzyme critical to metal metabolism. (McGinnis 2004)
- □ Helps support balanced blood sugar.
- □ Needed in neural development.
- □ Critical to transfer of genetic information.* (Pfeiffer 1987)

* Zinc fingers are appendages to the proteins that help turn genes on and off.

Physical effects benefitting mood

Helps counter dairy and grain sensitivity. (It's used by gut enzymes which break down casein and gluten).

Supports blood sugar balance, storage, insulin activity.

Counteracts excess copper, iron, heavy metals; helps prevent lead and cadmium absorption.

Supports methylation and homocysteine metabolism.*

Potent immune nutrient. (Maes)

Critical to action of thyroid on the cell.**

Supports circulation & creation of healthy blood cells.

Used in nucleus formation, DNA and RNA production, (Ferbabdez-Madrif 1973) and regulation.

Benefits certain types of headaches.

* Zinc helps B6 convert homocysteine to cysteine. The enzyme using betaine to methylate homocysteine to methionine, requires zinc.

** Supports thyroid activity and function, and receptor sensitivity to thyroid stimulation. Deficiency can damage receptors. (Rosenberg 1991)

Considerations (Murray 1996, Garrison 1985, Balch 1990, Page 1992, Quillin 1987, Lieberman 1990, Pfeiffer 1975, Walsh 1996, 2000, 02, 04ab)

Need may be suggested by

Difficulty with stress. Anxiety, irritability, hyperactivity, paranoia, mania. Depression, lethargy, apathy, fatigue. (Little 1989, Edwards 1980)

Memory impairment, learning disabilities, poor dream recall. (Pfeiffer 1975, 87, 88)

Problems with visual acuity and night vision.

Muted or distorted sense of taste* and smell, appetite loss* (Gold 1987, Slagle 1992), eating disorder. (Bryce-Smith 1984, Humphries 1989) Body and breath odor. (Walsh 2004ab)

Temperature dysregulation. Cold hands and feet (poor circulation), faintness, anemia. (Pfeiffer 1975, 87, 88)

Carbohydrate, gluten, casein, or chemical sensitivity. (Krohn 1991, Rogers 1997) Difficulty with anesthesia.

Frequent infections, immunodeficiency. Inflammation. Slow healing of wounds; leg ulcers, oral lesions. (Walsh 2004ab, 06) Increased susceptibility to shock. (Pfeiffer 1987, 88)

Fragile mucous membranes. (Ferbabdez-Madrif 1973) Abnormal bleeding. (Skalso)

Painful knee and hip joints. Tendency to malformed cartilege, bones.** (Pfeiffer 1987, 88, Kruesi)

Growth retardation, perhaps, dwarfism. (Prasad 1978, Pfeiffer 1987, 88)

Difficulty metabolizing protein (Ferbabdez-Madrif 1973), or EFAs.

Blood sugar problems (supports insulin).

Poor appetite, diarrhea, stomach pain.

Brittle hair, lacking pigment. Hair loss. (Pfeiffer 1987, 88)

Acne, skin rash, oily skin, eczema, stretch marks, psoriasis, other skin disorders. (Walsh 2004a)

Nails that are brittle,*** opaquely white, or show white banding, crosswise lines,**** or white spots.***** (Spot placement reflects periods of greater deficiency. Large spots grow out over 5-6 months, while small ones may resolve with therapy. Spots are especially likely on the index and fifth finger of the dominant hand, and may also be found on toe nails.) (Pfeiffer 1974, 75, 87, 88)

Delayed or absent menstrual cycle, suppressed ovulation, sterility. Extended pregnancy, toxemia, prolonged labor or premature delivery. Impotency (responsive to B6 and zinc), enlarged prostate. Impaired/delayed sexual development or viability. Birth defects.****** (Prasad 1978, Pfeiffer 1975, 87, 88, Walsh 2004ab, 06)

High blood pressure. Sickle cell or hemolytic anemia. Perhaps elevated homocysteine.*******

Headaches. Perhaps cirrhosis, arthritis.

* Zinc, B6, copper, and nickel support the sense of taste. (Henkin) Zinc also increases stomach acid and salivary secretion. (Gold 1987)

** With B6 and copper, zinc helps maintain and regenerate skin and cartilege. Zinc helps crosslink elastin chains to make collagen or elastin fibrils, (Skalso) and supports protein synthesis. It is thus important to cellular growth and repair, normal joint formation, (Ferbabdez-Madrif 1973) fetal development, and growth of long bones.

*** Women's nails are often more brittle due to higher estrogen. (Pfeiffer 1972)

**** Crosswise lines can be produced by zinc depletion during one week of fever, and take about a month to appear. (Pfeiffer 1972)

***** Especially, one week before menses (time of greatest depression), and with elevated estrogen (which increases copper, lowering zinc); (Pfeiffer 1972) and with extended fasting, psychosis, albuminuria, cirrhosis, or nephrosis. (Muerhcke 1956)

****** In some cases, cleft palate, malformed eyes, brain, heart, lungs, skeleton, genitals, other birth defects; or stillborn. (Hurley)

******* Helps convert homocysteine to cysteine. Required with the enzyme using betaine to methylate homocysteine to methionine.

Populations

Glacial or sandy soils. Constant farming, or use of manure from animals fed high copper.

Pyroluria. (Walsh 1997, 2006, Pfeiffer 1987, 88) (See pp.147-52.)

Malabsorption, anorexia, digestive problems, high sugar and fat diet. Diabetes. (Slagle 1992, Reuven 1991)

Type A blood (malabsorbs and responds slowly to zinc). (Pfeiffer 1972)

Prolonged stress (fatigue, illness, wounds, burns, infection, surgery, psychosocial stressors, etc). (Pfeiffer 1987, 88)

High estrogen (elevating copper), as in pregnancy, some cases of PMS. (Pfeiffer)

Excessive copper, iron or calcium. (Slagle 1992) Heavy metal toxicity. (Niklowitz 1973) Metal metabolism dysfunction. (Walsh 2004ab)

Newborn (if copper is elevated), growth spurts (especially in males), puberty, birth control pills. (Pfeiffer 1975, 87)

Longterm cortisone/steroids; some hypertensives, diuretics; perhaps penicillamine. (Gold 1987, Pfeiffer 1975, 87)

Considerations *continued*

Sickle cell anemia, (Reuven 1991) cirrhosis, cancer, senile confusion (if due to elevated copper).

Alcoholism, alcohol intolerance (alcohol dehydrogenase is zinc-dependent). (Reuven 1991)

Nutrient interactions

Important in B12 transport; (McLougin 1990) B1, phosphorus and protein metabolism; fatty acid and cholesterol synthesis. (Ferbabdez-Madrif 1973) Needed for B6 metabolism (in forming P5P). Chelates copper.

Lab (Rogers 1997, Little 1989, McLoughlin 1990, Nichols 1992, Slagle 1992, Walsh 2004ab)

Plasma zinc and zinc/copper ratio. *Avoid supplements 24 hrs before testing.*

Note: Zinc can show deceptively low or normal blood levels (due to homeostasis); or show high hair and urine levels due to inefficient use or high excretion. Consider clinical symptoms and therapeutic response.

Inability to correct low B6* or A suggest low zinc.

* Pyridoxal kinase is zinc-dependent.

Supportive nutrients (Slagle 1992, Walsh 2004ab)

Zinc absorption and use is supported by:

B6 — start before beginning zinc, to avoid mental symptoms, prevent seizure, or nausea.

Manganese — helps promote metallothionein function and copper excretion. May be especially indicated with hypoglycemia, pyroluria, high copper, or histapenia. *Can be inadvisable if prone to high blood pressure or histadelic.*

NAC — supports MT function, zinc absorption removal of excess copper. *Do not use at the outset.* (See *Metal metabolism*, p. 170-73.)

Antioxidants — C, E, A, etc. (Slagle 1992)

Antagonistic food, nutrients (Slagle 1992, Pfeiffer 1975, 88, Moyer 2003)

Food processing and boiling removes zinc. Hot dogs are low in zinc. Caffeine chelates zinc. (

Phytates in whole grains impair absorption, though leavening of breads or sprouting destroys phytates.

FD&C yellow #5 (tartrazine), found in soda, and some other artifical colors chelate (and deplete) zinc.

High phosphorus (in sodas, and heavy meat diets) also chelates zinc.

Competing metals. (Walsh 2004)

Sources (Balch 1990, Baumel, Slagle 1992, Braverman 1987, NutriCircles)

Herring, clams, seafood, liver, organ and red meat, egg yolk, dairy. Wheat germ and bran, nutritional yeast. Sunflower, pumpkin and other seeds, nuts. Legumes. Dairy. Sprouts, leafy greens (cabbage, watercress). Bee pollen. Modest amounts in carrots, beets, dates, bananna, asparagus, rutabaga, lettuce, potato, tomato, pineapple, currants, lemon, sweet potato, cauliflower, green beans, turnip greens, cherries, apricots, prune or citrus juice. Oysters, known for high zinc, aren't a good choice because of high copper and cadmium.

> Note: Zinc supplements can cause mild digestive symptoms, especially nausea, particularly in patients with pyroluria, or other B6-deficient conditions. The solution, in most cases, is to take zinc with B6 and food.

Supplements & dose (Slagle 1992, Braverman 1987, Jaffe 1992, Walsh 2006, 07)

Dose is that which normalizes tissue levels and decreases any copper overload. Usually 10-30 mg; 20-50 mg with histadelia; up to 50 to 100 mg, perhaps more, with pyroluria or very high copper.* Monitor response. (Walsh 2006, 07)

May need to introduce slowly, due to nausea, digestive effects, or other reactions. If metallothionein is too low, zinc may stimulate its genetic expression and, counterintuitively, MT may use up zinc, creating a deficiency. (Walsh 2007)

Give B6 for the first two days to avert depression or hallucinations.

Preferred supplements include zinc-gluconate, -picolinate, or -citrate.

* Even higher doses are sometimes used, only *if indicated,* e.g., in some cases with accompanying severe skin conditions, such as severe psoriasis or acne vulgaris. (Walsh 2006, 07)

Effects of excess, contraindications (Garrison 1985, Balch 1990, Page 1992, Lieberman 1990, Pfeiffer 1975, Murray 1996, Slagle 1992)

While zinc helps remit certain depressions, extended high doses can promote depression. (Additional manganese, copper, or B6 may help.)

Initially, may temporarily worsen hallucinations.

Excess zinc relative to manganese and B6 reduces the stability of neural membranes and may foster convulsive seizures, particularly in epileptics.

Gastrointestinal disturbances. (What isn't absorbed can induce diarrhea or vomiting.)

Increased perspiration.

Intolerance to alcohol.

Excess or deficiency can depress immunity.

At very high doses, incoordination, dizziness, lethargy, staggering, illegible handwriting; (Murphy 1970) over the long-term, may contribute to renal failure.

Chronic large doses (e.g., over 100 mg.) can deplete iron and copper, causing anemia, low HDL, etc.

Low-dose lithium-orotate

"[Lithium is] unmatched in research support for long-term clinical effectiveness against morbidity and mortality associated with bipolar disorders."

RJ Baldessarini, MD, 2000

"To date, only lithium is considered effective as a prophylactic. Studies on the other drugs are incomplete."

Peter Whybrow, MD, 1997

"Lithium is not the panacea it was once thought to be."

Mark Bauer, MD

Orotate (Dean 2006, Nieper 1973, Sartori 1986)

Lithium-carbonate (conventionally prescribed) and -citrate are poorly absorbed, and not efficiently transported within the cell, necessitating higher doses. As lithium accumulates with ongoing use, body load can approach-toxic levels. (Hence, the blood tests.)

Lithium orotate, on the other hand, increases bioavailability many-fold. Orotates more effectively transport lithium to the membranes of mitochondria, lysosomes, and glial cells, and help stabilize those membranes, preventing depletion of lithium and sodium. (Dean 2006) This allows for about a 7 to 8-fold lower dose of elemental lithium.* Most nutritionally-oriented practioners have been prescribing the orotate form for years.

* A 1979 study by Smith, discouraged work on lithium orotate. It found very high doses injected into rats produced much greater lithium concentration in kidney, serum and heart than equal quantities of lithium carbonate. Lithium orotate was thereafter assumed to posed greater potential for kidney damage. However, Smith's study was flawed, in that it had failed to compare *effectively*-equivalent doses, which would have involved a 1:7 ratio of lithium orotate to carbonate.

Lithium is an alkali metal, somewhat similar to sodium and potassium. Pfeiffer has suggested that it may be an essential trace mineral. An early epidemiological study by Dawson (1970) underscored the ability of naturally-occuring, trace quantities to alter mental function, tying high rates of mental disorder and crime with regions of Texas where lithium was not present in the water; low rates, where it was prevalent.

Pharmacological lithium (Ketter 2001, Brigham 2001)

Pharmacological dose lithium carbonate (typically starting at 600-900 mg., going as high as to 1800 mg. for some manias (Whybrow 1997)) has, for decades, been considered the gold standard in bipolar therapy. (Grof 1998, Kleindienst 2003) Improvement is generally held to occur in 50-80% of bipolars, (Gelenberg 1989, Baldessarini 2000) particularly in preventing and moderating mania. (Sachs 1998, Whybrow 1997) Research also suggests marked reduction in suicides and general mortality. (Balderessarini 2000, Mueller-Oerlinghausen 1991, 92, Ahrens 1995, Schou 1995)

Unfortunately, over many years, monotherapy relapse can become considerable; between-episode symptoms, substantial; (Werry 1991, Markar 1990, Grof 1998, Coryell 1997, Post 1993b, Maj 1989) and mood balance tends to shift toward depression, while damage to the liver, kidneys, or thyroid accumulates. (Ketter 2001) (See *Lithium,* p. 285.)

Warning: Nonetheless, discontinuation (or reductions) often leaves patients worse off, with increased new episodes, (Young 2006, Kukopulos 1995) and a precipitous increase in the risk of suicide to pre-treatment levels, or higher (typically, at least a sixfold increase, lasting a year or longer). (Zarate 2001)

Lithium orotate, nutritional doses

Many nutritionally-oriented physicians emphasize more biologically assimilable intake: both lower doses and use of lithium *orotate* (instead of carbonate). (*See sidebar.*) Though the initial benefit may not be as pronounced or rapid, use within the context of an individually tailored nutrient regimen creates a synergistic effect, increasing potency. Furthermore, low-dose lithium orotate resolves many of the above problems; it seems to be generally more sustainable over time, less suppressive of cognition, less likely to damage the kidneys and thyroid, etc.

Joan Matthews Larson, PhD, reports great success treating bipolars with low-dose, vegetable-based lithium orotate (e.g., 20 mg, 3x/day) (along with omega 3, B complex, ester C, and taurine).*(Larson 2001, 08) Similarly, Kruesi (1996) prescribes low-dose lithium orotate along with other nutrients for patients whose hair analysis shows less-than-detectable levels. Pfeiffer (1988) found small doses could even be strong enough to counter psychosis and facilitate reductions in neuroleptics, in certain patients (probably bipolar).

IMPORTANT: *This is not to preclude higher doses when medically relevant.* Any reductions should be undertaken *only if indicated, and under close medical supervision.* (See *Warning,* above, and, *If dose reduction is indicated,* p.289.)

Wright's list of cognitive & affective benefits from low-dose lithium

Jonathan Wright, MD, (2004) suggests possible benefits — most research is in early stages — of small quantities of lithium (10-20 mg elemental lithium chelated to aspartate or orotate).

Reduces depression and irrational anger, improves mood.

Reduces mental hospital admissions, violence, aggression, suicide, addiction, anorexia, cluster headaches.

May improve neural viability, and help repair signalling.

Increases bcl-2 (which regenerates axons).

Inhibits NMDA overactivity. Protects against excitotoxicity.

Protects against tardive dyskinesia.

Enhances neural DNA replication.

Protection from neural death due to mood-altering drugs or stroke.

May improve spatial memory. May improve Alzheimers.*

* Inhibits beta-amyloid secretion and prevents it from damaging the brain; inhibits tau protein and formation of neurofibrillary tangles; helps chelate aluminum.

Physical effects (Wright 2004)

Raises platelets, white and, possibly, red blood cell levels.

Lowers blood sugar in some diabetics.

May improve herpes, hyperthyroid, fibromyalgia, gout, Mediterranean fever.

See *Lithium side effects,* p. 285.

History (Whybrow 2001)

In the past, people journeyed far to drink and soak in lithium-rich waters. Lithium was also taken for gout in the mid 1800s, as a laxative in the early 1900s, a sleep-aid in the 1920s, and an anti-libido agent in the British army. In the 1930s and 40s, use as a salt substitute was suspended following heart and kidney problems and several deaths.

Dr. Manfred Anke first observed lithium could cause animals to lose muscle tone and lie dormant. Dr. John Cade (1949), used it to make the urine of psychotic patients soluble, then injected the combo into guinea pigs. Unexpectedly, instead of psychotic symptoms, the pigs became "extremely lethargic and nonresponsive to stimuli... without inducing sleep." Cade then tried lithium injections on agitated and manic patients. A chronic 5-yr manic improved in 3 weeks and, by 3 months, was discharged.

Within a decade, relatively substantial doses became the centerpiece of bipolar treatment in Europe; and then the United States.

Considerations

Need may be suggested by (Brigham 2001, Whybrow 1997)

Agitation, irritability, conduct disorder, simple mania, bipolar disorder.

Characteristics that help predict response (Grof 1993, Abou-Saleh 1990, Brigham 2001, Whybrow 1997)

No comorbid illness or substance abuse.

Fewer episodes, less deterioration.

Mania/depression/euthymic pattern.

No mixed episodes or rapid cycling.

Not schizoaffective. No psychotic manias.

Good thyroid function.

No neurological symptoms.

Poor response to VPA or CBZ.

Supportive nutrients

Wright (2004) recommends flaxseed oil [1T, 3x/day],* vitamin E [800 IU] to moderate blood pressure, tremors, nausea, protein in urine. These may be reduced later.

Folate may help counter any lithium related anemia (Prakah 1981), reduce morbidity, and support BH4 and serotonin creation. (Coppen 1982, 89) *Not helpful with histadelia.*

Lab (Kruesi 1996)

Less than detectable hair levels may indicate need.

Sources

Kelp, dulse, seafood, certain drinking waters.

Bipolar dosage (Pfeiffer 1988, Kruesi 1996)

Orthomolecular and naturopathic doses generally range from micrograms (Page 1992) to 5-20 mg. per day, and are often low enough to be available over the counter.(Kruesi 1996, Larson 2001 Wright 2004). Nonetheless, higher doses may be required (for instance, with intractable mania).

Prefered supplement: Lithium orotate. (Dean 2006, Kruesi 1996)

Outcome

Conventional doses can take 6 to 8 weeks to elicit complete response. (Ketter, Frye 2001) Physiologic doses may take longer. (See *Lithium side effects,* p. 285.)

WARNING: If you wish to alter your current dose of lithium, seek the advise of your physician. Extreme caution is warranted, as such changes involve life-threatening risk.

Biochemistry: Some conjectures as to how lithium moderates mood (Whybrow 1997, 2001, Pfeiffer 1988)

Selectively decreases stimulation — the most activated nerve cells are those most sensitive to lithium. (Hoffer 1989)

Modifies second messenger signalling — inhibits the enzyme (inositol monophosphatase) used in forming inositol, and modifies PLA2 signalling. (Horrobin) (See *Inositol, & EFAs,* pp. 86-97.)

Alters limbic neurotransmitter balances — influences acetylcholine, dopamine, serotonin, and GABA receptors in the limbic system and basal ganglia. (Pfeiffer 1988)

Decreases ionic conduction — forcefully shifts sodium and potassium levels, which are critical to conveying messages along the neural axon. May assist in sodium ion transport or substitute for sodium. (Rosenblatt 1981, Snyder 1980, Gold 1987, Baraban 1989)

Suppresses stimulating hormones — alters adrenal cortisol levels, and depresses the thyroid. (Pfeiffer 1988)

2. Seizural influences

This section briefly explores the possible role of subconvulsive limbic seizures in bipolar disorder, by looking at anticonvulsive mood-stabilizers, the relevance of kindling to bipolars, and other commonalities with epilepsy. It then goes on to inhibitory, anticonvulsant amino acids. These are among the most potent mood-stabilizing, mania-moderating nutrients.

"[Epilepsy] like lightning from a miniature thundercloud."

Wilder Penfield (1975)

"...an excruciating snatching of the body from the soul."

Gustav Flaubert

"There was a moment or two in his epileptic condition, almost before the fit itself, when... his brain seemed to catch fire at brief moments... His sensation of being alive and his awareness increased tenfold at those moments which flashed by like lightning. His mind and heart were flooded by a dazzling light. All his agitation... worries... composed in a twinkling, culminating in a great calm... full of understanding and knowledge of the final cause... an intense heightening of awareness."

Dostoyevsky, in *The Idiot*

History: Kindling in bipolars

Observations that intermittent electric stimulation of the amygdala increased sensitivity to seizures, and that young animals given cocaine (stimulating dopamine) became more prone to convulsions on maturity, led to a kindling theory of epilepsy.

Adopting the concept to bipolar disorder, Post (1986) proposed that repeated stressors, kindling nearby neuronal activation, could cause limbic and behavioral reactions. Arousal sensitization in vulnerable persons might lead to anxiety, insomnia, or mania, and eventually adaptive failure with exhaustion, depression, etc, creating a viscious feedback loop and increasing the frequency and precipitousness of affective cycles.

Although the kindling model, the changes in second messenger chemistry* and ion channel mechanisms, and the common therapies used in both disorders would seem to indicate a considerable relationship, Mazza (2007) notes that very little is actually known about the intersection of bipolar disorder and epilepsy,

*G proteins and PKC (p. 279), phosphatidyl inositols (pp. 95-97), calcium (pp. 122-25), etc.

Kindling (Post 1982, 89, 97, 2001, Ghaemi 1999, Bell 1992, Brewerton 1997)

Kindling was originally defined in terms of epilepsy, as a process by which repeated exposure to minor convulsive stimuli eventually increases the intensity and frequency of reactions. The threshhold for seizures falls progressively, over time, leading to apparently "spontaneous" episodes. (Post 1982)

Mood disorder may similarly be triggered or exacerbated by kindling. Stimulation (mania, rapid cycling, antidepressants, sugar, cocaine, amphetamines, allergens, junk food, hyperthyroid, environmental stressors) can elevate dopamine or norepinephrine. With excessive, continuous, or repeated stimulation, (Post 1982) receptors, gene regulators, and second messengers on excitatory pathways could become increasingly prone to react; less so, on inhibitory pathways. Minor cues might then overactivate signalling. Heightened exposures may create structural limbic lesions and permanently alter neurotransmitter reactions to certain stressors. Thus, sensitized limbic and frontal lobes may dysregulate mood and create mania. (Ghaemi 1999)

On the other hand, understimulation (depression, hypothyroid, sedatives, etc.), (Thierry 1976) can increase receptor number (Creese 1977) and sensitivity, cumulatively making mania more likely when stimulation occurs. (Bunney 1977) Mania may then go on to kindle further episodes.

Stoll and Severus (1996) suggest kindling and abnormal signal transduction (p. 279) may be a primary cause of bipolar disorder, interacting to induce mania and mood instability.

Consistent with a kindling etiology:

- ☐ Once mania occurs, further manias occur in 90-95% of cases.
- ☐ Over time, bipolar episodes tend to occur more frequently; and outcome, to deteriorate.
- ☐ Although triggers to initial mood episodes are usually readily identifiable, eventually, only minor instigation is evident, or none at all.
- ☐ All established mood stabilizers dampen excess signalling,* and so block kindling. (Stoll 1996) Most have anticonvulsive properties, which may, at least in part, be how they moderate mood. (Post 1997, Bauer 1996, Lane 1997, Ghaemi 1999, Bell 1992).

* Most inhibit calcium mobilization. Several interfere with creation of inositol- and choline-related second messenger signalling molecules, and/or inhibit kinase and G protein activity. (Stoll 1996)

See also, *Allergic kindling*, p. 208.

Anticonvulsant-properties in mood-stabilizing meds

The ability of anticonvulsive, anti-epileptic drugs to treat bipolars lends support to a subconvulsive seizure etiology, in at least some patients. — Peter Whybrow, MD, 1997

About two-thirds of bipolars respond best to carbamazepine (CBZ) or valproate (VPA); (Post 1996ab, Birkheimer 1985) two-thirds, to lithium. (Walden 1998) CBZ and VPA are anticonvulsant and antikindling, and generally more effective in patients with poor response to lithium.*(Coxhead 1992, Dilsaver 1996)

Neurological problems strongly suggest responsiveness to VPA or CBZ, lending credence to a seizural etiology in many bipolars. (Post 1996, 99) Both suppress transfer of calcium and sodium ions across the neural membrane, slowing nerve cell recovery and reducing messages conveyed. The consequent suppression of kindling and seizures (Yang 1998, Whybrow 1997), especially in temporal and limbic regions, may underly their antimanic benefits. (Weiss 1995a, Post 1992, 95a, Ketter 1994b) Further supporting this perspective, responders are more likely to show a history of seizures, head injury, or abnormal EEGs. (Stoll 1994)

Lamotrigene (a newer stabilizer, which seems to be more effective in countering depression) is also anticonvulsive. (Marano 2005)

Calcium channel blockers (used mainly as adjuncts to the above) (Brigham 2001, Ghaemi 1999) also seem to be anticonvulsant. (de Falco 1992)

Lithium shows minor anticonvulsive activity.

* And for mania rather than depression, (Emrich 1980, Pope 1991, Freeman 1992, Post 1996ab; McElroy 1992, Lambert 1992, Brigham 2001, Dilsaver 1996, Cullen 1991) especially severe, mixed state, (Whybrow 1997, Calabrese 1999, Walden 1998) rapid cycling, (Bowden 1997) or psychotic mania; (Post 87) Also for atypical bipolars (e.g, schizoaffectives), (Denicoff 1997) those with comorbid substance abuse, (Brigham 2001) or without close bipolar relatives.

Intersection with epilepsy

Epilepsy is a chronic condition characterized by sporadic and disorderly electric discharge of a number of hyperexcitable brain neurons. The sudden electric surges disorganize the brain and induce seizures. (Gold 1987)

It is often misdiagnosed as psychiatric illness. The neurologist, Norman Geschwind, MD, reports 30% of newly admitted mental hospital patients were found to have neurological disorders underlying the psychiatric symptoms. Kessler (1989) found seizure disorders in two of three treatment-resistant affectives with psychotic features. Moreover, sleep-deprived EEGs (a test for epilepsy) are sometimes used to confirm bipolar diagnoses. (Moore 1998) Pfeiffer finds pyrolurics particularly vulnerable.

Temporal lobe epilepsy (TLE)

Dr. Paul Spiers, a TLE expert, states that in the 1980's, up to one-third of TLE patients at Beth Israel Hospital had originally been diagnosed with a psychiatric illness. And according to Dr John Kuehne, many chronic back-ward psychotic patients nonresponsive to standard treatment, are actually TLE. (Pfeiffer 1983, LaPlante 1993, Galton 1979, Gold 1987, Davidson 1983)

Complex partial seizure disorder (temporal lobe & psychomotor epilepsy) is frequently misdiagnosed as bipolar disorder, atypical psychosis, or some other psychiatric disorder. (Gold 1987) Leis (1984), reports 50% of twelve consecutive bipolars had at least five major symptoms of psychomotor epilepsy. Similarly, a study by Negash (2003) finds a significant occurence in bipolars of a number of neurological soft signs , especially those which involve sequencing of complex motor activity.

Depression is estimated to occur in 19-50%, of TLEs, especially with left temporal involvement, (Mendez 1986) or hypometabolism between episodes (Victoroff 1994) (in which case, it is often complicated by delusions and suicidality. (Mendez 1986)).

Whybrow points out the similarity of TLE symptoms to mania and to a lesser degree, depression. TLE seizures can look like bipolar disorder with psychotic involvement. Emotions are frequently heightened. Ultra-good behavior may alternate with ultrabad. In some cases, the patient becomes violent to a person who had previously annoyed him, and then forgets the event. The TLE personality, as identified by the neurologist,

Van Gogh's epilepsy (Fieve 1975, Blumer 2002, Destaing 1972, Nagera 1967)

Vincent van Gogh's doctor believed his epilepsy may have been caused by oxygen deprivation during a difficult birth. The resulting scars on certain brain cells would explain the asymmetry of his face. Overindulgence in absinthe (which is neurotoxic) and his habit of eating paint (containing cadmium, lead, etc.) to avert starvation may have further destabilized neural function. He also was subject to periodic headaches and dizziness.

van Gogh intensely re-experienced early memories, and saw mystical visions and hallucinations. The villages called him "God's madman."

In 1888, he created 200 paintings. One day, while shaving, he heard a voice telling him to kill his friend and fellow artist, Gauguin. He walked to Gauguin's house, holding his razor. Gauguin, thinking him in a trance, sent him home. van Gogh complied, then sliced off part of his ear.

From then on, he was hospitalized repeatedly. As his symptoms increased, his art became more prolific and expressive, with intense, thickly painted colors and rapid, swirling brush strokes.

In 1890 he attacked a friend, Dr Gachet, with a gun, and two days later, shot himself.

Continued on next page

"Genius is a symptom of hereditary degeneration of the epileptoid variety."
Cesare Lombroso, 19TH century physician

Van Gogh *continued*

Scholars debate whether van Gogh had been schizophrenic or bipolar. Fieve claims the later, noting moods ranging from incapacitating depression to high energy, enthusiastic or violent mania, and severe paranoid rage. In the last two years of his life, van Gogh experienced recurrent psychosis.

Van Gogh's hypergraphia

"Sometimes I draw sketches almost against my will... the emotions are sometimes so strong that one works without knowing one works... One must strike while the iron is hot."

Vincent Van Gogh

Recommended Reading

LaPlante, Eve, *Seized*, 1993.
"Introduction to the Ketogenic Diet," 1997.

Norman Geschwind, suggests a mood syndrome: intense emotionality, imbuing of experience with deeply religious or moral significance, overattachment to social interaction ("stickiness"), hypergraphia (a compulsion to record thoughts through extensive writing, drawing, or other artistic expression) and, in some, increased sexual activity (though more often, reduced). (La Plante 1993, Schacter 1997)

Other seizural symptoms (Pfeiffer 1983, LaPlante1993, Galton 1979, Gold 1987, Davidson 1983)

Mild symptoms include: periodic deja vu episodes and amnesia, feelings of unreality or of detachment from the body, bright lights around objects, misperceptions of limbs.

Seizures can also involve sensory distortion, sound, odor and time dysperceptions (e.g. altered intensity), shape and distance distortions, irrational fear, jumbled thoughts, automatic thinking, intrusive repetitive ideas, alienation from reality, (Penfield 1954) illusions of significance, voices, hallucinations, and a series of automatic movements,* such as changing clothes. or dreamlike sequences which can last many days. (Gold 1987)

An average of fourteen years of seizures can cause permanent brain alteration, and psychotic behavior, even between seizures, in some TLE patients. Interpersonal relations and emotionality remain intense. Psychosis eventually occurs in almost 20%, especially if the focus is the left temporal lobe. 80% of psychotic epileptics display temporal abnormalities. Limbic involvement contributes to the psychosis. (Spiers, in LaPlante 1993, Gold 1987, Davidson 1983)

Considerations

Populations (Pfeiffer 1988, Geschwind 1954)

Causes include: heredity,* brain injury (including birth trauma), oxygen deprivation, brain tumor, heavy metal or other toxicity, high fever (especially in children), infection, metabolic error, abscess, stroke, hormonal imbalance, drug reactions, etc.

* It's transmitted by a dominant gene in 1% of the population. The gene may target specific structures (e.g, amygdala or hippocampus); or neurotransmitter/receptor/second-messenger/synapse activity, or metabolic enzymes. (Gold)

Lab: Electroencephalograms (Pfeiffer 1988)

The EEG often fails to detect epilepsy, especially between seizures. Sleep-deprived EEGs are more accurate. Peak discharges in the temporal region can be seen in light sleep. Brain waves may fluctuate, with wave shape more regular immediately before and during a seizure, taking the form of low frequency rectangular waves. Irregular EEGs can also occur in bipolars.

Nutritional approaches (Pfeiffer 1988, Balch 1990)

Nutrients are similar to those used in mood stabilization.

- □ Pfeiffer suggests supplemental glycine, taurine,* GABA,** B6, manganese, zinc*** to stabilize nerve cell membranes and prevent convulsions. (Pfeiffer 1988) (*Note: The balance among B6, manganese, and zinc is critical. Zinc is preventive, but excess can contribute to convulsions.*)
- □ Magnesium, B, B12, and choline may help. (Balch 1990)
- □ Hoffer finds high dose B3 reduces limbic kindling and anticonvulsive requirements.
- □ Melatonin helps stabilize electrical activity; and may reduce anxiety, panic, depression, mania, psychosis. (Lewis)
- □ Balance carbohydrate metabolism. Avoid sugar and other refined carbohydrates.
- □ Remove detrimental metals, through use of zinc, manganese, vitamin C, etc. (Pfeiffer 1988) (See pp. 170-83.)
- □ Herbs recommended by Balch (1990) include black cohosh, lobelia,**** and hyssop.
- □ Good diet, regular exercise, avoidance of recreational drugs, and stress reduction.
- □ Ketogenic diet — a diet promoting ketone formation. Usually involves 2-3 days of fasting, then 2 years of a specific, primarily fat diet, with enough protein to sustain growth, and severe carbohydrate restriction. High quality fats prevent other disorders from developing. While substantial benefit may occur in many childhood epilepsies, effectiveness in adults is unknown. (Charlie Foundation, 1997)

(Meds, as indicated.***** Anticonvulsive/antikindling drugs are estimated to help 75-90% of grand mal, but less than 35% of TLE patients. (LaPlante 1993))

Reminder: Full contraindications have not been included. Treatment must be tailored by the physician to individual biochemical requirements.

* Taurine may be especially helpful.

** The effectiveness of phenytoin-type anticonvulsives may be largely due to facilitating GABA messages and blocking glutamic acid activity.

*** Braverman suggests the tendency of certain seizure disorders to flareup during stress may reflect stress-induced depletion of zinc and B6.

**** Caution: too much lobelia can cause vomiting.

***** Note: Depletion of body stores of folate by phenytoin-type drugs may contribute to anticonvulsive effects, but, in some cases, foster depression or psychosis. Anticonvulsants may also produce deficiencies of vitamin K, magnesium and manganese. (Sullivan, 1979)

Inhibitory amino acids

Taurine, glycine and GABA are calming, membrane-stabilizing, sleep-promoting amino acids, as well as major inhibitory brain neurotransmitters They can be antidepressant, but primarily show promise as antimanic and mood-stabilizing agents.

Long-term depletion of these aminos promotes overstimulation and stress. A limbic/frontal imbalance may further compromise mood stability. Emotional intensity and reactivity could then spiral and become overwhelming, or evolve into confusion, mania, psychosis, or seizures. (SLAGLE 2000)

Inhibitory aminos (along with other mood-stabilizing nutrients) can be used as a base, upon which mood-specific therapies are layered. Thus, inhibitors would be used ongoing, for prevention. For mania, additional inhibitors and antimanics would be added. During depression, antidepressant nutrients would augment preventive doses of inhibitors. (BRAVERMAN 1987, ROSS 2002, LARSON 2001, SLAGLE 2000)

Aminos are best taken with B vitamins to support digestion and use.

Inhibitory potency (ROGERS 1997)

Taurine and GABA are both quite potent. Glycine is less so, but becomes more effective when combined with magnesium (as magnesium glycinate).

Strategies used by nutritionally-oriented practioners

□ Inhibitory aminos as secondary treatment — Aminos are potent, but can produce side effects (especially at higher doses, or with long-term use), may incompletely address underlying issues, and may interact with drugs. Some practitioners (e.g, ROGERS 1997, WALSH 2006, HOFFER 2008, LESSER 2008) generally focus more on minerals, vitamins, EFAs and phospholipids, and treatment of any biotype, allergic, toxic, or other health conditions — with whatever aminos that entails — *rather than* concentrating therapy on inhibitory vs. stimulating aminos. *In some cases, non-amino nutrients like magnesium, zinc, lithium, C, B3, B6, certain other B vitamins, EFAs, etc., seem to be sufficient.**

□ Inhibitory aminos as primary treatment — Other practitioners (e.g, SLAGLE 2000, ROSS 2002) emphasize aminos at the outset, especially with acute mood episodes, but also for ongoing prevention.

Appropritate treatment, of course, should always be determined by the patient's individual requirements.

* Perhaps, also, where indicated, increasing potency by IV administration.

Biotype considerations (WALSH 2007)

Inhibitory aminos are less useful for histadelia, which is characterized by severe depression, and already low levels of stimulating transmissions.

Relevance of free-form aminos

Individual indicated aminos, in free form, may be helpful, especially with malabsorption, gut oxidation, or dysfunction of digestive enzymes, as free form aminos do not need to be digested, and so are readily absorbed. However, free form amino *multis* are sometimes problematic, as they can compete for absorption, digestion and use with *specific* aminos most required for recovery. (WALSH 2007)

Taurine vs. GABA vs. glycine (WALSH 2007, BRAVERMAN 1987, SLAGLE, ROSS 2002, PFEIFFER 1975)

□ GABA — counters norepinephrine, benefits most histapenias, and is known to reduce anxiety, insomnia and general stimulation.

□ Taurine — may be especially relevant in bipolars with convulsive tendencies. (WALSH 2008) It excels at reducing stimulation in certain patients,(LARSON 2007) though intake may need to be reduced if it causes diarrhea. Another concern: Taurine decreases zinc absorption so can worsen symptoms in low-zinc, and/or high-copper patients, (WALSH 2008) unless good zinc levels can be maintained.

□ Glycine — is much less potent than taurine or GABA, though intake as magnesium glycinate enhances effectiveness. It may be most useful with pyroluria, and with histadelic agitation. Glycine also serves as a minor source of brain fuel.

Optimal treatment may involve intake, *several times* per day of:
□ one of these inhibitors
□ a mix of inhibitors *or*
□ different inhibitors over the day

See *Considerations* for each amino.

Cautions

When using significant quantities of mood-modifying aminos, watch for: (1) significant symptoms emerging before the next dose; or (2) patient resistance to taking aminos several times per day; or (3) inability to navigate PRNs.

In such cases, small (usually 100 mg) doses, or time-release aminos may be sufficient. Otherwise, at least temporarily, nutrient therapy may need to focus on other approaches, with only limited use of amino supplements, if at all.

Taurine

Mechanisms in mania moderation

Mechanisms that may help counter mania:

- □ Acts in brain regions which modulate mood.
- □ Moderates stress.
- □ Inhibits stimulating, and activates inhibiting, transmitters.
- □ Prevents glutamate elevation.
- □ Stabilizes membrane excitability. Anticonvulsive.
- □ Regulates electolytes.
- □ Modulates second messengers.
- □ Decreases thyroid and adrenal overactivity. Supports normal thyroid function.
- □ Reduces blood sugar, enhances use and storage.
- □ Helps regulate copper and iron levels.

See box, on the following page.

Taurine is the brain's second most abundant major inibitory neurotransmitter. It possesses a structure and metabolism similar to that of the other major inhibitors, GABA and glycine (all of which have anticonvulsive, sleep-promoting, sedative, mood-stabilizing properties). Braverman (1987) suggests minor tranquilizers may work via taurine (as well as GABA) in helping to calm mood and counter anxiety.

Mania & mood stabilization (BRAVERMAN 1987, BALCH 1990, PAGE 1992, LARSON 2001, SLAGLE 2000, BIRDSALL 1998)

Some practitioners report clinical benefit in hypomania and mania, (SLAGLE 2000, LARSON 2001) and in such related symptoms as anxiety, agitation, restlessness, irritability, hyperactivity, insomnia, obsessions, and seizures. (SLAGLE 2000, BIRDSALL 1998, BRAVERMAN 1987) Joan Matthews Larson, PhD, of the Health Recovery Center in Minnesota, has recommended taurine (500 mg, 3x/day) to dual diagnosis bipolars for years (along with other supportive nutrients), and finds it stabilizes mood as effectively as pharmacological lithium. (LARSON 2001) It may be especially indicated for bipolars with neurological symptoms. (WALSH 2007)

Depression

See *Taurine,* p. 118.

Biotype & low zinc concerns (WALSH 2007)

Taurine sometimes, counterintuitively, creates agitation and irritability, and generally increases symptom severity. Walsh (2007) suggests that such effects may be largely due to zinc depletion, as taurine blocks zinc absorption in the gut.

The practitioner might try optimizing zinc before giving taurine and during intake. However, in patients particularly prone to low zinc, or low zinc/elevated copper (e.g., in histapenia, pyroluria, and metallothionein imbalance), unless good zinc and B6 levels can be achieved and maintained, GABA may be the better choice.

Do not give zinc and taurine at the same time of day.

Levels in bipolars

Taurine tends to be low in bipolars (and some depressives), (TACHIKI 1977, STURMAN 1971, LARSON 2001) elevated in others, (FEEKES 1994) despite symptoms of deficiency.

Taurine & addiction

Taurine supports withdrawal and nervous system recovery from drug or alcohol addiction. (BIRDSALL 1998, BRAVERMAN 1987) It may increase alcohol's depressant effects, (BIRDSALL 1998) and may help reduce psychotic episodes. (BRAVERMAN 1987)

Taurine may also help block pleasant effects of opiates, and reduce the discomfort of withdrawal. (BRAVERMAN 1987)

Mechanisms likely to influence mood (SLAGLE 2000, BIRDSALL 1998, BRAVERMAN 1987) (SEE CORRESPONDING CHAPTERS FOR FURTHER DESCRIPTIONS)

Taurine regulates electrical and chemical communication between neurons, depressing the firing of brain cells, and reducing brain stimulation, and often, anxiety, insomnia and mania. Mechanisms include:

□ **Acts in brain regions which modulate mood** — Taurine is concentrated in the hippocampus (critical to memory), the pineal (light/dark response), and the olfactory lobe (taste, smell), regions variously implicated in bipolar disorder. (BRAVERMAN 1987)
See *Biorhythms*, pp. 259-62; and *Hippocampus*, p. 282.

□ **Inhibits stimulating, activates inhibiting transmitters** — Taurine suppresses release of dopamine, norepinephrine, glutamate, and aspartate (stimulating transmitters), and increases brain acetylcholine (which is mainly inhibitory). (SLAGLE 2000, BIRDSALL 1998, BRAVERMAN 1987) Taurine also may increase hippocampal histamine, which counterbalances dopamine. (BRAVERMAN 1987)
See *Catecholamines*, pp. 106-18; *Excitotoxins*, pp. 191-93; *Acetylcholine*, pp. 48-51.

□ **Prevents long-term glutamate elevation** — Taurine is an essential amino acid for the infant nervous system. It should be abundant in mother's milk. With early deficiency, glutamate can become permanently elevated,* creating chronic overstimulation and perhaps contributing to the development of bipolar disorder. Many researchers are now investigating the association of glutamate with mood disorder. (STURMAN 1971, 77, TACHIKI 1977, KRYSTAL 2002, MICHAEL 2003, KENDELL 2005)
See *Excitotoxins*, pp. 191-93.

□ **Moderates membrane excitability** — Taurine protects and stabilizes nerve cell membranes, dampening excitability and suppressing firing. (MURRAY 1991, BRAVERMAN)

□ **Electrolyte regulation** — Taurine controls the movement of electolytes (sodium, potassium, calcium) and water across the neural membrane.** This influences membrane stability, receptor activity, second messenger signalling, electrical communication along the axon,*** and chemical communication between cells, and may also lower catecholamines, all of which can modulate mania, anxiety, etc. (EL-MALLAKH 1993, SCHAFFER 2000, BRAVERMAN 1987)

□ **Modulates creation and activity of cAMP** — which helps initiate the second messenger cascade (which many researchers find pivotal to mood). (BRAVERMAN 1987, MARZ)
See *Second messengers*, pp. 279.

□ **Use of fat** — Taurine is important in fat absorption, metabolism, elimination.**** Membrane fats are critical to neural signalling. Fats (especially as cholesterol) are also the base for production of many hormones which affect mood. (SLAGLE 2000, BRAVERMAN 1987)
See *EFAs*, pp. 47, 52, 85-94.

□ **Balances thyroid** — In at least some bipolars, high thyroid fuels mania, low contributes to depression. In others, the thyroid is dysregulated and thyroid hormone can be elevated even in depression. One symptom of taurine deficiency is low thyroid, though some hypothyroids show elevated taurine. Taurine also helps some cases of overactive thyroid.***** (BRAVERMAN 1987)
See *Thyroid*, pp. 225-37.

□ **Moderates adrenal output** — Adrenal output is frequently distorted in bipolars. Taurine antagonizes cortisone, inhibits adrenalin release, and protects from adverse effects of excess adrenalin. This is part of why the brain uses more taurine during stress. (FEUER 1982, 83, BRAVERMAN 1987, SLAGLE 2000)
See *Adrenals*, pp. 238-40.

□ **Lowers blood sugar** — Blood sugar imbalances frequently contribute to bipolar moods. Taurine increases insulin release, (LAMPSON 1983) and enhances glucose use and storage as glycogen. (SLAGLE 2000)
See *Sugar*, pp. 214-22.

□ **Helps prevent chemical sensitivity & toxicity.**

□ **Regulates copper & iron** — Moderates levels of serum copper, and helps regulate iron metabolism.*****(SLAGLE 2000)
See *Copper, Iron*, pp. 135-37 and 171-73.

□ **Anticonvulsive** — Many of the above functions****** contribute to anticonvulsive effectiveness (often associated with mood-stabilizing properties). Taurine concentrates and acts in electrically excitable tissues such as the brain, and is reduced by as much as half in patients susceptible to seizures. Research suggests short-term antiseizure activity, but further study is needed to confirm long-term benefit. Taurine has been used alone, or with GABA, B6 and other nutrients held to counter seizures.*(SHIMADA 1984, BERGAMINI 1974, BONHAUSE 1984, BIRDSALL 1998, BRAVERMAN 1987)

* Taurine accelerates glutamate decarboxylase, the enzyme which breaks down glutamate.

*** Taurine acts on a number of ion channels and transporters, facilitating movement of sodium, potassium and perhaps calcium and magnesium ions. It blocks suppression of membrane sodium/potassium pumps, and is also involved in calcium metabolism. (Birdsall 1998, Slagle 2000)

**** Electrical messages arise as ions move in and out of the neuron. With instability of ion movement, the cell could fire rapidly, and erratically (as in some epilepsies).

**** Taurine is a key component of bile.

***** Excess brain iron promotes free radical destruction of neurotransmitters and other brain chemicals.

****** Including, osmoregulation, stress moderation, glutamate reduction, inhibition of excitatory and activation of inhibitory neurotransmitters, dampening of membrane excitability, modulation of second messenger activity, hormonal effects, etc.

Considerations (SLAGLE 2000, BIRDSALL 1998, BRAVERMAN 1987)

Need may be suggested by

Taurine is often low, as it's used continually in heart, immune, and retinal function.

Affective disorder. Anxiety, stress, insomnia, agitation, irritability, obsessions, hyperactivity, mania.

Depression, fatigue, lethargy.

Tingling, numbness, trembling, seizures. (SLAGLE 2000)

Vision problems.*(VOADEN 1982)

High blood pressure, (YAMORI 1983) rapid heart beat, other cardiovascular dysfunction, especially overstimulation.** (SLAGLE 2000, BIRDSALL 1988, AZUMA 1983, SEBRING 1983)

High cholesterol. Gall bladder disorders. Obesity.***

Suppressed lactation (it stimulates prolactin). Low sperm motility. Male infertility. Prematurity, failure to thrive, growth retardation. (BRAVERMAN 1987, BIRDSALL 1998, MARTIN 1974)

Immune problems. MSG sensitivity. Difficulty metabolizing alcohol. Increased tendency to Candida. Chemical sensitivity. Neurotoxicity. **** Migraine.

Temperature dysregulation (common in bipolars).*****

Blood sugar imbalances, especially diabetes. (BRAVERMAN)

Overactive adrenals.

Low thyroid and other thyroid imbalances. (SLAGLE 2000)

Tendency to gout, kidney dysfunction, (BRAVERMAN 1987) migraines. (SLAGLE 2000)

* Taurine is the most abundant amino acid in the retina and photoreceptors, and helps maintain retinal structure and function, and protect eyes from toxins and cataracts. It may benefit macular and retinal degeneration. (Voaden 1982, Birdsall 1998).

** Supports and protects heart contractibility, rhythms, and general function by: modulating cAMP, helping regulate calcium and sodium channels, electrically stabilizing heart cell membrane protein, and providing antioxidant protection. May also antagonize angiotensin and suppress renin (which increases blood pressure). (Braverman 1987, Birdsall 1998)

*** Supports fat absorption and metabolism. Supports gall bladder bile production. Inhibits cholesterol gall stones. (Braverman 87, Slagle 2000)

**** Protects cell membranes from oxidation. Helps control inflammation. Supports thymus development. (Braverman 1987, Slagle 2000) Stimulates immune function, increases natural killer cell activity & interleukin 2. Sulfur donor. Supports liver detox and conjugation of certain internal (e.g aldehyde) & external chemicals (chloride, hypochlorous acid, aldehyde, perhaps carbon tetrachloride). (Birdsall 1998) Helps decrease chemical sensitivity. (Rogers)

***** Taurine is cooling and helps the HPT regulate temperature.

Populations

Taurine is depleted by infection, chronic stress, trauma, institutionalization, inflammation, toxic exposure,* high-fat diets, vegetarianism, alcoholism, burns, surgery, radiation, muscle diseases, steroids, bacterial overgrowth in the gut, nursing (mothers), formula-feeding (infants),** certain metabolic disorders, or heightened genetic requirements. Thorazine® (an antipsychotic) and Chloroquine® (an antimalarial) reduce levels. (SLAGLE 2000, BRAVERMAN 1987) Depletion causes greater symptoms in females. (LARSON 2001)

* Toxic exposures divert cysteine (a taurine precursor) into creating glutathione, leaving less available to form taurine.

** It's in the placenta, and mother's milk, but low in cow's milk, and formula. (Hayes 1985, Erberdobler 1983)

Nutrient interactions

With glycine, supports formation of glutathione.

Supports absorption of fat soluble vitamins.

Supportive nutrients (BRAVERMAN 1987, SLAGLE 2000)

NAC — taurine is usually made from cysteine (but can be derived from methionine or sulfate).

P5P (from vitamin B6) — a cofactor in all three enzymes used in forming taurine.*

Zinc & manganese — build taurine, enhance neural effects, are closely bound to it in brain and retina.

Vitamin A — deficiency is associated with taurine loss.

Magnesium may also be helpful.

B vitamins support digestion and use.

Molybdenum — helps transform sulfite (a relatively toxic byproduct of taurine metabolism) to sulfate.

Antagonistic nutrients (BRAVERMAN 1987)

Glutamate (as in MSG) can decrease taurine.

Sources

Mother's milk, meat (including organ meats), fish (especially shark, abalone), poultry, eggs, dairy. (BRAVERMAN 1987)

Lab (FEEKES 1994, BRAVERMAN 1987, BONHAUSE 1984, BERGAMINI 1974)

Plasma taurine. Taurine may test normal or high, but still be needed.*

* Elevation may, in some cases, be due to increased demand (as in mania), or impaired transport or uptake.

Dose

To prevent rebound, take at least 2x per day or alternate with GABA over the day. Larson (2001) suggests 500 mg taurine, 2x/day orally,* to start, then 3x, if needed. Some patients may require a total of 1-2 gm, possibly more, (divided over 3-4 doses, e.g., 500 mg each). (SLAGLE 2000, BRAVERMAN 1987) Walsh, however, noting that taurine is metabolized slowly and tends to accumulate, finds the therapeutic effect can usually be maintained while gradually reducing the dose after approximately 2 wks, to about 500 mg/day. (Walsh 2006)

To minimize stomach acidity, take with food (dairy, if not sensitive to it) or lecithin and olive oil. (BRAVERMAN 1987)

* Taurine is water soluble, so doesn't readily cross fatty membranes or the blood brain barrier. Nonetheless, research suggests oral supplementation can correct brain deficiency. Transport may be impaired in epileptics. Homotaurine enters the brain in greater quantities. (Braverman 1987)

Effects of excess, contraindications

Interferes with gut zinc absorption, potentially worsening pyroluria, histapenia, metal metabolism dysfunction, agitation, anxiety, mania, irritability, etc. *Optimize zinc.*

Initially, agitation may occur as dosage wears off.

Decreases blood sugar. Exercise caution in unstable diabetes and hypoglycemia.* (See pp. 214-2.)

Reduces blood pressure. (ROSS 2002)

Can increase acidity, promote salicylate or other ulcers. *Avoid/limit if susceptible. Do not take with aspirin.* (SLAGLE 2000, BRAVERMAN 1987)

Laxative. *Reduce dose, increase GABA; modify diet.*

Diuretic, removing sodium and water.

High doses can decrease body temperature. (SLAGLE 2000)

GABA

Mood stabilization

GABA is critical in counterbalancing norepinephrine, and is like taurine, a major inhibitory neurotransmitter, controlling the speed and intensity of neural communication. It is the most abundant inhibitor in the brain,* and is present in up to half of all synapses. Depletion allows excitatory neurotransmissions to predominate. (Sahley 1995, Braverman 1987)

Again, like taurine, GABA promotes sleep and relaxation; and reduces stimulation, anxiety, and the tendency to seizures. Mood stabilization benefits are similar. (Christensen 1982, Emrich 1980, 81, Krystal 2002, Braverman 1987, Petty 1995,96. Taylor 2003, Shiah 1998)

Considerable evidence supports mood-stabilizing use for at least a subset of bipolars. Plasma GABA (which reflects brain levels) is often low during bipolar depression and mania. GABA agonists moderate mood. Successful treatment of mood episodes upregulates GABA receptors. At least part of the mechanism of action in some important mood-stabilizing drugs is through GABA. (Petty 1994, 95, Taylor 2003, Shiah 1998) Some studies point also to the importance of the GABA/glutamate balance in mood. (Kendell 2005, Brambilla 2003, Krystal 2002)

See box, *GABA activity in meds,* p. 42, and *Excitotoxins,* pp. 191-93.

* Especially in the cerebral cortex, substantia nigra, and thalamus.

Mania

Research suggests GABA or GABA agonists may benefit mania, (Emrich 1980, 81, Krystal 2002, Braverman 1987, Petty 1995, 96. Taylor 2003, Shiah 1998) as well as such related symptoms as anxiety, stress, nervous tension, excited repetitive speech, acute agitation, hyperactivity, insomnia, and psychosis. (Petty 1998, Braverman 1987, Slagle 2000, Pfeiffer 1988) Depletion has been associated with overexcitability, tremors, and hyperpragia (excess mental activity). (Post 1999, Petty 1998)

See also, *GABA,* p. 118.

Biotype indications (Walsh 2007)

Walsh finds GABA often useful in moderating norepinephrine overstimulation in histapenia, in copper-overload/MT dysfunction, and in pyroluria.

Histadelics, on the other hand, are less likely to respond to GABA, as norepinephrine is already overly repressed.

GABA levels in bipolars

Plasma GABA is often reduced in bipolars. (Petty 1994, 95, 96, Brambilla 2003) In one study, Petty found 30% of manic and 40% of depressed bipolars had levels below 95% of controls.*

Within patients, GABA can be (counterintuitively) higher in mania than depression. (Petty 1981, Post 1999, Gerner 1984) This may represent an attempt to address greater need, and still be insufficient, as manics often respond well to GABA, even when labs show adequate levels. So, a trial of GABA may often be indicated, and can be the most practical way to determine need. (Slagle 2000, Cousens 2000, Braverman 1987, Ross 2002)

* In fact, some researchers suggest low plasma GABA may be a marker for bipolar disorder, with low levels in both mania and depression. (Petty 1981, 92, 93ab, 94, 98, Berretini 1982, 84) However, between cycles, GABA has been observed to move toward normal. (Petty 1992, 98, Coryell 1992, Braverman 1987)

Brain effects & influence on mood

Antimanic effects

GABA is generally inhibitory, (Petty 1998), with low GABA activity* promoting excitatory neurotransmission. (Braverman 1987)

Counters norepinephrine — benefitting mania, and making it particularly helpful for histapenics. (Walsh 2008)

Counters dopamine — GABA decreases dopamine overactivity, particularly in the limbic system, contributing to its antimanic,** anti-psychotic, (Roberts 1976, vanKammen 1977) and anti-dyskinesiac effects. (Bartholini 1985)

* Or low GAD, the B6-dependent enzyme critical to GABA production.

** Silverstone (1985) suggests mania may result from dopamine/GABA/acetylcholine interactions in ventral tegmental regions.

Other effects influencing mood

Serotonin — GABA moderates serotonin activity. (Strahlendort 1988, Bartholini 1985, Schlicker 1984) Serotonin, in turn, increases GABAa receptor sensitivity to GABA. (Akasu 1988)

Acetylcholine — GABA also affects acetylcholine and may moderate hyperactive acetylcholine (e.g., in the striatum). (Bartholini 1985)

Antidepressant effects

See *Role of inhibitory aminos,* p. 118.

GABA activity in meds which counter mania

Benzodiazepines (used for anxiety, agitation, insomnia, acute mania) produce GABA-like effects, and are thought to work by activating GABA neurons and receptors. (POST 1999, BRAVERMAN 1987) Similarly, the major mood stabilizers, valproic acid, carbamazepine and lithium increase or mimic GABA messages. (EMRICH 1980, 81, PETTY 1996, MOTOHASHI 1992, BARTHOLINI1985) Neuroleptics, used to suppress mania, also increase GABA turnover. (BRAVERMAN 1987, EMRIC 1980, RING 1993, COUSENS 2000, BARTHOLINI 1985, PETTY 1993AB, 98)

Reaction to an extreme dose

To test the effects of high dose GABA, Pfeiffer took 10 gm. (The normal therapeutic range is generally between 500 and 3,000 mg, divided over the day. Breathing, heart rate, and blood pressure elevated. He wheezed, choked, vomited, fidgeted, couldn't sit still, and had a massive anxiety attack. He also experienced a constant flushing or tingling, possibly due to a neurologic reaction.

Other mental effects

□ Anxiety, agitation — GABA fills receptor sites and inhibits firing, so incoming anxiety and stress-related messages are less able to overwhelm cortex and motor centers. (SLAGLE 2000) GABA is often low in anxiety or panic disorder, and it has been successfully used, alone, or with B3, B complex, and inositol, as an alternative to benzodiazepines. (BRAVERMAN 1987, PFEIFFER 1988, SLAGLE 2000)

□ Insomnia — GABA produces a natural sleep inducer. (BRAVERMAN 1987) Moreover, the use of benzodiazepines for insomnia suggests GABA, itself, could be effective. (POST 1999)

□ Psychosis — Some schizophrenics show low brain GABA; and a small number recover on GABA. Braverman (1987) suggests megadoses may be needed, and that GABA may also help catatonia.

□ Intelligence — GABA (and glycine) have been observed to enhance in vitro dendritic growth and arborization, suggesting a possible benefit to intelligence. (BALOYANNIS 1983, CORYELL 1992, BRAVERMAN 1987)

□ Aggression — GABA can be low and may be helpful in some cases, (PETTY 1998, BRAVERMAN 1987, SLAGLE 2000, ROSS 2002, PFEIFFER 1988) perhaps especially with elevated copper or histapenia. (WALSH 2007)

Neurological

□ Epilepsy — Epileptics share many symptoms and much chemistry with bipolars. Taurine and glycine are usually decreased; aspartic and glutamic acids, increased. GABA is almost always depleted in epileptics. (CORYELL 1992, BRAVERMAN 1987, SLAGLE 2000) Many anticonvulsants (valproate, benzodiazepines, valium)** increase or mimic GABA. GABA supplements have been show to decrease neural stimulation and help control seizures, (CHRISTENSEN 1982, BARTHOLINI 1985, BRAVERMAN 1987) though getting enough GABA into the brain can be a problem. (LOSCHER 1984, SYTINSKY 1978). B6 may help. (BRAVERMAN 1987)

□ Other brain disorders — GABA activity can be low in Parkinson's, Huntington's, multiple sclerosis, action tremors, tardive dyskinesia, and Friedreich's ataxia, which may improve with intake. (SAHLEY 1995, BRAVERMAN 1987) GABA has also been used for pain relief.*(BIRD 1974, CHRISTENSEN 1982)

* Clinicians at the Pain and Stress Therapy Center, in San Antonio, report 750 mg free-form GABA dissolved in water mimics the analgesic effects of benzodiazepines within 10-12 minutes, without producing sedation or addiction. (Sahley 1995)

Benefits in alcoholism & substance abuse

□ Coryell (1992) suggests alcoholics may be genetically, and are clinically, similar to mood-disordered patients. Plasma GABA is reduced in both affectives and alcoholics. (MOSS 1990, CORYELL 1992, PETTY 1992) Low GABA may increase desire for alcohol in recovered alcoholics. (COUSENS 2000) GABA (with glutamine and tyrosine) is used in some treatments for substance abuse. (BRAVERMAN 1987, LARSON 2001, ROSS 2002)

Considerations: GABA

Need may be suggested by

Affective disorders, anxiety, agitation, tension, low tolerance for stress, aggression, insomnia. Pain.*(Braverman 1987, Ross 2002, Slagle 2000, Sahley 1995, Balch 1990, Petty 1998)

Numbness, tingling, seizures, other neurological symptoms. (Braverman 1987)

Muscle tension or stiffness. (Ross 2002)

High blood pressure. (Antonaccio 1984, Gillis 1984, Braverman 1987)

Immune and digestive symptoms.** Poor diet.

High blood sugar,*** alcoholism.****(Sahley 1995, Balch 1990, Petty 1998, Moss 1990, Coryell 1992)

Tendency to suppressed lactation, (Fuchs 1984) perhaps PMS, low sperm motility; low sex drive, enlarged prostate. (Braverman 1987)

* Reduces pain (typically at 750 mg). (Sahley 1995)
** GABA is important in the thymus and duodenum. (Braverman 1987)
*** Increases insulin's effects (Braverman 1987, Tews 1984).
**** May reduce withdrawal symptoms. (Slagle 2000, Coryell 1992)

Nutrient interactions

Supports use and metabolism of C. (Braverman, Bigelow 1984)

Lab

Plasma GABA but can be difficult to detect. (Braverman 1987) Levels presumably reflect what's in the brain, (Loscher 1981, 82, Ferkany Smith 1978b, Bohlen 1979) but not necessarily. (Ferkany 1978b, Loscher 1982, Tews 1984)

Ross (2002) suggests taking into account, high anxiety, panic, or insomnia. Also, checking for extremes of salivary cortisol, mercury toxicity, and elevated progesterone (which can reduce GABA).

Braverman (1987) suggests considering GABA when glutamic acid is high, glutamine deficient.

Sources of GABA

The brain stores glutamine, which it turns into glutamate (excess of which can be excitotoxic), as needed. Glutamate precurses GABA, but does not insure increased GABA, and is often counterproductive.

GABA alone may be difficult to absorb. Nutrients which support formation of GABA (B6, manganese, zinc, taurine) and enhance effectiveness (B3, C, magnesium, perhaps inositol) are important. (Cousens 2000, Sahley 1995, Braverman 1987)

Supportive nutrients (Braverman 1987)

B6 or *P5P* — a critical cofactor regulating GABA manufacture. (Cousens 2000)

Zinc — helps form, metabolize and regulate GABA. Deficiency decreases GABA. (Walsh 2008)

Manganese — can help correct low levels of GAD,* which helps form GABA from glutamate. (Braverman 87)

Taurine — increases breakdown of glutamate to GABA. Taurine, glycine and/or threonine, strongly enhance effectiveness, or can substitute for GABA. (Ross 2002, Sahley 1995, Larson 2008) *Be careful not to oversedate.*

B3 (niacinamide),** C, magnesium — optimize effectiveness. (Sahley 1995, Cousens 2000)

B vitamins — support digestion and use. (Braverman 1987)

Thymol, contained in thyme, potentiates GABA receptors. (Priestly 2003)

Inositol can also be helpful, but may overstimulate. (Braverman 1987)

Counteractive nutrients

Aspartic and glutamic acid counter or inhibit GABA activity. Aspartate inhibits absorption. (Braverman 1987)

See *Excitotoxins, Glutamate,* p.191-93.

Dose

To prevent rebound, give at least twice per day, or alternate with taurine, typically 100-500 mg., 2-3x/day, especially with stress, mania, agitation, etc. (Ross 2002, Cousens 2000, Slagle 2000) With high anxiety, Brain Bio Center gave 200 mg, 4x/day. (Braverman 1987)

Take with P5P (a form of B6). Slagle suggests separating intake from that of GABA by at least 5 hrs.

Effects of excess, contraindications

Reduces blood sugar. Decreases appetite. (Tews 1984) Take any hypoglycemia into account.*

If required in diabetics, introduce slowly and monitor blood sugar. (Braverman 1987)

May lower blood pressure.

Flaccidity and satiety. In some cases, even low doses can overtranquilize. High doses with niacinamide and inositol may magnify sedative effects, (Sahley 1995) Similarly, do not take GABA in IV form. (Ross, Larson 2008) Avoid alcohol and relaxants.

Avoid or, if indicated, use under cautious medical supervision if taking benzodiazepines, or certain other meds. (Sahley 1995, Braverman 1987)

Can worsen depression. (Petty 1995)

Not always sedative. (Braverman 1987)

* Though it may benefit hypoglycemia by preventing insulin spikes, be preventive, and support sugar balance (improve the diet, avoid sugar, provide chromium, manganese, etc. (Walsh 2007) See pp. 214-22.

Glycine (SLAGLE 2000, BRAVERMAN 1987, ROSS 2002, BALCH 1990, PAGE 1992. JAFFE 1992)

Location

Glycine is present throughout the central nervous system, especially in dopamine pathways. (BRAVERMAN 1987)

Mood stabilizers increase glycine

Initially lithium, valproate and other anticonvulsive mood stabilizers, increase glycine. (ROSENBLATT 1979, 82, DEUTSCH 1981, 82, 83, PESELOW 1982)

Depression

See *Role of inhibitory aminos,* p. 118.

Betaine (trimethylglycine)

Many of the effects of betaine are due to the triple methyl, rather than just the glycine.

See *Betaine,* p. 161.

Glycine is an amino acid and inhibitory neurotransmitter, less potent than GABA and taurine.

Mania

Very high doses of glycine can be antimanic. The Princeton Bio Center successfully treated two acute manics with 15 to 30 gms (a very high dose). (PFEIFFER 1988) Pearson and Shaw (1983) found 3-10 gm of glycine sedative. Glycine may also address various symptoms associated with mania: overstimulation, anxiety, agitation, aggression, hyperactivity, insomnia, and some cases of psychosis. (BRAVERMAN 1987, JAFFE 1992, PFEIFFER 1988)

High doses, however, are impractical. Eby (2001, 06) suggests using magnesium glycinate, which allows for lower doses of each component, and seems to have considerable antimanic, and mood-stabilizing effectiveness. See *Magnesium,* pp. 25-28.

Biotype indications (WALSH 2007)

Sometimes used with pyroluria, or histadelic agitation.

Levels in bipolars

Glycine may be reduced, (HENDLER 1989) as it often is in epilepsy, (BRAVERMAN 1987) or elevated, (ROSENBLATT 1979) perhaps, in some cases, reflecting attempts to moderate overstimulation. (BRAVERMAN 1987)

Brain/neurological effects

Enhances the activity of acetylcholine, can slow its breakdown, (TOMASZEWSKI 1983) and may stimulate its release in key mood-modulating regions (e.g. hippocampus). (BRAVERMAN 1987)

Weak methylator. Helps create SAM which methylates, activates, and recycles antidepressant neurotransmitters, (PFEIFFER 1988, BRAVERMAN 1987, HENDLER 1989) and cAMP. (SMYTHIES 1984)

Suppresses dopamine. (PFEIFFER 1988)

Helps form phospholipids —- including those of neural membranes and receptors. Phospholipids are critical to the flexible receptor response needed for mood stability. (SLAGLE 2000, BRAVERMAN 1987)

Minor source of brain fuel (as a substitute for glucose).

Has been used in treating epilepsy, and other conditions involving abnormal nerve firing (e.g., spasticity). May concentrate at epileptic foci. (BRAVERMAN 1987)

With arginine forms creatine, which slows nerve degeneration. (BRAVERMAN 1987)

Physical effects relevant to bipolars (BRAVERMAN 1987)

Helps balance blood sugar — increases both glucagon secretion (raising blood sugar) and sugar storage in the liver as glycogen.

Increases energy & stamina — Supports cell oxygenation. May lower blood lactic acid (associated with muscle fatigue and anxiety). *Though, high glycine may displace too much brain glucose, causing fatigue.*

Considerations

Need may be suggested by (BRAVERMAN 1987, PFEIFFER, 1988, BALCH 1990, JAFFE 1992, SLAGLE 2000, HERESCO-LEVY 1996)

Moodiness, depression, cognitive symptoms.

Fatigue. Slow metabolism.

Anxiety. Agitation.

Numbness, tingling, seizures, epilepsy. (BRAVERMAN 1987)

Hypoglycemia. Glucose intolerance.**

Immune, free radical, toxic susceptibility. Allergies.***

Pain, (BRAVERMAN 1987) perhaps arthritis. (YAMAMOTO 1981)

High blood pressure, poor circulation, homocysteinuria, other cardiovascular problems. (BRAVERMAN 1987)

Muscle weakness, slow repair, cramps, spasticity.**** (BRAVERMAN 1987)

Poor healing of wounds, aging skin, poor nails.

Poor growth. (KASAI 1980) Suppressed lactation. (BRAVERMAN)

Eye problems, perhaps cataracts. (BRAVERMAN 1987)

May benefit gout, kidney oxalate stones (*but not high doses*); low stomach acid; prostate problems, low sex drive; (SLAGLE 2000) starvation, rickets. (BRAVERMAN 1987)

* Helps liver store glucose as glycogen.

*** Supports immunity and liver function. May benefit fatty liver. Stimulates glutathione peroxidase. Helps form glutathione. Helps remove lead, detoxify benzoic acid, phenols, and ammonia. (Slagle 2000)

Considerations: Glycine *continued*

**** Precurses creatine which forms creatinine which promotes muscle repair and strength. (Braverman 1987)
***** Helps form collagen (which gives skin elasticity), keratine (which forms nails), and DNA. (Braverman 1987)
****** Helps stimulate growth hormone release. (Slagle 2000, Kasai 1980)
******* Increases urination. (Slagle 2000)

Testing

Plasma glycine (Jaffe 1992)
Low serum creatinine can suggest deficiency.(Braverman 1987)

Source (Braverman 1987)

Most protein foods: wild game, other meats, duck, turkey, poultry, dairy. Also, avocado, wheat germ, oats. Collagen (e.g., chicken bone gristle) is the richest source.

Supportive nutrients

Although considered a nonessential amino acid, brain glycine may depend on dietary glycine and threonine.* B vitamins support digestion and use.

* Glycine can be formed from threonine (perhaps most readily) or choline (->TMG->DMG->sacrosine->glycine). Serine degrades to glycine, but the opposite reaction is more likely, unless enough alanine is present to block serine formation. Glycine is also formed from endogenous glucose.

Therapeutic doses (Slagle 2000)

Suggested doses typically ranges from 100 to 500 mg. 2x/day.* Take with B complex or B6. Magnesium glycinate is useful for many bipolars.

*Braverman (1987) suggests higher doses may be needed for sedative effects since glycine does not readily cross the blood brain barrier.

Effects of excess, contraindications (Braverman 1987)

Nausea. Depression and fatigue.
Muscle weakness, possibly correctable with serine.
Growth depression (at 7% dietary glycine) due to glucagon and glucocorticoid deficiency.
May increase risk of ulcers.
Toxic levels create effects opposite to those of normal intake (reversable with arginine and methionine).

Threonine

Threonine, an essential amino acid, is important, with the help of B6, in the production of certain neurotransmitters, and also supports general nervous system health.

Mania

Threonine may provide some benefit to agitated states, such as mania, and anxiety, etc. It helps get the inhibitors, glycine* and GABA, into the brain. (Braverman 1987, Larson 2008)

* As threonine breaks down into glycine, serine and glucose.

Other potential benefits to bipolars (Braverman 1987)

- ☐ May help counter stress, irritability, agitated depression. (Braverman 1987)
- ☐ May benefit some cases of personality disorder (especially when levels are depleted). (Hendler 1989, Braverman 1987)
- ☐ Anticonvulsant properties. (Honda 1984)
- ☐ May help resolve confusion,(Braverman 1987) and improve neurological dysfunction.*(Honda 1984, Rogers 1980, Doolittle 1992, Blin 1989)
- ☐ Supports normal thyroid function.
- ☐ May reduce wheat gluten sensitivity. (Lotan 1980)
- ☐ Supports gut function, aborption, digestion, assimilation.
- ☐ Supports digestion of fats, reduces fatty buildup in tissue (and liver), perhaps especially when choline is low. (Fukuda 1990)
- ☐ Supports immune function.** (Lotan 1980)
- ☐ Helps maintain normal protein balance and uptake.
- ☐ Plays a minor role in sparing brain glucose.

* Animals on a low threonine diet develop neurological disorders and paralysis, reversible with threonine. (Rogers 1980) Researchers have looked at use for Lou Gehrigs, MS spasms, and ALS. (Doolittle 1992, Blin 1989)

** Antibody formation; thymus activity, growth; cellular immune defense; liver support.

Considerations (Braverman 1987, Pfeiffer 1988, Haas 2006)

Need may be suggested by

Depression, confusion.
Emotional agitation, irritability.
Stress; poor response to trauma.
Neurological dysfunction. (Honda 1984, Rogers 1980, Doolittle 1992, Blin 1989)
Immune weakness. (Lotan 1980)
Skin disorders. Poor structure to nails, tooth enamel, or bones.
Rigid or weak muscles, ligaments.*
Cardiovascular problems.
Problems digesting fat (Fukuda 1990) or protein.
Poor healing of wounds, injuries, or burns.

* Threonine is important in forming collagen and elastin.

Populations (Braverman 1987)

Levels can be low in depression, and epilepsy.
Stress increases urinary loss. (Braverman 1987)

Source

Legumes, most meats, dairy, eggs, moderate in wheat germ, some nuts, seeds and vegetables. Low in most grains and corn.

Lab (Braverman 1987)

Plasma threonine.

Effects of excess, contraindications

Can increase urea and ammonia.
Excess may disrupt liver function.
Pregnancy and nursing effects are unknown.

Serotonin

Some studies of tryptophan use in mania

Landry and Chouinard, 1991 — a double blind exploring maintenance use of tryptophan plus lithium in drug-resistant bipolars.

Chouinard, 1985 — a placebo-controlled clinical trial involving 24 patients reported improvement in acute mania with 12 gm L-tryptophan daily. In the second week, subjects who were switched to placebo deteriorated.

Prange, 1974 — In a small double-blind crossover, 6 gm free-form tryptophan per day improved mania, with results equal to, or better than, chlopromazine.

Murphy, 1974 — seven of ten acutely manic or hypomanic patients improved on an average of 9.6 gm per day, with three of the seven relapsing on placebo.

The amino acid, tryptophan, is metabolized into 5HTP, which precurses serotonin, a neurotransmitter popularly known for its antidepressant effects. (See pp. 100-05.) Serotonin also seems to benefit mania in some bipolars; trigger or worsen it in others. (GAYFORD 1973, ANNITTO 1979, BAUMEL 1995)

Permissive hypothesis

Coppen (1965, 1972) first suggested that low serotonin could play a role in mania. Prange later proposed a "permissive hypothesis" of bipolar disorder: Low serotonin permits extremes in stimulating (dopamine and norepinephrine) and inhibiting (acetylcholine) neurotransmitters to emerge, destabilizing mood. (PRANGE 1974)

Levels

Bipolars may underutilize serotonin. (SACHS 1989) Researchers have found low levels or activity in most affectives (and their families), (GOLD 1987) especially if violent or suicidal, (COPPEN 1988, MAES 1990, MARAZZITI 1991AB, SWANN 1983, 94, GOLDBERG 1999, BENKELFAT 1994) but even after remission. (COPPEN 1992, MALONE 1993, GOLDBERG 1999) Benkelfat (1994) suggests low intake of its precursor, tryptophan, augments genetic risk for affective disorder.

Serotonin can also be low in such mania-related symptoms as anxiety, insomnia, spontaneous aggression, psychomotor hyperactivity and sterotypy, and dysinhibition. (POST 1980, BRIGHAM 2001)

Possible mechanisms moderating mania (GOLD 1987)

Moderates neurotransmitters in the limbic system and other emotion centers. (GOLD 1987)

Generally inhibits or decreases dopamine and norepinephrine.* May alter MAO metabolism. (TAKAHASHI 1975, CHOUINARD 1983) Has parasympathetic action which moderates epinephrines.

Influences hypothalamus-pituitary-endocrine axis. (See pp. 223-40.)

Transmits messages which create a sense of security, relaxation, calm.

* High levels of tryptophan decrease tyrosine absorption, limiting dopamine and norepinephrine formation. Elevated 5HTP may displace neural dopamine and norepinephrine. (Gelenberg 1982)

Mood stabilization

Various studies investigate tryptophan or 5HTP as a preventive or mood-stabilizing treatment. (VAN PRAAG 1977, LANDRY 1991)

Mania

Anti-manic

Low serotonin is associated with increased susceptibility to mania and exacerbation of manic symptoms in some bipolars. (PETTY 1998) Research suggests tryptophan can be antimanic for some, (PRANGE 1974, GELENBERG 1982, SACHS 1989, CHOUINARD 1985, MURPHY 1974) either alone, or at low doses, adjunctive to lithium (which also increases serotonin). (BREWERTON 1983)

See box, upper left.

Pro-manic

Mood effects vary from one patient to another. (CHAMBERS 1978, NAYLOR 1978) In some bipolars, supplementation triggers hypomania, even during depression; and generally triggers or fuels mania. Some manics experience serotonin as a stimulant. (COLODNY, LANDRY 1991) Moreover, levels are sometimes higher in mania than depression. (GAYFORD 1973, ANNITTO 1979, BAUMEL 1995)

See *Serotonin*, pp. 100-105, for contraindications, etc.

3. EFAs & Phospholipids

Over time, the focus of bipolar research has largely shifted from neurotransmitters, themselves, to corresponding receptors and second messengers (SCHREIBER, PEREZ 1999, 00) — thus highlighting the importance of EFAs and phospholipids. This section discusses the effects of EFAs and phosphatidyl choline on mania and mood stabilization. For further information, especially as related to antidepressant effects, see *EFAs*, pp. 85-94; *Inositol,* pp. 95-97; *Serine,* p. 98; *Carnitine,* pp. 115-16.

Primer: Receptors, second messengers, & mood

Receptors

Neural receptors are locations on the nerve cell's membrane, which receive chemical information from other neurons. Neurotransmitters or other agonists (first messengers) bind to and interact with the receptor, then are released back into the synapse. Receptors initiate the transfer of information into the cell for response.

Oversensitive receptors within stimulating neurotransmitter systems foster mania; undersensitive, depression.

Second messengers (STOLL 2002)

Second messaging involves a cascade of biochemical events begun by the first-messenger/receptor interaction, and brought through the cell, altering activity and biochemistry and perhaps triggering electric potentials down the cell axon, which cumulatively provoke neurotransmission to other cells.

Many researchers believe that second messenger disturbances are central to bipolar illness: generally, overactive second messaging multiplies stimulation, promoting mania; underactive, suppresses communication, fostering depression.

The role of EFAs & phospholipids in mood

Essential fatty acids (EFAs)

Omega 3, particularly,* is key to brain communication, as it is essential to flexible receptor function, and in the initiation of second messenger activity.

Research suggests omega 3 (especially as EPA) may counter bipolar depression, while DHA may be helpful with mania, and the combo, with mood stability, mixed states, and rapid cycling. (STOLL 2002, WALSH 2008)

* Although an emphasis on arachadonic acid (best obtained via GLA) is often preferable for pyrolurics. (Bibus 2000) (See p. 92.)

Phospholipids

Phospholipids are fat/phosphorus* compounds which form the basic structural element of the neural membrane and its receptors. They serve as an important safe haven for EFAs (even during oxidative stress), (WALSH 2007) and thus are instrumental in conveying and activating neural response to outside messages. (ELKASHEF 1987, GUNDERMAN 1995)

Major phospholipids include phosphatidyl choline (discussed in this chapter) which is largely antimanic; and phosphatidyl inositol, phosphatidyl serine, and phosphatidyl carnitine which are largely antidepressant.**

* Hence, phosphorus is essential to neural signalling. Moreover, it serves as a component of cAMP (an important second messenger), ATP (which stores cellular energy), and DNA and RNA. Pfeiffer (1975, 88) finds that deficiency can produce almost any major neurologic or psychiatric disorder, minus hallucination (which can occur with excess). Nonetheless, he finds deficiency rarely implicated, as phosphorus is relatively abundant in the modern diet (it's prevalent in animal foods and some junk food (soda and some preservatives), with moderate quantities in nuts, grains, and beans).
On the other hand, the availability of optimal EFAs, is usually the critical consideration when trying to improve phospholipid function.

** Note: Choline, serine, and inositol are not, in themselves, phospholipids, but are discussed, along with their phospholipid forms, in the phospholipid sections of this book.

Choline (COUSENS 2000, ROGERS 1997, PFEIFFER 1975, 87, 88, MURRAY 1991, ROSS 2002, BRAVERMAN 1987)

Low choline symptoms

Early researchers found cholinergics could suppress spontaneous movement, rambling or pressured speech, verbal aggression, irritability, cheerfulness, and grandiosity; and produce apathy, lack of energy, drowsiness, confusion, slurring of speech, poor concentration, slowed thought, and emotional withdrawal. (CARROLL 1973, SHOPSIN 1975, JANOWSKY 1973)

Mania studies

Cohen, 1982 — In a small double blind, lecithin (rich in phosphatidyl choline) created significant improvement in five of six manic patients.

Schreier, 1982 — Case history of an agitated, aggressive, manic adolescent, treated with lithium. The addition of lecithin led to a remission which lasted two years. When lithium was withdrawn, the patient was able to maintain on lecithin alone.

Levia, 1990 — Successful treatment of ten manics with phosphatidyl choline. Improvements were sustained over a lengthy period.

Stoll, 1996 — Six consecutive rapid cyclers were given choline bitartrate augmentation of lithium. Manic symptoms were substantially reduced in five patients, all mood symptoms in four.

Choline is generally associated with the B vitamin family, and in the following forms, exerts important effects on brain function and mood:

□ **Phosphatidyl choline** — a key neural membrane phospholipid.

□ **GPC** (glycerophosphocholine) — serves as a choline reservoir. (CRAYHON 1998)

□ **Acetylcholine** — a major inhibitory neurotransmitter, which supports learning, (SITARAM 1978AB) memory, (SOLAMA 1990, WILLIAMS 1998) parasympathetic response, and nerve/muscle interaction. (COONEY 1999) (See box, below.)

Mania

A number of studies indicate choline or phosphatidyl choline can benefit mania and hypomania, in some cases, profoundly, (KATO 1998, LEIVA 1990, STOLL 1991, 96, HAMAKAWA 1998, ALARCON 1985, JANOWSKY 1972, 73, DAVIS 1978A, ROWNTREE 1950, RISCH 1984, COUSENS 2000, ROGERS 1997, COHEN 1980, 82) and perhaps particularly in histapenia. (PFEIFFER 1987, 88, WALSH 2007) (See *Mania studies,* at left.)

Levels

Brain choline is often low in mania. (SOARES 1996) Moreover, deficiency may increase the likelihood of mania. Thus, Stoll (1991, 1996) found four times as much mania as depression in bipolars with low red cell choline. With high choline, the number of manic and depressive episodes were approximately equal.

On the other hand, extended and, especially, pronounced elevation in choline activity can, in some cases, be stimulatory and antidepressant, (GROTH 1958) even to the extent of triggering or increasing hyperactivity, hypomania, or mania. (CASEY 1977, GERSHON 1961, SHOPSIN, ROWNTREE 1950) In the subgroup of manics with particularly elevated choline in Stoll's 1996 study, mania was more severe, less responsive to lithium, required more neuroleptics; and showed worse outcome at discharge.

Brain function: Acetylcholine (COUSENS 2000, ROGERS 1997, SLAGLE)

□ Essential to initiation of short-term memory, storage of memory, cognitive function and engagement. (WURTMAN 1983, 88)

□ Mainly acts on brain regions and neurotransmitters which depress or inhibit behavior and emotion. Conveys parasympathetic (calming, relaxing) messages, opposing sympathetic (fight or flight) stimulation. Counterbalances dopamine and norepinephrine.

□ Critical to nerve/muscle communication. Mediates motor coordination and tone, skeletal and smooth muscle activity, and involuntary nervous system reactions (e.g., moving your fingers away from a hot stove). (RISCH 1984)

□ Affects calcium channels (ALARCON 1985) and brain electrical activity.

Brain function: Phosphatidyl choline (KIDD 1996, ROGERS 1997)

□ Crucial component of neural membranes and receptors. Supports fluidity, structure, viability. (HIRATA 1978, KIDD 1996)

□ Protects omega 3 fats from oxidative stress. (WALSH 2006)

□ May play a key role in mediating transfer of signals into and through the neuron.* (MOORE 2000, LISCOVITCH 1993, NAKAMURA 1996)

□ Helps maintain cell homeostasis. (KIDD 1996)

□ Helps maintain the myelin sheath which protects certain nerve axons and facilitates rapid conduction. (COUSENS 2000)

□ Supports production of RNA and regulatory proteins.

□ May enhance creation of structural (dendritic) connections between neurons. (MERVIS 1987)

* The agonist/receptor interaction, via PLA2, PLC, or PLD, hydrolyzes phosphatidyl choline, creating a signalling cascade.

Choline helps form: (BRAVERMAN 1987, RISCH 1984, WURTMAN 1988, ROGERS 1997)

TAURINE & GLYCINE — inhibitory neurotransmitters.

CARNITINE — critical to cellular energy production.

METHIONINE & BETAINE — methylators.

CYSTEINE — component of GTF, MT, glutathione.

MYELIN — speeds neural impulses, protects neurons.

Mood moderation (COUSENS 2000, ROGERS 1997)

Modest doses of choline help moderate bipolar swings or rapid cycling in some patients (perhaps, often histapenic). (COUSENS 2000, ROGERS 1997, COONEY 1999)

Levels

Brain choline can be relatively low or somewhat elevated in bipolars, (STOLL 1991, HAMAKAWA 1999) often in specific brain regions, perhaps reflecting attempts of the brain to moderate mood. Deficiency can be associated with either mania or depression and, is often accompanied by memory problems. (COUSENS 2000, ROGERS 1997)

Mental symptoms (COUSENS 2000, ROGERS 1997)

Deficiency has been associated with, and may benefit, some cases of:

□ Anxiety, restlessness, stress, pain sensitivity, irritability. Insomnia.*

□ Racing thoughts, hypomania, paranoia, psychosis. (COUSENS 2000, ROGERS 1997, HITZEMANN 1985)

□ Cognitive dullness and fatigue, (COUSENS 2000) poor memory. (LEWIS 1973, 74AB)

□ Brain fog from chemical sensitivity, (ROGERS 1997) confusion, disorientation. (BARABEAU 1979, GROWDEN 1977, 87)

□ Hyperactivity. Learning and behavior disorders. (ROGERS 1997)

□ Tremor, incoordination, unsteady gait. (PFEIFFER 1975) Movement disorders, (CASEY 1977, MILLER 1974) tics, Tourettes, (FINNEY 1981) tardive dyskinesia. (DAVIS 1975, 76)

* Choline enhances and shortens the time til REM sleep and dreaming, especially in affectives and relatives; (Benedito 2001) and modulates SCN response to light and the sleep/wake cycle. (Pace-Schott 2002)

Caution: Bipolar sensitivity to choline

Affectives can be oversensitive to choline, which can destabilize mood. Cholinergic drugs can trigger or severely aggravate bipolar depression or contribute to symptoms of confusion or anxiety. High doses of choline, intake as DMAE, or sudden withdrawal has, in some cases triggered or worsened mania, or enhanced related symptoms (elation, behavioral inhibition, hostility, etc.). Some researchers suggest sensitivity to cholinergics may indicate an affective component to schizophrenia, personality disorders, and other disorders. (SWANN 1993, SOARES 1996, MANN 1993, JANOWSKY 1994, RISCH 1984)

Pay attention to dose, reactions during withdrawal, and ongoing clinical response. (COUSENS 2001) Histadelics are particularly vulnerable to excess (*see below*). (WALSH 2007)

Note: Choline compounds in certain regions of the brain (e.g., the anterior cingulate) may be altered in bipolars, with repercussions on neural signalling. (MOORE 2000)

Biotype considerations (WALSH 2006)

Choline or DMAE is often used for histapenia to counter the symptomatic anxiety, pacing, extroversion, and hypomania, and moderate the overstimulation due to any dopamine or norepinephrine elevation.

In the histadelic, choline is often already elevated, so intake is usually not needed, and can further reduce the already-low catecholamine activity, worsening the chronic depression, the tendency to silence, and other symptoms. Histadelics often instead require inositol.

Choline biochemistry (BRAVERMAN 1987, SLAGLE 2000, ROGERS 1997)

P-Eth --SAM--> PC --> Ach --> PC

SAM methylates phosphatidylethanolamine creating phosphatidylcholine (PC). Neurons (and other cells) acetylate choline into acetylcholine. Acetylcholine can then metabolize back into PC.

Lithium may moderate choline

Lithium may prevent enhancement of choline receptors in depression; dopamine receptors in mania:*(DILSAVER 1984)

□ It can triple choline. (JOPE 1980, STOLL 1996) Increased levels, (JOPE 1980, 93, STOLL 1996, 99, DOMINO 1985, UNEY 1986) activity and effects (SAMPLES 1977, 80, JUDD 1977, JOPE 1979, DILSAVER 1984) have been associated with manic improvement.**(SOLOSKI 1999)

□ When choline is excessive, lithium may block acetylcholine synthesis and release, and decrease cholinergic tone, thus countering depression. (JANOWSKY 1979, 81, 82, RISCH 1984, DOMINO 1985)

* Although some studies show no effect on choline compounds (Kato 1996, Mallinger 1984), or an effect uncorrelated with mood. (Kuchel 1984)

** Valproate may similarly promote cholinergic activity. (DeMet 1999)

Marijuana & choline

Marijuana increases cholinergic activity and behavior, (DUNCAN 1979) augments cholinergics, (ROSENBLATT 1972) and has been reported to moderate manic symptoms in some patients (DAVIS 1978B) (perhaps histapenic).

Nonetheless, it can play havoc with mood. It can trigger or worsen depression, (DAVIS 1978B) especially if oversensitive to choline (many bipolars), or if cholinergic activity is already elevated, and/or catecholamines, suppressed (as in histadelia). In one study, marijuana augmentation of physostigmine (a cholinergic) induced severe depression in two apparently healthy students. (EL-YOUSEF 1973) Conversely, abrupt withdrawal can trigger or worsen mania, especially if sensitive to choline/catecholamine balances (again, many bipolars).

Cognitive suppression with anticholinergics

Certain drugs (e.g. Parkinson's meds, or neuroleptics) and conditions (depression, allergies,or migraine) that deplete choline may promote dementia, especially in the elderly and other susceptible individuals.*(ROE 2002, TUNE 2001)

* Other anticholinergic effects can include dry mouth, urinary difficulty, excess perspiration, nausea, constipation, weight gain, anorexia, blurred vision, impotence, rapid heart beat.

Studies: Restrict inositol

Shaldubina, 2006 — Dietary restriction created a major reduction in illness severity, even in acute nonresponsive mania and in rapid cycling, within two weeks.

Also see, Berudsky, 1999.

Counterbalancing inositol overactivity in mania

Part of choline's antimanic effectiveness may be due to its ability to counterbalance hyperactive inositol signalling in mania. (STEEN 2002, AGAM 2002, KIM 2005, DUBOVSKY 1992, BROWN 1993, KATO 1998) Similarly, the three major mood stabilizers (lithium, carbamazepine, valproate) may, in part, work by selectively inhibiting inositol activity in mania, and stimulating it in depression. (DUBOVSKY 1992, WOLFSON 2000) Furthermore, some researchers suggest creating anti-manic drugs that focus on inositol suppression. Similar benefit may result from dietary restriction of inositol sources. (BERSUDSKY 1999, SHALDUBINA 2006)

See *Inositol*, pp. 95-97.

Cholinergic/Adrenergic Hypothesis of Mood Disorder (JANOWSKY 1972, 73, 94, LEIVA 1990, RISCH 1984)

This early hypothesis suggested that mania is due to underactive choline and overactive catecholamine transmission in brain regions regulating mood. Conversely, in depression, choline is overactive; catecholamines, underactive.* Thus:

Cholinergics

Acetylcholine (Ach)
Inhibiting, calming, fostering depression
Opposes dopamine, norepinephrine

Catecholaminergics

Dopamine, Norepinephrine, Epinephrine (DA, NE, E)
Stimulating, exciting, fostering mania
Opposes acetylcholine

Cholinergics fostering depression, countering mania

□ Chemicals (antipsychotics, reserpine, etc.) which oppose catecholamine activity generally increase choline activity and turnover, often have cholinergic properties, and can induce depressive symptoms. (SULSER 1964, STADLER 1973).

□ Cholinergic or acetylcholine dominance is often associated with depression and behavioral inhibition. (CHARLES 1994, SWANN 1993, SOARES 1996, JANOWSKY 1987, 94).

□ Cholinergics can benefit hypomania. (ALARCON 1985, JANOWSKY 1972, 73, DAVIS 1978A, ROWNTREE 1950, RISCH 1984, LEIVA 1990, STOLL 1991) Excess can create depression in bipolars, even if manic (SWANN 1993, SOARES 1996, JANOWSKY 1973, 94, MODESTIN 1973, DAVIS 1978ABC, ROWNTREE 1950) and, to a lesser extent, in people without affective disorder (CASEY 1979).

Catecholaminergics fostering mania, countering depression

□ Chemicals (L-dopa, amphetamines, etc.) which support catecholomine activity generally decrease choline turnover, output and activity. Low acetylcholine further promotes catecholamine dominance. (JANOWSKY 1973)

□ Anticholinergics often elevate mood and may cause euphoria or mania. Most antidepressants not based on serotonin, are adrenergic, suppress cholinergic activity, and can selectively induce mania, mixed mania, or rapid cycling in bipolars. (WEHR 1979, RISCH 1984, BECKMAN 1983, SWANN 1993)

However, note: Anticholinergic properties do not necessarily reflect antidepressant potency; and good antidepressants (such as, SSRIs) need not be anticholinergic.

* Current thought focuses more on receptors and second messengers, within such neurotransmitter systems.

Pharmaceutical rebound, choline/catecholeamine extremes, & rapid cycling

Withdrawal from norepinephrine and dopamine-based antidepressants can overactivate the cholinergic system, creating behavioral inhibition and depression.* Eventually norepinephrine and dopamine systems might compensate, triggering mania, which then seesaws back to a hypercholinergic state, as each system reacts against the other. (MANDELL 1971) perhaps leading in rapid cycling. (DILSAVER 1984)

Similarly, withdrawal from a cholinergic can produce catecholamine-mediated mania, (ROWNTREE 1950, SHOPSIN 1975) and then mood instability. Bipolars seem to be particularly susceptible, (JANOWSKY 1973) perhaps because the dopamine system is hypersensitive. (SHOPSIN 1975)

Considerations: Choline

Need may be suggested by

Memory, learning, or behavior disorders. Fatigue.

Anxiety, restlessness, insomnia, hyperactivity.

Movement abnormalities and disorders. (WURTMAN 1977, 79, DAVIS 1976, GROWDEN 1982, FINNEY 1981, CASEY 1977, MILLER 1974, D'ALDESSARIANI 1980)

Leaky cell membranes, altered cell homeostasis.*

Fat intolerance. High cholesterol.**(ALARCON 1985)

Weakened immunity. Cirrhosis, other liver damage. (KIDD 1996)

Toxicity.*** Chemical sensitivity. Increased reactivity to alflatoxin, pyrrolizidine (in comfrey), amanita, various synthetic chemicals, radiation. (KIDD 1996)

Hypothyroid. Adrenal issues. Endocrine dysregulation.

High blood pressure. Heart and kidney problems.

Deficiency may be due to allergies, intestinal malabsorption, low thyroid, liver toxicity (which can interfere with acetylation), or toxic chemicals.

* Choline acts as an osmoregulator. (Crayhon 1998)

** Choline supports fat transport and use and protects against lipid peroxidation. (Alarcon 1985)

*** Which reduces formation of acetylcholine, as acetyl groups get used up binding and eliminating toxins. (Kidd 1996)

Nutrient interactions

May support absorption of calcium, magnesium, manganese, and zinc. Enhances calcium-related learning. (EGOROV 1999) Increases RNA and protein synthesis.

Lab

Serum acetylcholine. (COUSENS 2000)

Sources (NUTRICIRCLES®1996, COUSENS 2000, SITARAM 1978AB, COONEY 1999)

Liver, kidney, eggs, meat, butter. Salmon, sardines, anchovies, other fish. Legumes, nuts, potatoes. Oats, corn, rice and other whole grains; wheat germ. Bee pollen, brewer's yeast. Tomato, orange, avocado, cabbage, leafy greens, cauliflower. Coffee contains a substantial amount, but doesn't significantly increase acetylcholine. *The more choline in the diet, the more acetylcholine is formed.*

Supportive nutrients

Activated B5 (pantethine) supports acetylation to acetylcholine. (ELKASHEF 2001) Formation is supported by B6, B1, B3, other B vitamins. Manganese helps make choline available to form acetylcholine.

Lithium and calcium* influence acetylcholine creation and release. (DILSAVER 1986C)

Choline works with inositol, C, E, zinc, EFAs.

Phosphatidyl serine with SAM and various cofactors, precurse phosphatidyl choline. (ROGERS 1986, CROOK 1991, KIDD 1996)

GABA may spare choline. (BARTHOLINI 1985)

Folic acid eliminates the fishy smell. (COONEY 1999)

* Calcium also decreases (muscarinic) receptor sensitivity to acetylcholine. (Egorov 1999)

Supplements

Effective supplements include choline citrate, phosphotidyl choline. (COONEY 1999) Also:

Lecithin is an excellent source, containing both phosphatidyl choline and phosphatidyl inositol, with the emphasis on choline. (WURTMAN 1977) The granulated form can be used as a dietary supplement, e.g., added, without cooking, to cereals, grains, yogurt, etc.

DMAE (dimethylaminoethanol) is more potent than choline, and more readily admitted through the blood brain barrier. (HAUDRICH 1975, WURTMAN 1977, ROGERS 1997)

Dose

Enough to reduce stimulation, but not so much that it causes anxiety (which occurs more readily with DMAE or Deanol). May need to introduce gradually. (PFEIFFER 1975, 87) The dose is lower for young people, or if taking other sources (e.g., betaine).

It may take up to nine months for choline plus supportive nutrients to correct imbalances . (COUSENS 2000)

Causes of excess

Agricultural exposure to certain pesticides* or contamination from food. Drugs which increase acetylcholine activity.

*Acetylcholinesterase inhibitors, which create damaging levels of acetylcholine. (Gershon 1961, 1982, Senakayake 1987)

Effects of excess, contraindications

Lethargy, fatigue, psychomotor retardation, decreased thoughts, social withdrawal. (JANOWSKY 1973)

Can initiate or worsen depression, sadness, feelings of uselessness, or tendency to suicide, especially in affectives. (JANOWSKY 1973)

Though it often benefits mania, very high levels, especially if taken as DMAE, or with cholinesterase inhibitors, can produce irritability, hypervigilence and, occasionally, trigger or worsen mania, or psychosis in susceptible persons.

Dizziness, nausea, vomiting, fishy odor in the sweat.

Can be detrimental in histadelia. (WALSH 2007)

Avoid with Parkinson's, or anticholinergics. (ROGERS 1997)

Essential Fatty Acids

"Omega-3 fatty acids with phosphospholipids... along with the antioxidants that naturally protect cell membranes, could complement (conceivably even supplant) lithium's proven signal transduction actions. Only after [such rational nutrient combinations] have been applied to maximum effectiveness would drugs have to be deployed. The next step would be the addition of low-dose lithium."

Paris M Kidd, PhD, 2004

Fiji island mountain people carried plants at night to a specified location, where they received seafoods from their enemies, the coastal natives. This exchange probably balanced the EFA intake of both peoples.

Dr. and Mrs. Price, as described in Rudin, MD, 1987

Omega 3

Omega 3, particularly EPA, an omega 3 fat found in fish, supports neural communication and flexible receptor response, helping to balance mood. EPA may be important in countering the neural overstimulation, disorganization, and miscommunication associated with mania and mood disorder in general. Preliminary results by Sublette (2007) suggest a relationship of manic severity with low EPA relative to omega 6 (AA). Benefit has also been reported for anxiety. (BUYDENS-BRANCHEY 2006)

On the other hand, high doses of omega 3 have been reported to worsen mania in some bipolars, (SU 2000, CHIU 2003, 05) so intake may need to be lower than that for depression, at least for certain subgroups.

Alternately, some researchers have found that manics seem to do better with DHA (another omega 3 fat found in fish) instead of EPA. DHA is often low during mania. (CHIH-CHIANG 2003, WALSH 2008)

GLA & biotype

Pyrolurics, especially with moderate-to-severe symptoms, often respond better to GLA.

See *GLA*, p. 92.

Supportive nutrients

Essential fatty acids should always be taken with antioxidants and B vitamins. Relevant phospholipids may also be helpful.

More on EFAs

See *EFAs*, pp. 85-94, for a more detailed description of the critical role of fatty acids in mood.

Functions of omega 3 which may help moderate mania

Omega 3 directly influences receptor/second messenger/nucleus interactions, thereby altering neurotransmitter and cell activity:

□ Supports receptor structure and fluidity. (STOLL 2002, HIRASHIMA 2004)

□ Inhibits second messenger signalling molecules (PLA2, (HORROBIN 1999)) PKC, G proteins, (SEUNG 2001) phosphatidyl inositol, (SPERLING 1999) moderating neural stimulation.

□ Interacts with ion channels, influencing electrical responsiveness and likelihood of transmission; and nucleus receptors, altering gene expression. (STOLL 2002)

Other functions influencing mood:

□ Protects brain cells and neurotransmitter systems from free radical assault and cell damage. (HORROBIN 1999)

□ Supports formation of serotonin, which helps moderate mood in some bipolars. (MAES 1995)

□ Opposes signalling changes due to inflammatory immune chemicals activated by stress or omega 6. (MAES 1995, MAESSMITH 1998, SMITH 1991, CONNOR 1998, STOLL 2002)

□ Helps balance thyroid function, exaggerated cortisol release, and other omega 6 hormonal effects (which can profoundly alter mood). (STOLL 2002)

4. Herbs

Herbs, in some ways, occupy a middle ground between drugs and nutrients. Benefits are generally more immediate than those of nutrients, though often not as rapid as those of drugs. The trade-off is that herbs are, in most cases, safer than drugs. And, many herbs are nutritive and, correctly chosen, support healing, rather than merely affecting symptoms.

The status of bipolar/herbal research

Not much is known about the use of herbs specifically for bipolars. Historical information does exist on "nervines," and the use of herbs for depression and "insanity." Researchers have also investigated herbs for specific symptoms (anxiety, insomnia, etc.), and confounding conditions (blood sugar imbalances, certain immune disorders, etc.). Some biotype research is now being conducted. More studies are needed which directly address herbs for bipolar disorder.

Valerian (MURRAY 1995, MOWREY 1986, KLOSS 1973, WEHRBACH 1994, LEATHWOOD 1982, DRESSING 1992, BOETERS 1969, LINDAHL 1989)

Valerian is strongly sedative. EEG readings confirm its tranquilizing effect on the nervous system. It has been used for hundreds of years to treat mental disorders, nervousness and pain. Reported benefits have included relief of anxiety, restlessness, mental strain, stress, overexcitement, exhaustion, headache, nervous stomach, tachycardia, spasms and tension. While calming the nervous system, it is reputed to improve concentration, energy levels, and coordination.

Murray states that valerian encourages a natural healing sleep, from which one wakes undrugged and refreshed. Valerian may be especially effective with insomnia due to anxiety, nervousness, exhaustion, headache or hysteria. One study found the combination of valerian and lemon balm promoted sleep as effectively as benzodiazepines, but with the added benefit of increasing deep sleep and not compromising daytime ability to concentrate.

Valerian is often helpful in histapenia. (WALSH 2007)

Side effects, contraindications

Increases agitation in a minority of patients (though many studies confirm its tranquilizing effect for most people).

Can overly potentiate sedation by barbiturates, benzodiazepines, opiates, alcohol. (D'ARCY 1993)

Scullcap (HOFFMAN 1990, MOWREY1986A, KLOSS 1973, STEIN 1992, MESHIKOVSKY, 1967, GAMMERMAN 1965)

Scullcap is classified as a tonic sedative and known to relax tension while revitalizing and rebuilding the central nervous system. It has been used in treating stress, depression, overexcitement, exhaustion, convulsions, insomnia, and pain.*

* It has also been reported to improve circulation, and strengthen the heart muscle.

Disclaimer

Just as with foods, a person may react adversely to a particular herb. Reactions to herbs can, however, be more intense. For this reason, many herbs are contraindicated for young children and the elderly; during pregnancy and lactation; and in fragile medical conditions. Some herbs may be contraindicated when taking specific psychiatric drugs or other meds.

Study the herbal literature to gain a more complete understanding of the actions of, and contraindications for, the various herbs. If you wish to be treated with herbs, you should seek the services of a knowledgeable physician, who will tailor treatment to individual needs (biotype, general biochemistry, response), and take into account potential interactions with meds.

Note: Some herbs need to be taken several times per day to avoid letdown.

A study investigating Valmane (a valerian-containing preparation) found improvement in 75% of 120 children with hyperactivity, anxiety and learning disabilities. Other studies show regulation of the autonomic nervous system, mild sedation, sleep enhancement, and relief of tension and restlessness (MURRAY, 1995)

Scullcap is known as a nervous system rebuilder. Kloss (1973), describes it as "one of the best nervines in the plant kingdom."

Kloss describes wood betony as "unsurpassed for insanity." Wood betony is reported to be beneficial to the liver, as well as the nervous system.

Wood betony (KLOSS 1973, HOFFMAN 1990, ZINCHERNKO 1962)

Wood betony is reputed to feed and strengthen the central nervous system, being sedative for children and mildly tranquilizing for adults. It is believed to act as a beta blocker. It contains B vitamins and manganese.

Wood betony has been used for nervous debility, tension, anxiety, pain, Parkinson's, palsy, convulsions, headaches and neuralgia. It is mildly stimulating to the heart. One study confirms its ability to loosen constrictive blood vessels, sometimes responsible for headaches and, perhaps, nervous tension.*

Warning: *Do not use with beta blocker medication. Exercise caution with sedatives, low blood pressure, cardiovascular and debilitated conditions.*

* It is also considered a blood purifier, and has also been used in treating liver disorders, inflammation, heartburn, gout, and colds.

Murray suggests kava may be an optimal alternative to benzodiazepines. Kava may also be helpful in preventing brain damage caused by reduced oxygen availability.

Kava (MURRAY 1995, 98, LINDENBERG 1990, KINZLE 1991, PITTLER 2001 03, CROPLEY 2002, PFEIFFER 1967, MALSCH 2001, FUGH-BERMAN 1999)

Kava is reported to reduce anxiety, stress, insomnia, nervousness, restlessness, dizziness, and headaches (as well as heart palpitations, chest pain, and gastric irritation). It is mildly anticonvulsant. Kava may also help prevent brain damage due to compromised circulation and decreased oxygen availability.

Murray suggests kava's sedative activity may provide an optimal alternative to benzodiazepines. Instead of binding to GABA/ benzodiazepine or opiate receptors, it may modify receptor domains, especially in the limbic system. Moderate doses do not appear to suppress general mental functioning, reaction time, or memory but, rather, improve vigilance, well-being and mood. At greater doses, it promotes sleep. Unlike benzodiazepines, which eventually require steadily increasing doses to get the same effect, tolerance does not develop.

Walsh (2006) finds kava useful in some histadelias.

Side effects, contraindications (CASS 2002, BLUMENTHAL 1998)

Increases sensory acuity (to sound, light, movement).

Can promote irritability or anger (perhaps an allergic reaction in some).

Chronic large doses can produce dry scaly skin, especially on the palms, forearms, soles of the feet, shins, and back; usually reversible once intake is discontinued.

Use with alcohol may be detrimental. (HERBERG 1993, STEVINSON 2002, JUSSOFIE 1994)

Liver damage has been reported, however most subjects in such studies drank or used drugs harmful to the liver. (ALMEIDA 1996, CASS 2002) Thus, a survey by Matthews (1988) suggests long-term high doses can be associated with liver, kidney, and spleen disorders, but does not control for the heavy use of alcohol and tobacco by participants. Dr Hyla Cass (2002) finds that for most patients, such problems do not occur, while anxiolytic drugs (benzos) *often* cause severe side effects. Nonetheless, til further research emerges, she suggests people with, or at risk for, liver damage probably should not use kava.

May be overly sedative for patients with slow cognitive function (low thyroid, very low blood pressure, dementias, etc.)

May potentiate adverse effects of antipsychotics, barbiturates, benzos.* (JUSSOFIE 1994, CUPP 1999)

May increase Parkinson's symptoms if L-dopa is being used. (CUPP 1999, BLUMENTHAL 1998)

* One case of coma occured with combined benzo/kava intake (Jussofie 1994).

Passion flower (MOWREY 1986A, KLOSS 1973, LUTOMSKI 1960, 81, AMBUEHI 1966, AKHONDZADEH 2001)

Passion flower (passifloraceae) is claimed to gently soothe the nervous system, without producing depression or disorientation. It has been reported helpful even with intransigent insomnia, and insomnia due to brain inflammation, producing a normal sleep with light easy breathing. It has been used in treating convulsive disorders and pain, and in easing withdrawal from sleeping pills and tranquilizers. (LUTOMSKI 1960)

Bach Rescue Remedy

Bach Rescue Remedy is formulated to manage stress in emergency situations. Some anecdotal reports suggest it may help (along with other therapies) in preventing mania, if caught when symptoms first emerge. Other Bach remedies such as Vervain, may also be appropriate.

See *The Bach Flower Remedies* by Dr. Edward Bach, and other related literature.

Theanine (LEKH 1999, KAKUDA 2000, YAMADA 2005, DHARMANANDA 1998, KOBAYAHI 1998, MASON 2001, ESCHENAUER 2006)

L-theanine (a constituent of green tea), increases GABA, blocks toxic effects of caffeine, and is a natural glutamate antagonist. Theanine reportedly benefits stressed, hyperexcited, anxious depressives, and may be of use for a subgroup of milder manias. It's tranquilizing — increasing alpha waves (which promote wakeful relaxation) — but not sedative. It increases thought concentration and focus, but doesn't change theta waves or interefere with the ability think or make decisions.

To limit stimulation, take theanine as a supplement, or drink decaf green tea.

RECOMMENDED READING

Mowrey, Daniel B, PhD, *Proven Herbal Blends,* and *The Scientific Validation of Herbal Medicine, 1986ab*

Murray, Michael, ND, *Stress Anxiety and Insomnia*, 1995

Werbach, Melvyn, MD, and Murray, Michael, ND, *Botanical Influences on Illness, 1994*

Christopher, John R, ND, *School of Natural Healing, 1976.*

Spinella, Marcello, PhD, *The Psychopharmacology of Herbal Medicine: Plant Drugs That Alter Mind, Brain, and Behavior.* .

Herbs sometimes used for anxiety, irritability, insomnia (KLOSS 1973, CHRISTOPHER 1976, MOWREY 1986AB, STEIN 1992, PAGE 1992, MURRAY 1995)

More potent herbs: scullcap,* valerian,* wood betony, wild lettuce, kava.**

Moderate: lady's slipper, passion flower.

Mild: hops, ginger, catnip, chamomile.

Calcium/silica sources:** horsetail, oatstraw.

Explore herbal literature for info on contraindications, formulas, etc., and consult with your physician as to appropriate therapy.

* Especially relevant with histapenia.

** Often indicated with histadelia or pyroluria.

4. Acute therapies

"Acute cases can be extremely challenging to manage in an out-patient setting... At times a hospital environment is necessary largely because of the controlled environment (and not necessarily because of the drugs). Having said this, it is possible to attempt controlling an acute manic episode if you have the proper support from family, friends, and physician (24 hour on-call care is vital). If not, I would not attempt such an intervention."

Walter Lemmo, ND

IV, IM, & other approaches for intractable mania

If optimizing the previous strategies is insufficient, consider the following approaches:

Lemmo's acute mania therapy

Walter Lemmo, ND, reports success with:

Individually-tailored, IV nutrients, a critical component. A good multi-vitamin/mineral, & extra B, ongoing.

Perhaps, one or more of the following, if indicated:

Tryptophan — 8,000-14,000 mg (oral). (*Contraindicated for bipolars [perhaps histapenic] in whom it fuels mania*).
Melatonin — 10 mg, 2x/day or more, orally.
Benedryl — 50 mg IM, every 2 hrs, *as needed.*

IV vitamin C

In high enough doses, C can act as a natural tranquilizing, antimanic, and antipsychotic agent. For acute cases, or where rapid response is needed, some practitioners use IV vitamin C. (COCCHI 1989, REBEC 1979, TOLBERT 1979AB, HOFFER 2007, LARSON 2008)

See *Vitamin C,* pp. 74-75.

High protein diet & psychotic mania

Michael Lesser, MD, has found a high protein diet, with red meat every hour or so, over a week or two, can reverse acute manic psychosis. The meat counters hypoglycemia, supports B3 receptors, and provides abundant B3, B6, B12, and needed aminos. If supplements are also taken (e.g., tryptophan GABA, B3 etc., *as relevant*), Lesser finds effectiveness further enhanced. (LESSER 2008)

See also, p. 268.

Myers (or Gaby-Wright) Cocktail (SALEEBY 2005, GABY 1998, 2002)

Gaby reports some success in treating bipolars (*though depressives tend to respond better than manics*) with a modified Myers Cocktail, a rapid (30 minutes or less) intravenous infusion of certain high dose vitamins and minerals. Rapid infusions are thought to force nutrient overloads into the cell, where they are "trapped," allowing effects to last several weeks.

It contains such generally antimanic nutrients as magnesium, B complex, B1, B3, C, and, also, B5 (which supports the adrenals), and B6. Trace minerals, or other relevant nutrients can be added. *Choice of ingredients and doses MUST be tailored to the patient's unique requirements, with meticulous attention to contraindications.*

Caution: May be overstimulating/detrimental to some manias. Further research is indicated.

Warning: Attention to contraindications and individual biochemical requirements is ABSOLUTELY CRITICAL with IV treatment. Consider biotype, response history, sensitivities, family history, etc.

I: Nutrient survey

b: Mania & depression

The following nutrients are generally helpful for *both* mania and depression (with some exceptions). *Requirements for specific nutrients vary with the individual.*

B vitamins — support brain communication and viability, and can be critical to mood stability. They are often low in bipolars, perhaps due to problems with absorption.

Antioxidants — protect brain neurotransmitter systems, neural membrane fatty acids, and overall brain health, with likely repercussions on mood regulation.

Cautions & reminders

This book is not intended as treatment sugestions for the general public. Individual biochemical requirements are not identical, and supplements helpful for one patient can be detrimental for another. Full contraindications, interactions with meds, dose information, etc. are not included. This material is presented for educational purposes only. Persons needing treatment for affective disorder, or other medical conditions, should seek the services of a knowledgeable physician, who will tailor dose, timing, and choice of nutrients to the patient's unique biochemical, symptomatic, and response profile.

I. B vitamins

Niacin, niacinamide (B3)
Pyridoxine (B6)
Choline/inositol
Folic acid & B12
Thiamine (B1)
Riboflavin (B2)
Pantothenic acid (B5)
Biotin, PABA

B vitamins, mood & related conditions (COUSENS 2000, LARSON 2001, SLAGLE 1993)

Add or remove B vitamins according to biotype and other individual requirements.

Mania — B1, B3, choline.

Bipolar depression — B2, B3, B6, B12, inositol, and often, folate (*but usually not if histadelic*).

Anxiety symptoms — B1, B3, choline or inositol (*check biotype needs*); often, B6.

Psychotic symptoms — B3, B6, B1; perhaps B12, NADH; folic acid (*if not histadelic*).

Allergic or adrenal involvement — B1, B2, B3, B5, B6, biotin.

Fatty acid deficiency/imbalance — B3, B6.

Histapenia (overmethylation) — B1, B3, B5, B6, folate, B12, choline.

Pyroluria — B1, B3, B5, B6, P5P.

Histadelia (undermethylation) — B1, B6, inositol, often methyl-B12, perhaps some B3. *Limit folic acid (which is usually overabundant), perhaps choline.*

B complex (COUSENS 2000, LARSON 2001, SLAGLE 1993)

B vitamins generally support neural health and communication, as well as, brain metabolism, energetics, and general viability. They are essential in producing and regulating neurotransmitters, and in fatty acid and hormone synthesis, all pivotal in mood. Both research and clinical results suggest profound influence on mood (with preventative, antimanic and antidepressant activity); also on memory, attention, personality, cognition and perception of reality.

Psychiatric symptoms are often the first signs of depletion, and can involve depression, mania, anxiety,* aggression, insomnia, restlessness, fatigue, or even psychosis. (SLAGLE 1993) Up to 80% of bipolars are low in B vitamins. Many are low in B12 and folic, with reduced uptake of inositol. Some may lack an enzyme used in absorbing B vitamins. (LARSON 2001, SLAGLE 1993, DUSTMAN 2005)

Larson 2001 claims B complex generally produces a lithium-like effect in the brain, and also works with lithium, reducing the need for high doses. She finds bipolars almost always benefit from B complex.

* Lactic acid, formed during exercise or certain metabolic activity, accumulates excessively when B vitamins (or oxygen) are low, promoting anxiety. (Slagle 1993)

Biotype indications

Walsh (2007), on the other hand, emphasizes that bipolars often preferentially require a specific pattern of B vitamins, to address unique requirements. Thus:

□ Histadelics usually should avoid B complex, multiples, or other supplements containing significant quantities of folic acid. On the other hand, they do well with B6 and inositol; frequently respond to methyl-B12; with voices or anxiety, often improve with some B3; and may require other individual B vitamins.

□ Histapenics usually require supplemental B3, B6, folate, B12, choline, and often, B1 and B5, perhaps along with a B complex (though inositol sometimes needs to be limited).

□ Pyrolurics commonly need substantial B6, and do well with B1, B3, B5, biotin, and, often, B complex.

Considerations (COUSENS 2000, LARSON 2001, SLAGLE 1993)

Nutrient interactions

B complex helps prevent deficiencies when taking single B vitamins.

Populations

Alcoholism, stress, mood disorder, psychosis, physical illness, excess perspiration, exhaustive exercise, pregnancy.

Dose

50-600 mg per day, *as relevant.*

Source

Legumes, organ meats, wheat germ, nutritional yeast, sprouts, whole grains, bee pollen, fresh fruits and vegetables, nuts, seeds.

Effects of excess, contraindications

Very high doses, over an extended period may oversupply certain B vitamins (e.g., inositol, B6, B12, folic acid), which, with susceptible chemistries, may foster mania. Monitor. Check biotype contraindications.

Niacin, niacinamide (B3)

Mania

B3 is often critical to mood, anxiety and psychosis, and is sometimes antimanic. This makes sense biochemically, as niacinamide, like the minor tranquilizers (sometimes used for mania), inhibits neural firing by activating GABA receptors. B3, moreover, supports formation of acetylcholine and COMT, which mute stimulation, and of serotonin, which does so for some (but not all) bipolars. (Hoffer 2005, Slagle 1993, Baumel 1995, Mohler 1979)

Anxiety (Strohle 2003ab, Curr Ther 1987, Osmond 1980, Hoffer 1983, Pfeiffer 1987, Mohler 1979)

Similarly, B3 helps moderate anxiety. Mohler (1979), in fact, suggests the sedative potency of relatively large doses can be equivalent to strong benzodiazepines (anti-anxiety drugs), but without the side effects.

Psychosis

B3 and C are usually the most important nutrients in countering voices, whatever the biotype. (Walsh 2007, Hoffer 2005) Numerous studies, including at least half a dozen double blinds, emphasize the importance of B3 in addressing psychosis, paranoia, dysperceptions, auditory and visual hallucinations, and schizophrenia, typically at gram doses. (Hoffer 1957, 64, 66, 67, 71, 73, 83, 87, Osmond 1962, 80, Pfeiffer 1987, 88, Ananth 1973, Wittenborn 1974, Patrie 1981, Jaffe 1992, Miller 2008)

See also, *Adrenochrome hypothesis,* p. 82, and *Manic psychosis,* p. 268.

Depression

B3 is critical to brain circulation, metabolism, and energy production; and, as NADH, supports formation of antidepressant transmitters. Improvement (sometimes dramatic) is reported in many cases of depression. (Strohle 2003ab, Tonge 1953, Sydenstricker 1941, Chouinard 1979, Green 1980) Niacinamide may be particularly potent for some, as it precurses NADH. (Birkmayer 1992, Hoffer 2005) (See *NADH,* p. 117.)

Biotype indications (Pfeiffer1987, 88, Jaffe 1992, Slagle 1993 95-6, Walsh 2007)

B3 fosters copper elimination, helps regulate dopamine and form histamine, and is antioxidant, making it particularly critical in histapenic, and metal-metabolism-disordered patients. It is also important in pyroluria, cerebral allergies, and sugar metabolism imbalance, especially with such symptoms as anxiety, voices, or insomnia; and may similarly help address such symptoms in histadelia, though at more modest doses.

Mental & neurological symptoms

- □ Mood disorders, depression, (see above studies) especially elderly depression, (Hoffer 1980) stupor, lethargy, (Sydenstricker 1941) alcoholic depression. (Kahan 1966, Wilson 1967, 68, Smith 1974, 78, 81)
- □ Anxiety, severe agitation, irritability. (above)
- □ Emotional lability, mania. Hyperactivity, aggression, violence, insomnia. (Patrie 1981, Hoffer 1983, 87, Slagle 1993, Jaffe 1991, Strohle 2003, Mohler 1979)
- □ Sensory dysperceptions (hypersensitivity to light, smell; dulled or salty taste distortions, etc.). Dread, suspicion, paranoia. Hallucinations, psychosis, schizophrenia. (above)
- □ Learning disorders, dementia. (Hoffer 1980, 83, 87, 94, Rimland, Sydenstricker 1988, Pfeiffer 1987, 88)
- □ Addictions, alcoholism. (Kahan 1966, Wilson 1967, 68, Smith 1974, 78, 81, Hoffer 1983, 87, 2005, Larson 2001)
- □ Headaches. (Velling 2003, Prousky 2005, Hoffer) Neurological symptoms, seizures. (Hoffer)

"Vitamin C and niacin (B3) (in dosages that provide a mild blushing sensation) provide almost instant relief to the overactive mind and help focus mental concentration."

Carl C Pfeiffer, PhD, MD

"B3 is great for many bipolars, producing especially dramatic improvement in histapenics."

William J Walsh, PhD, 2008

"If all the B3 were removed from our food, everyone would become psychotic within one year... They'd recover in a few months with B3 in the diet. But... many would be so damaged that only massive doses would alleviate their symptoms and this could be required for life. No one is ever cured of pellagra, for the dosage of B3 must be maintained."

Abram Hoffer, MD, PhD

Mechanisms

Antidepressant effects:

- □ Critical to brain metabolism, energy production, and circulation.
- □ Involved in creation of the antidepressant neurotransmitters, serotonin, dopamine, and norepinephrine.

Antimanic effects:

- □ Supports formation and release of histamine, which counterbalances dopamine.
- □ Promotes formation of acetylcholine, a key inhibitory transmitter; and serotonin, which is antimanic for some bipolars.
- □ Activates GABA receptors.
- □ Supports formation of the enzyme, COMT, which recycles catecholamines

Antioxidant effects: (McGinnis 2004)

- □ A strong antioxidant and free radical quencher. Some studies find it more effective than C.
- □ Forms NADPH which recycles glutathione.
- □ Protects lipids and proteins in mitochondria and neurons
- □ Blocks nitric oxide neurotoxicity.
- □ Low levels decrease metallothionein and increase brain cell death.

Considerations: B3 (Larson 2001, Hoffer 1980, 83b, Pfeiffer 1975, Balch 1991, Cousens 2000, Slagle 1993 95-6, Lieberman 1990, Garrison 1985)

Need may be suggested by

Mood and cognitive symptoms.
Anxiety, insomnia.
Confusion, memory loss.
Dizziness, weakness,* fatigue.
Nausea, bad breath, sore mouth, swollen gums, coated red-tipped tongue.
Poor appetite, gas, other gastrointestinal symptoms.
Skin disorders, burning sensations.
Poor body and brain circulation; cold hands, feet.
Muscle weakness or tension.
Cardiovascular weakness. High cholesterol and blood lipids.
Sugar imbalance (B3 is part of GTF). Allergies.
Increased vulnerability to toxins, chemicals.
Arthritis, certain porphyrias. Dementia, aging. (Hoffer 1980)

B3 may be depleted by (Gold 1987)

Anxiety, injury, chronic illness, *chronic* overexertion. Addiction, alcoholism. Aging. Liver disease. Histapenia, perhaps pyroluria. Psychotic and affective disorders. Excess caffeine, corn, refined sugar or starch. Anti-Parkinsonian drugs, antibiotics.

Nutrient interactions

Works with B1 in sugar oxidation. Degrades carbohydrates, fats, proteins. (Slagle 1993)

Useful diagnostic test (Jaffe 1992)

1NMethylnicotinamide (1NMN).

Sources (Pfeiffer 1988, 1987, Nutricircles, Slagle 1993)

Lean, organ, and other meats. Fish, poultry, brewer's yeast. Milk and eggs (which are also high in tryptophan, some of which the body converts to B3). Wheat germ, whole grains, mushrooms, potatoes, avocados, asparagus, tempeh, sesame and sunflower seeds, bee pollen, hot pepper, legumes.
B3 is destroyed in storage and cooking.

Supportive nutrients (Slagle 1993, Rudin 1983)

B, C, D, chromium, zinc. Tryptophan (*usually not if histapenic*), adequate protein, selenium and other antioxidants. Rudin emphasizes omega 3, especially in colder climates, as it acts as a substrate for B vitamins.

Supplementation (Jaffe 1992, Hoffer 1983ab)

Niacin or niacinamide are two forms of B3. The body changes some niacin into niacinamide. Patients may react better to one, or a combination of both. *Increase dosage slowly to avoid uric acid retention.*

For histapenics, doses typically involve 500 to 1300 mg, 3x/day. For others, the average psychiatric dose is 100 to 500 mg, 2x/day, perhaps higher with anxiety or psychosis. (Jaffe 1992, Hoffer 1983ab)

The niacin flush

Histamine is created and stored in cell granules, which, with enough niacin, release it. The sudden flood of histamine causes a "niacin flush" in many people: reddened skin, and a tingling, prickling, itching, or burning sensation. The flush can be extensive, especially in redheads, (Pfeiffer 1987, 88) but is temporary, and not harmful. (Rogers 1997) All bipolars flush, perhaps especially during flareups. (Werbach 1991, Horrobin 2000ab) (See *Flush test,* p. 91.)

To limit flushing

Introduce niacin slowly, e.g. increase 25-50 mg at each stage. Give several times per day (e.g., every 6 hrs) to deplete histamine granules. If a dose is missed, granules fill up, so the next dose should be lower. Flushing often stops with consistent intake over several weeks. *Dosage should be kept below that which produces nausea or other side effects.* Also:
Niacinamide is less likely to produce a flush, but can't be taken in as large quantities. (Hoffer 1983)
C helps metabolize the histamine. (Rogers 1997)
B3 preparations with chromium or inositol eliminate or minimize flushing. Inositol hexaniacinate also helps prevent glucose tolerance and changes in liver enzymes. (Head 1996)

Effects of excess, contraindications (Hoffer 1983ab, Cousens 2000, Slagle 1993, Pfeiffer 1975, 87, 88, Werbach 1991, Lieberman 1990, Garrison 1985)

Over 500 mg niacinamide, in some cases, fosters depression.
May be overstimulating. (Case report of one patient, given B3 with B6, who became manic. (Chaturvedi 1988))
High doses can be counterproductive in histadelia.
Often produces a flush (see box, above).
Sudden high doses can produce uric acid retention (B3 competes for excretion) and exacerbate gout; or water retention (ankles may swell during warm months). Lower the dose or switch forms.
Niacin can slightly raise blood sugar. High doses may create glucose intolerance.
Nausea or digestive disturbances usually indicate dose should be reduced. Nausea may indicate liver dysfunction.
Jaundice (.05%) or liver dysfunction. Usually reversible when B3 is discontinued. Time-release B3 is more likely to cause liver problems. Liver enzymes should be checked periodically with doses of 1 gm or more (e.g., once per month til optimal dose is reached, then every three months for a year, then, every six.)
May sharply lower blood pressure.
Areas of temporary skin discoloration, or rash.
With ulcers, niacinamide may be preferable.
May be contraindicated in, and should be carefully monitored if used with glaucoma, diabetes, pregnancy, liver problems, or peptic ulcers.

History of the use of B3 for pellagra (HOFFER 1973, 83AB, PFEIFFER, 1975, 87, 88)

This history provides an early example of the "curing" with nutrients of often-severe mood symptoms in a condition previously considered exclusively a "mental" illness.

Pellagra has been characterized by "the four D's:" Dermatitis, Diarrhea, Dementia, and Death. Physical symptoms include: itchy, inflamed, red-to-brown patches of skin (especially where exposed to sun); these spread, the edges darken, and the skin eventually roughens and thickens. The tongue may become red, sore, and swollen, particularly if B2 is also low. Other symptoms: lethargy, muscle wasting, fatigue; various gastrointestinal complaints, especially diarrhea; palpitations; motor changes (rarely, paralysis).

Mental symptoms may appear first, and often involve: depression, crying spells, melancholia; also, nervousness, tension, restlessness, irritability, agitation, giddiness, severe anxiety, insomnia. Other symptoms can include: crippling mental fatigue, confusion, memory loss (perhaps resolving into dementia); hyperacute or dulled senses, illusions, hallucinations (eventually, perhaps, psychosis); burning sensations or numbness; intense headaches.

The corn scorge (pellagra) (HOFFER 1973, 83AB, PFEIFFER 1975, 87, 88, RUDIN 1983, GREEN 1971)

Over thousands of years, native Central Americans developed a wild grass into corn (through five mutations of the plant), and thrived on it.* Others, however, did not do so well when corn became the mainstay of their diet:** Hence, 1500 years ago, innumerable Northern Mound People of the mid-plains and Mississippi Valley lost their lives to a mysterious illness. Similarly, in the early eighteenth century, many Europeans died of "rose sickness" (*mal de la rosa*), or "rough skin" (*pelle agra*). In the early twentieth century, in certain impoverished regions of the southern US, pellagrins occupied up to half of all mental hospital beds (approximately 200,000 people total); one third died of pellagra.

* Their ability to do well on a corn-based diet may been due to (1) genetic adaptation; (2) use of lime water, which releases B3, to cook corn tortillas; (3) the warm climate, which created less need for omega 3.

** Perhaps because, in corn: (1) B3 is bound tightly, and not readily released; (2) B6, needed to convert B3 to NAD, is low; (3) Tryptophan (which precurses serotonin, B3 and NAD) is very low; (4) Omega 3, a substrate for the B vitamins, is very low; (5) The amino acid, leucine, is excessive relative to isoleucine, causing urinary loss of B3.

Search for a cure (HOFFER 1983, PFEIFFER 1975, SPIES 1938, 40, GREEN 1971, JOLIFFE 1939, PATTON 1984)

Joseph Goldberger first suspected pellagra was due to a nutrient deficiency, and in 1928, linked it to black tongue disease in dogs, then treated with liver. Elvehjem, in 1937, isolated the active component, B3. Tom Spies then pioneered the B3 remedy to hospitals and hillfolk alike.

At least 10% of Southern mental patients recovered within weeks with approximately 600 mg. per day. Patients who recovered readily with B3 were retroactively diagnosed pellagrins. (HOFFER, NUTR 1983)

Populations (HOFFER 1973, 83B, SPIES 1938)

Although niacin has been added to flour in the US since the 1940s, pellagra still can occur if high-quality protein is sparce; or corn, pork, or junk food, oversupplied. It also sometimes surfaces in drug addicts, alcoholics, and the elderly; in patients on anti-Parkinson's drugs; and people with liver disease, carcinoid, or inflammatory bowel disease; and still plagues Asia.

Treatment (HOFFER 1973, 83B, PFEIFFER 1975, 87, 88, RUDIN, 1983)

B3 and tryptophan are critical. B6, B2, B complex, sufficient protein, and omega 3 (with antioxidants) are also important. B3 sources include lean meat, liver, fish, and wheat germ. Pfeiffer further suggests: beans (for molybdenum, B3), eggs (sulfur, selenium, B3, tryptophan), and milk (calcium, B3, tryptophan). *Avoid corn, processed foods (which deplete B), peanuts, hydrogenated oils, and meat toxins. Restrict omega 6 oils and pork.*

"If poor people subsist on a diet of cornbread, cane syrup, and pork fat, they will inevitably get sick."

Joseph Goldberger, MD

"The Pellagrosi affords a melancholy spectacle of physical and moral suffering... [they] seem under the influence of an invincible despondency; seek to be alone; scarcely answer the questions put to them; and often shed tears without any obvious cause. Their faculties and senses become alike impaired and the progress of the disease, where it does not carry them off from debility and exhaustion of the vital powers, generally makes them incurable ideots [sic], or produces occasionally maniacal affections, which terminate eventually in the same state. Attempts at suicide are frequent... particularly... by throwing themselves in the water."

Sir Henry Holland, 1817

"The mind begins to suffer... the feeling of anxiety and despondence is very strongly marked, and later the anxiety, watchfulness and moral depression of the patient is rapidly augmented."

Joseph Goldberger, MD

"I could not accept the concept that their brains were irreparably damaged; It seemed that the cells were waiting listlessly and would function again at full efficiency when we gave them the required nutrients."

Tom Spies, MD, 1940

"I'd found this young woman, violently insane they said. They had to keep her tied down... back home she had suddenly grabbed the axe and tried to kill her husband; would've too, if he hadn't been too fast for her. Just to think, I've sent people like this home, well and happy, all with fifteen cents worth of nicotinic acid."

Tom Spies, MD

B6 (pyridoxine, pyridoxal)

Brain functions (HOFFER 1983, PFEIFFER 1975, 87, 88, SLAGLE 1993 1993, QUILLIN 1987)

Supports mood-modulating neurotransmitter pathways:

□ Critical to serotonin activity; a cofactor in enzymes converting tryptophan to serotonin; slows tryptophan destruction; helps unclog kynurenine pathways.* (MURRAY 1996, 98, GREEN 1983, COUSENS, ROGERS, HOES 1982)

□ Necessary in metabolism of phenylalanine to tyrosine to dopamine to norepinephrine; and phenylalanine to phenylethylamine (ROGERS, BUKREEV 1978)

□ Supports creation of acetylcholine, and GABA, important inhibitory transmitters.

□ Used in forming MAO, which breaks down monoamine transmitters in the synapse.

Other functions which influence mood:

□ Supports the thyroid.

□ Used in cerebral detox. Decreases toxicity to the brain of acetaldehyde from Candida. (KAKUMA 1976)

□ Used in RNA and DNA synthesis.

Antioxidant activity (MCGINNIS 2004):

□ P5P (a potent form of B6) is strongly antioxidant and required in creating glutathione, MT, CoQ10 and heme, all antioxidant.

□ Helps maintain glutathione peroxidase

□ Required in forming GAD, which blocks excitotoxicity.

Some depression studies

Benton, Hallert, 1995 — Double blind. Mood improvement in females was associated with increased B6.

Adams, 1983 — Double blind. Depressed women taking oral contraceptives responded to B6.

Hallert, 1983 — Coeliac patients with symptomatic depression did not respond to a year without gluten, but then improved significantly on 80 mg B6 per day for six months.

Pfeiffer, 1975ab, 87, 88ab — Reports substantial clinical response, backed up by often extensive labs, of pyroluric depressives to B6, zinc and manganese.

B6 is often critical to mood regulation. Depletion is frequently associated with affective disorder, (CARNEY) and compromises production of mood-mediating neurotransmitters.

Depression

B6 plays a key role in antidepressant neurochemistry. (DAKSHINAMURTI 1982) Deficiency is common in depressives, and estimated to occur in up to 75%, (NOBBS 1974, RUSS 1983, STEWART 1984, BELL 1992, SHILS 1988, CARNEY 1979, 82) especially females with elevated estrogen. (ADAMS 1974, WYNN 1975, GUNN DOLL 1989, BERMOND 1982, BRUSH 1985, KENDALL 1987) Supplements often improves depression (BERNSTEIN 1990, SHILOH 2001, HOES 1982, BELL 1992, DEIJEN 1992, BENTON 1995, HALLERT 1983) (including hormonal depressions (ADAMS 1973, 74, WYNN 1975, GUNN, BERMAN 1982, WYATT 1999)), sometimes dramatically, (BUKREEV 1978, SHILOH 2001, HALLERT 1983, COUSENS 2000) particularly in pyrolurics. (PFEIFFER 1975AB, 87, 88AB)

Mania

Depletion can be associated with mania, and such manic symptoms as agitation, hyperactivity, irritability, aggression, and insomnia, (BRENNER 1982, BERNSTEIN 1990, BUIST 1984) *however, in some cases, excess promotes mania.*

Biotype indications

Vitamin B6 is essential in pyroluria, a condition found in many schizoaffectives and bipolars. It also benefits histamine (methylation) imbalances. (PFEIFFER 1975, 87, 88)

Other indications

Check for cyclical symptoms, female hormone imbalance, digestive problems, hypoglycemia, and convulsive disorders* (especially in children). (TOHOKU 1983, BRAVERMAN 1987, PFEIFFER 1975AB, 87, 88AB)

* Thus, B6-inhibiting drugs can be potent seizure inducers (Braverman 1987)

Mental and neurological symptoms

B6 may provide support in the following conditions, especially if cyclical:

□ Depression. (SHILOH 2001, BERNSTEIN 1990, HOES 1982, BELL 1992, DEIJEN 1992, BENTON 1995, HALLERT 1983, BUKREEV 1978, PFEIFFER 1975, 87, 88, WALSH 2000, 02)

□ Agitation, insomnia, sensitivity to sound, irritability, aggressive behavior, mood disorder, mania. (BUIST 1984, BERNSTEIN 1990)

□ Learning disabilities, confusion, hyperactivity, nervousness, anxiety. (BERNSTEIN 1990, BRENNER 1982)

□ OCD. (RUSS 1983)

□ Autism (with magnesium, B6 may benefit 50% of cases). (RIMLAND, MARTINEAU 1985, HALLERT 1983)

□ Schizophrenia, psychosis, childhood schizophrenia. (BROOKS 1983, PFEIFFER 1975AB, 87, 88AB, WALSH 2000, 02, 06, ANANTH 1973, PATRIE 1981, JOSHI 1982, SHILOH 2001)

□ Cerebral allergies, cerebral toxicity. (HALLERT 1983)

□ Symptoms of low serotonin, catecholamines, or other transmitters. (GREEN 1983, COUSENS, HOES 1982)

□ Brain wave abnormalities, seizures (especially in children). (PFEIFFER 1975, 87, 88)

Considerations

Need may be suggested by (LARSON 2001, SLAGLE 1993, LIEBERMAN 1990, KROHN 1991, GARRISON 1985, PFEIFFER 1987, 88)

Cyclical symptoms.

Mood and cognitive symptoms. (*See previous page.*)

Poor dream recall, insomnia, amnesia, dizziness.

Pallor, anemia,* weakness, fatigue.

Neurological symptoms. Numbness, tingling shock-like sensations in the limbs, carpal tunnel, childhood convulsions, seizures, temporary limb paralysis.

Sensitivity to sound.

Joint pain, muscle weakness. Hand and foot cramps, Arthritis. (ROGERS 1997)

Female hormone imbalances. PMS. Postpartum depression.**

Digestive system problems. Poor appetite. Nausea (morning nausea, motion sickness, nausea of pregnancy). Low hydrochloric acid.

Carbohydrate intolerance, diabetes, hypoglycemia.

Allergies, addictions, alcoholism. (BAKER 1975)

Cheilosis (small lesions in the mouth or cracks at the corner of the lips), glossitis (inflammation of the tongue). Cavities.

Acne, eczema, dermatitis, striae, other skin problems. Hair loss. Pale skin and hair, relative to genetics.***

Water retention, urinary problems, kidney stones.

Tendency to infection and chronic illness.**** Prone to asthma, arteriosclerosis, stillbirths, melanoma.

* B6 helps form hemoglobin from iron and red blood cells, prevents B6-deficient anemia, may benefit sickle cell anemia

** B6 is used in estrogen degradation, steroid synthesis.

*** B6 is needed to form elastin and collagen, skin and hair pigment

**** B6 supports immune activity, including antibody production, B and T-lymphocyte activities, and thymus and spleen function.

Populations (QUILLIN 1987, BALCH 1990, GARRISON, SLAGLE 1993, ROGERS 1997, BAKER 1975)

Levels can be reduced by pyroluria, stress, aging, high metabolism, toxicity, malabsorption, gastrointestinal disorders, pregnancy, nursing, uremia, Down's syndrome, immunosuppressant diseases, radiation exposure, heart failure, liver cirrhosis, alcoholism,* smoking. Also: diets involving high protein and fat, overprocessed or overcooked foods; prolonged B vitamin imbalances. And, extended use of certain pharmaceuticals, e.g., estrogen-based contraceptives, L-dopa, MAOIs, penicillamine, isoniazide; certain antihypertensives and antibiotics.

* Which compromises use of B6, folate, and B1.

Nutrient interactions

Enhances B12 and magnesium absorption.

Helps regulate the sodium/potassium balance.

Used in carbohydrate and fat metabolism, glycogen conversion.

Helps remove homocysteine and form cysteine.

Critical to amino acid absorption, metabolism, and transport.

Useful diagnostic tests (B6) (JAFFE 1992, WERBACH 1991)

Erythrocyte glutamate/oxalate transaminase (EGOT).

Red cell pyridoxal-5-phosphate.

Urinary pyrroles.

Deficiency is suggested if the upper finger joints can't bend the fingers enough to touch the palm of the hand without bending the knuckles.

Sources of B6 (LIEBERMAN, 1990, BALCH 1990, NUTRICIRCLES® 1996)

Salmon, herring and other fish, organ and other meats, poultry, eggs, butter. Brewer's yeast, blackstrap molasses, bananas, walnuts, potatoes, bee pollen, royal jelly, wheat germ, brown rice, avocados, watermelon, spinach, nuts, flax, sesame and sunflower seeds, yams, tempeh, mangoes, grapes, prunes, squash, carrots, pears, other vegetables, fruits, and whole grains. Unfortunately, bioavailability is often limited.

Supportive nutrients

Zinc and magnesium are used in B6 metabolism; manganese is needed for the magnesium to work. (ROGERS 1997)

B, C, E, chromium, cobalt, and potassium work with B6. (So do sodium, copper, and phosphorus, but they are usually not lacking; also, linoleic acid (which is not usually depleted, except in pyroluria.) (SLAGLE 1993)

Therapeutic dose range (JAFFE 1992, SLAGLE 1993, PFEIFFER 1987, 88)

Typical doses are 15-100 mg; in some pyrolurias, 500 mg or more, depending on need.*

B6 forms P5P, which is more potent.** The P5P dose varies from 10 to 50 mg, and may go higher in pyroluria.

Both B6 and P5P may be indicated, at correspondingly lower doses.

* In pyroluria, B6 intake must compensate for the rapid depletion rate, but not be so high that it overshoots need and becomes detrimental.

Effects of excess, contraindications (SLAGLE 1993)

One gram or more per day may cause signs of sensory nerve damage* (e.g, numbness or tingling in the extremities), (SCHAUMBERG 1983) *usually reversible if dose is decreased or discontinued. Intake of other B vitamins may help, as may switching to P5P, at a lower dose.*

Very high B6 decreases methyl availability by converting excess homocysteine to cysteine rather than methionine. (See *Histapenia, Histadelia*, pp. 153-67.)

Can be overstimulating.

* Schaumberg (1983) reports neurological side effects in a few individuals taking 1 to 6 gm over two to forty months. This reversed when B6 was discontinued. Though perhaps due to excess B6, such effects could have been caused by lack of other B vitamins (which were not supplied), low magnesium, or too much of the pyridoxine form of B6.

Inositol

May improve bipolar depression, panic disorder, OCD, (Levine 1997) or insomnia, (Pfeiffer) in some patients, particularly if histadelic. (Walsh 2007) *Manics (especially if histapenic (Walsh 2007)) may overact to inositol.*

See *Inositol*, pp. 95-97, for further discussion, including references.

Choline

May improve unresponsive mania, and also benefit insomnia and anxiety, particularly in histapenic (Walsh 2007) patients. *Bipolars (especially if histadelic (Walsh 2007)) are often hypersensitive to choline, too much of which may trigger or worsen depression.* (Cohen 1982, Leiva 1990, Stoll 1996, Janowsky 1972, 73b, 84, Risch 1984)

See *Choline*, pp. 48-51, 97, for further discussion, including references.

B12 & folic acid

Mood biochemistry (Baumel 1995, Slagle 1993)

Interaction with neurotransmitters (Abou-Saleh 1986, Crellin 1993)

Serotonin, dopamine, norepinephrine — B12 and folate (via BH4) play a critical role in forming these antidepressant transmitters. (Coppen 1989, Leeming 1982, Curtis 1982, 83)

Acetylcholine, taurine — B12 and folate, via methionine, help form choline, which precurses acetylcholine (a parasympathetic, inhibitory transmitter), and taurine (another inhibitor).

Support for brain viability

Help maintain the myelin sheath.

Essential to nervous system function and repair.

Important in RNA/DNA replication (which is critical to the transfer of genetic information).

Metabolize homocysteine. (Fava 1997, Papakostas 2004, Tiemeier 2002. Reutens 2002, Duthie 2002, Bottiglieri 2000, Tolmunen 2004, Morris 2002)

Mental symptoms (Slagle 1993, Gold 1987, Pfeiffer 1975, 87, 88)

B12 and folic acid work together in the brain, profoundly influence mood and cognition, and are commonly depleted in affectives. *Psychiatric symptoms frequently become apparent before physical, and may include:*

☐ Depression, apathy, fatigue. Loss of alertness, drive, confidence, and independence. Social withdrawal. Mental lethargy, which may resolve into stuporous depression. (Coppen 2005, Zhang 2006, Howard 1975, Alpert 1997, 2000, Penninx 2000, Tiemeier 2002, Morris 2003, Bell 1991, Pfeiffer)

☐ Nervous irritability, insomnia, moodiness, severe agitation, anxiety, hostility, mania. (Hasanah 1997)

☐ Auditory hallucinations, psychosis (often histapenic). (Bottiglieri 1996, Godfrey 1990, Alpert 1997, Abou-Saleh 1986, DeLiz 1979)

☐ Anxiety. Delusions of persecution, paranoia. (Bottiglieri 1996, Godfrey 1990, Joshi 1982)

☐ Confusion. Memory loss. Concentration and learning difficulties. Delirium. Dementia. (Rita 2004, Mesulam 1985, Hilsson 1998, Crellin 1993, Howard 1975, Thornton 1977)

☐ Headaches. Incoordination. Neurological symptoms and eventual degeneration. (Ravakhah 1995, Bottiglieri 1995)

Biotype indications

B12 and folate deficit can, even by itself, lead to histapenia, or histapenic mania. Intake improves histamine production and reduces homocysteine (which is often elevated in histapenics (Walsh 2007)). (Tiemeier 2002, Fava 1997, Papakostas 2004, Duthie 2002, Bottiglieri 2000, Morris 2002)

In some cases of histadelia, B12, especially methyl-B12, improves the constant depression (though B12 alone is sometimes counterproductive). Significant folic acid supplements (including content in many multivitamins and B complex supplements) are usually contraindicated for histadelics, as folate tends to already excessive (as it is not being utilized in methylation). (Pfeiffer 1976, 87, 88, Walsh 2007)

Important: B12 should usually be supplemented at least several months before adding folate.

Folic acid

Folic acid supports formation of antidepressant transmitters (dopamine, norepinephrine, serotonin (COPPEN 1982, BOTEZ 1979, ENGSTROM 1999) and of COMT, and raises brain SAM. (CRELLIN 1993, ABOU-SALEH 1986) Depletion is common worldwide, particularly in psychiatric patients, (CARNEY 1967, 78, 79, 90, HUTT 1997, HOWARD 1975) and prevalent in bipolars, (COPPEN 1986) especially with neurological symptoms.

Mania

Red cell folate is reduced in some manics (HASANNAH 1997) and in most histapenic bipolars (who are prone to hypomania and psychosis). (WALSH 2006) Deficiency has also been associated with such manic symptoms as irritability, hostility, obsessions, paranoia, and psychosis. (HASANAH 1997 HERMEST 1988, CARNEY 1967, 78, 79, 90, HUTTO 1997, BOTEZ 1977, PROCTER 1991, GODFREY 1990)

Depression studies

Low folate is frequently tied to depression, (BJELLAND 2003, MORRIS 2003, LEE 1998, REYNOLDS 2002, TOLMUNEN 2003, WOLFERSDORF 1995, ZHANG 2006, TIEMEIER 2002, FAVA 1997, PAPAKOSTAS 2004, HOWARD 1975, GHANDRIAN, ALPERT 2000, 03) which is the most common symptom of deficiency. (MURRAY 1996, GOLD 1987) Folate is insufficient in an estimated 31% (CRELLIN 1993, CARNEY 1990, REYNOLDS 1970) to 75% of depressives; (LEE 1992) especially in the elderly depressed. (PFEIFFER 1975, 87, THORNTON 1977, ABALAN 1984, BELL 1990, 91) Low levels also occur in lithium-treated patients. (LEE 1992)

Low folate has been correlated with greater severity, (ABOU-SALEH 1989, CRELLIN 1993, GHADIRIAN 1980) episode duration, (LEVITT 1989) length of hospitalization, (BELL 1990) and affective morbidity; (COPPEN 1998) and with nonresponse to antidepressants and lithium. (LEE 1992)

Folic acid trials are positive for many. (TAYLOR 2004, COPPEN 2005) Benefit has been noted in lithium-treated patients, (HASANAH 1997) in unipolars with low levels, (GODFREY 1990) and in elderly (PASSERI 1993, GUARALDI 1993) and alcoholic depressives. (DIPALMA 1994) Alpert (1997, 03) finds folate levels predict antidepressant response in the elderly.

Megadoses of methylfolate, a potent form, show significant antidepressant benefit for many patients, (GUARALD 1993) possibly equivalent to pharmaceuticals. (CRELLIN 1993)

Folate also can augment antidepressant (LEVITT 1998, FAVA 1997, COPPEN 2000) and lithium response. (COPPEN 1986, LEE 1992, PRAKASH 1981) Recovered depressives with high folate are less likely to relapse. (ABOU SALEH 1986, SING 1992)

Biotype indications (JAFFE 1992, PFEIFFER 1979, 87, 88, WALSH 2000, 07)

Because it stimulates histamine production, folic acid is particularly indicated for histapenic patients, and is reported to improve such histapenic symptoms as anxiety, paranoia, and psychosis.

It also helps some pyrolurics (*if not also histadelic*).

Histadelics generally accumulate too much folic acid. Supplements can worsen, perhaps severely, histadelic depression and other symptoms.

Mental & neurological symptoms

Folic acid may provide support in the following conditions:

- ☐ Depression. (TAYLOR 2004, COPPEN 2005, HASANAH 1997, GODFREY 1990, ALPERT 1997, 2003, PASSERI 1993, GUARALDI 1993, DIPALM 1994, CRELLIN 1993)
- ☐ Paranoia, OCD, psychosis, irritability, hostility, some manias. (HASANAH 1997, HERMEST 1988, CARNEY 1967, 78, 79, 90, HUTTO 1997, BOTEZ 1977, PROCTER 1991, GODFREY 1990)
- ☐ Cognitive or neurological impairment. Weakness, apathy, memory problems. Headache. (RITA 2004, BOTTIGLIERI 1995, BOTEZ 1977)

"Psychiatric patients tend to have low folate."

Mark Gold, MD

BH4 (Tetrahydrobiopterin)

BH_4 is a critical coenzyme in forming serotonin, norepinephrine and other antidepressant neurotransmitters. It has been used by itself in treating depression, and can be dramatically effective. (MURRAY 1996)

Reduced levels have been associated with recurrent depression. (CURTIS 1982, 83). Hasimoto (1990) suggests bipolars may have problems with BH4 metabolism.

Synthesis is stimulated by folic acid, B12, and SAM;* and C. (COPPEN 2005, LEEMING 1982)

* That is, synthesis depends on the status of the brain's folate/methyl balance. (Walsh 2006)

Interactions with meds (PFEIFFER 1997, 88)

Pfeiffer reports primary B12/folate-deficiency is not responsive to neuropleptics.

Dilantin® (used for epilepsy) depletes folic acid.

Folate/B12 anemias (GOLD 1987, PFEIFFER 75, 87, GARRISON 1985, LIEBERMAN 1990, READING 1975)

A serious deficiency of B12 causes pernicious anemia. 80% develop neurological changes; 60%, personality changes. CNS changes are often the first sign of illness; nerve cells can be permanently destroyed before other symptoms become evident.

A folic acid or B12 deficiency can cause megaloblastic anemia, a condition characterized by reduced quantities of red blood cells, enlarged in size (megaloblasts).

Treatment of either anemia involves both vitamins, *starting with B12.*

Considerations (folate)

(GOLD 1987, SLAGLE 1993, PFEIFFER 1975, 79, 87, 88, BALCH 1990, LIEBERMAN 1990, GARRISON 1985, HOFFER 1983B, REYNOLDS 1984, GODFREY 1990, JAFFE 1992, WERBACH 1991, ABOU-SALEH 1989, HOWARD 1975, CARNEY 1978, 79, 90)

Need may be suggested by (GOLD 1987, PFEIFFER, 1975, 87, 88, GARRISON 1985)

Depression, isolation, other affective symptoms.

Poor memory, confusion, cognitive difficulties.

Apathy, fatigue, lethargy, weakness. (HOWARD 1975, 92)

Irritability, increased sensitivity to pain.

Neurological symptoms. Lesions in corners of the mouth, sore tongue, graying hair.

Anemia.* Vascular fragility. Palpitations. Cardiovascular symptoms. Homocysteinuria. (TIEMEIER 2002, FAVA 1997, PAPAKOSTAS 2004, DUTHIE 2002)

Gluten intolerance, allergies, prone to infection.*

Burning feet, restless leg syndrome. Spasticity numbness, stiffness, muscle atrophy.

Digestive problems, nausea, diarrhea, constipation, anorexia, weight loss. Prone to celiac disease.

Prone to toxemia of pregnancy, premature births, birth defects, low estrogen. (SLAGLE 1993)

Low adrenal steroids.

B12 deficiency symptoms.

Populations (GOLD 1987, PFEIFFER 1975, 87, GARRISON 1985, MORRIS 2003, SLAGLE 1993)

Aging, poverty, illness.* Poorly-nourished pregnant, postpartum and nursing mothers.** Prolonged stress. Malnutrition, eating disorder, overcooked and processed foods, reducing diets. Alcoholism (alcohol interferes with folate metabolism), caffeine, antibiotics, anticonvulsants, barbiturates, birth control pills, aspirin, and certain other medications.

* 2/3 of those unable to care for themselves are folate-deficient.
** Deficient maternal folic acid may cause miscarriage, retardation or congenital malformations, and is a major cause of neural tube defects, such as spina bifida.

Nutrient interactions

Needed in assimilating pantothenic acid.

Works with B12 in metabolizing carbohydrates, fats, and proteins, and in forming proteins.

Sources (NUTRICIRCLES® 1996)

Deep green leafy vegetables, e.g, kale, chard (the term "folic" derives from foliage). Whole grains, germ and bran, nutritional yeast. Liver, kidneys, eggs, lean and organ meats. Asparagus, legumes (peas, beans), cabbage family (broccoli, cauliflower, etc.), beets, sweet potatoes, artichoke. Bananas, oranges, cantaloupe, papaya, bee pollen. Also in sunflower seeds, almonds, filberts, walnuts, oats, rye, poultry.

Folate is sparse in root vegetables, corn, light greens, dairy, pork, and starchy foods low in iron (e.g., rice). It dissipates in storage. Cooking severely reduces folate content. C and iron may partially inactivate folate.

Lab (JAFFE 1992, SLAGLE 1993, WERBACH,1991)

Red blood cell folate.

Urinary formiminoglutamate (FIGLU).*

Response to treatment.

The degree to which treatment normalizes:

Plasma homocysteine.

Urinary methylmalonic acid.

Neutrophilic segmentation index.

* A histidine metabolite, which correlates inversely with folate/B12. Readings may be elevated in liver disease.

Supportive nutrients (SLAGLE 1993)

B, B12, C.

Iron or copper, *but consider potentially adverse effects.*

Dose folic acid (SLAGLE 1993, GARRISION 1985, BORIDA 2001)

Some patients testing normal for folic acid improve further with supplementation. Keeping folate at the high end of normal or beyond may minimize depression, *unless histadelic.* (WALSH 2007)

Dose is typically 400 mcg to 2 mg* per day depending on specific needs. Some physicians recomend up to 10 mg. for specific conditions for a short time. (BORIDA 2001)

* Note: Multiples and B vitamins typically contain 400 mcg, sometimes 800 mg. Other supplements containing folate further increase daily levels.

Effects of excess, contraindications (SLAGLE 1993, MURRAY 1996, PFEIFFER 75)

Folate can mask B12 deficiency. Although folic acid deficiency can undermine mental functioning, effects are generally reversible. Lack of B12, on the other hand, can demyelinate nerve cells and cause irreversible neural damage (and compromise access to stored folic acid). Folate supplements cannot prevent such damage, but mask it. So B12 is often prescribed first. After several months folic acid may be added.

Histadelics usually have excessive folic acid. Supplementation can increase the severity of their depression or other symptoms.

Prolonged intake and/or high doses can overstimulate, producing irritability, insomnia, euphoria, hyperactivity, mania, or even a rebound histadelia in the low histamine patient. Watch for muscle restlessness or jerking (usually at doses over 5 mg). Symptoms often reverse when intake stops or decreases.

Folate reduces anticonvulsant efficacy and can worsen seizure problems. (HOMMES 1979, ROSCHE 2002) On the other hand, certain anticonvulsives, such as Dilantin, decrease folic acid (which may be part of how they work), so some physicians supplement small doses. (SLAGLE 1993)

Excess can deplete zinc. Additional zinc may be helpful, especially during pregnancy or estrogen intake.

Gastrointestinal effects.

Usually contraindicated with any tendency to hormone-related cancers (though sometimes used to make up for blocking of folic metabolism by chemotherapy).

Vitamin B12

Levels

Deficiency is common in psychiatric patients. (*ACTA MED SCAND* 1965, KALLSTROM 1969, HUNTER 1967) Neurological and psychiatric symptoms can occur long before physical symptoms of pernicious anemia.

Depression

At least 10-30% of depressives are low in B12. (BELL 1991, CARNEY 1978, DOMMISSE 1991, BAUMEL 1995, ZHANG 2006) Deficiency frequently leads to depression, (HOLMES 1991) is prevalent in patients institutionalized for depression, (WOLFERSDORF 1995, BELL 1990, 91) and especially related to depression in the elderly.*(KIVELA 1989, PENNINX 2000).

Thiemeler (2002) suggests B12 is more important than folate in countering depression. Elevated B12 is often associated with good treatment outcome. (HINTIKKA 2003) Mood can improve dramatically with repletion. (LINDENBAUM 1988, SCHILLING 1971, COPPEN 2005, MURRAY 1996)

Mania

Mania can occasionally be directly due to B12 depletion.*(HECTOR 1998, GOGGANS 1984, HASANAH 1997) Deficiency has also been associated with such manic symptoms as irritability, agitation, OCD, hallucinations, paranoia, and acute psychosis. (HOFFER 1978, HEMEST 1988, HECTOR 1998, SLAGLE 2003, DELIZ 1979, PFEIFFER 1979, 88, JOSHI 1982, *BR J PSYCHIAT* 1988, JAFFE 1992) *On the other hand, excessive B12 can be overstimulating, and promote mania.*

* In fact, originally, an X chromosome segment, associated with low B12 and red/green color blindness, was thought to be associated with dominant inheritance of bipolar disorder in some patients. (Reading 1979, Gold 1987)

Biotype indications (PFEIFFER 1979, 87, 88, JAFFE 1992)

B12 benefits histapenia.

It supports methylation, benefitting some (but not all) histadelic patients. With significant oxidative stress, histadelics often preferentially need methyl-B12.

Mental symptoms (LINDENBAUM 1998, HESEKER 1992, EDWIN 1965, DOMMISSE 1991, SHORVON 1980, CARNEY 1978, HUTTO 1997, BRAVERMAN 1997, PFEIFFER 1979, 87 88, JAFFE 1992)

B12 can be low in, and may benefit the following conditions:

- ☐ Mood changes, moodiness, depression. (HINTIKKA 2003, LINDENBAUM 1988, SCHILLING 1971, COPPEN 2005, HOLMES 1991, BELL 1990, 91, KIVELA 1989, PENNINX 2000)
- ☐ Irritability, agitation, mania. (GOGGANS 1984)
- ☐ OCD. (HEMEST 1988) Preoccupation with guilt.
- ☐ Mental fatigue, slowed cognition, memory problems, lack of focus/attention, confusion, dulled senses, dementia. (KARNASE 1990, WHYTE 2002, EASTLEY 2000, LARNER 1999, RITA 2004, ENGELBORGHS 2004)
- ☐ Delirium, delusions, hallucinations, paranoia, acute psychosis. (HOFFER 1978, HECTOR 1998, SLAGLE 1993, DELIZ 1979, PFEIFFER 1979, 88, JOSHI 1982, *BR J PSYCHIAT* 1988, JAFFE 1992)

Neurological symptoms

Chronic depletion can cause severe and permanent neurological damage, including, spinal cord changes,. Demyelination of nerves may at first appear as intermittent numbness, tingling or weakness in arms and legs, diminished tendon reflexes, dizziness, unsteady gait, disruption of fine movement in the hands, spasms. If unchecked, it may lead to spinal cord degeneration, cerebral and optic nerve degeneration, and cerebellar atrophy, leading to difficulty walking, speaking, seeing, or thinking, and spastic paralysis.

"A vitamin B12 deficiency may be a possible diagnosis in the majority of psychiatric patients."

JG Handerson, MD

"Depression can occur even without anemia."

JM Holmes, MD, 1991

"Even without obvious deficiency, [B12] injections have improved mood."

FR Ellis, MD, 1973

Some depression studies

Penninx, 2000 — Epidemiological study. Serum B12 was significantly lower in 122 severely-depressed, physically-disabled elderly women living in the community, as compared to 478 nondepressed women in the same situation. B12 deficit was twice as likely with severe depression.

Tiemeier, 2002 — Controlled study. In 112 depressives, depression related to homocysteinemia, low B12 and, to some degree, low folate. Adjustment for disability and heart disease reduced the association of folate and homocysteine, but B12 was independent, suggesting a causal relationship with depression.

B12 functions in the brain (GOLD 1987, PFEIFFER 1987)

- ☐ Support for nervous system metabolism.
- ☐ Supports methylation and homocysteine metabolism. (FAVA 1997, PAPAKOSTAS 2004, TIEMEIER 2002)
- ☐ Role in histamine formation. (PFEIFFER 87, 88)
- ☐ Role in EFA and folic acid metabolism and balance. (COUSENS 2000)
- ☐ Support for melatonin secretion and regular sleep rhythms. (OHTA 1992)
- ☐ May help prevent excitotoxicity due to homocysteine/NMDA interactions.*
- ☐ Maintenance of the functional integrity of myelinated nerve fibers.**

* Which is more likely if B12 is low during stroke, head trauma, etc. (See *Excitotoxicity*, p. 191-93.)

** Demyelination can occur, for instance, on exposure to nitrous oxide (e.g., in dental treatment), if B12 is low. (Gold 1987)

Considerations (B12)

(*Br J Psychiat*, 1988, *Lancet* 1984, Joshi 1982, DeLiz 1979, Godfrey 1990, Pfeiffer 1979, Jaffe 1992, Werbach 1991, Zucker 1981, Ghadirian 1980, Abou-Saleh 1989, Howard 1975, Coppen 1989, Carney 1979)

Need may be suggested by

(Pfeiffer, 1975, 1988, Lieberman 1990, Krohn, 1991, Garrison, 1985, Hoffer, 1983, Cousens 2000, Slagle 1993)

Mood swings, depression, apathy. Irritability, agitation, mania. (See studies on previous page.)

Confusion. Memory or concentration problems. Dementia.

Paranoia, hallucinations, psychosis. (Joshi 1982, DeLiz 1979, *Br J Psychiat* 1988)

Weakness, fatigue, dizziness. (Ellis 1973)

Light or noise intolerance. Numbness, tingling, pain. Unsteady gait. Eventually, difficulty walking or speaking, leg paralysis, neurological deterioration.

Sore or burning tongue. Hair loss. Skin disorders.

Gluten intolerance, allergies, low resistance to infection (poor antibody formation).

Poor appetite or digestion. Weight loss. Diarrhea.

Chest pain, rapid heart beat, heart palpitations, shortness of breath. Homocysteinuria. (Tiemeier 2002, Fava 1997, Papakostas 2004, Duthie 2002)

Inflammation of small joints. Rheumatoid arthritis. (Slagle 1993)

Pernicious anemia.*

Increased tendency to diabetes, MS, infertility, suppressed bone marrow formation, organic brain disease, gout, liver dysfunction, alcoholism, hangovers, TB, certain cancers. (Slagle 1993)

Severe untreated deficiency can be fatal.

* Not coincidentally, the structure of B12 is similar to that of hemoglobin, except with cobalt instead of iron in the center.

Populations (deficiency)

(Pfeiffer 1975, 87, 88, Gold 1987, Garrison 1985)

The elderly (especially if isolated, ill, depressed, or not eating much), people undergoing chronic stress, (Slagle 1993) vegetarians (especially vegans), alcoholics, hypothyroid patients, (Levitt 1993) the malnourished (e.g., due to dieting, eating disorders, poverty, institutionalization, chronic illness, etc.). Pregnant, postpartum, or nursing mothers;and women with elevated estrogen.

Prolonged exposure to certain antibiotics (can deplete intestinal bacteria which manufacture B12), oral contraceptives, barbiturates, analgesics, phenytoins (e.g, phenobarbital), laxatives, or alcohol.

Difficulties with absorption

(Gold, 1987, Newbold, 1989, Garrison, 1985, Lieberman 1990)

B12 or folate deficiency is often due to problems with absorption, digestion, or transport. Such problems increase markedly with age. To absorb B12, the body requires:

Intrinsic factor (found in gastric juice) — which is crucial, and diminishes with aging and various conditions.*

Sufficient hydrocholoric acid and pepsin.

Adequate thyroxine.

Sufficient C, B1, B5, folic acid, biotin; perhaps, A, E.

Adequate protein. Effective calcium and sugar metabolism. Restriction of dietary sugar.

Attention to any GI conditions that block absorption.**

* Perhaps due to damage to the cells which create it, or to autoimmune interference.

** Celiac sprue, fish tapeworm, blind-loop syndrome (B12-greedy bacteria), gastrectomy, steatorrhoea, or ileitis.

Nutrient interactions

Helps metabolize carbohydrates, fats, protein.

Used in carotene absorption and conversion to A.

Plays a role in EFA and folic acid metabolism.

Sources

(Nutricircles® 1996)

The liver normally stores 3-5 years worth of B12 (2-5 mg). It's depleted with low intake, or poor absorption.

B12 is prevalent in meats, fish, chicken, organ meats, seafood (lobster, scallops, crabs), salmon, sardines, flounder, swordfish, egg yolk, cheese; less so, in poultry and milk. Some cultures derive B12 from insects.

It's debatable whether enough B12 can be absorbed from solely non-animal sources (seaweeds, nori, (Bagnelie 1991), nutritional yeast, mushrooms, Concord grapes, sunflower seeds, bee products, ferments (tempeh, miso).

Supportive nutrients

B1, B5, folic acid, biotin, choline, inositol, B complex, A, E, C, calcium, iron, copper, phosphorus, potassium (food sources), some sodium, adequate protein. (Slagle 1993)

Lab

(Jaffe 1992, Werbach 1991)

B12/B12 binding capacity, or formiminoglutamate.

The degree to which treatment normalizes plasma homocysteine, urinary methylmalonic acid, and/or the neutrophilic segmentation index.

Note: Because of the possibility of irreversible brain damage, discerning B12 requirements is critical. Blood tests may reflect recent intake, or homeostatic mechanisms, and miss localized brain or nervous system deficiency. (van Tiggelen 1983) So even with negative labs, a trial of B12 may be advisable with symptoms that suggest deficiency (e.g., low-energy depressives with neurological symptoms). (Geagea 1975, Newbold 1989, van Tiggelen 1983, Ellis 1973, Slagle 1993)

Supplemental B12

Sublingually, 250-2000 mcg, in the morning.

With high oxidative stress, histadelics often need methyl-B12.

With absorption problems, B12 may work better mixed with intrinsic factor, or taken as a nasal spray. (Pfeiffer 1975, 87) In some cases, injections* are indicated, (Ellis 1973, van Tiggelen 1983) typically 1 mg., 1-4x/month. (Newbold 1989) Eventually, some may be able to switch to 1 mg/day sublingually, though others need injections lifelong. (Ellis 1973)

* Note: Cyanocobalamin contains cyanide, to which some patients are intolerant, and which can cause optic atrophy, so hydroxycobalamin, which sustains blood levels longer, may be preferable. (Pfeiffer 1975, 87)

Effects of excess, contraindications

Helpful in some histadelias, not others.

Can be overstimulating.

Thiamine (B1)

Thiamine is important in countering anxiety and supporting mood. A 1985 survey found 30% of psychiatric patients low in thiamine. Mental symptoms can occur before physical. (CLIN NEUROPHARM 1985)

Mania

Research suggests sedative effects. (OSTERMAN 1959, MCCONACHIE 1958, 88) Deficiency can increase stimulation and has been associated with such manic-type symptoms as anxiety, agitation, hypersensitivity, insomnia, irritability, aggression, and psychosis. (FATTAL-VALEVSKI 2005, BOWMAN 1939, BROZEK 1957, LERBOULLET 1958, SLAGLE 1993)

Depression (ROGERS 1997, SLAGLE 1993)

Carney suggests about one-third of depressives may be at least mildly deficient. (CARNEY 1979, 82, BROZEK 1957) B1 is often indicated for depression. (ROGERS 1997) Research suggests it can improve mood and cognition, (BENTON 1995, 97, 99, SMIDT 1991) and enhances antidepressant response (along with B2 and B6). (BELL 1992)

Mental & neurological symptoms (QUILLIN 1987, PFEIFFER 1975, THIESSEN 1978, JAFFE 1992, WERBACH 1991, BROZEK 1957)

- ☐ Anxiety, aggression, irritability, agitation, restlessness, apprehension, insomnia, night terrors, mania.
- ☐ Low mood, apathy, depression, suicidal thoughts. (LONSDALE 1980, SLAGLE 1993, BENTON 1997, 99, ROGERS 1997)
- ☐ Memory problems, difficulty focusing attention, confusion.
- ☐ Numbness, tingling,neurological symptoms. (SLAGLE 1993, BROZEK 1957)
- ☐ Sensitivity to noise, personality change, psychosis.
- ☐ Weakness, dizziness, exhaustion, chronic fatigue.
- ☐ Alcohol-type nervous system damage, beriberi, Korsakoff's psychosis, Wernicke's encephalopathy,* MS-like symptoms. (GOLD 1987)

* Wernike-Korsakoff syndrome, commonly due to alcoholism and loss of B1, is characterized by apathy, confusion, personality change, profound depression, and eventual nervous system damage.

Some B1 studies

Benton, 1995 — Double blind. A year of low B1 in female university students was associated with low mood (POMS), improving over 3 months with B1 intake. With a year of B1, sleep also improved.

Smidt, 1991 — Double blind. B1 given to 80 elderly Irish women with marginal deficiency, significantly improved well-being, activity, energy, fatigue, appetite, low weight, and sleep patterns, suggesting benefit to depression.

Brain function

- ☐ Helps regulate a number of neurotransmitters. Contributes to acetylcholine synthesis. Inhibits MAO. (CONNOR 1981)
- ☐ Supports brain repair. (COUSENS 2000) Deficiency can induce neural swelling and damage, altering communication. (WILLIAMS 1943)
- ☐ Megadoses can be a neural stimulant. (SLAGLE 1993, NEWBOLD 1975, HOFFER 1987, ROGERS 1997)

Considerations (LIEBERMAN 1990, MURRAY 1996, GARRISON 1985, QUILLIN 1987, PFEIFFER 1975, THIESSEN 1978, JAFFE 1992, WERBACH 1991, BROZEK 1957)

Need may be suggested by (LARSON 2001, SLAGLE 1993, ROGERS 1997)

Depression, confusion, fatigue, apathy, memory loss.

Anxiety, restlessness, irritability, aggression, mood disorder, emotional lability, personality change, psychosis.

Night terror, insomnia. Sensitivity to sound.

Pain. Headaches.

Trembling, tingling, numbness or burning in hands and feet. With severe depletion, seizures, paralysis.

Sugar craving, appetite loss,* anorexia, nausea, acidity, constipation, other GI issues. Difficulty metabolizing drugs. Water retention.

Vulnerability to toxins and infection.**

Muscle weakness, numbness, or atrophy.

Heart palpitations, shortness of breath, chest pain.

Stress, heavy exercise, alcoholism, smoking, delirium tremors, drug addiction, high metabolism, hyperthyroidism, illness, high fever, surgery, aging. Pregnancy, nursing, birth control pills. Excess junk or overcooked food, carbohydrates, caffeine, shellfish, raw fish. (LONSDALE 1984) Yeast overgrowth.*** (ROGERS 1997) Sulfa drugs, prednesone.

* B1 supports appetite, GI tone; creation of HCl, carbohydrate metabolism.
** Protects from free radicals, acetaldehyde, and lipid peroxidation. Helps maintain the thymus and stimulates the immune system.
*** B1 inhibitors (formed by some yeast) occur in raw & shell fish.

Nutrient interactions (BAUMEL 1995, SLAGLE 1993)

Helps metabolize brain glucose, and absorb and use magnesium.

Useful diagnostic tests (JAFFE 1992, WERBACH 1991, LONSDALE 1980)

RBC transketolase; or RBC thiamine diphosphate.

Supportive nutrients

B, C, E, manganese, magnesium, sulfur. (SLAGLE 1993)

Sources of thiamine (NUTRICIRCLES® 1996, SLAGLE 1993)

Brewer's yeast, wheat germ and bran. Sunflower, flax, sesame and chia seeds. Oats, other whole grains. Garlic, potatoes, leafy greens. Pine, Brazil and pistachio nuts. Tuna, salmon, other fish, liver, eggs, dairy. Legumes, watermelon, mushrooms, blackstrap molasses.

Dose (JAFFE 1992, MURRAY 1996, WERBACH 1991)

When indicated, 100-500 mg, perhaps with B complex.

Effects of excess, contraindications (WERBACH 1991)

Rarely, itching, flush, nervousness, perspiration, shortness of breath, rapid heart beat.

Riboflavin (B2)

Trends toward affective improvement

Bell 1992 — randomized, placebo-controlled double blind. 14 depressed geriatrics were given 10 mg each B1, B2, B6. Supplementation significantly improved B2 and B6 enzyme activity and created trends to greater improvement in depression and cognitive scores.

Riboflavin supports neural metabolism and is critical to brain cell energy production and response to stress. It is often low in affectives.

Mood issues

B2 is often low in affectives, especially during depression (CARNEY 1982, STERMER 1973, HESEKER 1992, BELL 1991, SLAGLE 1993), and may enhance antidepressant response. (BELL 1992, MIHAKE 2006, SLAGLE 1993)

Deficiency can also occur in hypomania. (SLAGLE 1993)

Mechanisms

- □ Supports response to stress.
- □ Used in tryptophan metabolism. (BALCH 1990)
- □ Supports methylation and thyroid function. (BELL 1992B)
- □ Critical to brain cellular energetics. (SLAGLE 1993)
- □ Supports transport and use of oxygen, and red blood cell formation. (BALCH 1990, SLAGLE)

Mental symptoms (ROGERS 1997, SLAGLE 1993, HESEKER 1992, BENTON 1997, 99, BELL 1992, SMIDT 1991, CARNEY 1982, SACKS 1988, THIESSEN 1978, WERBACH 1991, GOLD 1987)

B2 may benefit the following conditions:

- □ Depression, fatigue, lethargy, mental sluggishness. (PFEIFFER 1975, 88, MURRAY 1998, 96, BALCH 1990, STERNER 1973)
- □ Moodiness, heightened susceptibility to stress. Irritability, aggression, hysteria, mood disorder, insomnia. (PFEIFFER 1975, MURRAY 1998)
- □ Personality change, occasionally psychosis. (SLAGLE 1993)

Considerations (LARSON 2001, SLAGLE 1993, MURRAY 1996, BALCH 1990, PFEIFFER 1975, 87, ROGERS 1997, QUILLIN 1987, WERBACH 1991, LIEBERMAN 1990, GARRISON 1985, TENNEY 1987)

Need may be suggested by (SLAGLE 1993, PFEIFFER 1975, 87, 88, MURRAY 1996, 98, BALCH 1990)

Depression, mental slowness, dizziness, fatigue, lethargy. Weakness, trembling.

Susceptibility to stress,* irritability.

Patches of flaking, cracked, or oily skin. Red, scaly skin around nose, ears, eyelids, forehead, lips, mouth, genitals (perhaps fungal infection). Dry chapped lips; narrowing upper lip. Premature wrinkles.

Red/purple discoloration or inflammation of the tongue. Discomfort swallowing. Poor digestion. Compulsive eating.

Bloodshot, itchy or burning eyes, sensitive to light, perhaps ulcerated. Eye fatigue. Blurred vision. Cataracts.

Increased vulnerability to allergies, infection,** fungal infection. Migraines.

Poor digestion. Compulsive eating.

Perhaps, thyroid dysfunction, hypoglycemia, undermethylation. (BELL 1992)

Problems with growth and repair, carpal tunnel, malformations, muscular function.

* B2 supports creation of adrenal cortisol.

** Helps form mucoproteins and antibodies. Helps maintain mucus membranes. (BALCH 1990)

Contributory conditions (SLAGLE 1993)

Stress, high metabolism, fever, pregnancy, nursing. Liver disease. Alcohol. Diets high in sugar, starch, or protein. Malnutrition, vegetarianism. Antibiotics, phenothiazines.

Nutrient interactions (MURRAY 1996, 98)

Needed in metabolizing fatty acids, protein, carbohydrates. Supports metabolism of folate and B6, and handling of iron. Helps regenerate glutathione. Supports methylation and helps remove homocysteine.

Useful diagnostic test (JAFFE, 1992)

Erythrocyte glutathione reductase (a B2-dependent enzyme).

Supportive nutrients (SLAGLE 1993)

B, C, A, iron, copper, phosphorus.

Sources (NUTICIRCLES® 1996, SLAGLE 1993, COUSENS 2000)

Organ and lean meats. Brewer's yeast, royal jelly, bee pollen. Goat cheese, yogurt, other dairy. Fish, poultry, eggs. Almonds, wheat germ, dark leafy greens, legumes, seeds, nuts, grains, blackstrap molasses.

Effects of excess, contraindications (SLAGLE 1993)

Mildly contraceptive. Limit in pregnancy, especially second trimester.

Excess may be detrimental to cataracts.

Pantothenic acid (B5)

Pantothenic acid is needed in converting (i.e., acetylating) choline to acetylcholine (an inhibitory, antimanic neurotransmitter, important to memory and movement). It also provides critical support to the adrenals in handling stress, (Casentini 1956, Amrich 1956, Hodges 1958, Thornton 1955) and may reduce norepinephrine levels. (Vesci 1990) The brain has a high concentration of B5. Levels plummet with chronic stress, and are often low in affectives.

Mood

Deficiency can create a profound depression, typically accompanied by fatigue and exhaustion. (Hodges 1958) Low levels have also been associated with such manic symptoms as irritability, aggression, restlessness, insomnia, hyperactivity. (Brenner 1982, Tohoku 1983, Thornton 1955)

Mental & neurological symptoms (Pfeiffer 1975, Slagle 1993, Murray 1996)

B5 may provide support in the following conditions:

- ☐ Depression, sullenness, listlessness, fatigue. (Hodges 1955, Gensini.1985, Early 1969, Thornton 1955, Fry 1976)
- ☐ Chronic stress. Adrenal exhaustion. (Casentini 1956, Amrich 1956, Hodges 1958, Fry 1976, Thornton 1955, Early 1969)
- ☐ Nervousness, restlessness, ADD, hyperactivity, insomnia. (Casentini 1956, Amrich 1956, Brenner 1982) Irritability, anger, aggression. (Thornton 1955)
- ☐ Epilepsy. (Tohoku 1983, Vesci 1990) Cerebral (and other) allergies.

Biotypes (Pfeiffer 1987, 88, Walsh 2006)

Often benefits histapenia and pyroluria.

Physical functions supporting mood

Critical in adrenal moderation of extreme stress. (Thornton 1955) Helps produce cortisol and adrenal steroids. (Slagle 1996)

Decreases norepinephrine (Vecsci 1990).

Important in preventing allergies, including cerebral allergies; (Vecsci 1990, Slagle 1996) antihistamine in large doses.

Supports EFA functioning and metabolism. (Cousens 2000, Early 1969) May increase EPA and DHA, decrease AA. (Gensini 1985) Helps move fatty acids to and from mitochondria (which make energy). Lowers cholesterol and triglycerides. (Gensini 1985) (High cholesterol can cause depression. (Rogers 1997))

Antioxidant properties.

See *Allergies, Hypoglycemia,* pp. 207-18.

Chemistry

Pantethine --> CoA --> cystaeamine.

Considerations (Lieberman 1990, Balch 1990, Garrison 1985, Werbach 1991, Murray 1996, Larson 2001, Slagle 1993, Rogers 1997, Tenney 1987)

Need may be suggested by (Larson 2001, Thornton 1955, Vecsci 1990, Fry 1976, Early 1969, Slagle 1993)

Depression, increased vulnerability to stress, sullenness. Avoidance behavior.

Overstimulation, irritability, restlessness, insomnia.

Numbness, tingling, sore or burning limbs. Kindled seizures, pain.

Compromised adrenal function.

Fatigue, weakness, exhaustion.

Muscle cramps, headaches.

Allergies, hypoglycemia, susceptibility to infection, especially respiratory infections.

Hair loss, eczema, poor healing of wounds.

Low blood pressure, high cholesterol, atherosclerosis, cardiovascular conditions.

Vomiting, diarrhea, constipation, other digestive complaints.**

Levels may be depleted with ulcers, duodenal and kidney disorders, arthritis, anemia,*** alcoholism, prolactin-secreting adenomas, Huntington's, Parkinson's, chronic illness, injury, aging. Also by processed food, tobacco, caffeine, estrogen and sulfa drugs.

Nutrient interactions (Gensini 85, Pfeiffer, Early 1969, Thornton 1955, Fry 76)

Helps metabolize carbohydrates, proteins, fats, and maintain EFA balance.

Sources (Lieberman 1990, Balch 1990, Nutricircles 1996, Rogers 1997)

Most foods (*pantos* means all). Prevalent in: brewer's yeast, royal jelly, bee pollen, organ meats, herring, other fish, eggs. Also found in: dairy, poultry, flax, bran, sesame and sunflower seeds, nuts, shiitake mushrooms, potatoes, yams, legumes (soy, lentils), green vegetables (broccoli, collard greens, avocado), papaya, watermelon, banana, whole grains.

Supportive nutrients (Slagle 1993)

B, C, chromium, zinc.

Lab (Rogers 1997)

There's no readily available way to measure B5, except by trial (especially in depressives with high cholesterol and difficulty handling stress).

Form (Rogers 1997)

Pantethine is the preferred, more active form of B5.

Effects of excess, contraindications

Joint and teeth sensitivity. Diarrhea.

More B vitamins

Biotin (Lieberman 1990, Garrison 1985, Murray 1996, Jaffe 1992, Balch 1990)

Physical effects supporting mood

Supports energy metabolism.
Helps prevent blood sugar elevation.*
Supports fatty acid synthesis.
Promotes intestinal flora and may help counter Candida. (Yamaguchi 1974)

* Enhances insulin secretion and response, and helps the liver convert glucose to glycogen.

Mood

□ Deficiency can be associated with depression, anxiety, lethargy, and fatigue, as well as such manic symptoms as irritability, insomnia, and hallucinations. (Levenson 1983, Shirayama 2002)

□ Helpful in pyrrole disorder (as it's often depleted). (McGinnis 2004, 08)

□ Helps produce serotonin and fatty acids, and counter Candida.

Note: Anticonvulsives (most mood stabilizers) can deplete biotin.

Considerations (Lieberman 1990, Krohn 1991, Garrison 1985, Murray 1996, Jaffe 1992)

Need may be suggested by

Anxiety, panic, irritability, perhaps hallucinations.
Depression. Extreme fatigue, numbness, weakness.
Pale smooth tongue, dry greyed skin, scaly dermatitis, hair loss. Other skin, nail, and hair changes. (Pawlowski 1966, Haneke 1994)
Nausea, appetite loss. Low intestinal flora.
Carbohydrate intolerance. Allergies. Mild anemia.*
Muscle pain, chest pain. Headaches.
Tendency to hypertension, alcoholism.
Compromised fetal development, increased birth defects.

* As biotin is used in hemoglobin production.

Populations (Murray 1996)

Deficiency can occur with chronic stress, or pyroluria. Also, extended use of anticonvulsives (most mood stabilizers), (Mock 1998) antibiotics, sulfa drugs; and high intake of raw egg whites;* possibly, long-term high-dose B5.

* Which contain avidin, which prevents biotin absorption.

Nutrient interactions

Supports fatty acid synthesis. Required in fat, carbohydrate and protein metabolism.

Useful diagnostic test (Jaffe 1992)

Carboxylase.

Sources of biotin (Balch1990)

Cheese, organ meats, nutritional yeast, cauliflower, royal jelly, liver, egg yolk, fish, lamb, meats, nuts, dairy, legumes (soy, chick peas, lentils), whole grains (barley, oats, rice, wheat). Biotin is also made by intestinal bacteria.

Supplementation & supportive nutrients

30-100 mcg. Supportive nutrients include B complex, manganese, C, CoQ10, carnitine. (Murray 1996, Slagle 1993)

Effects of excess

May foster a blood sugar drop.

PABA (Lieberman 1990, Krohn 1991, Garrison, 1985, Balch 1990)

Physical effects supporting mood

Stimulates gut bacteria to form folic acid (needed in forming norepinephrine and serotonin), and B5 (for acetylcholine).

Helps maintain intestinal flora, and prevent some allergies.

Mood

PABA is prescribed in China as an antidepressant.

Deficiency has been associated with depression, irritability, nervousness, fatigue, increased susceptibility to stress, and symptoms of low B5 or acetylcholine.

Considerations (Lieberman 1990, Krohn 1991, Garrison 1985, Balch 1990)

Need may be suggested by

Irritability, anxiety, depression, fatigue. Headaches.
Eczema, other skin disorders.* Hair loss, or greying.
Constipation, other digestive complaints.
Possibly, anemia** allergies, overactive thyroid.
Chronic antibiotic use (which may deplete PABA).

* PABA also helps protect skin from UV rays.
** It's involved in blood cell formation.

Nutrient interactions

Helps metabolize protein, and form folate and B5.

Sources

Liver, kidneys, nutritional yeast, whole grains, mushrooms, molasses, legumes, spinach. Also made by gut bacteria.

Supplementation & supportive nutrients

50 mg or more. Supportive nutrients: C, B, folate.

Effects of excess, contraindications

Excess is stored in, and may damage the liver.
Malaise, nausea, anorexia. Skin rash. Fever.
Decreased white blood cells.
Can temporarily reduce female fertility.

2. Antioxidants

"[In] mitigating neuronal injury... antioxidants [are]... a no-brainer, as oxidative stress, especially when toxic substances are in contact with cells, is always an issue." — Charles Gant, MD, 1991

Vitamin C	Glutathione
Herbs, foods	Lipoic acid
Bioflavonoids	NAC
Vitamin E	Molybdenum
CoQ10	Vitamin A
Selenium	Carotenes
Enzymes	Miscellaneous

The brain is particularly susceptible to oxidative damage due to vulnerable neurotransmitter systems, high levels of fats, and of oxygen and other oxidizing agents (e.g., iron, copper, excitotoxins, PLA2, etc.), and the difficulty of neuronal repair. Antioxidants protect cells from oxidative damage by slowing oxidation, and scavenging free radicals (neutralizing them by donating an electron). They thus protect the following brain constituents associated with mediation of mood:

□ EFAs, phospholipids and other brain fats — thereby, receptor and second messenger function, blood brain barrier and myelin integrity, and prostaglandin formation. (Emerit 1989, Ernster 1991, Kut'ko 1996, Kogolu 2002, Aleksandrovskii 1988, Ranjekar 2003)

□ Neurotransmitters and mechanisms for their creation — catecholamine pathways (often antidepressant) are particularly vulnerable, as is the catecholamine/GABA balance (important to mood stability). (Cohen 1984, Graham 1978, Hoffer 1990)

□ Neurons — otherwise oxidative assault could disorganize neural activity, destroy the cell, or make it so unrecognizable, that it provokes an autoimmune attack. (Horrobin 2000, Kogolu 2002)

□ Brain enzymes, metabolism, and access to energy.

Since antioxidants protect brain structure and function, benefit to mood and cognition should not be suprising.* Oxidative stress is, in fact, prevalent in bipolars.

Mental health research thus far has focused on vitamins C, E, selenium, glutathione, NAC, zinc, B3, B6, lipoic acid, melatonin, and nutrients supporting metal metabolism and methylation, though other antioxidants may also be important. (Leng 1998, Ranjekar 2003, Larson 2001, Abdalla 1986, Kuloglu 2002, Benton 1991, Altschule 1955, Hoffer 1990, Mahadik 1996, Reddy 1996, 91, Kutlo 1996, Walsh 2006, 08, Horrobin 2000)

* In fact, early "megavitamin" therapies began, in 1954, with Hoffer's free-radical "adrenochrome hypothesis" (that oxidized catecholamines might foster schizophrenia), leading to the development of a successful, largely antioxidant, niacin/vitamin-C therapy (later expanded). Hoffer (2008b) recently suggested oxidation of the profuse catecholamines of mania may similarly underly psychotic mania. Schizophrenia and bipolar disorder share many pro-oxidant triggers (stress, allergies, stimulants, PLA2 overactivity, excitotoxicity, metal toxicity and other mineral imbalances); while antioxidants, such as C, B3, NAD, B6, E and zinc, address both psychosis and mood. (Hoffer 1990, Graham 1978, Mathews 1985, Pfeiffer 1975) (See pp. 82, 268.)

Free radicals (Emerit 1989, Capel 1988)

Free radicals are highly reactive molecules with at least one unpaired electron. Such electrons readily transfer to other molecules, oxidizing and altering them.

Free radicals are produced and used by the body, and are also naturally present in the environment. At normal levels, the body can neutralize them efficiently. Overexposure, however, can overwhelm and inactivate coping mechanisms, creating profound damage to the brain or other organs, to DNA patterns, and immune and cardiovascular function; and generally accelerating aging. (Masoro 1984, Gaev 1988, Ku 1993, Sohal 1994, Stram 1990) Free radicals can also destroy key gut enzymes (e.g., those which break down casein and gluten), and alter absorption and digestion (creating diarrhea, cramps, multiple food sensitivity, etc.), with repercussions on brain activity in vulnerable persons. (Walsh 2002, 04ab, 06)

Free radicals multiply in overcooked, processed, and, especially, fried, microwaved or irradiated food. Oxidative stress is magnified by MT dysfunction and high levels of pro-oxidant metals (e.g., copper, iron), homocysteinuria, various hormone imbalances, physical illness, sugar, tobacco, alcohol, certain drugs, pesticides, other pollutants, etc. Significant exposure to ionizing radiation or intake of radioactive materials creates massive quantities of free radicals, which can severely alter and destroy tissue, perhaps fatally.

The extent of the damage depends on the nature of the exposure, diet, antioxidant and nutritional status, patterns of protective enzymes, fatty acid levels and membrane integrity, MT function, methylating activity, endocrine balances, stress, age, genetic factors, etc. (Capel 1988) Peroxidation seems to be directly correlated with emotional stress. (Aleksandrovskii 1988)

Importance of taking multiple antioxidants

Taking a variety of antioxidants, along with those particularly indicated, enhances effectiveness, as:*

□ Different antioxidants are specific to given free radicals, and to distinct stages of detox.

□ Antioxidants are oxidized in neutralizing free radicals, and then may act as free radicals, themselves, unless specific antioxidants are available to recycle them to their original (reduced) state: (Beyer 1994, Ohlen1994, Ketterer 1983, Gotz 1994, Kagen 1990)

— Glutathione (GSH) helps restore CoQ10, E, NAD. (Ohlenschlager 1994, Ketterer 1983)

— Anthocyanins help regenerate glutathione. (Ohlenschlager 1994)

—Lipoic acid helps spare or recycle CoQ, GSH, E, C. (Gotz 1994, Kehrer 1993, Packer 1997, Murray 1996)

— Beta carotene, C, CoQ, & GSH help recycle E. (Kehrer 1993. Kagen 1990)

* But consider contraindications, e.g., if copper is elevated or MTs suppressed, until resolved, lipoic acid, certain SODs, and certain copper-rich antioxidant herbs may need to be limited. Also see *Lipoic acid issues,* p 178; *Side effects* (cysteine & NAC), p. 166; etc.

"Vitamin C and niacin (B3) (in dosages that provide a mild blushing sensation) provide almost instant relief to the overactive mind and help focus mental concentration."

Carl C Pfeiffer, PhD, MD

"I have found a lot of depressive and manic symptoms have responded to a combination of vitamin C and magnesium supplements....several grams of vitamin C via powder with bioflavonoids and ... magnesium...to calm the nerves and... [hold] back mania. My mood has picked up, sleep and concentration is improved, I socialize better and am more motivated in the day... I am a lot better now."

Anonymous

History: Vitamin C & scurvy (MURRAY 1996)

Scurvy is caused by an extended vitamin C deficit. Depression and irritability often occur early. Other symptoms can include fatigue, weakness, apathy, aches and pains. Eventually, gums bleed, teeth fall out, wounds fail to heal, and coiled hairs may appear in leg sores. (GOLD 1987) Exhaustion intensifies. Hysteria, hypochondria, profound depression often develop and, in some cases, psychosis. Without treatment, many die. (HODGES 1971)

Until the nineteenth century, epidemics of scurvy killed countless sailors on lengthy sea voyages, as well as Europeans enduring long winters without fresh food.

In 1742, James Lind proposed a dietary cause, and in a study showed lemon juice produced recovery. A quarter of a century passed before Captain James Cook, in 1768 and 1779, introduced citrus to his crew's rations. After another 25 years, the British navy began to regularly carry citrus (earning its sailors the nickname "limies").

In 1928 Albert Szent-Gyorgyi identified vitamin C as the active principle.

RECOMMENDED READING

Irwin Stone, *The Healing Factor: Vitamin C against Disease*, 1974

Emmanuel Cheraskin, *The Vitamin C Connection*, 1983

Thomas Levy, *Vitamin C, Infectious Diseases, & Toxins: Curing the Incurable*, 2002

Vitamin C (ascorbic acid)

Research suggests vitamin C benefits both mania and bipolar depression, and may be critical for bipolars. (TOLBERT 1979AB, MILNER 1963, NAYLOR 1981, 84, KAY 1984, HOFFER 1983, 87) Its ability to counter scurvy, support histamine balance, help form serotonin, decrease vanadium toxicity, and reduce allergic sensitivity contribute to its effectiveness. (SUBOTICANEC 1984, PFEIFFER 1975, BEAUCLAIR 1987, COCCHI 1989)

Levels

The second highest concentration of vitamin C occurs in the brain (the highest is in the adrenals). C is often so low in psychiatric patients as to approach levels found in scurvy.*(MILNER 1963, VON LEITNER 1956, SHORAH 1983) Moreover, anxiety, excitement, and stress use it up, increasing need. (MAAS 1961, BAUMEL 1995)

* In a study by Milner (1963), most of 465 psychiatric patients took 6 days to achieve vitamin C tissue saturation as compared to 1-2 days in normals; 10% took over 7 days. This degree of depletion is found in borderline or clinical scurvy, and the above patients, not suprisingly, showed signs of scurvy. Similarly, Leitner (1956) found average plasma C in 885 psychiatic patients less than 60% of control levels; in one third, less than 40% (i.e., below 35 mg/100ml). Depletion was associated with immune and behavioral changes.

Mania (TOLBERT, 1979, REBEC 1985, PAULING, SUBOTICANEC 1984, 86, MILNER 1963, VANDERKAMP 1966, CHERASKIN 1983, GOLD 1987, QUILLIN 1987)

Vitamin C may be a natural tranquilizer-antipsychotic-antimanic agent. (MILNER 1963, REBEC, 1985) Hoffer (2005) reports it effective, even by itself, in countering psychosis in some patients. Preliminary work by Tolbert suggests it occupies the same (dopamine) receptor sites as phenothiazines (antipsychotics, also used for mania), and can be equally as powerful in blocking receptors, minus the drug's side effects. Relatively large doses of C are required because, as a nutrient, it does not cross the blood brain barrier as readily as meds (against which nature has not had much opportunity to develop a defense). (TOLBERT 1979, SUBOTICANEC 1984) Orthomolecular recommendations for a tranquilizing effect cluster around 10 grams and up, either divided into hourly portions [0.5-1.5 gm/hour], or with time-release C, perhaps every two hours [e.g., 2 gm/2-hrs].

Some practitioners administer IVs, which, though more cumbersome, are generally more potent, more effective acutely, and sidestep absorption problems. (COCCHI 1989, LARSON 2008) (For contraindications, etc., see pp. 56, 144.)

Depression (TOLBERT 1979, REBEC 1985, MILNER 1963, HODGES 1971, CHERASKIN 1983, SLAGLE 1992)

Vitamin C is also antidepressant. It helps form both serotonin and norepinephrine, key antidepressant transmitters. And depletion causes depression. In fact, depression is usually among the presenting symptoms of scurvy (chronic lack), persisting until C is repleted. Cousens (2000) finds 95% of his depressive clients need more vitamin C.

Other symptoms (PFEIFFER 1987, SLAGLE 1992, BAUMEL 1995)

- ☐ Problems with mood, cognition, socialization, isolation, well-being, lethargy. (VANDERCAMP 1965, 66, GOLD 1987, KANOFSKY 1989, BEAUCLAIR 1987, MILNER 1963)
- ☐ Anxiety, severe tension, stress. (TOLBERT, 1979, REBEC 1985, MILNER 1963)
- ☐ Psychosis, paranoia, voices, schizophrenia. (SUBOTICANEC 1984, 86, TOLBERT 1979, PFEIFFER 1975, 87, HOFFER 1987, 2005)

Antioxidant & immune function (PFEIFFER 1987, SLAGLE 1992, BAUMEL 1995, PAULING)

C is an important antioxidant, protecting cells, hormones, E and enzymes from free radical assault. It also stimulates the immune system; increases resistance to stress, infection and inflammation; helps eliminate toxins and heavy metals; (VANDERKAMP 1966, HOLLOWAY 1984) and (buffered with minerals) is important in neutralizing allergic reactions. (PHILPOTT 1984) Such functions may help stabilize mood indirectly, by protecting brain integrity.

Possible mechanisms underlying mood benefits (COUSENS 2001, SLAGLE 1992, PFEIFFER 1975, 87, REBEC 1985, NAYLOR 1984, KAY 1984)

MANIA
Blocks dopamine receptor sites.
Helps form serotonin (via BH4).
Helps form COMT, which breaks down epinephrines in the synapse.
Anti-anxiety, antipsychotic.

DEPRESSION
Helps form NE and Ser.
Protects catecholamine pathways. Helps prevent NE breakdown.
Supports removal of neural sodium. Decreases vanadium toxicity.

STABILIZATION
Supports histamine balance.
Benefits cerebral allergies.
Supports immunity.
Antioxidant.
Helps remove heavy metals, toxins.

Considerations (CHERASKIN 1983, GOLD 1987, QUILLIN 1987, PFEIFFER 1975, REBEC 1985, LIEBERMAN 1990, KROHN 1991, HOFFER 1983, BALCH 1990, RUDIN 1987, WERBACH 1991, TENNEY 1987, GARRISON 1985)

Need may be suggested by (SLAGLE 1992)

Moodiness, depression, fatigue, apathy, confusion, weakness, listlessness.

Mania, paranoia, psychosis. Irritability, tension.

Rough skin, easy bruising, slow healing of wounds or burns, bleeding gums, nose-bleeds, other bleeding.*

Aches, pain, edema.

Recurrent infections, allergies. (ANDERSON 1984)

Reduced appetite, constipation, digestive problems.

Weak adrenals. Hypothyroid. Inefficient use of iodine. Other endocrine problems. (HOLLOWAY 1984)

Tendency to drug-induced delirium, drug sensitivity, addictions. Alcoholic psychosis.

Prone to accumulate metals.

* Generally weak blood vessel walls. C is critical in forming collagen and connective tissue.

Conditions promoting depletion (SLAGLE 1992, BAUMEL 1995)

Illness, high fever. Prolonged stress (bipolars, depression, anxiety, pyroluria, etc.). Adrenal exhaustion, hyperthyroid. High estrogen, pregnancy, nursing, oral contraceptives. Inflammation, surgery, burns, allergies, Candida. Excess copper, iron, protein, or junk food. Toxicity (chemicals, mercury, lead, cadmium, radiation, alcohol, tobacco, street drugs. Chronic antibiotics, salicylates (e.g., aspirin), barbiturates, amphetamines, cortisone. Deficit is common in the elderly, the malnourished, psychiatric and institutionalized patients, alcoholics.

Nutrient interactions

Contributes to metabolism and use of EFAs, iron, folic acid, amino acids.

Sources (NUTRICIRCLES ® 1996)

Fresh, uncooked fruits and vegetables. Peppers, kale, kiwi, lemon, lime, satsuma, kumquat, orange, black currant, strawberry, acerola cherry, tomatoe, parsley, sorrel, pomegranate, guava, mango, papaya.

Useful diagnostic test (JAFFE, 1992)

White blood cell ascorbate.

Therapeutic doses (JAFFE 1992, WERBACH 1991, STONE 1979, CHERASKIN 1983)

Primates are among the few animals that don't create C internally. Linus Pauling has estimated that relative to what most animals produce, the human dose should be 2-19 grams (in the higher range with stress).

Therapeutic doses vary from 100 mg to 5 gm, 2-4x/day. When maximal doses are indicated, they are often set just below that which produces diarrhea. Any reductions (if indicated) should be gradual.

C should be taken at least twice daily, to prevent fluctuations and deficiency reactions. Sustained-release C (two or more per day) may also help.

In patients dealing with toxicity, dose is sometimes temporarily lowered to reduce toxic release.

Forms

Buffered C (before meals) is often helpful, but the minerals may reduce the amount of C that can be taken. C from sago palm, etc., can be used for patients allergic to corn (of which most supplements are made). Powdered C may increase absorption. Ester C enhances effectiveness.

Effects of excess, contraindications (LIEBERMAN1990, KROHN 1991, HOFFER 1983B, WERBACH 1991)

Nausea or diarrhea if dosage is to high.

Occasionally, 1-2 gm, over months, can cause a burning sensation on urination, or a skin rash.

Rarely, people of Asian or Mediterranean heritage have an enzyme deficiency which causes red blood cell destruction on exposure to large doses of C.

High doses, in rare cases, decrease white blood cell antibacterial activity.

Excessive intake (probably as *sodium* ascorbate) may exacerbate kidney disorders.

As *ascorbic acid* may, rarely, activate peptic ulcers.

Antioxidant herbs

Grape seed extract, rosemary, turmeric, milk thistle, bilberry, amla fruit, pine leaf, green tea, ginger root, rose hips, hibiscus, lemon grass, golgi berries, noni, acai, resveratrol, etc.

Antioxidant foods

Raw vegetables, berries and fruits. (Deep colors (e.g., dark leafy greens, beets, blackberries, yams) usually indicate high antioxidant content.) Sprouts and grasses. Seeds and nuts, preferably sprouted.

Bioflavonoids

(Pfeiffer 1975, 87, Lieberman 1990, Krohn 1991, Balch 1990, Casey-Smith 1983, 86, Bland 1984, Tolbert, 1979, VanderKamp 1966, Cheraskin 1983, Beauclair 1987, Ohlenschlager 1996, Makhtar 1992)

"I believe a leaf of grass is no less than the journeywork of the stars....And the running blackberry would adorn the parlors of heaven..." — Walt Whitman, *Song of Myself,* poem XXXI

Bioflavonoids are water soluble phenol-type phytochemicals, linked to the coloring matter in fruits and vegetables. Bioflavonoids are strong antioxidants. They play a critical role in the absorption, use and storage of C, and protect adrenalin and C from oxidation. Bioflavonoids work with C as antioxidants and immunity agents, and may similarly contribute to its mood-moderating, anti-anxiety, and antipsychotic effects.

□ **Rutin** — seems to exert a combined sedative/stimulant effect and has been found helpful for depression and high blood pressure.

□ **Quercetin** — known for its beneficial effects on allergies; helps prevent histamine loss,* improving histapenic depression, anxiety, and other symptoms. It also helps block release of inflammatory chemicals (leukotrienes) associated with depression.

□ **Anthocyanidins**—flavonal-type bioflavonoids, second only to melatonin in antioxidant potency. They support vitamin C activity, help protect glutathione and C from oxidation, help recycle C and E, and relieve symptoms of oxidative stress such as fatigue. (Ohlenschlager 1996)

□ **Catechins** — may help protect the liver from oxidative stress. (Makhtar 1992)

* Quercetin has a strong affinity for mast cells and basophils, both of which store histamine; it also stabilizes the cell membrane, preventing histamine loss.

Considerations

Need may be suggested by

Depression, fatigue, anxiety.

Inflammation. Allergies. Infections. Liver toxicity.

Bruising, capillary fragility, varicose veins, psoriasis, dental problems. Other collagen disorders.

Arthritis (anthocyanidins).

Tendency to clots, high blood pressure, high cholesterol, insufficient oxygen. Cardiovascular problems.

Prone to bladder disorders, cataracts, diabetes, or high estrogen.

** Bioflavonoids, especially anthocyanidins, support the interweaving of collagen molecules, strengthening skin, tendons, ligaments and bone.

Sources of bioflavonoids (Balch 1990, Bland 1984)

Citrus (especially the white portion of citrus peels and pulp), grapes, plums, black currants, apricots, cherries, blackberries, elder flowers, lemon balm, rose hips, and other fresh fruits and vegetables.

□ Rutin — buckwheat

□ Hesperidin — lemons and sweet oranges.

□ Quercetin & epicatechins — blue-green algae, onion, rinds and barks of wild fruits and trees, clover blossom, eucalyptus, pansies, and green tea (catechins).

□ Anthocyanidins — red-purple fruits and vegetables, e.g., bilberry, red cabbage, purple grape skin, cranberries, blackberries.

Vitamin E

(Quillin 1987, Pfeiffer 1975, 87, 88, Lieberman 1990, Krohn 1991, Hoffer 1983, Rudin 1987, Werbach 1991, Tenney 1987, Garrison 1985, Cousens 1990)

"We didn't make vitamin E so versatile. God did. Ignore its mercy at your peril." — Evan Shute, MD

Depletion has been associated with a greater degree of depression. (Owen 2005, De Vos 1995) In a study by Morishita (2000), E augmentation created significant improvement in six of nine patients experiencing prolonged depressions.

E is abundant in the brain/pituitary/adrenal axis (which mediates anxiety and stress), and is reported to interfere with transmission of anxiety impulses from the emotional (limbic system) to the thinking brain (cerebral cortex). (Lieberman 1990) Low levels are associated with increased susceptibility to stress. (Aleksandrovskii 1988)

Vitamin E has also been used to treat moodswing, hostility, and pellagra, and has shown benefit to concentration, memory, attention span, alertness, motivation, cognitive impairment. (BiolTrace El Res 1985, Cousens 2001) It is often used in orthomolecular treatment of schizophrenia. (Pfeiffer 1987, Hoffer 1978, DeLiz 1975) It also supports brain circulation, can block porphyrin activity (see), and may help preserve neurological function. (*Can J Neuro Sci* 1984, *Free Rad Biol Med* 1989, Muller 1986, Barak 1998)

Antioxidant function

Vitamin E is an important antioxidant. It protects fatty acids, (Beyer 1994, Kogolu 1986 Stork 2005) hormones, and vitamins A, C and K. Tocopherols (components of E complex) sit on the cell membrane, where they identify free radicals and neutralize them, by donating an electron.

Considerations (vitamin E) (Quillin 1987, Pfeiffer 1975, 87,88, Lieberman 1990, Krohn 1991, Hoffer 1978, 83ab, Tenney 1987, Garrison 1985, Cousens 2001, Slagle, Murray 1996, Kuloglu 2002, Muller 1986, Stork 2005, DeLiz 1975, Balch 1990)

Need may be suggested by (Cousens 2001, Murray 1996)

Depression, anxiety, restlessness, insomnia, hostility, mood swing. (*BioTrace El Res,* 1985)

Perhaps, neurological symptoms. (*Can J Neuro Sci* 1984, *Free Rad Biol Med* 1989, Muller 1986, Barak 1998)

Muscle weakness. Fatigue.*(Stork 2005)

High cholesterol. Cardiovascular disorders.

Reproductive disorders, menopausal symptoms. (Murray 1996)

Dry dull hair; hair loss. Dry skin, scarring; other skin problems. Poor wound healing.

Immune vulnerability. Allergies. Inflammation.

Diabetes. (Murray 1996, Cicero 2004) Gastrointestinal problems.

Eye problems. (Berson 1993)

Aging. (Cousens 2001, Murray 1996)

Tardive dyskinesia. (Murray 1996, Barak 1998)

* E is essential to muscle, cardiovascular, and skeletal health; and enhances oxygen use and athletic performance. (Cousens 2001)

Nutrient interactions (Murray 1996)

Protects fatty acids and influences prostaglandin activity.

Helps maintain RNA and DNA function.

May support B12 activation.

Sources (NutriCircles® 1996)

Seeds, nuts, nut butters, fish and fish oil, wheat germ, purslane, grain germs, sprouted grains and beans, whole grains. Some in leafy greens, sweet potatoes.

Supportive nutrients

Selenium supports vitamin E activity. Beta carotene, CoQ10, glutathione and C regenerate oxidized E.

Therapeutic dose range (Wehrbach, 1991)

Dosage often start at 100 IU and may increase to 400-600, (Cousens 2001) in more extreme cases, 800-1600. Dose increases should be gradual. High doses should not be taken indefinitely, as E is less readily eliminated than water-soluble vitamins. With heart conditions or diabetes, the water miscible form is often preferable, with doses introduced gradually and, perhaps, kept low.

Effects of excess, contraindications

Sudden or sustained high doses can raise blood pressure and triglycerides, and may play a role in blood clots.

Monitor for reduced insulin requirements.

High doses (e.g, over 1200 IU) may increase the time needed for blood to clot.

High doses may cause palpitations, fainting, dizziness, nausea, gas, or diarrhea.

Megadoses may decrease thyroid hormone levels.

Extremely high doses (e.g, over 4,000 IU during pregnancy, may foster malformations.

Coenzyme Q-10 (ubiquinone)

CoQ10 may help support mood, particularly in individuals requiring enhanced cellular oxygenation and energetics, and antioxidant protection. (Stork 2005, Kato 2000, Konradi 2004, Dager 2004, Schweitzer 2004, Prabakaran 2004, Quiroz 2004) Researchers have explored benefit to depression, anxiety, mental lethargy, fatigue, memory, attention difficulties, certain schizophrenias and some neurodegenerative conditions (M.S, Alzheimer's). (Eikasbef 1994)

Antioxidant function (Murray 1996, Beyer 1994)

CoQ-10 resembles E and is an even stronger antioxidant, important in protecting the mitochondria (which produce cellular energy), and cell membranes.

Considerations (Eikasbef 1994, Lieberman 1990, Krohn 1991, Balch 1990, Garrison 1985, Murray 1996, Cousens 2001)

Need may be suggested by

Anxiety, difficulty focusing, poor memory.

Lethargy, depression, fatigue.*

Immune weakness, Candida.

Asthma, allergies, high histamine. High blood sugar.

High blood pressure. (Gaby 1996) Cardiac hypofunction.

Muscle weakness, lack of endurance. Muscular dystrophy. (Murray 1996, Folkers 1995)

Periodontal disease.

*Helps cells use oxygen and create energy. Catalyzes production of ATP.

Sources

Sardines, salmon, mackerel, cold-water fish, spinach, whole grains. Modest amounts in most foods. Also made in body cells. Plasma levels in vegetarians are over twice that in meat eaters. (Lieberman 1990, Murray 1996)

Supportive nutrients

B, C, and E help produce CoQ10. It works with carnitine and B5. (Kagen 1990)

Dose

10-125 mg, typically 30-75 mg.

Effects of excess, contraindications

Gastrointestinal disturbances (nausea, diarrhea, etc.)

Suddenly stopping intake can contribute to congestive heart failure. (Cousens 2001)

Selenium (Se)

Research, including at least one double blind crossover, suggests supplementation improves depression, especially in those with low selenium. (BENTON 1990, 91, 2002) Mood benefits may be due to improvement in thyroid status (SHER 2001, GARDNER 2002) as well as antioxidant activity, and general immune support. (SHER 2002AB, TATUM 2004)

Berry has proposed that with environmental insult, low selenium (and consequently, glutathione peroxidase) can disregulate the dopamine system, allowing dopamine-containing cells to burst. Reduced dopamine levels could then lead to such symptoms as social withdrawal, apathy, emotional flatness, poverty of speech and thought, anhedonia, and brain damage; while excess could overstimulate, perhaps triggering mania or psychosis. (BERRY 1992, 93)

Selenium may also improve anxiety, fatigue, alertness, motivation, general well-being, self-care, (BRAVERMAN 1987, BENTON 1991, HOFFER 1983AB) and may help preserve cognitive function. (AKBARALY 2007)

Antioxidant function

As an antioxidant, selenium helps protect fatty acids, cell membranes, and mitochondria from oxidation. It is a key component of glutathione peroxidase, a major endogenous free-radical-scavenging enzyme.

Considerations (GARRISON 1985, BALCH 1990, PAGE 1992, LIEBERMAN 1990, KROHN 1991, PFEIFFER 1975, 87, 88, BRAVERMAN 1987, WERBACH 1991)

Need may be suggested by (ROGERS 1997, MURRAY 1996, PFEIFFER 1975, 88)

Ambivalence, anxiety, depression, moodswing.

Hypothyroid. Low blood pressure.

Immune vulnerability.* Increased susceptibility to illness, heavy metals, other toxins, cancer. Problems with antibody production.

Fatigue, weakness. Incapacitated by hot weather.

Liver, pancreatic, or heart dysfunction

Arthritis, skin disorders, muscular dystrophy, chromosome breakage. Inflammatory disease. Cataracts.

Levels are low in bottle-fed infants,** malnourished children, people who eat too much processed food.

* Se may inhibit replication of strains of AIDs, hepatitis, and other viruses.

** Nursing infants receive six times the selenium (and twice the E) of infants fed cow milk. Low E and Se may contribute to crib deaths. (Pfeiffer)

Nutrient interactions (ROGERS 1997)

Works with glutathione and metallothionein against oxidative stress and metal overloads. (Walsh 2008)

Selenium protects fatty acids and E from oxidation, enhances the effectiveness of E, supports vitamin C activity, and is used in producing CoQ-10. It also helps metabolize EFAs and synthesize proteins.

Sources (NUTRICIRCLES ® 1996, PFEIFFER)

Seafoods (tuna, salmon, etc., kelp). Animal foods. Brazil nuts, poultry, sunflower seeds, brewer's yeast, grains, mushrooms, onions, garlic, tomatoes, eggs, liver. Reflects soil content (e.g., depleted in glaciated regions).

Dose

100-200 mcg.

Effects of excess, contraindications

Garlic odor in breath, urine and sweat (usually, at 500 mcg or more). (HARR 1972)

Nausea. (MURRAY 1996)

Irritability, behavior disorders, emotional instability.

Depression, fatigue. (MURRAY 1996)

Altered composition of enamel during tooth formation. Tooth decay. (HADJIMARKOS 1973)

Thick fragile fingernails, eczema, dermatitis, hair loss. (PFEIFFER 1975, HADJIMARKOS 1973, MURRAY 1996)

Convulsions, progressive paralysis. (MARLOWE 1986)

Acute poisoning (e.g., industrial) can produce fever, rapid breathing, gastroenteritis, myelitis (spinal cord and bone marrow inflammation), anorexia, death.

Avoid the selenite form, which increases free radical creation.

Antioxidant enzymes

Endogenous (made by the body) antioxidant enzymes protect immune and neurological function. Levels in bipolars are often depleted. (RANJEKAR 2003) Selenium, manganese, zinc, etc., support respective enzyme formation.

Key antioxidant enzymes include:

Glutathione peroxidase — a selenium-based enzyme. Levels may be reduced in depression. (STOKLASOVA 1990AB) Chronic depletion has been linked to increased ventricle size and brain atrophy in negative-symptom, nonparanoid schizophrenia, (STOKLASOVA 1986, 90AB, BERRY 1992, BUCKMAN 1987, 90, REDDY 1991) and in some chronic bipolars.

Superoxide dismutases (SODs) — copper/zinc, or manganese-dependent enzymes. Low red blood cell superoxide dismutase has been correlated with neurological soft signs. (REDDY 1993) Excess, however, with relatively low levels of the other antioxidant enzymes, can increase peroxidation. (ABDALLA 1986, REDDY 1991, 93. BERRY 1992AB)

Catalase — an iron-based enzyme, catalyzes reduction of hydrogen peroxide to water and oxygen.

Sulfur-containing antioxidants (pp. 79-80)

Sulfur-containing antioxidants include: glutathione, lipoic acid, NAC, methionine and various phytochemicals.* NAC is critical with MT disorder and histapenia; glutathione and methionine, in histadelia; (Braverman 1987, Walsh 2000, 04ab, Pfeiffer 1987) lipoic acid, when mercury is elevated. (Cutler 2000)

* Such as the following thiols: Glucosoinolates (found in broccoli), which protect specific tissue and activate liver detox enzymes, cytokines, and white blood cells; allylic sulfides (in garlic), which protect the heart and immune system from oxidative stress; and indoles, which increase glutathione, and inactivate toxins.

Glutathione (GSH)

GSH production is depleted in many bipolars. Altschule (1955, 95) suggests it may have antidepressant activity.

Role in methylation may help counter depression (Walsh 2007)

□ Chronically low glutathione can compromise methylation,* potentially fostering a prolonged, perhaps severe, depression. (See pp. 155-8.)

* GSH is needed to connect B12 to methyl, which goes on to convert homocysteine to methionine. (Walsh 2006, 07, 08)

Antioxidant mechanisms which may support mood

□ Helps recycle/spare other antioxidants.

□ Supports metal metabolism, thereby countering oxidative stress. Glutathione allows MTs to work, and enhances zinc's effectiveness. However usable levels of GSH are limited, after which MTs take over. (Walsh 2008)

□ Protects mitochondria, membranes, and general neural integrity. (Kidd 1997, Tateishi 1981, Saez 1982, Ohlenschlager 1994, Ketterer 1983, Gotz 1994, Levy 1991, De Leve 1991, Pal 1994, Altschule 1955)

□ Decreases glutamate. Helps protect from NMDA-mediated toxicity. (Levy 1991)

□ Source of non-oxidized cysteine (which otherwise auto-oxidizes and can be excitotoxic). (Tateishi 81, Kidd 97, Saez 82)

□ Critical to phase II liver detox (e.g., from heavy metals, radiation, pesticides, fungicides, plastics, nitrates, cigarettes). (Ketterer 1983, DeLeve 1991, Sumanthi 1996, Bland 1997)

Other mechanisms which may support mood

□ Acts as a neurotransmitter.

□ Supports prostaglandin metabolism.

□ Benefits allergies, including cerebral allergies.

□ Supports brain carbohydrate metabolism. (Altschule 57)

□ May support cerebrospinal healing. (Ketterer 83, Levy 91, De Leve 91)

Considerations

Need may be suggested by

Depression, perhaps psychosis.
Immune dysfunction. Low zinc. Toxicity. Allergies.
Kidney and liver dysfunction. (Ketterer 1983, Levy 1991, De Leve 1991) Cirrhosis. Problems with blood cell formation.
Low energy ** Perhaps hypothyroidism (Engin 2005).
Tendency to cataracts, arthritis, cell proliferation

Nutrient interactions

Cysteine and glycine help form glutathione.
Helps recycle CoQ10, E, NAD.
Works with MT, selenium, zinc. And GSH peroxidase.
Supports protein and DNA synthesis and repair

Effects of excess

Detox reactions (fatigue, muscle aches, slight fever).

Lipoic acid

Lipoic acid has shown some benefit to depression, (Salazar 2000) memory, (Stoll 1993) nerve damage, (Altenkirch 1990) and neurotoxicity. As a disulfide it is highly effective in detoxifying and chelating certain heavy metals. (See *Mercury*, pp. 174-80.) It also helps create cellular energy, (Murray 1996) and improves glucose use (perhaps benefitting diabetic neuropathy and alcohol toxicity). (Tritschier 1995, Gotz 1994, Grunert 1960, Muller 1990, Sumathi 1994ab, 96)

Antioxidant function

Protects neurotransmitter systems and brain structures. Widely effective, as it works in both fat and water soluble tissue, in both its oxidized and reduced form. (Suzuki 1991, Murray 1996) Recycles or spares E, C, (Podda 1994, Murray 1996, Packer 1997) glutathione, beta carotine. (Gotz 1994) Helps protect the brain when taking stimulating supplements or foods (e.g., carnitine, phenylanine, SAMe). (Crayhon 1998)

Considerations

Need may be suggested by

Depression, poor memory. Neurotoxicity/degeneration.
Excess lactic acid. Fatigue (low ATP). (Murray 1996)
Reduced muscle mass. Failure to thrive. (Murray 1996)
Alcohol toxicity, (Passwater 1995) diabetic neuropathy. (Nichols 1997) Immune dysfunction. Liver disorders. (Murray 1996)
Heavy metal poisoning, (Tritschier 1995, Grunert 1960, Muller 1990, Sumathi 1994, 96) chemical sensitivity; exposure to radiation, (Rogers 1997) venom, (Lorano 1994) amanita. (Murray 1996)
Cataracts, aging. Heart conditions. (Murray 1996)

Food sources (Murray 1996)

Small quantities in: potatoes, yeast, spinach, broccoli, tomatoes, peas, brussel sprouts, red meat, kidney, liver.

Cautions

IMPORTANT: Whatever the purpose in supplementing lipoic acid, it will chelate metals, which — since metal toxicity is so common — *poses serious risks, unless proper chelation protocols are followed.* (Cutler 1999, 04) See pp. 177-8.
If giving high doses, correct for low B1, (Gal 1965) suboptimal zinc, or high copper. (Cutler 2000)

N-acetyl-cysteine (NAC) (PFEIFFER 1987, BRAVERMAN, 1987, WALSH 1997, 2000AB, JAFFE 1992, BEYER 1994)

Mood

NAC has shown occasional benefit to bipolar depression or psychosis. Improvement can be due to its role in creating glutathione, or to benefits to histapenia or metal metabolism. (PFEIFFER 1987, BRAVERMAN 1987, WALSH 2000, JAFFE 1992)

Biotype issues (PFEIFFER 1987, BRAVERMAN 1987, WALSH 1997, 00AB, JAFFE 1992)

NAC is often very useful, *but only after several months of supportive nutrients,* in histapenia (which is often associated with anxiety, mania, depression, or psychosis), and in metal metabolism disorders. See *NAC,* p. 165.

Antioxidant & immune function

Protects the brain from toxins (alcohol, tobacco, etc.)

Chelates metals. A critical component of metallothioneins (which remove excess copper and other divalent pro-oxidant metals). (PFEIFFER 1987, WALSH 2000, JAFFE 1992).

Generally stimulates the immune system, and supports lymphocyte function. (TATEISHI 1981, SAEZ 1982, VAN ZANDWIJK 1995)

Oral NAC effectively and rapidly increases glutathione (which is critical to detox, and protection against infection and chronic inflammation). (TATEISHI 1981, SAEZ 1982, VAN ZANDWIJK 1995)

Considerations (PFEIFFER 1987, BRAVERMAN, 1987, WALSH 1997, 2006, JAFFE 1992, VAN ZANDWIJK 1995, TATEISHI 1981, SAEZ 1982)

Need may be suggested by

Histapenia, metal metabolism disorders, affective symptoms, seizures.

Toxicity, heavy metal accumulation, immune dysfunction, inflammation, infection.

Sources

Nuts, seeds, grains, poultry, eggs, legumes.

Supportive nutrients

B6 supports cysteine formation from methionine. Selenium may allow slightly higher doses of NAC.

Lab

Serum cysteine.

Dose

As NAC. 500 mg 2x/day. Introduce gradually. Correct first for low plasma zinc, folic acid, taurine.

Warning & supportive nutrients

Cysteine readily oxidizes, and can cause excitotoxicity, so is best taken as NAC (which allows cysteine to be formed as needed), along with antioxidants. *Avoid if undermethylated (histadelic).* Also, see *Biotype issues,* above, left.

Effects of excess, contraindications

Indigestion. Cystine gallstones. Aggravates cystinuria.

Supports metal metabolism, but can increase toxic metal levels if taken too early in MT therapy.

Molybdenum (SLAGLE, GARRISON 1985, BALCH 1990, PAGE 1992, HOFFER 1983, JAFFE 1992, PAPAIOANNOU 1984, PFEIFFER 1975, 87, PANNEERSELVAM 2004)

Levels are altered in some bipolars.

Bioype indications

Interferes with copper absorption, benefitting histapenia, metal metabolism dysfunction, and some pyrolurias.

Other effects which may influence mood

Mediates some neurotransmitter & hormonal activity.

Contributes to carbohydrate metabolism.

May reduce fatigue.

When indicated, may help counter allergies.

Regulates acidity, profoundly influencing the blood's ability to carry oxygen, thereby, perhaps, helping to counter anxiety and depression.

Frees liver iron, so it can carry oxygen to body cells, supporting metabolism and ability to burn fat.

Antioxidant & detox function

Note: The effects of molybdenum are not well studied, and it is somewhat of a stretch to classify it as an antioxidant, though note the following functions:

Enhances the use of sulfur amino acids critical to immune and antioxidant protection.

Essential to cellular use of vitamin C.

Helps decrease and detox copper, thus limiting free radical formation.

May decrease iron absorption, with similar results.

Helps turn nitrogenous waste to uric acid, a potent antioxidant.

Supports degradation of sulfite (a fairly toxic product of taurine metabolism) to sulfate.

Considerations

Lab (JAFFE 1991)

Molbydenum loading. Elevated urinary sulfite; low sulfate. Look for pronounced allergies.

Sources (NUTRICIRCLES® 1996)

Legumes (soy, pea, lentil, lima), cauliflower, spinach, garlic, yam, sunflower seeds, liver, kidney, eggs, fish, brewers yeast, wheat germ, buckwheat, barley, oats. *Reflects soil content.*

Effects of excess, contraindications

Can inhibit iron and copper absorption, and interfere with copper metabolism.* Copper depletion decreases angiogenesis (and so can suppress growth in children), creates anemia, and can promote diarrhea.

Excess can suppress the thyroid or contribute to gout.

* On the other hand, elevated copper can deplete molybedenum.

Vitamin A (QUILLIN 1987, LIEBERMAN 1990, KROHN 1991, GARRISON 1985, PFEIFFER 1975, 1987, WERBACH 1991, COUSENS 2001, MURRAY 1996)

Vitamin A and carotenes alter mood mainly when allergies, environmental sensitivities, or immune disorders are contributing to affective symptoms. Fatigue, insomnia, increased vulnerability to stress, and autism (see pp. 274-75) may also occur with deficiency.

Antioxidant function: Protects the cell membrane, and its hormone and neurotransmitter receptor sites.

Considerations (COUSENS 2001, MURRAY 1996)

Need may be suggested by

Fatigue, insomnia, increased susceptibility to stress.

Allergies. Leaky gut. Fragile mucous membranes.

Vulnerability to respiratory or other infection, or toxins.

Poor color vision, night-blindness, dry eyes.

Reproductive dysfunction.

Hyperthyroid, diabetes, other endocrine imbalance.

Loss of the sense of smell.

Weight loss or growth impairment.

Acne, dry dull hair, rough dry skin, fragile nails, compromised tooth enamel, slow healing of wounds.

Prone to alcoholism, migraines, arthritis, kidney stones.

Nutrient interactions

Needed for fatty acid and protein metabolism, and absorption of vitamins B, C, E, and K.

Sources (NUTRICIRLCES 1996)

Liver, fish liver oil, salmon, halibut, other fish, dairy, eggs.

Supportive nutrients

Zinc, E, mixed carotenes, other antioxidants.

Antagonistic factors

Chronic psychic or immune stress depletes A. Certain drugs or alcohol may compete with A for metabolism.

Effects of excess, contraindications

Especially with over 25-50,000 IU, long-term:

Restlessness, emotional instability, fatigue, fainting

Cracked bleeding lips, mouth fissures, dry skin, hair loss.

Joint pain, muscle incoordination.

Intracranial pressure (headaches, nausea, vomiting).

Gastrointestinal disturbances, anorexia.

Growth irregularities. Congenital abnormalities.

Retinal hemorrhages, blurred vision, sore eyes.

Enlarged spleen, liver, lymph nodes.

Fragility and thickening of long bones.

Chronic high doses can be fatal.

Pregnant women should not take high doses.

Carotenes (QUILLIN 1987, LIEBERMAN 1990, KROHN 1991, GARRISON 1985, PFEIFFER 1975, 87, WERBACH 1991, COUSENS 2001, MURRAY 1996)

Carotenes are terpene phytochemicals, often found in orange-red fruits, yellow-orange or green vegetables (especially when intensely-colored), and create A-type benefits. Improved mental function is mainly via protection from cerebral and other allergies.

Antioxidant function

Carotenes provide antioxidant support to body fats; spare E, CoQ10, and glutathione so they can be recycled; and help temper the free radical proliferation that can occur with high copper (as in histapenia).

Considerations

Need may be suggested by

Eye problems, immune dysfunction, allergies.

Tendency to chemical toxicity, debilitation.

Nutrient interactions

Carotenes supports EFA metabolism.

C, zinc, protein and thyroid help carotene convert to A.

Sources (NUTRICIRCLES® 1996)

Yams, pumpkin, squash, carrots, spinach, peppers, apricots, tomatoes, dark leafy greens (kale, beet greens), dense greens (spirulina, blue green algae, barley grass).

Effects of excess, contraindications

Low thyroid, diabetes, or liver disorders can obstruct conversion of beta carotene to A. (*Take A instead.*)

Two studies suggest chemical beta carotene, taken alone, may increase lung cancer risk in smokers. (LEO 1999)

Elevated levels can produce an itchy, orange skin discoloration, reversible when intake is reduced/stopped.

Isolated beta carotene may accelerate phase 1 liver detox only, and contribute to tremors, irritability, depression, nausea, rash. (CUTLER 2000, 07, HUGGINS, 1982, 93)

More antioxidants (WALSH 2007)

□ **Nutrients which support metal metabolism** (See pp. 170-73.)

□ **Nutrients which counter excitotoxicity** (See pp. 191-93.)

□ **Nutrients which counter high homocysteine** — which can produce profound oxidative stress. (See pp. 157, 167.)

□ **Carnitine** — a major means of protecting mitochondria from oxidative stress. (See pp. 115-16.)

□ **Vitamin D** — an excellent antioxidant. (See pp.119-20, 262.)

□ **Melatonin** — an extremely potent antioxidant. (See p. 261.)

□ **Methionine** — precurses cysteine, NAC, and glutathione; *contraindicated if histapenic.* (See pp. 157, 161.)

□ **Resveratrol** — a potent antioxidant; may counter glutamate, moderating mania. (See pp. 191-93.)

Antioxidants in biotype therapy (MCGINNIS 2004)

Some antioxidants not yet discussed, and important in biotype therapy include:

□ **Zinc** — induces metallothionein, a potent antioxidant enzyme critical to metal metabolism. (*See pp 29-31, 170-71.*).Zinc also protects sulfhydryls and lipids; and helps maintain levels of A, glutathione, E, glutathione peroxidase, and superoxide dismutase, all antioxidant.

□ **P5P** — a potent form of B6, is strongly antioxidant and required in creating glutathione, metallothionein, CoQ10 and heme, all antioxidant. P5P also helps maintain levels of glutathione peroxidase and, with zinc, is required in forming GAD, which helps block excitotoxicity. Oxidative stress can destroy B6 and impairs many B6 enzymes.

□ **Vitamin B3** — recycles glutathione; protects lipids and proteins in mitochondria and neurons; and blocks nitric oxide neurotoxicity. Low levels decrease metallothionein and increase brain cell death. Some studies find B3 more effective an antioxidant than C.

□ **Manganese** — a cofactor in some superoxide dismutases, antioxidant enzymes produced by the body to nseutralize superoxide radicals.

Antioxidants used in biotype therapies

□ **Pyrrole disorder** — B6, zinc, B3, manganese, C, E, selenium, other antioxidants; often, nutrients countering excitotoxicity; and in some cases, nutrients supporting metal metabolism.

□ **Overmethylation** (histapenia) — B6, zinc, B3, manganese, C, E, selenium, NAC; in many cases, nutrients which support metal metabolism; and, in some cases, nutrients which counter homocysteinuria.

□ **Undermethylation** (histadelia) — glutathione, selenium, E, zinc, B6, C, methionine, SAMe, and other nutrients supporting methylation.

Antioxidants & the adrenochrome hypothesis (HOFFER 1954, 2008, FOSTER & HOFFER 2004AB, SMYTHIES 1997, 98, 02, SMYTHIES & GALZIGNA 1998)

Hoffer's adrenochrome hypothesis, originally developed for schizophrenia, suggests that oxidation of dopamine, norepinephrine, and/or epinephrine,* creates chrome indoles (e.g., adrenochrome) which are hallucinogenic, and may underly the perceptual changes in schizophrenia (HOFFER 1954) and psychotic mania. (HOFFER 2008) *He finds the following antioxidants highly effective in preventing that oxidation and resulting symptoms:*

□ **Vitamin B3** — a potent adrenalin antagonist.

□ **Vitamin C** — which can convert some of the adrenochrome to leuco-adrenochrome (5,6, dihydroxy M-methyl indole), which helps counter anxiety and tension.

□ **Sufficient sleep** — a major means of removing chrome indoles.

See also *Bipolar delusions & psychosis,* p. 268.

* Typically elevated in histapenic, MT dysfunction, and many pyroluric patients. (Walsh 2008)

I: Nutrient survey
c: Bipolar depression

"Suppose the looking-glass smashes, the image disappears, and the romantic figure with green of forest depths all about it is there no longer, but only that shell of a person which is seen by others."

Virginia Wolf, *The Mark on the Wall,* 1921

"You do not get the time back. It is not tacked on at the end of your life... The minutes ticking by as you experience the illness are minutes you will not know again. No matter how bad you feel you have to do everything you can to keep living, even if all you can do for the moment is to breathe. Wait it out and occupy the time of waiting as fully as you can. That's my big piece of advice... Hold onto time."

Andrew Solomon, *The Noonday Demon,*
speaking from experience

See also:
Mania & Depression, p. 57-83.

The following framework roughly brings together some of the nutritional approaches described throughout this book. Although definitive cures do not exist, the physician or researcher may find these perspectives helpful in evaluating therapeutic options. For the general public, the material in this book is presented for strictly educational purposes, to facilitate understanding, and should not be construed as treatment suggestions. *Persons needing treatment for mood disorders or other health conditions should consult a knowledgeable physician who will tailor treatment to unique individual biochemical requirements.*

Framework 3: Depression (REFERENCES CAN BE FOUND IN RELEVANT CHAPTERS)

General nutritive approach

□ Biotype requirements and contraindications, and other nutritive needs, as dictated by the patient's unique biochemical profile. If more is needed:

□ Ongoing mood stabilization (see pp. 21-58), tapering any clearly depression-promoting components (possibly choline, melatonin, etc.), at a pace dictated by mood status, health, etc., carefully monitoring reactions.

□ The least stimulating antidepressant therapy that works. Too extreme or prolonged a regimen can promote a switch to mania. Weigh the need for the more potent antidepressant nutrients and herbs,* in terms of symptom severity vs the likelihood of triggering mania over time.

A note on the research: Bipolar depression is relatively understudied. Though almost 40% of those initially diagnosed with major depression are eventually rediagnosed bipolar, not all data on major depression is applicable.(MARANO 2005) Moreover, many studies do not distinguish bipolar from unipolar depression, and few specifically target bipolars. (COMPTON 2000)

* Relatively milder choices may generally include tyrosine, tryptophan EPA (or GLA if pyroluric), noni, B, C, antioxidants, calcium, chromium, manganese, etc. Phenylalanine, SAMe, 5HTP, rhodiola, Korean ginseng, etc. are generally more potent.

Biotype therapies

Biotype imbalances are often the overriding consideration. Treat pyroluria, methylation imbalances, or metal metabolism disorders, as relevant.

See pp. 145-68; 170-83.

Nutrients which may benefit depression

Dose, timing, and choice of nutrients should be tailored to unique biochemical requirements, taking into account daily variations in symptom intensity, and ongoing response.

□ **OMEGA 3** (especially EPA) — especially critical in bipolar depression (usually with higher doses needed than during maintenance or mania). May also help with anxiety and psychosis. Benefits histamine (methylation) biotypes. *Pyrolurics tend to do better with GLA.*

□ **PHOSPHATIDYL INOSITOL** — critical to signalling; especially indicated with histadelia. *Usually not helpful with histapenia, or mania.*

□ **ANTIDEPRESSANT NEUROTRANSMITTER PRECURSORS** — Patients may respond better to precursors and cofactors of serotonin, or norepinephrine, or both, or a free form amino acid complex. SAMe is very helpful for a subset of depressives (usually histadelic).

□ **MINERALS** — Calcium, especially with histadelic depression; magnesium, especially with irritability; chromium, especially with blood sugar issues; manganese, particularly with pyroluria (*but not with histadelia or high blood pressure)*; perhaps potassium (*preferentially from food sources*); zinc, if low, or low relative to copper, and especially with pyroluria, and histapenia; iron, if low. Possibly, germanium, rubidium, or cesium.

□ **B VITAMINS** — support brain activity, communication, energetics, and general viability, and can be antidepressant. *Depending on patient chemistry and biotype, consider:* B3 or NADH (critical to brain metabolism); B6, folic acid, and B12 (which support formation of antidepressant neurotransmitters); B5 (which supports adrenal function); B complex, etc., *as relevant.*

□ **VITAMIN C & BIOFLAVONOIDS** — supports histamine balance; benefits cerebral allergies and vanadium toxicity; can improve depression, anxiety, psychosis.

□ **VITAMIN D** — helps maintain natural biorhythms; supports production of serotonin, dopamine and norepinephrine; supports normal thyroid function, promotes proper use of calcium, protects neural membrane fats from peroxidation; counters SAD and probably other depressions.

□ **ANTIOXIDANTS** — full spectrum, plus individual supplements, *as indicated* (e.g., selenium, E, CoQ-10, reduced glutathione, etc.).

□ **SUPPORT FOR BRAIN ENERGETICS** — Acetyl-L-carnitine (with antioxidants), CoQ10, NADH, pyruvate, thyroid or methylation support, *as indicated.*

□ **FREE FORM AMINO MULTIS, OTHER MULTIPLES** — *only* if not contraindicated due to biotype, mood state, competition with key required nutrients, etc.

□ **OTHER NUTRIENTS**, *as relevant.*

□ **ANTIDEPRESSANT HERBS** — e.g., St. John's wort, ginseng, ginkgo, goji, gotu kola, noni, etc.), *if indicated.*

See pp. 86-144.

Attend to physical health

- □ Malabsorption. Candida. Sugar metabolism.
- □ Allergies, sensitivities.
- □ Malnutrition, eating disorders, vegetarianism (unless consuming enough B3, B6, B12, zinc, protein).
- □ Thyroid, adrenal, and other endocrine imbalance.
- □ Convulsive and other neurological disorders.
- □ Metal toxicity. Chronic free radical or excitotoxic exposure. Pesticides, chlorine, fluorine, other toxins.
- □ Problems with caffeine, tobacco, alcohol, street drugs.
- □ Reaction to medications.
- □ Porphyrias, anemia, polycythemia vera, blood pressure problems, other cardiovascular illness.
- □ Immune dysfunction. Autoimmunity. After-effects of viral illness, liver cirrhosis. Certain other illnesses.
- □ Childbirth, nursing, puberty, aging.

See pp. 169-250.

Optimize diet

Tailor diet to biotype, blood sugar balance, allergic considerations, and other physical needs.

The optimal diet generally includes plenty of fresh vegetables, fish, beans; some seeds and nuts, whole grains, fresh fruit, and (if not vegetarian) high quality animal food. Six to eight glasses of water per day.

Avoid allergens, sugar, white flour, detrimental fats, fried foods, processed food, MSG, aspartame; too much salt (increases water retention), caffeine, dried fruit and processed fruit juice. Limit vanadium sources.

Superfoods may include freshly made vegetable juices, nutritional yeast, blue green algae, spirulina, chlorella, bee pollen, barley grass, seaweed, sprouts.

See pp. 254-56.

Lifestyle support

- □ Exercise, deep breathing, outdoor light, fresh air, light therapy if indicated, etc.
- □ Adjust daily activity to natural biorhythms. Morning walks; regular sleep, meals, etc.
- □ Psychosocial support, stress reduction techniques, cognitive exercises.
- □ Meaningful work and/or creative outlet.
- □ Extra support during seasonal change, illness, injury, emotional or other stresses.

See pp. 251-62.

Monitor

Monitor carefully for early signs of mood changes and adjust treatment accordingly.

If depression will not remit

If depression is severe and does not remit, the more potent choices may be indicated. These involve more risk. Too much or too extended a treatment can trigger mania. Introduce gradually. Use the lowest effective dose.

- □ Check for overlooked nutrient, health, and environmental factors. (e.g.biotype, thyroid, allergies, anemia, mood stabilization, antidepressant herbs etc.)
- □ IV or IM treatment, *if indicated.* (See p. 144)

Medication as prescribed. Consult with your physician.

Cautions

Antidepressant nutrients, particularly aminos and herbs — like meds (but usually to a lesser extent) — can contribute to mania. The physician might do well to aim for the lowest dose needed to provide optimal benefit. Monitor assiduously, and fine tune. Inhibitory nutrients should be increased, antidepressant nutrients reduced/ stopped, with any sign of mania.

Individual biochemical requirements are not identical, and supplements helpful for one patient can be detrimental for another. Full contraindications are not included. Amino acids and herbs, particularly, can interact with meds. Inappropriate dose reduction or withdrawal from mood-stabilizing drugs can be life-threatening.

1. EFAs & Phospholipids

Essential fatty acids and phosphoplipids are critical to neural messaging, with profound effects on mood. See also *Primer,* p. 94, *Second messengers,* p. 279.

See also, *Carnitine*, pp. 115-16.

Essential fatty acids (Rudin 1981, 87, *Prosta Leukot EFAs* 1996, Horrobin 1979, 80, 83, 89, 98, 99, Vaddadi 1979, Dunbar 1975, Mathe 1981, Maes 1998, Passwater 1981, 87, Elkashef 2001, Smith 1998)

The brain is 60% fat. Essential fatty acids are prevalent. High quality dietary sources include local fish, seeds, and nuts and, more modestly, legumes, grains, roots, and sea plants.

EFAs include omega 3, 6, and 9, so named for the position of their double bonds. DHA (an omega 3 fat) and AA (omega 6), *each* constitute 8% of the brain. EFAs are integral to brain communication and viability:*

- □ Key to receptor function and interaction with neurotransmitters.
- □ Interact with cAMP, and ATPase, initiating second messenger cascades.**
- □ Interact with the sodium potasium/pump, which constructs the action potentials that conveys messages along the neural axon.
- □ With their double bonds, support neuroplasticity.
- □ Essential to membrane structure and permeability. EFAs transport certain biomolecules in and out of the neuron (and across the blood brain barrier). Some molecules are kept out entirely, or prostaglandins may be produced to convey their messages into the neuron.)
- □ Influence brain development, metabolism, energetics, oxygenation.

This section focuses on omega 3 and GLA. Omega 3 is especially needed by methylation imbalance patients; GLA tends to be more important to pyrolurics.

* They are also important in creating certain enzymes, steroids, and lipoproteins; in helping nourish the thyroid and adrenals; and in supporting immune function, hemoglobin production, and blood clotting. (Elkashef 2001)

** Which bring biochemical messages through the cell and into its nucleus, changing cell activity and perhaps leading to new transmissions. (See p. 279.)

Phospholipids

Phospholipids are fat/phosphorous compounds which play a critical role in neural receptor and membrane function and include:

- □ Phosphatidyl inositol — a critical second messenger, which generally enhances signalling, and can be important in certain bipolar depressions (particularly in histadelics). (See pp. 95-7.)
- □ Phosphatidyl serine — becomes particularly relevant in depression in older persons. (See p. 98.)
- □ Phosphatidyl carnitine — protects mitochondria from oxidative stress, and may be needed for depressives showing slowed cognition and ongoing mental fatigue.

This section focuses on inositol and serine. Carnitine is discussed under *Brain energetics* (pp. 115-16). Choline, which is primarily stabilizing and, for some, antimanic, is discussed in Part Ia (pp. 48-51).

Omega 3

Omega 3 in the brain (HORROBIN 2000AB, STOLL 2002)

Omega-3 is highly concentrated in nerve endings, receptors and other neural membrane structures. It supports neural communication, receptor function, membrane permeability and structure, and myelin formation. It also imparts flexibility to the membrane and its receptors, enabling them to more accurately convey messages into the neuron. On the other hand, hydrogenated fats (as in margarine), and excess saturated fats or cholesterol reduce fluidity, impairing communication.

Low omega 3 in modern diets (RUDIN 1981, 82, 87)

The majority of nerve cell membrane lipids should be omega 3, with the optimal body ratio of omega 6 to omega 3 at approximately 4:1; and 1:1 in the brain.

Our ancestors ate mostly omega 3-rich leafy greens, wild game, and fish, generally meeting the 1:1 ratio; contrast that to the 10 or 20 to 1 ratio in the modern US diet. Current intake of omega 3 is about one-fifth that of 100 years ago. And omega 6-rich sources (vegetable oils, margarine) are widespread. (The ratio in corn oil, for instance, is 75 to 1.)

Moreover, healthy fats are typically overshadowed by a plethora of overheated, fried, rancid, and hydrogenated fats, which threaten cognitive, affective, and physical health. Avoid!

Omega 3 countering depression

Population studies find that the more omega 3 in the diet (especially omega 3-rich fish), the less the incidence of depression. (HIBBELN 1995, 97, 98AB, TIMONEN 2004) Blood analysis frequently associates depression with low omega 3 (particularly EPA), and low omega 3 relative to omega 6 and saturated fats.*(ADAMS 1996, MAES 1996, 99, SEKO 1997, PEET 1998, EDWARDS 1998, MAIDMENT 1990)

Research suggests omega 3 may be a remarkably promising nutrient for bipolars, especially during depression, and perhaps particularly for medication-resistant patients. (STOLL 2002) (See: *Stoll studies*, and *Further studies*, on the next page.)

Treatment with omega 3 also counters the omega 6 immune and inflammatory effects often associated with, and perhaps contributing to, the depression. (LEONARD 1996, CONNOR 1998, SMITH 1991, MAES 1998, HORROBIN 2000, 03)

Fish-based omega 3 is optimal

To optimally support mood, the brain requires the longer-carbon-chain omega 3* (EPA or DHA) present in fish, rather than the shorter chain found in flax seeds, nuts and greens. Though the body can lengthen the plant-based chain, many bipolars, especially as they get older, lack the nutrients, or the properly functioning enzymes required for efficient conversion.

Fish oil supplements optimize availability, making them especially useful during depressive episodes.

* Unless significantly pyroluric — see pp. 147-51.

"It takes the wires out of my head."

Rudin's patient, explaining why he wanted to resume EFA treatment.

"Epidemiological studies in various countries and in the United States in the last century suggest that decreased omega-3 fatty acid consumption correlates with increasing rates of depression."

Jerry Cott, PhD

"There appears to be little reason to withhold omega-3 fatty acids from most patients with bipolar disorder... The risks are low, and the benefits can be striking."

Andrew Stoll, MD, 2002

Early trials (RUDIN 1981, 82, 87, 96)

The earliest trial was by Donald O Rudin, MD, of Eastern Pennsylvania Psychiatric Institute in Philadelphia. He has suggested deficient membrane omega 3 might sometimes play a role in bipolar disorder, schizophrenia (especially with negative symptoms) and anxiety, as well as food intolerance and, perhaps, seizures.*

* Also arthritis and hypertension.

Mania from high doses

In an open label trial, Rudin (1981) gave over 50 gm flax seed oil per day to 3 bipolars (and other psychiatric patients). This was a high dose, five times that in the Stoll study. All three developed hypomania or mania, and increased cycling.

Similarly, Stoll (1999) mentions another study involving 22 bipolars (given what Kidd (2004) estimates to have probably been 7 gm flax seed oil/day), which also led to several hypomanias or manias.

The Stoll studies on omega 3 (STOLL 1999, 2002)

In a 1993 literature review associated with Harvard Medical School, Doctors Andrew Stoll, MD, and W Emmanuel Severus, MD noted that most mood stabilizers act on second messenger systems, and suggested that omega 3 (like lithium and valproate) may block the abnormal signalling associated with bipolar disorder. It also offered the potential to increase serotonin, possibly dopamine; replenish the neural membrane lipids; and directly alter gene expression in the nucleus. (STOLL 2002)

Stoll at Brigham and Woman's Hospital in Boston, and Lauren B Marangell, MD, at Baylor College of Medicine in Houston, subsequently began a double blind trial (STOLL 1999) which was to bring omega 3 treatment into the mainstream limelight.

The study involved thirty patients with unstable, treatment-resistant bipolar disorder, and high risk of relapse. 40% were rapid cyclers. Twenty-two were taking mood-stabilizing drugs. Eight were unmedicated (due to poor response, side effects, or personal choice).

Patients were randomly assigned to receive just below 10 gm per day (ten .96-gm capsules) of "Omega-Brite," (a tasteless supplement containing 92% omega 3, with over 70% EPA, 10%,DHA), or an olive oil placebo.

After four months, Stoll found dramatic improvement in the omega 3 group on almost all measures, and every affective scale. Depression had decreased substantially, remission was lengthy. Only 14% (2/14) relapsed.

Subjects who initially were not taking pharmaceuticals, did especially well, suggesting some bipolars may maintain on EPA alone. Stoll (2002) suggests the brain may need sufficient omega 3 to respond to antidepressants, so EPA may particularly benefit drug-resistant patients.

In controls, depression increased, and 80% (13/16) relapsed. Nine of the thirteen were hospitalized or needed major medical intervention.The difference from the experimental group was highly significant.

The study ended early, at month four, when supplement manufacture stopped. Controls who accepted the remaining Omega-Brite improved dramatically. Some subjects began a high-DHA omega 3, but deteriorated, until they switched to high EPA.

Stoll states he has subsequently consulted with hundreds of bipolars. He finds EPA augmentation of stabilizers often provides striking results; and that recovery or great improvement frequently occurs with omega 3 alone — without drugs — in patients with mild and, occasionally, severe bipolar disorder. (STOLL 2002)

Further studies

Frangou, 2006 — Twelve-week randomized double-blind placebo-controlled study. 24 bipolar depressives received 1 gm/day of EPA; 25 received 2 gms; 26, placebo. Both omega 3 groups experienced similar and significant improvement, as compared to controls. EPA was well-tolerated.

Osher, 2005 — Open label trial involving twelve bipolar I depressed patients on taking medication. They were given 1.5 to 2 gm EPA daily, and assessed monthly via HamD, for up to 6 months. Eight of the ten who completed at least one month experienced at least a 50% reduction in depression scores; a ninth patient, by two months. The tenth showed a 26% reduction. Hypomania did not get triggered, and no adverse reactions were reported.

Nemets, 2002 — Double blind. EPA added to ongoing antidepressants created highly significant improvement by week three.

Peet, 2002 — Double blind. 70 treatment-resistant depressed patients were given 1, 2 or 4 gms of EPA per day over twelve weeks, in addition to medication. Results suggest 1 gm is optimal.

Puri, 2001 — Case study of a patient experiencing seven years of severe, unremitting, suicidal depression, unresponsive to treatment. One month of adjunctive EPA produced sustained improvement in severe suicidal ideation, social phobia, and other depressive symptoms. Niacin response and neuronal phospholipid turnover increased. Lateral ventricular volume decreased (suggesting an increase in brain size).

Confounding factors in omega 3 research (WALSH 2006, 07)

□ Pyroluria — especially common in rapid cyclers. Omega 3 is often counterproductive, particularly in moderate to severe cases, where GLA is usually what's needed (along with B6, zinc, etc). (BIBUS 2000, WALSH 2007)

□ Low or depleted B vitamins — which critically interact with omega 3.

□ Oxidative stress — e.g., with pronounced histapenia, metal metabolism dysfunction, extended excitotoxic exposure, deficient phospholipids or antioxidants, chronic severe illness, etc. If not redressed, significant EFA intake will *increase* free radical proliferation, aggravating symptoms.

□ Lack of phospholipids — which shield EFAs.

□ Poor quality omega 3 — rancid, contaminated (e.g., mercury in tuna oil), exposed to light or heat, etc.

Other mental benefits

Many researchers find EPA (a long-chain omega 3 fat, found in fish) may benefit not only bipolar disorder, (PEET 1998, WALSH 1998, HORROBIN 2000 STOLL 2000) but also unipolar, (MAIDMENT 1999) psychotic, (MAHADIK 1996) and postpartum depression; (ADAMS 1996, MAES 1996, SEKO 1997, PEET 1998, EDWARDS 1998, HIBBEIN 1995,97,98AB,) schizophrenia (WALSH 1998, HORROBIN 1998) hyperactivity, (STEVENS1995, 96, WALSH 1998) behavior disorder, (STEVENS 1995) violence, (HIBBELN 1996, WALSH) alcoholism, (HORROBIN 1980) anxiety, (LEONARD 1996) and MS. (HORROBIN 1999) *Note: Moderate-to-severe pyrolurics may do better with an emphasis on GLA.* (WALSH 2006)

Possible mechanisms by which omega 3 moderates mood & stress (STOLL 2002)

- □ Supports receptor structure and plasticity. (STOLL 2002)
- □ Inhibits second messenger signalling molecules (PLA, (HORROBIN) inositol-related PLC, PKC, (HOLIAN 1992) and G proteins. (SEUNG 2001)) See *Second messengers,* p. 279.
- □ Activates nucleus receptors, altering gene expression.
- □ Interacts with binding sites on ion (calcium, sodium, potassium) channels, modulating electrical responsiveness and likelihood of neurotransmission. (STOLL 2002) Blocks L-type calcium channels. (ASCHERIO 1995)
- □ Mediates neurotransmitter and cell activity.
- □ Supports creation of serotonin (associated with contentment) and, possibly, dopamine (motivation). (MAES 1995)
- □ EPA, particularly, opposes inflammatory and immune chemicals activated by stress or omega 6.* Such chemicals can alter signalling and create severe depression. (MAES 1995, SMITH 1998, SMITH 1991, CONNOR 1998, STOLL 2002, MURCK 2004)
- □ EPA counters omega 6 and stress-related hormones (e.g, altered thyroid function and heightened cortisol release, (MURCK 2002)) which can profoundly influence depression, mania and immunity. (LEONARD 1996, CONNOR 1998, STOLL 2002)
- □ Enhances insulin, (COONEY 1999) and helps counter Candida. (TRUSS, TROWBRIDGE, HORROBIN 1999)
- □ Helps balance histamine levels, reduce homocysteine (see biotypes). (COONEY 1999, BIBUS 2000, WALSH 2000C)
- □ Often improves conditions associated with bipolar chemistry: learning and memory problems, hyperactivity, behavior disorders, (STEVENS 2005, 06) stress, (LEONARD 1996, CONNOR 1998, MURCK 2002, 04) psychosis. (KAIYA 1984, PEET 1994, 97, 98, 2000, PURI 1998AB, 2000AB, MELLOR 1998, HORROBIN 1991, 2000, BIBUS 2000, YAO 1994, MUKHERJEE 1994)

* Such as omega 6 cytokines (which in excess can promote inflammation or cancer), interleukins 2 and 6, tumor necrosis factor, and cox 1 and 2 enzymes (which create inflammation and pain). (Lieberman, Stoll 2002).

EFA status helps explain the association of certain physical conditions with depression (MAES, SMITH 1998, CONNOR 1998)

Altered phospholipid metabolism and signal transduction may, for many patients, be a primary cause of uni and bipolar depression as well as common co-occuring illnesses: diabetes, cardiovascular illness, MS, osteoporosis, cancer, aging.

David Horrobin, PhD, 1999

Candida/EFA link

Candida overgrowth is prevalent in bipolars. Candida toxin interferes with EFA metabolism, (TROWBRIDGE) which may one of the means by which Candida worsens bipolar symptoms. The lack of EFA may in turn contribute to the chemical sensitivity typical in Candida, and its repercussions on mood. Truss (1984) suggests successful resolution of Candida, tends to normalize desaturated EFAs, and improve mood. (See *Candida*, pp. 202-06)

EPA lack may tie cardiovascular illness to depression

Lifetime prevalence of depression in heart patients is 50%. (CARNEY 1997) Risk, (FRASURE-SMITH 1993), and 6-month mortality following heart attack (PRATT 1996) may be four times greater in patients also depressed. (KOLATA 1997)

Depression is often associated with many risk factors for heart disease: hyperarousal, insomnia, malnutrition, elevated cortisol,* rapid heart beat unrelated to activity, high blood pressure, and blood clots. These common symptoms also occur with omega 3 deficit and omega 6 elevation, which may contribute to both conditions.* (GOLD 1983, STOLL 2002)

In countries where fish is rarely eaten, the risk of heart attack is up to 50 times greater than in countries where it is a mainstay of the diet. (BAREFOOT 1996, HIPPISLEY 1998) Over many years of depression, the risk of heart attack gradually increases three to seven-fold, (KOLATA 1997, PRATT 1996, CARNEY 1988) conceivably reflecting progressive EPA and DHA depletion. (HORROCKS 1999, FUGH-BERMAN 1999)

In fact, many researchers suggest EPA is beneficial. It has been reported to prevent sudden cardiac death, normalize heart rhythm, improve peripheral circulation, decrease triglycerides, (MUR) and lower homocysteine. (HAGLUND 1993) It is prescribed in Japan to 150,000 heart patients per year.** (MURRAY 1998)

* Which promotes the abdominal fat associated with heart disease, increases LDL, and worsens arhythmias.

Depression & low omega 3 in other conditions

Besides cardiovascular illness, depression is often associated with diabetes, immunological disorders, MS, cancer, osteoporosis, aging, etc., outcome of which is worse in depressed patients. As with depression, these conditions have also been associated with impaired phospholipid metabolism and signal transduction, and low omega 3. (HORROBIN 1999) Deficiency may also play a role in arthritis, intestinal inflammation, cellulite, bone and joint weakness, skin and kidney problems, and poor salivation. Thus, EPA may be the common denominator in such conditions and the accompanying depression. (PEET 1997, HORROBIN 1999, LEONARD 1996, MAES 1999)

Phospholipid hypothesis (HORROBIN 1994, 98, 2000AB, GLEN 1996, YAO 1994, PELLEGREW 1993, GATTAZ 1990, PROSTA LEUKOT EFAs 1996)

The late David Horrobin MD, PhD, has been a key investigator, over the past decades, of the role of EFAs in mental illness. What follows is condensed from Horrobin's Phospholipid Hypothesis (2000AB) which see, for further details, as well as other cited references.

Structure

A large part of the brain consists of thousands of variations of phospholipids, e.g, phosphatidylcholine, phosphatidylinositol. These are fat/phosphorus compounds, water permeable in one portion, fat permeable in another. In the neural membrane they line up and interlock, forming a double layered matrix, critical to the membrane's role as gatekeeper to the cell.

Fats and amino acids give phospholipids unique properties. Phospholipids should be especially rich in long-chain, omega 3 (as in fish) and other highly unsaturated fatty acids, which give the membrane flexibility. If unavailable, saturated fats (as in meat or butter) are used instead, but at a cost to receptor and transmitter activity, neural vitality and communication.

Splitting membrane phospholipids: "PLAY vs. FACULTY"

With sufficient stimulation, nerve cells release neurotransmitter across a synapse (gap) to bind to the phospholipid membrane receptors of the neurons with which it is communicating. This activates the enzyme phospholipase A2, also called PLA2. (Horrobin suggests the nemonic, "PLAY.") PLA2 splits membrane phospholipids into lipophospholipids and long chain unsaturated fatty acids (such as EPA and AA), (HORROBIN 1999, PEET 1996, ROSS 1999, GATTAZ 1990) which rapidly activate the cell. They alter gene expression, calcium movement, cyclic nucleotide function, and protein and enzyme activity. Memories may be formed, neurotransmitter release triggered, neural receptivity altered, etc. (AXELROD 1990, DENNIS 1991, HORROBIN 2000AB)

Seconds later, another enzyme, FACL4 (think "FACULTY"), should reunite the highly unsaturated fatty acids (HUFAs) with lipophospholipids, thus regenerating phospholipids and suppressing neural activation, i.e, "FACULTY" stops "PLAY." Thus:

phospholipids —**PLA2**—> lipophospholipids + HUFAs —> activation

HUFAs + lipophospholipids —**FACL4**—> phospholipids

Phospholipid functions

*Phospholipids are critical to the structure and function of membranes of the neuron and its organelles.** (HORROBIN 1996). *They:*

- ☐ Are critical to receptor activity in forwarding neurotransmitter messages. (GATTAZ,1996, AXELROD 1990. L'HIRONDEL 1995, WILLIAMSON 1996)
- ☐ Activate cAMP and other second messengers. (GUNDERMAN 1995)
- ☐ Impart fluidity to receptors.
- ☐ Convey admissable molecules into the cell.
- ☐ Influence membrane electrical properties (e.g, sodium/potassium pumps) and fluidity, modifying density and binding affinity of neurotransmitters and neurohormones. (5HERON 1980, ERNSTER 1991, REDDY 1996)
- ☐ Alter neurotransmitter synthesis, uptake, signalling, and MAO activity. (MAHADIK 1996, GATTAZ 1996, HERON 1980, L'HIRONDEL 1995, HIRATA 1980, RAFALOWSKA 1989, SCHWARTZ 1988, STROSZNAIDER 1994, OLIVEIRA 1994)
- ☐ Form a supportive matrix within the neural membrane, in which receptors, ion channels, second messenger systems, and proteins, are attached to or embedded. This matrix supports communication, and balance with the external environment. (HORROBIN 1996).
- ☐ Are indispensable to membrane metabolism; cell-based immune reactions; cell differentiation, proliferation, and regeneration. (GUNDERMAN 1995)

* Including the nucleus (which contains the genetic information), mitochondria (which produce energy), lysosomes (which eliminate waste), and synaptic vesicles (which store neurotransmitter).

Phospholipid chemistry & its influence on mood (HORROBIN 2000AB)

Sn1: fatty acid — CH_2O
|
Sn2: fatty acid — CHO
|
Sn3: headgroup — Ph — CH_2O

Most phospholipids contain a three-carbon glycerol backbone. Fatty acids connect to carbons 1 & 2 (at Sn1 & 2).

Phosphorus is attached to carbon 3 (at Sn3), and linked to head groups (proteins or fats), which impart specific properties and influence how information is processed.

Fats at Sn2 may be particularly important in some mental disorders. Here, the brain should place long-chain, highly unsaturated fats, with highly flexible double bonds (e.g, EPA). These help maintain appropriate neural membrane structure and accurate signalling.

When EFAs are lacking, saturated fats are used instead, but at the price of suboptimal receptor function (GATTAZ 1996, AXELROD 1990, DENNIS 1991, WILLIAMSON1996, REDDY 1996) and mood-modulating neurotransmitter activity; (GATTAZ 1996, HERON 1980, HIRATA 1980, HERON 1980, RAFALOWSKA 1989, SCHWARTZ 1988, STROSZNAIDER 1994, OLIVEIRA 1994) and compromised neural energetics, waste elimination, and viability. (MAHADIK 1996) Communication deteriorates, altering cognition and mood.

Phospholipid hypothesis *continued*

"PLAY" overwhelming "FACULTY" in bipolars (HORROBIN 1999)

Horrobin suggests PLA2 overactivity could be a critical abnormality in bipolars. The elevated PLA2 would increase fatty acid turnover, heightening susceptibility to free radicals, and altering neurotransmitter systems and neural membranes. Nerve cells would become overstimulated and disorganized, causing miscommunication, and cell damage or destruction. Eventually HUFAs would become less available, compromising receptor flexibility.

Horrobin notes that although FACL4 is probably relatively active in bipolars (as suggested by the tendency to niacin flush — see box, below), it may be unable to keep up with rampant PLA2.

A study by Rintala (1999) suggests PLA2 may be one of lithium's primary targets — with its potent inhibition of PLA2 (CHANG IN HORROBIN 1999) profoundly altering signal transduction, and so stabilizing mood.

Interactions with antidepressant neurotransmitters & omega 6

The increased dopamine and, in some cases, serotonin, which can occur in and contribute to mania, help drive PLA2 activity. (HORROBIN 1999, KIDD 2004)

Elevated PLA2, in turn, increases the activity of norepinephrine, dopamine and serotonin, promoting mania; (HIBBELN 1987, 89) conversely, in depression.

Excess PLA2 would also increase release of AA, and omega 6 prostaglandins, perhaps thereby further aggravating mood. (ABDULLA 1975, KIDD 2004)

The EPA solution (HORROBIN 1994, 2000)

EPA inhibits PLA2, activates FACL4, moderating mood

EPA, an omega 3 fat found in cold-climate fish may present a ideal solution:

(1) It is crucial to neural membrane properties, cell signalling and brain regulation.

(2) It inhibits PLA2 and activates FACL4, suppressing phosphoinositide splitting and signal transduction (perhaps especially benefitting depressive cycles).* (HORROBIN 2000AB, BARTON 1975, SPERLING 1999, STOLL 1999, MEDINI 1990, 94, PURI 2000AB)

(3) It helps quench free radicals, protecting membrane chemistry, and may help reverse the ventricle enlargement that can occur in chronic bipolars. (PEET 1993, 98, 99, 2000B, PURI 2000AB, LAUGHARNE 1996, MELLOR 1998)

* Lithium and valproate may act on the same pathway. (Rintala 1999, Berridge 1982, Chen 1993, Manji 1996, Stoll 1996b)

EPA from fish oil is generally optimal

Again, fish-derived omega 3 is the most direct source, and usually preferable. Conversion of the plant-based, 18-carbon LNA to the longer-chains tends to be too slow to counteract PLA2/ FACL4 abnormalities, and requires enzymes and nutrients which may be lacking. Since current research shows EPA superior to DHA in bipolar and treatment-resistant depression,* EPA becomes optimal,** (PEET 1993, 97, MELLOR 1998, STOLL 1999, KAPLAN 1999) perhaps, ideally, at 2 gm/day. (STOLL 2000)

* And schizophrenia. (Peet 1992, 98, Laugharne 96, Mellor 98, 99, Puri 98)

** Both the Horrobin and Stoll studies went one step further, using purifed EPA, as omega 3 contains constituents which partly counter EPA benefits.

B3 flush test, Omega 6, FACL (GLEN 1996, HORROBIN 2000AB)

Horrobin, Glen, et al., developed a niacin-response test, which helps distinguish bipolars from schizophrenics.* Four niacin patches of increasing concentration are applied to the forearm for one minute. Normals exhibit graded flush responses. All bipolars flush to the same or a greater degree than normals. 60% of schizophrenics do not react, except perhaps with a mild flush at the most concentrated patch. Thus, people who flush minimally are most likely not bipolar, and could be schizophrenic. (GLEN 1996)

Glen 1996 found flushing tied to affective symptoms and elevated omega 6 (red cell AA); and suggests further investigation may link increased flushing to bipolar flareups. Horrobin points out that since virtually all bipolars flush, and FACL needs to be present to flush, FACL is probably relatively adequate in bipolars (see above *Hypothesis*). (HORROBIN 2000AB)

* Ten independent groups confirm this approach, including psychiatric genetic researchers at University of Colorado; and a World Health Organization group in Perth, Western Australia, both of whom use the niacin flush test to track inheritance.

RECOMMENDED READING

Peet M, Horrobin DF, *Phospholipid Spectrum Disorder in Psychiatry,* 1999.

Prostaglandins, Leukotrienes and Essential Fatty Acids, 7-8/1996, and 3/1999:141-67.

Rudin, Donald O, MD, *The Omega 3 Phenomenon,* 1987.

Stoll, Andrew, MD, *The Omega 3 Connection,* 2002.

Erasmus, Udo, PhD, *Fats that Heal, Fats that Kill,* 1995.

Davis, Donald R, PhD, "Omega 3 fatty acids in clinical practice," *J Adv Med,* 8(1):5-35; 1995.

DHA & mania

Though useful through all phases in histamine axis patients, several studies suggest that higher doses of omega-3 are not necessarily helpful to bipolar I manics. (CHIU 2005, SU 2000, STOLL 1999, RUDIN 1981) The problem may actually be the high EPA, which may be more effective in countering depression than mania.

On the other hand, DHA, a longer-chain omega 3 fat, also derived from fish, may be the best choice for mania.*(WALSH 2008) Further research into these distinctions is needed.

* DHA has also been suggested for hyperactivity and other learning disorders; and to support brain growth and development in the infant, and maintain brain function in the adult). (Horrocks 1999, Fugh-Berman 1999)

EPA-plus-DHA therapies

Some mixed state and rapid cycling bipolars do well with the right ratio of both omega 3 fats. (STOLL 2002)

Walsh finds many patients who cycle between histapenia and histadelia as they move from mania to depression and back, respond to concurrent intake of both EPA and DHA, as the *major focus* of treatment. (WALSH 2008)

Biotype/EFA studies (WALSH 2006)

Dr. William J. Walsh and Dr. Douglas M. Bibus originally suspected fatty acid requirements for the different biotypes might be distinct, and that attention to specific requirements could improve therapeutic effectiveness. In a pilot study analyzing plasma fatty acid profiles, they found over and undermethylated patients were *both* (unexpectedly) low in omega 3, while arachidonic acid (AA), a key long-chain omega 6 fat, was normal. (BIBUS 2000) In subsequent lab assessment of thousands of methylation imbalance (histapenic and histadelic) patients Walsh found profiles again showed low omega 3, with supplementation generally beneficial. (WALSH 2000C)

In pyrolurics, on the other hand, the Bibus/Walsh study found AA significantly low,** while EPA, (a long chain omega 3) was insignificantly elevated. Similarly, pyroluric labs showed low AA. (WALSH 2000C) The response of severe pyrolurics to evening primrose oil, a rich source of GLA (omega 6) was excellent, the response to omega 3, negative. (BIBUS 2000)

Nonetheless, omega 3 was slightly low in some mild to moderate pyrolurics, who responded to small doses, along with the primrose oil. (BIBUS 2000)

GLA & pyroluria (BIAGI, HRELIA 1991, ERASMUS 1995, *PROSTA, LEUKOT EFAs 1996,* HORROBIN 1999)

GLA is an intermediate in the formation of longer-chain omega 6. Nonetheless, dietary intake (e.g., as primrose or borage oils), in appropriate doses, generally produces omega 3-like benefits (e.g., countering pain and stress). On the other hand, excess (*relevant to individual biochemistry*), or intake when omega 6 is already overabundant, can contribute to the latter's inflammatory and degenerative effects.

Biotype needs: Omega 3 vs. GLA (BIBUS 2000, WALSH 2006)

Not all bipolars do well with omega 3. Research by Walsh and Bibus (see box), as well as extensive biochemical and outcome data on over 1800 bipolars, generally points to the following subgroups (*though, therapy, as always, should be fine-tailored to unique individual biochemical requirements*):

☐ Histamine imbalance patients (*both* under and over-methylated), an estimated 60% of bipolars — respond best to omega 3.

☐ Severe and some moderate pyrolurics* — do better with evening primrose oil (GLA), exclusively.

☐ Mild to moderate pyrolurics — some may need a modest quantity of omega 3 along with the primrose oil.

* B6 and zinc, the key deficiencies in pyrolurics (who probably represent 18-20% of bipolars), are critical to forming higher-chain EFAs. (Walsh 2006)

Oxidative stress issues

The brain is highly vulnerable to oxidative stress. It is exposed to higher levels of oxygen than the rest of the body, and contains significant quantities of transition metals (e.g, iron, copper), which promote creation of free radicals. Metal metabolism disorders, malnutrition, toxicity, immune disorders, etc., compound the risk.

The brain's abundant lipids are particularly vulnerable. Significant assault on EFAs in neural membrane phospholipids compromises PGE synthesis, dopamine/GABA balances, and hippocampal pyramidal cell transmission, (RAFALOWSKA 1989, OLIVEIRA 1994, LEVIN 1961, REDDY1996) and has been associated with CT scan abnormalities, neurological damage, negative symptoms in schizophrenia, (REDDY1996) and tardive dyskinesia. Thus, generous antioxidant intake is always indicated when supplementing EFAs. (See pp. 73-83)

Considerations Omega 3 (Stoll 2002, Rudin 1987, Erasmus 1995 Davis 1996, Bibus 2000, Walsh 2000, Kruesi 1996, Horrobin 2000ab)

Subtypes

LNA or ALA (alpha-linolenic acid) is a shorter chain EFA, found in cold climate seeds and nuts and other plant sources

EPA & DHA (eicosapentaenoic and docasahexaenoic acids), rich in fatty fish, are longer chain omega 3 fats, crtical to the brain.

EPA seems to be more important to neural function, DHA to membrane structure.

Need may be suggested by

Depression. Other mood and cognitive symptoms. Poor memory. Learning and behavioral changes.

Possibly anorexia. (Ayton 2004) Growth retardation.

Weakness. Incoordination. Tingling arms and legs.

Dry, dull hair. Hair loss. Dandruff.

Soft, peeling, striated, or brittle nails. Slow growth.

Dry skin, psoriasis.

Vision problems. Profuse ear wax.

Allergies. Craving for fatty or fried foods.

Blood sugar imbalance. (Kruesi 1996) Perhaps, Candida.

Increased thirst and urination.

Methylation imbalances.

Elevated cholesterol, triglycerides, blood pressure, blood clotting. Various cardiovascular disorders.

Inflammatory disease (e.g. lupus, arthritis, tobacco-induced lung conditions). Autoimmunity.

Certain types of migraines. PMS. Breast pain. Menstrual cramps.

Slow metabolism. Weight gain.

Sources

LNA, the shorter chain omega 3, is found in flax, walnut, chia, pine nut, sesame seeds, and more modestly in kidney, navy, and pinto beans, purslane, squash, kale, blue green algae. Flax oil has 60% ALA.

EPA & DHA, the longer chain omega 3s, are found in fatty cold-water fish, such as salmon, herring, tuna, swordfish, sardines, oysters, halibut.

Lab (Kruesi 1996, Davis 1996)

Plasma & red cell membrane EFAs. (Davis 1996, Walsh 2006)

ELISA to assess PLA2 in red cell enzymes. (Horrobin)

Delta-6-desaturase — low levels can signal EFA deficiency; or indicate slow EFA metabolism, but reasonal availability. (Kruesi 1996, Davis 1996)

Clinical response. (Davis 1996)

Take the demands of climate into account. (Horrobin 1979)

Biotype indications

Individuals with histamine imbalances (especially when depressed*) usually require omega 3 (Bibus 2000, Walsh 2000c) with high EPA content. (Horrobin 2000ab)

* Or with signs of neurodegeneration.

Mechanisms which deplete EFAs (Hrelia 1991, Vaddadi 1989, Glen 1994, Peet 1994, 95, Mahadik 1995, Gattaz 1995, 1990, Axelrod 1990, Dennis 1991, Farooqui 1992, Schwartz 1988, Hudson 1996)

- ☐ Poor diet.
- ☐ Free radical assault, insufficient antioxidant defense (Capel 1988, Abdalla 1986, Reddy 1991,93,96, Buckman 1987,90, Peet 1993, Mahadik 1995, Kut'ko 1996, Rafalowska 1989, van Kammen 1989, Ernster 1991, Oliveira 1994, Stoklasov 1986, Aruoma 1987, Sohal 1990,94, Ku 1993, Masoro 1984, Pall 1987, Stram 1990, Szabo 1983, Bates 1996, Emerit 1989)
- ☐ Increased PLA2, decreased FACL4. (See pp. 90-91.)
- ☐ Decreased delta-4, -5 or -6 desaturase (enzymes involved in EFA metabolism).

Individuals with pyroluria, especially if severe, often preferentially require GLA (Bibus 2000, Walsh 2000) Mild pyrolurics may respond to GLA plus omega 3.

Fat ecology

To obtain optimal benefit, fats should be non-oxidized, non-hydrogenated (which rules out margarines), non-rancid and, preferably, organic. Also: fresh, unfried, uncooked (if appropriate), and unprocessed. Oils are best expeller-pressed, as even cold-pressed oils may have been processed, i.e, subject to deodorizing (with temperatures up to 500° F), bleaching (230° F), degumming and alkali refining (which removes lecithin, chlorophyll and minerals). Oils should be stored in opaque bottles and refrigerated to prevent rancidity.

Supportive nutrients

A full range of antioxidants to protect EFAs, including bioflavonoids, reduced glutathione, antocyanins, NAC, grape seed extract, optimal doses of C (as mineral ascorbates) (Mahadik 1995, 96, Horrobin 1989, Rudin 1981, Fleischman 1975) carotenes, A, selenium (Rudin 1981. Fleischman, 1975) Modest caloric restriction can further enhance antioxidant enzymes. (Sohal 1990, 94, Ku 1993, Masoro 1984)

B complex — act on omega 3 fats and support prostaglandin formation. Rudin *Check biotype restrictions.* (Horrobin 1989, Rudin 1981, Fleischman, 1975)

Cofactors in conversion into PGEs — sufficient zinc, magnesium, vitamin C, B3 and B6, folic acid. (Erasmus 1995, Rudin 1981, Fleischman, 1975)

Fiber — to help regulate gut cholesterol metabolism.

Adequate exercise and stress reduction.

Avoid refined sugars (Rudin 1981) — Sears finds a diet which supports glucagon,* rather than insulin, production promotes beneficial EFA metabolism.

Phospholipids (e.g, phosphatidyl choline) — incorporate omega 3 into the cell membrane. (Elkashef 2001)

Flax oil — some researchers suggest flax oil in addition to fish-derived omega 3 (Elkashef 2001, Kruesi 1996)

* Small meals, sufficient protein, healthful fats, moderate carbohydrates (mainly from vegetables), minimal sweets, adequate protein, etc. (Horrobin, 1979).

Common doses (Stoll 2002, Rudin 1987, Erasmus 1995, Larson 2001)

500 to 1200 mg/day or fish 2-3 times per week. Some studies suggest 2 gm/day. (Stoll 2000, Osher 2005)

Considerations Omega 3 *continued*

Effects of excess, contraindications (RUDIN 1981, ERASMUS 1995, MAHADIK 1995, 96, SOHAL1990, 94, KU 1993, MASORO 1984, FLEISCHMAN 1975)

May contribute to racing thoughts or hypomania. (RUDIN 1980) Manics may not need as high a dose. (CHIU 2003, 05, SU 2000)

Usually counterproductive with significant pyroluria. (BIBUS 2000, WALSH 2006)

Fish aftertaste (not with plant-based omega 3), burping, mild diarrhea.

With low B vitamins, may worsen B-deficiency symptoms (sleepiness, ringing in the ears, mild headache, skin and hair problems, muscle or joint discomfort, etc.)

With insufficient antioxidants, can produce fatigue and other signs of oxidative stress.

Can increase blood sugar and decrease insulin secretion. Diabetics should work with their physician. (COONEY 1999)

May thin blood excessively, especially if already taking blood thinners. Increases risk if prone to hemorrhage. (COONEY 1999)

May augment drugs taken concurrently.

Mercury issues (MOZAFFARIAN 2006)

Mozaffarian claims the health benefits of eating omega 3 fish, twice weekly, generally outweigh the risks of mercury content, especially if large ocean fish (e.g., tuna) are limited or avoided. Restriction becomes more critical in pregnant and nursing mothers.

Considerations GLA (STOLL 2002, RUDIN 1987, ERASMUS 1995, DAVIS 1996, BIBUS 2000, WALSH 2000, 06, KRUESI 1996, SLAGLE, LARSON)

Note: Though GLA often provides omega 3-type benefits, (BIAGI, HRELIA 1991) *too much can contribute to omega 6 predominance and accompanying adverse effects.*

Need may be suggested by

Pyroluria, porphyrria. Hyperactivity. Behavior symptoms, difficulty with stress, learning disorders.

Rough, dry, scaly or flaky skin. Dull patches. Psoriasis. Back of upper arms dry, with raised nodules. Dry hands. Cracking or peeling fingertips, toes.

Craves fatty or fried food. Diabetes, alcoholism. Colitis.

Hypertension, MS, inflammation, pain, heart conditions.

Sources

Evening primrose, borage, and black currant seed oils.

B6, zinc and magnesium support GLA formation.

C and B3 help create PGE1.

Effects of excess, contraindications

Exacerbation of mania. (HORROBIN 1980, 1983, ABDULLA 1975)

Too much can create symptoms of excess omega 6.

Considerations Omega 6 (STOLL 2002, RUDIN 1987, ERASMUS 1995, KRUESI 1996, COONEY 1999, DAVIS 1996, BIBUS 2000, WALSH 2000, KRUESI 1996)

Need may be suggested by (ERASMUS 1995)

Motor incoordination.

Very dry skin; dry eyes, hair, glands. Eczema. Hair loss.

Profuse perspiration. Excess thirst. Crave fatty/fried food.

Slow immune & inflammatory reactions & wound healing.

Fatty liver, kidney degeneration.

Male sterility, female miscarriage. Growth retardation.

Arthritis, irregular heartbeat, circulatory problems.

Populations

Intake is usually excessive in industrial countries. Deficit is rare except with pyroluria, starvation, hydrogenated and rancid fat diets (fried or canned fats, margarine), or post-gall bladder removal.

Sources

Warm-climate seeds and nuts (cashews, pecans, Brazil). Some in black, mung, garbanzo beans; black-eyed peas, lentils. *Present in vegetable oils (corn, cottonseed, safflower, etc.) and mayonnaise, which are are not recommended.* Meat, butter, poultry and dairy contain long-chain omega 6.

Effects of excess, contraindications

Mood and cognitive symptoms.

Blood sugar imbalances. High cholesterol.

Skin conditions. Vision problems.

Hypertension. Certain types of migraines. PMS.

Increased risk of inflammatory (e.g. lupus, arthritis, tobacco-induced lung conditions) and degenerative disease (cancer, cardiovascular disorders).

Primer: EFAs: Omega 3 & 6, GLA; & Prostaglandins (PGs) (ERASMUS 1995, *PROSTA, LEUKOT EFAs 1996*, HORROBIN 1999, DAVIS)

Omega 3s include LNA (alpha-linolenic acid), which is found in plants; and EPA and DHA (eicosopentaenoic and docosahexaenoic acids, respectively) found in fish. Omega 3 forms PGE3s (series 3 prostaglandins), which are largely beneficial.

Omega 6 fats are common in the modern diet, and include LA (linoleic acid), GLA (gamma linolenic acid), DGLA (dihomogammalinolenic) and AA (arachidonic acid). Omega 6 generally forms PGE 2, which facilitates rapid immune and inflammatory reactions, and becomes detrimental in excess.

GLA (gamma-linolenic acid) can be an intermediate product in omega 6 metabolism to PGE2, or (often), when obtained from the diet, a precursor to PGE1.

PGE3 (from omega 3) and PGE1 (from GLA) have similar effects (though important differences exist).

Omega 3: LNA —> EPA —> DHA —> PG3s
Omega 6: LA —> GLA —> DGLA —> AA —> PG2s *or*
GLA —>DGLA —> PG1s

Inositol

Inositol is generally considered a B vitamin, and is also a sugar. It is slowly formed from glucose in the brain, (AUKEMA 1994) and can, itself, provide some fuel for the brain.

Phosphatidyl-inositols constitute a substantial portion of substances bound to the neural membrane. They protect it and are essential to its activity. Inositols are critical to response to mood-modulating neurotransmitters (including acetylcholine, serotonin, norepinephrine), second messenger signalling, and mobilization of stored calcium, stimulating neurotransmitter release. (HERTZ 1992, COLODNY 1998, EL-MALLAKH 1993, DRUMMOND 1989)

Depression (JOPE 1996, DUBOVSKY 1992)

Levels may be low in bipolar depression, (SHIMON 1997, BANKS 1990, BARKAI 1978) with signalling reduced in specific regions. (JOPE 1996)

Recent studies (which have generally involved high doses) suggest inositol can be an effective antidepressant for some bipolars, (LEVINE 1995AB, 1997, HARDAN 2000, EDEN 2006) perhaps especially, histadelics. (WALSH 2000, 02, 06, 07) Augmentation studies also suggest antidepressant benefit, (CHENGAPPA 2000) though perhaps not in mixed state patients. And animal studies indicate antidepressant properties. (EINAT 1999, 2001, 02)

Mania (STEEN 2002, AGAM 2002, KIM 2005, DUBOVSKY 1992, BROWN 1993, KATO 1991, 98, SOARES 1996, BERSUDSKY 1999, SHALDUBINA 2006, WOLFSON 2000, WALSH 2000, 02, 06, 07)

Supplementation can worsen mania, perhaps especially in histapenics. (WALSH 06, 07) (See *Inositol,* p. 50.)

Biotype indications (PFEIFFER 1987, WALSH 2000, 02, 06, 07)

Inositol is often useful in histadelia, but can be less than helpful with histapenia, and many non-histadelic manias.

Other mental effects (COLODNY 1998)

- □ Supports memory.
- □ Benefits some cases of anxiety, perhaps especially if depression-related, (LEVINE 1997) or histadelic. (WALSH 2000, 06, 07, COUSENS 2001)
- □ Reported effective in unipolar depression.
- □ Reported helpful in promoting sleep, as it is mildly sedative, but can worsen insomnia in many bipolars. (PFEIFFER)
- □ Has been investigated for use in panic disorder, OCD, (FROLOV 2001, LEVINE 1997, COLODNY 1996) and TD. (JACKSON 1979, GELENBERG 1979, 90)
- □ May benefit Alzheimer's, in that it seems to counteract message inhibition by aluminum. (BARAK 1996)
- □ Can be used to replete inositol reduced by lithium,* and help address certain lithium side effects, e.g., psoriasis, and excess urination and water-drinking. *However, too much can foster mania.*

* Decreasing inositol availability may be one of the means by which lithium works.

Some depression studies

Levine, 1995ab — a controlled double blind, giving 12 gm inositol/day (more than ten times normal dietary intake*), over 4 wks. Depression (HAM-D) improved significantly in11/13 patients, versus no improvement or deterioration in placebo. Side effects were minor** and did not include mania. Discontinuation produced rapid relapse in half the responders — like what happens when antidepressants are stopped abruptly.

Eden, 2006 — nine depressed bipolars were given inositol (with valproate or lithium) over 6 wks. Four experienced at least a 50% reduction in symptoms (HRSD); controls did nto improve. The two patients who at baseline showed greater irritability, hostility and unkempt appearance (suggesting mixed state) worsened on inositol.

Chengappa, 2000 — pilot study. Twelve bipolars were given 12 gm inositol plus antidepressant meds. Six showed at least a 50% reduction in depression measures (HAM-D), and much to very much improved CGI, as compared to 30% in controls on meds alone. Eight had at least a 50% reduction in MADRS, as compared to 3 in placebo.

* Levine (1993) found no significant benefit with 6 gm, and notes that for many patients, the lower doses may be less effective, in that 7-8 gm/day can be lost via the kidneys, so large doses may be necessary to get enough into the brain.

** Nausea, flatus. In a few, mild increases in serum glucose.

Mechanisms for influence on mood

Signalling

Phosphotidylinositol levels and signaling are abnormal in bipolars. (DUBOVSKY 1992, BANKS 1990, JOPE 1996, KATO 1998, BROWN 1993) In mania, inositol (and calcium) signaling may become hyperactive, increasing stimulation. (DUBOVSKY 1992, KATO 1991, BROWN 1993, STEEN 2002, AGAM 2002, KIM 2005) In depression, levels can be low, (SHIMON 1997, BARKAI 1978, BANKS 1990) and signalling reduced in specific regions. (JOPE 1996)

Osmoregulation

Inositol influences the sodium/potassium pump and cell osmosis, (LENOX 1994) thereby influencing signaling and receptor interactions, hence, mood. (EL-MALLAKH 1993) Sodium feeds back, regulating inositol levels.

Lithium & other stabilizers working via inositol

Mood stabilizers may work, in part, by modifying inositol activity — reducing uptake when inositol is already high, increasing uptake when low — thus balancing extremes in inositol and calcium messaging. (DUBOVSKY 1992, SOARES 2000, WOLFSON 2000)

Berridge (1982, 1989) had originally suggested lithium may act by inhibiting inositol formation in overstimulated systems (e.g., during mania), thereby suppressing the phosphoinositide second messenger system. Many studies now confirm that chronic lithium decreases brain inositol.* (RICHARDS 1996, JENKINSON 1994, CASEBOLT 1987, BATTY 1995, EINAT 1998)

Lithium is thought to inhibit inositol creation from glucose, and from IP3 degradation. It most strongly inhibits the enzyme (*IMPase*) which degrades IP to inositol. (GREIL 1991, NEMANOV 1999, FAROUX 1999, JOFMAN1993, SJOHOLT 2000)

IP - - *IMPase* - -> Inositol

Reduced levels of inositol mean less inositol phosphatides and phosphoinositols will be formed, and the inositol-phosphate/phosphoinositide cycle will be suppressed. (SOARES 1999, EL-MALLAKH 1993, LENOX 1994, ATACK 1996, MOORE 1999). IP3 and DAG become less available. Second messenger response to norepinephrine, serotonin, acetylcholine, etc., is thus blunted, and gene expression may be altered. (MOORE 1999, BELMAKER 1996,98, DRUMMOND 1989)

* Although some question the suppressive effect on inositol (Agam 1995, Shaldubina 2001, Sherman 1986, Honchar 1990), possibly because lithium moderates, rather than just suppresses, inositol activity.

INOSITOL PHOSPHATIDE/PHOSPHATIDYLINOSITOL CYCLE (COLODNY 1998)

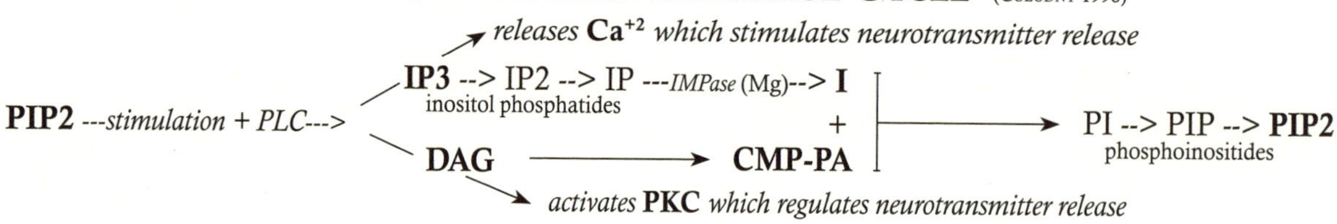

(1) **PIP2 --> IP3 & DAG** — Neurotransmitter stimulation causes the enzyme, *PLC,* to break down PIP2* to second messengers, IP3 and DAG.

(2a) **IP3 releases Ca^{2+}** — IP3** moves from the membrane to the cell's endoplasmic reticulum where it mobilizes stored calcium, *or*

(2b) **IP3 --> Inositol** — IP3 progressively degrades into IP2, IP, and then, through *IMPase* (*inositol monophosphatase*), a magnesium-dependent enzyme, into inositol (I). (COLODNY 1998, BERRIDGE 1982, DRUMMOND 1986, 89, RAGAN 1990, FISHER 1992)

(3a) **DAG activates PKC** — DAG*** activates PKC (protein kinase C) *or*

(3b) **DAG-->CMP-PA** — DAG (when condensed by *cytidine triphosphate*) forms CMP-PA****

(4) **Calcium & PKC increase signaling & transmitter release** (COLODNY 1998) — Both calcium and PKC regulate cell and membrane phosphorylation, cell metabolism, ion channels, and transporter activation. They generally increase cell excitability and stimulate neurotransmitter release. In mania, calcium signaling may be overactive, (KUSUMI 1992, DUBOVSKY 1989, 91A, 92B, COUSENS 2001, PFEIFFER 1987, 88) and PKC, elevated. (MANJI 1999B, SCHREIBER 1991A, WANG 1999) (See p. 279.)

(5) **Inositol & CMP-PA form PIP2** — Inositol combines with CMP-PA to form phosphatidyl inositol (PI). Phosphorylation then forms PIP, PIP2, etc.

*phosphatidylinositol-4,5-biphosphate **inositol triphosphate ***diacylglycerol/diacyltriglyceride ****cytidine monophosphoryl-phosphatidic acid

Considerations (Inositol) (COLODNY 1998, COUSENS 2001, COONEY 1999, MURRAY 1996, BALCH 1990, WALSH 2000, 02, 06, 07)

Need may be suggested by

Depression, confusion, OCD, anxiety, panic, sleep and memory problems. Histadelia.

Tendency to liver cirrhosis (COONEY 1999), diabetes, galactosemia, kidney dysfunction (BANKS 1990), multiple sclerosis, chronic retinal injury (Greil 1991), leaky cell membranes. Also, neural tube defects, pediatric respiratory distress.

Nutrient interactions

Helps regulate cellular sodium, potassium and water. (LENOX 1994)

May help absorb calcium, magnesium, manganese, and zinc.

Supports activity of folates, choline, B6, B12, betaine, and methionine.

Reduces the niacin flush.

Helps mobilize fat.

Lab

Even with elevated CSF inositol, supplementation may benefit depression. (LEVINE 1996)

Sources of inositol (BALCH 1990, LIEBERMAN 1990, COUSENS 2001)

Citrus (oranges, grapefruit, lime, etc.), cantaloupe, other fruits, nuts, whole grains, beans, cabbage, milk, meat, brewer's yeast. Lecithin, is an excellent source, but contains more choline than inositol.

Supportive nutrients

Works well with C, E, zinc, and EFAs.

Use with choline may help balance effects, for some.

Dose

Too high a level could trigger mania; too abrupt a withdrawal, depression.(COUSENS 2001) Walsh (2006, 07) notes histadelic (undermethylated) patients tend to do well with inositol, while histapenics respond better to choline.

Walsh (2006, 07) suggests 500-1500 mg, as per patient requirements. Cousens (2001) uses 500 to 1000 mg for sleep or anxiety.*

The preferred form is usually phosphatidyl inositol.

* Though bipolar depression studies have used up to 12 gm, (Levine 1995a) working on the premise that larger quantites may be needed to get enough inositol across the blood brain barrier (only 5% of intake gets to the brain), and into glial cell storage, so it can be used as needed. (Spector 1975, Robinson 1997) Nonetheless, many practitioners find *extended* intake of the lower doses seems to suffice, and entails less risk of triggering mania.

Effects of excess, contraindications

Discontinuation can produce rapid relapse. Stop gradually. Monitor.

High doses, especially, can trigger or worsen mania. (HARDAN 2000)

Gastrointestinal effects, e.g., nausea, flatus.

Occasionally, mildly increased serum glucose. (LEVINE 1995)

May be detrimental in AHDH. (LEVINE 1995)

Can stimulate uterine contractions, premature delivery.

Restricting choline in bipolar depression

Choline or phosphatidyl choline (described in more detail on pages 48-51) generally suppresses stimulation, and can trigger depression or increase severity in many bipolars, who tend to be particularly sensitive to it (perhaps especially if histadelic (WALSH 2006, 07)).

A number of studies suggest choline receptor disregulation in depression. Hamakawa (1999) notes MRIs often show increased basal ganglia choline compounds in depressives. Moreover, the antidepressant effectiveness of sleep deprivation — which tends to be more successful in patients with relatively greater initial cholinergic activity — may be partly due to its suppression of acetylcholine. (COUSENS 2001, ROGERS 1997)

Nonetheless, in certain cases of depression, modest doses of choline may be helpful, particularly with signs of deficiency, (GROTH 1958) or if histapenic. (WALSH 2006, 07) Improvement may be indirect, reflecting increased alertness and mental energy, (COUSENS 2001) catecholamine compensation, or a reduction in chemical sensitivity and brain fog. (ROGERS 1997)

In cases where choline is indicated, monitor ongoing clinical response, and reactions during withdrawal.

More on choline

See Choline (pp 48-51), for further information, references, and contra-indications.

Serine

Brain functions (KIDD 1996, 05, ELKASHEF 1987)

Critical to receptor function. Helps convey messages into the neuron, and activate neural reponse. Influences neurotransmitter production and release.

Provides structural support in the neural membrane. Supports membrane proteins essential to specialized cell functions, homeostasis, and maintenance.

Helps integrate brain waves.

Plays a part in the hypothalamic-pituitary-adrenal axis, and the daily rhythms of hormone release, commonly disordered in bipolars.

Serine, a nonessential amino acid, abundant in the brain, supports mood stability and cognitive function. (ELKASHEF 1987, KIDD 1996). It precurses acetylcholine, which is critical to memory and mood stability.

As phosphatidyl serine, it is a major component of the neural membrane, supporting membrane structure and receptor function, and moderating neurotransmitter release. (ELKASHEF 1987, KIDD 1996, 05)

Antidepressant & cognitive benefit in older patients

Levels often decrease with age. Depletion has been associated with elderly depression, which often improves with supplementation. (MAGGIONI 1990, BRAMBILLA 1996, KIDD 1996, 05, BROIDA 2001)

Serine also supports memory, learning, vocabulary, concentration, sociability, alertness and other functions which tend to decline with age. (KIDD 1996, 05, ELKASHEF 1987) Robert Crayhon, PhD (1998, 2008) suggests serine often works well with acetyl-L-carnitine and GPC (a form of choline) to protect and support brain function.

Biotype indications

Supports methylation of homocysteine, via vitamin B6, into cysteine.
See callout, p. 157.

Supports metal metabolism.
See pp. 170-71.

Considerations (KIDD 1996, 2005, PFEIFFER 1988, BALCH 1990, PAGE 1992)

Need may be suggested by (KIDD 1996, 2005)

Depression.
Confusion, poor memory, reduced cognitive function. (CROOK 1991)
Immune vulnerability. (Serine helps create antibodies.)
Weak muscles, arteriosclerosis.

Nutrient interactions

Supports fat metabolism.
Precurses choline.*

* Note: Though it can also form glycine, the reverse reaction is much more rapid. (Kidd 1996)

Source (KIDD 1996)

Serine is made from glucose and aspartate. It's prevalent in animal food (particularly, processed meat (e.g., sausage, luncheon meat), *which is not recommended*).

Supplements

Phosphatidyl serine supplements were previously obtained only from cow brain, but are now available from a soy lecithin concentrate. (KIDD 1996)

Effects of excess, contraindications (PFEIFFER 1988, YANIA 1986, PEPPLINKHUIZEN 1980, WILCOX 1985, WAXMAN, 1983, WSAZIRI 1983)

Elevation may occasionally be associated with psychosis.

2. Antidepressant aminos

Major antidepressant amino acids discussed in this section include tryptophan, tyrosine, and phenylalanine.

Amino acids versus more broad-spectrum protocols

A primary focus on antidepressant aminos* (especially when emphasizing the more potent choices, e.g., phenylalanine, 5HTP or SAM), plus inhibitors, may (if relevant to patient needs) be one of the more *acutely* effective counters to depression, and also may, if started early, help avert a looming depression. (Slagle 1992, 99)

On the other hand, treatments whose primary focus includes relevant vitamins, minerals, EFAs, etc. (perhaps with some key aminos), *may be more sustainable and get closer to the root of the illness;* and are usually less likely to trigger mania or promote cycling. (Hoffer, Larson, Walsh 2007)

Or biotype issues may be the predominant concern, e.g., histadelics, though they often respond to antidepressant aminos, fundamentally require methylation-support; histapenics may do well on inhibiting aminos, but better still when methylation is reduced; inhibitors may temporarily calm the pyroluric, but ultimately be less potent than B6 and zinc. (See pp. 145-68.)

Optimal therapeutic choices will come down to the unique biochemical, symptomatic, and response profile of the individual.

Distinctions between antidepressant aminos

Tyrosine, phenylalanine, tryptophan, 5HTP (Slagle 1992, 99, Walsh 2006, 07)

Tyrosine and phenylalanine (with cofactors, B6, B12, C, iron, etc.) precurse catecholamines (dopamine, epinephrine, and norepinephrine). Tryptophan and 5HTP (with B6) precurse serotonin. Some bipolars respond better to the former; others, the later; still others, to both (e.g., tyrosine AM, serotonin PM), or neither.

Methionine, carnitine, serine (Pfeiffer 1988, Slagle 1992, 99)

□ SAMe or methionine — as methylators, activate the above antidepressant neurotransmitters. *Many advise against bipolar use of SAMe, as it can readily trigger mania.* Walsh, however, emphasizes they SAMe and methionine are key therapeutic nutrients for most undermethylated (histadelic) bipolars, who do not become manic on them, when used appropriately. *For histapenics, on the other hand, they are contraindicated and highly detrimental.* (Walsh 2006, 07)

□ Acetyl-L-carnitine — especially with fatigue and poor stamina. Take with alpha lipoic acid. (See pp. 115-16, 178)

□ Serine — especially with memory problems. (See p. 98.)

General amino considerations (Pfeiffer 1988, Slagle 1992, 99)

Check biotype and other biochemical requirements, contraindications, drug interactions. Amino multiples may be detrimental if they compete for absorption with key required aminos.

Monitor. With the slightest hint of mania, discontinue stimulating aminos, increase stabilizing nutrients, decrease environmental stimulation, etc.

Reminder: If considering amino acid therapy, consult a knowledgeable physician. Particular caution is advised for pyrolurics, diabetics, pregnant women; cardiovascular, liver, or kidney patients; persons on psychiatric or certain other meds; other susceptible persons.

Catecholamines versus serotonin

Check for neurotransmitter and metabolite levels, and for relevant symptoms. Consider history of response to related meds. Also, potential interactions with drugs.

Catecholamines (Beckman 1979, 83, Gibson 1983, Bell 1988, Sabelli 1986, Buist 1983, Gold 1987)

Deficit is suggested by low MHPG, prior response to tricyclics, MAOIs, etc., and such symptoms as exhaustion, ambivalence, apathy, low libido, slowed thoughts and movement.

Biotype indications: Catecholamine precursors are often useful in histadelic depression, but not in histapenia. (Walsh 2007)

Phenylalanine, particularly, can trigger/worsen mania. Depressives are sometimes allergic to it. Avoid completely with PKU.

Catecholamines are usually inadvisable if already elevated, and contraindicated with hyperthyroid, high blood pressure, tendency to melanoma, MAOI intake, and most cases of liver damage, serious illness, or pregnancy. (See *Contraindications*, p. 112.)

Serotonin (Zmilacher 1987, Werbach 1991, McGrath 1990, Chouinard 1983, 1985, Prange 1974, Delgado, Branchey 1984, Pope 1985, Young 1989, Buist 1983)

Check plasma levels. Low serotonin is also suggested by depression with high MHPG, prior response to SSRIs, and such symptoms as dysphoria, pain, anxiety, agitation, aggression, guilt, low self-esteem, recurrent thoughts of suicide and death, insomnia.

Biotype indications: Serotonin precursors often benefits B6-depleted pyroluric irritability and depression. Modest doses may be helpful in histadelia. Benefits some agitated histapenic depressions, but usually not helpful for histapenia.

Serotonin can worsen certain depressions, and contribute to mania in some bipolars. Contraindicated with MAOI's, SSRI's; and in severe liver disease. (Also, see *Side effects*, & *Legal issues*, p. 105.)

Both

Use of precursors and cofactors of both is helpful in some cases, (van Praag 1984, Axorin 1990, Meyers 2000) perhaps especially in histadelia. (Walsh 2007)

Interactions (Raleigh 87, Mongeau 97, Foote 95, Geracoti 97)

Serotonin and catecholamines interact. High serotonin may reduce catecholamines and *vice versa*, in some regions of the brain, but not necessarily in depressives.

Serotonin

Definitions

Serotonin — an antidepressant neurotransmitter.

Tryptophan — amino acid precursor of serotonin.

5HTP — intermediate in metabolism of tryptophan to serotonin. It's five to ten times as potent.

5HIAA (5-hydroxyindoleacetic acid) — metabolic byproduct of serotonin breakdown by MAO.

Serotonin, a brain and gut neurotransmitter, influences sensory perception, learning, memory, and attention span; and may contribute, with dopamine, to motivation and reward dependence. (BLUNDELL 1984, BENJAMIN 1997, COMINGS 1984, 90) Serotonin conveys messages which create a sense of security, relaxation, and contentment; (GOLD 1987, KNUTSON 1998) and helps impart confidence, humor, optimism, and flexibility. (ROSS 2002) Thus, not suprisingly, it's often elevated in people in leadership positions. (Similarly, in the dominant monkey, serotonin levels can be double that of his followers.)

Levels

Serotonin is low in most affectives (COPPEN 1988) (and their families (GOLD 1987)), especially if violent or suicidal, (ASBERG 1976ABC, 84, AGREN 1980, 91, LIDBERG 1985, COPPEN 1988, MAES 1990, MANN 1986, 89, 90, MARAZZITI 1991AB, SWANN 1983,94, GOLDBERG 1999 BENKELFAT 1994) and even after remission. (COPPEN 1972, MALONE 1993) Imaging studies frequently indicate low serotonin activity. (MALISON 1998, DREVETS 1999, STOCKMEIER 1998) Tryptophan can also be low; (MAES 1990, COPPEN 1968, 74, GRONIER 1993) or tryptophan transport (GRONIER 1993) or 5HTP uptake (AGREN 1991) may be compromised.

Alternately, serotonin levels and activity can appear normal, but be low relative to competing aminos (MAES 1990) and mood-altering neurotransmitters; (MANN 1986, DAVIS 1986) or, serotonin may be underutilized. (SACHS 1989)

Serotonin synthesis (NISHIZAWA 1997) and availability (MAES 1990) may be somewhat higher in males.

Mechanisms for influence on mood (DELGADO 1990)

- □ Moderates neurotransmitters in the limbic system and other emotion centers. May alter MAO metabolism. (TAKAHASHI 1975, CHOUINARD 1983)
- □ Works with norepinephrine to alleviate depression. (VAN PRAAG 1984, BRAVERMAN 1987, BRIGHAM 2001)
- □ Influences hypothalamus-pituitary-endocrine interactions. (PORTER 2004) May increase growth hormone and thyroid secretion. (KHALZALI 2006)
- □ 5HTP increases beta endorphins, promoting a sense of well- being. (MAES 1996, BAUMEL 1995)
- □ Reduces overall stress. Challenges (such as stress, or low tryptophan) to either the adrenal axis or the serotonin system may impair the other, and lead to depression. (POLDINGER 1990, 96, PORTER 2004)

Mania & mood stabilization

For some bipolars, serotonin precursors (and serotonin, itself) help stabilize mood, (CHOUINARD 1979, 85, BRAVERMAN 1987, PRANGE 1974, MURPHY 1974, CHAMBERS 1978, BREWERTON 1983, BEITMAN 1982, BYERLY 1987, ZMILACHER 1988, VAN PRAAG 1981) but they fuel mania in others. (COLODNY, LANDRY 1991, CHOUINARD 1978).

See *Mania*, p. 46; and *Responders & Biotype indications, p. 102.*

History (BAUER 1996)

Ashcroft (1960), noting low 5HIAA, a serotonin metabolite, in some depressive psychoses, developed the hypothesis* that low serotonin may induce depression. Coppen (1965) suggested it might also induce mania.

Prange later proposed a "Permissive" hypothesis of bipolar disorder: Low serotonin allows dopamine, norepinephrine,** and acetylcholine*** fluctuations to become more extreme, destabilizing mood. (PRANGE 1974, JANOWSKY, GOLDEN 1988, NEWMAN, GOODWIN 1990, MENDELS 1974, GOLDBERG 1999, LUNCHINS 1976)

Prior to SSRIs (introduced in late 1980), tryptophan was widely researched & prescribed, especially to stabilize mood and augment tricyclics. The 1989 toxicity issue (see p. 105) sharply reduced use, until 5HTP became popular.

Most current mainstream antidepressants stimulate serotonin activity, at least to some extent, (COPPEN 1988) as does lithium. (CONLAY 1989) SSRIs, which focus primarily on serotonin, are the most widely-used antidepressants for bipolar adults. (GOODWIN 1990, COPPEN 1972, BAUER 1996)

See *SSRI side effects*, p. 287.

Researchers continue to investigate and prescribe tryptophan*** or 5HTP. (JANOWSKY , GOLDEN 1988, MURRAY 1996, 98, BENKELFAT 1994, FERRIER 1990, HENNINGER 1992, SALOMON 1993, BHATTI 1998)

* Indoleamine hypothesis of affective disorder.
** Stimulating neurotransmitters, with antidepressant activity
*** An inhibitory, calming, and parasympathetic neurotransmitter, with antimanic properties.
*** Though in the US, it is usually available only through compounding pharmacies.

Depression

Serotonin is popularly perceived as antidepressant, (ROGERS 1997) and depleted serotonin has been shown to promote depression. (BENKELFAT 1994) Thus: (1) tryptophan depletion (or sudden SSRI withdrawal) produces relapse (sometimes, in hours); (FERRIER 1990, MORENO 2000, BELL 2001, MILLER 1992, SMITH 1997) (2) a tryptophan-deficient diet or amino acid drink induces depression in affectives, (HENNINGER 1992, SALOMON 1993) and depressed mood in normals; (YOUNG 1985, BHATTI 1998) (3) drugs which decrease tryptophan can produce depressive symptoms even in patients on antidepressants; (SHOPSIN 1976) (4) low CSF levels of 5HIAA, a serotonin metabolite, often reflect depression severity. (ASHCROFT 1966, DENCKER 1966, MENDELS 1972, BRIDGES 1976)

Tryptophan & depression (MALONE 1993, BAUMEL 1995)

Benkelfat (1994) suggests low dietary tryptophan augments genetic risk of depression. Numerous studies find tryptophan decreases depressive symptoms, (LINDBERG 1979, COPPEN 1978, VAN PRAAG 1984, WOOD 1977, CHOUINARD 1977, 78, 79A, BOMAN 1988, BAUMEL 1995, QUADBECK 1984, DELGADO 1994, PRICE 1998, SHAW 2006) and some show precursors producing equivalent benefit to antidepressants, (CHOUINARD 1975, VAN PRAAG 1982, BYERLEY 1987, DELGADO 1994) or effective augmentation. (COPPEN 1972, 74, WALLINDE 1976, VAN PRAAG 1981) Some practioners find tyrosine, AM, and tryptophan, PM, particularly helpful. (COUSENS 2001, BUIST 1983)

Other studies report mixed results for depression, (GOODWIN 1990, SHAW 2006, BROIDA 2001, DOERFLER) though tryptophan may be more effective in bipolar than other depressions. (BRAVERMAN 1987) Thus, Farkas (1976) suggests many of the more positive studies probably included a greater proportion of bipolars. Enhancing tryptophan availability with B6* and other supportive nutrients may increase effectiveness. (MOHLER 1983, BRAVERMAN 1987)

Braverman points out that, over time, drug effectiveness wanes, side effects increase, and serotonin levels drop; as contrasted to supplemental tryptophan,** which, even if less *acutely* potent, provides steady nourishment supporting serotonin activity.

Guard against interactions with medications. (BRAVERMAN 1987)

* Though B6 usually should be taken at a separate time to prevent conversion to serotonin in the body instead of the brain.

** With the proper dosing schedule and relevant cofactors.

5HTP

5HTP may be up to ten times as potent as tryptophan for depression, (SANO 1971, 72, STOCKMEIER 1997, PERSSON 1967, TAKAHASHI 1975, QUADBECK 1980, 84, NARDINI 1983, VANHIELE 1980, VANPRAAG 1980, 83, 84, KAHN 1985, 87, ZMILACHER 1988, BYERLY 1987, MAES 1992). Several studies report equivalent benefit to pharmaceuticals. (NOLEN 1988, POLDINGER 1991, ANST 1977)

5HTP has also been used in the past to augment antidepressants, (ALINO 1976) a practice now largely abandoned, due to an increased risk of triggering mania or serotonin syndrome.

In fact, many researchers warn against bipolar use of 5HTP because of the relatively high risk of triggering mania.

Moderating SSRI withdrawal

Some physicians supply conservative increments of *tryptophan* to spare patients from suicidal depression and other severe symptoms on SSRI withdrawal, often with the goal of eventually replacing the drug. (CASS 2001) *Note: Such procedures, if indicated, should be cautiously administered and monitored by a knowledgeable physician, and tied to indications of serotonin depletion.* (See *Contraindications, Serotonin syndrome,* p. 105.)

Some of the studies

Poldinger, 1991 — the benefit associated with 5HTP was equivalent to fluvoxamine. HAM-D, and investigator and subject impressions, showed both groups improving significantly at 2, 4, and 6 weeks. Depression scores decreased 50% by 6 weeks. The most common side effects were initial gastrointestinal symptoms. More treatment failures (4:1) and more severe side effects occured in the drug group.

Brewerton 1983 — Double blind. Five bipolars who received 3 gm L-tryptophan, 3x/day, with lithium carbonate, showed significantly greater improvement than the four bipolar controls on lithium alone.

Related pharmaceuticals

Many antidepressant medications stimulate serotonin activity (COPPEN 1988), particularly SSRIs, which are held to be effective in approximately two-thirds of depressives, (VANPRAAG 1983, FARKAS 1976) (and have also been used for anxiety, panic, insomnia, OCD, alcoholism, pain, and aggression).

Of mood stabilizers, lithium promotes serotoninergic transmission during depression, and carbamazepine also raises tryptophan. (SACHS 1989, BRAVERMAN 1987)

Serotonin pathways (GOLD 1987, BRAVERMAN 1987)

Serotonin tracts begin and cluster in the raphe nuclei* and connect to most of the brain, perhaps focusing on the hypothalamus (which governs the endocrines).

Deficit in depression may be specific to regions related to symptoms (e.g., frontal and parietal cortex, caudate nucleus). (YOUNG 1994)

Low serotonin & depression in chronic illness

"Immune activation is associated with enhanced degradation of tryptophan. As a consequence, availability of tryptophan for the biosynthesis of serotonin in reduced [during illness], and may represent the basis for the development of depressive disorders in patients with various immunopathologies, especially in chronic diseases."

B Widner, 2002

Tryptophan & carbohydrate craving (MURRAY 1996, 98)

Serotonin regulates feeding. (BAUMEL 1995, STEIGER 2004) SSRIs, as well as 5HTP and tryptophan, are commonly used to decrease appetite, and moderate compulsive eating and drinking (e.g., in bulimia). (BRAVERMAN 1987, LOPEZ 1992, BAUMEL 1995, BLUNDELL 1984) Since serotonin promotes satiety and contentment, and reduces the desire for sweets and starches in order to feel good, (WURTMAN 1988, 89) it can, at least initially, facilitate weight loss. (SOULAIRAC 1977, CANGIANO 1992, SCHWEIGER 1986)

Dietary factors (MURRAY 1996, 98, BRAVERMAN 1987, GOLD 1987)

Approximately 1-3% of serum tryptophan gets into the brain. The more the tryptophan in the diet, the greater the uptake across the blood brain barrier. Increased tryptophan in the brain, increases neural production of serotonin

Large neutral amino acids* compete with tryptophan for active transport into the brain. (JANOWSKY 1988, SCHWEIGER 1986) Whole food complex carbohydrates, by stimulating gradual and prolonged insulin secretion, support preferential uptake of tryptophan.

With low insulin (as in diabetes), serotonin's competitors gain relatively greater access to the brain, increasing the likelihood of serotonin depletion, and consequent depression, irritability, and carbohydrate craving.

* Tyrosine, phenylalanine, valine, leucine and isoleucine.

Likelihood of response (BRAVERMAN 1987, COUSENS 2000, POLDINGER 1991)

Researchers have estimated that between one and two-thirds of depressives improve with serotonin support (tryptophan or 5HTP, plus B6). (VAN PRAAG 1983, BUIST 1983, FARKAS 1976, POLDINGER 1991) Response is most likely in individuals with:

- ☐ Bipolar depression.
- ☐ Low serotonin, elevated catecholamines.
- ☐ Agitation, anxiety, tension, aggressive symptoms, phobias, or insomnia, along with depression. (WALSH 2007)
- ☐ Pyroluria, especially with very low B6. (BRAVERMAN 1987, WALSH 2007)
- ☐ Many histadelias. (WALSH 2007)

The typical profile for a poor responder

- ☐ Unipolar depression, flat affect, low energy.
- ☐ Low catecholamines, elevated serotonin.
- ☐ Unresponsive to SSRIs.
- ☐ Perhaps, histapenic.

Biotype indications

Histapenia — Serotonin can be excessive in some histapenias, and overmethylation may further magnify serotonin activity, so intake of precursors is usually *not* indicated. (WALSH 2007) Occasionally, though, the characteristically low B3 (and, often, B6) reduces serotonin levels. High catecholamines relative to serotonin, or agitated depression, may also suggest need. (BRAVERMAN 1987, PFEIFFER 1987, 88)

Histadelia — Serotonin is often low; and tryptophan, often helpful. (WALSH 2007) Pfeiffer advises to keep doses modest, as the rapid metabolism of the histadelic may create a 2-3 hour blush, cardiovascular reaction, and overstimulation. Methionine can then help reduce the elevation (and is often, in any case, more important for the histadelic). (BRAVERMAN 1987, PFEIFFER 1987, 88)

Pyroluria — Serotonin support is commonly needed by pyrolurics, as low B6 decreases its formation. (PFEIFFER 1987, 88, BRAVERMAN 1988) Supplements may improve the irritability and depression, especially when B6 is particularly low. (BRAVERMAN 1988)

Other mental benefits (YOUNG 1986, REUVEN 1992, VAN PRAAG 1986, POLDINGER 1991, 96)

Depending on individual chemistry, serotonin precursors may benefit:

Other depressions — Major depression, melancholy, (MAES 1990) suicidal preoccupation. (PRANGE 1974, COUSENS 2000)

Seasonal Affective Disorder — Serotonin seems to be important, especially in winter.*(NEUMEISTER 1997, LAM 1997, MCGRATH 1990)

* Some studies: A double blind by McGrath (1990), finds improvement on tryptophan/B6/C equivalent to that produced by light therapy. Similarly Lam (1997) reports good response in 64% on 1 gm tryptophan, 3x/day.

Anxiety —Low serotonin patients are prone to greater agitation, anxiety, (BAUMEL 1995) and panic. (DAVIS 1986) Rapid depletion worsens such tendencies. (REILLY 1997) Tryptophan, or moderate intake of 5HTP, (KAHN 1985) is frequently beneficial, with optimal effect within several weeks. (VAN PRAAG 1988) Serotonin support generally promotes tranquility, emotional stability, and well-being. (COUSENS 2000, GOLD 1987, KNUTSON 1998) (SSRIs: BALLENGER 1998, MUNDO 1997, DEAKEN 1998)

Sleep (BAUMEL 1995, LARSON 2001, MELTZER 1987) — Serotonin is involved in normal sleep; sleep onset; slow wave (HAURI 1974) and REM sleep; and general maintenance of sleep patterns. (JOUVET 1969, HARTMAN 1974, 77, BRAVERMAN 1987) Melatonin, which initiates and sustains sleep is a serotonin metabolite; thus low tryptophan (common in bipolar depression) reduces melatonin, making sleep elusive. (HUETHER 1992)

Tryptophan often benefits insomnia (particularly when serotonin is low), (STOCKMEIER 1997, COUSENS 2000, URSIN 1976, SCHNEIDER-HELMET 1986) without distorting sleep physiology. 5HTP benefits mild insomnia in some, (LOEW 1997) but is too stimulating for others. (COUSENS 2000, BRAVERMAN 1987, BAUMEL 1995)

OCD — Tryptophan or 5HTP (as well as SSRIs) has been used to treat compulsive shopping, eating, (BAUMEL 1995, BLUNDELL 1984) drinking, and gambling; (LOPEZ-IBOR 1992) obsessions, and OCD. (COLODNY, MAES 1990, BAUMEL 1995, LUCCA 1992,YARYURA-TOBIAS 1977, LOPEZ-IBOR 1992) *Such treatment is not always successful, particularly in histadelia, where other nutrients can be more important.* (WALSH 2006)

Aggression — Numerous studies tie low tryptophan, serotonin or 5-HIAA to increased irritability, hostility, aggressive behavior, or violence, (BRAVERMAN 1987, MALONE 1993, AGREN 1980, POLDINGER 1998) perhaps especially in affectives. (GOLD 1987) Low levels have been found in personality disorders; (GOLD 1987) and in criminals who are aggressive or violent, or have poor impulse control, (LINNOILA 1992) or are violent and have double-Y chromosomes. (BROWN 1982, VAN PRAAG 1984)

Tryptophan-deficient dietary formulas increase male aggression and hostility, with the greatest aggression correlating with the least tryptophan. (COLLINS 1996) Rapid depletion worsens such symptoms. (REILLY 1997) On the other hand, tryptophan repletion modifies aggressiveness in many persons with low levels. Aggressive individuals may be especially responsive and sensitive to tryptophan. (CLEARE 1994)

Suicide — Some suicides may have low levels or impaired serotonin metabolism. (ASBERG 1976AB, LLOYD 1974 BOURNE 1968, PARE 1969, BRAVERMAN 1987, PFEIFFER 1985, VAN PRAAG 1984, 86, KITAHARA 1987) Low dietary tryptophan is also common. (KITAHARA 1987) Attendant symptoms of violence, aggression, agitation, and impulsivity further suggest serotonin deficit. (DAVIS 1986, ASBERG 1976AB, BROWN 1982, VAN PRAAG 1984)

Warning: When taking precursors, serotonin levels may wear off over the day (even more likely with SSRIs (see p. 287)), leading to potentially life-threatening symptoms. Prevention may entail divided doses, with the dosing schedule optimized to symptom pattern & daily biochemistry. Monitor.

Psychosis — The benefit of serotonin precursors to psychosis varies with the patient. Low tryptophan, 5HIAA, or serotonin is, in some cases, associated with visual and auditory hallucinations, (BRAVERMAN 1987, POST 1975) perceptual illusions, (YARURA-TOBIAS 1977) depersonalization, paranoia, (BRAVERMAN 1987, SLAGLE 1999, COMINGS 1984, 90) delusions, (BRAVERMAN 1987) other psychotic symptoms, (KIRSTEIN 1976) and schizophrenia. (PRANGE 1974)

On the other hand, elevated tryptophan and/or serotonin may contribute to psychosis in some.**(BENDER 1983) Abnormal and hallucinogenic metabolites of tryptophan have been found in some schizophrenias. (BRAVERMAN 1987)*

* Serotonin is 5-hydroxytryptamine. N-methylated tryptamines are hallucinogenic. Urinary NN-dimethyltryptamines have been found in some schizophrenics. (Braverman 1987)

** Perhaps mainly when certain glutamate-regulating receptors are also compromised. (Sealfon 2008)

Other conditions — Supports learning, memory, and attention span; (COMINGS 1990) and may benefit ADD, confusion, dementia. (GILKA 1975, THOMAS 1986, SLAGLE 1992, MELTZER 1998) Also, phobias, epilepsy, (PRATT 1984, SLAGLE 1992, BRAVERMAN 1987) Tourette's, (COHEN1978, COMINGS 1990) or Down's. (AGARWAL 1984) Has been used in alcoholism (BRANCHEY 1984) and alcoholic depression. (BUYDENS-BRANCHEY 1989, SLAGLE 1992, ASHEYCHICK 1989)

Serotonin precursors & pain

Tryptophan and 5HTP decrease perception of pain. (LIEBERMAN, SLAGLE 1999) They increase endorphins, which dull pain, (MURRAY) and are important in the pain-modulating raphe nuclei. (BRAVERMAN 1987) Dietary deficiency can increase pain sensitivity. (BRODERICK 1984)

Tryptophan has been used extensively in treating chronic pain, (POLLOCK 1986, SELTZER 1983, BLUNDELL 1984, BAUMEL 1995, SLAGLE 1999) including migraine, (POLLOCK) fibromyalgia,*(BAUMEL 1995) and dental pain.**

* Low blood tryptophan (Russell 1989, Moldofsky 1978) or inhibition of serotonin formation (Goodnick 1993) may play a role in the pain sensitivity and insomnia of fibromyalgia, which often responds to 5HTP. (Caruso 1990, Puttini 1992).

** Electrical dental pain inhibitors are thought to work by converting tryptophan to serotonin. Over time they lose effectiveness unless tryptophan is replenished. (Seltzer 1983)

"When you are kind to someone, both you and the person you are kind to end up with a good feeling, a real increased level of serotonin, the calming, feeling-good hormone… the witnesses to this act of kindness also feel good, and their serotonin levels increase as well."

Dr. Wayne Dyer, 2004

Tryptophan deficiency conditions (GOLD 1987)

Pellagra

Pellagra is a tryptophan and B3 deficiency condition, usually due to poor diet (e.g., too much corn and pork). (See p. 61.)

Hartnup's Disease

Hartnup's Disease is a congenital disorder of tryptophan (and perhaps alanine, serine, or methionine) metabolism. Bacteria break down tryptophan in the small intestine, compromising absorption. Symptoms are similar to pellagra, perhaps with cerebellar involvement.

Considerations

Need may be suggested by (Braverman 1987, Cousens 2000, Baumel 1995, Slagle 1999, Ross 2002)

Depression, SAD, low self-esteem, negativity, shyness, suicidality, moodiness.

Anxiety, panic, OCD, PTSD, obsessions, phobias, impatience, irritability, aggression, rage.

Late hours, insomnia.

Confusion, dementia. (Gilka 1975, Thomas 1986, Slagle 1999, Meltzer 1998)

Heat sensitivity, temperature dysregulation. (Baumel 1995)

Skin eruptions, dry scaly skin, etc.

Gastrointestinal disorders. (Baumel 1995, Cousens 2000) Uremia.

Low blood sugar.* Cravings, especially in the later part of the day, for carbohydrates,* fat, chocolate, tobacco, marijuana, or alcohol. (Ross 2002)

Pain (PMS, migraine, fibromyalgia, TMJ, etc.). (Baumel 1995, Ross 2002)

Endocrine imbalances.**

Cardiovascular symptoms.***

* As tryptophan can raise blood sugar, increase sugar available to the brain, decrease appetite. (Braverman 1987)

** Helps regulate the hypothalamus-pituitary endocrine axis. (Braverman 1987) A primary activator (with dopamine) of pleasure and sexual centers. (Cousens 2000, Slagle 1999) Influences growth hormone, prolactin. (Charnet 1982, Baumel 1995)

*** Supports the cardiovascular system. Regulates heart output, blood vessel contraction, blood clotting. (Cousens 2000, Baumel 1995)

Populations (Braverman 87, Baumel 95, Gilka 1975, Miller 1975, Bender 1983)

Conditions associated with low serotonin include:

Stress, starvation, anorexia, obesity, malabsorption (e.g., celiac sprue). Puberty, PMS, pregnancy, lactation, oral birth control (depletes B6), menopause. Hyperthyroid, hypopituitary, high cortisol, Cushings. Pyroluria, histadelia, pellagra, nicotinic acid encephalopathy, porphyria. Fever, liver disease, aging. Low B6, B3, B2; too much copper; Wilson's disease; too much corn. Caffeine, amphetamines, other stimulants.

Nutrient interactions

Forms niacin.

May support zinc absorption. (Evans 1980)

Lab

Plasma — the most practical test, and directly correlated with brain levels. (Braverman 1987, Murray 1996, 98)

Serum serotonin — often low in depressed, agitated, anxious, or insomniac patients. (Slagle 1999)

Platelet serotonin. (Murray 1998, Gold 1987)

Urinary 5-HIAA — a metabolite (though levels can vary with diet, drugs, stress). (McIntyre 1984, Murray 1998)

Tryptophan loading — measures absorption. (Gilka 1975)

Also check for low B6 or pyroluria (which can strongly suppress serotonin), methylation imbalance, estrogen. (Ross 2002)

Sources (Broida 2001, Cousens 2000, Braverman 1987)

Brain serotonin is proportional to dietary tryptophan, (Wurtman 1971, 78) *which is not particularly abundant. Sources include:*

Good quality protein (wild game, beef, anchovies, other meats, eggs) and dairy (milk, Swiss, parmesan, and other cheeses). Also in: bananas, pineapple, walnuts, sunflower and pumpkin seeds, cashews, almonds, lentils, soy. Complex carbohydrates (legumes, potatoes, sprouted breads, etc.) support absorption.

Dose

Tryptophan* — Doses have started at 250 (Hartmann 1979) to 500 mg, (Cousens 2000) perhaps increasing over time to 1.5 (Ross 2002) to 2 gm; (Slagle 1999) with max possibly 4 gm for bipolar depression, 3-6 gm for mania, 1-3 gm in augment-ing lithium to reduce switching, (Slagle 1999, Braverman 1987) *as dictated by individual need,* and with *doses divided over the day.*

* Note: Sale of tryptophan is legally restricted in the US.

5HTP — Doses start low, perhaps 25 mg at meals, and may increase to 150-200 mg total, (Cousens 2000, Rogers 1997) with no more than 300 mg for depression, 600 mg for mania, (Cousens 2000) *with doses divided doses over the day, and total quantity tailored to individual need.*

Monitor. High doses can be counterproductive. (Gelenberg 1982)

Since 5HTP may interfere with sleep, Cousens (2000) prescribes 5HTP in the day; tryptophan, one hour before bed, with complex carbohydrates or without food. Ross (2002) suggests adding melatonin before bed if insomnia persists.

Adjust dose and timing as needed, to prevent periods of low serotonin with irritability, depression or other symptoms. Rogers (1997) suggests that if the patient is too sleepy in the day, tryptophan can be concentrated at night (*except when also needed through the day for mania, agitation, anxiety, pain, food or alcohol craving*).

Benefits may not be evident for 2-3 weeks. (Cousens 2000)

Supportive nutrients

B6 (or *P5P*) — *critical* to conversion to serotonin. Research emphasizes its benefit to serotonin-depleted conditions, such as depression, chronic pain, headache, aggressive behavior. (Bernstein 1990) *Do not take at the same time as tryptophan.* Can be counterproductive if 5HTP is used.* (Larson 2001)

* Otherwise conversion to serotonin may take place in the body, instead of the brain. Some practitioners advise separating B6 (and perhaps other nutrients which promote metabolism to serotonin) 6 hours from precursors, and taking tryptophan in preference to 5HTP, especially in persons prone to gut or heart reactions. (Larson 2001)

B3 — supports tryptophan metabolism to serotonin instead of niacin. Forms NAD, a cofactor in tryptophan metabolism. (Chouinard 1978, 83, Gilka 1975, Young 1974, Green 1980abc)

B12, folic acid, C, SAM — support formation of biopterin (BH4), which stimulates serotonin synthesis. (Young 1991, Coppen 1982, Botez 1979, Gilka 1975, Braverman 1987) The proper folate/methyl ratio is important. (Walsh 2007)

Other cofactors: Iron, calcium, magnesium, zinc.

B1, B2, biotin, inositol, chromium, or manganese may be supportive. (Larson 2001, Gilka 1975, Slagle 1999)

A high-complex-carbohydrate/low-fat diet maximizes uptake into the brain. (Pollock 1986, Wurtman 1988, 89)

D3 (or, exposure to sunlight, especially AM; or to blue light) seems to increase brain serotonin. (Lambert 2002, Cannell 2007, Glickman 2006)

Considerations *continued*

Aerobic exercise can also be helpful. (CONLAY 1989).

C, E, Mg, fish oil may help protect the heart. (LARSON)

Thyroid may foster serotonin activity. (CLEARE 1996)

Curcumin may reduce serotonin breakdown.

Effects of excess, contraindications (POLDINGER 1990, BYERLEY 1987)

Agitation, dysperceptions, hypomania. (GAYFORD 1973, BRAVERMAN 1987)

Aggression can occur in 1%, and may, in some, remit with co-nutrients, or small divided doses. (LARSON 2001)

Decreased libido (mostly at high-dose 5HTP).

Drowsiness, grogginess, bizarre dreams. Headache. (LARSON 2001, COUSENS 2000)

If too much converts in the blood instead of the brain, serotonin could increase blood pressure, promote coronary artery spasm, clotting, etc., countermanding use with cardiovascular disease. (LARSON 2001, COUSENS 2000, BAUMEL 1995)

Creation to serotonin in the gut can produce cramps, nausea, diarrhea, constipation, gastric irritation, vomiting. Conversion by gut bacteria to methyl tryptamines may promote malabsorption, celiac sprue, constipation, diverticulosis, or psychotic symptoms. (BROIDA 2001)

High levels of tryptophan, or interaction with carbidopa, may cause skin problems. (SLAGLE 1999)

See *Biotype indications*, p. 102.

Note: 5HTP is much more likely than tryptophan to convert to serotonin before it reaches the brain (especially when taken at the same time as B6), potentially leading to severe side effects. Larson's clinic will not even prescribe it. (Larson 2001)

Serotonin availability

Serotonin availability is influenced by diet, heredity, circulation, sensitivities,* and receptor and hormonal response. And by the status of tryptophan uptake, storage, release, reuptake, and breakdown.

* e.g., wheat and dairy may compromise intestinal absorption.

Competition with kinurenine pathways (MURAY 1996, 98)

Tryptophan may form kinurenine instead of serotonin, especially with too much estrogen, sugar, or stress, and low B6 and B3. Kinurenine then competes with tryptophan for transport to the brain. (MULLER 1989) B6 is particularly important in reducing kinurenine levels. (GREEN 1980ABC, 1983, JANOWSKY 1988)

Avoid 5HTP with carcinoid, ulcers, Crohns or other GI disease; severe liver disease; (BACHMANN 1983, GILKA 1975) perhaps, pregnancy, asthma, lupus, scleroderma. (COUSENS 2000)

Tryptophan in broiled or burnt food can form potent carcinogens. Increased tryptophan metabolites have been found in some cancers. On the other hand, melatonin, a tryptophan metabolite and potent antioxidant, has been researched as an anticancer agent. (PANZER 1998)

Do not take with SSRI's unless so advised by (and under the care of) a knowledgeable physician.

Caution: Serotonin syndrome (NULAND 1994)

High levels may lead to confusion, fever, fatigue, shivering, sweating, nausea, diarrhea, impotence, rigidity, incoordination, exaggerated reflex, severe agitation, hypomania, rapid heartbeat, low blood pressure, violent muscle twitching/ contractions, seizures, loss of consciousness, death.

It's usually due to interactions of drugs which block serotonin metabolism (especially SSRIs; also tricyclics, MAOIs, pain meds); rarely, to drug interactions with natural agents.*

* SSRIs steadily deplete tryptophan, (Moore 1998) then become less effective, (Delgado 1990) leading to higher doses. If 5HTP, St. Johnswort, or tryptophan (Pope 1985) is suddenly added, magnification of SSRI potency and serotonin activity could increase the risk of serotonin syndrome. Melatonin similarly increases serotonin availability and therefore risk. Some practioners suggest waiting ten days after discontinuing antidepressants before starting natural agents. Nonetheless, to reduce severe depressions from tapering SSRIs, others (Moore 1998, Rogers 1997, Cass 2007) recommend gradually introducing tryptophan (separating the two by at least 6 hrs (Ross 2002)). Such approaches mandate ongoing monitoring, and educating the patient to immediately report suspicious symptoms. (See also, *SSRIs*, p. 287.)

Legal toxicity issues

Originally tryptophan was widely researched and prescribed by mainstream physicians, especially to stabilize mood and augment tricyclics. (SLAGLE 1999) In 1989, two years after introduction of the first SSRI, one manufacturer, trying to short-cut tryptophan formation, inadvertently created a toxic contaminant. (BRYCE 1992) 1500 people became seriously ill with eosinophilia-myalgia syndrome; dozens died.*(BELONGIA 1990, SLUTSKER 1990) The FDA then banned US tryptophan sales.**

5-HTP, which is more potent than tryptophan, remains legally available. (BAUMEL 1995) Tryptophan can still be obtained by prescription at compounding pharmacies. (ROGERS 1997)

* Catterall (1988) suggests metabolizing nutrients could have been helpful. ** The FDA now claims uncontaminated tryptophan may cause EMS in animals, or the rare sensitive patient, and cites a few high-dose studies.(Blauvert 1991) 5-HTP has been implicated in 3 cases. In two of these, patients were taking carbidopa, which increases tryptophan reaching the brain. (Sternberg 1980, Lampert 1992, Bryce1992). Case 3 may not even have involved 5HTP. (Farinelli 1991)

Serotonin chemistry (SLAGLE 1999, MURRAY 1996, BRAVERMAN 1987, ROGERS 1997, LARSON 2001, GILKA 1975, COPPEN 1982, BOTEZ 1979, BERNSTEIN 1990, GREEN 1983, YOUNG 1974)

L-tryptophan + *BH4* (folate + B12 + C + SAM) + O_2 via *tryptophan hydroxylase* (cofactors: Fe + Ca + B3) --> 5-HTP

5HTP via *5-hydroxytryptophan decarboxylase* (cofactors: B6 + Mg + Zn + C) --> serotonin

Serotonin -- via *MAO* (which is copper dependent) --> 5HIAA

□ Tryptophan, in the presence of oxygen, *biopterin* (whose activity depends on the folate/methyl balance), and the enzyme *tryptophan hydroxylase* (cofactors: iron, calcium, B3), becomes 5HTP.

□ 5-HTP via *5-hydroxytryptophan decarboxylase* (cofactors: B6, magnesium, zinc, C), becomes serotonin.

□ Other supportive nutrients: D3, some B vitamins (B1, B2, biotin, inositol), complex carbs, chromium, omega 3.

□ On firing, presynaptic storage vesicles release serotonin. After interacting at the postsynaptic receptor, some serotonin is taken back into the presynaptic neuron. Some is inactivated by synaptic *MAO* (a copper-dependent enzyme) which oxidizes it to 5HIAA, which is released to the CSF, and then the blood and urine.

□ Melatonin (which promotes sleep) is also a metabolic product of serotonin.

Catecholamines

Catecholamines are a class of stimulating and antidepressant neurotransmitters, including norepinephrine and dopamine. They are formed from the amino acids phenylalanine and tyrosine,* with the help of B12, folic acid, and SAMe;** vitamins B6 and C; and iron and copper. Further support may be provided by B3, magnesium, biotin, and other nutrients. The sequence proceeds thus:

PHENYLALANINE --> TYROSINE --> DOPAMINE --> NOREPINEPHRINE --> EPINEPHRINE

* Tyrosine also precurses thyroid hormone, which interacts profoundly with catecholamines, and has important antidepressant activity. (See pp. 225-37.)
** Optimizing the folate/methylation ratio. (Walsh 2007) (See pp.153-67.)

Dopamine (Snyder 1974, Beckman 1979, Pfeiffer 1987, Cousens 2000)

Dopamine is a major stimulating neurotransmitter and catecholamine. Dopamine connects the frontal (cognitive) lobes with the limbic (emotional) system and deeper regions of the brain, integrating experience with memory, thought and emotion. It exists in a dynamic balance with histamine, acetylcholine, and GABA. (Snyder 1974, Beckman 1979, Pfeiffer 1987, 88,· Hoffer 1983)

Dopamine functions (Cousens 2000, Jaffe 1992, Braverman 1994, Pfeiffer 1987, 88)

- Critical to abstract thought, creativity, logic, will, and judgment.
- Essential to concentration, learning, and intelligence. Mediates short-term memory.
- Reinforces positive feelings & reward-seeking.
- Stimulates the pleasure center of the brain.
- Affects sexuality and sexual arousal.
- Mediates eating and drinking behavior.
- Mediates activation, exploration, and fine motor movements.
- Mediates hormonal response.

Depression

Dopamine activity may be suppressed in depression and suicidal depression.*(Roy 1992, Bowden 1997) Especially with indications of low activity, precursors and cofactors may benefit unipolar, (Kapur 1992, Muscat 1992, Nierenberg 1998, Grunder 1993, Benkert 1992) and probably, bipolar depression. (Perugi 2001, Durval 2000)

* And with chronic neuroleptic intake.

Biotype indications (Hoffer 1983, Jaffe 1992, Braverman 1994, Fischer 1973)

Dopamine activity tends to be reduced when undermethylated (histadelic). In histapenia, high levels contribute to anxiety, psychosis, mania, and other symptoms.

Treatment

See *Phenylalanine, Tyrosine,* pp. 111-14.

Dopamine, reward, & addictions: The effect on mood

Reward-seeking & mania

Dopamine reinforces the positive feelings and reward-seeking,*(Crow 1981) which are enhanced in manics.

Adverse experiences impairing reward-response, fostering depression

Adverse experiences, especially those over which the individual has no control, may inhibit ongoing nucleus accumbens dopamine release and impair response to reward, (Cabib 1996) increasing the tendency to depression.

Dopamine craving, addiction, & mood instability

Chronic dopamine overactivity (as may occur in mania) can eventually reduce dopamine messaging and so lead to depressed mood, lack of motivation, suppressed cognition, and difficulty feeling pleasure. The tendency then is to turn to substances which stimulate catecholamines (coffee, chocolate, cocaine, etc.), creating a vicious cycle of addiction and furthering mood instability.

Function & brain anatomy

Dopamine projects mainly to the nucleus accumbens and forebrain; nigral dopamine, mainly to motor areas. (Ressler 1999)

Wires thought to emotion — via frontal/ limbic connections. (Snyder 1974, Beckman 1979, Pfeiffer 1987)

Cognitive, language & social learning — at mesocortical regions. (Moore 1978)

Mediates pleasure & reward seeking — especially in the nucleus acumbens (in the mesolimbic system). (Cousens 2000, Crow 1981, Cabib 1996, Chronister 1982)

Basic drive (arousal, sleep, appetite) — at midbrain and hypothalamic regions.

Motor mechanisms — at striatal, and mesolimbic regions. (Moore 1978, Costal 1977, Cools 1977)

Contribution to mania

Dopamine (and norepinephrine) messages may elevate just before the switch, and during mania. (GOODWIN 1970, BUNNEY 1972, BOND 1972, SHINFUKU 1961, GREENSPAN 1970, JONES 1973, POST 1980) A number of studies find increased dopamine metabolites in mania, (SLOANE 1966, STROM-OLSEN 1958, MESSIHA 1970) reduced in depression. (ROY 1992, BOWDEN 1997 BOWERS 1976) Levels may be greater during acute mania (decreasing over time), (POST 1975) and even higher with manic psychosis.*

Research now finds enhanced second messenger signalling and receptor sensitivity on dopamine and other excitatory pathways may be more important to mania than absolute neurotransmitter levels.** (PARK 2005, BEAULIEU 2005, POLLACK 2004, *SCI STKE* 2005). (See p. 279.)

Thus, as mania escalates, dopamine messages may dominate limbic pathways, producing overstimulation, intense agitation, disorganization, confusion, and psychosis; (GOODWIN 1974) and fueling such manic symptoms as impulsivity, irrational behavior, irritability, aggression, insomnia; addiction to pleasurable activity, novelty and reward-seeking; (BENJAMIN 1997) and increased libido, assertiveness, mental and physical activity, energy, strength, and vibrancy of thought and emotion. (GOODWIN 1990, COUSENS 2000)

* Elevated dopamine activity is associated with schizophrenia, hallucinations, voices, schizoid avoidant behavior, and probably contributes to the accompanying emotional agitation, dysperceptions, distorted thinking, fragmented speech, etc. (Bunney1972 abc)

** Thus, pharmaceutical studies suggest that though increases in absolute levels of dopamine may transiently trigger and modulate mania, they probably do not sustain it. The response lag of two to three weeks with antidepressants, and several days or more with antimanics, (Gerner 1976) does not support neurotransmitter etiologies, but rather, may reflect the time needed to alter receptor number and sensitivity, (Nathanson 1977) and second messenger systems. (Ansseau 1990, Wybrow 1984) These profoundly influence mood-related catecholamine messages, explaining contradictory studies. Most researchers now posit receptors, second messengers, and the signalling cascade as the more critical players. (Park 2005, Beaulieu 2005, Pollack 2004, *Sci STKE* 2005).

History: Catecholamine hypothesis

This hypothesis, developed in the 1960s, suggested elevated levels of catecholamines (norepinephrine and dopamine) may cause mania; low levels, depression. (AXELROD 1975, PRANGE 1964, BUNNEY 1977, DAVIS 1965, SCHILDKRAUT 1965, WHYBROW 1984)

It was supported by observations that drugs which increased dopamine and norepinephrine synthesis, release, or synaptic accumulation were often antidepressant, (ANNITTO, SHOPSIN 1979, GOODWIN 1971, 78, MURPHY 1972, RANDRUP 1977) and sometimes induced mania; (BUNNEY 1977, WHYBROW 1984) while drugs which inhibited synthesis, or blocked receptors (e.g. neuroleptics, lithium), decreased manic symptoms and promoted depression. (POST 1978, WHYBROW 1984)

Considerations (HOFFER 1983, JAFFE 1992, PFEIFFER, 1987, 88, BRAVERMAN 1987)

Need may be suggested by:

Depression, lack of motivation, apathy, ambivalence. Learning and memory problems. General cognitive impairment.

Lack of appetite, suppressed sexuality. Reduced hormonal response. Fatigue. Somnolence.

Difficulty with fine motor movements. Reduced muscle tone, coordination, motor activity and fluidity.* Movement disorders. (COUSENS 2000)

Less ability to repair damaged cells. (COUSENS 2000) Compromised immunity.

* Dopamine counterbalances acetylcholine in governing nerve/muscle interactions, and is highly concentrated in the substantia nigra and basal ganglia, which coordinate movement. Excess dopamine has been associated with chorea; deficiency, with Parkinsons (and characteristic muscle tremors, rigidity, and shuffling walk).

Populations (deficiency)

Drug addiction, chronic neuroleptic use, prolonged stress, histadelia, Candida, hypothyroidism, alcoholism. *Depletion may be due to overuse, insufficient precursors or accessory enzymes, or problems with re-uptake.* (FISCHER, 1973)

Populations (elevation)

Elevation can occur with lead toxicity, (WALSH 1986) histapenia, high copper, puerpureral psychosis, (CHECKLEY 1994) high estrogen, (PFEIFFER 1987) migraine, hypertension, hyperthyroid or too much supplemental thyroid, schizophrenia, sympathetic tumors, L-dopa treatment,* phenylketonuria,* liver disease. Dopamine is stimulated by caffeine, cocaine, other stimulants.

* Especially if taken with carbidopa, which prevents L-dopa breakdown.

Lab (JAFFE 1992, ROSS 2002, PFEIFFER 1987, 88)

Platelet dopamine, or urinary homovanilic acid.
Histamine and methylation balances.
Folate, copper, zinc. Metal metabolism.
Thyroid and adrenal function.

Norepinephrine (NE) (noradrenaline)

NE functions (Whybrow 1984, Ressler 1999)

- Mental acuity, intellectual performance, learning ability, attention, alertness.
- Fight-or-flight sympathetic activation.*
- Important in fear reactivity. (Golden 1986, Janowsky 1988)
- Increases sensitivity to the external environment. (Janowsky 1988, Gold 1987)
- Enhances visual acuity and response. (Ressler 1999)
- Mediates mood, arousal, anxiety, pleasure. (Gold) Helps associate reward with stimulus.
- Important interactions with endocrines.
- Modulates dopamine** and serotonin release.***
- Supports subtle complex motor tasks.

* It's a major sympathetic transmitter. (Janowsky 1988)

** Potentiates firing of ventral tegmental dopamine neurons which connect to the limbic system. (Kasamatsu 1984, Greenhoff 1993, Waterhouse 1988)

*** Moderates raphe nuclei serotonin firing. Low and very high norepinephrine decrease serotonin response. (Foote 1995). Serotonin, in turn can inhibit or activate locus coeruleus NE. (Mongeau 1997, Ressler 1999)

Anatomy (Ressler 1999, Janowsky 1988, Levitt 1984, Gold 1987, Descarries 1984, Lindvall 1984, Golden 1986, Potter 1993)

NE neurons are concentrated in the locus coeruleus of the brainstem, and project through the hippocampus to the cortex and the rest of the CNS. (Ressler 1999)

Locus coerleus NE organizes behavioral state, in part by decreasing Purkinje cell spontaneous firing, increasing the strength of reactions to stimuli.

Hypothalamic NE mediates arousal and attention in response to the environment, and governs hormonal activity via the pituitary. NE also connects hypothalamic pleasure centers with the limbic system, and projects to an emotion center in the cortex. Fear may be mediated through NE hypothalamus/locus-coeruleus/cortex interactions.

Thalamus/cortex NE enhances arousal and sensory and motor gating.

Hippocampal NE mediates learning and memory. Connections to the amygdala pair memory with emotion.

Effects of rate of firing (Foote 1995, Aston-Jones 1991,91a)

During alert, awake, orienting, focused attention, or arousal behavior, NE firing is rapid and complex til accomodation occurs. Firing is extremely rapid during hyperarousal or distractibility; low, during sedation. Locus coeruleus and thalamic firing stops during REM.

Norepinephrine is a major stimulating neurotransmitter, and a catecholamine. It is found in the adrenals and sympathetic nervous system, as well as the brain.

Bipolar fluctuations (Ressler, Nemeroff, 1999)

The effectiveness of norepinephrine-related nutrient precursors and cofactors (and of NE-stimulating pharmaceuticals) in many depressions, along with norepinephrine's generally activating and alerting properties, and its role in emotional gatekeeping, suggest increased NE messages in mania (perhaps especially at the switch to mania); decreased, in depression.

A number of studies show increased absolute levels in mania, (Muscettola 1984, Schatzberg 1989, Schildkraut 1978, Potter 1993) decreased in depression, though not all studies confirm this. However, researchers are finding changes in norepinephrine receptor sensitivity, (Spyraki 1980, Charney 1981, Meana 1992, Piletz 1986, Karege 1991, Matussek 1980, Siever 1992, Schatzberg 1995, Mann 1985, DePARMENTIER 1990, Hosada 1993, Ordway 1994b) second messenger activity, (Nibuya 1996, Durman 1997, Ressler 1999) and neurotophic factors, (Nibuya 1996, Ressler 1999) all of which may be more primary to the influence on mood.*

* And through their influence on norepinephrine homeostasis, help explain some of the counterintuitve findings on absolute levels. (Werstiuk 1990, Pande 1979, Biegon 1988, Mann 1985, Halper 1988, Ebstein 1988, Ressler 1999, Belmaker 1981)

Depression (Ressler, Nemeroff, 1999)

Depression is often associated with norepinephrine/locus coerleus dysregulation, (Ressler 1999, Berman 1996, Charney 1998, Heninger 1996,. Leonard 1997, Owens 1997, Potter 1993, Schatzberg 1995) and/or low norepinephrine metabolites (Potter 1993, Karege 1991, Blomberg 1980) (though, again, metabolites sometimes test high,* or non-specific). (Post 1966, 80, 89, Willner 1985, Roos 1969, Bowers 1969, Sjostro 1972, 73, Goodwin 1971, 73, Ashcroft 1977, Morris 1974, Roy 1988, Christensen 1980, Berrettini 1985, Leonard 1997))

Depletion is known to trigger depression in vulnerable persons. (Muller 1955, Schildkraut 1965) And norepinephrine pathway suppression by drugs** sometimes creates severe depression, (Freis 1954, Muller 1955, Spector 1965, Charney 1998) especially in affectives responsive to norepinephrine-based antidepressants (but not usually in normals). (Heninger 1996, Charney 1998) Such depressions are reversible when NE suppression ends, or norepinephrine activity is enhanced. (Schildkraut 1970, Sulser 1975)

Many antidepressant drugs target the norepinephrine system, but deplete norepinephrine, and so become less effective over time unless stores are repleted. (Charney 1998, Delgado 1990)

However, concurrent intake of precursors risks overstimulation, mania, cardiovascular damage, etc., and so, if not contraindicated altogether, requires cautious medical supervision.

* Perhaps due to: anxiety, adrenal dysregulation (Potter 1993), physical activity (Potter 1993), hospitalization (Post 1984), pharmaceuticals (Karki 1956), aspirin, steroids (Curzon 1970), amphetamines (Schildkraut 1970), antipsychotics (Guldberg 1968), receptor mechanisms (e.g., very high levels of NE might allow alpha 2 inhibitory receptors to take over, producing inhibition, while somewhat lower levels activate alpha 1 receptors and BARs, creating stimulation, (Foote and Aston-Jones 1995, Ressler 1999), etc.

** Reserpine, for example, can create a severe depression.

Contribution to mania

NE hyperactivity can trigger or sustain mania and produce:

- ☐ Mood elevation. Euphoria. Increased drive, ambition, initiative.
- ☐ Enhanced memory. Hyperpragia. (GOODWIN 1990)
- ☐ Intrusive curiosity. (GOODWIN 1990) Alertness, vigilence. Grandiosity.
- ☐ Increased brain sensitivity to stressors and other stimuli. (Stress activates NE neurons). (POST 1978C) Insomnia.*
- ☐ Anxiety, restlessness, agitation. Irritability, anger, aggression.
- ☐ Paranoia. (HANSEN 1973, HOKFELT 1970, SLAGLE 1992)

* With enough light, acetylcholine causes the SCN in the hypothalamus to transmit norepinephrine to the pineal, which then inhibits melatonin production, compromising sleep.

Therapies

Depression: NE cofactors and precursors, *if indicated.** (SLAGLE 1992)
Mania: Hamner (1999) suggests using serotonin to counterbalance NE, rather than trying to inhibit it with drugs. (Similarly, acetylcholine, taurine, GABA, and glycine help counter norepinephrine.)

* Note: Sufficient brain NE is needed for related drugs to work optimally, however, NE supplements (especially with sudden or high-dose) may dangerously enhance drug effects.

Norepinephrine promotes emotional intensity

The anterior cingulate acts as a gatekeeper for emotional and behavioral reaction to conditioned stimuli (e.g., fear). Hamner proposes that mania may occur when high norepinephrine from the locus correleus overcomes that gating, intensifying emotional and behavioral response; depression, when low levels support gating, dampening emotional response.* (ADLER 1990, HAMNER 1999)

* Other disorders: Hamner (1999) points out that PTSD, common in bipolars, probably involves a more constant cingulate inhibition. Adler (1990) suggests the relatively continuous cingulate suppression in schizophrenia, and perhaps other psychoses, probably involves dopamine (rather than norepinephrine).

Medication-based evidence (RESSLER 1999)

*Ressler points out that the mechanisms of most antidepressant drugs suggest abnormal NE activity in depression.**

MAOIs — These inhibit the enzyme (*monoamine oxidase*) which breaks down intracellular NE (and other monoamines). (MAOI effectiveness led to the original catecholamine hypothesis of affective disorders.) (LOOMER 1957, SCHILDRAUT 1965, BUNNEY 1972ABC, PRANGE 1964)

Tricyclics — The antidepressant effectiveness of imipramine and other tyricylics depends on the extent to which they inhibit NE reuptake. (AXELROD 1961, GLOWINSKI 1964)

SSRIS — Serotonin reuptake inhibitors downregulate some NE receptors, (VALENTINO 1995, MONGEAU 1997) and reduce production of the rate-limiting enzyme in creating norepinephrine. (BARON 1988, NESTLER 1990) At least one SSRI is a relatively potent norepinephrine reuptake inhibitor. (OWENS 1997)

Newer antidepressants — Many powerfully influence the NE system. (ASCHER 1995,SCHATZBERG 1995, OWENS 1995, DEBOER 1996, ANDREWS 1996, MUTH 1986, SCHWEITZER 1994)

Possible mechanisms contributing to depression (RESSLER 1999)

- ☐ Disordered NE activity.* (BERMAN 1996, CHARNEY 1998, HENINGER 1996, LEONARD 1997, OWENS 1997, POTTER 1993, SCHATZBERG 1995)
- ☐ Cellular damage to the NE system (DURMAN 1997) in the locus coeruleus, (CHAN-PALAY 1989, ARANGO 1996) cortex, (KITAYAMA 1997, VALENTINO 1995, KLIMEK 1997) limbic system, (DREVETS 1998) etc.; (perhaps due to stress,**(HENINGER 1996) adrenal overactivation, (ARBORELLUS 1999) NATHAN 1995, PLOTSKY 1998) or toxic assault).
- ☐ Difficulty forming *tyrosine hydroxylase*, the rate-limiting enzyme in creating NE. (RESSLER 1999, ORDWAY 1994, WANG 1998, BIEGON 1992)
- ☐ Effects of NE depletion on attention, concentration, memory, socialization and arousal, distorting response to stress and new stimuli, and indirectly altering mood. (ROBBINS 1995)

* This may manifest as (Ressler 1999):
— NE firing extremes, with little relation to stimuli, altering receptor sensitivity and neurotropin levels, causing neural degeneration or axon pruning. (Durman 1997, Kitayama 1997)
— Uncoupling from serotonin, (Mongeau 1997, Geracioti 1997) brainstem GABA, glutamate, enkephalin, CRF, or neuropeptide (Roy 1992, Cleare 1997) systems, compromising postsynaptic NE modulation.

** Especially in the young, prolonged stress and NE secretion which doesn't shut down, creating longterm limbic/frontal tendencies to overreact (possibly leading to shyness, mood disorder, etc.). (Yahuda)

Considerations (COUSENS 2000, SLAGLE 1992, GOLD 1987)

Need may be suggested by

Depression, hopelessness, anhedonia, apathy, isolation, distractibility, indecisiveness, cognitive suppression.

Exhaustion, fatigue. Craving for stimulation. Muted response to stress.

Narcolepsy, caffeinism. (LEONARD 1997AB, NUTT 1997 PLAZNIK 1991)

Low libido. Low blood pressure, slow heart beat. (HANSEN 1973, HOKFELT 1970, SVENSSON 1977)

Low energy, increased appetite and weight.*(COUSENS)

* Due to slow conversion of glucose to energy.

Deficiency may be promoted by

Overuse (as in stress), insufficient precursors or relevant enzymes, disturbed* re-uptake (as in Candida, hypothyroid, alcoholism).(HOFFER 1983B, FISCHER 1973)

Supportive nutrients

Precursors: phenylalanine or tyrosine.

Cofactors: B6, folate, SAMe, C, B12, iron, copper.

Lab

Platelet, plasma (or CSF) NE or normetanephrine.

Urinary MHPG or vanilmandilic acid.

Consider thyroid, adrenals, and methylation status. (ROSS)

Cautions

Excess NE activity can trigger mania.

Usually inadvisable with antidepressant meds. Can pose severe cardiovascular risk. *Check with your physician.*

Phenylethylamine (PEA)

A study of antidepressant benefit

Sabelli 1996 — 12 of 14 major depressives, some unresponsive to meds, responded rapidly to 10-60 mg PEA/day (plus a drug which slows its degradation), and were still improved, at the same dose, 20-50 weeks later, apparently without side effects.

PEA is present in chocolate and marijuana, and may be the chemical most responsible for the feeling of "being in love." PEA, like amphetamines, stimulates norepinephrine activity. It is also structurally similar to amphetamine, and too much can similarly produce psychosis, often involving paranoia. (Baumel 1995, Sabelli 1986, Janssen 1999)

Depression

PEA powerfully elevates mood. (Sabelli 1995, 96) It is often deficient in bipolars, especially in bipolar depression, as well as in major depression (and perhaps ADD). (Mann 1980, Janssen 1999, Sabelli 1995) Some suggest defiency may play a primary role in depression. (Sabelli 1986, Wolf 1983, Baumel 1995) Decreased urinary levels normalize with antidepressant therapy. (Mann 1980)

Contribution to mania (Sabelli 1995, 96)

PEA may be excessive in, and contribute to, some manias. Low MAO (see *Enzymes*, below), found in some patients, allows PEA to build up, perhaps contributing to symptoms. PEA also promotes manic symptoms, increasing energy, attention and activity, and sometimes fostering aggression, and possibly psychosis.*

* Thus, phenylacetic acid (the main PEA metabolite) is increased in schizophrenia and in schizoaffective an disorder. (Janssen 1999)

Considerations

Source

For antidepressant use, many physicians use D-phenylalanine (which most readily converts to PEA) or DLPA (a 50/50 mix of D- and L-phenylalanine).* (Janssen 1999)

Exercise also increases PEA. (Szabo 2001)

* Precursors are needed since PEA is not stored, and degrades rapidly.

Caution

Can trigger mania. *May be contraindicated for many bipolars.*

Especially within the first two hours of intake, can raise blood pressure.

Enzymes which recycle catecholamines

Monoamine oxidase (MAO) (Pfeiffer 1988, Gold 1987)

MAO is a copper-containing enzyme, popularized by MAO inhibitor antidepressants. MAO is found in the cell body or nerve terminal, on the mitochondrial membrane. It degrades neural dopamine, norepinephrine, serotonin and PEA.

□ **Mania** — Low MAO allows antidepressant neurotransmitters to accumulate, (Farley 1978) and has been associated with thrillseeking, impulsivity, and paranoia. (Gold 1987, Pfeiffer 1988) Several studies have related low platelet MAO to some cases of mania and bipolar disorder. (Gold 1987, Belmaker 1976) Generally lower MAO in men may contribute to a higher incidence of paranoia and more extreme manias. (Krauthammer 1978)

□ **Depression** — Elevated MAO lowers excitatory neurotransmitters (norepinephrine, dopamine, etc.) and is associated with depression and anxiety. MAO increases with age, (Robinson 1972) and is higher in women, perhaps contributing to the increased incidence of depression, particularly in older women.

□ **Conditions that may be associated with low MAO** — Mood disorder, alcoholism, iron deficiency anemia, paranoid schizophrenia, certain antihypertensives. (Belmaker 1980, Pfeiffer 1988)

□ **Lab** — Platelet MAO. (Gold 1987)

Catechol-O-Methyltransferase (COMT)

COMT is an enzyme which breaks down catecholamines (norepinephrine, dopamine, etc.) in the synapse. Imbalanced COMT can contribute to mood shifts.

Phenylalanine

Ninety per cent of dietary L-phenylalanine is metabolized into tyrosine, which produces catecholamines (epinephrine, norepinephrine and dopamine); and thyroid hormone; all of which are generally antidepressant. D- or DL-phenylalanine forms PEA, a particularly potent antidepressant. Phenylalanine also discourages breakdown of certain endorphins and enkephalins which mildly elevate mood (FOX 1985) (and may help alleviate pain). (BRAVERMAN 1987)

In general, phenylalanine is a nervous system stimulant and creates the effects produced by the above neurotransmitters, supporting memory, alertness, and awareness of the environment; and enhancing mood and thought. Excess increases vigilence and irritability. (COUSENS 2000) Deficiency promotes lethargy, fatigue, immobility, exhaustion (LARSON 2001)

See *Dopamine, Norepinephrine,* previous pages.

Depression

A number of studies find phenylanine highly beneficial in depression,* (KRAVITZ 1984, SPATZ 1975, BECKMAN 1977, 78, 79, 80, SABELLI 1983, DA DIEH 1992) (especially in patients with diminished catecholamine or endorphin activity (GIANNINI 1989, MEYERS 2000, COUSENS 2000, BAUMEL 1995)), and bipolar depression.** (SABELLI 1986, 91, SIMONSON 1985) Patrick Darby, MD, (2006) finds phenylalanine alleviates approximately 75% of cases of bipolar depressions.* It can, however, trigger mania.

Catecholamine vs serotonin support

Consider symptoms, diet, history of response to aminos and other nutrients, antidepressant drugs, and lab findings.

A combo of precursors and cofactors of both transmitters (e.g., tyrosine plus 5HTP) is helpful in some cases, (VAN PRAAG 1984, AXORIN 1990, MEYERS 2000) perhaps especially in histadelia. (WALSH 2007)

See also, *Catecholamines vs serotonin,* p. 99.

Some of the studies

Beckman 1979 —Double blind. 13 depressives on DL-phenylalanine for 30 days improved equivalently to 14 on imipramine.The later was sometimes a little better for anxiety and sleep.

Beckmann 1983 — DL-phenylanine was equal to or better than low dose imipramine for depression.

Birkmayer 1984 — 69% of 155 treatment-resistant depressives recovered on low dose LPA, another 15% improved.

Yaryura-Tobias 1974, 76 — the majority recovered by 2 weeks, most by 2 months.

Simonson 1985 — 50% of depressed bipolars recovered rapidly on low-dose LPA.

Sabelli 1986 — 31 of 40 depressives responded to doses up to 14 gm/day.

Sabelli 1991 — 9 of 10 bipolar depressives, unresponsive to medication, responded to phenylalanine.

Chemistry & supportive nutrients (ROGERS 1997, HASHIMOTO 1983, SLAGLE 1992 ,WURTMAN 1974)

(1) **L-PHENYLALANINE** --> TYRAMINE *or* **TYROSINE** *or* **DL-PHENYLALANINE** --> **PEA**
(2) **TYROSINE** --> **L-DOPA** --> **DOPAMINE** *or* **TYROSINE** --(iodine)--> **THYROXINE**
(3) **DOPAMINE** --> **NOREPINEPHRINE** --> **EPINEPHRINE**

Cofactors in catecholamine formation: Vitamin B6, copper (*DBH*), C, B12-folate/SAM balance (*BH4*), and iron support formation of tyrosine, dopamine and norepinephrine.

Other support for catecholamine activity: B3 (*NADH* stimulates *BH4*, and DA formation), D (increases the rate-limiting enzyme), magnesium (can increase SAM and perhaps, DA synthesis), B complex (for B1, B2, B3, biotin). Also, CoQ10 and carnitine (metabolic support); omega 3, calcium and inositol (second messenger support); and attention to thyroid, pancreas, and adrenal function. (BUKREEV 1978, PFEIFFER, LARSON, COUSENS) (Manganese and zinc* are largely regulatory.)

Antioxidants: C, E, glutathione or NAC, melatonin, CoQ10, etc., help protect the catecholamine system.

Considerations: Phenylalanine (Cousens 2001, Baumel 1995, Broida 2001, Larson 2001, Slagle 1992, Rogers 1997, Gold 1987, Sabelli 1986)

Need may be suggested by

Depression, boredom, lack of drive, trouble concentrating, low mental and physical energy, too much sleep, difficulty waking, cold-intolerance, cold fingers and toes. Prone to overeating; or attracted to stimulants, alcohol, diet soda, caffeine, chocolate, sugar, tobacco, or marijuana. (Ross 2002) Low thyroid, (Slagle 1992, Braverman 1987), conditions involving pain, Parkinson's. Low dopamine, norepinephrine, or PEA.

Populations

Severe stress (depletes catecholamines), (Wurtman, Banderet) as does overuse of stimulants (including coffee). (Gelenberg 1982, Braverman 1987) Hypothyroidism. Plasma PA is low in about 10% of depressives. (Braverman 1987, Pfeiffer 1975, 87)

Supportive nutrients (Bukreev 1978, Pfeiffer, Larson 2001, Cousens 2000, Ross 2002)

B3, B6, C, folic acid/SAM, B12, iron, copper, support metabolism to catecholamines. (To a lesser degree, magnesium, D, B complex (for B1, B2, biotin, etc.).

Source (Cousens 2000, Slagle 1992, Pfeiffer)

The richest sources are red meat and wild game. Also found in: ricotta or cottage cheese, other dairy, eggs, poultry, fish, wheat germ, soy, nuts, seeds. (Very little in grains, vegetables, fruits, oils.)

Dose

Start low (e.g., 100-250 mg) and gradually increase* to target dose, divided into several times per day (perhaps 1/2 hour before meals, and not past mid afternoon. (Cousens 2000, Braverman 1987) Cousens (2000) suggests a total over the day between 350-1500 mg, depending on patient need. Take with B6, C. Slagle suggests using tyrosine too, allowing for lower doses of phenylalanine. If potent enough, tyrosine alone is preferable. Full benefit may not occur for several weeks or more. (Braverman 1987, Larson 2001)

* In some patients, doses must be kept low (e.g. 100 mg). C helps prevent excess accumulation. (Braverman 1987)

Warning

Antidepressant drugs that focus on catecholamines typically exhaust stores of both neurotransmitters and precursors. When effectiveness diminishes, the drug dose is usually upped. Adding phenylalanine replenishes raw materials, but can magnify the action of the drug, and especially with abrupt high doses, may cause mania, cardiovascular complications or death.

Effects of excess, contraindications (all forms)

Overstimulation. Hypomania or mania. Agitation, anxiety, insomnia.

Constipation, nausea, headaches.

High blood pressure (especially in the first 2 hrs), perhaps hypertensive crisis or stroke. *Avoid if vulnerable.*

Not recommended for children or nursing mothers.

Avoid with any tendency to melanoma.

Avoid with phenylketonuria, psychosis, schizophrenia.

Not recommended with antidepressants, antihistamines, ADHD or Parkinson's meds.

D or DL-Phenylalanine

Need may be suggested by (Ross 2002, Braverman 1987, Slagle 1992)

Cries easily. Depression, anhedonia. Low endorphins.

Craves reward, comfort, carbohydrates, chocolate, tobacco, marijuana, alcohol, caffeine, certain foods.

Intractable, (Budd 1983) acute, (Halpern 1986) and chronic pain, (Fox 1985) as in arthritis, joint and back pain, menstrual cramps, whiplash, migraine. (Fox 1985, Beckmann 1979, Heller 1978, Budd 1983)

Dose

Typically, 500 mg, 2 to 3x/day, not past mid-afternoon, possibly somewhat more. The D form is less stimulating. (Ross 2002) Increase, slowly, cautiously, and only if necessary. Take with B6. (Braverman 1987) *May trigger or worsen mania. Monitor for agitation, overstimulation.* See *Contraindications*, above.

Reminder: Consult with your physician as to appropriate care.

Phenylketonuria (PKU) (Braverman 1987, Pfeiffer 1988)

Phenylketonuria is an inherited difficulty in forming tyrosine from phenylalanine (usually a problem with the enzyme *phenylalanine hydroxylase*).

Intelligence** shows some correlation with the ability to make tyrosine, and can be somewhat stunted, even with mild illness. The severe condition is often associated with profound retardation, and/or inability to talk or, in some, to walk. Many are hyperactive, aggressive, microcephalic and prone to seizures. Adults show serious psychiatric disorder.

PKU is rare, though mild cases are more common, and often missed. Bessman (1979) advises testing light-featured children with peculiar postures and gaits, learning and developmental problems, hyperactivity, tremor, skin conditions.

Lab

Markedly elevated phenylalanine (urine and blood can be several hundred times normal). Normal to low tyrosine.

Perhaps, low blood serotonin, low hair magnesium and calcium, urinary B6 excretion, abnormal EEGs.

Treatment

Treatment is best begun at birth, and typically includes avoiding foods containing phenylalanine, and supplementing tyrosine, perhaps B6 and tryptophan.

Tyrosine (Braverman 1987)

Tyrosine is a precursor to catecholamines and thyroid hormone, and is important in enkephalins (which influence immunity, inflammation and mood) and other peptides.

Intake promotes mental effects attributable to catecholamines and thyroid hormone, including increased mental (and physical) energy, clarity of thought, alertness, and stimulation. (Rogers 1997, Cousens 2000, Young 1996) It is also critical in the striatal region of the basal ganglia, where it helps mediate movement.

Depression

Tyrosine levels, (Goodnick 1980) activity, and metabolism (Hale 1991) can be suppressed in bipolar depression. Besides depression, deficiency can produce such related symptoms as lethargy, immobility, fatigue, and excess sleep. (Larson 2001, Hendler 1989)

Various studies have investigated tyrosine's effectiveness in major (Gelenberg 1980, 82, 83, 90, Goldberg 1980, Gibson 1983, Buist 1983) and bipolar depression. (Takahashi 1968, Benkert 1979) Some report equivalence to pharmaceuticals in mild depression. Most non-SSRI antidepressants prolong the action of tyrosine metabolites. (Braverman 1987)

For more severe episodes, higher doses create greater benefit; or phenylalanine might be used. (However, tyrosine, because it is less potent, is generally less likely to lead to mania.) (Cousens 2000)

Serretti (1998) suggests a gene for *tyrosine hydroxylase*, the rate limiting enzyme in forming catecholamines, may play a role in mood disorder.

Stress: Depleted tyrosine & hormonal changes worsen depression

Tyrosine is used up in forming catecholamines to cope with intense or prolonged stress. Less tyrosine is then available to replenish norepinephrine and dopamine (which counter depression), and thyroid hormone (which mediates mood and energy); (Wurtman 1988, Banderet 1989, Salter 1989) and to suppress cortisol. (Reinstein 1985) The combination of diminished catecholamines with adrenal and thyroid exhaustion or overresponse may then trigger or worsen mood episodes. (Braverman 1987, Gelenberg 1983, Baumel 1995)

Biotype indications

Catecholamine precursors can be helpful for the histadelic (undermethylated/high folate) patient (though support for methylation is more directly effective), and detrimental for the histapenic (in whom dopamine and norepinephrine tend to be excessive). (Walsh 2007)

Reminder: This book is presented for educational purposes only. If you need treatment for mood disorder, phenylketonuria, tyrosemia, or any other medical condition, please seek the services of a knowledgeable physician.

Phenylalanine vs tyrosine (Cousens 2000, Larson 2001, Slagle 1992)

Tyrosine is less likely to contribute to racing thoughts, insomnia, irritability, headaches, increased blood pressure, and exacerbations of Parkinson's. It can be particularly helpful for hypothyroid patients.

Phenylalanine is generally a more potent antidepressant, as it can be absorbed over five times more readily, and it precurses PEA (see p. 110). The risk of triggering mania is also greater, though, especially with chronic pain, phenylalanine (especially the DL form) is often preferentially indicated. (Braverman 1987)

A double blind

Gelenberg 1990 — four-week, controlled, double blind. Among 65 unipolar outpatients, the difference in antidepressant effectiveness between tyrosine and imipramine was only 5%. Moreover, tyrosine produced less clinical deterioration or other side effects.

Addictions

Low levels of catecholamines can contribute to drug cravings and addictions (Larson). Tyrosine and/or phenylalanine have been used to help repair neurotransmitter damage by cocaine, amphetamines, and alcohol; and help wean depressives off caffeine, tobacco, and other drugs. (Goldberg 1980, Lancet 1980, Gibson 1983, Wojcik 1982, Wurtman 1974)

Tyrosemia (Braverman 1987)

Tyrosemia is a genetic defect, associated with extreme accumulation of tyrosine. It can produce mild retardation, neurological damage, seizures, and pigment problems (melanin is a tyrosine metabolite).

Transient tyrosinemia is common in premature infants, usually causing lethargy and feeding problems. Insufficient maternal vitamin C (especially if protein intake is high) may play a role, impairing tyrosine oxidation.

Considerations: Tyrosine

Need may be suggested by:

Major and bipolar depression, (Goodnick 1980) postpartum depression, (Maes 1992) apathy, boredom, attention disorders, (Ross) too much sleep, hypothyroid, (Slagle 1992, Braverman 1987) low metabolism, (Cousens 2000) low sex drive, tendency to overeat. (Cousens 2000, Reeves 1984)

Check labs for DA, NE, PEA.

Conditions fostering deficiency (Cousens 2000)

Drug abuse (especially stimulants), overuse of coffee or alcohol. In some cases, birth control pills.

Starvation, low birth-weight infants, sexual dysfunction, chronic kidney disorder (which also decreases other aminos).

Phenylketonuria, even if mild.

Nutrient & hormonal actions

Used in forming various amino sugars and lipids, catecholestrogens, and thyroxine.

Supportive nutrients & hormones (Cousens 2000, Larson 2001, Gold 1987, Braverman 1987, Mandel 1978, Rogers 1997, Ross 2002, Puchacz 1996)

B12, folate, SAM;* and copper, iron, C, B3 (*NADH*), B6 *(P5P)*, and B complex support formation and metabolism to catecholamines. (Magnesium, D, manganese, and zinc, and antioxidants may provide further support.)

Normal thyroid activity allows for greater conversion of tyrosine to catecholamines (otherwise it may be diverted to form thyroid hormones). Adrenal support is similarly helpful.

* In proportions that create an effective folate/methylation ratio.

Counteractive nutrients

Tryptophan, valine, leucine, norleucine, and branched chain aminos compete for absorption, and/or lower or inhibit tyrosine.

Source (Cousens 2000)

Meat, eggs, fish, legumes, wheat germ, dairy, poultry, almonds, sesame and sunflower seeds, spirulina.

Dose

Dose often starts low (e.g., 100 mg), (Larson 2001) with gradual increases. (Cousens 2000) 500 mg, 2-3x/day is typical, skewed to the beginning of the day (e.g, before breakfast and lunch, early afternoon). (Cousens 2000, Braverman 1987) The upper limit may generally be 1 gm 3x /day.*(Cousens 2000, Braverman 1987, Larson 2001) In some patients, doses must be kept low (e.g., 100 mg). Vitamin C helps prevent accumulation. (Braverman 1987) Over time plasma levels tend to increase, often allowing for lower doses. (Braverman 1987)

Absorption is better on an empty stomach, though mild gastric distress may occur. (Cousens 2000) N-acetyl-L-tyrosine or tyrosine dipeptide with glycine may be best absorbed. (Cousens 2000, Braverman 1987)

* Lower if also taking phenylalanine.

Effects of excess, contraindications (Cousens 2000, Rogers 1997, Larson 2001, Baumel 1995, Broida 2001, Slagle 1992, Braverman 1987)

Can exacerbate mania; increase adrenaline, fear, stress, overstimulation, insomnia.

May worsen psychosis or schizophrenia.

Excess may eventually inhibit the enzyme used in creating neurotransmitters from tyrosine.

Migraine (more often with phenylalanine). Tryptophan may help.

High blood pressure (though tyrosine is less likely than phenylalanine to cause hypertensive crisis, or stroke).

Adults with limited tyrosine-metabolizing enzymes can accumulate high levels, which can cause neurological damage, pigment dysfunctions, perhaps mild retardation or seizures.

Contraindicated in breastfeeding, pregnancy, and with any tendency to melanoma.

Not recommended with MAOIs, tricyclics, other antidepressants, antihistamines, ADHD or Parkinson's meds, except under medical supervision.

Considerations: Tyramine

Source

Tyramines are produced in tyrosine or phenylalanine metabolism. Food sources include: hard cheeses, processed meat, pork, chicken, liver, other animal foods, certain food additives, avocado, lima beans, lentils, snowpeas, certain other legumes, nuts, bananas, beer, ale, wine (especially Chianti), ergot (a mold sometimes present in rye).

Cautions (Cousens 2000, Larson 2001, Broida 2001)

Limit exposure when taking MAOIs, antihistamines, tricyclics, Parkinson's meds. Signs of toxic reactions include headaches and severely high blood pressure. Toxicity can be life-threatening. Avoid with liver damage, overactive thyroid, melanoma. Patients with serious illness should alert their physicians.

3. Role of cellular energetics

"Oxidative stress, poor energetics and excitotoxicity are fundamentally inter-related. The three conditions both cause and effect one another." — Woody McGinnis, MD, 2004

Kato (2000) first suggested that altered energy metabolism and calcium uptake, due to mitochondrial* dysfunction, may underly bipolar changes. Several studies since find disturbed mitochondrial activity; (KONRADI 2004, DAGER 2004, SCHWEITZER 2004) reduced frontal lobe or basal ganglia metabolism and blood flow, and suppressed cellular energetics, (MODICA-NAPOLITANO 2004, KATO 2000) particularly in depression. (MAYBERG 1994, KENNEDY 2001, DREVETS 2002, SHAPIRA, LEVINE 2007, KATO 2000, QUIROZ 2004) Relevant nutrients discussed on the following pages include ALCAR, creatine, and NADH. Also see: *CoQ10* (pp. 77, 117), *B6* (pp. 62-63), *B3* (pp. 59-60), *B2* (p. 70), *Magnesium* (pp. 25-28, 126), *Excitotoxicity* (pp. 191-93).

Acetyl-L-Carnitine (ALCAR) (CRAYHON 1998)

L-carnitine, an amino acid primarily found in red meat, supports body energetics. Acetyl-L-carnitine (ALCAR) crosses into the brain more readily, and so more effectively supports brain energetics.

ALCAR helps create and store neural energy, and is the only means to transport fat into the neuron's energy-producing mitochondria, where it serves as a major fuel source. And it serves as a mitochondrial antioxidant. (WALSH 2007)

It also helps boost the antidepressant effects of the thyroid, (BRAVERMAN 1987, FURLONG 1996) and may have a role, as a minor methylator, in helping to activate the antidepressant neurotransmitters, dopamine and norepinephrine. (ROGERS 1997)

Research suggests it may clear or markedly improve certain depressions, especially in fatigued or older patients. (CALVALLINI 2004, TEMESTA 1987, GECELE 199, BELLA 1990, ROGERS 1997, PETTEGREW 2000, GARZYA)

ALCAR also affords the brain some protection from stress-related damage, and low oxygen. And it promotes acetylcholine and melatonin activity (associated with mood moderating, anti-insomnia benefits).

Benefits with age

Acetyl-L-carnitine promotes brain health, slows brain aging, and protects against age-related receptor loss. (CRAYHON 1998) It supports the ability to learn and interact positively, (KOHJIMOTO 1988) and protects against senile brain degeneration and memory loss,* and Alzheimers dementia. (BROOKS 1990, SALVIOLI 1994, CALVANI 1992, BODIS-WOLLNER 1990, RAMPELLO 1992). Thus, it may be especially indicated for depressed patients over forty, with impaired cognition or alertness, (CRAYHON 1998, ROGERS 1997) poor stamina, and low thyroid or adrenals. (CALVALLINI 2004, TEMESTA 1987, GECELE 1991, BELLA 1990, ROGERS 1997, PETTEGREW 2000, GARZYA 2000)

* One mechanism: ALCAR increases and enhances hippocampal response to nerve growth factor (which preserves neurons, especially acetylcholine neurons, but declines with age). (Rampello 1992, Agnelucci 1988)

Biotype indications

Walsh (2007) notes low energy and oxidative stress may suggest a trial of carnitine. For histadelics, ALCAR is the preferred form, and may improve brain methylation. For histapenics, L-carnitine, which increases physical function, is ususally more helpful.

Carnitine vs Tyrosine (CRAYHON 1998)

Carnitine tends to be a less potent antidepressant than tyrosine, but generally protects the heart, and can be taken with MAOIs, and by melanoma patients.

Functions supporting mood

- □ Crucial component (as phosphatidyl-carnitine) of neural membranes, influencing signal transmission and reception. (HIRATA 1980, TOMMASO 1990, BRAVERMAN 1987, PETTEGREW 2000, ROGERS)
- □ Helps create and store neural energy. Transports fat to mitochondria, where it provides the main source of energy for ATP (which stores energy). (ROGERS 1997)
- □ Critical as a mitochondrial antioxidant. (WALSH 2007)
- □ Helps preserve mitochondrial genetic info; thus, ability to produce energy. (GADALETA 1990, CRAYHON 1998, PETTEGREW 2000)
- □ Protects the brain from free radicals, (ROGERS 1997, AMENTA 1989, CRAYHON 1998) low oxygen, (Rampello 1992, PATTI 1988) and stress-related damage. (ROGERS 1997) Reduces damage to fats and may help prevent lipofuscin formation. (AMENTA 1989) Supports glutathione creation. (BRAVERMAN 1987)
- □ Helps the brain get energy from lipids or ketones when glucose is low (before meals, in hypoglycemia, etc.). (AURELI 1990) May benefit hypoglycemia. (ROGERS 1997) Helps regulate insulin. (BRAVERMAN 1987)
- □ Increases physical energy and stamina. Thyroid effects on metabolism may be partly via carnitine.* (LEIBOWITZ 1984)
- □ May help prevent loss of brain glucocorticoid receptors. (PATACCHIOLI 1989)
- □ Spares methionine, and activates catecholamines, improving mood in undermethylated patients. (ROGERS)
- □ Helps maintain acetyl CoA (an intermediary in creating energy from aminos, fats, carbohydrates.)
- □ Precurses and increases activity of acetylcholine. (WHITE 1990)
- □ Supports melatonin release, regulating sleep. (ROGERS)
- □ Prevents loss of substance P (which reduces pain, and may have some effect on mood). (DI GIULO 1992)
- □ Decreases acidity (and aciduria). (BRAVERMAN 1987)
- □ Helps maintain the myelin sheath (which speeds transmission in certain neurons). (CRAYHON 1998)

Considerations: Carnitine (CRAYHON 1998, BRAVERMAN 1987)

Need may be suggested by

Depression, lack of focus, cognitive impairment, memory loss, learning problems, autism (COOK 2004).

Low energy, weak muscles, fatigue. Poor endurance and stamina. Sugar craving.

Low thyroid symptoms.* (BRAVERMAN 1987)

Elevated triglycerides, cholesterol, blood ketones.**(ROGERS 1997, BRAVERMAN 1987)

Atherosclerosis. Weak heart. (ROGERS 1997)

Difficulty accessing stored fat or carbohydrates. Obesity, cravings. (BRAVERMAN 1987) Liver cirrhosis. (BRAVERMAN 1987)

Reduced sperm motility. (BRAVERMAN 1987)

* Carnitine also may protect heart and bone calcium in hyperthyroids, and in patients given high-dose thyroid. (Pettegrew 2000)

** Due to incomplete fat oxidation, as in diabetes, high protein or fat diets.

Populations

Levels decrease with age, toxicity, stress, worry, depression. Low serum carnitine can occur with low thyroid, pituitary or adrenals, (CRAYHON 1998) and in many autistics. Also, during pregnancy or nursing (it's used in breast milk and colostrum), and in preterm babies. (BRAVERMAN 1987)

Supportive nutrients (ROGERS 1997, BRAVERMAN 1987, CRAYHON 1998)

Glutathione, lipoic acid,* or other potent antioxidants — *critical* when taking carnitine to help protect the brain from the increased energy. (CRAYHON 1998)

* However, consider *Lipoic acid issues*, p. 178.

Phosphatidyl serine, (CRAYHON 1998) phosphatidyl choline, (CORREDOR) and C help balance carnitine.

For further support in countering depression, Crayhon (1998) suggests considering phosphatidyl serine, EPA, B, B6, B12, folic acid, C, E, magnesium, calcium, zinc, selenium and, if low, NADH.

To support carnitine synthesis, consider lysine, methionine, B, B3, C, iron, manganese. (BRAVERMAN 1987)

Source

Red meat is the richest source. (BRAVERMAN 1987)

Dose (BRAVERMAN 1987)

Doses have ranged from 500 mg, up to 1000 mg 3x / day (which is high). Determine actual need.

Introduce gradually.

Skew dosage toward the early part of the day.

Effects of excess, contraindications (BRAVERMAN 1987)

If epileptic or manic, brain cell energy may already be too high, making carnitine inadvisable.

Adjust dose if dreams become over-vivid. (CRAYHON 1998)

High doses (3 gm/day) may deterimentally affect triglyceride platelet aggregation in uremics.

Do not use with antidepressants or hyperactivity meds, except under medical supervision.

Creatine

Brain functions: Creatine (KIDD 1996)

Critical to receptor function. Helps convey messages into the neuron, and activate neural reponse. Influences neurotransmitter production and release.

Provides structural support in the neural membrane. (ELKASHEF 1987) Supports membrane proteins essential to specialized cell functions, homeostasis, and maintenance.

Helps integrate brain waves.

Plays a part in the hypothalamic/pituitary/adrenal axis, and daily rhythms of hormone release, commonly disordered in bipolars.

Creatine supports brain energy balance and probably oxygen use, (PERSKYBRAZEUA 2001) and buffers neural ATP (which stores cellular energy). (WYSS 2000)

Depression

MRS studies show significantly reduced phosphocreatine with severe (versus mild) depression. (KATO 1992) Similarly, in depressed and mixed state bipolars, brain imaging suggests severity is inversely correlated with creatine levels. (DAGER 2004)

One open study of creatine augmentation of antidepressants finds significant benefit to resistant depression. (ROITMAN, BRAVERMAN) Doctors Baruch Shapira, Boris Nemetz, Joseph Levine in Israel are at the initial stages of a 4-week randomized double blind trial of adjunctive use of creatine in depression.

Researchers have also explored use in anxiety, mental lethargy, fatigue, memory and attention difficulties, certain schizophrenias, MS, and Alzheimer's.

Supportive nurients

SAM and ALCAR increase phosphocreatine. (SILVERI 2003, PETTEGREW 2002)

Cautions (ROITMAN)

Introduce gradually.

Too much can trigger mania. Do not use with antidepressants or ADHD meds except under medical supervision.

Can cause mild nausea or gas.

NADH

NADH* is a coenzyme form of niacinamide (B3), continuously formed in the body. It is crucial to brain respiration and metabolism/energy production,** (Hoffer 1964, 73, 83) and stimulates catecholamine synthesis. (Birkmayer 1989abc, 1993, Kuhn 1996, Vrecko 1997) It's also a potent antioxidant.

* Nicotinamide adenine dinucleotide with hydrogen.

** And helps synthesize ATP.

Depression

Research suggests excellent anti-depressant activity. (Birkmayer 1991, 92, 96b) Cousens (2000) claims 85% of his clients improve.

Note: NADH is generally not recommended during mania.

Psychosis (Hoffer 1995, 2005)

A preliminary study by Hoffer, with a supplement formulated to prevent breakdown of NADH in the stomach (a critical factor), suggests even greater benefit to schizophrenia than from B3.

Mental symptoms

Deficiency may foster, and NADH intake may help correct the following conditions:

- □ Depression and related symptoms. Low dopamine.
- □ Schizophrenia, psychosis. (Hoffer 1995, 2005)
- □ Reduced alertness and mental activity. Compromised cognition and memory. Dementia. (Birkmayer 1993, 96abc)
- □ Poor psychomotor performance. Parkinson's. (Birkmayer 1996)
- □ Low energy, chronic fatigue. (Birkmayer 1993,1989bc 1996a, Kuhn 1996)

Biotypes

May benefit histapenics, perhaps even more than B3, (Hoffer 2005) and pyrolurics, especially if psychotic or anxiety-prone. (Walsh 2007)

See *Vitamin B3*, pp. 59-60.

Brain functions

- □ Works with bipopterin to create dopamine and norepinephrine. (Vrecko 1997, Birkmayer 1989a, Kuhn 1996)
- □ Critical to brain respiration, metabolism and energy production. (Hoffer 1973, 83)
- □ Potent antioxidant.

A NADH study

Birkmayer 1991 — open label trial. 93% of 205 patients with various forms of depression responded to NADH (orally, IM or IV) over 5 to 310 days.

Predator response, violence & addiction (Cleary 1986)

Dr. John Cleary, MD, postulates that when early humans encountered a scarcity of meat (a major source of B3), the uncovering of niacinamide/NAD receptor sites aroused the predator instinct. So the more avid hunters may have been those most susceptible to B3 or NAD deficiencies.

10% of the population is severely NAD deficient. Cleary suggest that, instead of predation (which is no longer socially acceptable), NAD-deficient individuals may now unconsciously turn to nicotine, alcohol, drugs, or the endorphins generated by prolonged exercise to cover their receptor sites. When unavailable, violence may ensue. The successful clinical use of B3 to reduce craving for, and counteract, alcohol, tobacco, and various addictive drugs lends weight to this hypothesis.

Considerations

Need may be suggested by (Birkmayer 1996b)

Depression, anhedonia.

Memory problems, suppressed cognition, dementia.

Low mental or physical energy, especially with age. Slow reaction time and motor activity. Suppressed motor skills.

Overweight. Compromised oxygen uptake.

Prone to free radical toxicity, high blood pressure, chronic fatigue, Parkinson's, Alzheimer's.

Source

Meat, poultry, fish, fresh vegetables, nutritional yeast.

Low in most foods; easily degraded by humidity, water, heat, light, oxygen.

Dose

5-10 mg, perhaps more. May feel results within 3 wks, increasing over 6 months to a year. (Cousens 2001)

Side effects

Can be more pronounced than those of B3 (p. 60).

CoQ10

CoQ10 helps protect and energize brain cells. Crayhon (1998) suggests 50 to 100 mg may help support mood, particularly in individuals requiring enhanced cellular oxygenation, antioxidant protection, and support for cellular energetics. (See *CoQ10*, p. 77.)

4. Inhibitors as antidepressants

Inhibitory aminos are often continued during bipolar depression (though the dose may change some) to maintain mood stability. Interestingly, they also can be antidepressant for some patients.

Taurine

Taurine may have some antidepressant activity,* especially if used with catecholamine agonists.**(Seidl 2000, Machado-Viera 2001, Warburton 2001, Slagle 1992) It is significantly reduced in some depressives, (Braverman 1987, Tachiki 1977, Sturman 1971, Larson 2001) and low levels are associated with certain hereditary depressions. (Braverman 1987, Tachiki 1977)

Dr JA Sturman (1971) comments on a family in British Columbia with a hereditary flaw in taurine metabolism and extremely low levels in blood, brain, and cerebrospinal fluid. Initially symptoms were similar to those of Parkinson's, and included depression, lethargy, fatigue, sleep disturbance, weight loss, and impaired depth perception.***(Braverman 1987)

Deficiency can also be associated with fatigue, lethargy, and low thyroid (which depletes taurine and promotes depression), (Sturman 1971) especially in women. (Braverman 1987)

See *Taurine,* pp. 38-40, for further details, including contraindications.

* Perhaps because it helps regenerate the nerve cell after firing, making it receptive to further stimulation.

** Or, it may facilitate higher doses of stimulants.

*** Eventually speech, swallowing and breathing became difficult, and respiratory failure caused sudden death.

GABA

Both too little and too much GABA can induce depression. (Ring 1993)

On the other hand, GABA is sometimes facilitory, (Petty 1998) stimulating serotonin (Akasu 1988, Bartholini 1985, Francois-Bellan 1988, Strahlendort 1988, Gray 1987) or norepinephrine* release. (Bonanno 1987ab, Petty 1993a) Like taurine, it also helps depolarized neurons recover after transmission, preventing neural fatigue and increasing receptiveness to ongoing stimuli. (Braverman 1987)

GABA may sometimes be an effective mood booster for a subset of bipolars. Agonists have been shown to reverse some animal and human depressions. (Petty 1995) And Cousens (2001) has found it helpful, especially for depressives who are GABA-deficient.

GABA has also been used alone, or with B3, B complex and inositol, as a natural tranquilizer to address the anxiety and stress that often accompany depression. (Petty 1993, 98)

Some of the pharmaceutical support for antidepressant activity

Drugs promoting GABA activation tend to have antidepressant effects, while those that decrease activation can promote depression. (Cousens 2000, Bartholini 1985) In fact, antidepressants may work, in part, through GABA. (Krystal 2002, Kendall 2005) A number of them (including MAOIs, atypicals, GABA-mimetics, SSRIs) stimulate GABA release and/or increase GABA receptor density (and so, sensitivity to GABA). (Lloyd 1983, 89, Suzdak 1986)

See *GABA,* pp. 41-43, for further details, including contraindications.

* Including release in the limbic system, the seat of deep emotions. (Suzdak 1985ab, Petty 1993a, Bartholini 1985).

Glycine

Glycine may improve some cases of bipolar depression, (Braverman 1987) especially in patients with low serum levels (Heresco-Levy 1996) It may also benefit such depression-related symptoms as anxiety, fatigue, social withdrawal, emotional flatness, apathy, and cognitive dysfunction, (Heresco-Levy 1996) however, too much can induce depression. (Braverman 1987, Slagle 1992)

Glycine helps form SAM, which activates (methylates) antidepressant neurotransmitters and second messenger systems (such as cAMP), (Smythies 1984) countering depression. Dimethyl and trimethyl glycine, particularly, (but probably more due to the methyl) increase methylation, helping with histadelic depression.

See *Glycine,* pp. 44-45, for further details, including contraindications.

Threonine

Threonine can be low in depression (Hendler 1989). In some patients, depletion is associated with severe or agitated depression, which may respond to supplementation.* (Braverman 1987, Pfeiffer, Baumel 1995)

Doses used for depression in low threonine patients have varied from 250 mg (Haas 2006) to 1 gm, 2x/day. (Braverman 1987)

See *Threonine* , p. 45, for further details, including contraindications.

5. Vitamin D3

Vitamin D is variously considered a vitamin or a hormone. It is critical to the effective use of calcium, magnesium, and other minerals, and the maintenance of biological rhythms.

Role in mood

Vitamin D may be important in countering depression. (CANNELL 2007) Deficiency may contribute to SAD, (GLOTH 1999) and probably other depressions, (VIETH 2004, LANDSDOWNE 1998, GLOTH 1999) as well as to nervousness, insomnia, irritability, and learning disorders. (KOZIELEC 1994, STAROBRAT-HERMELIN 1998)

Activity in the brain

□ Supports creation of catecholamines (by increasing the rate-limiting enzyme). (PUCHACZ 1996)

□ Like exposure to sunlight, it increases brain serotonin. (LAMBERT 2002, CANNELL 2007)

□ Protects membrane fats from peroxidation, perhaps even more effectively than vitamin E. (SARDAR 1996, WISEMAN 1993)

□ Increases glutathione and antioxidant enzymes. May otherwise support brain detox. (CANNELL 2007, GARCION 2002)

□ Conceivably, plays a role in the nucleus of neurons and glial cells.* (CANNELL 2007)

* Which contain receptors for vitamin D.

Physical functions supporting mood

Vitamin D's role in producing thyroid hormone, supporting calcium absorption and use, balancing blood sugar,* (SULLIVAN 2000) and counteracting allergies and seizures may contribute to its antidepressant effects. (CANNELL 2007)

* Reduces sugar craving, increases synthesis and release of insulin, counters glucose intolerance; protective for both type I and II diabetes. (Sullivan 2000)

Levels

In one study, levels in depressives were 80% of that in normals. (SCHNEIDER 2000) Another study found mental health scores in functional older adults directly reflected levels of vitamin D. (KENNY 2003)

Also see, *Biorhythms,* pp. 259-62.

"The healthy 'primitive' peoples that Dr [Weston] Price observed not only had broad, round, 'sunny' faces, they also had sunny dispositions and optimistic attitudes towards life in spite of many hardships. Typical intake [of vitamin D now found in people living indigenously] ranged from 3000 IU to 6000 IU. [Intake in industrialized countries] 'is paltry by comparison.'... The first step to redress... depression... road rage... cavities... osteoporosis [and other modern plagues] would be to get more light... Vitamin D adds sunlight... [and is one of] the strongest markers of health and longevity."

Krispin Sullivan, RN, 2000

RECOMMENDED READING

Sullivan, Krispin, RN, *Sunlight and Vitamin D,* at: www.sunlightD.org

Some of the studies

Vieth, 2004 — Randomized comparison study. Of 130 adults with normal levels of D,* those deemed most likely to develop depression were given 600 or 4000 IU per day, summer through winter. Both groups achieved 40ng/mL. Mood improved with increasing D. Instead of worsening, they felt better in the winter. The group taking 4000 IU showed the most benefit.

Gloth, 1999 — a small study involving a one-time oral dose of 100,000 IU. Improvement in depression was better than produced by light therapy in SAD patients, and significantly correlated with 25(OH)D levels.

Landsdowne, 1998 — Randomized double blind, involving 44 healthy subjects. 400 or 800 IU significantly improved mood over 5 days in late winter, as compared to placebo.

* 24 ng/mL in summer, generally dropping to 16 in winter.

Considerations: Vitamin D (Cannell 2007, Zitterman 2003, Sullivan 2000, Quillin 1987, Lieberman 1990, Krohn 1991, Garrison 1985, Pfeiffer 1987)

Need may be suggested by (Sullivan 2000)

Depression. SAD. Learning and behavior disorders.

Exhaustion, low thyroid. Low adrenals. Sugar craving.

Allergies. Gluten intolerance.

Burning sensation in mouth or throat. Prone to cavities.

Psoriasis, other skin disorders. Muscle weakness. Pain.

Bowed legs, poorly formed bones and crooked teeth (rickets), other bone disorders. (Zitterman 2003, Dawson-Hughes 2004)

Obesity,* low temperature, weak metabolism, thyroiditis.

Calcium deposits** (e.g., in arteries (leading to high blood pressure), (Zitterman 2003) coronary arteries, (Watson 1997) joints, kidney, perhaps brain).

Osteoporosis, (Bettica 1999) perhaps arthritis. (Zitterman 2003, Dawson-Hughes 2004, Watson 1997) Peripheral neuropathy.

High cholesterol. High blood pressure. Cardiovascular disorders, worsening in winter.

Infertility, low estrogen, PMS, menstrual migraine, polycystic ovaries.

Immune and autoimmune problems*** (perhaps MS, chronic fatigue, fibromyalgia symptoms, Parkinson's, diarrhea, Crohn's). (Cantorna 2000, Vogelsang 1989, Cannelll 2006)

Perhaps, myopia, senile cataracts. (Zitterman 2003)

May help reduce risk of cancer. (Garland 1999, 2007, Lappe 2007, Miller 1998, Kleibeuker 1995)

Has been used in diabetes, alcoholism. (Zitterman 2003, Sullivan 2000)

* D and calcium inhibit fatty acid synthase, which turns calories into fat

** D regulates calcium binding proteins which take calcium where appropriate, and protect cells from free calcium.

*** D enhances NK and T cell production, reducing autoimmune and inflammatory reactions.

Nutrient interactions

Supports assimilation of A, metabolism and transport of calcium and phosphorus, absorption of magnesium, iron, zinc. (Sullivan 2000) Controls circulating calcium levels; regulates binding proteins (which take calcium where it's needed and protects cells from free calcium) and counters coronary calcification. (Watson 1997)

Populations

People with SAD, or limited exposure to outdoor light, (e.g., chronically hospitalized patients, prisoners, people working night shift or living in cold climates, the elderly (who are less able to form D on their skin). The US population shows generally low levels.

Supportive nutrients

Moderate levels of A help reduce toxicity. (Sullivan 2000) Omega 3 and saturated (butter, coconut) fats support absorption. Omega 6 (e.g., vegetable oils), and polyunsaturated fats (PUFAs) do not.

Sources (Vieth 2004, Sullivan 2000, Glerup 2000, Lieberman 1990, NutriCircles 1996)

At least 20-30 minutes of mid-day summer sunlight (rich in UV-B), on sufficiently oily skin, is a major source of vitamin D, creating 20,000 IU. Unfortunately, UV-B rays can burn skin, and ozone depletion has magnified the risk of skin cancers, especially in ozone-sparse regions of the world. Breaking up the 20 minute exposure into shorter time chunks may help, as may exposures at safer times of the day. *Physician and patient should carefully weigh relative risk.*

> *"I would say that anyone in North America should be able to walk into any drug store and buy 1,000 IU vitamin D supplements. And if you consume those supplements every day, you should feel better."*
>
> Reinhold Vieth, PhD, in a comment to WebMD

D is also present in animal tissue exposed to light (e.g. skin) and animals which eat foods rich in vitamin D (e.g., plankton, oily fish (e.g., herring, oysters, catfish, sardines, mackerel, wild salmon, shrimp, halibut, tuna, cod), as well as fish liver oils, shiitake mushrooms, butter, fortified dairy, egg yolk, sunflower seeds.

Lab (Sullivan 2000)

25(OH)D (25-hydroxy-vitamin D) — the best measure.

Low hair calcium, despite artery deposits, might suggest low D.*

* Vogelsang (1989) found D increased hair levels, while levels fell back when D was discontinued.

Supplements

D3 (cholecalciferol), found in animal food, is preferable to D2.* (Trang 1998, Cannel 2007, Vieth 2004) [Dose may range from 400-1000 IU/day, perhaps, in some cases, up to 4000 over the winter, if depleted and prone to depression. Check labs (above). (Glerup 2000, Vieth 2004ab)]

2 teaspoons of cod liver oil provide 1000 IU, *but may supply too much A for some.* (See *Contraindications*, p. 81.)

* D2 (manufactured from irradiated ergosterol) is considerably less potent and less well utilized, and may encourage calcium deposits in blood vessels.

Effects of excess, contraindications (Sullivan 2000, Saul 2003)

Excess (usually over 25,000 IU/day, long-term) may cause:

Weakness, depression, dizziness, headache.

Restlessness. Tetany. May worsen hyperthyroid.

Thirst, frequent urination, nausea, appetite loss, diarrhea.

D2, especially, can promote calcium deposits in soft tissue, irreversible calcification of lungs or kidneys, arthritis, atherosclerosis.

Kidney or liver damage.

Lipid oxidation.

May worsen sarcoidosis.

If calcium is insufficient, too much D may contribute to bone demineralization and loss, and heart disease.

If calcium magnesium and phosphorus, and certain other minerals, are inadequate, elevated D may increase uptake of lead, cadmium, aluminum, strontium, etc. (Pfeiffer 1975, 87)

6. Minerals

The following minerals may, depending on individual requirements and contraindications, help counter bipolar depression: (SUPPORTIVE STUDIES ARE LISTED IN RESPECTIVE CHAPTERS.)

□ Calcium — antidepressant, supports neurotransmission, counters fatigue. Especially indicated in histadelia.

□ Iodine — often helpful, especially if thyroid dysfunction or low metabolism accompanies the depression. (See pp. 235-37.)

□ Chromium — especially with blood sugar issues.

□ Manganese — supports membrane stability, critical in pyroluria, useful in histapenia. Can be detrimental for histadelics.

□ Vanadium ***restriction*** — often critical in bipolar depression

□ Potassium — often low. Check balance with sodium. *Food sources, unless supplements are clearly indicated, and then, dosage usually must be conservative.*

□ Iron or copper — only if low or if increased need is anticipated. Can be useful for a subset of depressives.

□ Selenium — antioxidant; used in forming glutathione. (See p. 78)

□ Organic germanium sesquioxide — may be useful in Candida and conditions where more oxygen is required.

□ Possibly, rubidium, or cesium.

The following minerals generally help stabilize mood and so are typically indicated ongoing. For some bipolar depressives, increased quantities may help elevate mood, or may be indicated to support stability when taking antidepressant nutrients.

□ Magnesium — need is suggested by such symptoms as irritability, anxiety, insomnia, mood instability. Used in forming SAMe. Often indicated with pyroluria, histadelia, or autism.

□ Zinc — especially if low. Critical in pyroluria. Also supports histamine balance and sugar metabolism. Too much can be sedative.

□ Lithium — can be antidepressant in some bipolars, though too much can cause depression.

"I had suffered from more than 20 years with a serious and incurable" case of bipolar II depression... My psychiatrist had ultimately prescribed twenty different medications over a one year period of time... I missed months of work and... My family were absolutely devastated.

I finally stumbled onto several articles... I started [using] seafood [daily] and full spectrum trace minerals... Within four months, and to the absolute disbelief of my doctors, I was able to stop taking all mediations, and have been quite fine for well over a year."

A.P.

Calcium/Magnesium balance

"The alert physician can fingerprint a person's mood on the basis of his or her calcium level"

Mark Gold, MD, 1987

Calcium (Ca)

Calcium is generally stimulating. It activates neural functioning, regulates cell conduction and membrane permeability, and is critical in conveying and enhancing neural communication. It also stimulates ACTH secretion, and may contribute to adrenal elevation in bipolars. (HADEN 1999, COLODNY 1998)

Various researchers have drawn attention to the influence of calcium on mood. (GOLD 1987, MANNA 1991, POST 1999) A large study, (SKLAR 2008) pooling international data on over 4000 bipolars, found the second most robust genetic association in bipolars is to a gene regulating calcium channels.

A number of studies report abnormal calcium activity, and hyperactive calcium signaling.*(BOWDEN 1988, KUSUMI 1992, DUBOVSKY 1989, 91A, 92B) Also, increased cellular calcium, particularly during acute episodes. (DUBOVSKY 1989, 91, 92B) Emamghoreishi (1997) finds highest levels in bipolar 1 males, then females, then bipolar II, depressives, controls. Unusual extracellular serum calcium has also been associated with disturbed mood, cognition, and arousal. (CURRIER 1998)

* Thus, Okamato (1995) finds calcium response to serotonin greater in bipolars, sustained longer, and decreased by lithium.

Calcium generally enhances neural communication

Intracellular calcium mediates synthesis and release of dopamine, norepinephrine, and serotonin. These antidepressant neurotransmitters increase calcium activity which, in turn, increases neurotransmitter activity. (DUBOVSKY 1983, POLLACK 1987, BERK 1994)

Calcium can also increase the number of active neural receptors, thereby enhancing sensitivity to neurotransmitter stimulation.**(COUSENS 2000)

Though very high levels can be inhibitory

As calcium levels increase, type 1 IP3 receptors become more sensitive, *increasing* neural stimulation. *However,* at even higher levels, calcium (like lithium and magnesium), inhibits the enzyme which converts IP to I, thereby *decreasing* stimulation.*(COLODNY 1998)

See *Inositol*, p. 96.

How calcium facilitates neurotransmitter release

Levels of calcium inside the neuron are usually kept 5,000-10,000 times lower than outside by membrane calcium pumps and the endoplasmic reticulum. With enough stimulation of neural receptors, second messengers release IP3 into the cell, stimulating the endoplasmic reticulum to release stored calcium. If axonal electrical activity is sufficient, calcium causes the synaptic vesicles in the neuron's terminal branches to fuse with the cell membrane, releasing their neurotransmitter content into the synapse. Enzymes then decrease calcium mobilization, enabling the cell to respond to further stimulation. (COLODNY 1998)

Depression

Both deficient (WINTER 1988, ALVIR 1991) and elevated calcium (JIMERSON 1979, THAKAR1985, PAVLINAC 1979, LEVINE 1999) can occur in depression. (EDWARDS 1980, BROIDA 2001, BAUMEL 1995)

Deficiency & need for calcium

Deficiency can contribute to mood swing and chronic depression (as well as fatigue, poor concentration, anxiety, insomnia). (GOLD 1987, LARSON 2001) Supplemental calcium is particularly needed by histadelic bipolars, who are subject to a virtually constant suicidal depression. (WALSH 2000, 2002)

Note: Elevated readings can be deceptive: (KUSUMI 1992, DUBOVSKY 1992B)

(1) Blood and CSF calcium may rise while tissue calcium is depleted.*(ALVIR 1991, WHYBROW 1987) Pfeiffer notes an effective antidepressant therapy, pioneered by Dr. Flach of Cornell Medical Center, based on *increasing calcium retention* and *reducing serum levels.* (FLACH 1964, 70)

(2) High levels may represent the body's attempt to compensate for undersensitivity or ineffectiveness.

* Due, for instance, to: bipolar disorder and its etiology, (Whybrow 1987) hyperparathyroid or thyroid disorder (Klein 1998, Baastrup 1978, Hojo 1997), or chronic lithium or certain other meds. (Abdullah 1999, Baastrup 1978)

Calcium elevation

Even though calcium is generally stimulating, elevation (perhaps especially, if elevated relative to magnesium (LEVINE 1999)) seems to contribute to some depressions, particularly in bipolars, (DUBOVSKY 1990, 91) with calcium supplements further worsening mood. (CARMAN 1984) Possibly calcium is so high as to be inhibitory (COLODNY 1998) (*see box, above, left*), or perhaps it's aggravating depressive irritability, insomnia, or agitation. *Rule out deceptive readings (as above).*

Mania

Calcium hyperactivity and sensitivity in mania

The status of calcium *signalling*, rather than absolute levels, probably gives the most accurate reflection of the influence of calcium.* (Kusumi 1992, Dubovsky 1992b) Hyperactive signalling heightens norepinephrine and other stimulatory messaging, so may fuel mania. (Kusumi 1992, Dubovsky 1989, 91a) (also, agitation, anxiety, neural toxicity or dysfunction. (Cousens 2000, Gold 1987)).

Moreover, manics may overact to calcium. Thus, Dubovsky (1989, 91) finds reactivity to free intracellular calcium** greatest in untreated manics (then bipolar depressed, unipolars, controls).

Many stabilizing and mania treatments lean toward *reducing* cellular calcium activity, e.g., with magnesium supplements, calcium-restricted diets, (Carman 1984) or medications. Similarly, calcium channel blockers, (Dubovsky 1991) lithium, (Pavilinac 1979, Okamoto 1995) and other major mood stabilizers are thought to act, in part, by moderating calcium's second messenger activity — see box, below).

* Extremes of which have long been suspected of triggering or contributing to mania, with studies reporting both low, (Bowden 1988, (CSF) Dubovsky 1983, Post 1980, Carmen 1979, Jimerson 1979) and high (Groat 1980, Manna 1991, Dubovsky 1990, 1991, Swartz 1990) levels. (Gold 1987)

** Which is more important to excitability than calcium outside the cell, and may be more sensitive to subtle changes.

Underactive calcium in mania

Some manics, nonetheless, clearly manifest low calcium activity, with intake helping to stabilize mood, (Baumel) and support sleep. (Cousens 2000, Felberg 1957, Veal 1971) See, for instance, *Biotype*, on the following page.

"[With too much calcium] nerve impulses may multiply to the extent that organization deteriorates."

Carl C Pfeiffer, MD, PhD

Case study: Calcium triggering mania

Groat 1980 — Rapid IV calcium, given to a 35-year-old depressive, character-disordered woman with low levels (hypocalcemia), led to racing thoughts, euphoria, exaggerated feelings of power, pressured speech, hyperactivity, insomnia, and other manic symptoms. Six days after the calcium IV was stopped, symptoms resolved.

Ca pump instability may be greater in bipolars

Calcium pumps* help maintain an appropriate ratio of calcium outside the nerve cell to that within. This ratio (typically 4: 1) is an important influence on neuronal activity and mood. (Dubovsky 1983) Research suggests greater fluctuation of pump activity in bipolars, greatest in bipolar I, and greater in mania than depression.*(Linnoila 1983, Meltzer 1988)

* CA2+ATPase

Psychiatric meds & calcium (Meltzer 1986, Manna 1991, Okamoto 1995, Dubovsky 1992, 93)

A number of mood-stabilizing pharmaceuticals may act, at least in part, by normalizing calcium activity:

Lithium — decreases platelet intracellular calcium ion concentrations (Dubovsky 1991b) in actively ill patients* and shows significant similarity to calcium antagonists, (Manna 1991, Sarfati 1996) perhaps contributing to its effectiveness. (Meltzer 1986, Manna 1991, Okamoto 1995, Murphy 1992) Baseline calcium elevation has been highly associated with initial responsiveness to lithium. (Smigan 1985)

Calcium channel blockers — modulate calcium hyperactive cells, and are useful in some manias, especially in patients responsive to lithium. (Dubovsky 1993)

Phenothiazines & other psychotropics — influence calcium channels. (Dubovsky 1983, 1986, 1992, Himmelhoch 1986, Johnson 1993, Wood 1985)

Beta blockers and calcitonin — lower free intracellular calcium, and sometimes decrease agitation in manics. (Carman 1984, Dubovsky 1986)

* Blood calcium increases correspondingly during the first few months of treatment. Then, if depression responds, serum levels decrease, and urinary excretion increases. (Smigan 1985, Carmen 1979, Dubovsky 1983, Pfeiffer)

Parathyroid & calcium (Gold 1987, Pfeiffer 1988, Konig 1989)

Parathyroid hormone raises circulating calcium by increasing gut absorption, inhibiting kidney excretion, mobilizing bone calcium, and decreasing plasma phosphate.

Hyperparathyroidism & high calcium (Gold 1987, Pfeiffer 1988, Joborn 1986, Alarcon 1984, Pang 1996)

Hyperparathyroidism* is characterized by excess blood calcium, in some cases due to severe hyperthyroidism, stress, or too much vitamin D. Psychiatric symptoms, especially depression or anxiety, may occur in up to 25%, and are more likely in older patients. Other symptoms:** apathy, memory lapses, confusion, cognitive dysfunction, delusions, severe emotional disturbance, hallucinations, paranoia, psychosis, organic brain syndrome. (Whybrow 1987, Joborn 1986, Alarcon 1984)

Peterson found mental dysfunction related more to the increased calcium than to the hormone. (Whybrow 1987)

* A hormonal disorder, typically caused by a parathyroid tumor, but can be due to kidney or liver disorders, or other factors. Frequency is one in 800 adults; 3:1, females to males. (Morgan 1989)

** Physical symptoms can include weakness, appetite loss, nausea, constipation, abdominal pain, thirst, excess urination, urinary tract stones, bone and kidney damage, ulcers, arthritis, heart problems.

Hypoparathyroidism & low calcium (Joborn 1986, Alarcon 1984, Pang 1996)

Hypoparathyroidism* is marked by low blood calcium. Disturbed cognition and depression are common. Other symptoms** can include: psychosis, irritability, anxiety, emotional lability, neurosis, dementia, retardation, delirium, perhaps convulsions. Surgical hypoparathyroidism can cause organic brain syndrome. (Denko, Whybrow 1987)

Treatment may include supplements of calcium, magnesium, boron, silicon, vitamins C, D3, and other nutrients supporting calcium use and absorption. (Pfeiffer 1988, Morgan 1989)

* A hormonal disorder caused by autoimmunity or thyroid operations. It occurs in one in 50,000 people, especially women. (Morgan 1989)

** Physical symptoms include brittle finger nails, dry scaly skin, patchy hair, cataracts, poor formation of tooth enamel (children), cramps, muscle spasms (especially in the fingers and toes, but also the face).

Some key considerations

Biotype (Pfeiffer 1987, Walsh 2000, 02, 07)

Calcium is typically elevated in histapenia (calcium releases histamine, fostering its elimination), and increases catecholamine stimulation, and the tendency to mania. Magnesium, counterbalancing calcium, is usually beneficial.

In histadelia, tissue calcium tends to be low (with osteoporosis, and other symptoms of depletion, common). In such patients, increased calcium usually helps address the prevailing depression.

Role of sugar, caffeine, inactivity, stress, menopause

Calcium depletion and greater risk of depression (and osteoporosis) increases in women around the time of menopause and beyond; people over 45; and persons indulging in sugar, (Yudkin 1973) caffeine,* (Hollingbery, Heaney 1982) alcohol, (Spencer 1985) stimulants, etc, and/or lacking reasonable physical activity.* Stress can also deplete calcium.

* Too much sugar and caffeine (as in colas) has been tied to bone loss and fractures, (Saffar 1981, Hernandez-Avila 1991, Gaby 1994, Johnson 2001, Wyshak 2000. Ericsson 1990, Fitzpatrick 2003) as well as mood instability. (See pp. 185-89, 214-15).

Dairy issues (Weintraub 1995, Rogers 1997)

Dairy is typically a highly effective source of calcium, but is counterproductive for some: sensitivity reactions may impair absorption; an overly protein-rich dairy/meat diet can deplete calcium; or pasteurized dairy may be difficult to metabolize.

Nonetheless, though various studies suggest populations whose diets avoid dairy but contain other calcium sources (e.g., greens, especially cabbage family), and who lead physically strenuous lives, have considerably less osteoporosis, Hu (1993) found that within such populations, those who consume dairy show greater bone density.

Effective supplements

Look for *absorbable* forms of calcium (e.g., citrate, ascorbate, malate, etc.) plus supportive nutrients and herbs (vitamins C and D3, boron, manganese, silicon, magnesium, horsetail, oatstraw, etc. For peri and post-menopausal females, consider vitex, licorice, dong quai, etc., *as relevant to individual requirements*.)

Considerations

Need may be suggested by (Pfeiffer 1975, 88, Larson 2001, Gold 87)

Anxiety, irritability, nervousness, tension, obsessions, compulsions, insomnia, mania.

Chronic depression, fatigue, poor concentration.

Rickets. Tendency to fractures, backaches, bone pain, osteoporosis, osteomalacia (bone softening).

Tooth decay, peridontal disease.

Limb numbness, cramps, muscle spasms.

Palpitations, excess urination, acidity.

Tendency to accumulate lead, cadmium, or mercury.

Populations (Pfeiffer 1975, 88, Gold 1987)

Stress. Physical exhaustion/overexertion, lack of physical activity, too much sleep.

Diet rich in sugar or other refined carbs. Blood sugar imbalance. (Johnson 2001, Wyshak 2000, Ericsson 1990, Fitzpatrick 2003)

Overindulgence in protein, processed or overcooked foods. Overeating or malabsorption.

Overuse of alcohol, caffeine, stimulants or tobacco.

Low magnesium, vitamin D, or boron.

Too much phosphorus (e.g., from a diet rich in meat and sodas) relative to calcium. (Pfeiffer)

Too much oxalic acid (spinach, beet greens, sorrel) or phytates (as in uncooked grains).

Allergies, which often decrease hydrochloric acid, compromising calcium absorption.

High metabolism, reducing circulating calcium (e.g., as in histadelia, hyperthyroid).

Parathyroid imbalance.

High calcitonin (a thyroid hormone which inhibits calcium release from bones, lowering blood levels).

Kidney disease, leukemia, fluoride toxicity.

Neuroleptics, lithium, certain other drugs.

Nutrient interactions (Pfeiffer 1975, 88)

Supports proper use of phosphorus, magnesium, and vitamin D; and B12 absorption

Excess may interfere with vitamin K in clotting blood, or reduce zinc absorption and transport.

Lab (Jaffe 1992)

Ionized calcium.

Calcium distribution & deposits

Calcium is not always sent where it's needed, e.g., blood levels may be elevated while calcium is depleted from bones, perhaps deposited in blood vessels or joints; or blood levels may be insufficient, altering mood.

Supportive nutrients & life-style factors

Magnesium, manganese, zinc, boron, silicon, vitamins B6, C, horsetail, oatstraw, taurine. (Birdsall 1998)

Vitamin D3 is critical to calcium absorption and use; it regulates calcium binding proteins (which take calcium to where its needed), and protects cells from free calcium.* (Sullivan 2000)

For women near or past menopause, attention to hormonal balances. (Nieves 1998, Heaney 1989) (Consider vitex, licorice, dong quai, etc., *as relevant to individual requirements, with meticulous attention to risk.*** (Mattarello))

Physical exercise, particularly if weight-bearing, (Nieves 1998, Heaney 1989) but not to the point of exhaustion.

Enough (but not too much) sleep. Adequate sunlight.

* Reduces urinary calcium loss.

** Too little estrogen depletes calcium; too much may promote cancer. Consider the balance with progesterone, family history of cancers, etc.

Sources (Cousens 2000, Larson 2001, NutriCircles 1996))

Dairy, salmon, other fish, dark leafy greens (kale, parsley, watercress, collard green), cabbage family (broccoli, cauliflower, etc.), almonds, tahini, sesame and sunflower seeds, seaweeds, legumes.

Supplements (Cousens 2000)

High quality sources are important. Look for absorbable calcium, with a good balance of synergistic nutrients. Preferred forms include calcium-citrate, -ascorbate, or -hydroxyapatite.

Calcium carbonate and -phosphate are not well absorbed and promote calcium deposits (especially if vulnerable, e.g., low magnesium, hypothyroid, etc.)

Absorption is greatest at night, and most efficient with moderate intake (200-250 mg) several times per day skewed to the later part of the day. Do not take at the same time as zinc (which competes for absorption) or inositol (to avoid overstimulation).

Conditions associated with elevated calcium (Cousens 2000, Pfeiffer 1988, Larson 2001)

Bipolar disorder, insomnia, hypoglycemia,* slow oxidizer,** hyperparathyroid.

* Pfeiffer finds circulating calcium and magnesium often elevated in hypoglycemics, perhaps in an attempt to substitute for the manganese, chromium and zinc used up in sugar metabolism.

** Difficulty processing calcium, may elevate blood levels and promote deposits.

Effects of excess, contraindications (Cousens 2000, Pfeiffer 1975, 88)

Agitation, anxiety, mania, depression, personality change, delusions, disorientation, hallucinations, psychosis. (Gold 1987) Neural overstimulation and malfunction. Neurotoxicity. (Cousens 2000, Pfeiffer 1988)

Inability to regulate water and maintain soft stool. Overstimulation of gastric acid secretion.

Bone and tissue calcification, (Larson 2001) kidney stones. (Pfeiffer)

In some, depressed neural and muscular function. (Pfeiffer 1975, 87, 88)

"My depression was... accompanied by... anxiety, hypomania, fibromyalgia, infrequent panic attacks, anger, stress, overwhelming emotional feelings, night-time muscle spasms, paranoia, asthma, prickly sensations in hands, arms, chest and lips. My lips felt that they were going to vibrate or tingle off my face! I even saw a spider disappear into my arm once... I had very low energy, mental fogginess, depression with strange suicidal thoughts... Now, I can recognize these "mental" symptoms as symptoms of magnesium deficiency...

"I was put on nearly every antidepressant drug known and had severe side effects to all of them and felt sicker and sicker. None worked...

"Now [with 200 mg magnesium glycinate, 4x/day] my depression is completely, totally, absolutely gone!... I am active and can function mentally, emotionally, and physically at my best again."

George Eby 2006

Magnesium (Mg)

Depression

Practitioners report benefit in some bipolar depressions, particularly in patients with anxiety, irritability, or other symptoms of deficiency.* (EBY 2006, HASHIZUME 1990)

ML Robinet (1934) found magnesium depletion in local soil strikingly related to suicides.* Other researchers have found reduced levels in some depressions. (KIROV 1990, BERUBE 1992, ANANTH 1979) The relation to calcium levels may be a key factor. (LEVINE 1999, RAMUSSEN 1989)

An NIH study found low magnesium associated with more depressive symptoms, and perhaps a higher rate of suicide in hospitalized patients. (COUSENS 2000, MASON) Widmer (1992) notes red cell magnesium often normalizes with clinical improvement.

Nonetheless, magnesium elevation can also occur,** and researchers find not all bipolar depressives require more magnesium. (GOLD 1987, WIDMER 1992, ANANTH 1979, LINDER 1989, BJORUM 1972, FRAZER 1983)

Lab tests, symptom profile, and clinical response can help determine requirements. Symptoms of excess include oversedation, nausea, diarrhea, overly slow heart beat, very low blood pressure, etc., but should be distinguished from medication effects.

* Ubell (1966) also notes that completed suicides are often preceded by highly elevated adrenalin, which may provide some of the drive, or may act via its depletion of magnesium.

** Although some such cases may be compensatory, with additional magnesium still needed.

Biotype indications

Walsh (2007) finds that magnesium usually benefits all biotypes, improving histadelic depression, pyroluric irritability and stress, and histapenic anxiety and hypomania.

Mental symptoms (GOLD 1987, PFEIFFER 1975, 87, 88, EBY 2006)

Magnesium can also be low in, and may provide benefit for, such depression-related symptoms as:

☐ Increased vulnerability to stress; difficulty with social interactions.

☐ Irritability, anxiety, fear, insomnia, conduct disorder.

☐ Rigid personality, uncooperativeness. Autism. (RIMLAND)

☐ Depression. Seasonal depression.

☐ Apathy, weakness, drowsiness, stupor. (RASMUSSEN 1989)

☐ Confusion, disorientation, perhaps psychosis. (RASMUSSEN 1989)

☐ Concentration problems, neuroses, attention deficit. (MOUSAIN-BOSC 2006, BOSC 2004, NIZANKOWSKA-BLAZ 1993, STARABRAT-HERMELIN 1997, 98)

See *Magnesium*, pp. 25-28, for considerations, further discussion and references.

Possible mechanisms

Role in second messenger system.

Used in forming SAMe, thus supporting methylation (and often, histadelia).

Helps counter excitotoxicity.

Calcium channel blocker.

Anticonvulsive.

Also see p. 26.

Chromium (Cr)

Depression

Chromium may support mood stability, and improve depression, (COHEN 1994, GARETZ 1976) especially in patients whose symptoms deteriorate with exposure to sugar, refined starches, or alcohol; (COUSENS 2001) or who experience weight problems and/or pronounced food cravings and appetite. (JONATHAN 2003, MALCOLM 2000, MCLEOD 1999, 2000, DOCHERTY 2005)

Sugar/mood/chromium cycle (ROGERS 1997, DUFY 1975, BUCKLEY 1978, MOORE 1998, PRANGE 1987, GOLD 1987, MURRAY 1995, 96, PFEIFFER 1975, 87)

Chromium is a key component of glucose tolerance factor (along with niacin, zinc, and glycine). Persistent intake of refined sugars and starches depletes chromium, triggering depression and mood swings, along with blood sugar swings, all of which tend to increase the craving for sweets, creating a vicious cycle. Chronically disordered blood sugar fosters Candida, hypoglycemia, diabetes, calcium depletion and other health complications which multiply the threat to mood stability.

See *Blood sugar imbalances*, pp. 214-22.

Neurotransmitter effects (MCCARTY 1994, ATTENBURROW 2002, MALCOLM 2000)

Insulin supports antidepressant neurotransmissions. It is important in preferentially transporting tryptophan across the blood brain barrier, increasing brain serotonin. And it may also intensify norepineprhine and dopamine activity, as insulin receptors are particularly concentrated in catecholamine terminals.

McCarty notes depressives often develop insulin resistance (perhaps due to elevated cortisol), which may then go on to suppress catecholamine activity, and further dampen mood.

Thus part of the mechanism by which chromium improves depression in sugar-imbalanced patients may involve enhanced sensitivity to insulin, which then promotes norepinephrine and serotonin activity. Similarly, aerobic exercise, and avoiding detrimental or excessive fats may be helpful.

Symptoms: low chromium & sugar imbalance (GARETZ 1976, COHEN 1994, ROGERS 1997, DUFY, 1975, MOORE 1998, BUCKLEY 1978, SCHRAUZER 1992, CHRISTENSEN 1988, PRANGE 1987, MURRAY, 1995, 96, PFEIFFER 1975, 87, CURRIER 1979, ROSS 1974, 89, GOLD 1987, BENNETT 1974, LARSON 2001)

- ☐ Late afternoon blues, uncontrollable crying, depression.
- ☐ Confusion, difficulty concentrating, indecisiveness, poor concentration and memory, dementia.
- ☐ Social withdrawal, low motivation and energy, fatigue.
- ☐ Fear, anxiety, tension, irritability, anger, hostility. Difficulty with stress.
- ☐ Nightmares, insomnia. Headaches related to sugar imbalance.
- ☐ In extreme cases, personality changes/disorders, visual dysperceptions, periodic paranoia, psychotic episodes, suicidal depression, symptoms of dementia. (COHEN 1994)
- ☐ Can trigger allergies and sensitivities, compounding the problem.
- ☐ Sugar imbalance may eventually create nerve damage.

Some studies

Docherty, 2005 — 8-week, double-blind, multi-center, placebo-controlled trial. Subjects with various depressions were given chromium picolinate (containing 600 mcg elemental chromium). In the 75 subjects who took at least 80% of the nutrients, the greatest benefit occurred in atypical depressives with severe carbohydrate craving. Appetite and cravings also improved.

Jonathan, 2003 — 8-week placebo-controlled double blind trial. 400-600 mcg chromium picolinate per day. Depressive symptoms decreased more than 66% in 7/10 atypical depressives with co-occurring weight gain, fatigue, and carbohydrate cravings at baseline. Improvement was significant. No side effects occurred and no additional meds were needed. None of the five placebo patients responded.

McLeod, 2000 — Case series. Chromium was given to eight chronic refractory mood disorder patients (including bipolar II); most with carbohydrate craving and overly hearty appetites. All recovered, and returned to productive functioning. Self-reports of improved depression and food cravings were dramatic. Side effects were minor (e.g. enhanced dreaming, mild psychomotor activation). Authors suggest benefit may be due to enhanced insulin use, alone, or also, promotion of tryptophan availability and norepinephrine release.

McLeod, 1999 — Chromium (especially chromium picolinate) augmentation of antidepressants in five chronic dysthymic patients produced a rapid antidepressant response.

Considerations (chromium) (GOLD 1987, MOORE 1998, COUSENS 2001, SHRAUSER 1992, MURRAY, 1995, 96, PFEIFFER 1975, 87, GARETZ 1976, COHEN 1994, ROGERS 1997, DUFY, 1975, BUCKLEY 1978, CHRISTENSEN 1988, PRANGE 1987, CURRIER 1979, ROSS 1974, 89, BENNETT 1974, LARSON 2001)

Need may be suggested by (ROGERS 1997, SCHRAUSER 1992, MURRAY 1995, 96, ROSS 1989, PFEIFFER 1975, LIEBERMAN 1990, PHILPOTT 1980, 87, WEINTRAUB 1995, COUSENS 2001)

Moodiness, insomnia, confusion, anxiety, irritability.

Hypoglycemia. Diabetes.* (ROGERS 1997, COUSENS 2001, ATTENBURROW 2002)

Hunger, food binges, sugar-craving, bulimia, obesity.

Headaches, fatigue.

Allergies. Increased vulnerability to infection.

Arterial plaque. Cardiovascular symptoms.

* Chromium enhances sensitivity to insulin. (ATTENBURROW 2002)

See *Blood sugar imbalance*, pp. 214-22.

Populations (ROGERS 1997, PFEIFFER 1975, 1987)

In industrialized nations, chromium is highest in infants and decreases with age.* In more land-based societies, levels are maintained through old age.

Depletion occurs with mental stress, physical exhaustion, and sugar/white flour consumption.**

Larson (2001) finds slow oxidizers with sugar metabolism disorders are particularly likely to need chromium.

* A US Department of Agriculture survey, for instance, found chromium inadequate in 90% of Americans. Chromium can decrease 50% with each pregnancy, first creating intolerance to alcohol, then glucose.
** Also, post-operative glucose IVs can deplete chromium precipitously.

Nutrient interactions (ROGERS 1997)

Critical in sugar metabolism.

Supports amino acid and cholesterol metabolism. Aids in synthesis of fatty acids.

Helps stabilize nucleic acid structures.

Sources (NUTRICIRCLES 1996, PFEIFFER 1975, 87)

Brewers or nutritional yeast, liver, broccoli, potatoes, beef, turkey, shellfish (oysters, shrimp), haddock, tomatoes, whole grains, legumes, butter, mushrooms, basil, cloves, apples,* grapes,* beets,* bananas,* oranges,* carrots,* black pepper.**

* Some of the chromium is used up metabolizing these sweet foods.
** Note: Chromium is also high in eggs, but not very biologically available as GTF. (Pfeiffer 1975)

Advisability of more than one dose per day

Single doses of chromium may lead to sugar craving, hunger, and mood symptoms 6 to 8 hours later. So, some patients may need to take chromium-rich foods at that point, or take two or three doses of chromium (lowered accordingly) over the day.

Supportive nutrients (MURRAY, 1995, 96, PFEIFFER 1975, 88, ROGERS 1997)

Niacin, glycine, zinc — with chromium, support formation of glutose tolerance factor.

B6 and other B vitamins — to support carbohydrate metabolism.

C, magnesium, manganese, potassium, carnitine, and other nutrients and herbs can be important.

See *Blood sugar*, pp. 214-22, for uses, contraindications, etc.

Supplements (ROGERS 1997, COUSENS 2001)

Chromium picolinate or polynicotinate.

Effects of excess, contraindications (COUSENS 2001, MOORE 1998, PFEIFFER 1975, 87)

Too much may trigger mania.

High doses may inhibit insulin activity. (COUSENS 2001)

It is especially important for diabetics to seek the aid of their physician in determining requirements and monitoring intake.

Manganese (Mn)

Depression

Various investigations offer some support for antidepressant use with other nutrients, especially in cases involving high copper, pyroluria, (PFEIFFER 1987, 88, WALSH 2006) low magnesium, or low thyroid* and perhaps other endocrine hypofunction. (SLAGLE 1992)

Moreover, industrial toxicity is known to create a "mania" (*see callout*), suggesting possible antidepressant benefit.

Unfortunately, research targeting manganese alone is sparse.

* On the other hand, significant excess may suppress the thyroid.

Manganese mania

"Manic excitement, incoherent speech, irritability, insomnia, refusal of food, spontaneous laughing; also depression, crying — these are the symptoms of 'manganese madness' [a condition caused by repeated respiratory exposure to manganese dust, as when working in manganese mines, steel foundries, etc.]. *"*

Dr. Penalver, 1955

Mental & neurological symptoms

Manganese may benefit, and be lacking in the following conditions and symptoms, especially if not histadelic:

- □ Irritability, stress (manganese supports parasympathetic activity).(ROGERS 1997)
- □ Mood or cognitive symptoms. Psychosis. (PFEIFFER 1972, 75AB, 83, 88, 87, SLAGLE 1992, ROGERS 1997, JAFFE, 1992, ENGLISH 1964, BALCH 1990, HOSKIN 1934, LARSON 2001)
- □ Memory problems. Fatigue. Dizziness. (PFEIFFER 1975A, BALCH 1990, GARRISON 1985, QUILLIN 1987, LIEBERMAN 1990)
- □ Incoordination, tardive dyskinesia. (HAWKINS 1989, KUNIN 1976, NORRIS 1977, HOFFER 1977, TKACZ 1984)

Anticonvulsive effects

Low levels may trigger seizures. (SAMPSON 1977, HURLEY 1963) In some studies, patients with the lowest levels show the most seizure activity.*(CARL 1986, DUPONT 1985, SOHLER 1979) Moreover, manganese, balanced against zinc, B6, magnesium, etc., has shown some anti-convulsive benefit. (PFEIFFER 1976, 87, 88, BALCH, CARL 1986, SAMPSON 1977, MURRAY 1998)

* Seizure-susceptible rats also show low levels, and brain waves typical of epilepsy. (Hurley 1963)

Biotype indications

Manganese counters dopamine, so is often helpful for histapenics, perhaps at one-fifth the dose of zinc. (WALSH 2008) It's also useful with concurrent metal metabolism disorders and high copper. (PFEIFFER 1975A, 87, 88, WALSH 1991, 96, 2000, 07, 08)

In pyrrole disorder, low zinc often means metallothioneins are low, similarly suggesting a need for manganese to stimulate MT synthesis. (WALSH 2008)

On the other hand, Walsh (2007) finds manganese is generally *not* helpful for histadelics, as it can reduce dopamine (which already tends to be underactive), thus increasing depression and certain neuromuscular (e.g. Parkinsonian) effects. It may also downregulate serotonin, destabilizing mood and reducing sociability.

Possible antidepressant mechanisms (SLAGLE 1992, PFEIFFER 1987, 88, ROGERS 1997, BALCH 2001, MURRAY 1998)

Neurotransmitter effects

□ Helps form and regulate histamine. (See 152-66.)

□ Influences dopamine levels (KONTUR 1988, ALI 1985, SHIRANI 2000, SUBHASH 1991) and, perhaps, serotonin. (KIMURA 1978, NEFF 1969)

□ Helps form glutamine.

□ Supports creation and metabolism of fatty acids.

□ Critical to neural and neuromuscular communication. (ROGERS 1997)

□ Helps make choline available to form acetylcholine. (ROGERS 1997)

Support & protection for brain function

□ Supports energy metabolism. (LARSON 2001)

□ Some antioxidant activity.*

□ Supports use of B and C, and amino acid formation. (LARSON 2001)

□ Antiseizure activity, (DUPONT 1985, CARL 1986, SAMPSON 1977, SOHLER 1979) suggesting possible bipolar benefit.

* Manganese is a cofactor in some superoxide dismutases (which help prevent cell damage and inflammation), and is used in producing glutathione peroxidase. (McGinnis 2004, Murray 1998, Rogers 1997)

Endocrine balance (LARSON 2001, SLAGLE 1992)

□ Promotes normal pituitary, thyroid, and adrenal function. Supports formation of thyroxine, and oxytocin secretion. (EDER 1996, BUTHIEAU 1983)

□ Supports sugar tolerance and metabolism. Helps stabilize blood sugar. Needed in insulin regulation. (NUTR REV 1968, ROGERS 1997, LARSON 2001)

Allergies

□ May benefit brain and body allergies, and certain autoimmune disorders. (KROHN 1991)

Considerations (Pfeiffer 1975a, 87, 88, Slagle 1992, Rogers 1997, Jaffe 1992, Balch 1990, Larson 2001, Murray 1998, Garrison 1985, Quillin 1987, Lieberman 1990)

Need may be suggested by

Depression, ambivalence, poor memory, fatigue.
Dizziness, fainting. Trembling, numbness, seizures.
Histapenia, MT dysfunction (high copper), pyroluria.
Balance problems, incoordination. Tardive dyskinesia and other movement disorders.
Immune and antioxidant dysfunction. Allergies, sensitivities, autoimmune disorders. (Rogers 1997, Slagle 1992)
Glucose intolerance, diabetes. (Nutr Rev 1968, Rubinstein 1962, Rogers 1997) Weight loss.
Low blood phospholipids, fats. (Slagle 1992)
Thyroid (Eder 1996, Buthieau 1983, Kawada 1985, Misiewicz 1993) or pituitary dysfunction.
Difficulty healing. Inflammation. (Murray 1998)
Poor bone growth. Bone pain. Disc degeneration, osteoporosis. (Saltman 1993, Rico 2000) Cramping. Rheumatism. Malformed or painful joints, muscle weakness.*
Slow growth of hair, nails. Skin disorders.
Irregular heart beat, hypertension, atherosclerosis.
Ringing in the ears, hearing loss.
Reduced fertility, low libido, miscarriages, suppressed lactation, birth defects.** Low oxytocin.***
Carpel tunnel syndrome, lupus, MS, myasthenia gravis.
Severe deficiency in children may lead to deafness, blindness or paralysis.

* Mn is used to form collagen, bones, joints and cartilage.
** Needed in fetal development.
*** The hormone underlying maternal love and protectiveness.

Populations (Pfeiffer 1975a, 87, 88, Slagle 1992, Rogers 1997)

Malnourished, e.g., junk food (refined flour and sugar, sodas, etc.), iron deficiency, food grown in depleted soil or soil with relative excess of lime. Pregnant or nursing mothers. Older males. Repeated phenothiazines.

Nutrient interactions (Pfeiffer 1975a, 87, 88, Balch 1990, Slagle 1992, Rogers 1997)

Augments molybdenum and zinc in decreasing copper and promoting urinary excretion.
If too low, magnesium deficiency won't correct. (Pfeiffer)
Activates various enzymes involved in using C, B, B1, choline, and biotin.
Supports iron metabolism, and formation of vitamin K.
Used in synthesis and metabolism of fatty acids.
Required in creation and breakdown of protein and nucleic acids. Activates arginase.
Plays a role in oxidative phosphorylation.

Useful diagnostic test (Jaffe 1992)

Loading test.
Hair manganese (first rule out content in hair dyes).

Nutrient interactions

Excess iron or copper (possibly, also, calcium or zinc), can deplete manganese.

Sources (Larson 2001, NutriCircles®1996)

Mussels, snails, coconut, sunflower, other seeds, walnuts, other nuts, wheat germ, leafy vegetables, barley, rye, buckwheat, oat, millet, other whole grains (especially germ or bran), pineapple, soy, split peas, seafoods, organ meat, potatoes, legumes, blueberries, avocados, olives, raspberries, persimmons, carrots, eggs, lamb, tomatoes, cantalope. Alkaline soil and lime decrease manganese.

Supplements (Jaffe 1992, Pfeiffer 1988)

Manganese citrate, ascorbate, or gluconate. [Dose is that which normalizes tissue levels and decreases copper overload.]
Supportive nutrients include choline (e.g., lecithin), and vitamins C, B1, E, and K.

Counteractive nutrients & foods (Pfeiffer 1975a, 87, 88, Slagle 1992, Rogers 1997)

Phytates bind manganese in whole grains, unless sprouted or cooked with yeast.
Too much calcium, phosphorus, copper, zinc, cobalt, iron or soy may inhibit absorption.
Tannin (as in tea) decreases availability.

Sources of excess

Pronounced toxicity occurs mainly through industrial pollution, usually respiratory exposure, e.g., in mining; steel foundries; ore-crushing plants; dry battery and match manufacture; construction, cement, rubber, and iron work; electric welding; coloring on glass or ceramics, fungicide creation, or application, etc.

Effects of excess, contraindications (Pfeiffer 1975a, 87, 88, Slagle 1992, Rogers 1997, Larson 2001, Gold 1987, Penalver 1955, Donaldson 1981, 82, Crawte 1984, Stauber 1989, Barceloux 1999, Gottschalk 1991, Montes 2001, Cook 1974, Casdorph 1995, Walsh 2007)

With mild excess:
Overstimulation, insomnia, irritability.
Sleepiness, appetite loss, weakness.
Neuromuscular symptoms. Increased stiffness in Parkinsons. Worsens tics. (Walsh 2007)
May alter B1 metabolism, deplete copper, or contribute to iron-deficiency anemia.
Can raise blood pressure and produce hypertensive headaches in susceptible persons. (Stop intake, add zinc).
Detimental if dopamine or copper is too low (e.g., in histadelia.)

With pronounced toxicity:
Acute exposure: Shortness of breath, fever, chills; incoherence, manic excitement, compulsions, emotional lability, violence, insomnia, personality change, hallucinations. (Barceloux 1999, Gottschalk 1991). Confusion, depression, memory loss, learning disability (Colipp 1983), headaches. (Gold 1987)
Chronic toxicity:
Neurological deterioration which eventually becomes permanent. Dopamine depletion may induce a Parkinsonian syndrome with tremors, muscle rigidity, irritability, impotency, mask-like face, monotonous voice. Asthma, allergy to manganese, lung damage. Low thyroid, or goiter. (Eder 1996, Kawada 1985, Misiewicz 1993, Buthieau 1983)

Zinc (Zn)

(Garrison 1985, Pfeiffer 1972, 75, Br Med 1984, Hoffer 1983b, Jaffe 1992, Werbach 1991, Watts 1988, Crawford 1974, Sohler 1987, Walsh 1996, 2000, 02, 04, 06)

Depression

Zinc helps integrate thought, memory, and emotion. It can be low or high in depression (Rogers 1974) and often moves toward normal with recovery. (Little 1989, McLoughlin 1990, Schlegel-Zawadzka 2000, Nichols 1992, Narang 1991)

Lack of zinc can be associated with or cause some depressions. (Schlegel, Maes, Nowak 2002, 03, 1999, Hansen 1983, Markovits 1990, Narang 1991, Khan 1989) In fact, serum zinc is often low in severe drug-resistant depressions, and, according to Maes, is a sensitive predictor of poor response to medication. (Maes 1994, 2003)

Biotype indications (Pfeiffer 1987, 88, Walsh 2000, 02, 04, 06)

Lack of zinc can cause a profound depression in pyroluria, where it's critical to treatment. Zinc is also essential in histapenia and metal metabolism disorders (especially when copper is overloaded), where it may benefit some depressions. And it may be needed by histadelic (undermethylated) patients (often severely depressed).

Other mental symptoms (Pfeiffer 1975, 87, 88, Prasad 1978, 83, Jaffe 1992, Kimura 1965, Hoffer 1983a, Murray 1992, NIH)

Zinc may be low in, and provide benefit for, these depression-related symptoms:

- ☐ Seasonal depression. Apathy, indifference. (*Am J Clin Nutr* 1985, Prasad 1978)
- ☐ Anxiety, panic, paranoia, insomnia, increased vulnerability to stress. (Szewczyk 2002, Kroczka 2001, Ossowska 2002)
- ☐ Irritability, behavior disorder, rigid personality; difficulty with social interactions and cooperation. (NIH, Gold 1987, Prasad 1978)
- ☐ Memory impairment, learning disabilities, confusion, disorientation. (Constantinidis 1991, Prasad 1978, Pfeiffer 1975)
- ☐ Psychosis. (Pfeiffer 1972, 73, 83, 87, 88, Kimura 1965)
- ☐ Headaches, fainting, weakness.

Potential mechanisms (Pfeiffer 1975, 87, 88, Jaffe 1992, Braverman 1987)

- ☐ Anticonvulsive.
- ☐ Benefits pyroluria, metal metabolism disorder, histapenia.
- ☐ Counters and helps eliminate copper.
- ☐ Role in neurotransmitter creation.
- ☐ Antagonism to NMDA receptors & excitotoxicity. (Blaylock 1995)
- ☐ Supports blood sugar balance and metabolism.
- ☐ Immune and anti-inflammatory activity.* (Maes 1997)
- ☐ Some antioxidant activity.
- ☐ Benefits anxiety, insomnia.

* Inflammation is often associated with depression. (Maes 1997)

Treatment

Supplementation can be helpful, (Bryce-Smith 1984. Pfeiffer 1975) especially when depleted, (Narang 1991, Nowak 2003, Maes 1997) but also in some patients with normal labs. (Bryce-Smith 1984, Pfeiffer 1975) Zinc also may produce some adjunctive benefit. (Szewczyk 2002, Nowak 2003, Kroczka 2000, 01)

Very high levels, if not required, can be sedative, and can eventually foster depression in some. (Pfeiffer 1988, Braverman 1987)

Depression & zinc malabsorption

In acrodermatitis enteropathica, a rare genetic disease, zinc absorption is severely limited, causing a periodic disabling depression (the only presenting symptom in 50% of patients). (Edwards 1980, Pfeiffer)

Some studies

Little, 1989 — Eight of 21 depressed women and one of nine depressed men were zinc-deficient, including two of the three most severely depressed. Other studies confirm the tendency of depressed women particularly, to show low levels. (McLoughlin 1990, Nichols 1992)

Animal studies suggest antidepressant benefit. (Ossowska 2003, Szewczyk 2002, Nowak 2003, Kroczka 2001, 2000)

Further info

For effects on mania, and mood stabilization, and for considerations, see pages 29-31.

Potassium, sodium, & vanadium

(JOFFE 1992, TOLLEFSON 1986, BARTOSZEWICZ 1973, BAER 1970, WIDMER 1992, RYBAKOWSKI 2000, HIYAMA 2002, PFEIFFER 1975, 87, 88)

The sodium/potassium balance regulates cell permeability, i.e. controlling what goes into and out of the cell. This balance is often compromised in bipolars. In some, sodium — which should be mostly outside the cell — increases within the cell during mania, decreases some during depression. Others show high intracellular sodium with low potassium in depression, as well. (COX 1971, BAUMEL, WEBB 1981)

Low potassium depressives tend to improve on diets rich in fresh vegetables and their juices, salads, soups, and other major sources of potassium, while restricting soy and other vanadium sources (which inhibit sodium pumping). (HARLAND 1994, MURRAY 1995, NAYLOR 1981, 87, DICK 1981, 82, JANDHYALA 1983, NAYLOR 1981)

Mechanisms which may support mood

- □ Critical to the action potential which forwards messages down the neural axon.
- □ Helps regulate membrane permeability, receptor activity, cell access to nutrients, and waste elimination.
- □ Supports fluid balance.
- □ Releases minerals so ATP can create energy.
- □ Helps sustain alkalinity.
- □ Supports adrenal function, and glandular secretions.
- □ May help reduce blood sugar.
- □ May help protect against allergies.
- □ May reduce some lithium side effects (e.g., thirst, tremor. (BHASKARA 1990 CATER 1986)

Potassium (K)

"Potassium made my hypomania noticeably worse... my depressive state, noticeably better." — Allen Darman, 2002

"Lithium displaces sodium so you'd think potassium might benefit bipolar." — Tom Lane, 1997

Potassium can be antidepressant, especially if deficient. Low levels are frequently associated with depression, apathy and, in some cases, insomnia, apprehension, suicide attempts, or an organic brain syndrome. (WEBB 1981, BAUMEL 1995)

Caution: Supplements may upset the sodium/potassium balance, perhaps posing significant risk (see *Side effects*, below). Food sources are usually preferable (and bolster health) (e.g., fresh vegetables, dark leafy greens, potatoes, legumes, papaya, currants, avocado, squash, banana, seaweeds, citrus, sprouts, whole grains, sunflower and other seeds, nuts, fish, wheat germ, plums, tomatoes). (NUTRICIRCLES® 1996, LARSON 2001)

Considerations (LARSON 2001, PFEIFFER 1975, 88, MURRAY 1995, GARRISON 1985, BALCH 1990, PAGE 1992, QUILLIN 1987, LIEBERMAN, 1990)

Need may be suggested by (LARSON 2001, GOLD 1987)

Depression, apathy, apprehension, weakness, fatigue.

Allergies. Headache. Nausea, vomiting, constipation.

Edema, thirst. Acidity. Kidney or liver disease.

Adrenal dysfunction, diabetes.

Muscle cramps or spasms, Joint pain.

High blood pressure. Irregular or racing pulse, chest tightness, hyperventilation, heart disease. (LARSON 2001)

With severe deficiency, slows body activity, perhaps leading to irregular heartbeat, heart failure or paralysis. (GOLD 1987)

Populations

Malnutrition. Diets high in refined carbohydrates, salt,* denatured fats. Alcoholism, anorexia, other eating disorders. Prolonged vomiting or diarrhea. Overuse of diuretics,** CCBs, laxatives. Hypothalamus problems. Stress. Injury. Steroid use. High vanadium in bipolar depressives (altering sodium pump activity).

* High sodium causes potassium excretion, and can exhaust adrenals.

** Diuretics (e.g. used in hypertension) deplete both potassium and magnesium, promoting elevated lipids (Rayssiguier 1981), arteriosclerosis, and arrhythmias. If CCBs are then prescribed, magnesium is further depleted, reducing potassium uptake, perhaps increasing blood pressure still more, in a viscious cycle. (Ebel 1980, Pfeiffer 1975, 88)

Supportive nutrients

Magnesium is critical to uptake of potassium.

To support membranes and sodium/potassium pumps: EFAs, relevant phospholipids, avoid detrimental fats.

Useful diagnostic test

Plasma potassium. (JAFFE 1992)

Dosage

Potassium-rich foods are safer than supplements.

Effects of excess, contraindications

Apathy.

Increased vulnerability to infection.

Potassium tablets may cause stomach irritation and pain; enteric-coated tabs, small intestine ulcers. (LARSON 2001)

Severe excess can cause renal disturbances, adrenal insufficiency, irregular pulse, muscle and heart weakness, heart failure, death.*

* Kidney failure, dehydration, or cardiac arrest can cause toxic elevation. (Larson 2001)

Sodium (Na) issues

Sodium lowers magnesium, alters neurotransmitter levels, and increases neural excitability. Prounced excess (especially when potassium is low), besides destabilizing mood, can compromise physical health (see *Side effects*, below).

Mania

Sodium may be significantly higher than in depression, (Tandon 1988, Larson 1992) and accumulate within the nerve cell, with too much potassium without, stimulating mania. (Demers) With severe sodium/water imbalance, psychosis can occur.

Depression

Significant deficiency can lead to depression, (Rybakowski 2000, Gold 1987) especially when depleted gradually; rapid depletion is more likely to produce agitated delirium or psychosis. (Goggans 1980)

On the other hand, elevation also fosters depression, with potassium foods and sodium restriction improving mood. (Beard 1982 Baumel 1995, Lesser)

Sources (NutriCircles® 1996)

Salt,* seaweed, meats, fish, many cheeses, olives. Modest quantities in celery, Swiss chard, spinach.

* Celtic or sea salts are preferable, supplying various minerals, besides sodium.

Sodium/potassium pumps (NA+K+ATPase) (Reddy 1992, Thakar 1984, Rybakowski 2000, Hiyama 2002, Linnoila 1983, Naylor 1985, 87)

Sodium is normally concentrated outside the neuron; potassium, within. The transfer of neural messages depends on a consecutive exchange of sodium and potassium ions along the neural axon. This forwards a wave of electrical potential to the axon terminal, where neurotransmitter release occurs. Communication is most precise if, when the cell is at rest, potassium is primarily within; sodium, without.

Effects on mood

Sodium/potassium pumps remove sodium from the cell, moderating signalling, excitability and mood; (Xie 1998) and may also regulate calcium channels, influencing calcium signalling. (Birdsall 1998)

Bipolars may be less able to create new sodium pumps as needed,*(Naylor 1981, Thakar 1984, Reddy 1992) thereby allowing sodium and calicum to accumulate inside the neuron, heightening stimulation. In fact, lithium, (Naylor 1981) lamotrigine, (Gold 1987) carbamazepine, (Naylor 1985, 87) and taurine (Birdsall 1998) increase pump activity, which may be one means by which they stabilize mood.)

* Perhaps due to disturbed hypothalamic control of pump activity, (Rose 1986) or oversensitivity to vanadium. (Naylor 1987)

Considerations (Larson 2001, Garrison 1985, Balch 1990, Page 1992, Quillin 1987, Lieberman, Cox 1971, Eby 2001)

Excess sodium: Populations (Beard 1982, Baumel 1995)

Tension, stress, irritability, overstimulation, mania.
Bipolars with high vanadium.
PMS. Inflammation, muscle spasms. Hypertension.
Abnormal thirst, dehydration.

Effects of excess, contraindications

Overstimulation, mania, perhaps, depression.
Water retention and tissue swelling.
High blood pressure. Liver, kidney, or heart disorders.
Acidosis, dehydration, diarrhea, nausea, vomiting.
Frequent urination, muscle tremors, spasms.
If severe, tissue atrophy, convulsions. Can be fatal.

Need may be suggested by (Ohsawa 1992, Lieberman 1990)

Some depressions. Memory loss, poor concentration. Apathy, confusion, psychosis. Anorexia.
Weak, fatigued, heat-sensitive. Low blood pressure.
Edema. Extended vomiting, diarrhea. Excess diuretics.
Too much water. Possibly with low salt, high potassium.
Porphyria. Certain kidney, adrenal, pituitary, thyroid, brain, heart, lung or liver disorders.

Hyponatremia: too little sodium relative to water (Pfeiffer 1988, Gold 1987, Webb 1981, Oshawa 1992, Jose 1979, Blum 1984ab)

Hyponatremia (like its opposite, dehydration) alters mental state and can be life-threatening. Mental/neurological symptoms can include depression, irritability, restlessness, confusion, impaired concentration, disorientation, lethargy, loose associations, paranoia, auditory hallucinations, psychosis, tremors, twitching, convulsions, major motor seizures, stupor, coma, brain damage. (Physical symptoms include frequent and profuse urination, diarrhea, increased salivation, frothing, nausea, vomiting, cerebral and body edema.)

Iatrogenic causes — Water retention may occur after ECT. Phenothiazines (antipsychotics), and other medications can make the mouth dry, or otherwise promote thirst. Post-operative fluid retention (more common in women) can cause life-threatening hyponatremia. Antidiuretics can cause water retention, while diuretics decrease sodium.

Other causes — Caffeine depletes electrolytes. Smoking promotes water retention. Hypothyroidism, Addison's disease, acute intermittent porphyria, and certain neurological disorders may increase pituitary ADH release, causing water to be retained. Pain, endurance exercise, sudden high-dose niacin (which can promote water retention), postpartum shock, tumors, infections, fungal infestations, and aneurisms can also reduce the sodium/water ratio.

SIWIS (Self-Induced Water Intoxication & Schizophrenic Disorders) — insistent intake of potentially toxic quantities of water, from any source. Note: About 25% of sufferers have psychiatric diagnoses other than schizophrenia.

Treatment — Non-acute treatment usually involves fluid restriction, balancing electrolytes, and gradually increasing serum sodium. Acute water toxicity requires emergency medical treatment. Delay can cause irreversible brain damage or death. (Pfeiffer 1988, Gold 1987)

"Vanadium toxicity is known to produce depression and melancholia."
D Witkowska 1979

Restrict vanadium (Va)

Although required for sugar metabolism, and other functions, (MURRAY 1995, PFEIFFER 1987, 88) too much vanadium can aggravate bipolar disorder, particularly bipolar depression. (YUNG 1984)

Levels

Vanadium tends to be elevated in both depression and mania. Mood symptoms, especially depression, (KAY 1984) have been associated with elevated plasma, serum and whole blood vanadium, (NAYLOR 1984AB, 1987, DICK 1981, 83) generally normalizing with recovery.

Treatment

Many (perhaps most) bipolar depressives show particular sensitivity to vanadium, and should probably minimize intake. (KAY 1984) They do well with substances which reduce its toxicity. The effectiveness of high dose vitamin C in bipolar depression may, in part, be due to its moderation of vanadium toxicity.*(LARSON 2001) Similarly, EDTA, methylene blue, exercise, and other therapies which decrease vanadate, have elevated mood.** (NAYLOR 1981-83, 1984AB)

Vanadium may be somewhat less of a problem in mania. In one study, bipolar depressives responded more to substances which neutralize vanadium than to lithium; manics responded more to lithium. (KAY 1984)

See *Sodium/Potassium*, pp. 132-33; *Inositol*, pp. 95-97; *Vitamin C*, pp. 74-75.

*It reduces the more toxic vanadate (+5) ion to vanadyl (+4), a less potent sodium pump (NA+K+ATPase) inhibitor.

** Smoking also decreases vanadium (perhaps partly accounting for its popularity), but the detrimental health effects, and nutrient depletion, make it a poor choice.

Possible mechanisms for influence on depression

"Vanadium may help characterize intracellular signalling and inositol phosphate metabolism."
— M Bencherif 1992

□ Vanadium strongly inhibits sodium pump activity and recovery, (HARLAND 1994, MURRAY 1995, 98, NAYLOR 1981, DICK 1981, 82, JANDHYALA 1983) and may contribute to sodium transport changes in bipolars. (NAYLOR 1987) The suppressed pump allows too much sodium to accumulate within the neuron, and too little potassium to enter. This compromises the ability to create an electrical potential upon transmitter stimulation, and so decreases neural responsiveness.

□ Vanadium increases inositol triphosphate (IP3) accumulation, perhaps by restricting metabolism to inositol, thus interfering with the signalling cycle. (BENCHERIF 1992)

□ Elevated vanadium may promote irregular cortical activity. (HARVEY 1992)

□ Vanadium may alter brain serotonin, norepinephrine, and dopamine. (WITKOWSKA 1979)

Pharmaceuticals which support sodium pump activity

Countering vanadate's suppression of the sodium pump may be part of the means by which certain meds alter mood. (NAYLOR 1981, 82, 85, HARLAND 1994) *Consider that:*

Lithium response coincides with increased pump activity. (NAYLOR 1981, HARLAND 1994, MURRAY 1998)

MAOIs and phenothiazines catalyze vanadate reduction by NADH to vanadyl, which is less able to inhibit pump activity. (NAYLOR 1982, 1983, LARSON 2001)

Considerations

Need may be suggested by

Glucose intolerance, insulin sensitivity.*

Demineralized bones, poor development. (HARLAND 1994)

High cholesterol. (HARLAND 1994, MURRAY 1995)

Suppressed lactation, infant mortality

Compromised endocrine, cardiovascular, reproductive and kidney function. (MURRAY 1995)

* Improves or mimics insulin activity (Murray 1995, 98, Harland 1994, Cohen 1995, Brichard 1995.

Sources (MURRAY 1995)

Fats. Soy (tofu, etc.), fish, shellfish, dill, olives, meat, radish, snap peas, buckwheat, other whole grains, black pepper, parsley, mushrooms. Smaller amounts in safflower and sunflower oil, oats, olive oil, sunflower seeds, corn, green beans, peanut oil, carrot, cabbage, garlic.

Effects of excess

Mood symptoms, especially depression. (WITKOWSKA 1979, YUNG 1984)

Decreased CoA and CoQ10.

Compromised cell energy production.

At higher doses, cramps, diarrhea, increased blood pressure.*

* Toxic exposure is uncommon, but occurs in some workers in steel, oil, and other heavy industries. (Jandhyala 1983)

Lab

Serum and whole blood (but not hair) vanadium strongly correlate with each other. (NAYLOR 1984AB)

Iron & copper – only if needed

Iron and copper are essential to mood and health, however, if chronically oversupplied, can contribute significantly to brain hyperstimulation and oxidative stress, so Pfeiffer (1987, 88) suggests that, in most cases, they be given only when clearly needed.

Iron (Fe)

Depression with deficiency

Low iron can produce depression,*(MAES) and such related symptoms as fatigue, listlessness, (GOLD 1987) irritability, malaise, odd behavior, anxiety, (BEARD 2002, ESEH 2005) hyperactivity, reduced attention span, memory difficulties, and learning disorders. (KONOFAL 2004, YOUDIM 1982, 1984, 2000, COUSENS 2000, TUCKER 1984)

If depleted, supplementation may be antidepressant, (HEATH 1999, 2001, 2003) though not necessarily, even in low-iron (but nonanemic) women. (SWAIN 2006) *Take with antioxidants.*

* E.g., in iron-deficient anemia.

Depression or mania with excess (HEATH 2003, RICHARDSON 1992, CUTLER)

Overload fosters free radical proliferation, which can compromise neurological function. With prolonged excess, a scurvy can occur, causing depression or, possibly, mania or psychosis. The dose must then be reduced or stopped to facilitate response to vitamin C.

See *Vitamin C*, pp. 74-75.

Biotype indications (PFEIFFER 1987, 88)

If low, iron is sometimes helpful in treating histapenia.

Functions influencing mood (TUCKER 1984, COUSENS 2000, SLAGLE 1992)

□ Important to activity of key mood-modulating neurotransmitters. (SLAGLE 1992)

□ Supports (with NADH) metabolism of tyrosine to L-dopa and dopamine. (COUSENS 2000)

□ Concentrated in dopamine structures. Deficiency reduces dopamine receptor binding sites, downregulating dopamine activity (thereby, compromising attention and learning ability,* and fostering hyperactivity in children). (YOUDIM 1982, 84, 2000, BEARD 2002)

□ Supports acetylcholine transmission and synthesis, and GABA and serotonin function. (COUSENS 2000)

□ Important in metabolism of B vitamins, which are critical to neural function.

□ Required in brain oxygenation (and the ability of hemoglobin to carry oxygen). (SLAGLE 1992)

□ Helps produce mitochondrial energy.

□ Supports immunity. (MAES 1996)

* Perhaps, reversible with nutritional support. (Politt 1993, 00)

Iron-deficient anemia (PFEIFFER 1975, 88, BRAVERMAN 1987)

Iron is critical to the ability of blood to carry oxygen.*

Heterozygous beta-thalasemia, a microcytic anemia, commonly due to iron deficiency, occurs in an inordinate number of bipolars; (BOCCHETTA 1990, 1993) 16%, in a study by Brodie (2005).

Microcytic anemia typically causes depressive symptoms, pallor, fatigue, loss of sex drive, appetite loss, constipation and, eventually, difficulty swallowing or breathing, and heart palpitations with activity. If untreated, the patient may go into shock, or succumb to congestive heart failure. (PFEIFFER GOLD 1987. COUSENS 2000, TUCKER 1984, YOUDIN 1989)

* Plasma iron, with copper as a catalyst, is combined with protein, in the bone marrow, to form hemoglobin, the oxygen-carrying component in red blood cells. (Braverman 1987)

NOTE: Other nutrient-deficient anemias can appear similar, but require different nutrients: (PFEIFFER, ROGERS 1997, BRAVERMAN 1987)

COPPER-DEFICIENT ANEMIA — iron, instead of copper, may worsen the illness or create iron toxicity.

B6-DEFICIENT ANEMIA — iron is sometimes already too high (and bone marrow hemosiderin, increased).

B12-DEFICIENT PERNICIOUS ANEMIA — iron, instead of B12, can allow irreversible neurological damage to develop.

Hemosiderosis (PFEIFFER 1975, 88)

Hemosiderosis, most common in males over 40, primarily involves accumulating deposits of iron oxide, due to chronic overload (e.g., with iron injections, excessive content in certain supplements or tonics, food or alcohol stored in iron containers,* iron-rich red wine, repeated blood transfusions, hemolytic or aplastic anemia, or acute hepatitis). Oversaturated transferrin then becomes unable to bind all absorbed iron.

Early symptoms include headache, shortness of breath, fatigue, dizziness, weight loss, greyish skin (due to deposits). Elevated tissue iron oxidizes vitamin C, promoting a scurvy (typically producing depression and other mood changes), which vitamin C can't reverse until iron is decreased. With enough iron in liver, lungs heart, pancreas, etc., deterioration occurs. (PFEIFFER)

* In northern South Africa, Bantus use storage containers made of iron, which eventually leaches into their contents of beer or sour porridge.

Hemochromatosis (PFEIFFER 1975, 88)

Hemochromatosis is a genetic disorder which promotes accumulation of iron, creating a characteristic bronze cast to the skin, and eventually compromising the liver, bone marrow, pancreas (causing diabetes), or other organs.

Considerations: Iron

Need may be suggested by (SLAGLE 1992, GARRISON 1985, BALCH 1990, PAGE 1992, QUILLIN 1987, HOFFER 1983, LIEBERMAN 1990, PFEIFFER 1975, JAFFE 1992, CASDORPH 1995, PARKER 1984)

Depression, learning and attention difficulties, irritability, odd behavior, poor memory.

Weakness, fatigue, lethargy, dizziness, headaches, general malaise.

Numbness, tingling.

Sore or burning tongue. Ringing in the ears.

Craving for salt, dirt, paint or ice.

Pallor, cold hands and feet, low energy, anemia.

Increased suceptibility to infection, allergies.

Appetite loss, constipation.

Shortness of breath, difficulty swallowing. Heart palpitations. Elevated blood and liver lipids.

Growth suppression.

Brittle or sparse hair. Spoon-shaped, brittle, flat, or vertically-ridged nails.

Conditions which promote deficiency (COUSENS 2000, SLAGLE 1992, GOLD 1987, PFEIFFER 1975, 88)

Increased blood volume, e.g., during rapid growth in children, teens, pregnant women. (PFEIFFER)

Protein deficiency, vegetarianism,* junk food diet, illness, aging, athletic overtraining. Poor digestion, Candida, low stomach acid, stomach surgery.

Iron-free vitamins, especially with iron-poor diet or if prone to depletion.

Menstruation, pregnancy, nursing. (Thus, deficiency is more likely in females.)

Excessive bleeding.

Low thyroid. (LEEDMAN 1996, BEARD 1989, 90, 97, ARTHUR 1999)

Kidney or liver failure, infections, herpes, rheumatoid arthritis, cancer, other chronic illness. (PFEIFFER)

Phytates (in grains), tannic acid (in black tea), caffeine, antacids, or tetracycline. (Due to interference with absorption.) (COUSENS 2000)

Pronounced excess of calcium, phosphorus, zinc, E, B. Depleted copper or C.

* Cousens, however, points out that though iron from animal sources is presumably better absorbed, anemia is more common in meat eaters.

Useful diagnostic test (Fe) (WERBACH 1991, JAFFE 1992, PFEIFFER)

History.

TIBC/% saturation — total iron storage (ferritin)/iron binding capacity of transferrin.

Serum iron.

Sources (PFEIFFER 1975, COUSENS 2000, SLAGLE 1992, NUTRICIRCLES 1996)

Liver, lean and organ meats, beef, clams and other shellfish, salmon, turkey, egg yolks. Dulse, kelp, dark green leafy vegetables, deeply colored fruits, legumes, dried fruit, blackstrap molasses, pumpkin and sesame seeds, walnuts, almonds, sunflower seeds, whole grains.

Iron in foods cooked or stored in cast iron is not readily absorbed, and may deposit.

Supportive nutrients (COUSENS 2000, SLAGLE 1992)

C, copper, B12, folic acid, amino acids. Vitamin C aids absorption. Antioxidants reduce free radical formation, *however, too much E or zinc may interfere with absorption.*

Supplementation (WERBACH 1991, PFEIFFER 1975, 88)

Use amino acid-chelated iron.

Iron should not be taken at the same time of day as nutrients increasing cellular oxygenation (e.g., germanium, ginkgo) or hydrogen peroxide formulas (sometimes used in treating Candida).

Avoid ferrous sulfate, which is less tolerable to the digestive system and more likely to deposit.

Though iron is essential to mental and physical functioning (e.g. immunity, oxygenation), too much can be damaging. Supplements are best given only when, and to the extent that, iron is actually deficient.

Conditions promoting elevation (PFEIFFER 1975, 88)

Extensive blood transfusions. Acute hepatitis.

Excess iron-rich red wine, tonics. Iron storage containers. Over-supplementation (oral or injections).

Elevation is more likely in males.

Effects of excess, contraindications (COUSENS 2000, ROGERS 1997, PFEIFFER 1975, 88, CASDORPH 1995)

Depression or mania.

Free radical damage. Brain lipid peroxidation.

Fatigue.

Grey or bronze discoloration of skin.

Gastrointestinal effects (common).

Depletion of zinc, manganese. (NUTR 1993)

Can eventually create liver cirrhosis or toxicity.

May promote bacterial growth during infection.

May promote cardiovascular disease, rheumatoid arthritis, dementia.

Prolonged elevation can cause hemosiderosis and can be fatal in hemochromatosis, thalassemia, or sickle cell anemia.

Copper (Cu)

(HOFFER 1983, PFEIFFER 1972, 75, *BR MED J* 1984, JAFFE 1992, SOHLER 1987, CASDORPH 1995, WALSH 2000, 02, 04AB, 06)

Copper increases catecholamines, and brain oxygenation and energy production, and so can be antidepressant. It is known to benefit some depressives, e.g., copper-deficient anemics, some histadelics, some hypothyroid depressives, etc.

On the other hand, chronic excess generally overstimulates, and can create considerable oxidative damage in the brain, both of which can distort cognition and affect. Copper can thus be harmful (and is often already excessive) in many manias, female hormonal depressions, learning and behavior disorders, schizophrenias, cases of anxiety, etc. (PFEIFFER 1975, 87, 88)

See, pp. 171-73.

Biotype indications (PFEIFFER 1972, 75, 87, 88, JAFFE 1992, HOFFER 1983, WALSH 2000, 2002)

Histapenia — copper is typically elevated, especially if metal metabolism is also disordered. *Further intake (even the 2 mg in most multivitamins) can be detrimental to devastating.*

Pyroluria — symptoms usually worsen with copper (though after lengthy treatment with high-dose zinc, Pfeiffer found *small* doses of copper sometimes helpful to encourage more efficient use of the zinc).

Histadelia — copper can be low. Small doses are occasionally helpful, *but usually not with appreciable oxidative stress* (prevalent in histadelics).

Other indications

Consider copper status, balance with magnesium (ZIEBA 2000, SIWEK 2005) and zinc, (PFEIFFER 1975, 87, 88) and metallothionein function. (WALSH 2004, 06)

Potential antidepressant mechanisms (PFEIFFER 1975, 87, 88, BALCH 1990, HOFFER 1983)

Increases CNS stimulation:

□ Supports conversion of tyrosine to dopamine to norepinephrine.

□ Increases electrical potential of the neuron (perhaps by enhancing movement of sodium).

□ Supports cellular energy production (electron transport).

□ Supports brain oxygenation (e.g., iron absortion and use to form hemoglobin).

□ Helps maintain the myelin sheath which increases the speed of transmission in certain neurons.

□ Like iron, supports thyroid activity, *though too much copper is counterproductive.* (ARTHUR 1999)

□ Regulates and degrades histamine, sometimes benefitting histadelic depression.

Role in the hippocampus

□ With zinc, its concentrated in the hippocampus, a brain region critical to mood (and short-term memory and behavior). (WALSH 2004)

Supports brain viability:

□ Supports vitamin C metabolism.

□ Detoxifies the superoxide radical.

Considerations (GARRISON 1985, BALCH 1990, PAGE, 1992, QUILLIN 1987, PFEIFFER 1972, 75, 87, 88, LIEBERMAN 1990, HOFFER 1983B, JAFFE 1992, CASDORPH 1995)

Populations

Celiac/sprue, long-term antacids, serious malnutrition (as in anorexia or other eating disorders), long-term parenteral nutrition, exclusive cow's milk diet in infants.*

* Note: Pfeiffer found deficiency rare in psychiatric (mainly schizophrenic) patients, and then, the result of very high doses of zinc.

Need may be suggested by

Apathy, depression.

Fatigue,* weakness. Chronic fatigue.

Neurological symptoms. (STRAUSAK 2001) Myelin disorders.

Frequent infections, breathing difficulty, allergies.

Increased tendency to chemical toxicity, and oxidative stress from superoxide radicals.**

Dulled taste sensitivity.

Steely, faded or greying hair. Hair loss. Pallor.***

Nausea, vomiting, diarrhea, stomach pain.

Skin sores, gum disease, stomach ulcers, blood vessel fragility. Osteoporosis, other bone and joint problems.****

Low thyroid or other dysfunction. Premature aging.

Iron-deficiency anemia,***** low white blood cells, high cholesterol, low LDL, arteriosclerosis, irregular heart beat, cardiovascular disorders.

* Copper supports respiration and energy production.
** Key component of superoxide dismutase.
*** Copper is needed in forming melanin.
**** Critical to formation and integrity of collagen and elastin, cartilege and bone development, maintenance, and repair.
***** Supports iron absorption and use, helps regulate and form hemoglobin

Nutrient interactions

Copper supports C and fatty acid metabolism, and absorption and use of iron. Lipoic acid mildly increases copper.

Food sources of copper (NUTRICIRCLES)

Organ meats, shellfish, other seafood, liver. Dark leafy greens, carob, squash, oranges, eggplant, tomatoes, beets, red pepper, avocado, seeds and nuts, legumes, mushrooms, potatoes, ginger, radish, garlic, turkey. Wheat germ, bran, yeast, oats, barley, other whole grains.

For reactions and populations associated with excess copper, counterbalancing nutrients, nonfood sources, lab, and side effects, see pp. 171-73.

Trace minerals

The following minerals are less well known but, in some cases, may provide that critical component that reverses a depression.

Boron

May provide some antidepressant support, due to benefits to pyroluria. (McGinnis 2004) Can increase mental alertness. (Slagle 2000) Helps maintain magnesium and calcium levels. In low-magnesium, post-menopausal women, improves estradiol and testosterone levels. (Nielsen 1987) Further research is indicated.

Sources

Found in fresh fruits and vegetables.

Cesium

Cesium, a mineral related to lithium, alkalinizes body tissue, increasing access to oxygen. It is reported to be antidepressant for some, even when everything else has failed. (Missiha 1973, 75, 77) It may also speed recovery from alcohol and pharmaceuticals with depressive side effects. (Missiha 1975, 77, 84) Unfortunately, it can be expensive and difficult to obtain, and requirements can be difficult to assess. Thus caution is advised, e.g., start at the lowest dose, keep dosage modest, etc. (Ali 1985, Rogers 1997)

Rubidium

Various studies have noted rubidium's stimulating and antidepressant activity. (Brundusino 1996, Torta 1993, Placidi 1988, Williams 1987, Malek-Ahmadi 1984, Paschalis 1978, Carolei 1975) Fieve (1989) suggests it may be most helpful in slowed, apathetic depressions.

Warning

Rubidium can trigger mania and increase the length of manic cycles. These effects can be long-lasting as rubidium has a long biological half-life. *It may be contraindicated for most, if not all, bipolars.* (Paschalis 1978, Fieve 1989)

Lithium (Missiha 1984)

Nutritional lithium may provide some antidepressant benefit, perhaps largely due to its ability to reduce cycling.

Germanium (Asai 1977, Tanaka 1980, Levine 1986ab, Balch 1990, Lieberman 1990, *J Pharmacobio-Dynamics* 1983, *Microbiol Immun* 1985)

Organic germanium sesquioxide increases cellular oxygenation, which may make it useful in some bipolar depressions, especially if accompanied by low oxygen availability, anxiety due to lactic acid buildup, Candida (which is prevalent), or general acidity. Dr. Asai, who pioneered dietary use of germanium, claims it can successfully alleviate psychotic depression.*(Asai 1977, 80, 84) Similarly, Dr. Tanaka, head physician at Chofu Hospital in Japan, finds it can improve depression and insomnia. (Tanaka 1980)

* He also notes the following reactions: general cheerfulness, increased mental acuity, and improved sleep.

Populations (Asai 1977, Tanaka 1980, Levine 1986ab, Balch 1990, Lieberman 1990, *J Pharmacobio-Dynamics* 1983, *Microbiol Immun* 1985)

Anxiety. Muscle fatigue. Anemia. Low oxygenation. Candida. High blood pressure. Pain. Liver dysfunction. Low interferon.

Supportive mechanisms (Asai 1977, Tanaka 1980, Levine 1986ab, Balch 1990, Lieberman 1990, *J Pharmacobio-Dynamics* 1983, *Microbiol Immun* 1985)

Benefits Candida.

Antioxidant. Increases glutathione formation. Helps remove heavy metals.

Increases oxygen uptake (and readily reacts with hydrogen and free radicals, sparing oxygen).

Prevents lactic acid buildup, benefitting some cases of anxiety and panic attacks.

Supports glandular function.

Helps counter mercury poisoning.

Sources

Germanium is found in a number of herbs and foods reputed to promote longevity, e.g., ginseng, garlic, suma, angelica, tea leaves, bamboo, chlorella, reishi and shiitake mushrooms, onions, aloe, and certain health-promoting mineral waters.

Side effects, toxicity

May cause a skin rash (or just an initial feeling of warmth and a healthy glow to the skin).

May soften the stool.

CAUTION: Use only **organic germanium sesquioxide**. Germanium *dioxide* can cause kidney failure and should be avoided.

7: Antidepressant herbs

If an antidepressant herb is considered in the treatment of bipolar disorder, take into account:

□ The degree the herb might be contraindicated due to biotype or general biochemistry.
□ Whether the herb may trigger to contribute to mania.
□ The effect on neurotransmitters, second messengers, and regulatory enzymes involved in symptoms.
□ Interactions with medication.
□ The extent to which the herb is addressing contributory factors, or temporarily suppressing symptoms.

More cautions

□ Tailor formulas to individual needs. Supply relevant stabilizing nutrients. Monitor for any hints of mania.
□ Consider dose schedule. (E.g.: (1) some herbs may need to be taken more than once daily, to avoid letdown; (2) stimulating herbs, taken later in the day, may inhibit sleep.)
□ When the depression ends, most antidepressant herbs should be gradually discontinued. Exact timing varies per individual. Suddenly stopping may reinvoke depression, increase cycling, or trigger mania (usually less so than meds).
□ Many herbs are contraindicated for children, the elderly, persons with fragile medical conditions, and during pregnancy or lactation.

Reminder: Not all contraindications are known or listed. Study the literature to get a more complete idea of the effects of these herbs. This information is presented for educational purposes only. If you wish to receive herbal treatment, or need help for a medical disorder, please consult a knowledgeable physician.

St John's wort (MOWREY 1986, MURRAY 1995, 98, SOMNER 1992, COTT 1998, 2001, MULDNER 1984)

St John's wort (i.e., *hypericum*, not the ornamental plant) has been used for certain types of anxiety and sleep disorders, hysteria, nerve pain, headaches (especially with excitability).

Use for mild and moderate depression is supported by multiple studies including a number of randomized controlled double blinds. Results find it equal to or better than SSRIs, tricyclics, and other antidepressants. (LINDE 1996, 2002, KIM 1999, HARRER 1999, BRENNER 2000, STOLL 2001) Several studies find it more effective than fluoxetine in mild to moderate depression; (SCHRADER 2000, FAVA 2005) and at least one shows improvement in severe depression. (SZEGEDI 2005)

St John's wort increases levels of antidepressant transmitters, especially serotonin, but also dopamine, norepinephrine and GABA. (SUZUKI 1984, BLUMENTHAL 1998, ERNST 1999, KLEPSE 1999)

Mania has been reported. (NIERENBERG 1999) Uneven intake may destabilize mood. Some bipolars, probably, especially, histapenic, do not do well with serotonin support. Do not use with antidepressants unless so directed by a knowledgeable physician.

Some of the studies

Linde, 1996 — Review of 23 randomized trials, over 1757 patients. The herb was as effective as antidepressants, and significantly more so than placebo. Side effects occured in 20% versus 52% in those on meds. Dropouts due to side effects were 0.8% on the herb, 3% on meds.

Fava, 2005 — Randomized double blind after 1-wk washout. The herb was significantly more effective than fluoxetine, and appeared safe and well-tolerated.

Szegedi, 2005 — Randomized double blind. 251 moderate-to-severe depressives from 21 practices, were given 900 mg (divided over the day) or 20 mg paroxetine. If response was not forthcoming, doses were doubled. The herb was at least as effective as the drug, and better tolerated.

Considerations (MOWREY 1986, MURRAY 1991, 95, SOMNER 1992, COTT 1998, 2001, MULDNER 1984, SUZUKI 1984)

Need may be suggested by

Depression. Irritability. Certain types of anxiety. Hysteria. Sleep disorders. Headaches with excitability. Nerve pain. Jaundice, gall bladder issues, irregular menses, urinary suppression.

Dose (STOLL 2001)

Stoll typically uses 300 mg (.3% hypericin), 2x/day, increased after 3-4 days to 3x/day; with no response by 3 wks, perhaps, 600 mg 2x/day.* If it's going to work, some response should occur by 2-6 weeks.

Contraindications, side effects

Overstimulation, agitation, insomnia, occasionally mania (in bipolars), (NIERENBERG 1999) or psychosis.

Mild stomach upset, nausea. Photosensitivity. Skin rash, sunburn. May interact with tyramines.

Rarely, serotonin syndrome (especially if taken with SSRIs), (ERNST 1999) usually mild. (GORDON 1998, LANTZ 2000, MILLER 2000)

Interactions with pharmaceuticals

Many researchers recommend at least a two-week buffer around antidepressant use, (GORDON 1998, BLUMENTHAL 1998, CUPP 1999, KERB 1996) though Dr Hyla Cass (2007) and others use the herb cautiously to ease antidepressant withdrawal symptoms.

May interact with some drugs used for depression, psychosis, cardiovacular disorders, asthma, HIV, blood thinning and chemotherapy. Avoid with amphetamines, stimulants. Caution in administering with L-dopa. (CESARIN 1999) As a potent inducer of P450 enzymes, it may decrease effectiveness/availability of anticonvulsants, oral contraceptives, anti- organ-transplant-rejection meds, etc. (RUSCHITZKA 2000; FETROW 1999, ROBY 1999, BON 1999 IN FUGH-BERMAN, 2000)

Gotu kola (Chen 2003, 05, Balch 1990, Murray 1995, Kloss 1973, Mowrey 1986, Crayhon 1998)

Gotu kola (*Centella asiatica*) is a central nervous system stimulant, believed to be a nerve and glandular tonic. Animal studies, (Chen 2003, 05) historical use, and anecdotal reports suggest some antidepressant effectiveness. It stimulates acetylcholine release, which may account for its reported ability to decrease fatigue and depression and help manage stress.

It is held to benefit insomnia, anxiety, and senility and to increase mental activity and alertness. Mowrey (1986) states it slowly builds mental stamina and neurological health, and is an excellent treatment for nervous breakdowns. It is used traditionally in India to support memory and longevity.

Considerations (Chen 2003, 05, Balch 1990, Murray 1995, Kloss 1973, Mowrey 1986)

Need may be suggested by

Insomnia, anxiety.

Depression, slowed cognition. Memory issues.

High body temperature. Fluid retention.

High blood pressure. Blood acidity.

Some adrenal, liver, heart, and immune disorders.

Contraindications, side effects

Large doses may induce mania.

May be contraindicated with blood pressure medication, or significantly low blood pressure; or with diuretics, or with excessive urination.

Rarely, some are allergic to gotu kola.

Interactions with psychiatric medications are not well explored.

Ginkgo biloba (Murray 1991, 95, Mowrey 1990, Werbach 1994)

Possible antidepressant mechanisms

Increases blood flow, and so, the oxygen and glucose available to the brain. (Peter 1968, Etiene 1982, Auget 1982, 86)

Fosters dopamine and norepinephrine synthesis, stimulates epinephrine and norepinephrine release. (Racagni 1986, Murray 1995, 98, Mowrey 1990)

Increases cholinergic receptors,* and inhibits histamine.** (Racagni 1986, Murray 1995, 98, Mowrey 1990)

Protects serotonin (1A) receptors (Bolanos, Jimenez 1995).

Neuroprotective. (Kniegistein 1995) Antioxidant.

* Not necessarily antidepressant, especially not for bipolars.

** Making it antidepressant in high histamine individuals, but inadvisable for histapenics.

Depression

Several studies confirm ginkgo's effectiveness for depression. It may prove especially beneficial for poor-circulation, and dopamine-depleted depression, depressions in the elderly, (Schubert 1993) and depressions accompanied by dementia or cerebral dysfunction. (Gaby 1996)

Memory

Ginkgo especially benefits memory (and often, memory for numbers), (Schubert 1993, Peltov 1993) and cognitive function. (Gebner 1985) One double-blind reports ginkgo decreases the brain's theta rhythms (associated with a diffuse, unfocused mental state) and increases alpha (alertness). Researchers are investigating use for dementia. (Kanowski 1996, Kleijnen 1992, Hofferberth 1989) Itil (1995) finds benefits comparable to many cognitive activator and antidementia drugs.

Ginkgo, lactic acid and anxiety (Mowrey 1990)

Ginkgo is known to be sedative for some individuals. Its ability to increase oxygen availability may make it particularly useful in treating certain cases of lactic acid-sensitive anxiety.

Considerations (Murray 1991, 95, Mowrey 1990, Werbach 1994)

Need may be suggested by

Depression, memory problems. Anxiety.

Poor cerebral circulation, dementia.

Fatigue, toxicity, immune weakness, inflammation.

High blood pressure. Excessive blood clotting. (Braquet 1991, Kleijnen 1992)

Sexual dysfunction (e.g., from SSRIs). (Cohen 1996, 97, 98)

Possibly, asthma, cyclic edema. (Gaby 1996)

Vascular tinnitus. Acute cochlear deafness. Vertigo. Macular degeneration. (Gaby 1996)

Contraindications, side effects (riverhouse.com...)

May trigger mania. Monitor.

Can worsen dizziness and low blood pressure.

May increase symptoms brought on by caffeinism,* or elevated catecholamines or choline.

Avoid if prone to bleeding disorders or stroke.

* With caffeine it may cause subdural hematoma. (Rowin, Lewis 1996)

Drug interactions

Augments action of, and usually should not be taken with, blood thinners, aspirin, antihypertensives, and certain psych meds.

Ginseng (Karman 1988, Vogler 1999)

Ginseng is a direct central nervous system stimulant. (Pefkov 1961) It increases brain monoamines (dopamine, norepinephrine), (Farnsworth 1985) and enhances brain circulation. (Kehara) It has been used for depression, insomnia, and various neuroses.

Siberian and American ginsengs are reported to strengthen the nervous system. They nourish the adrenals and pituitary, thereby increasing resistance to stress. (Hal 1979, Fulder 1981) Korean (Panax) ginseng is more stimulating, and definitely contraindicated in mania, mixed states and rapid cycling, and with symptoms of anxiety or agitation, and may be contraindicated entirely for some bipolars.

Considerations (Karman 1988, Volger 1999, Farnsworth 1985)

Need may be suggested by

Depression, fatigue, suppressed cognition, susceptibility to stress. Poor endurance.

Weak cardiovascular and immune function (Siberian and American ginseng). Aging.

Adrenals and pituitary hypofunction. (Hal 1979)

Poor health. Sexual dysfunction (Panax). (Lee 1987)

Contraindications, side effects

WARNING: Panax (Korean ginseng), particularly, can increase overstimulation, exacerbating or triggering mania or psychosis, particularly if catecholamines are already elevated (as in histapenia, especially if acute), or if used as an adjunct to antidepressant treatment. (Gonzalez-Seiji 1995, cited in Ayd 2000) High doses (less so, with other ginsengs), may induce insomnia, irritability, anxiety, or melancholy. Individuals with rheumatic heart disease might experience headaches, increased blood pressure, or pericardial pain.

Drug interactions

Can potentiate caffeine (Klepser 1999) and stimulants. (Blumental 1998, Fetrow 1999, Inst Ntnl Prod Res 1999) May potentiate MAOIs. (Shader 1988, Stockley 1994 cited in Wong 1998) With Nardil may produce headache, tremor, mania, insomnia, irritability, visual hallucinations. (Shader 1988) May potentiate haldol catalepsy. (Klepser 1999, Mitra 1996 cited in Wong 1998) May interact with barbiturates. (Farnsworth 1985, Medon 1984, Getrow 1999, Wong 1998)

Noni la'au

Noni (*Morinda citrafolia,* also called, Indian mulberry) is an evergreen plant found in India, Southeast Asia, Malaysia, and Hawaii. Components include zeronine and prozeronine, which seem to work together to stimulate cell function and initiate cell repair (Heinicke 1985 2001). It also contains caprillic acid (which counters Candida), and various antioxidants (selenium, tepenes, anthraquinones).

Noni is traditionally given for central nervous system disorders, and to support immunity. (Atkinson 1956, Busnell 1950, Leach 1988, Rai 1975, Hirazumi 1994, 96ab, Solomon 1998, 99) It also helps activate thyroid, encourages thymus growth, and has been used for allergies, (Abbot 1985) and pain. (Solomon 1999, 2001)

Noni is reputed to benefit depression, (Elkins 1997, Solomon 1998, Langford 2002, Henicke 1985ab) perhaps due to its effects on neurohormones and transmitters. (Harrison) but also, perhaps, to improvement in Candida, allergies, thyroid activity, immunity, fatigue, digestion, oxidative stress, and general health.

Noni & bipolar II

"I have suffered with Bipolar II illness for more than 20 years... I loaded with Noni juice... Within 6 weeks [4 oz per day, eventually 3 oz] I began to become a totally new person... after about a year...[I] was able to cut my antidepressant medication in half and still feel wonderful."

Judith Dawn Whyte

"People are crazy about this plant."

Dr Isabella Alona Abbot, Professor of Botany, U Hawaii.

Considerations

Need may be suggested by (Abbot 1985, Heinicke.1985ab, Solomon 1998, 99, 2000, 2001, Wang 2002, Elkins 1997)

Depression, agitation, anxiety, memory issues, dementia. Addictions.

Allergies. (Abbot 1985) Candida, other digestive issues.

Slow-healing injury. Ulcers. Immune dysfunction. (Atkinson 1956, Busnell 1950, Leach 1988, Rai 1975, Hirazumi 1994, 96ab, Solomon 1998, 99)

Asthma and other respiratory conditions. (*Am Chem Soc* 2000)

Possibly, diabetes, arthritis, menstrual cramps, chronic fatigue, pain, (Solomon 2001) cancer (Issel, Hiazumi 94, 96ab) hypertension, vascular problems, aging. (Abbot 1985, Heinicke 1985a)

Contraindications, side effects (Mueller 2000, Saxema 2003)

High potassium content makes noni diuretic, and mandates caution with dosage, particularly for persons prone to hyperkalemia.

"Goji makes it impossible to stop smiling."

Gojibook, 2008

Note

Antidepressant effects of goji and noni can be relatively mild at first, but increase over time.

Goji berries (MINDELL 2005, *HEALTH MAG* 2006, YU 2005, *GOJIBOOK* 2008)

Proposed benefits influencing mood include:

Antidepressant. Promotes a cheerful attitude. Known in Asia as "happy berry."

Adaptogen, increases stamina, energy, and ability to handle stress.

Improves memory (contains betaine which converts to choline).

Benefits sleep quality. Counters fatigue.

Potent antioxidant. Fights inflammation.

Helps balance blood sugar and supports insulin response.

Increases testosterone, which besides enhancing libido, has antidepressant activity.

Counters headache or dizziness.

Considerations (MINDELL 2005, *HEALTH MAG* 2006, YU 2005)

Need may be suggested by

Memory problems, depression. Neurotoxicity. (YU 2005)

Oxidative stress.*(YU 2005, LI 2007, WU 2006)

Candida; immune dysfunction. (LEE 2005, HE 2005)

Dry cough.

Menopause. Infertility. Morning sickness.

Weak muscles and bones.**

Circulation problems. High cholesterol and blood pressure.***(JIA 1998) Certain kidney problems.

Hypoactive stomach cells. Poor conversion of food to energy, increasing fat formation.

Night blindness, blind spots, macular degeneration, (CHENG 2005) cataracts, glaucoma. (CHAN 2007)

DNA issues.****

* Rejuvenates blood and protects it from free radicals. Contains flavonoids, anthocyanidins. Increases formation of SOD which counters lipid peroxidation.

** Stimulates growth hormone release

*** Contains a sesquiterpene which supports the heart and blood pressure; anthocyanins, which benefit blood vessel integrity; beta sitosterol, which lowers cholesterol.

**** Its polysaccharides and betaine help restore and maintain DNA.

Rhodiola rosea

Rhodiola rosea (also called arctic or golden root) is found in Europe, Asia and the Arctic, and has been used for centuries. It's considered an adaptogen (acting to improve general health, and normalize imbalances), (BREKMAN 1969, MAMEDOV 2005) and is used in Russia for chronic fatigue and neurological conditions; and to support attention, memory, learning, ability to work, immunity, and resistance to stress. (BROWN 2002) It's also part of standard medical treatment in Sweden and Denmark. (vrp.com)

It's a relatively strong antidepressant, and dramatically enhances mental energy and performance, (BROWN 2002, RAMAZANOVE 2003, DARBINYAN 2000, MARMEDOV 2005) motivation, and optimism. It is reported to improve memory, and reduce stress, anxiety and fatigue. (KELLY 2001, MAMEDOV 2005)

Mechanisms which may underly benefit to mood

Activates the cerebral cortex and limbic system. (BROWN 2002)

Increases serotonin up to 30%, increases dopamine and norepinephrine, may reduce COMT. (DARBINYAN 2000, KELLY 2001)

Influences opioid peptides e.g., beta endorphins. (KELLY 2001)

Enhances thyroid functioning without causing hyperthyroidism. Increases adrenal reserves. (RAMAZANOVE 2003)

Stimulates ATP (key energy source) and creatine phosphate (energy reserve) production, and breakdown and transport of fat. (RAMAZANOVE 2003)

Antioxidant.

Need may be suggested by (RAMAZANOVE 2003, KELLY2001, DARBINYAN 2000, MAMEDOV 2005, BROWN 2002)

Depression. Forgetfulness. Attention problems.

Neurological conditions.

Low thyroid or adrenal activity

Fat accumulation.* Lipid peroxidation.

Poor physical performance and recovery. Low-stamina, muscle energy, protein synthesis.

Low energy, exhaustion.** Fatigue. Chronic fatigue. (BROWN 2002)

Stress-induced damage to the heart. Recovering from cardiovascular illness.

Liver toxicity. Thymus shrinkage.

Erectile dysfunction. Premature ejaculation.

* Activates fat breakdown and mobilizes fat.

** Stimulates production of ATP and creatine phosphate

Cautions

Give early in the day, as it can overstimulate. Avoid caffeine or other stimulants.

Important: Some researchers *warn against any use of rhodiola by bipolars,* because of the risk of triggering mania or destabilizing mood. Others believe conservative use in severe, nonresponsive bipolar depression can be acceptible, *if indicated.* See *Reminders,* next page.

Other possibilities

Green tea (perhaps decaf)— mildly stimulating and antidepressant; at the same time, calming and antioxidant. (COOPER 2005, MITCHER, ESCHENAUER 2006) Contains theobromine* and theanine. (See *Theanine,* p. 55.) (LEKH 1999, KAKUDA 2000, YAMADA 2005, DHARMANANDA 1998, KOBAYAHI 1998, MASON 2001)

Cacao nibs — from the bean from which chocolate is produced* (but without the added sugar and detrimental fats). Mildly stimulant, with anecdotal antidepressant (JORM 2002) and anti-anxiety (DALLARD 2001) benefits. Claimed to be helpful, for some, in breaking chocolate and coffee addictions. *Warnings: The patient must restrain themselves to a small pinch per serving. Too much can overstimulate, and may contribute to mania. Not recommended if copper is overloaded relative to zinc (as in MT dsyfunction, pyroluria, and many histapenias).*

* Cacao and green tea contain theobromine, which produces both mildly stimulating and calming effects. Cacao also contains antidepressant neurotransmitter precursors, including phenylethylamine, the "love neurotransmitter" (see p. 110); canabanoid-like chemicals (anandamide analogues); (Bruinsman 1999) epicatechins, which are potent antioxidants; and magnesium.

Bacopa monnieri (also called water hyssop, or brahmi**) — grows in Asia, Asia Minor, and southeastern US, in damp conditions. It promotes brain protein synthesis, cell repair, and dendrite growth. Studies suggest it improves memory, curiosity, concentration, and cognitive ability in general; may counter anxiety and epilepsy; is antioxidant and particularly effective at protecting fats; supports digestion and counters parasites. (STOUGH 2001, ROODENRYS 2002) It may help resolve resistant bipolar depression, *or be entirely contraindicated* — see *Reminders,* below.

** But don't confuse it with Centella asiatica.

Suma — a South American plant, known as an adaptogen. It is claimed to oxgenate cells, increase circulation, enhance memory, calm nerves and restore function; and may counter anxiety, stress, pain, inflammation, exhaustion, and perhaps chronic fatigue. (BARTRAM, RAIN-TREE.COM/SUMA.HTM) *May be entirely contraindicated* — see *Reminders.*

Physical claims: Supports hormonal function. Estrogenic. Increases libido. Benefits PMS, menopause. Minimizes birth control side effects, inhibits blood clots. Supports endurance; strengthens and builds muscles. Enhances immunity, neutralizes toxins. Antifungal, antibacterial. Held to inhibit leukemia, cancer, tumor growth. Reduces cholesterol. May benefit sickle cell anemia.

***REMINDERS** — To the patient: Seek the advice of your physician on the use of antidepressant herbs.*
To the physician: Many practitioners warn against giving moderate-to-strong antidepressant herbs to bipolars. If nonetheless indicated (possibly in countering certain severe, nonresponsive depressions), be conservative about dose, and wary of triggering mania, or increasing cycling, or otherwise worsening short or long-term outcome. Monitor. Taper carefully as depression ends. Educate patients about countermeasures and advise them to contact you immediately with any problems. Such herbs will probably be entirely contraindicated with any tendency to mixed states, rapid cycling, extreme manias, other instability. Check herbal and bipolar literature for further contraindications.

Approaches to antidepressant herbal formulations (KLOSS 1973, MURRAY 1995, 98, MOWREY 1986, 90, CHRISTOPHER 1976, BALCH, CRAYHON)

Herbal formulations may include some of the following categories, as tailored to individual biochemical requirements:

SEROTONIN SUPPORT — St John's Wort.

MILD ANTIDEPRESSANTS — lemon balm, mint, borage, lavender, lime blossom, lemon grass, peppermint, cinnamon.

MODERATE ANTIDEPRESSANT HERBS — Siberian or American ginseng, ginkgo, gotu kola, goji, noni, acai, green tea.

MORE POTENT ANTIDEPRESSANTS — *only if required due to nonresponsive depression, & carefully tailored to individual biochemical needs, with attention to preventing mania* — rhodiola, bacopa, Korean ginseng, suma. *May be entirely contraindicated.*

CHLOROPHYLL SOURCES — barley or wheat grass, spirulina,* chlorella,* *may benefit fatigue, anemia, blood sugar imbalance, depression, but check for sensitivity reactions, and consider effects of copper content.*

NUTRITIVE SOURCES — Alfalfa, horsetail, yellow dock, nettles, red clover, watercress, parsley, dandelion, etc.

ANTIOXIDANT/IMMUNE HERBS — rosehips, rosemary, milk thistle, reishi, bilberry, grape seed, wild cherry bark, *to protect heart and brain from pro-oxidant effects of the formula.*

ADRENAL SUPPORT — licorice, ginseng, etc., *if indicated.*

THYROID SUPPORT — Irish moss; kelp, dulse or other seaweeds, *if indicated.*

B VITAMINS — bee pollen,** nutritional yeast (also a great souce of chromium).***

ANTI-ANXIETY & MOOD-MODERATING HERBS — hops, catnip, scullcap,**** lady's slipper,**** valerian,**** wood betony,**** kava,**** *as indicated, to support balanced mood.*

"SMART" HERBS***** — capsicum, lobelia,****** perhaps, ginger.

* Algae may be overstimulating in some manias, or in some individuals prone to violence, perhaps especially in persons with elevated copper (e.g., in histapenia, MT dysfunction, pyroluria). Algae occasionally contains lead or other impurities.
** But check for sensitivities (especially in persons with hayfever).
*** May cause bloating or gas (acidophilus may help). Can be contraindicated with Candida.
**** These can, in some cases, especially with high intake, contribute to depression.
***** Dr. Christopher's designation for herbs which he claimed help bring the formulation to where it's needed in the body.
****** Given judiciously, because too much, or any amount in a sensitive individual, can be emetic.

"By appropriate use of these injectables, I personally believe that the Center has helped untold numbers of patients who would otherwise be unresponsive."

Robert Carson, MD

Myers cocktail, history (GABY 2002)

Dr. John Myers, MD, originally developed a relatively high dose, vitamin/mineral rapid IV infusion (focusing on magnesium, B, C, calcium, and B5) as part of the treatment of certain medical conditions. Dr. Alan Gaby, who inherited many of his patients, has since administered some 15,000 IVs to at least 900 persons. He estimates over 1000 US physicians now use Myers-type coctails; more, worldwide.

Infusion case study

Gaby describes a man, aged 46, with anxiety and depression since childhood, and poor response to drugs or nutrients. He was taking a diuretic (which depletes magnesium), and symptoms were aggravated by alcohol (which reduces levels further).

Treatment involved relatively high doses of magnesium, with B, B1, B5, B6, B12 (but no calcium). * Infusion rate was gradually increased til optimal. By year four, the need for injections decreased to no more than one per month.

8. Injection therapies

Injection therapies may be helpful for some depressives nonreponsive to oral therapies, perhaps especially malabsorbers. Such therapies are usually *not* advisable for mixed state or relatively rapid cyclers.

Myers (or Gaby-Wright) Cocktail — Quick infusions are believed to force high quantities of nutrients into the cell,* where they are retained up to several weeks. Gaby (2002) finds a modified Myers Cocktail, containing C and B vitamins, and emphasizing magnesium,** benefits some bipolars, perhaps especially during depression. Some depressives with high vulnerability to stress, alcoholism, or chronic pain (SHEALY 1997) have also improved. This approach may also benefit the following conditions (which often accompany bipolar disorder): chronic fatigue, fibromyalgia, MS, dementia, asthma, migraines, seasonal allergies, hyperthyroid, and various immune, respiratory, cardiovascular and other conditions. It has also been used post chelation. (SALEEBY 2005)

Some patients improve to the extent that the need for IV treatments diminishes; others respond, but require ongoing IVs. (GABY 2002)

* The heightened serum levels facilitate markedly greater tissue uptake than with oral supplements. (Shealy 1997, Gaby 2002)

** Gaby generally increases magnesium (up to 10-fold) and C (especially with allergy or infection), while eliminating folate (which tends to form a precipitate) and, for some, calcium, and does not use hydrochloric acid. He adds nutrients relevant to patient chemistry (e.g., B6, B12, small doses of trace minerals, zinc). Separate injections might include: reduced glutathione (buffered), adrenal cortical extract, or an active component from licorice, etc. (Saleeby 2005)

Other IV nutrient therapies — The Olive White Garvey Center, in Kansas, the clinic of the late Dr. Hugh Riordan, MD, has used IV nutrition (or IM, which is absorbed more slowly) for decades in treating psychiatric disorders, to forestall relapse, to accelerate healing, or to circumvent malabsorption. (Riordan (1995) found that after approximately 100 days, digestion often improves enough to switch to oral nutrients.) The Fryer Research Center in New York, and the Health Recovery Center in Minnesota (LARSON 2008) also use IV therapies.

Gaby-Wright formula (SALEEBY 2005, GABY 2002))

MAGNESIUM. Gaby usually doesn't use calcium,* unless indicated.

B COMPLEX, PLUS EXTRA B1, B3, B5, B6, B12.

VITAMIN C.

Additions, as indicated by patient biochemistry, might include trace minerals, zinc; or separate injections of reduced glutathione (buffered), adrenal cortical extract, etc.

Components are gently mixed in sterile water, and administered over 5-30 minutes.

Children, and elderly and frail patients are given lower doses. Initial treatments may be best done in two stages to observe cardiovascular effects.

See Gaby or Saleeby for doses.

WARNING: Select patients carefully. Give meticulous attention to contraindications to nutrients and other components, and to precise biochemical requirements. Reactions to contraindicated nutrients can be severe. Pace, dose and choice of nutrients must be customized to biochemistry. Adjust overall treatment to prevent rebound as dosage wears off.

* Which can be contraindicated for elderly or cardiac patients.

Contraindications, side effects (GABY 2002, SALEEBY 2005)

Sudden high concentrations of certain nutrients (e.g., B6, B12, calcium) may trigger mania.

Use with psychiatric medication is relatively unstudied.

Hypotension, lightheadedness (especially with rapid infusions). Contraindicated for some with low blood pressure.

Calcium may pose a risk to cardiac patients

The elderly often need lower doses, or IM injections instead.

Muscle cramps or heart arrythmias, especially if potassium is low (e.g., with certain diuretics, glucocorticoids, beta agonists, diarrhea, vomiting, poor diet). *Oral* potassium before and after treatment may help. *Do not include it in the IV. Keep potassium dosage modest, and match to patient requirements.*

Phlebitis.

Burning sensation at injection site, or heat, typically starting in the chest. [*Reposition the needle and/or dilute.*]

Rare risk of anaphalactic shock from B1.

Uneasiness, perhaps due to preservatives.

Enhanced visual acuity, color perception, for up to 2 days.

See also, *Warning,* p 56.

II: Major biotypes

The following biotypes were initially developed for the treatment of schizophrenia through research headed by Carl C Pfeiffer, PhD, MD, in New Jersey, and Abram Hoffer, MD, PhD, in Canada. This work has been continued and extended by numerous practitioners across the world. (Walsh 2006, Lesser 2008, Schuitemaker 2000, Larson 2008, Jaffe 1992, Kruesi 1996, Riordan 1995, Holford 2000, etc.)

Psychiatric databases

In the following decades, Pfeiffer's Brain Bio Center developed a biochemistry database of over 20,000 patients, which strongly tied biotype improvement to specific nutrients. Dr. William J Walsh, PhD, has expanded this work, creating extensive databases detailing biochemistry (typically, with a minimum of 90 distinct lab assays per person) and response to nutrients in another 20,000 patients. Together, this data has charted dramatic improvement in tens of thousands of psychiatric patients, with various disorders, in response to biotype therapy.

Biotypes in bipolars (Walsh 2006, 07)

From data on over 1800 bipolars, Walsh reports three main biotypes:

- □ **Pyrrole disorder** (pyroluria) — 18-20% of bipolars, or more.
- □ **Brain undermethylation/high folate** (histadelia) — 35%
- □ **Brain overmethylation/low folate** (histapenia) — 25%

Note: Pyroluria can overlap with methylation-imbalance biotypes. Methylation status may cycle with mood in approximately 5% of patients.

Pyrrole disorder

Histamine & Methylation

Histadelia

Histapenia

Comparison chart

Biotype outcome data (Walsh 2007)

In Walsh's preliminary internal outcome study conducted to determine whether biotype-based treatment might work for bipolars, 65-75% of families reported improvement (as compared to 85% with schizophrenia).

Since that time, the data on biochemical analysis and treatment of over 1800 bipolars suggests that of those who stick with their biotype-based nutrient program, 70% achieve substantial improvement, with approximately 50% of those treated recovering to the extent that they eventually no longer require medication (usually, as determined by their physicians).* In others, meds cannot be reduced completely, but usually can be lowered enough so that side effects are substantially minimized or absent.

Walsh states that histapenics and pyrolurics do extremely well, especially when biotype treatment is begun relatively early.** Histadelics also do well if they keep taking their nutrients.

Similar positive results with biotype treatment are reported by other practitioners. (Larson 2008, Lesser 2008, Riordan 1995, Kruesi 1996, etc.)

* Note: This doesn't mean that meds are suddenly stopped. Typically, dosage is maintained for at least three to four months, until significant improvement with biotype treatment becomes evident. Then *gradual* reductions are instituted (*if indicated*), and *tailored to patient status.*

** However, if decades elapse without biotype nutrients, treatment often becomes more difficult (perhaps reflecting cumulative oxidative and excitotoxic damage, and repeated distortions of brain homeostasis by both pharmaceuticals, and the illness, itself). (Walsh 2007)

Role of individual biochemistry

An intricate interplay often exists between biotype and:

Other nutrient needs (Part I)

- □ Receptor & second messenger support.
- □ Electrolyte balances.
- □ Neurotransmitter precursors, cofactors and regulatory enzymes.
- □ Anticonvulsive nutrients.
- □ Assorted nutrient dependencies, deficiencies, or overloads.

Toxicity issues (Part III)

- □ Metal metabolism dysfunction (prevalent in pyrolurics and histapenics).
- □ MT overactivity (common in histadelics).
- □ Oxidative stress (ubiquitous).
- □ Other neurotoxicity (excitoxicity, overuse of caffeine or sugar, substance abuse, reactions to drugs, etc.).

Further health issues (Part IV)

- □ Malabsorption, Candida, allergies, sensitivities.
- □ Blood sugar issues. Thyroid, adrenal and other endocrine imbalances, often fluctuating with mood.
- □ Autoimmune, immune, and chronic illness.
- □ Lifestyle factors (stress, altered biorhythms, poor diet, etc.)

Therapy integrates requirements and limitations of all components.

Considerations

Applicability

These biotypes may be a primary influence on symptoms in most (but not all) bipolars.

The intricacies of therapeutic indications

Intra-biotype variability — any given individual may not require all biotype-related nutrients, while other nutrients may also be needed. Optimal dosage can vary considerably between patients. And it can also change over time, as can the required balance between nutrients.

Multiple biotypes — a person may belong to more than one biotype and so need a combination of treatments relevant to both conditions, including elimination of contraindicated factors.

Additional factors — see previous page.

Conditions obscuring diagnosis — e.g., high copper in a histadelic; hyperthyroidism in a histapenic; methylation (histamine) balances changing with mood (e.g. overmethylated during mania, undermethylated with depression); cycling hormone levels; a subfunctional enzyme, requiring high levels of a nutrient that otherwise tests sufficient; elusive physical illness or toxicity issues; etc.

Further information on listed nutrients

For more complete information on mental and physical effects, sources, diagnostic tests, contraindications, references, etc., refer to separate listings for each nutrient, and the relevant literature.

Appearance & physical tendencies

Beside mental function, disordered biochemistry influences appearance and other physical characteristics, especially in those who have had biotype imbalances since childhood. Such effects help confirm results of biochemical tests and therapeutic trial (and are sometimes clear enough* to indicate diagnosis without further tests. (Walsh 2007))

* However, beware. Biotype is not always obvious. Patients often show traits which do not correspond to their biotype, or lack others that do.

Reminder to the patient: Persist

□ Take it easy. Even the most astute physician may not instantly arrive at the perfect regimen. And even once determined, improvement can take time.

□ When recovery does occur, don't stop. Discontinuing nutrients often leads to relapse (though not always right away). As a general rule, nutrients are good for you, make you happy, and prolong your life. So keep it up! *But do bring any concerns to your doctor.*

Dose listings

Doses listed in this section are average requirements, as used by the physicians cited, and are given in brackets.

Recommended reading

Pfeiffer, Carl C, PhD, MD, *Nutrition and Mental Illness,* 1987.

Pfeiffer, Carl C, PhD, MD, *The Schizophrenias: Ours to Conquer,* 1988.

Hoffer, Abram, MD, PhD, *Orthomolecular Medicine for Physicians,* 2008.

Jaffe, Russell, MD, PhD, Kruesi, Oscar, MD, "The biochemical immunology window: A molecular view of psychiatric case management," *J Appl Nutr*, 44(2); 1992.

Recommended websites

www.alternativementalhealth.com
www.walshinstitute.org
orthomed.org
www.orthomolecularvitamincentre.com

Reminder: The material in this book is intended for educational purposes only. It is not meant to replace medical diagnosis or prescription and should not be construed as treatment recommendations or other medical advice. If you need treatment for mood disorder or any other medical illness, please consult a knowledgeable physician. This may entail seeking the services of a nutritionally-oriented or orthomolecular physician.

1. Pyrrole disorder (Pyroluria)

Pyroluria is a stress disorder associated with profound anxiety, and a tendency to severe mood symptoms and rapid cycling. Stress (physical or emotional trauma, illness, lack of sleep, and even minor problems) leads to devastating reactions. Symptoms usually first emerge in teens under stress. (McGinnis 2004, Walsh 2007)

Walsh reports that of more than 1800 bipolars, 15 to 20% were primarily pyroluric, with some overlap into methylation imbalance groups.* Of the few hundred who were rapid cyclers, many were severely pyroluric.

* Pyroluria in other psychiatric disorders: Hoffer finds pyroluria in approximately 20% of depressed, anxious, or addicted adults, and behavior or learning disordered children. For schizophrenia, pyroluria may be primary in 15-30% (Hoffer 1979, 95), and present in up to 70% (McGinnis 2004, O'Reilly 1962). McGinnis also reports pyroluria in 50% of autistic, 30% of ADHD, 80% of alcoholic, and 70% of Downs patients. Pyroluria may occur in 10% (Hoffer 1983a) to 43% (McGinnis 2004) of patients with chronic illness or undergoing other prolonged physical stress.

Chemistry

Pyroluria is caused by abnormalities in forming hemoglobin, (Walsh 2006) perhaps due to pronounced oxidative stress, (McGinnis 2004) elevating a specific pyrrole, which then binds to and eliminates circulating zinc, (Walsh 1992) and often impairs B6 function, (Sohler 1974, Irvine 1969, Pfeiffer 1975, 76, 83, 87, 88, Walsh 2006) and reduces arachidonic acid (an omega 6 fat). (Bibus 2000, Walsh 2006)

Neurotransmitter and oxidative effects

- □ Increased dopamine — facilitated by depleted zinc and B6.*
- □ Low serotonin — pyrolurics cannot make serotonin efficiently due to low B6, which is required in the final step in creating serotonin. (Walsh 2002bb, 06)
- □ Anemia, excitotoxic stress, and severe metal-mediated oxidative stress, are common and alter neural function. (Walsh 2006, McGinnis 2004)

Sara (Pfeiffer 1987, 88)

Sara was the first patient treated for pyroluria. She came to Pfeiffer for help as a teen, in 1971. He describes her walking slowly "with feet wide apart as if following a hand plough drawn by tired oxen." Her knees hurt; the cartilage was malformed. Her left side would occasionally spasm with "foot clawed and fist doubled, arms and legs making wild flaying motions." Her breath smelled fruity and she was constantly nauseous. Menstruation had ceased. She was subject to seizures, amnesia, and periodic loss of contact with reality. She repeatedly tried to hang herself. Urinary kryptopyrrole was seven times normal. Symptoms were aggravated by tranquilizers.

Zinc and manganese helped her cartilage and tendons repair. B6 remitted the anemia, nausea and convulsions, and helped her body detoxify from psychiatric drugs. Zinc and B6 stopped the dysperceptions and restored endocrine balance. Manganese and B6 ended the depression and fatigue. After treatment, Sara finished college, and went on to work in New York.

Characteristics

Listed below are associated mental symptoms, physical conditions, and appearance characteristics. These are not definitive but, if many are present, lend weight to the results of laboratory tests. Pyrolurics do not necessarily manifest all these traits, especially if complicating conditions exist. Also, an individual can exhibit a number of these traits and not be primarily pyroluric.

Mental/neurological tendencies (Pfeiffer 1975, 76, 83, 87, 88, Jaffe 1992, Walsh 1991, 1997abc, 2006, 07)

Again, only some of these symptoms may be present.

- □ Low tolerance for stress, which worsens symptoms, and can be devastating. Overwhelmed by criticism. Adverse to changes in routine. Pessimistic.
- □ Profound anxiety. Fear. Severe internal tension; nervous exhaustion. Irritable, tense. Violatile, over-reactive.
- □ Explosive temper, episodic rage. Prone to assaultive behavior.
- □ Moodswings, rapid-cycling, labile emotions, histrionic behaviors, mania.
- □ Predominant depression, often severe.

History

In the 1950s, Abram Hoffer, MD, PhD, et al, discovered that, in many schizophrenias, urinary analysis with paper chromatography revealed a mauve (lilac) spot near the top of the paper. Patients who recovered with Hoffer's B3-based treatment no longer showed mauve factor. If B3 was discontinued and the patient relapsed, it reappeared. (Hoffer 1963) Researchers also found mauve factor in behavior and learning-disordered children, criminals, and others.

Irvine (1969) identified mauve factor as a pyrrole.* (Pyrroles are the basis for the heme** in hemoglobin, the component of the blood which carries oxygen, giving blood its red color.) The "mauve factor" condition was thus redubbed "pyroluria." A year later, Arthur Sohler discovered a strong association with zinc and B6 depletion. Carl C Pfeiffer, PhD, MD, and colleagues then added high dose zinc and B6 to the treatment, allowing for lower doses of B3, and developed a simpler test.

* At first thought to be kryptopyrrole (literally, a "hidden pyrrole"), (Irvine 1969) but later determined to be a similar molecule, OHHPL (hydroxyhemopyrrolin-2-one). (Graham, Audhya, McGinnis 2004)

** Heme also: supports immunity; helps form antioxidant enzymes; helps sustain zinc, C, melatonin and, probably, biotin and glutathione levels; and supports cell differentiation and response to growth factors.

Bipolar vs Pyroluric

Mental symptoms in bipolars often suggest pyroluria but can, in some cases, be misleading. Check labs.

- □ Dysperceptions, delusions. In some, hallucinations or paranoia.
- □ Periodic loss of contact with reality, but relatively good insight (the pyroluric knows she is ill).
- □ Underachievement, slowed thought processes, reduced learning abilities, reading disorders.
- □ Poor short-term (but, often, good long-term) memory. Periodic spells of amnesia. Difficulty recalling events and people.
- □ Lethargic, sometimes apathetic. More alert in the evening.
- □ Difficulty sleeping; rarely sleeps long. Poor dream recall, or nightmares.
- □ Prone to teenage delinquency and suicides.
- □ Tendency to hyperactivity if copper or lead is elevated.
- □ Prone to social withdrawal and isolation, especially with age. Uncomfortable with crowds and strangers. Tendency to become dependent on, and build one's life around, a single person.
- □ Neurological signs are common. In some, convulsive seizures.
- □ Oversensitivity to light, sound, odor.
- □ Cluster headaches.

Pyroluria: Some Tendencies and Symptoms

These characteristics, taken with other mental and physical symptoms, tend to indicate pyroluria. However, characteristics may be atypical, and not fit well into these guidelines and, conversely, people with a number of these traits aren't always necessarily pyroluric.

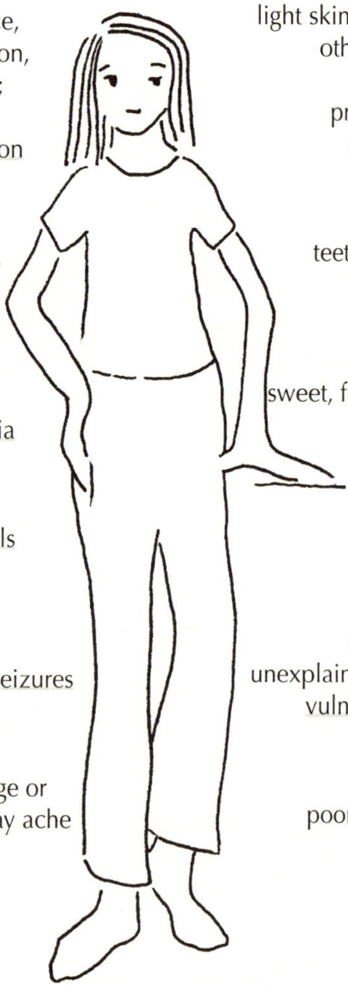

Creativity (Pfeiffer 1987, 88)

Pfeiffer states pyrolurics are among his most original patients and finds that many great people were pyroluric, despite the mental anguish and physical deterioration caused by the illness.

Physical tendencies (Pfeiffer 1975, 76, 83, 87, 88, Jaffe 1992, Walsh 1991, 1997, Ross 2002)

- □ Sweet fruity acetone breath and body odor,* especially with stress or illness.
- □ General loss of appetite. Tendency to avoid breakfast and protein (especially animal protein).
- □ Nausea (often in the morning). Motion sickness. Morning or treatment-resistant constipation.
- □ Poor sense of smell or taste. Preference for spicy or strongly-flavored food.
- □ Intolerance/sensitivity to some proteins, alcohol or drugs. Allergies.
- □ Problems with sugar metabolism.
- □ Easily fatigued.
- □ Eye pain.
- □ Joint pain or swelling. Knees may ache, crack, or cause pain. Impaired collagen synthesis may compromise cartilage and tendon development, causing malformed joints.
- □ Stunted growth. Improves after age sixteen. (Walsh 2006)

- ☐ Tingling sensation in limbs. Tremors may evolve into severe muscle spasms or convulsive seizures.
- ☐ Cold hands and feet. Unexplained chills and fevers.
- ☐ Dry skin. Tendency to stretch marks, herpes, acne, eczema, or psoriasis.
- ☐ Poor healing of wounds.
- ☐ Poor immune function; frequent colds and infections. With chronic untreated pyroluria, Pfeiffer finds increased tendency to cancer. (PFEIFFER 1987, 88)
- ☐ Altered glandular function, with delay of puberty, irregular or absent menstruation, or impotency.
- ☐ Sore adrenals.
- ☐ Upper left quadrant (spleen) pain and sensitivity, especially with stress.
- ☐ Stitch in the side when running.
- ☐ *Highly prone to* oxidative and excitotoxic stress. (MCGINNIS 2004)
- ☐ Tendency to macrocytic, low-B6 anemia and eosinophilia.
- ☐ Sensitivity to gluten (in wheat, rye, etc.) and casein (in dairy) due to low zinc.

Appearance (PFEIFFER 1975, 76, 83, 87, 88, JAFFE 1992, WALSH 1991, 1997, 2006)

- ☐ Usually female.
- ☐ Often has the lightest skin and hair in the family. Hair tends to grey prematurely (zinc and B6 are needed in forming pigment). Eyebrow hair may be coarse.
- ☐ Pallor may impart a "China doll" appearance. Skin tends to be dry, and to itch or burn in the sun, rarely tan, may not even get red. Face may swell during significant stress.
- ☐ Nails are typically pale, soft, easily-broken. White spots are common, and often reflect periods of low zinc or protein.
- ☐ Upper front teeth are usually crowded, and overlap, unless they were corrected by braces. Tooth enamel tends to be poorly formed, prone to decay; gums, inflamed and retracted.
- ☐ May limp due to malformed joints.
- ☐ Wrists and ankles may be thin, with body weight concentrated in the midsection.

Family & congenital history (PFEIFFER 1987, 88)

The tendency to pyroluria is genetic. In one case, *all* fifteen children of a severely pyroluric mother were pyroluric. (PFEIFFER 1987, WALSH 2008)

Other family tendencies may include cluster headaches, depression, fatigue, sensitivity to cold, anemia, nausea, lack of dream recall, and suicides.

Pfeiffer finds the pyroluric mother tends to have mainly female children, who look remarkably alike. He notes that males are often miscarried or stillborn, perhaps, at least partly due to insufficient zinc, which is needed by developing male organs.

Zinc deficiency also affects RNA and DNA protein synthesis, brain lipids, hippocampal size, cerebellar development, axonal transport of neuronal tubulin, and neurotubule synthesis and assembly. Fewer neurons develop. Brain size may be reduced.

Emily Dickinson

*"Take all away from me, but leave me Ecstasy,
And I am richer then than all my Fellow Men"*

Emily Dickinson,
from one of her last poems

Professor John F McDermott (2001), of the University of Hawaii, suggests Dickinson was mildly bipolar. Most of her work was written between ages 28 and 35. During the first four of these years, her moods (and letters) showed a seasonal pattern,* tending to a creative hypomania in the spring and summer when she did most of her writing. From sleepless, exuberant, "intoxicating" summers, she fell into hopeless winters, plagued by self-doubt. Her winter poems are cold and despondant.

The onset of the second four years was marked by emotional crises. Dickinson wrote of enduring a "Terror." She went on to a prolonged hypomanic phase, writing all day (half her poems were written during this period), and magnifying what she saw in a radically new poetic style. Time went by "in a blur."

* Rosenthal suggests SAD.

Dickinson's pyroluria

"The Soul selects her own Society — Then — shuts the Door —"

Emily Dickinson, c. 1862

Pfeiffer (1987, 88) suggests Emily Dickinson may have been pyroluric. She was easily upset by criticism, and prone to nervous prostration. Great drive and creativity alternated with depression, cluster headaches, and fatigue. Her eyes were hypersensitive to light, and subject to incapacitating pain.

Dickinson was highly dependent on her family and devastated by her father's death. She grew terrified of change, and increasingly reclusive. She wouldn't venture outside, except when she had someone close to her to hold her hand. Strangers often triggered palpitations. She ran for cover when the doorbell rang, and eventually retreated completely to the house she shared with her sister, maintaining outside contact only by letter.

"We all stopped froze, didn't move a muscle, and were passed over for dead. We all became cells of a larger organism. There were billions of us. One of us would breathe and then another; each holds the spark of life for an instant and then passes it on. Playing a shell game with our precious ember that would bring us all back to full being as soon as the danger passed. What a brilliant strategy."

A delusion experienced by Mark Vonnegut, believing that life on earth was being extinguished. He received treatment for pyroluria, and later became a physician.

Primrose oil (BIBUS 2000, WALSH 2000, 06)

A pilot study by Drs. Douglas M. Bibus and William J. Walsh examined plasma fatty acid profiles for the different biotypes. In pyroluria, arachidonic acid (AA), a long-chain omega 6 fat, was significantly depressed; EPA (omega 3), insignificantly elevated. This study suggested pyrolurics might have less need for omega 3, and perhaps do better with GLA.

Walsh reports that lab results for thousands of pyrolurics since have confirmed low omega 6, especially in severe cases, with very good response to GLA, especially evening primrose oil.

Drugs (PFEIFFER 1987, WALSH 2000)

Pfeiffer observes that pyrolurics are often intolerant of barbiturates, neuroleptics, etc., with the sedation worsening symptoms, perhaps, in part, due to problems metabolizing and eliminating the drugs. He warns that abnormal EEGs with single convulsions can occur with initial neuroleptic treatment. He finds, in most cases, any intake must be decreased or eliminated. Walsh notes that though pyrolurics seem to respond to SSRIs, if given long-term, pyroluric vulnerability to side effects can be prohibitive, while for most, nutrients alone produce a relatively rapid and substantial response.

Treatment (PFEIFFER 1974, 75, 76, 83, 87, 88, JAFFE 1992, WALSH 1991, 95, 97, 2000, 02, 06, ROSS 2002, WALLWORK 1981, KIMURA 1965)

Treatment focuses on vitamin B6, zinc and manganese. According to Pfeiffer (1987), pyroluria is easily treated, and patient improvement is directly related to decreases in urinary pyrrole.

Average doses used by Pfeiffer (1987, 88) or Jaffe/Kruesi (1992) are in brackets. Dose varies with the patient. Treatment choices must reflect individual biochemical requirements. See nutrient descriptions in Part I.

☐ **Zinc** — constant depletion often compromises metal metabolism and augments oxidative stress. [Start with 25 mg, increase in 25 mg steps.* May need to go up to 50-100 mg, perhaps more. (WALSH 2007, 08) Divide intake, so zinc is given at least twice per day. (PFEIFFER 1987, 88) (Zinc picolinate, -gluconate, (WALSH 2004) or -citrate)]

* May need to start with a few days of B6, then stepwise introduction of zinc, to avert depression, nausea, digestive effects, or other reactions. (Walsh 2007)

☐ **Vitamin B6** [Taken sufficiently to enable the individual to recall her last dream of the night; or to the point at which EGOT activity normalizes. Dose might start at 100 mg, 2x/day. Total should not exceed 2 gm. If fingers or toes become numb, pyridoxal-5-phosphate may be indicated instead, at one-tenth to one-fifth the B6 dose. (PFEIFFER 1987, 88)]

☐ **Manganese** — supports MT synthesis, and counters elevated catecholamines [Approximately 10 mg., twice daily. (PFEIFFER 1987) The ratio to zinc may need to be fine-tuned. *Check contraindications.* (WALSH 2004)]

☐ **Magnesium** — often necessary with the increased zinc and B6. Irritability can signal a need for magnesium.

☐ **Evening primrose oil** — which provides GLA. In severe cases, GLA alone is usually indicated. (See callout, *Primrose oil.*) Omega 3 can be less than helpful,* except in some milder pyrolurias, and then usually should be given with GLA. (Thus for moderate-to severe pyroluria animal fat may be preferable to cod liver oil.) Check labs. (BIBUS 2000, WALSH 1997, 2000, 06)

* Since it competes with GLA for metabolic enzymes (delta 5 and 6 desaturases).

☐ **B3 (niacinamide)** — helps correct pyroluria, (MCGINNIS 2004) and is especially indicated with symptoms of anxiety or voices. (HOFFER 2005)

☐ **Vitamins B5, C** — support adrenals and immune function.

☐ **Vitamin E, selenium, glutathione, & other antioxidants** — to combat the typically severe oxidative stress, compromising neurological and immune function. Probably, most importantly, replenish zinc and support metal metabolism (See pp 170-73). Restrict exposure to free radicals, excitotoxins, and other implicated factors. Also, methyl B12 and glutathione may be needed to reverse any homocysteine accumulation (caused by the oxidative stress, and further worsening it).

☐ **Boron, biotin** — may be helpful, especially if depleted. (MCGINNIS 2004, WALSH 2007)

☐ **Tryptophan or 5HTP** — *if indicated.* Pyroluria can strongly suppress serotonin, due to the B6 depletion. (ROSS 2002))

☐ **Inhibitory nutrients** — if further support is needed for anxiety, etc., consider glycine, perhaps glycinated minerals (e.g. magnesium glycinate), and/or GABA.* Inositol or choline (depending on methylation status) may also be useful.

* Unless zinc levels can be kept up, taurine may not be helpful. (Walsh 2007)

☐ **Support balanced blood sugar** (chromium, etc.) (See pp. 127, 214-5.) (Walsh 2007)

☐ **Carnitine** — a great antioxidant, focusing on the mitochondria. A trial may be indicated in patients with low energy and signs of oxidative stress. (Walsh 2007)

☐ **Restrict copper** — initially, copper tends to be much too high relative to zinc, so environmental and supplemental sources should be restricted. Eventually, however, copper can become deficient due to zinc megadoses. Jaffe/Kruesi (1992) find that after six months, in some cases, modest doses of copper may be needed. Also, in some unresponsive patients, Pfeiffer found a small amount of copper might stimulate zinc uptake. (*Note: Zinc and copper compete for absorption, so should not be taken together, and may need to be given on alternate days.*)

Prevention (Pfeiffer 1987, 88)

Increase nutritional support in anticipation of reactions to emotional trauma (love affairs, leaving home, leaving for college, joining the military), physical illness or injury, sleep deprivation, etc.

Diet (Pfeiffer 1987, 88)

Pyrolurics usually do better initially on a relatively vegetarian, whole-foods diet, as low zinc and B6 make protein difficult to handle. Organic food can be helpful, due to poor processing and elimination of toxins.

Avoid

☐ Refined foods such as sugar and white flour. B6 is reduced 80% in refined carbohydrates. Also, avoid fried and hydrogenated fat.

☐ Allergens. Heavy metals. Alcohol and street drugs. Other toxins. Unnecessary stress.

Outcome (Pfeiffer 1987, 88, Walsh 1991, 2004a, 06)

Walsh finds bipolar pyrolurics usually improve quickly on zinc, B-6, primrose oil, and augmenting nutrients, often with some response evident within a few weeks, and optimal stabilization within three to six months, longer if confounding conditions (e.g., metal metabolism dysfunction or methylation imbalance) also require treatment. Response is also slowed by growth spurts, injuries, illness, stress, malabsorption, or Type A blood.

To avoid relapse, nutrient therapy should be ongoing, *and increased if stressors increase.* If zinc and B6 are discontinued, serious symptoms often recur within two to fourteen days.

Zinc, manganese & B6 primer (Braverman 1987, Walsh 1997)

Zinc helps moderate moods, supports intellectual functioning, promotes resistance to stress, and is required in neural development and normal thyroid function. Deficiency has been associated with paranoia, memory problems, irritability, episodic anger, behavior disorders, histapenia, pyroluria, and MT dysfunction. Also, muted sense of smell, distorted taste, immune weakness, carbohydrate intolerance, joint pain.

Manganese is antidepressant, and important to memory (and makes choline available to form acetylcholine). It supports thyroid function, and helps prevent allergies and autoimmune disorders. Deficiency has been associated with fatigue, dizziness, glucose intolerance, joint malformation, incoordination, seizures.

Vitamin B6 supports formation of key neurotransmitters: serotonin, dopamine, norepinephrine, acetylcholine, and GABA, and has been used in treating hyperactivity, autism, epilepsy, depression, agitation, cerebral allergies or toxicity, pyroluria, and histapenia. Deficiency can induce nausea, tingling shock-like sensations in the limbs, and childhood convulsions. B6 is also essential to the production of hemoglobin, and supports immune activity, thyroid function, DNA and RNA synthesis, and metabolism of carbohydrates, fats, and amino acids.

Pyroluria nutrients as antioxidants (McGinnis2004)

Pyrrroles create significant oxidative stress. B6, zinc, manganese and B3, all critical in treating pyroluria, are also powerful antioxidants. (See p. 82.)

See *B6*, pp. 62-63; *Zinc*, 29-31; *Manganese*, 129-30; *B3*, pp. 59-61 for more information on benefits, side effects, contraindications, references, etc.

Reminder: This information is presented for educational purposes only. If you need treatment for bipolar disorder, pyroluria, porphyria, or any other medical condition, please seek the services of a knowledgeable physician.

Considerations: Pyroluria

Lab (PFEIFFER 1974, 75, 76, 83, 87, 88, JAFFE 1992, WALSH 1991, 06, SOHLER 1974, RIDGES 1972)

Note: Pyroluria can be difficult to distinguish from the methylation axis biotypes by signs and symptoms, alone.

Urinary pyrroles. Normal is 4-8 mcg/dL; 20-50 is moderate pyroluria (which can be a serious condition); over 50 is severe; below 3 suggests samples may have been handled improperly.* Levels can vary over the day.

EGOT (erythrocyte glutamate/oxalate transaminase) — a key B6-dependent enzyme. Reflects B6 levels.

Zinc — blood, serum, or hair may be high or low.**

White spots on nails may roughly map periods of zinc deficiency*** (nails take about 5-6 months to grow in).

Red cell membrane EFAs.

Toxic metals and metal metabolism assays.

Other nutrients or related enzymes may be low.

EEGs may be abnormal, with occasional slow waves and isolated voltage spikes.

Serum IgA may be depressed.

* Samples should be frozen immediately and kept well below 32 degrees in shipping. Keep away from light.

**Low hair and plasma zinc almost always correlate, though very high hair zinc can occur with low serum levels and high urinary excretion. (Walsh 2006)

*** But can be due to other causes.

Contraindications, side effects (PFEIFFER 1987, 88)

While zinc may help depression, psychosis, etc., chronic elevation can promote such conditions, perhaps due to relative insufficiency of manganese, copper, or B6.

Excess zinc relative to manganese reduces neural membrane stability and may lead to convulsive seizures. Epileptics are particularly at risk.

Excess zinc can cause nausea and other digestive symptoms, profuse perspiration, intolerance to alcohol.

Excess manganese relative to zinc may foster mania.

If also histadelic, manganese may need to be limited. (WALSH 2007)

Manganese can increase stiffness in Parkinson's, and aggravate tics.

Excess manganese may elevate blood pressure in persons over 40, and cause hypertensive headaches.

Excess B6 relative to magnesium or zinc may be associated with adverse mental reactions.

High B6 (usually over 2 gm) has, in a few cases, caused sensory nerve damage, reversible when intake was stopped. Damage may be indicated by numb or tingling fingers or toes (but can be due to other causes, e.g., low B12).

See each nutrient (Part I), for further contraindications, etc.

Porphyria (PFEIFFER 1988, GOLD 1987)

Porphyria is a rare inherited disease, caused by excess porphyrins* or their precursors. Some porphyrias are bone-marrow based; others, liver. Neurological symptoms are common in three liver-based porphyrias.

* Porphyrins are used to create heme, which is used in forming hemoglobin, the oxygen-carrying molecule in blood.

Relation to pyroluria — A ring of linked pyrroles form the basic structure of the porphyrin molecule. Both pyroluria and porphyria involve urinary zinc loss. Acute intermittent porphyrinuria, and coproporphyrinuria (common with chemical sensitivity) can produce a pyroluric syndrome, with low zinc, B6, serotonin; high dopamine; and attendant symptoms. (LANE 1997)

Symptoms — Can attack any part of the nervous system. May produce depression, mood swings, and body pain, with no other signs. Other mental symptoms can include psychosis, neurosis, seizures, convulsions, paralysis, an organic brain syndrome, altered consciousness, confusion, delirium, hallucinations, irritability. Between attacks, depression is common.

Physical symptoms: Characteristic port-colored urine and feces which darken on exposure to light. Aches, pains, weakness. Light sensitivity, vision loss. Vomiting, diarrhea, constipation. Acne. Altered fat metabolism. Paralysis.

Populations — Porphyrinuria seems to be more common in psychiatric patients. (One study of 2500 patients found 1.5% with acute intermittent prophyria.) Inbreeding has increased incidence in certain populations (e.g., in European royal families; the white population of South Africa, where it may affect 10%); and Sweden, due to first-cousin marriages).

King George III's porphyria (PFEIFFER 1988)

"If he [George Washington] refuses to be king, he is the greatest man alive." — King George III

George III, King of England during the American Revolution, had acute intermittent porphyria, perhaps contributing to the creation of the Stamp Act, etc. In 1788, his first severe attack involved abdominal cramps, nausea, constipation, weakness, profuse perspiration, hoarseness, rambling speech, visual distortions, insomnia, excitement, vertigo, convulsions. He relapsed in 1801, 1804, and 1810, deteriorating physically and mentally, and losing his vision. He was eventually deemed insane and replaced by the Prince of Wales. His latter years were relatively calm, interspersed with episodes of painful convulsions.

Pfeiffer's suggestions for management (PFEIFFER 1988)

- ☐ Support immunity. Correct electrolyte, nutritional and biochemical imbalances.
- ☐ A diet rich in unrefined complex carbohydrates.
- ☐ Relatively high doses of zinc and B6.
- ☐ E (which blocks porphyrin activity; may counter anxiety).
- ☐ B3 (especially for psychosis and anxiety).
- ☐ Do not fast. Fasting is detrimental.
- ☐ Correct any imbalanced testosterone metabolism.
- ☐ Avoid triggers: drugs, alcohol, toxic chemicals, faulty poor diet, refined carbohydrates. Barbiturates, estrogenics and other meds which cause flareups, *if medically feasible.*

2. Histamine, methylation, & biotype

In 1966, Dr. Carl C. Pfeiffer, MD, PhD, at the New Jersey Neuro-Psychiatric Institute, first noted abnormal blood histamine levels in schizophrenic patients, with improvement occuring as histamine was brought toward normal. He coined the term, *histapenia*, to describe the low histamine biotype; *histadelia*, for elevated histamine, and achieved great success in treating thousands of schizophrenics, depressives and other patients who fit into these biotypes. (See p. 145.) Subsequently, Dr. William J. Walsh found such biotypes critical to symptoms in 60% of 1800 bipolars.

Histamine vs Methylation axis

The major means of regulating and removing histamine is methylation. Thus, chronic undermethylation leads to histamine accumulation, (Cooney 1999) i.e. histadelia; overmethylation, to histamine depletion, i.e. histapenia.

In fact, Walsh notes that current research suggests that brain methylation may be more primary to histapenia and histadelia than histamine status. Supporting this view, Walsh has occasionally seen psychiatric recovery with nutrient therapy for methylation imbalances, *even when histamine parameters remain unchanged.* (Walsh 2007)

Nonetheless, histamine extremes contribute significantly to symptoms. And histamine levels remain one of the best determinants of methylation status — to which they are almost always inverse. (Cooney 1999)

Role of methylation/folate balance (Walsh 2006, 07)

Methylation involves the attachment of methyl (CH_3) to a molecule. All body cells have the same DNA, but genes may or may not be expressed, thus bringing out unique characteristics. Methylation is one of several key influences, usually acting to selectively suppress genetic expression of various amino acids. (Walsh 2008)

Methylation is essential to normal brain chemistry, and profoundly influences the activity of neurotransmitters and other key mood-altering brain chemicals, and the communication of mood and cognitive messages. (Cooney 1999) The proper methylation/ folate ratio, in particular, is critical to the formation of BH4, the rate-limiting enzyme in creating norepinephrine, dopamine, and serotonin.

Thus, the key target in treating histapenia and histadelia, becomes the status of *brain* methylation,* especially, as related to folate levels.

* Irrespective to that in the rest of the body, which will not necessarily be the same.

A note on nomenclature

This book retains Pfeiffer's original "histapenia" and "histadelia" designations, as well as using "overmethylation" and "undermethylation," along with the more accurate, but wordy, "brain overmethylation/ low folate," and "brain undermethylation/ high folate," respectively.

Effects of histamine on the brain

Histamine is found in blood basophils and mast cells, and all nerve cells (stored in nerve endings). (Pfeiffer 1988, Green 1978ab, 87, Schwartz 1977, 91, Hough 1988, Wada 1991) It is popularly known for instigating mucus reactions that cause sneezing and sniffling, in response to allergies and infections. It also stimulates tears, saliva flow, and inflammation; (Pfeiffer 1987) and accelerates metabolism, increasing body heat.

Histamine is also an important brain neurotransmitter and neuroregulator, strongly influencing mood and cognition. (Prell 1995)

One important mechanism may be its role in counterbalancing catecholamines and serotonin in key mood-modulating regions.*

* E.g., it influences release of dopamine, serotonin, and norepinephrine in the hypothalamus (which governs the endocrines, fight-or-flight emotions, and eating, drinking, and sleep), (Phillipu 1984, Blandina 1989, Pilc 1979) and probably counterbalances dopamine in the nucleus acumbens (which filters incoming sensory information, and produces feelings of reward). (Chronister 1982, Pfeiffer 1988) Conversely, dopamine and epinephrines modulate histamine release in the hypothalamus (Prast 1991, 93) and cerebrum. (Hill 1988, Gulat-Marnay 1989)

Overview: Undermethylation, Overmethylation (Walsh 2006, 07)

Note: These biotypes will be described in more detail in the following chapters.

Brain undermethylation/high folate (Histadelia)

Walsh reports that of over 1800 bipolars, undermethylation was primary in approximately 35%. Severe cases are associated with obsessions, compulsions, and constant suicidal depression.

Undermethylation/high folate inhibits formation of antidepressant transmitters, serotonin, dopamine and norepinephrine, along with many aspects of brain metabolism, leaving the brain underactive and fostering depression. It also decreases creation of SAM, compromising methylation further. Such patients deteriorate when supplemented with significant folic acid.

Relation to histamine levels

Undermethylation/high folate increases histamine and impedes its elimination,* promoting "histadelia." The high histamine, in turn, decreases methyl.

* Histamine N-methyltransferase (which is the main regulator of histamine), requires SAM as a methyl donor. Depletion of SAM (due to undermethylation) thus allows histamine to accumulate.

Intersection with metal metabolism status (Walsh 2006, 07)

If metal metabolism is disordered, it tends to be overactive, usually depressing copper.

Brain overmethylation/low folate (Histapenia)

Walsh has found overmethylation primary in approximately 25% of 1800 bipolars. Overstimulation, anxiety, and depression are typical, and, in severe cases, profound panic disorder, paranoia, psychosis, and/or mania.

Overmethylation/low folate promotes the creation of serotonin, dopamine, and norepinephrine, and generally overstimulates brain activity, fostering hypomania, etc.* Increased production of SAM further increases methylation. Such patients deteriorate when supplemented with methionine, SAMe, DMG, TMG, or copper.

* Also see *Methylation effects,* in the box, below.

Relation to histamine levels

Overmethylation/low-folate removes histamine,** promoting "histapenia."

* And also decreases folate, B3, and B12, while increasing copper, methionine and SAMe, all of which worsens histapenia further.

Intersection with metal metabolism status (Walsh 2006, 07)

Underactive metal metabolism function is common, and worsens histapenic chemistry, typically allowing copper to increase, intensifying oxidative stress, and promoting more severe symptoms, such as thought disorder, paranoia, and hallucinations. (Wada 1991, Green 1978)

If methylation status cycles (Smythies 1984, Walsh 2007)

Walsh's data shows at least 5% of bipolars cycle from over- to under-methylation and back, as they move from mania to depression to mania, often making typical biotype treatment difficult. He finds that such patients tend to respond to therapy focused on a mix of long-chain omega 3 fats: *both* EPA, to counter depression, *and* DHA, to counter mania. (See *Essential Fatty Acids,* p. 86-94.)

Methylation effects (Cooney 1999)

Mechanisms which may contribute to effects of methylation on mood include:

- □ Activates, helps produce and release dopamine, norepinephrine, serotonin, and other mood-modulating transmitters. (The methyl/folate ratio regulates *BH4,* a key enzyme in producing these transmitters.)
- □ Helps metabolize, detoxify and eliminate* histamine.
- □ Increases MAT which produces SAM. (Smythies 1984)
- □ Increases neural membrane fluidity, improving regulation of electrolyte flow. Methylates membrane phospholipids. Increases coupling of receptors to adenylate cyclase. (Smythies 1984)
- □ Helps maintain and protect neural (and body) DNA* and chomosome integrity. Regulates genetic expression of many neurochemicals.
- □ Helps repair brain and other proteins, benefitting some cases of seizures, other neurologic disorders and perhaps dementias.
- □ Supports melatonin creation (thus, sleep). (Meck 1987)
- □ Helps reduce overall toxicity, in that it is used in phase II liver detox.
- □ Required in maintaining myelin, which helps conduct neural messages and is reduced in some depressions.

* Methyl attaches to DNA, and methylation patterns are transferred to daughter strands, thereby controlling gene activation and expression. Undermethylation is associated with breaking, unwinding and decondensing of chromosomes, which may result in birth defects, aging, cancer, heart conditions, or autoimmune disorders. (Cooney 1999)

3. Undermethylation/high-folate (Histadelia)

Undermethylation of neurotransmitters and other brain chemicals, accompanied by high folate, is a genetic disorder, usually diagnosable by elevated blood histamine and, often, elevated basophils. Activation of mood-modulating neurotransmitters and other brain systems is usually suppressed; serotonin is typically low; similarly, dopamine and norepinephrine. And copper is often low. Walsh reports that out of over 1800 bipolars treated via biotype therapies, this condition was primary in 35%.

Typical symptoms include compulsions, phobias, obsessions, addictions, perfectionism, severe inner tension, and chronic suicidal depression. Common diagnoses include: schizoaffective, bipolar or unipolar depressive, OCD, and delusional or oppositional defiant disorder. Early detection is important, due to the constant threat of suicide. (PFEIFFER 1975, 87, 88, WALSH 97AB)

> *"Many depressives are undermethylated and respond to increased methylation."*
>
> Craig Cooney, PhD, 1999

Characteristics

Not all the following characteristics will necessarily manifest. For example, extended antipsychotic intake may cause obesity; overexposure to copper may temporarily produce symptoms of overmethylation. On the other hand, a person may exhibit a number of suspect traits and not be undermethylated.

Mental symptoms (PFEIFFER 1975, 87, 88, WALSH 97ABC, 2006, JAFFE 1992, HITZEMANN 1985)

- ☐ Often, severe depression; may show a seasonal cycle. Cries easily, compulsively suicidal.
- ☐ Overstimulated, somewhat manic.
- ☐ May sit silently, without moving, apparently calm, for hours, while enduring extreme internal tension.
- ☐ Strong will. Aggressive. Perfectionist. (WALSH 2006)
- ☐ Difficulty getting to sleep, easily woken. Insomnia can be severe.
- ☐ Obsessive rituals, ruminations, compulsions, phobias. Prone to OCD; eating, shopping/gambling, or oppositional/defiant disorders; trichotillomania.

UNDERMETHYLATION: SOME TENDENCIES AND SYMPTOMS

These characteristics, taken with other mental and physical symptoms, tend to indicate undermethylation. However, characteristics may be atypical, and not fit well into these guidelines and, conversely, people with a number of these traits aren't always undermethylated.

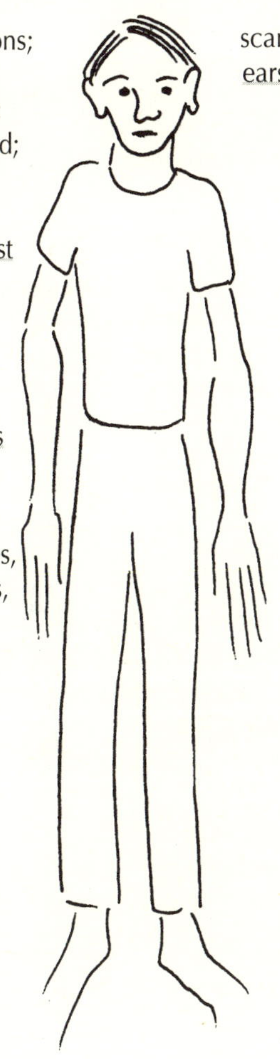

Nijinsky's last dance (NIJINSKI 1934)

"[He] picked up a chair, sat down on it facing the audience, and stared at them, as if he wanted to read the thoughts of each... for half an hour... [then he made a cross the length of the room, and] stood at the head of it with open arms, a living cross himself. 'Now I will dance you the war, with its suffering, with its destruction, with its death. The war you did not prevent and so you are also responsible... '

"[His dancing was different, like] that scene in Petroushka when the puppet tries to escape his fate... He seemed to fill the room with horror stricken humanity... His gestures were all monumental, and he entranced us so that we almost saw him floating over corpses... [He was] a tiger let out from the jungle who in any moment could destroy us... taking his audience with him to war... destruction... suffering and horror, struggling with all his steel like muscles, his agility, his lightning quickness, his ethereal being, to escape the inevitable end. It was the dance for life against death."

Nijinsky's last dance, as described by his wife, Romola Nijinsky

Soon after, Professor Bleuler found him incurably insane.

Pfeiffer suggests Nijinsky may have been histadelic.

For the rest of his life, Nijinsky was prey to catatonic episodes, which could last months; violence, especially when away from the asylum; and persistent visions of dying World War I soldiers and sounds of gunfire. He periodically refused to eat, particularly meat.

His memory remained intact, and he could recall every movement in his dances, but never danced again, and never recovered. When his former employer, Diaghileff, asked if he would dance for him once more in the Russian ballet, Nijinsky replied: "I cannot, because I am crazy."

- □ Episodes of blank mind, dysperceptions, delusions, thought disorder. Severe cases can lead to delusional thinking and a distorted sense of reality. Hallucinations are relatively rare, but may be diagnosed schizoaffective.

Note: Bipolar mental symptoms can misleadingly suggest this biotype. Confirm with labs.

Creativity (PFEIFFER 87, 88, WALSH 2006, 07)

Often shy and oversensitive as a teenager. The adult can be perfectionist, competitive, compulsively productive and creative, highly accomplished; and frequently excels in science, business, and right brain activity.

Physical symptoms (PFEIFFER 1975, 87, 88, WALSH 1997ABC, 2006, JAFFE 1992, HITZEMANN 1985, BRAVERMAN 1987, COONEY 1999)

- □ High incidence of seasonal, respiratory allergies; asthma;* autoimmune disorders.
- □ Rapid metabolism. High body temperature. Needs little sleep.
- □ Pulse can often be heard against the pillow when resting.
- □ Abundant production of fluid secretions. Profuse perspiration. Heavy salivary flow (e.g., may often wipe saliva from his mouth). Frequent colds. Prone to asthma.* Easy, well-sustained orgasm and high sex drive. Plentiful gastric juices, and a tendency to heartburn and nausea; perhaps, Crohn's or ulcerative collitis.
- □ High tolerance for, and tendency to, addictions to drugs, sugar, or alcohol.
- □ Low pain threshhold. Frequent headaches (perhaps migraines (LOW 2003)), backaches, bellyaches muscle cramps.
- □ Prone to osteoporosis, arthritis, cataracts, MS, lupus, perhaps, early aging, birth defects, or cancer.**

* Which is more likely in bipolars. (Goodwin 2003)

** Rogers see cancer as "the ultimate methyl deficiency disease," reflecting damage to chromosomal integrity. (Cooney 1999)

Appearance (PFEIFFER 1975, 87, 88)

- □ Typically male, with a lean build, despite a hearty appetite.
- □ To dissipate heat, his body may have formed an enlarged nose and ears, and elongated fingers and toes, with the second toe longer than the first. Veins may be highly visible.
- □ Body hair is usually sparse.
- □ Teeth tend to be in excellent shape. Incisors may be prominent.

Family history (PFEIFFER 1987, 88)

The undermethylation biotype is usually hereditary. Family history may include suicide, depression, allergies, alcoholism, headaches, insomnia, hives, etc. The undermethylated mother usually gives birth to male children (thin copious vaginal secretions foster creation of males).

Treatment (PFEIFFER 1975, 87, 88, WALSH 97ABC, 2006, 07, JAFFE 1992)

Average doses used by Pfeiffer (1987, 88) or Jaffe/Kruesi (1992) are in brackets. Actual dose and treatment choices must reflect individual biochemical requirements.

Walsh (2007) states the key is optimizing methyl, while keeping homocysteine low to protect the heart.

- ☐ **SAMe** — known as an effective and relatively rapid (usually within one to three weeks) antidepressant, for the appropriate patient, (BELL 1988, CARNEY 1988) probably, mostly histadelic (i.e., since SAMe rapidly increases methylation). (WALSH 2006) Walsh suggests introducing it cautiously (low, gradually-increasing doses). Clear improvement by one to two weeks helps confirm* undermethylated status. Once improvement is established, SAMe often can be slowly tapered, while substituting methionine, to reduce expense to the patient. (WALSH 1997ABC, 2000B, 06)

* This is critical, for if the patient is actually overmethylated (histapenic), SAMe worsens the imbalance, and can cause mania and other harmful reactions. (Walsh 2007)

- ☐ **Methionine** — offers a methyl group, which increases molecular weight and promotes excretion of histamine (also copper, iron and zinc). Works with calcium. [500 mg., 2-4x/day, (PFEIFFER 87, 88, JAFFE 92) typically up to 2,000 to 3000 mg, total. *Check labs, as some histadelics show normal methionine.* (WALSH 2006, 07)]
- ☐ **TMG** (trimethylglycine or betaine) — sometimes beneficial, improving well-being, and increasing methionine formation, especially in cases where homocysteine is high, folic acid low, and pathway (i) (*see callout*), compromised. In such cases, pathway (ii) may compensate. *However, if folate is elevated, TMG can decrease homocysteine conversion and worsen oxidative stress.*
- ☐ **B6** — Helps metabolize homocysteine to cysteine. Supports serotonin and metallothionein formation. [enough to induce recall of one dream per night — no more; (PFEIFFER 1987, 88) perhaps, start with 20-50 mg. and go up from there, *as indicated.**]

* But keep the upper limit below that at which pathway iii predominates, converting homocysteine to cysteine rather than methionine, and so reducing methyl availability.

- ☐ **Magnesium** — critical in metabolizing methionine to SAM. Often pivotal in stabilizing mood. *Take absorbable forms, avoiding magnesium-aspartate or -glutamate.*

Methylation biochemistry (WALSH 1997, 2006, 07, COONEY 1999)

METHIONINE ---Mg + ATP---> SAM

SAM ---> METHYL + SAH

SAH ---> HCY

Dietary methionine and SAMe provide new methyl groups to brain and body.

- ☐ **Methionine** (via **magnesium**, ATP, MAT,* and water) metabolizes to SAM.
- ☐ **SAM** readily yields SAH** and methyl, which is used in neurotransmitter metabolism, neural activity, DNA regulation of proteins, etc.
- ☐ **SAH** degrades into **homocysteine.**

* Methionine-adenosyl-transferase.
** S-adenosylhomocysteine.

Methionine, homocysteine, SAM and SAH signal methyl metabolism status to cell enzymes. This helps regulate and accelerate chemical reactions, prevent misfires, and counter disease.

Neutralizing homocysteine (HCY)

Via the following 3 pathways:

(i) **HCY --folate + B12 + GSH--> METHIONINE**
HCY is methylated with the help of folates,* B12, and glutathione into methionine. *This is the primary pathway.*

* Via *5-methyl-tetrahydrofolate/B12)*

(ii) **HCY --TMG--> METHIONINE + DMG**
Betaine (TMG) methylates HCY, *but only if B12 and folate are too low for path (i). In some people, path (ii) is relatively ineffective.*

(iii) **HCY --- B6 ---> CYSTEINE**

Increasing brain methylation in histadelic subtypes: Walsh's strategies for each subtype (WALSH 2006, 07, 08)

"For most undermethylated persons, folate and B12 are critical to therapy. However, psychiatric patients with abnormal levels of norepinephrine, dopamine, or serotonin *are an exception to this rule.* They represent a special case, in which *the methyl/folate ratio in the brain* becomes the predominant concern."

WILLIAM J WALSH, PHD, 2008

"Most mentally ill histadelics are low in everything, homocysteine, SAM, methionine, etc, & what they need is more methyl

1 **VERY SLOW SAM CYCLE** (B12 & FOLATE ARE INEFFICIENT IN CONVERTING HCY TO METHIONINE ((i), *above*). FOLATE TENDS TO ACCUMULATE, AND TRAP METHYL.) (*Hereditary & common in histadelics*) — Use **SAM** or **methionine** to add new methyl.

2 **SEVERE OXIDATIVE STRESS** (CREATING SAH & PERHAPS SOME HCY ACCUMULATION) — Supply **glutathione** to create homocysteine from SAH, and to attach methyl to B12 so it will convert HCY to methionine ((i), *above*). Or, **methyl-B12** may need to be provided directly. Address also, any **metal metabolism** dysfunction, or other factors worsening oxidative stress.

3 **MALABSORPTION OR LOW PROTEIN DIET** — Increase sources of methyl and nutrient cofactors. Support absorption.

4 **CAN'T MAKE SAM** (EVEN WITH ENOUGH BETAINE OR METHIONINE) (*Genetic enzyme disorder in a small number of histadelics*) — give **SAM,** perhaps **magnesium**. Methionine and TMG are of little benefit.

" — unless homocysteine is high, and needs to be brought down to protect the heart." — *WILLIAM J WALSH, PHD, 2008*

5 **EXCESS HOMOCYSTEINE** (Not common in histadelics) — Instead of adding more methyl from methionine or SAM, protect the heart by recycling HCY with **betaine**, **B6**, and **serine** ((ii) & (iii), above). Keep folate low to encourage the betaine pathway ((ii)). Also, address oxidative stress.

CAUTION: Make sure methylation does not start or stop abruptly. Do not give SAMe or methionine to histapenics.

Drugs (PFEIFFER 1987, 88)

Lithium — Pfeiffer finds low-dose lithium sometimes helps, and may moderate histamine levels. (ISSIDORIDES 1981, RICHELSON 1982)

Dilantin, Benedryl — Pfeiffer states judicious use of Dilantin® (an anticonvulsant which decreases folate) or Benedryl® (an antihistamine) may afford some relief from severe depression or compulsions, but can eventually cause serious side effects; while methionine, calcium, zinc, etc., are usually sufficient.

Antipsychotics — Pfeiffer (1987) finds histadelics don't respond well to antipsychotics (or ECT) and may become immobile/catatonic on Prolixin.® Antipsychotics deplete magnesium, which the histadelic needs.

SSRIs — Walsh (2002B, 07) states that though SSRI's may help, side effects can be prohibitive, while nutritive support for underlying imbalances can be at least as effective.

Meds tend to be rapidly metabolized, necessitating adjustments in dose and dosing schedule. (WALSH 1991, JAFFE 1992)

Recreational drugs (PFEIFFER 1987, 88, JAFFE 1992)

The tendency to compulsive behavior can make it difficult to reduce drug use. Street drugs may be perceived as suppressing symptoms more effectively than nutrients. Since alcohol is a light histamine releaser, the histadelic may tend toward hard drinking. Opioids (e.g., heroin, morphine, opium, codeine, methadone) may be sought as strong histamine releasers; stimulants (e.g., amphetamines, caffeine, sugar) to moderate depression.

Over time, such drugs steadily compromise stability, and wind up promoting those very symptoms they once temporarily relieved, making the histadelic feel much worse.

Fortunately, effective nutrition-based withdrawal therapies are emerging. (LARSON 1997, 2008)

□ **Calcium** — releases and so, lowers, histamine. Deficiency can directly cause histamine elevation. Supports catecholamine release into the synapse. Calcium is often depleted.* [500 mg, 2x/day; (PFEIFFER 1987, 88, JAFFE 1992) up to 2000 mg, total, *if indicated.* (WALSH 2006, 07)]
See also, *Osteoporosis issues*, p. 235.

* Note: Histadelics are prone to osteoporosis and calcium stones, representing the body's attempt to cling to what calcium is available by binding it with oxalates. (Walsh 2007))

□ **Zinc** — Counters overstimulation. Supports homocysteine metabolism to cysteine or methionine. [Typically, 20-50 mg; (WALSH 2008) preferably as zinc-citrate or -picolinate.]

□ **B12** — if depression doesn't respond, a moderate-dose trial may be indicated. B12 supports methylation, and creates dramatic improvement in some patients, but worsens others. With considerable oxidative stress, *methyl*-B12 usually helps.* (WALSH 2007)

□ **Inositol** — may reduce anxiety, promote sleep. (JAFFE 1992, WALSH 2006) Critical to signalling. Counterbalances choline. Supports folates, B6, B12, betaine and methionine. [250-500 mg; Walsh, in some cases, suggests 1 gm, 3x/day; or, for sleep, up to 2 gm, depending on need, 30-60 minutes before bed (WALSH 2006))] *Too much may promote anxiety or panic in some bipolars, but not usually histadelics.*

□ **Omega 3** — supports methylation. (BIBUS 2000) [600-1200 mg, or fish 2-3x/week].

□ **Niacinamide** — modest amounts, introduced gradually, with attention to reactions. If voices occur, B3 usually becomes crucial. Anxiety may also signal greater need. (HOFFER 2005, WALSH 2007)

□ **Kava** — calms limbic activation, but overstimulating for some.

□ **Serotonin support** (e.g, St Johnswort, tryptophan, 5HTP) — modest intake may help balance mood, *especially if depleted.* (HOFFER, WALSH 1997A, 2007, JAFFE 1992). (See *Cautions*, p. 105.)

Antioxidant support

With undermethylation, and especially if metallothionein is low, oxidative stress becomes prevalent, and further compromises methylation pathways and depletes neurotransmitter precursors. Consider using:

□ **Glutathione** — needed to methylate B12, so it can turn homocysteine to methionine. Depleted by oxidative stress.

□ **Selenium & E** — work with glutathione.

□ **Vitamin C** — antioxidant; decreases histamine; moderates stimulation; antidepressant. [enough to keep urinary excretion over 100 mg./dl; perhaps 1 gm, twice daily, preferably, buffered, time-release (PFEIFFER 1987, 88, JAFFE 1992)]

□ **A** — antioxidant; counters seasonal allergy.

□ **Acetyl-L-carnitine** — a great mitochondrial antioxidant; need *may* be suggested by low mental energy. (WALSH 2007)

□ **Other antioxidants**, *as relevant.*

Other nutrients, sometimes indicated (PFEIFFER 1987, 88, WALSH 2006, 07)

□ **Copper** — supports dopamine and norepinephrine formation,* decreases histamine.** In histadelics, MT disorders tends toward overactivity, decreasing copper. If so, small doses, in some cases, may become useful (*but not if it worsens oxidative stress*).

□ **Tyrosine** — or possibly phenylalanine (which is stronger), may temporarily help counter the depression, especially if depleted, at least until methylation increases.

* Via *dopa beta hydroxylase* and *dopa decarboxylase*.
** By activating *diamine oxidase* which lowers histamine.

Restrictions (WALSH 1997B, 2006, 07)

- □ Folic acid, which is already excessive relative to methylation status, usually must be significantly restricted. (See note, p. 157.)
- □ Choline (which generally counterbalances catecholamines) and, especially, DMAE, may worsen histadelic depression, so may need to be limited. Similarly, GABA is not likely to be helpful during low-catecholamine depressions.

Diet

Eat whole foods. A high protein diet with quality animal proteins (preferably fish from mercury-free waters; organic meats, free-range poultry) provides methionine.* The diet should also include complex carbohydrates, adequate vegetables (though intake of greens, in some cases where folate is too high, needs to be moderated), fruits, and healthy fats. *Minimize/avoid immunoreactive foods.* Dairy provides calcium, which the histadelic needs, but is commonly an allergen (if so, consider goat dairy, zinc requirements, and *Therapies*, p. 213). *Avoid sugar, white flour, fried and hydrogenated fat.*

* Animal proteins also contain histidine, which is why Pfeiffer originally suggested they be avoided. However, Walsh (2007) suggests the benefits accruing from the additional methyl far outweigh any minor increases in histamine that might result from their histidine content.

Psychosocial support (PFEIFFER 1987, 88)

Undermethylated patients may find it difficult to continue taking vitamins and avoiding addictions, and may then succumb to depression and compulsions. Suicide can be a constant threat. Friendship can be lifesaving; as can living with a supportive relative or good friend.

Outcome

Noncompliance is always an issue with histadelics (who tend to be adverse to most treatments). If therapy is followed, prognosis is good. When treating with methionine, some improvement often occurs at six to eight weeks, though full benefit typically requires six to twelve months. SAMe works much faster, with benefit apparent within a couple of weeks. Depression and blank mind usually improve first. Eventually, compulsions and obsessions diminish. Abnormal fears are the most resistant to treatment. (PFEIFFER 1987, 88, WALSH 2006, 08)

Reminder: This information is presented for educational purposes only. If you need treatment for histadelia, bipolar disorder, or any other medical condition, please seek the services of a knowledgeable physician.

Considerations

Lab (PFEIFFER 1987, 88, JAFFE 1992, WALSH 1997AB, 2002, 06, 07, 08)

Whole blood histamine* — Normal is 40-70 ng/dL) Over 70 is high, and suggests undermethylation. (WALSH 2006)

Absolute basophils* — less sensitive, but help confirm histamine elevation. Normal is 30-50. Over 50 suggests high histamine, and undermethylation. (WALSH 2006)

The best methylation test would be the SAH/SAMe ratio,** but this test is still under development. (WALSH 2007)

SAH and methionine*** are also good tests. (WALSH 2007)

Homocysteine tests are not helpful. (WALSH 2007)

If methylation status is still unclear, Walsh finds a 1-2 wk trial of SAMe (cautiously!) often resolves the matter.

* Note: Antihistamines or antigens lower histamine, altering results.
** That is, elevated SAH relative to SAM points to undermethylation.
*** Though methionine is not always low in such patients.

Also check for:

Red cell, serum or plasma folate — usually high.
Serum copper — often low, unless masking symptoms.
Generally, low calcium, magnesium, B6.
Serotonin, dopamine, norepinephrine — often low.
Respiratory allergies — common.
Lead — histadelia in children can be due to high lead.
Methylation status cycling with mood.

Side effects, cautions (PFEIFFER 1987, 88, WALSH 2002B, 06, 07)

Too much, or too prolonged a dose of SAMe or, secondarily, methionine, can trigger or aggravate mania in many bipolars, though for histadelics, such reactions are rare, unless introduced too abruptly. So proceed gradually, and make sure the patient is not actually histapenic (overmethylated).* (WALSH 2007, 08)

* Methylation status is not always apparent. Check labs and symptoms meticulously. If ambiguous, clear improvement on a 1-2 wk trial of SAM or methionine helps confirm undermethylation (histadelia). Determine, also, whether methylation is cycling with mood (see p. 154). (Walsh 2008)

Methionine, in some cases, increases homocysteine production.

Folate, usually already very high, can cause symptom flareups, as (along with B12) it can increase the trapping of methyl molecules. Thus undermethylated/high folate patients (histadelics) need to restrict folate (i.e., limit sources from multiples, B complex, etc., and, in some cases, leafy greens). (WALSH 2006)

Too much tryptophan may induce a 2-3 hour blush and cardiovascular reaction, due to rapid conversion to serotonin. Rule out interactions with medication. Serotonin may overstimulate some patients.

Melatonin may overstimulate or otherwise worsen symptoms.

Choline, and especially, DMAE, is more likely to produce side effects than in histapenia. (WALSH 2006)

Manganese lowers dopamine, so can be harmful for histadelics (or with tics, or Parkinson's). (WALSH 2007)

See further contraindications, listed for each nutrient.

Three major methylating nutrients

(1) SAMe (S-adenosyl-L-methionine)

"Personally I believe the use of SAMe is the quickest way to help an undermethylated person." — Walsh 2006

SAM readily gives up methyl, making it the most important neurotransmitter methylator, critical to proper function of antidepressant neurotransmitters, (BELL 1988) and improvement in histadelia.

Benefit to depression

Natural levels, in some cases, decrease in depression, increase in mania.* (SMYTHIES 1984) CSF levels are sometimes significantly lower in severe depression. (COUSENS 2001, BOTTIGLIERI 1994)

Studies find SAM benefits up to 70-80% of depressions,** (AGNOLI 1976, CARNEY 1988, KAGAN 1990, ROSENBAUM 1988,90, LIPINSKI 1984 SALMAGGI 1993) often within 3-7 days, (ROSENBAUM 1988), LIPINSKI) especially when intravenous,* (*however IV use commonly triggers mania in bipolars*). Response is often equivalent, (BRESSA 1994) or better than that to pharmaceuticals. (BELL 1988) SAM can also accelerate response to antidepressants. (BERLANGA 1992)

* Similarly, in some depressives, the Vmax of MAT (methionine adenosine transferase, which produces SAM) is decreased, and in some manics increased. (SMYTHIES 1984)

** In one such study (Kagan, 1990), a randomized double blind, completed by 15 (of 18) major depression patients, test scores indicated a significant decrease in depression in the group which received SAM (2x/day for 21 days), as compared to placebo. One patient became manic. Otherwise, side effects were few, and minor.

Biotype indications (WALSH 2007)

Walsh (2007) finds SAMe highly beneficial for most histadelic (undermethylated/high-folate) patients, while it can readily trigger mania or other adverse effects in the overmethylated (histapenic). (*Consider that histadelics are more prone to severe depression; histapenics, to mania.*)

SAM: Mechanisms influencing mood

Mechanisms by which SAM influences mood (mostly via methylation) may include:

- □ Can increase key antidepressant (serotonin, dopamine, norepinephrine, carnitine) and antimanic (acetylcholine, taurine) transmitters.*(BIDARD 1977, BELL 1988, 94, BRAVERMAN 1987, COUSENS 2001)
- □ May alter cell signalling. (STOLL 2002) Methylates G-proteins.
- □ Important in membrane phospholipids. Helps form phosphatidyl choline and phosphatidyl serine. (COUSENS 2001) Supports membrane fluidity. (STOLL 2002)
- □ Methylates myelin basic protein.
- □ Helps clear and eliminate histamine. (COUSENS 2001)
- □ Helps make melatonin from serotonin, benefitting sleep.
- □ Helps regulate hormones. (YOUNG 1993)

* Also supports formation of: betaine, creatine, normetanephrine, nucleic acids; and some methylated glycines, tyramines, methionines, nicotinamides, and lysines. (Cooney 1999)

Considerations

Need may be suggested by

Chronic depression. Suicidality. Schizoaffective. (PFEIFFER 1988, FREDERICKS 1982)

Histadelia/ undermethylation.

Low energy.*

Allergies. Immune dysfunction. Low glutathione. (ROGERS 1997) Heavy metal toxicity. (COUSENS 2001)

Difficulty eliminating estrogen. (COUSENS 2001)

Poor cartilage/joint formation and repair.

Age-damaged proteins. (COUSENS 2001)

Migraine, PMS, drug dependency, chronic pain (PFEIFFER 1988, WURTMAN 1988, GOODNICK 1993), cirrhosis, other liver disorders, arthritis, MS, fibromyalgia, Parkinson's.

Lack of relevant nutrients.

** SAM is critical in cell energy production and storage (produces carnitine which delivers fat to mitochondria; and creatine (which stores muscle energy). (Cousens 2001)

Dose

100-200 mg orally, several times per day, possibly more if no side effects occur. (STOLL 2002) Potency varies. Take with antioxidants (including C, E, glutathione), magnesium, omega 3, B3, B6, and other relevant nutrients..

Side effects, cautions (ROSENBAUM 1988, KAGAN 1990, BRESSA 1994, STOLL 2002)

Nausea, dry mouth, restlessness, mild anxiety.

Usually not helpful in people who respond poorly to antidepressants. (ROSENBAUM 1990)

Cardiovascular risk, perhaps less than methionine.

Some researchers warn against any use by bipolars, due to a high risk of mania.*(KAGAN 1990, LIPINSKI 1984) It may be especially detrimental for rapid cyclers. (STOLL 2002) Stoll says "[SAM] might be considered if other treatments are unsuccessful [however] only with the supervision of [an experienced] psychiatrist." He notes bipolar II poses somewhat less risk. If used, he advises extreme caution, dedicated monitoring, and low doses, accompanied by mood stabilizers, especially with newer patients.**

Entirely contraindicated in overmethylated (histapenic) patients, as it feeds the imbalance, and readily triggers mania. (WALSH 2006, 07)

On the other hand, Walsh (2007) states that both SAM and methionine have been used successfully for years to treat undermethylated patients (histadelics), and that in histadelic bipolars, it should not trigger mania, though it still should be introduced gradually, with relevant cardio-protective and mood-stabilizing nutrients.

* The original studies in Italy used up to 1600 mg/day, which may have contributed to the high rate of switching (up to 50% in 2-3 weeks. Similarly, estimates of bipolars switching on antidepressants without mood stabilizers ranged from 25 to 50%. (Post 2003) (See *Antidepressant side effects,* p 287.)

(2) Methionine

The amino acid, methionine, is also a major methyl donor (though generally slower), and is required in forming SAM.

Depression benefits

Pfeiffer's Brain Bio Center found half their patients with low plasma methionine, had a history of major depression. (BRAVERMAN 1987) Walsh uses methionine in many undermethylated (usually depressed) patients, after initial treatment with SAM, as a less expensive substitute, or as an adjunct to SAM.* (*See p. 157.*)

Mood influences availability, influences mood (SAHLEY 1995)

Like other methyl donors, methionine is depleted in activating and eliminating transmitters involved in fear, panic, sadness, anger, and worry; so becomes less available to form stabilizers (taurine, acetylcholine) and antidepressants (SAM, serotonin, carnitine).*

* Also, antioxidants such as cysteine, which supports MT function, and glutathione, which supports methylation, both thereby influencing mood.

Mechanisms influencing mood (ROGERS 1997, CRAYHON 1999)

Methylating agent. Increases histamine breakdown, benefitting histadelia.

With ATP, creates SAM. (CONLAY 1989)

Increases serotonin (less so, dopamine and norepinephrine).

Used in making choline. Sometimes increases taurine. (antimanics) (ROGERS 1997)

Supports cellular energy. Used in making acetyl CoA (which makes ATP), and carnitine (which bring fats to the mitochondria).

Component of methionine enkephalin (a pain-relieving peptide), and various endorphins, which may influence mood.

Helps regulate insulin.

Forms glutathione.

Considerations

Need may be suggested by

Depression, mood symptoms, anxiety.

Allergies, asthma, stunted growth.

High cholesterol. Insulin dysregulation. (ROGERS 1997)

Toxicity issues. Aging. Perhaps cancer. (SAHLEY 1995)

Problems with methylation, and alkylation.

Populations

Ongoing stress: mood disorder, rage, chronic illness, toxic accumulation. Dietary lack of quality proteins.

Sources

Eggs, wild game, turkey, duck, ricotta or cottage cheese, fish, avocado, wheat germ, sunflower seeds.

Dose

Cousens (2001) suggests 0.5-2 gm, divided doses, with nutrients which foster creation of SAM (Mg, B6, NADH, etc).

Side effects, cautions

If conversion to SAM is compromised, homocysteine can accumulate and cause cardiovascular symptoms. (DE VANNA 1992)

Chronic high doses (especially without supportive nutrients) may cause hyperactivity, uneasiness, and a roller coaster rise and fall of homocysteine and SAM. (COONEY 1999)

May increase calcium excretion (BRAVERMAN 1987)

Loading can increase urination and palpitation, perhaps due to imbalances with other aminos. (BRAVERMAN 1987)

Appetite and growth suppression, gas. (BRAVERMAN 1987)

Low hemoglobin and hematocrit; iron accumulation. (BRAVERMAN 1987)

Damage to the pancreas, liver and spleen. (BRAVERMAN 1987)

High doses may worsen psychosis. (BRAVERMAN 1987)

Do not use with histapenia (overmethylation). (PFEIFFER 1987, WALSH 2006)

(3) Betaine (trimethylglycine or TMG) (BRAVERMAN 1987, SLAGLE)

TMG generally supports well-being and stamina, due more to its methyl than its glycine.

TMG is a direct methyl donor. It converts homocysteine to methionine when folic acid is low, thus protecting the heart, and promoting methylation activity.

Increased oxygenation may reduce lactic acid-caused anxiety.*

* May also benefit fatty liver (as in alcoholism) and, perhaps, allergies.

Biotype indications

May be helpful in some cases of histadelia (see *TMG*, p. 157), but should *not* be used with histapenia.

Sources

Beets, spinach, other vegetables, depending on soil content. Also, seafood.

Dose

750-1000 mg/day. Can increase gastric acidity, so take with food.

4. Overmethylation/low-folate (Histapenia)

Overmethylation with low folate, produces chronically low blood histamine and absolute basophils. Methionine, SAM, serotonin, dopamine, and norepinephrine, are usually elevated; niacin and B12, low. With dysfunctional metal metabolism and high copper, symptoms become more intense. Walsh has found that of over 1800 bipolars treated with biotype therapies, this condition was primary in 25%. (WALSH 2002)

Overview (WALSH 2007)

Symptoms typically involve anxiety and depression.

Co-occuring MT disorder often leads to paranoia, mania, or psychosis.

The main biochemical considerations are copper, methyl, and folate.

Causes

Role of methylation (COONEY 1999, WALSH 1997AB, 2000AB, 2006)

Walsh suggests that overmethylation, rather than low histamine, is probably the primary imbalance in the histapenia biotype.

Methylation markedly clears and eliminates histamine (COONEY 1999, WALSH 2006). It also uses up nutrients (folate, B3 and B12) that would otherwise help correct histapenia, and increases nutrients (copper, methionine and SAMe) that worsen it. And it activates dopamine, norepinephrine, serotonin and other brain chemicals, increasing stimulation.

OVERMETHYLATION: SOME TENDENCIES AND SYMPTOMS

These characteristics, taken with other mental and physical symptoms, tend to indicate histapenia. However, characteristics may be atypical, and not fit well into these guidelines and, conversely, people with a number of these traits aren't always necessarily

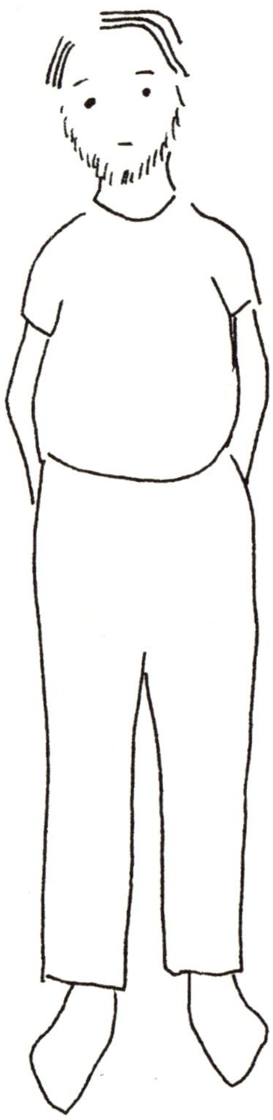

Role of niacin & vitamin C (HOFFER, 1957, 64, 66, 67, 71, 73, 83, 87, 2005, OSMOND, 1962, 80)

The original megavitamin treatments for schizophrenia, pioneered by Dr. Abram Hoffer, MD, PhD, emphasized megadoses of B3 and C* (and later, zinc, B12, folic acid, etc.). This approach has turned out to be especially relevant for patients (with various diagnoses) who respond to therapies which address histapenia (overmethylation). (PFEIFFER 1987, 88)

Role of metal metabolism & high copper (PFEIFFER 1972, 75, 83, 87, 88, WALSH 1997AB, 2000AB, 02, 04AB, 06, 07, JAFFE 1992)

Anxiety and depression are usually the main manifestations of overmethylation. Walsh (2007), however, finds that, if accompanied by metal metabolism dysfunction (see pp.170-73), and marked overloads of copper or toxic divalent metals, brain tissue becomes subject to potentially severe oxidative stress, aggravating symptoms, perhaps resolving into profound anxiety and panic disorder, mania, paranoia, psychosis, or schizophrenia.

In depressives, copper overload is less common, except as a consequence of female hormone imbalances. (WALSH 2006)

Role of allergies (PFEIFFER 1987, 88)

Allergic reactions occasionally disrupt histamine storage in blood basophils enough to create a histapenic syndrome.

Characteristics

These physical and mental characteristics are not definitive, but point to the possibility of histapenia, and lend weight to the results of laboratory tests. Histapenics usually will not manifest all these traits, especially if complicating conditions exist (e.g., a hyperthyroid histapenic will have high metabolism). Also, an individual can exhibit a number of these traits and not be primarily histapenic (e.g., in hypothyroidism).

Mental tendencies (COONEY 1999, WALSH 1997AB, 2000ABC, 02, 04AB, 06, 07, PFEIFFER 1972, 83, 87, 88, JAFFE 1992, HOFFER 1983, 87)

- ☐ Pronounced anxiety, panic attacks, overstimulation.
- ☐ Depression. Despair. Low motivation.
- ☐ Hypomania, grandiosity.
- ☐ Childhood learning disabilities or hyperactivity, underachievement.
- ☐ Insomnia; turning day into night.
- ☐ Less prone than histadelics to severe depression and blank mind.
- ☐ Obsessions, but not compulsions. (WALSH 2006)

Symptoms become more severe if metal metabolism is also disordered:

- ☐ Suspicions, delusions of persecution, paranoia. Mania.
- ☐ Severe dysperceptions of time, body, self, others.
- ☐ Thought disorder. Problems with abstractions. Racing thoughts, pressure of speech. Ideas of reference. Thought withdrawal or insertion.
- ☐ Withdrawal from reality. Auditory hallucinations, voices, evil spirits, psychosis, schizophrenia.

Creativity

Artistic or musical interest/creativity. (WALSH 2006)

Physical tendencies (COONEY 1999, WALSH 1997AB,2000AB, 02, 04AB, 06, 07, PFEIFFER 1972, 83, 87, 88, JAFFE 1992, HOFFER 1983, 87)

- ☐ Often very allergic or sensitive to foods. Can have severe chemical sensitivities. Walsh finds over 90% are sensitive to perfume, and a small percentage are especially sensitive to metals. (WALSH 2006)
- ☐ Slow metabolism. Easy fatigue or frustration. Sparse perspiration.
- ☐ High pain and shock threshold.
- ☐ Headaches, colds, and seasonal allergies are uncommon (due to minimal histamine response).
- ☐ Stuttering, ringing in the ears. Dry eyes.
- ☐ Poor dental health, due to the lack of secretions in the mouth.
- ☐ Difficulty reaching orgasm. Low libido.
- ☐ Prone to upper body pain (shoulder, upper back, head, neck).
- ☐ Tendency to tremors, restless leg syndrome, obsessional or hyperkinetic movement.
- ☐ Estrogen sensitivity. Tendency to postpartum and menopausal depression, and PMS.
- ☐ Prone to hypertension, cardiovacular disease, high homocysteine.

Appearance

- ☐ Young looking. Plentiful body hair.
- ☐ Often overweight.
- ☐ Teeth tend to be in poor shape.

Histapenic paranoia

"I imagined people were talking about me and my unpardonable sins. I... imagined one friend was actually trying to poison me... that the village had set up a special 'vigilante' group to hound me... [that] people were wearing different colored clothes according to a predetermined secret color code and that I was getting personal messages from the television and the radio. I was convinced that I was being followed by the plain clothes police when I was out driving, and obsessionally noted down car numbers to try to prove this.

Diane Walker, 1986

Influence of methylation on psychosis

Methylation is known to create hallucinatory substances, e.g., methylated catecholamines, and ergosterol. (SMYTHIES 1984) Overmethylation has long been noted in some schizophrenias,* (BRUEN 1962; BIDARD 1977, REYNOLDS 1984) and is the most common biotype (occuring in an estimated 50%). (PFEIFFER 1987, 88, WALSH 2006) And if methionine or SAMe, which increase methylation, is given to the already-overmethylated patient, it often triggers or aggravates psychosis, psychotic mania, or mania, especially if copper is also elevated. (WALSH 2006, 07, BRAVERMAN 1987)

Initial deterioration (Pfeiffer 1987, 88)

Especially when metal metabolism dysfunction and copper overload are involved, patients may get worse during early treatment. Pfeiffer advises caution to start, as substantial copper may be liberated from the muscles and liver, and trigger life-threatening symptoms, such as severe paranoia, making rapid elimination critical. Zinc shouldn't be used alone, but should be accompanied by other nutrients which foster elimination, (e.g., C, B3, manganese, molybdenum, etc., *as relevant*). Even so, over the first three months, blood copper may fail to reach acceptable levels. In the rare extreme case, penicillamine or other chelators may be required, temporarily, to speed elimination and moderate symptoms.

Drugs & meds (Pfeiffer 1987, 88)

Drinking, drug use, or eating may take on a binge pattern.

Due to slow metabolism, tolerance for many medications is low, and side effects, common.

Pfeiffer states that: Histapenics tend to do poorly on SSRI's. They may initially respond to benzodiazepines or antipsychotics, though benefits dwindle with time. In consideration of risks, he suggests antipsychotics only when unavoidable (e.g. when paranoia edges into violence, or when the histapenic cannot be treated or cared for any other way), and then, preferably, just one, and only at bedtime, with the dose minimal, and slowly tapered,* as nutritive healing takes effect.

See *Withdrawal*, p. 289.

*The mainstream protocol generally suggests *atypicals* for nonresponsive or psychotic mania, tapered after the episode ends. Many bipolars, however, wind up on chronic antipsychotics, perhaps due to a heightened tendency to rebound psychosis or mania following attempts to reduce intake.

Treatment (Hoffer 1983, 87, 2005, Pfeiffer 1972, 83, 87, 88, Walsh 1997ab, 2000ab, 02, 04ab, 06, 07, Jaffe 1992)

Treatment focuses on decreasing methylation, increasing histamine activity, supporting metal metabolism (if disordered), and counterbalancing dopamine and norepinephrine. Key nutrients include niacin, B6, B12, folic acid, B complex, C, zinc, selenium, manganese, omega 3. Average doses used by Pfeiffer or Jaffe/Kruesi are in brackets. Actual individual biochemical requirements vary.

- □ **Vitamin B3** — traps methyl molecules (which block histamine activation). Essential to cerebral circulation and metabolism, histamine production, and copper elimination. A strong antioxidant. Supports metallothionein function. Tranquilizing; usually the most critical nutrient in reducing voices and other psychotic symptoms. *May produce a flush* (see p. 60). [Typical dosage increases gradually to 500 to 1500 mg., as indicated, 2-3x/day. (Hoffer 1983, 87, Pfeiffer 87, 88, Jaffe 1992)]
- □ **Vitamin C** (preferably, buffered, time-release) — promotes copper excretion, protects brain tissue from oxidation. Antidepressant. Tranquilizing; counters mania and psychosis; useful with overstimulation or paranoia. [Up to 2-5 gm or more, distributed over the day. (Hoffer 1983, 87, Pfeiffer 1987, 88, Jaffe 1992)
- □ **Folic acid & B12**— low in many depressions, and some manias. (Hasanah 1997) Antidepressant for the overmethylated patient.* Counterbalances and traps methyl; (Walsh 2006) converts homocysteine to methionine. Important in forming BH4, which helps produce histamine. [Folic acid is typically suggested at 0.5 to 2.0 mg. Walsh (1995) uses up to 5 mg/day in certain severe histapenias. 1-2 mg. B12 is typical, sublingually or combined with intrinsic factor; if ineffective, injections may be required, perhaps weekly. (Hoffer 1983, 87, Pfeiffer 1987, 88, Jaffe 1992)]
- □ **Zinc** — with manganese, inhibits absorption and promotes bile excretion of copper, and facilitates normal histamine storage in blood basophils. Important in countering oxidative stess. Helps maintain GABA levels. Used in metabolizing homocysteine. [Dose is that which normalizes tissue levels and decreases copper overload. (Pfeiffer 87, 88, Jaffe 1992) Preferred forms: zinc picolinate or citrate.]
- □ **Manganese** — especially helpful to high-copper histapenia. Lowers dopamine. Suports MT function. Makes choline available to form acetylcholine. [Histapenics may need a ratio of 5:1, zinc to manganese. Dose is that which normalizes tissue levels and decreases copper overload. Preferred forms: manganese citrate, gluconate, or ascorbate. (Pfeiffer 1987, 88, Walsh 2008)]
- □ **Molybdenum**, with sulfur, is important in copper metabolism and can correct copper overload. (Walsh 2007) It is often especially indicated in cases of pronounced allergies or elevated urinary sulfite. [500 mcg, 2x/day. (Pfeiffer 87, 88)] *May be contraindicated for children.*
- □ **Vitamin B6** — helps form GABA, glutathione, CoQ10. Antioxidant. Supports B12 absorption and zinc metabolism. High doses, may decrease methyl availability by converting homocysteine to cysteine, and may reduce agitation and depression. [50-100 mg, or enough to induce recall of one dream per night, no more. (Pfeiffer 1975, 1987)]
- □ **DMAE** or **choline** — important in countering dopamine and norepinephrine, and reducing hyperactivity and stimulation. (Walsh 2000c) DMAE gets more effectively past the blood brain barrier, then converts to choline and acetylcholine in the brain.
- □ **Vitamin E, selenium, other antioxidants** — help protect against peroxidation due to elevated copper and metal metabolism dysfunction; may also reduce anxiety.
- □ **Omega 3** (EPA & DHA) — helps lower homocysteine, supports membrane and receptor function. (See *EFAs*, pp. 85-94.)

- ☐ **Pantothenic acid** (B5) — helps keep copper low. Supports adrenals and ability to handle stress.
- ☐ **B complex** — helps prevent deficits due to high doses of specific B vitamins. [50-100 mg of most components, (JAFFE 1992) up to 2-3 x/d.]
- ☐ **GABA** — tends to be low, and is highly effective in countering elevated norepinephrine. (WALSH 2007)
- ☐ **Valerian** — if needed, for anxiety and insomnia. (WALSH 2002B, 1997BC, 2007, PFEIFFER 1988)
- ☐ **Iron** — use only if deficient. (As ferrous citrate.) (JAFFE 1992)

Additional aminos, sometimes needed. Rule out drug interactions.

- ☐ **Isoleucine** — helps prevent B3 loss. While usually not needed, Hoffer found it rapidly clears symptoms in some acute B3-deficient patients, especially when leucine is excessive. (HOFFER 1983, PFEIFFER 87)
- ☐ **Carnitine** — mitochondrial antioxidant; may be indicated with low physical energy. (WALSH 2007)
- ☐ **Tryptophan** — though usually overloaded, and *not* indicated, it is sometimes needed due to malabsorption or dietary issues.
- ☐ **Taurine** — only if zinc is sufficient. (WALSH 2007)

Address any concurrent metal metabolism suppression (WALSH 2004AB, 06, 07)

Metal metabolism disorder aggravates histapenia. Typically, overloaded copper then increases norepinephrine and dopamine, worsening anxiety, agitation, paranoia, mania, psychosis, etc. Therapy generally includes:

- ☐ Zinc, a critical component, introduced over several weeks, often in 25 mg steps, up to a total, perhaps, of 75 mg/day.
- ☐ Manganese and often, molybdenum.
- ☐ B6 (and *P5P*) — support MT function.
- ☐ B3 & B5 — decrease copper.
- ☐ C — supports removal of certain metals.
- ☐ E, selenium, milk thistle, other antioxidants.
- ☐ Serine, *if depleted.*
- ☐ *If needed to reduce stimulation,* GABA, valerian, lecithin, glycine, or taurine, *as relevant.*
- ☐ NAC (and perhaps other amino components of MT) — introduced slowly and only after about three months of zinc, etc. NAC is *critical,* but can cause severe symptoms if given too soon. See *Copper* and *Metal metabolism,* pp. 170-73, for further details.

Pfeiffer found the nutritive approach sufficient for almost all patients. However, in extreme (and rare) cases (e.g., life-threatening paranoia), he sometimes recommended penicillamine, a copper-chelating agent. To decrease side effects, he emphasized minimal effective dose, perhaps only on alternate days, (JAFFE 1992) *while replenishing zinc, molybdenum (mainly for adults), manganese, etc.*

Avoid

Avoid methionine, SAMe, TMG, DMG, copper, perhaps inositol. These supplements will increase stimulation, and aggravate symptoms (e.g., anxiety, insomnia, irritability, mania, psychosis, or violence).

Diet (WALSH 2007, PFEIFFER 1987)

Focus on whole foods, organic (if possible). Abundant folic acid-rich vegetables are recommended. Omega 3 fish is helpful. The optimal balance of meat versus complex carbs, depends on individual reactions and biochemistry.* *Avoid fried and hydrogenated fat, allergens, sugar, alcohol, white flour and other refined carbohydrates.*

* On the one hand meat provides B3 and may increase B3 receptor sensitivity. (Miller 2008) It may also be helpful for any hypoglycemia (which is common, but in some patients better addressed with beans and other complex carbs). And it supplies B6, B12, L-carnitine, and some histidine (the histamine precursor). (Pfeiffer 1987) On the other hand, meat substantially increases methionine, which is detrimental to the overmethylated (histapenic) patient. Moreover, its histidine can worsen zinc deficiency, making histamine storage more difficult. (Walsh 2008)

Outcome (PFEIFFER 75, 87, 88, WALSH 2000B, 02AB, 04AB, 06)

Over the first three weeks or so, as copper is released into the bloodstream, some patients worsen, but by week four, improvement should be evident, and usually increases steadily over two to four months, (WALSH 2006) as over-methylation, metal metabolism dysfunction, high copper, folate deficiency, and other imbalances correct. Sweaty hands, racing thoughts, insomnia, and hypomania usually disappear within a month. Hallucinations continue longer. Obesity and paranoia take perhaps a year to resolve, assuming there are no confounding factors.

Histapenic catecholamines & copper

"Copper regulation is a big problem in catecholamine chemistry. You need enough glutathione, metallothionein, and selenium."

— William J Walsh, PhD, 2007

See *MT dysfunction, & Copper,* pp. 170-3.

Considerations

Lab (HOFFER 1983, 87, PFEIFFER 1972, 83, 87, 88, WALSH 1997AB, 2000AB, 02, 04AB, 2007, JAFFE 1992)

Whole blood histamine* — a crucial determination (but available in only a limited number of labs. Normal is 40-70ng/dL. To be accurate, other polyamines** must be excluded. *Antihistamines or antigens alter results and worsen symptoms.* (PFEIFFER, WALSH 2006)

Absolute basophil count — blood basophils and mast cells are the main storage sites for histamine outside the nervous system. Mast cells tend to be scarce in the skin of low histamine patients, and increase with therapy. (PFEIFFER 1972, 83, 87, 88) The basophil count confirms results of the blood histamine test. Normal is 30-50. (WALSH 2006)

Folic acid & B12 — may test low. Check red cell, serum or plasma folate, neutrophillic segmentation, methylmallonic acid.

Instead, SAH & methionine to test methylation status. (WALSH 2006) (SAH/SAMe would be ideal. (J AMES))

Hair & serum copper — usually elevated, suggesting MT dysfunction.

Serum zinc — may test low, but not necessarily.

Mercury — high levels may keep copper high, even with enough zinc. (CUTLER)

Other heavy metals — check for overload or sensitivity.

Fatty acid profile.

Food and environmental allergies.

Potassium & magnesium — may be low and accompanied by metabolic acidosis.

Homocysteine status — see following page.

Additional nutrient imbalances — may result from the depressed metabolism.

Thyroid, estrogen, and other hormone balances.

* Note: Clinical work with histapenia and histadelia is based on blood histamine, and has established a strong correlation between moderation of blood levels and improvement in symptoms. Blood levels do not necessarily correspond to levels in the brain. (Prell 1995)

** Spermidine (which gives indications concerning cancer, B6 deficiency, liver, skin and digestive tract conditions); and spermine (which is low in senility, recent memory disorders, and nutritional hypoglycemia, and high in patients recovered from psychotic breaks). (Pfeiffer)

Side effects, cautions

Avoid methionine, SAMe, TMG, DMG supplements — which increase methylation, trigger mania, and otherwise worsen symptoms. Low folic acid multiplies the risk. (WALSH 1997A, 2002)

Restrict copper exposure. Make sure supplements (e.g. multiples) contain little or no copper. Use bottled water, if appropriate; limit copper-rich foods (shellfish, chocolate, carob, etc.) and exposure to copper sulfate anti-algae agents (e.g., in some swimming pools, jacuzzis), etc. (PFEIFFER 1987, 88, WALSH 2004AB)

Inositol may overstimulate, worsening symptoms.

B3 (niacin, niacinamide) should be introduced gradually to avoid urinary suppression and elevated serum uric acid (symptoms can include nausea, vomiting, gout).

Niacin, may initially cause a flush. This can be limited by intake more than once per day, and with food (but not warm liquids). Non-flush niacin is available, but usually contains inositol. Niacinamide reduces flushing, but is more likely to produce liver toxicity at high doses; and may induce depression in some patients (reversible when intake is stopped).

Molybdenum depletes copper, reducing angiogensis (which may then suppress growth in children).

Manganese increases rigidity in Parkinson's, is not helpful with tics, and can increase blood pressure.

Iron shouldn't be used unless deficient.

Do not use cysteine, which can be excitotoxic. Take NAC instead, cautiously, and not before at least 3 months of nutrient therapy. Watch for signs of excess toxic metal release, excitotoxic effects, etc. Prescribe only to the extent needed.

Too much choline or DMAE may foster depression (though usually not in histapenics).

SSRI's, and St Johnswort often produce adverse reactions, (WALSH 2002B) (perhaps due to low folate (SAVA))

Too much dairy can deplete zinc (a zinc-dependent enzyme is required in metabolizing casein).

Hydrazine-containing dyes in processed foods decrease zinc, and should be avoided.

Dilantin,® an anti-epileptic drug, depletes folic acid, and can thereby worsen histapenia. An alternate anticonvulsive, may be preferable, if medically indicated. (PFEIFFER 1987, 88)

Reminder: This information is presented for educational purposes only. If you need treatment for histapenia, bipolar disorder, or any other medical condition, please seek the services of a knowledgeable physician

Homocysteinuria

Homocysteinuria is caused by problems in methyl metabolism, which allow homocysteine to accumulate, with renown cardiovascular complications. Though the severe genetic illness is rare (and usually evident in childhood), the milder form is more common, especially in males, post-menopausal females, and histapenics.*

* Other contributory factors include: hypothyroidism, malabsorption (particularly of B12 and folate, putting the elderly at risk), other dietary factors, pernicious anemia, GI disorders, alcoholism, chronic renal disorders, extended intake of certain anticonvulsants or immunosuppressants.

Role of oxidative stress

High homocysteine fosters profuse oxidative stress,* which compromises homocysteine metabolism further.**

* And which Walsh (2007) suggests may more directly harm heart function than the homocysteine itself.

** By decreasing the availability of glutathione which is needed to attach methyl to B12, a critical step in converting homocysteine to methionine.

Interaction with histapenia & mood

Walsh (2007) finds homocysteine elevation most likely in histapenia — despite overmethylation— but, largely due to histapenic lack of folate and B12.** Low B6 is also detrimental. And any metal metabolism dysfunction, common in histapenics, further worsens homocyteinuria by multiplying the oxidative stress.

The low folate and B12, the extreme oxidative stress, along with the effects of any MT dysfunction, damage brain lipids, myelin, cells, and circulation (Miller 1997) worsening mood. (Walsh 2007)

* Which are essential in the major pathway which converts homocysteine to methionine.

Mental & neurological effects*

Effects vary with degree of homocysteine elevation: (Morris 2002)

Depression (often drug-resistant) — which is pervasive. (Tiemeier 2002, Fava 1997, Papakostas 2004, Tolmunen 2004, Reynolds 1984)

Paranoia, psychosis, or other psychiatric conditions.

Neural tube defects, poor mental development, mental retardation, dementia. (Pfeiffer 88, Regland 1995, Reutens 2002, Duthie 2002)

Abnormal gait, sleep apnea, seizures.

Increased tendency to alcoholism.

Higher risk of Parkinson's, Alzheimer's, MS. (Reutens 2002)

Excitotoxicity, due to interaction with NMDA receptors. (Lipton 1997)

* Physical effects: elevated blood lipids, artery calcification, hypertension, and blood clots, leading to heart attacks, strokes, and brain and lung obstructions; abnormal glucose tolerance, elevated insulin, diabetes; damage to bones and joints, osteoporosis, rheumatoid athritis, scoliosis; gout, renal failure; detached or abnormal optic lens; placental abruption, spontaneous abortion. (Pfeiffer 1988, Miller 1997)

Effects on nutrients

Decreased coenzyme A; (Miller 1997) altered levels of glutathione, taurine, epinephrines, cysteine, glycine, other transmitters, melatonin, CoQ10, carnitine, phosphatidyl choline, polyamines. (Miller 1997, Bottiglieri 2000)

Lab (Cooney 1999)

Fasting plasma homocysteine; abbreviated methionine loading test for plasma homocysteine (assesses efficiency of homocysteine recycling); red cell, serum or plasma folate; blood SAM and methionine; DNA methylation.

General approach (Pfeiffer 1988, Walsh 2007)

Walsh suggests that for the histapenic with homocysteinuria, the focus should be on converting available homocysteine, rather than supplying additional methyl, which would worsen the histapenia, as well as, promoting further HCY buildup. Thus, methionine, SAM, and betaine supplements are contraindicated. Other nutrients supporting homocysteine metabolism are used instead, usually targeting the B12/folate pathway (see p. 157).

Nutrients (Walsh 2007, Pfeiffer 1988, Miller 1997, Narath 1995, Bottiglieri 2000, Ubbink 1993, Morris 2002, Tiemeier 2002, Fava 1997, Papakostas 2004, Duthie 2002)

Pfeiffer (1988) suggests that if defects are mild, nutrients may boost enzymes enough to reverse the condition.

- □ B12 and folic acid.
- □ Glutathione, E, and other antioxidants.
- □ Nutrients addressing any MT dysfunction (which otherwise increases oxidative stress).
- □ B6, zinc, serine, perhaps B2 (Bell 1992).
- □ Relevant EFAs.

For approaches for the histadelic, see *Excess homocysteine*, p. 157, #5.

Diet

EFA-rich fish, seeds, and nuts. Limit saturated, and avoid hydrogenated and trans fat. (Pfeiffer 1988)

Focus on complex carbohydrates, especially vegetables and fruit (grains and corn are less helpful); avoid refined carbohydrates, and high-glycemic-index foods. (Pfeiffer 1988)

Avoid coffee, (Nygard 1997) alcohol, (Cravo 1996, Hultberg 1993) tobacco, stimulants.

Comparison of Pyrrole Disorder, Histadelia, & Histapenia

Most of the characteristics below are tendencies, and not diagnostic. The presence of a number of such traits helps point to a particular biotype, but biotypes can be atypical, as various confounding factors can influence listed characteristics. An individual may also belong to more than one biotype. Other conditions (e.g., hypothyroid, Candida) may alter characteristics. This chart is an outline, and doesn't include all items in each category. (PFEIFFER 1987, JAFFE 1992, WALSH 1997, 2002, 04AB, 06, 07, SAHLEY 1995, ETC.)

Pyrrole disorder (Pyroluria) (18%)	Brain undermethylation/high folate (Histadelia) (35%)	Overmethylation/low folate (Histapenia) (25%)
Mood symptoms		
depression predominates	pervasive, severe depression	depression, despair
profound anxiety	compulsively suicidal	anxiety, prone to mania
mood swings, rapid cycling	often schizoaffective or bipolar	prone to schizophrenia
cyclic symptoms, labile emotions	may cycle with seasons	
Consciousness – typical symptoms		
teenage amnesia, no dream recall	blank mind	racing thoughts, thought disorder
better contact with reality, insight	delusions	hallucinations, psychosis
severe stress	phobias, obsessions, compulsions	paranoia, obsessions
Typical appearance		
thin wrists, ankles; midsection weight	lean build	tendency to obesity
pale nails or white spots on nails	elongated fingers, toes	stubby fingers
pale or "China doll" appearance	scant hair	plentiful hair
Physical tendencies		
fatigue, morning nausea	fast metabolism	slow metabolism
poor dental enamel	great teeth, bathed in saliva	dental carries, low salivary flow
impotent, delayed sexual development	easy prolonged orgasm	difficulty achieving orgasm
joint pain/malformation; spleen pain	headaches, sensitive to pain	upper body pain
allergies, difficulty w. proteins, toxins	seasonal & respiratory allergies	food and environmental allergies
prone to look-alike female offspring	tendency to male offspring	
sweet (acetone) breath & body odor		
Lab findings		
elevated pyrroles, low EGOT	elevated histamine & basophils	low blood histamine & basophils
	high folate, undermethylated	low folate, overmethylated
high or low serum & hair zinc	low copper	often MT dysfunction, high copper
low Ser, elevated DA	low DA, NE, Ser	elevated DA, NE, perhaps Ser
Typical supplements		
B6, C, B3, B5, biotin	B6, C, perhaps methyl B12, some B3	B3, NAD, B6, C, folate, B12, B5, B
magnesium, boron	calcium, magnesium	magnesium, molybdenum
zinc, manganese, selenium	zinc, selenium	zinc, manganese, selenium
GLA, antioxidants	omega 3, glutathione, antioxidants	omega 3, NAC, E, other antioxidants
often, tryptophan, 5HTP, glycine	SAMe, methionine, TMG, tryptophan	GABA
St John's wort, inositol or choline	inositol, St John's wort, kava	choline, valerian
Potentially harmful supplements for this biotype		
copper, especially at the outset	folic acid, omega 6, Mn	methionine, SAM, PA, TMG, DMG, omega 6
omega 3 is not always helpful	DMAE, perhaps, choline	copper, perhaps, 5HTP or inositol

III: Neurotoxins

"Neurotoxic substances can cause a variety of adverse health effects, ranging from impairment of muscular movement to disruption of vision and hearing, to memory loss and hallucinations."

U.S. Office of Technology Assessment, 1990

Neurotoxins* often contribute to mood symptoms; critically, in some cases. Neurotoxicity can also be important in anxiety and behavior disorders, psychosis, retardation, dementia, etc. Neurotoxic effects on the brain include:

- □ Distorted message transmission. Changes in crucial neurotransmitter balances, synthesis or secretion; or in electrical balances along the axon. (Atchison 1988)
- □ Disruption of brain biochemical activity, causing neural inflammation, acidity, or destruction.
- □ Compromised cerebral circulation, damage to glial cells, and general obstruction of brain access to oxygen, energy, and nutrients. (Nutritional imbalances then go on to increase susceptibility to neurotoxins.)

Aside from metal overload, potentially mood-disturbing neurotoxins include: caffeine, tobacco, certain alkaloids, pesticides, solvents, and such other chemicals.

Reminder: The material in this book is presented for educational purposes only. It should not be used in place of medical diagnosis and treatment. Treatment descriptions are merely sketched in. If you need treatment for toxic exposures, mood disorder, or any other medical condition, you should consult a knowledgeable physician.

* For the purposes of this text, we expand the term, *neurotoxin,* to refer not only to the classic toxins (e.g., solvents, pesticides, certain metals, etc.), but also, other substances toxic to neural function or viability, as listed at right.

Metals

See also:
Vanadium, p. 134.

Other toxins

See also:
Sugar imbalances, pp. 214-22
Free radicals, p. 73

1. Metal toxicity

Even minerals essential to health can be damaging, if overloaded. Vanadium is critical to sugar metabolism, but significant intake often worsens bipolar depression. Copper supports catecholamine formation, counters certain anemias, and is crucial to blood vessel, joint and bone integrity, but cumulative excess often plays a major role in anxiety, psychosis, and mood symptoms. And electrolytes (potassium, sodium, magnesium, calcium) are crucial to neurological messaging, but significant imbalances challenge mood stability.

Heavy metals, such as lead and mercury, are toxic at any level, and can impair fetal brain development, stunt intelligence, and create behavior and learning problems in children, psychiatric syndromes in adults. Lead toxicity, for instance, can be mistaken for mental retardation, and causes learning difficulties and behavior disorder. Mercury can create profound depression, dementia, or psychosis.

Metal metabolism dysfunction in bipolars

"Metals compete for participation in chemical reactions. Which one is used depends on local concentration and relative position in the chemical activity series. Too much of one metal can displace others."

— William J Walsh, PhD, 2004

MT support vs. chelation

Walsh suggests the preponderance of cases of metal toxicity in bipolars can be reversed by glutathione and nutrients which support MT function, while chelation is useful mainly for short-term relief with severe exposure (less than 1% of cases), in conjunction with ongoing MT therapy. Once severe issues are addressed, he finds ongoing problems usually respond to MT support and other nutrients which promote elimination and protect tissue, along with measures which limit future exposure. He states that IV chelation removes zinc (which is critical to handling metals), and has toxic effects; and the typical protocol involves numerous chelations, since response generally lasts only a few weeks, *as chelation does not correct what for most patients is the primary problem: difficulty processing metals.* (WALSH 2004, 06, 07, 08)

Cutler, on the other hand, finds *high mercury* underlies many mineral transport disorders (see pp. 174-83), so often is the focus of therapy. He generally finds most people with enough mercury toxicity to contribute to severe psychiatric symptoms need chelation, since mercury does not leave the brain on its own. He emphasizes *oral* chelation (DMPS or DMSA, later adding alpha lipoic acid).* (CUTLER 1999, 2004)

See Cutler 2004 for other heavy metals protocols.

* And finds IV chelation indicated mainly for people not expected to regain consciousness soon, or whose entire GI tract has been removed.

High copper relative to zinc is a relatively good marker for metal metabolism dysfunction. While Walsh's work shows only a small number of depressives with this imbalance, it pervades bipolars who lean toward mania, and is common in histapenics and pyrolurics, creating marked sensitivity to toxic metals, profuse oxidative stress, (WALSH 2004AB, 08) and cumulative neural dysregulation and destruction. (SCHEUHAMMER 1985, STOHS 1995)

Metallothioneins (MTs) (WALSH 2002, 04AB, 2006, 2007)

The liver and kidneys form small proteins, called metallothioneins (MTs), which bind to, transport, regulate, and eliminate divalent metals. They modify harmful (ionic or elemental) forms of such metals and use them to support health, and they remove toxic or overloaded metals. And they bolster blood, brain, and intestinal toxic metal barriers. Thus, use of zinc, manganese, and copper is facilitated and excess removed; and lead, mercury, cadmium, etc., are eliminated.

MTs are also important in the development of brain cells and neural connections over the first three years of life. And they support immune function, counter oxidative stress, regulate intestinal bacteria, help destroy Candida, and reduce food sensitivities, all of which can influence mood.

Conditions associated with MT dysfunction (WALSH 2004AB, 06)

- ☐ Often, a major role in manic-dominant bipolar disorder, hormonal depressions, schizophrenia (especially histapenias), autism (especially post vaccine or post thalidomide).
- ☐ Certain learning and behavior disorders, hyperactivity, memory loss.
- ☐ Pronounced oxidative stress.
- ☐ Nutrient and enzyme imbalances. Hypersensitivity to toxic metals.
- ☐ Multiple food sensitivites. Dairy and gluten intolerance.* Candida overgrowth. Leaky gut. Low stomach acid. Other GI symptoms.*
- ☐ Chemical sensitivity (perhaps severe, especially in histapenics.)
- ☐ Immune dysfunction.

* Zinc depletion (due to MT dysfunction) tends to compromise the zinc-dependent gut enzyme (DDP-IV) which breaks down casein and gluten, creating sensitivities to wheat and dairy. Moreover, oxidative stress caused by elevated copper, iron, etc., can destroy such enzymes, and also interfere with absorption and digestion, promoting sensitivities, diarrhea, digestive cramps, and other GI symptoms. (WALSH 2006)

Contributory factors. The role of biotypes. (WALSH 2007)

Dysfunction seems to be genetic, though exacerbated by lack of required nutrients, and by toxic exposures. Metallothioneins tend to be subfunctional in histapenics, increasing copper and, thus, norepinephrine; overactive in histadelics, lowering copper.

Considerations (MT underactivity) (WALSH 2002, 04AB, 08, PFEIFFER 1987)

Lab

Elevated serum copper. Copper/zinc ratio over 1.2.
Under 85-90% serum copper bound to ceruloplasmin.
Plasma zinc and manganese depletion.
Elevated hair mercury, cadmium, lead, antimony, etc.
Possible deficiency of B6, cysteine, or serine.
Increased, perhaps severe, reactivity to elevated metals.
Typically, high norepineprhine.
Chemical sensitivities (especially in histapenics).
Milk/wheat hypersensitivity/intolerance. Candida.
History of metal exposure.

Therapy

Walsh (2004ab) suggests a gradual increase in relevant supplements over 4 weeks, with particular caution the first 10 days, to avoid sudden toxic metal dumping, worsening symptoms, and kidney damage. Even so, symptoms may slightly deteriorate at first, but then improve steadily over 2-3 months. Gluten/casein sensitivity may also respond.

- ☐ Zinc (picolinate or gluconate) — stimulates MT and counters oxidative stress. [Walsh (2004ab) suggests: Start with 25 mg in the evening; increase gradually to 2x, then 3x/day, etc, *as relevant*).]
- ☐ B6 — supports MT function.
- ☐ C — supports removal of certain metals; antioxidant.
- ☐ Selenium, E — antioxidant, required in MT function.
- ☐ Glutathione — antioxidant and liver nutrient. Key MT component. Enhances MT and zinc effectiveness. Critical to mercury and fat-soluble heavy metal elimination. With MT, helps gut and blood brain barrier restrict uptake.
- ☐ Additional antioxidants to limit oxidative stress.
- ☐ Manganese (*but not with histadelia*), molybdenum (*especially with high copper*) — also stimulate MT.
- ☐ Serine — an MT component. *Useful if depleted.*
- ☐ Limit exposure to implicated metals.
- ☐ NAC* — Walsh (2000) suggests postponing, til after at least 3 mo. of zinc, B6, C, etc., and til adverse metals have diminished, then slowly introducing small doses.**
- ☐ Full MT constituents**— all 14 component aminos, in the correct ratio, plus zinc, GSH, selenium, E, etc. *Instead of NAC alone, but with the same restrictions as above.* (WALSH 2008)

Removal of some metals from bones or brain may be slow, requiring extended therapy, perhaps including additional support for binding and elimination, and densensitizing the body.

* Cysteine is a major component and potent stimulator of MT, but can be excitotoxic, so is best taken as NAC.

** Too much, too soon, can release a flood of toxic metals into the blood, exacerbating symptoms, promoting sensitivity, and making elimination more difficult (and fostering tinnitus and hypertension).

Caution (BIOCHEMICAL-BEHAVIOR.COM/NEWINFORMATION, WALSH 2007, 08)

Only treat if indicated. Excess MTs (as in many histadelias) deplete copper and require a different set of therapies.

Copper overload

Copper & mania

The most common manifestation of metal metabolism dysfunction is high copper and low zinc. This decreases histamine, and allows norepinephine and dopamine to accumulate. The elevated copper and catecholamines, along with the low zinc and histamine, magnify neural excitation, destabilizing mood. Pfeiffer and Goldstein (1984) found equivalent doses of copper could stimulate the brain to the same extent as dexedrine, an amphetamine, known for inducing mania or psychosis in some.*

Dr. Walsh reports that over 90% of 1800 bipolars show below-median zinc, with 30% clinically deficient (below 70 mcg/dL). And where mania is predominant, most show either high serum copper (and low ceruloplasmin), suggesting MT dysfunction, or pyrrole disorder (which depletes zinc relative to copper).

An elevated copper to zinc ratio is also commonly associated with grandiosity, psychosis, hyperactivity, insomnia, and other manic symptoms, (PFEIFFER 1988) as well as schizophrenia, autism, ADHD, fear, paranoia, anxiety, learning difficulties, stuttering, restlessness, behavior dyscontrol,* and episodic violence.** (WALSH 2004AB)

High copper/ low zinc is prevalent in histapenia and pyroluria.

* As evidenced by characteristic flattened brain waves on 5 mg doses of either.

* In many males with low zinc to copper, intellectual ability and behavior control improve at about age 20, when growing stops and zinc is no longer used so rapidly. (Walsh 2004ab)

** Walsh (2004ab) identifies type A violent behavior by episodic outbursts, followed by remorse, and tied to high copper to zinc and to sodium ratios, high lead, and histamine imbalance. (p. 266)

Factors promoting high copper to zinc (WALSH 2004AB)

MT dysfunction — primary in most cases of copper accumulation. (WALSH 2004AB, 06)
Pyrrole disorder — severely depletes zinc.
Histapenia — the low histamine allows copper to accumulate.
Blood type A or AB — associated with a tendency to sequester copper. (PFEIFFER 1975, 87)
Insufficient bile — promotes copper and mercury accumulation. (CUTLER 1999, 2004, 07)
Wilson's disease (*See box, next page*)
Elevated estrogen in females raises copper (e.g., with puberty, pregnancy, hormone treatments).
Puberty or growth — depletes zinc.

Such factors are exacerbated by:
Overexposure to copper, or mercury.
Poor diet or malabsorption of counterbalancing nutrients, e.g., of B3 (depleted in histapenia, anxiety), C (in scurvy, severe mental illness), zinc (in pyroluria, histamine imbalances).
Emotional stress.

Means by which copper may destabilize mood (WALSH 2004AB)

Elevates catecholamines,* increasing stimulation, facilitating mania or psychosis.

Increases the electrical potential of the neuron (perhaps enhancing sodium activity), increasing stimulation. (FRERREIRA 1970, PFEIFFER, 1987)

Increases electron transport (energy production).

Decreases histamine,** furthering copper accumulation, in a vicious cycle. (PFEIFFER 1980, SOHLER 1980)

Concentated in the hippocampus, a region critical to mood, behavior and memory.

High levels can create profuse oxidative stress, compromising neural viability and function.

Can deplete zinc, B3, C, and other mood modulating nutrients. Can distort glycolysis, reducing brain access to fuel and energy. (PFEIFFER 1988)

May promote depression via MAO. (See p. 110.)

The zinc/copper balance may influence brain laterality (see p. 283), (PFEIFFER) thereby altering mood. (GEORGE 1993, DREVETS 1992, GUR 1995, ROBINSON 1988, 89, STARKSTEIN 1988, 89, 90, MIGLIORELLI 1993)

* *Dopa b-hydroxylase* and *dopa decarboxylase*, copper dependent enzymes, metabolize tyrosine to dopamine and norepinephrine.

** The copper-containing enzymes, *histaminase* and *ceruloplasmin*, regulate histamine. Copper also activates *diamine oxidase*, which lowers histamine.

Copper overload in depressed & postpartum women

Depression, copper, estrogen — Of depressions resulting from copper overload, Walsh reports 93% occur in females, 7%, in males, suggesting a tie to female hormones. In fact, increased estrogen (which doubles in pregnancy, or with estrogen-dominant birth control or menopause meds) elevates copper, and has been associated with mood changes, especially in bipolars. (WALSH 2006, 07) Thus, Crayton (2007) finds significantly elevated serum copper in postpartum depression as compared to other depressions and controls.

Postpartum mood — Postparum depression is ubiquitous in affectives, much more likely than in the general postpartum population,* and more severe. And the risk of mania to bipolars may be over 50%.**(BRIGHAM 2001) Pfeiffer (87, 88) notes that copper is elevated just post-birth due to the high estrogen*** (more than double nonpregnant levels), and readily triggers/ worsens histapenic or pyroluric symptoms in vulnerable persons.

* Whose rate (2-8%) is already high, even higher in women aged 22-28 within two weeks after a first birth, particularly if the baby is male.

*** Though, in the next few months, copper should slowly decline, improving symptoms.

*** And ceruloplasmin, a major copper-containing enzyme.

Biotypes & copper (PFEIFFER 1987, 88, SOHLER 1980)

Histapenia — increases anxiety and promotes psychosis.

Histadelia — may be low. Moderate doses are in some cases helpful, *but not if subject to significant oxidative stress.*

Pyroluria — aggravates imbalance with zinc, worsening symptoms (though small doses are sometimes needed after extensive zinc).

B3 & C inverse to copper (PFEIFFER 1987, 88)

B3 deficiency (as in pellagra) increases copper, while high copper decreases B3. (KRISHNACHAVI) Similarly, low dietary vitamin C increases copper, high copper destroys C. (HITIER 1976)

Walsh/Pfeiffer approach (PFEIFFER 1983, 87, 88, WALSH 2000, 02, 04AB, 08, NICHOLSON 1966)

Generally: (1) Raise zinc; (2) Restict copper intake; (3) Support metal metabolism; (4) other therapies which eliminate tissue copper. In the first month, nutrient doses are increased *gradually*, to avoid sudden dumping of metals, (which can worsen symptoms and damage the kidneys).

□ **Zinc** — counterbalances copper, reduces absorption; stimulates MT. [If copper is very high, the dose may need to go up, in 25 mg increments, to 100 mg or more. Monitor response. (PFEIFFER 1987, 88, WALSH 2008)]

□ **Molybdenum** — like zinc, counterbalances copper and helps correct copper overload. Supports excretion.

□ **B6, P5P** — Support MT function and copper elimination. Before introducing zinc, a couple of days of B6 may help avert depression and gastrointestinal side effects.

□ **B3, C** — antioxidant; support copper elimination.

□ **B5** — helps lower Cu and support adrenals, reducing stress.

□ **Glutathione, E, selenium, & other antioxidants**, — counter oxidative stress and support MT function. GSH is critical, but only so much can be used til MT takes over. (WALSH 2008)

□ **Manganese** — supports MT function; lowers dopamine.

□ **Folate** (*if not histadelic),* **B12** — reduce anxiety, depression.

□ **GABA, magnesium** — *if needed* to counter norepinephrine.

□ **Restrict sources of copper.**

□ **NAC** or full **MT constitutents** (NAC, serine, etc.) — after about three months, once zinc is built up.

OUTCOME: *Though at first, blood copper may increase, perhaps creating mild deterioration*, levels soon diminish, and improvement typically emerges by week 3, increasing steadily, perhaps strikingly, over several months. (WALSH 2000) (See also, *Therapy,* p. 171.)

Wilson's disease (KRAUTHAMMER 1978, AKIL 1991, BREWER 1995, GOLD 1987)

Wilson's disease is a genetic copper metabolism disorder. Impaired copper excretion leads to toxic accumulations in the liver, brain, and other organs. A gold/brown or gray/green ring forms around the cornea. Nerve cells are destroyed, with neurological symptoms by about age 21. These include difficulty speaking and coordinating fine motor movement; tremor, rigidity, odd gait, and dystonias. Psychiatric symptoms occur in approximately 75%, often before other symptoms. Affective syndromes are common, with depression in 20-30% or more. Other symptoms include mania, anxiety, hyperactivity, hysteria, cognitive impairment, irritability, aggression, psychosis, personality changes, dementia. May be reversible if treated at onset. Otherwise, serious disorders of the eye, kidney, liver, immune or nervous system develop and can be fatal.

Cutler's approach (CUTLER 1999, 2004)

Cutler similarly suggests: (1) Zinc, molybdenum; (2) Restrict copper; (3) Various supportive nutrients (magnesium, B complex, B12/folate, EFAs, antioxidants, and other vitamins and minerals. See, *Cutler's supportive nutrients*, p. 178.). His suggestions involve *less complete intake of MT constituents*, but do include: (4) Liver support (milk thistle extract, lecithin, glycine, taurine) — *Note: The liver is a major site of MT production.* Good improvement is typical by 3-4 months.

NOTE: The differences in approach may, in part, reflect different targets: Walsh works with a relatively wide range of psychiatric disorders, often entailing profound nutrient needs; Cutler, with metal toxicity in the general population, along with a focus on autistic children; i.e., people whose liver may respond more readily.

Penicillamine issues

With severe symptoms (e.g., life-threatening paranoia), Pfeiffer occasionally used small doses to rapidly reduce high copper. (PFEIFFER 1987) *Too much penicillamine, or inadequate support, can drastically impact symptoms.* (CUTLER 2007)

Antidepressant effects

Walsh (2004) finds hypercupremic depressives often deteriorate on antidepressants.

Considerations: Excess copper

Potential effects (PFEIFFER 1972, 74, 75, 87, 88, WALSH 2000, 04AB)

Memory and attention difficulties. Hyperactivity.
Restlessness, insomnia. Hypomania, mania.
Grandiosity. Fears, paranoia, psychosis.
Behavior dyscontrol, episodic violence
Depression, fatigue.
In females, estrogen intolerance, postpartum psychosis, mood symptoms during hormonal events.
Oxidative stress, and consequent neurological damage.
Worsens histapenia and pyrrole disorder.
Headache, vertigo, fatigue. Tremor, stuttering. Tinnitus.
Symptoms of decreased C, B3, zinc, and histamine.
Nausea, diarrhea, abdominal pain.
If MT is disordered, skin and other sensitivity reactions to cumulative toxic metals.
With chronic overload, eye, kidney, liver, immune or nervous system disorders. Extreme excess can be fatal.

Populations (WALSH 2004AB)

High levels are relatively uncommon in the general population, but found in many mania-dominant bipolars, mood-disordered high-estrogen women, schizophrenics, pyrolurics, histapenics, people with blood types A and AB, autistics, and in senility. Underlies Wilson's disease.

Can be aggravated by poor diet, malabsorption, emotional or physical stress, zinc depletion (e.g. pubertal growth spurts), overexposure to copper or heavy metals.

Counterbalancing nutrients

C, B3, zinc, histamine. Metallothionein support.

Common sources of copper (WALSH 2004AB)

Contamination is widespread. Sources:

Most multiples contain 2 mg copper, or more. Multis with minimal to no copper are available, and may be acceptible for some, if not otherwise contraindicated.

Tobacco, herbicides, pesticides, IUDs, jewelry, cookware, dental fillings.

Some anti-algae agents in jacuzzis or pools.

Soft water (e.g., in the US East coast and the Northwest), leaches copper from copper plumbing. (Hard water lines pipes with minerals, offering some protection.)

Benefits (GARRISON 1985, BALCH 1990, PAGE 1993, LIEBERMAN 1990, KROHN 1991)

Pfeiffer warned that most persons with mental health issues tend to be overloaded in copper and need to limit intake. (PFEIFFER 1987, 88)

Nonetheless, copper is an essential trace element, and not always detrimental, e.g., supplements may be indicated to elevate catecholeamines and counter depression, as in some cases of histadelia.* (See p. 137.)

* Though enhancing methylation is more directly effective. (Walsh 2008)

Mining, welding, brazing, metal-joining.

Food dyes with hydrazine, which depletes zinc.

Elevated estrogen (e.g., with puberty, pregnancy, PMS, perimenopause, environmental exposure, many birth control and menopause meds).

If after concerted therapy, and limiting the above sources, dietary changes are still needed, start with sugars (blackstrap molasses, dry fruit, oranges, and chocolate) and copper-enriched foods. (See *Food sources*, p. 137.) Restriction of copper-rich proteins, vegetables and herbs is usually unnecessary, but if indicated, *should be weighed against need for specific health benefits they convey.*

Lipoic acid mildly increases both copper and zinc (p. 178)

Lab (WALSH 2004AB, 06, 07) (Also see *MT, Lab*, p. 171)

The copper/zinc balance is a critical consideration.

Plasma Cu/Zn. Over 1.2 suggests excess unbound copper.

Elevated serum copper.*

Under 85-90% serum copper bound to ceruloplasmin (suggesting MT underactivity and oxidative stress).

Elevated norepinephrine or NE/dopamine ratio.

Hair copper — often reflects tissue burden. *Elevated readings, however, can be due to hair dye or other environmental factors not removed by washing.*

Toxic metals in hair — suggest MT dysfunction.

Low B3, C, zinc, or selenium — can elevate copper.

Mercury overload — can alter the copper/zinc ratio, and increase reactivity to copper. (CUTLER 2007)

History of exposure.

* Though deceptively low serum and ceruloplasmin may be due to Wilson's disease, where copper is extremely elevated, but mainly unbound.

Mercury (Hg)

Mad hatters, etc. (GOLD 1987)

In the nineteenth century, felt hat makers, who dipped furs into mercury vats, often developed tremors, incoherent speech, loose teeth and mental disabilities. Many spent the rest of their lives in insane asylums. Mirror makers and goldsmiths also worked with mercury, and were similarly afflicted.

Dentists

Dentists or dental personnel who use mercury experience chronic exposure. As compared to other occupations, they have been reported to have the highest suicide rate (US), and twice the brain tumors (Singapore). Also, a divorce and heart attack rate 50% above average; and 3.5-times average sterility, stillbirths, and miscarriage. (WOODRUFF 1995, KUPSINEL 1984)

Minimata Bay disease

In 1953, in Minimata Bay, Japan, mercury contamination produced a multiple sclerosis-like illness, "Minimata Bay disease," in a large portion of the population. A plastic-producing plant had dumped mercury waste into the bay. Many who ate local fish stumbled around, had difficulty speaking, and sustained neurological damage. Babies were born deformed and retarded. Hundreds of people were permanently disabled.

Mercury exposure (HUGGINS 1982, PFEIFFER 1972, MUIR, 1997, GOLD 1987, CUTLER 1999, 2004, WEINER 1996. APPLEGARTH 1976, LOB 1975)

Mercury may be present in food and water contaminated with industrial wastes, fungicides, or pesticides. Other important sources include silver amalgam dental fillings, thimersol in vaccines and some allergy injections, and certain antiseptics (e.g., merthiolate or mercurochrome (which is 1% readily absorbable mercury)). It is also present in certain paints, wood preservatives, floor waxes, douches, skin creams, diuretics, fabric softeners, talc, laxatives (e.g., calomel), fluorescent lights, and thermometers.

Mercury toxicity produces affective symptoms, and can contribute, as well, to cerebral allergies, Candida, thyroid imbalance, pancreatic dysfunction, and other biological conditions that often play a role in bipolar disorder.

Potential mental effects (CUTLER 1999, 2004, 07, STOCK 1983, JAENSCH 1926, HUGGINS 1982, 93, FASCIANA 1986, GOLD 1987, PFEIFFER 1972, 88, J ORTHOMOL PSYCHIAT 1975, 82, TAYLOR 1988, MARLOWE 1986, ZIFF 1984, 87, 97)

- □ Profound depression. (GOLD 1987) Mood changes.* Manic depression.
- □ Agitation, tension, intense anxiety, panic, painful inner unrest.
- □ Low stress tolerance, lack of self-control, severe irritability, fits of anger, emotional instability. Difficulty getting along with people.
- □ Disturbed sleep, insomnia.
- □ Shyness, reduced self-confidence, fear of strangers, self-consciousness. Social withdrawal.
- □ May contribute to autism. (CUTLER 1999, 2004, BERNARD 2000, HALSEY 1999)
- □ In some cases, dysperceptions. Hearing thoughts or voices, taste distortion, hallucinations, psychosis.
- □ Drowsiness, fatigue. Lack of energy and ability to do work, especially intellectual work.
- □ Difficulty thinking, or reading. Confusion, brain fog, memory loss, intellectual impairment, attention deficit and other learning disabilities. Cognitive deterioration may eventually evolve into permanent dementia. May play a role in Alzheimer's. (GODFREY 2000, CASDORPH 1995)

A rapidly changing progression of mental symptoms may occur, as if the patient is pretending.

Potential neurological effects (STOCK 1983, JAENSCH 1926, HUGGINS 1982, 93, PFEIFFER 1972, 88, J ORTHOMOL PSYCHIAT 1975, FASCIANA 1986, TAYLOR 1988, MARLOWE 1986, ZIFF 1984, 87, 97)

- □ Damage to the blood brain barrier. (STEINWALL 1977)
- □ Interference in the metabolism of nerve endings, especially acetylcholine metabolism.
- □ Tingling toes, lips and nose. Tremors or numbness of hands, face and limbs. Twitching, spasms, seizures.
- □ Reduced muscle coordination and reflexes. Difficulty writing or walking. In some severe cases, partial paralysis. (CUTLER 2004)
- □ Dizziness, headaches, pressure in the head. Neuralgia.
- □ Narrowed field of vision, double vision, dimming of vision. Large pupils and light sensitivity. Trouble seeing close up, or focusing at all distances. (CUTLER 1999, 2004)
- □ Ringing in the ears, earaches. Impaired speech. Suppressed hearing and sense of smell; altered sense of taste and smell.

Physical symptoms (STOCK 1983, JAENSCH 1926, HUGGINS 1982, 93, J ORTHOMOL PSYCHIAT 1975, FASCIANA 1986, PFEIFFER 1988, TAYLOR 1988, WOODRUFF 1995, SILVERUD 1990, ZAMM 1990, PLEVA 1983, KUPSINEL 1984, ZIFF 1984, 87, 97, SALONEN 1995, GOLD 1987, CUTLER 1999, 2004)

- □ Food and chemical allergies and sensitivities. Impaired gluten and gliadin digestion.
- □ Candida, which may fail to respond unless mercury is removed from the brain. (CUTLER 1999, 2004)
- □ Craving for sweets. Blood sugar disorders.
- □ Low body temperature.
- □ Low levels of thyroid and other hormones, with attendant symptoms, or false normal labs.*
- □ Increased urination and sweating. Night sweats.

- □ Recurrent infections. Respiratory swelling, irritation, difficulty breathing. Throat inflammation, persistent cough.
- □ Dry mouth, metallic taste, bad breath, excess salivation. Swollen, receding, bleeding gums.
- □ Diarrhea, cramps, heartburn, appetite loss, anorexia, nausea, constipation, ulcers.
- □ Dermatitis, skin lesions, edema. Tissue pigmentation issues.
- □ Slowed movement, fatigue, exhaustion. Chronic fatigue.
- □ Joint pain, cramps, arthritis, fibromyalgia. Physical deterioration.
- □ Rapid heartbeat, hypertension, chest pain. Interferes with heart contractibility. May promote atherosclerosis, blood clots, heart attacks. (FLEISCHER, BOLGER 2002)
- □ Mucocutaneous lymph node syndrome (swollen glands, joint pain, fever, lethargy, sore throat, anorexia, irritability, sensitivity to light, elevated white blood cells and IgE, heart conditions). (KUPSINEL 1984)
- □ Growth irregularities, birth defects.**
- □ Tendency to anemia, colitis, infertility, menstrual disorders, lupus, asthma, immune dysfunction, (WOODRUFF 1995) MS, leukemia, other cancers. (KUPSINEL 1984, BIESEL)
- □ Symptoms may mimic various natural diseases.

* Cutler (1999, 2004) points out that mercury concentrates in the hypothalamus and pituitary, suppressing formation of stimulating and releasing factors. Many endocrine tests then give false normal readings.

** Mercury inactivates the mitotic spindle (which mediates cell reproduction), causing chromosomal damage. (Silverud 1990)

Vulnerability

Although mercury is universally toxic, some people are less able to eliminate it (particularly with concurrent metal metabolism dyfunction, low thyroid, or immune weakness); or are hypersensitive (e.g., those with nervous system fragility, Candida, allergies or environmental illness). Maternal exposure puts the fetus at risk (infants take in two to threefold more mercury than the mother). The elderly are also highly susceptible. Exposure and, often, reactivity may be increased by overuse of alcohol, tobacco, various drugs; gum chewing; (MUIR, 1997) salivary acidity; bacterial overgrowth in the mouth; and electrical charge due to the interaction of diverse metal fillings. (CUTLER 1999, 2004)

Treatment

Treatment choices must be tailored to individual biochemical requirements. Check nutrient and biotype considerations.

Support metal metabolism

Optimization of MT activity reduces the toxic load, helps prevent further accumulation, and improves symptoms. (See pp. 170-71.)

Dental treatment (HUGGINS 1982, 93, FASCIANA 1986, PFEIFFER 1988, TAYLOR 1988, KUPSINEL 1984, ELY 1994, ZAMM 1990, PAGE 1992, LARSON 1992)

Amalgam removal issues (ELY 1994, FASCIANA 1986, TAYLOR 1988, KUPSINEL 1984)

In many cases, attempts at correction cannot remove enough of the brain and body burden, unless all sources of exposure, including amalgams, are eliminated. (PFEIFFER 1988, HANSON) Thus, if serious symptoms cannot be sufficiently redressed with nutritive support, amalgam removal may be indicated. Otherwise, vulnerability increases with cumulative exposure, especially in persons with numerous fillings, and may eventually cause considerable damage to the brain and other soft tissue.

Dental fillings (STOCK 1983, JAENSCH 1926, HUGGINS 1982, FASCIANA 1986, TAYLOR 1988, WOODRUFF 1995, PLEVA 1983, KUPSINEL 1984, SVARE 1981, EGGLESTON 1984)

Early amalgam fillings contained copper and cadmium. Most now consist of approximately 50% mercury, 35% silver, and up to 3% copper, 13% tin, and 1% zinc.

Dentists are generally taught that mercury stays locked in the fillings. Cumulative mercury loss in old amalgams, however, averages 30-40%. (KUPSINEL 1984) And University of Calgary researchers report 10% of amalgam mercury eventually accumulates in body organs. (WOODRUFF 1995)

Mercury is continually released from amalgam fillings, more rapidly with certain activities. Svare (1981) found the mercury in respired air after eating increased about fifteen-fold, and proportionally to the number of mercury fillings. Gum chewing creates a lengthy exposure. Tooth-brushing also increases mercury release, (PATTERSON 1985) as do hot drinks.

Inhaled mercury can travel through the nasal cavity directly to the brain. Schiele and Eggleston (1984) claim brain mercury correlates with number of amalgams.

In acknowledgment of the danger, Degussa, previously one of the largest European manufacturers of mercury amalgams, stopped producing them. The government of Sweden has instituted a complete ban on mercury amalgams and apologized for any harm they might have caused. Amalgams are also prohibited in Germany.

Mercury hypersensitivity & amalgams

Several studies find up to a 16% rate of hypersensitivity to mercury among individuals with amalgam fillings. (DJERASSI 1969, N. AM. CONTACT DERM GP 1973, NEBENFUHRER 1984) Hypersensitivity is most common in individuals who have the greatest number of fillings. Miller (1985) reports a 44% rate in persons with 10 or more amalgams. The age of fillings also plays a role.

Removing amalgams: Risks to bipolars

"Bipolars are unusually sensitive to mercury, but sudden removal can be awful, producing mental breakdowns in maybe one in fifty."

William J Walsh, PhD, 2008

Difficulty removing brain mercury (HANSON, ZIFF 1984, 87, 97, CUTLER 1999, 04, 07)

Organic mercury (found in certain vaccines, fungicides, contaminated food, etc.) and mercury vapor (from chewing, removing amalgams, broken fluorescent lights, etc.) penetrates readily into the brain. There, it gradually converts to inorganic mercury, which does not easily pass back through the blood brain barrier. Mercury can thus stay in the brain for decades, or lifelong, unless effectively treated. Over time, brain damage becomes more difficult to reverse.

Mercury sources

Bottom feeders (shrimp, lobster and other shellfish; catfish) and large ocean fish (tuna, shark, swordfish) tend to accumulate mercury.* Other potential sources: mercury-pesticides on apples; poultry and eggs raised on fish meal.

The most significant source is chronic mercury release from dental amalgams. (HANSON, ZIFF 1997) Sugar increases exposure by feeding mouth bacteria which foster mercury release from fillings.

* Levels are usually considerably lower in salmon, halibut, mackerel, herring, sardines, cod.)

Dietary mercury & metal metabolism

Walsh (2006) points out that we commonly eat 15-20 mcg of mercury. Large ocean fish contains even more, up to 60-80 mcg. Typically, 5% of intake enters the bloodstream, less than 1% gets through to the brain. With metal metabolism dysfunction, however, "all bets are off." Large quantities can be absorbed, and hypersensitivity is likely.

Oxidative damage by mercury

(FLEISHER, BOLGER 2002, DEAN 2002ABD, SILVERUD 1990)

Increases free radicals and lipid peroxidation, compromising fats, DNA, enzymes with sulfhydryl groups, etc.

Binds selenium, preventing its use as a cofactor for glutathione peroxidase.

Inactivates antioxidant properties of GSH, catalase, superoxide dismutase.

Affects inflammatory response.

Other neurotoxic mechanisms (SILVERUD 1990)

Compromises membrane activity.

Binds to thiol (SH^-) groups, disturbing function of sulfur aminos, enzymes, etc.

Alters immune function. Stimulates antibodies, represses T-lymphocytes. May foster autoimmune illness, allergies.

Suppresses pituitary and hypothalmus. Alters pancreas and thyroid function.

Nonetheless, many practitioners contend that the importance of mercury amalgams in psychiatric symptoms varies from patient to patient. Moreover, even if done correctly, amalgam removal is stressful, and can increase brain exposure. For some bipolars, it can be disastrous. (See *Risks to bipolars,* callout, previous page.) (WALSH 2008)

Replacement fillings (KUPSINEL 1984)

Unfortunately, all types of fillings currently available carry some health risk. Gold may be the least toxic, but can increase corrosion and mercury release if any segments of amalgam fillings remain in the mouth. This does not occur with enamel and dentin bonding composites, which are electric insulators, but they instead present their own toxicity issues. Ceramics and fired inlays use little of the sometimes-problematic resin found in other white fillings. Various tests (e.g., the Clifford blood test) may help rule out dental materials which trigger immune reactions.

Preliminary nutritive support until amalgams can be removed

Nutrients are discussed more fully on pages 178-9. Various practitioners have suggested the following nutrients before fillings are removed:

☐ High-dose C. (KUPSINEL 1984, ROSS)

☐ Large quantities of additional antioxidants, 3-4x/day. (CUTLER 1999, 2004, 07, KUPSINEL 1984, ZIFF 1984, 87, 97)

☐ Metal metabolism support, *as relevant.* Address any copper elevation. (CUTLER 1999, 2004)

☐ EFAs, to replace rapid use. (CUTLER 1999, 2004)

☐ B vitamins, B1. Magnesium, zinc. (ZIFF 1984, 87, 97)

☐ Lactobacillus, fiber (e.g., pectin). (KUPSINEL 1984, ZIFF 1984, 87, 97)

☐ Hanson suggests activated charcoal immediately before and after removal to absorb and help prevent recirculation of mercury. (PFEIFFER 1988)

☐ NAC, garlic, reduced glutathione and other sulfur sources can be very useful (KUPSINEL 1984, ZIFF 1984, 87, 97) for some, harmful for others. (CUTLER 1999, 2004)

See also *Cutler's supportive nutrients,* p. 178.

During removal (CUTLER 1999, 04, 07)

☐ High dose, or IV vitamin C. Increase antioxidants and B complex.

☐ Continue MT support. Avoid copper.

☐ Restrict sulfur to prevent loose binding to the mercury in amalgam dust and release back into body tissue.*(CUTLER 1999, 2004)

☐ Continue EFAs, probiotics, and fiber.

☐ Zinc [50-100 mg/day] and magnesium [500-1000 mg, divided doses], chromium picolinate [200 mcg with meals], molybdenum [1000 mcg/day].

* Instead, allow the mercury in the amalgam dust to be eliminated in the feces, which is a relatively safe and effective route. (Cutler 1999, 2004)

Removal procedure (ZAMM 1990, ZIFF 1984, 87, 97, HUGGINS, 1982, 93, FASCIANA 1986, KUPSINEL 1984)

A fan is centered on the patient to dissipate vapors in the mouth area. The patient is given oxygen or compressed air to breathe, and IV vitamin C [up to 50 gm]. Clothes and body are covered. A rubber dam in the mouth offers some protection against ingesting particles of the filling. A high speed water coolant spray is used (Dr. Joseph Pipkin uses catalyst water, which binds mercury and strengthens the immune system). (KUPSINEL 1984) Some practioners advocate removing fillings according to their electrical charge (negative, high positive, then, low positive) to lessen symptoms. (CASDORPH 1995) Even so, some brain exposure may occur, and symptoms may worsen following treatment.

For further info, see "Safe removal of amalgam fillings" at IAOMT.org

If chelation is required: Cutler's protocols (CUTLER 1999, 2004, 07)

Our bodies do not know how to remove mercury from the brain, so with significant acute toxicity, or serious chronic symptoms, DMSA / lipoic acid chelation may be indicated. Andrew Cutler, PhD, PE, author of "Amalgam Illness: Diagnosis and Treatment of Mercury Poisoning," and "Hair Test Interpretation: Finding Hidden Toxicities," describes the following approach to chelation.

Summary

The goal is to remove, bind and eliminate mercury from brain and body, minimize reabsorption, and limit toxic effects. Cutler's protocol focuses on relatively small oral doses, given regularly, at the half-life of the chelator, several days at a time, then resting.

One of his key concerns, is to limit mercury release into the circulatory system from which it can recontaminate soft tissue (e.g., the brain and nervous sytem) causing substantial additional damage. He therefore strenuously warns against IV or IM administration of chelators or sulfur sources (e.g., NAC or GSH), against excessive oral doses or irregular dosing, and against using monothiols instead of true chelators.

Before removal & throughout therapy (CUTLER 1999, 2004, 07)

Attention, both before dental mercury removal and replacement, and ongoing, up until the patient has stabilized post chelation.

□ Reduce copper levels *if elevated,* and limit sources. (Copper has similar characteristics to mercury and excess often worsens symptoms in mercury-toxic patients. Alpha lipoic acid, the centerpiece of this protocol, may mildly limit copper excretion. (See p. 178, and *Copper* pp. 171-73.)

□ Zinc 50 mg or more, *as relevant,* divided over 3-4 doses/day, to limit copper absorption, and to support mercury removal.

□ Treat insufficient bile, *if relevant.* (Low bile can cause both mercury and copper accumulation.) Cutler suggests taurine, glycine, lecithin, and milk thistle to encourage bile formation and secretion.

□ Treat any metal metabolism dysfunction (*perhaps lifelong* (WALSH 2004, 06)).

□ Ongoing intake of supportive nutrients is essential.

Step 1: DMSA

Indications: ***If the body load of mercury is above that of the brain*** (especially following significant recent exposure*), DMSA is usually started, alone, as it only lowers *body* mercury. (If lipoic acid, which lowers brain levels, were used here, it would distort the balance of mercury pressure maintained between body and brain, encouraging mercury migration into the brain.)

Procedure: Wait at least four days after the final filling removal or acute environmental exposure. Start with a low dose of oral DMSA.** A *strict* dosing schedule is important to prevent mercury release into the blood stream, posing further damage to the nervous system and body tissue. DMSA is given at its half-life, i.e., every four hours, day and night*** (waking up in the night to continue intake).**** Typically it's taken three consecutive days per week (or per fortnight),***** for 3 to 10 cycles.

* Despite preventive efforts, the breaking up of mercury fillings during removal, often heightens respiratory and circulatory exposure.

** Cutler mentions 2.5 to 10% of the mainstream 10 mg/kg dose, but since he suggests dosing twice as often, that comes to a total of 5-20% of the conventional total.

*** If doses are mistakenly taken too closely, do not wait beyond the half life for the next dose.

**** If symptoms recur intermittently during treatment, mercury is reentering the bloodstream. (Especially common are mouth inflammation, headache, dizziness, sensitivity to any external mercury exposure, and a one degree reduction in body temperature.)

***** That is, 3 days on, 4 off. Or 3 on, 11 off. If copper is increasing, breaks could be lengthened, e.g., 3 days on, 18 or 25 off.

Chemical chelators will not remove brain Hg

DMSA and DMPS, the most used chemical chelators, remove only extracellular mercury and whatever body tissues throw off. (CUTLER 1999, 04, 07) They do not effectively remove brain mercury (DMSA enters the brain in rat studies, but not in humans; (BUCHET 1989)) and by increasing circulatory levels, can increase the mercury absorbed into the central nervous system. (EWAN 1995)

DMPS vs. DMSA (CUTLER 1999, 2004, 07)

Cutler warns that the common high doses (including large oral challenge doses), as well as IV intake, of either chelator is harmful and inadvisable. Even more reasonable doses, if not given on the half-life, can encourage mercury release into the bloodstream, where it can re-poison tissue, creating serious symptoms.

Though injected DMPS can create particularly severe side effects,* Cutler finds modest oral doses (every 8 hrs), are more benign than oral DMSA. However DMPS is expensive, and available in the US by prescription only.

Since DMSA is rarely injected, Cutler suggests it has mistakenly gained a reputation for comparatively less toxicity, but it does (though, rarely) produce neutropenia (typified by rashes and neutrophil depression), which can be life-threatening.

Chelation pitfalls (CUTLER 1999, 2004, 07)

What to avoid:

Sulfur foods or supplements, unless deficient (see *Elimination test*, p. 180).

DMPS or DMSA challenge — can cause permanent disability or death, and overproduces false positives. (DMPSBACKFIRE.COM)

Single doses of chelator — instead, take equal doses, strictly at the half-life, several consecutive days,* then break (e.g., 3 days on, 4 or 11 off). Repeat, til done.

Do not use EDTA or penicillamine.

Do not use time-release chelators.**

Do not inject sulfur compounds (DMPS, DMSA, ALA, NAC or GSH).

Further cautions, side effects:

DMPS or DMSA (especially high doses or injected) can damage the liver.

Avoid hyperbaric oxygen therapy in mercury-toxic patients. (onibasu.com/archives)

Chelation can cause fatigue or temporarily upset hormone balance.

ALA may stimulate the gut and growth of gut bugs. Double probiotics! Yeast can usually be treated while chelating.

* Every 3 hrs for ALA, 4 for DMSA, 8 for DMPS.

* They may release unevenly. And, absorption may be limited to a specific part of the intestines, compromising extended release and the quantity absorbed.

Lipoic acid issues

Importance of chelation protocols

Besides being a strong chelator, lipoic acid is a potent antioxidant — but whatever it's used for, it will chelate metals, and can do permanent damage (as most people, these days, have some degree of metal toxicity), unless proper chelation protocols are followed. (CUTLER 1999, 2004)

Copper /zinc balance

Though lipoic acid can mildly increase copper, it also increases zinc, so in most cases does not significantly alter the balance.(CUTLER 2007) (See *Before Removal,* p.177.) *Nonetheless, the effect on copper may need to be considered in susceptible individuals.*

Lipoic acid: food sources

Lipoic acid is found, in very small quantities, in the mitochondria of plant leaves and red meat, usually bound to lysine. Sources include, potatoes, yeast, spinach, broccoli, tomatoes, peas, brussel sprouts, red meat, kidney, liver, and skeletal muscle.

Note: Such sources are too minor to produce any significant chelating activity. (CUTLER 1999, 2004)

Cutler's supportive nutrients (1999, 2004)

□ Good multi-vitamin/mineral without iron or copper.
□ B50 or B100, 1-2x/day.
□ Buffered C — 4 gm/day* or to bowel tolerance. Divided doses.
□ Magnesium — 100 mg, 4x/d. Increase to 200 mg in a few weeks.* With meals, perhaps at bed. Increase to bowel tolerance. (Magnesium-citrates, -malates, or -amino chelates. Avoid -oxides.)
□ Calcium — enough to keep the Ca/Mg ratio somewhere between 1:2 and 2:1.
□ If can't get enough Mg in, try adding taurine, up to 500-1000 mg,* with meals.
□ E — up to 1600 IU.*
□ CoQ10 — 75-200 mg/d.*
□ Zinc picolinate.
□ Flax oil — 2T; or CLO — 1/2-1 tsp.*
□ Borage oil — 1-2 tsp.*
□ Milk thistle — 1-2 caps/meal.*
□ Folate — 400-800 mcg.*
□ Selenium — 50-400 mcg total.* (Selenomethionine, selenocysteine or Se-yeast. No selenite or selenium citrate.
□ Perhaps lecithin, choline, B12.

* Scale to body weight, especially in children.

Step 2: Alpha lipoic acid

Indications:

□ ***Once body mercury is reduced enough*** (usually after about three months of DMSA, perhaps sooner) for brain/body mercury across the blood brain barrier to equilibrate, ***add alpha lipoic acid, or***

□ ***If body levels are sufficiently lower than those of the brain, start with lipoic acid, and skip the DMSA*** (e.g., in *some* cases where body mercury has decreased enough with time).

Procedure: *Once body mercury is lower than brain levels,* alpha lipoic acid* is taken by itself (*if indicated*), or with the DMSA, every 3 hours, for 3 consecutive days per week or per fortnight (longer if copper is too high), and continued til done. People often initially feel energized for 3-4 months, then fatigue might set in for another 4-8 months, before steady gradual improvement sets in. Sufficient improvement can take one to three years, perhaps longer (look for absence of symptoms, reasonable use of minerals by the cells, etc.).

Rationale: Lipoic acid is a natural antioxidant, and a disulfide. In the body, it becomes a dithiol (a molecule with two sulfur groups). Dithiols bind (and remove) mercury much more strongly than monothiols (many of the better known sulfur sources).** Moreover, researchers find lipoic acid — a water and fat-soluble compound, and the only chelator known to cross the blood brain barrier — is effective in getting inorganic mercury out of the brain. (DOMANSKA 1987, LESKOVA 1979, TRAKHTENBERG 1974, GREGUS 1992). At the same time, it protects neurons from glutamate toxicity, (BIEWENGA 1997, TIROSH 1999) and oxidative damage,*** and promotes recuperation.

See Cutler 1999 and 2004 for protocol details.

A note on cilantro — Dr. Y. Omura claims that cilantro, another disulfide, is also a strong mercury chelator. Unfortunately, lack of knowledge about the half-life of the active ingredient, and the varying potencies, depending on the plant, makes it difficult to keep levels of disulfide relatively constant. Inconsistent levels pose a risk of redistributing body and nervous system mercury, creating mercury-poisoning symptoms. (CUTLER 1999, 2004)

* Cutler suggests 50-100 mg, or 1/8 to 1/2 mg alpha lipoic acid, per lb body weight, per dose.
** "Chelator," was originally defined by *two or more* binding groups in one molecule.
*** And also regenerates other antioxidants (C, E, glutathione), and increases reduced gluathione.

Nutritive support (FASCIANA 1986, KUPSINEL 84, ELY 94, ZAMM 90, PAGE 92, TAYLOR 88, MUIR97)

Supportive supplements recommended by various practitioners. (See callout, at left, for Cutler's recommendations.)

□ **Metal metabolism support** — ongoing, *as relevant.* (See pp. 170-71.)

□ **Optimized antioxidant protection:**

Vitamin C — mobilizes mercury from its bound state in the cells. Mercury decreases C. Kupsinel uses up to 12 gm/day in divided doses, for up to 90 days (ZIFF 1984) Ross suggests a weekly drip of 30-50 gms of vitamin C, with minerals (but minimal calcium), for up to 3 months. (CALABRESE 1980, LEVANDER 1980, SOLOMON 1980)

E — antioxidant, works with selenium. (CALABRESE 1980, LEVANDER 1980, ZIFF 1984, 87, 97, CUTLER)

Selenium — availability is decreased by mercury. Selenium binds tightly to free mercury and neutralizes it, helps form glutathione peroxidase, and is used in the enzyme which converts T4 to T3, the more active thyroid hormone (thyroid is important in toxic elimination). [Selenomethionine, 1-2 mcg/lb body weight. (CUTLER, KUPSINEL 1984)] (MAGOS 1991, CHIMELNICKA 1983, IMURA 1985, WHANGER 1992)

CoQ-10 — also supports oxygenation. (KUPSINEL)

Generous intake of a good full-spectrum antioxidant (e.g., with lycopene, pycnogenols, milk thistle, anthocyanidins, resveratrol, moderate vitamin A and mixed carotenes, etc. (CUTLER, HUGGINS, 1982, 93, ZIFF 1984, 87, 97, APOSHIAN 1983, MUIR, 1997)

□ **B complex** [4 x/day, up to 100 mg total], plus, in many cases, extra B1 [up to 250mg.], niacinamide [to 1 gm], B6 [to dream recall], folate,** and pantothenic acid (B5) (which is often depleted or blocked by mercury) — May help restore psychiatric and neurologic function. (CUTLER 1999, 07, ZIFF 1984, 87, 97)

* Huggins (1982, 93) suggests avoiding high dose B12* during detox because, as a methylator, it promotes formation of methyl mercury (which is about 100-fold more toxic than inorganic mercury). He also suggests counterbalancing B12 with enough folic acid. Too much SAMe or methionine may also be problematic. [Consider individual biotype and other biochemical requirements.]

□ **EFAs** — often depleted or obstructed, especially with dry skin. Fish oil, flax seed, and/or GLA. (CUTLER 2007) *Consider biotype and other requirements.*

□ **Beneficial minerals ongoing:**

Magnesium — divided over the day. *Decrease dose if diarrhea occurs.* (ZIFF 1984, 87, 97, CUTLER 1999, 2007)

Zinc — increases metallothionein, which stores and neutralizes mercury; and decreases copper. [up to 0.5 mg/lb] (ZIFF 1984, 87, 97, CUTLER)

Molybdenum — especially with sulfation problems. Decreases copper, improves sulfur production, supports metal metabolism, may increase urinary mercury excretion and reduce kidney levels. [5-20 mcg/lb] (ZIFF 1984, 87, 97, CUTLER) See *Sulfur Indications,* at right.

Manganese, potassium (food sources), chromium; perhaps, germanium, iron, some calcium — *as relevant to individual chemistry.* (CHOWDHURY 1987)

□ **Monothiols** — this form of sulfur (contained in *Sources*, at right) binds too loosely to mercury, redistributing it, rather than effectively chelating (unlike lipoic acid — see pp 177-8). Cutler finds monothiols detrimental in 50 to 70% of people with significant toxicity issues, with restriction advisable at all stages, and even more strictly during lipoic acid treatment. On the other hand, another subgroup requires lots of sulfur sources all the time, except during amalgam removal, when it should be restricted for everyone (see *During removal,* p. 176). (CUTLER 1999, 2004)

□ **Support bile formation** — by which mercury is excreted. (CUTLER 99, 04) *If indicated.* Consider milk thistle (which is also antioxidant and increases glutathione creation) [4x/day, about 20-80 mg total]. And taurine, choline (e.g., from lecithin), and glycine (all three of which may also help moderate anxiety, insomnia, agitation, etc.). *Note: Taurine can be laxative.*

□ **Miscellaneous support**

Sunflower seed husk preparations — a recent study reports prevention of mercuric chloride accumulation, reducing levels over 25-fold in rabbit kidney, and almost 5-fold in muscle, as compared to controls. (DONTSOV 2000)

Thyroid and pituitary glandulars, *if relevant.*

Probiotics (e.g., lactobacillus, bifidobacteria) — to replenish beneficial bacteria injured by mercury, correct any imbalances due to lipoic acid, and generally address GI symptoms. (ZIFF 1984, 87, 97)

Dulse and other seaweeds (excellent source of iodine and other minerals) *May be contraindicated with manics.* Check *Sulfur Indications* at right.

Chlorophyll sources — may help detoxify mercury. Check *Indications.*

Digestive enzymes (KUPSINEL 1984) and/or fiber (e.g., pectin) (TRAKHTENBERG 1980), as relevant, to address gastrointestinal symptoms.

Fresh air, good diet, organic vegetables, herbal teas. At least two quarts of water daily. (ROSS 2002)

Treat gluten, casein, soy, and other allergies. (CUTLER 1999, 04, 07)

Melatonin — *only if needed,* for sleep problems. (CUTLER)

Colonics, *if needed to reduce side effects* (weekly, monthly, or PRN). (MURAN, IN ROSS 2002)

Sulfur issues

Indications

Sulfur foods are helpful for some, (KUPSINEL 1984, ZIFF 1984, 87, 97, ROSS 2002) (e.g., if deficient, or if kidneys tend to dump sulfur) to maintain healthful body function, but in significant quantities, may be detrimental for the majority of mercury-toxic individuals (enabling mercury to recontaminate tissue). (CUTLER 1999, 2004)

See *Monosulfides,* in the main column, at left and *Plasma cysteine & sulfate,* p. 180.

Sources

Garlic, chives, onion, leek, horseradish, yeast extract, turmeric, curcumin, chlorella, chlorphyll, seaweeds. Legumes (tofu, bean sprouts, beans, carob, chocolate, coffee, soy foods, green beans, lentils, peas, miso). Cabbage family (asparagus, bok choy, broccoli, brussels sprouts, cabbage, cauliflower). Jerusalem artichokes. Sesame seeds. Collard greens, daikon radish, jicama, kale, radish, rutabaga, spinach, turnip Eggs. Casein foods: cheese, cream, milk, sour cream, whey). Some: papaya, pineapple.

Note: Sulfur aminos in meat are not readily absorbed.

Besides such foods, *some* low sulfur patients need supplemental support to maintain adequate body function. Cutler suggests NAC, in such cases. NAC increases glutathione, and supports metal transport and elimination. (CUTLER 1999, 2004) *However, Walsh advises against use until toxic metals have decreased sufficiently* (see pp. 170-1).

Alternately, reduced glutathione, a systemic antioxidant, critical to liver detox, may be helpful, *if absorbed.* It may work with lipoic acid to eliminate fat-soluble heavy metals (and bind to methyl mercury, copper, cadmium, and zinc, facilitating bile excretion). (ZIFF 1984, 87, 97, KUPSINEL 1984, ROSS 2002)

RECOMMENDED READING

Cutler, Andrew, PhD, PE, *Amalgam Illness: Diagnosis and Treatment of Mercury Poisoning,* 1999, and *Hair Test Interpretation: Finding Hidden Toxicities,* 2004. www.noamalgam.com

Ziff, Sam, DDS., *Silver Dental Fillings: The Toxic Time Bomb,* 1984

Fasciana, Guy, MD, *Are Your Dental Fillings Poisoning You?* 1986

Taylor, Joyal, DDS, *The Complete Guide to Mercury Toxicity from Dental Fillings,* 1988.

Huggins, Hal A, DDS, *It's All in Your Head,* 1993.

"I have seen really dramatic results [in children] from... [the] proper nutritional/ supplement intervention that corrects the defects mercury causes."
Andrew Cutler, PhD, 2007

Sweating (exercise, saunas, etc.) foster further elimination. (Ross) *Avoid infrared saunas, which heat the body unevenly.*

Drainage formulas — Suggested by Ross to support kidney, liver and lymph drainage, starting at least two weeks before treatment.

Avoid: sugar, alcohol, (FASCIANA 1986, TAYLOR 1988, LARSON 1992, ROSS 2002) hydrogenated fat, excess copper, high-mercury fish, other contaminated food. (CUTLER 1999, 04)

Considerations: Lab (HUGGINS 1982, FASCIANA 1986, TAYLOR 1988 KUPSINEL 1984, CUTLER 1999. 07, PFEIFFER 1988)

"Response is the ultimate guide." — Andrew Cutler, PhD

Tests suggested by various practitioners

Check history of mercury amalgam fillings; exposure to fungicides, contaminated fish, or other sources.

Urinary tests: 24 hour mercury.* Specific gravity and pH. Albumin (intermittent traces). Vitamin C.

Whole blood mercury — for inhalation exposure.

T-cells — often compromised.

B12-deficiency anemia (blood count).

White blood cells — according to Dr. O. Pinto of Brazil, a count over 11,000 for 3 mo. suggests mercury toxicity. Post-elimination, it should lower to 5000-7000.

Neutrophil count — may be altered by DMSA.

Elevated lactate and, especially, pyruvate — carbohydrate metabolism byproducts, which may accumulate due to interference by mercury (or other heavy metals) with mitochondrial activity. (CUTLER)

Copper, zinc, and metal metabolism status. Copper, needs to be kept low enough to use lipoic acid. Elevated copper which doesn't decrease with zinc intake may be due to kidney impairment.

Trial of nutrients that counteract mercury. Alfred Zamm, MD, (1986, 90) gives B1, selenium, zinc, etc., and considers amalgam removal if Candida, allergies, or other mercury-related symptoms improve.

Urine organic acids.

Plasma aminos.

Complete blood chemistry.

Creatinin clearance — if kidney issues are suspected.

Electrocardiogram.

* Using potassium persulfate as a preservative. Measures excretion only.

Hair analysis (CUTLER 1999, 04, 07)

Hair, blood, or urine mercury are rarely accurate, due to mercury's volatility.*(CUTTLER 1999, 2004)

Disordered elements** are often a significantly more accurate sign of toxic levels of mercury — which damages the ability to transport minerals in and out of cells (e.g., tin, aluminum, perhaps bismuth, arsenic, antimony, titanium, or nickel, may test high; calcium, very high; essential elements scattered or low; lithium, very low.***) If minerals are generally normal, high copper may be the problem. (See Cutler 2004.)

Or, high cadmium, lead, antimony, etc., and high copper with low zinc, may suggest MT issues alone. (WALSH 2006)**

* Though slightly more indicative if these tests are considered together.

** Because mercury alters mineral transport, and may interfere with cell surface transport proteins causing the abnormal element levels. (Cutler 2004)

*** And hair metals (except lead) may not necessarily reflect the body load.

Plasma cysteine & sulfate – Therapeutic implications (CUTLER 2004)

Plasma cysteine indicates thiol levels, but accurate tests are currently unavailable. Try an elimination diet: low-sulfur foods for one week, followed by high-sulfur meals.

— ELEVATED SULFUR (thiols): *Such individuals initially feel energized, then lethargic and depressed. High sulfur in the bloodstream allows mercury to readily move from tissue to blood and back, multiplying symptoms.* A low sulfur diet is indicated.

— DEPRESSED SULFUR: *The individual experiences sustained improvement on the high sulfur meals.* Sulfur-rich foods (beans, dairy, etc., see previous page) and, in some cases, even NAC, is needed to maintain normal body function.

Plasma sulfate can be reliably tested.

— IF LOW: supplement orally and through the skin (possibly, epsom salt baths, *but not if mixed with certain meds or other factors which risk oversedation and drowning.*)

— IF ELEVATED: metabolism may be blocked, and sulfate not utilized.

Either way, consider dietary effects. Foods containing phenols or salicylates require sulfate for processing, and may be poorly handled. Limit such foods one week. Then reintroduce, one at a time to determine which provoke symptoms, and so require ongoing dietary restriction.*

* Such tests may be contraindicated for certain patients.

High cysteine relative to sulfate suggests a possible need for molydenum to support conversion.

Porphyrins (CUTLER AT: ONIBASU.COM/ARCHIVES/AM/552.HTML)

*Porphyrins make hemoglobin and are contained in certain enzymes. High levels occur when liver metabolism is compromised (often by toxic metals or other toxins). Elevations in fractionated urine porphyrin may thus help suggest detrimental levels of metals.**

COPROPORPHYRIN — elevation suggests a rare inherited condition, liver disease, certain drug effects; or lead, mercury (which may triple levels), or arsenic toxicity.

UROPORPHYRIN — Mercury sometimes raises levels.

ELEVATIONS IN BOTH — more definitely point to mercury.

* However, porphyrins are highly sensitive to heat, light, and agitation, yielding abundant false negatives from most labs, though positives tend to be accurate.

Challenge tests with DMPS or DMSA are inadvisable

Challenge tests force mercury into the kidneys for elimination (instead of the stool), (WALSH 2008) and recontaminate tissue, potentially causing acute mercury poisoning, possibly resulting in partial paralysis or death.*(CUTLER 2004)

See *Chelation pitfalls*, callout, pp. 178, & dmpsbackfire.com

* And can be inaccurate: lack of negative response is no insurance it won't occur on the next test, as Hg is suddenly released from organ compartments.

Lead

Potential mental effects (GOLD 1987, MOORE 1975, PAPAIOANNOU 1978, PFEIFFER 1988, CASDORPH 1995, CAMPBELL 1970, GORDON 1978, SACHS 1979, STERN 1969)

Chronic elevation can significantly compromise mood, cognition, and behavior:

- □ Listlessness, tears, depression, suicide. (TOWNSEND 02, MARLOWE 83, EMORY 99)
- □ Irritability, restlessness, insomnia. Mania, hallucinations, psychosis. (TOWNSEND 2002, MARLOWE 1983A, EMORY 1999)
- □ Disinhibition, difficulty with stress, childhood behavioral problems; increased anger, aggression, or violence; criminal behavior; other personality and behavioral changes. (WALSH 2006, LEVITON 1993 EMORY 1999, BROCKEL, NEEDELMAN 1996, NEVIN 1999, ARCH PED 2001, STRETESKY 2001, BURNS 1999, PIHL 1990)
- □ Hyperactivity, (WALSH 1986) other attention and learning disabilities; memory loss, intellectual deficit, dementia, other cognitive or neurological changes. (MARLOW 1983B, THATCHER 1982, SAVERHOFF 1973, OLIVER 1977, PIHL 1977)
- □ Lead toxicity (also mercury or arsenic) can cause porphyria. (GOLD 1987, CUTLER 2004)
- □ Sometimes associated with histadelia in children. (WALSH 2000, 04A)

Effects of lead on the central nervous system

- □ Disrupts neurotransmitter synthesis. Decreases acetylcholine activity. (GORDON 1978) Acutely, increases dopaminergic effects; (WALSH 1986) eventually, reduces dopamine levels. (SAVERHOFF 1973)
- □ Inhibits calcium-mediated release of neurotransmitters. (PFEIFFER 1988) Interferes with the calcium ion channel. (PFEIFFER 1988)
- □ Alters trace mineral levels. (WALSH 2004)
- □ Alters hippocampal activity. (PETIT 1983)
- □ Interferes with nerve myelination and myelin transmission. (KUPSINEL 84)
- □ Can compromise sensorimotor performance, especially visual motor skills; can cause optic atrophy.
- □ Can cause numbness or tingling in the extremities, muscle tremors, headache, convulsions, epilepsy, peripheral nerve disorders (note dropping of wrists, ankles). (GOLD 1987)
- □ Can cause muscle incoordination, weakness, wasting, poor balance, abnormal gait.
- □ May foster encephalitis, recurrent cerebral palsy, cerebral vascular disease, or brain tumors. (BIESEL)

Treatment (PAPAIOANNOU 1978, PFEIFFER 88, LARSON 1992, CASDORPH 1995, MUIR 1997, KESSEL 1997)

- □ Avoid exposure. Too much D or sunlight *during exposure*, facilitates bone absorption and storage (thus poisoning cases increase in the summer.)
- □ Calcium competes with lead, limiting absorption.
- □ Determine whether MT dysfunction is compromising elimination. (Therapy typically involves zinc, C, B6, selenium, E, glutathione, etc., and after a few months, NAC. (See pp. 170-71.)) (WALSH 2004)
- □ Pfeiffer emphasizes vitamin C and zinc to support lead excretion; B3 and B6 to help restore mental functioning.
- □ Larson suggests B1; injected, if nonresponsive.
- □ Casdorph and Walker (1995) emphasize antioxidants and relevant minerals, hyperbaric oxygen, and restricted fats.
- □ Trakhtenberg (1995) suggests pectin helps bind and remove lead.

Chelation (LARSON 1992, CASDORPH 1995, PFEIFFER 1988)

Brain lead can be eliminated in weeks. However, 95% is stored in the bones, where its half-life is 22 years. Entry into the bloodstream can recontaminate the brain. Thus, chelation may be indicated, especially when serious symptoms are involved.

Sources (GOLD 1987, CASDORPH 1995, PFEIFFER 1975)

Lead-based gasoline (now largely phased out in the US), battery terminals and casings. House paint (especially older or exterior paint), and burning of painted materials. Lead solder (often found in water coolers or tanks, tin cans, electrical devices), lead glaze on some cookware or other ceramics, moonshine from lead stills. Certain bonemeal supplements, most liver. Some insecticides.

Water is a common source. Lead leaches from solder, leaded brass or bronze pipes. To minimize, drink water from the cold faucet only and run it til cold, and use household water purifiers. If too contaminated, bottled water, if lead-free, may be preferable.

Industrial exposure: ammunition, pipes, solder, cables, lead shielding, some pigments, lead-containing smelter fumes, manufacture of brass or bronze, some chemicals and processed metals, waste incineration.

Children are particularly vulnerable (BRYCE-SMITH 1972, GOLD 1987, US CONGRESS 1990)

The child's high metabolism enhances susceptibility to lead. Moreover, children spend a lot of time on the ground, where their hands may come into contact with oxidized lead (a fine powder), and bring it into their mouths. And children are often attracted to lead paint chips, which taste sweet.

Goyer (1986) finds children absorb 40% of inhaled or ingested lead (as compared to 5-15% in adults) and retain 30% (adults, 5%). Lead periodically moves from growing bones to the bloodstream, and gains easier access to the brain, through the child's incompletely-developed blood brain barrier. Lead is particularly damaging to the developing brain.

Lead toxicity has been associated with childhood learning disabilities, hyperactivity, autism, convulsions, mental retardation. Severe poisoning can damage brain capillaries enough to cause irreversible encephalopathy.

RECOMMENDED READING

Cutler, Andrew, PhD, PE, *Hair Test Interpretation: Finding Hidden Toxicities,* 2004. www.noamalgam.com/hairtestbook.html and *Amalgam Illness: Diagnosis and Treatment of Mercury Poisoning,* 1999.
Casdorph, Richard H, MD, PhD, *Toxic Metal Syndrome,* 1995.
Lawson, Lynn, MA, *Staying Well in a Toxic World,* 1993.

In such cases, Cutler recommends low dose *oral* DMSA, every 4 hrs, 3 consecutive days, once per month,* until lead is completely removed (which can take years). He also suggests B, C, magnesium, zinc, antioxidants, EFAs, and a multiple, *as appropriate to individual requirements.*

Walsh emphasizes that once lead (or other toxic metal) levels are low enough, a focus on glutathione and metal metabolism becomes critical in preventing ongoing accumulation, and will probably avert years of IV chemical chelation with attendant side effects, and ongoing depletion of critical nutrients. (WALSH 2004) (See pp. 170-71.)

* As once the blood is clear, you have to wait til more lead leeches from the bones.

Considerations (lead toxicity)

Physical effects (GOLD 1987, PFEIFFER 1988, CASDORPH 1995)

Ashen hue to the face. Pale lips. Lead line on gums.
Metallic taste in mouth, nausea, vomiting, intestinal spasms, cramps, constipation, occasionally, diarrhea.
Fatigue,* weakness, discomfort. Anemia.** Altered blood pressure. Cardiovascular disorders.
Kidney dysfunction. Gout. (KIM 1996, MARDEN 2003, LIN 2003)
Bone and muscle pain.
Inhibition of sulfhydryl enzymes.
Low libido. Poor fertility. (LUSTBERG 2002)
Increased susceptibility to cancer. (LUSTBERG 2002)

*Lead alters mitochondrial energy processes.
** Lead depletes iron and represses hemoglobin synthesis.

Lab (PFEIFFER 1988, PIHL 1977)

Blood lead.
Upper limit erythrocyte protoporphyrin.
Decreased hemoglobin.
Hair analysis for lead and other heavy metals.
Perhaps, increased serum and whole blood copper, serum uric acid; increased blood spermine; decreased serum inorganic phosphate.

More metals

Sources of aluminum (CASDORPH 1995, GOLD 1987)

Kidney dialysis has been a significant source.* Aluminum cookware and foil (especially watch out for leaching by acid foods). Aluminum is also found in some deodorants (including "natural crystal" types), many baking powders and toothpastes, most salt (in the anti-caking agent). Also, water treated with alum (an aluminum salt) or aluminum fluoride (which is readily absorbed into the brain). And, certain aspirins, antidiarrheal meds, antacids, processed cheeses, nonherbal teas, soy-based infant formulas, pickling salts, self-rising flours, cake mixes.

* In one study, instead of addressing the cause, i.e., aluminum, 86% of dialysis dementia patients were treated with antidepressants. (Gold 1987)

Sources of cadmium (CASDORPH 1995)

Cigarettes are a major source (cadmium is usually in the fungicide used on tobacco). Passive smoking also exposes the lungs.

Other sources may include coffee, black teas, instant coffee and tea, refined carbohydrates, evaporated milk, processed meats, organ meats, oysters, other shellfish, contaminated fish, food grown in high-cadmium soil or with superphosphate fertilizers, rice irrigated with cadmium-contaminated water, soft drinks from certain vending machines.

Aluminum (DEAN 2002ABCD, CASDORPH 1995, PFEIFFER 1988, GOLD 1987)

Aluminum accumulation has, in some cases, produced profound depression, hyperactivity, learning disorders, memory lapses, mental deterioration/ dementia, motor incoordination, seizures, hallucinations, or coma; and can be fatal. (CRAPPER-MCLACHLAN 1973, 75, RIFAT 1990, BOWDLER 1979)

Mechanisms: Brain aluminum can inhibit acetylcholine, catecholamine, and other neurotransmissions; (BANKS 1983, LAI 1980, 81, HETNARSKI 1980) increase neurotransmitter breakdown; and stimulate crosslinking of proteins. (CRAPPER-MCLACHLAN 1973, 1975, RIFAT 1990, BOWDLER 1979)

Therapies: Avoid exposure. Support metal metabolism (pp. 170-71). Magnesium malate is reputed to be beneficial, as it readily crosses the blood brain barrier and chelates aluminum. Other forms of magnesium may also be helpful, as may plentiful antioxidants, particularly vitamin C and, possibly, calcium. Support for the thyroid, and for cerebral circulation (e.g., ginkgo, niacin) is probably indicated. (CASDORPH, 1995) Check for underlying mercury toxicity, causing aluminum retention. (CUTLER 2004)

Cadmium (CASDORPH 1995, WEINTRAUB 1995)

Cadmium toxicity may contribute to learning and behavior disorders, memory and cognition problems, fatigue, irritability, violence, neurotoxicity, and various mental disorders.* (MARLOWE 1983, THATCHER 1982, JIANG 1990, BURNS 1999, HART 1990, PHILPOTT 1990, WALSH 2006)

Nutrient interactions: Cadmium interferes with the metabolism of calcium (leading to bone disorders) and zinc; and the absorption of iron, copper and manganese; and also causes sodium retention. (SMITH 1989, STEWART-PINKHAM 1989)

* Physical symptoms can include yellowing teeth, mouth lesions, dry scaly skin, hair loss, appetite and weight loss, lower back and leg pain, sore joints, impotence, decreased lactation, loss of the sense of smell. Urinary sugar and proteins. An increased tendency to immune dysfunction, high blood pressure, anemia, cerebral hemorrhage, cardiovascular disorders, kidney and liver disorders (Sumathi 1996), and rheumatoid arthritis. (Casdorph 1995, Petering 1971)

Nutrients: High hair levels may be an artifact of mercury toxicity. If actually elevated (very high, other minerals relatively normal), it's difficult to clear. (Cutler 2004) Helpful nutrients may include C, zinc, calcium, selenium, trace minerals; support for MT function (pp. 170-71); high protein diet; *as relevant; and* copper and iron, *only if needed.* (Fox 1974, Hill 1963, Suzuki 1969, Maji 1974) Lipoic acid to help protect the liver. (Sumathi 1996) See protocol in Cutler 2004.

Arsenic (Gold 1987, Pfeiffer 1988, US Congress 1990)

Mental or neurological symptoms: Depression, crying, apathy, agitation, paranoia, visual hallucinations, psychosis. Dizziness, confusion, disorientation. Anorexia. Chronic headache, or pain. Encephalopathy. Paralysis. Cutler suggests it may contribute to Asperger's.**

Therapies: Cutler finds lipoic acid highly effective in removing arsenic. (Every 3 hrs for 3 days, skip 4 days. Repeat until eliminated.) Methylation support may help. Check for underlying mercury toxicity. (Cutler 2004)

* Physical symptoms: Burning feeling in the throat, gastrointestinal complaints. Skin thickening or darkening, hair loss. White line across fingernails. Liver damage. Depressed respiration. Can be fatal.
** And reports on primary arsenic toxicity in 3 cases.

Bismuth (Gold 1987, Pfeiffer 1988, US Congress 1990)

Sporadic psychiatric symptoms generally emerge early, and can include depression, apathy, slowed thinking, anxiety, antisocial behavior, delusions, or hallucinations. Symptoms can evolve into widespread confusion, involuntary behavior, tremors, and death.

Other heavy metals (Gold 1987, Pfeiffer 1988, US Congress 1990)

Overloads of nickel, antimony, etc., as well as metal metabolism dysfunction, itself, has been associated with affective, cognitive, and neurological symptoms.

See Cutler 2004 for a detailed discussion of sources, effects, and therapies.

General approaches (miscellaneous heavy metals)

Lab (Gold 1987, Pfeiffer 1988)

MT. Hair mineral and heavy metals, urine and blood tests. Nutrients.

Therapies (Pfeiffer 1988, Jaffe 1992, Lawson 1993, Casdorph 1995)

Treatment choices must be tailored to individual biochemical requirements.

- ☐ Optimize metal metabolism function. (Walsh 2007) (See pp. 170-71.)
- ☐ Vitamin C sufficient to maintain urinary levels above 100 mg/dl.
- ☐ B vitamins, to restore brain function. (Cutler) *Check biotype issues.*
- ☐ Glutathione and other antioxidants (E, carotenes, lycopene, luteine, anthocyanidins, etc.) to protect brain tissue.
- ☐ Beneficial minerals — zinc, magnesium, etc. (Cutler) Mineral-rich, alkaline diet. Supernutrition. Avoid junk food, allergens.
- ☐ Flax or fish oil, (Cutler) and/or GLA. *Check biotype requirements.*
- ☐ Supplement deficient nutrients.
- ☐ Glandulars, *if appropriate.*
- ☐ Reduce exposure to implicated metals and other toxins.
- ☐ Nutrient-based chelators, *as relevant.* Appropriate chemical chelators, *only if indicated.* (Casdorph 1995, Muir 1997, Kessel 1997, Pfeiffer 1988)

Natural chelators or competitors for specific metals (Larson 1992, Casdorph 1995)

- ☐ Lipoic acid protocol — arsenic, (Muir1997) cadmium, (Kessel 1997, Sumathi 1994) mercury, (Keith 1997) platinum, thallium, antimony, possibly brain lead. (Cutler 04)
- ☐ Perspiration — especially in removing nickel and body mercury.
- ☐ Methylation support — helps remove antimony & arsenic. (Cutler 2004)
- ☐ Magnesium malate — reputed to chelate aluminum.
- ☐ Calcium competes with lead, helping prevent absorption. (Cutler 2004)
- ☐ Zinc may compete with mercury & cadmium.

Sources of cadmium *continued*

Acidic soft water running through galvanized pipes. Black rubber (e.g., tires, carpet backing), burned motor oil.

Sometimes in pesticides, fungicides, certain dental prosthetics, dust. And certain paint pigments, ceramics, plastic tapes, polyvinyl plastics, sewage, silver polish.

Industrial exposure can occur in manufacturing cadmium alloys, fungicides, jewelry, nickel-cadmium batteries, and lead. Also in process engraving, soldering, copper refining, rustproofing of tools and marine hardware, polymetallic ore smelting, electroplating, and through contamination of air and water.

Sources of nickel (Casdorph 1995, Gold 1987)

Some refined foods, hydrogenated fat, fertilizers, metal cooking utensils. Leaching by acidic foods heated in stainless steel cookware. Some coins, eyeglass frames, jewelry, appliances, scissors, hair clips, dental crowns, braces. Oil refinery exposure (nickel carbonyl), other industrial exposure. Most cigarettes.*

* 15 such cigarettes per day, for one year, can be sufficient to induce lung cancer.

Sources of arsenic (Casdorph 1995, Gold 1987)

Certain insecticides, herbicides, rat poisons, anti-amoeba drugs. Preservative in pressure-treated wood. Well water in certain regions (arsenic leaches readily).

Sources of bismuth (Gold 1987, Cutler 2004)

Some cosmetics, gastrointestinal tract products, skin-lightening creams, and diaper rash balms. (Gold 1987)

Sources of antimony (Casdorph 1995, Gold 1987)

Fireproofing in bed clothes and bedding (can be reduced by multiple cleanings with sodium carbonate washing soda). Industrial exposure. Certain injections. Tropical parasites.

Importance of antioxidants & MT support

"[IV chemical] chelation may occasionally be helpful for lead or heavy metal poisoning. But depletion of glutathione, and MT is often the problem. [IV] chelation is usually unnecessary for bipolars. Less than 1% need [chemical] chelation."

William J Walsh, PhD, 2008

2. Other common neurotoxins

Tobacco

Insidious health effects

Karl Humiston, MD, notes the first cigarette makes most people sick. With continued exposure, tolerance develops, obscuring symptoms. Discomfort occurs mostly when too much time passes before the next cigarette. The immune system is thereby subjected to chronic and largely unnoticed stress. Health is constantly undermined. (PHILPOTT 1977, HUMISTON 1993)

Nicotine increases cortisol, heart rate, blood pressure, and respiration rate; and increases free radicals and carcinogens, cumutatively placing the heart and lungs at risk. It can also cause diarrhea, vomiting, headache, dullness and drowsiness; and impair physical skills. (HUMISTON 1993, MURRAY 1995, MUNRO 1997)

Perceived benefits (PHILPOTT 1977, HUGHES 1986, HUMISTON 1993, HOFFER 1983, AM J ADDIC 1993)

Cigarettes are ubiquitous in most mental hospitals. Estimates hold that 75-95% of mental hospital patients smoke. Many claim cigarettes ease symptoms, and have reported enhanced concentration and mental clarity, increased relaxation, reduced tension, and escape from some of the suppressive effects of antimanics and antipsychotics.

Mechanisms: Tobacco may provide short-term relief by occupying vitamin B3/endorphin/opiate receptor sites, (HOFFER 1983) or by decreasing vanadium. And, by mimicing acetylcholine, nicotine may help calm mania; while increased dopamine and cerebral circulation may produce a mild, antidepressant effect.

Damage to mental function

Such benefits last minutes to a few hours, but may, cumatively, produce substantial deterioration. Nicotine is known to increase adrenal stress homones, commonly implicated in anxiety and affective disorders. (MURRAY 1995) And it significantly depletes C, E, B1, folic acid, and other nutrients critical to brain function. Chronic use promotes nervousness, agitation, emotional lability, loss of concentration and judgment, (HUMISTON 1993, MUNRO 1997, HANDELMAN 1996) and, in some, paranoia, psychosis and other extreme symptoms. (HUGHES 1986) As a antidiuretic, it may also contribute to self-induced water intoxication and psychosis. (VIEWEG 1986) Nicotine may also promote earlier onset, and double dementia risk. (OTT 1998)

A data analysis by Dr. Wesley Boyd finds almost double the incidence of smokers in persons currently mentally ill,* possibly because smoking contributes to mental illness.**

* Of 4411 persons, 41% of those with mental illness (broadly defined) in the past month were smokers, 34.8% of those who ever had mental illness; only 25% of those with no history of mental illness. (Boyd 2000)

** Or because they are more prone to smoking.

Allergy or sensitivity to tobacco (PHILPOTT 1977, 80, 87)

Sensitivity to tobacco can produce anxiety, fatigue, tension, perceptual distortions, paranoia, delusions, hallucinations, weakness, dizziness, nausea; neurological symptoms; eye, throat, lung, gastrointestinal, or circulatory symptoms. (PHILPOTT 1977, 80, 87, HUGHES 1986, HUMISTON 1993)

In allergy tests, some patients must resume the pretest regimen (or avoid solanine foods) three days after a trial of tobacco, to clear reactive symptoms. In some, tobacco distorts judgment to the extent that the patient cancels further testing. (PHILPOTT 1977, 80, 87)

Withdrawal

Hoffer warns to withdraw gradually. Walsh (1993) suggests linking reductions to stages in nutritional healing. Support may include: B6, C, B3, (HOFFER1983) GABA, magnesium, zinc, B complex, (LARSON 1992) E, ginkgo, (MOWREY 1990) antioxidants and liver support (e.g., milk thistle, glutathione), perhaps, lecithin or tyrosine. Also, exercise, and a healthful diet. (DOUGLAS 1985) Philpott (1977, 80, 87) uses sodium bicarbonate to counter allergic reactions and reduce acidity. *Consider indications for mood, biotype, and individual biochemistry.*

Philpott's withdrawal strategies (PHILPOTT 1980, 87)

William Philpott, MD, starts treatment with a three to four day withdrawal period in which patients fast (if not contraindicated), or avoid foods to which they are allergic (as some allergens increase craving for tobacco). When patients experience an urge to smoke, they're given up to 1 tsp (3-4 gm) vitamin C powder, perhaps, up to 20-30 gm/day, to bowel tolerance. Small doses of B6, *if indicated*, may also be included.

Philpott finds tobacco cravings reach a peak by three minutes, so postponing five minutes allows the urge to subside, especially if also actively engaging in a positive practice (e.g., a vigorous walk, a behavioral drill, eating healthy nonallergic food, taking vitamin C).

Philpott's behavioral drill: (1) Close your eyes, relax, think of the urge to smoke and hold your breath. The oxygen deficit causes the brain to lose contact with the image, lessening the urge. (2) Connect the image of the urge to smoke with an unpleasant situation. (3) Recall a situation in which you like to smoke and imagine not smoking. Give yourself credit. Then think of an especially pleasant situation, or take three deep breaths and hear yourself being praised for not smoking. Relax, and repeat. (4) Every three seconds, starting from the feet, up, command a part of the body to feel heavy, warm, relax. Relax all over.

Repeat these steps, 15-30 minutes at a time, 6-8x/day.

Note: Some patients cannot give up tobacco until nutritional/psychiatric improvement becomes substantial. (HOFFER 1983)

Caffeine

Perceived benefits

Patients may use caffeine to counteract depression and medication, or to enhance mania. In most mental hospitals, coffee is freely available, and used profusely. In the short-term, coffee may increase concentration, energy and alertness, but it can also worsen irritability, mood lability, mania and, in the longer term, depression.

Potential mental effects (GREDEN 1976, 85, MCMANAMY, MIKKELSEN 1978, 80, GALTON 1979, CHRISTENSEN 1988, KREITSCH 1988, BOLTON 1981, CASDORPH 1995, HOFFER 1983)

Caffeine is a central nervous system stimulant. Extreme intake, long-term, can produce a syndrome like that seen with amphetamine addiction.* Caffeine can thus exacerbate or trigger hypomania or mania (MOORE 1998) or psychosis in susceptible individuals.** Several studies indicate that the greater the use of caffeine, the more pronounced the psychiatric symptoms, the more severe the depression, (GREDEN 1976, 85, MCMANAMY, CHRISTENSEN 1990) and the greater the likelihood of psychosis. Patients in the worst shape generally consume the most caffeine. (GREDEN 1976, MCMANAMY) Bipolars may be particularly prone to overindulge. (NEIL 1978)

Other effects: irritability, apprehension, restlessness, anxiety (LEE 1988, ROBERTSON 1978, LEVI 1967, BRUCE 1989, UHDE 1984) (perhaps, severe,*** (BOULENGER)), panic disorder, and chronic insomnia. Nervousness may lead to barbiturate or tranquilizer abuse.

With initial withdrawal (or skipped coffee breaks): severe headache, lethargy, depression, confusion, light-headedness, fatigue. (SILVERMAN 1992, HUGHES 1991)

* Zander (1982) finds the neurological stimulation from 200 mg caffeine comparable to 10 mg amphetamine sulfate (known for its ability to induce psychosis or mania with extended use).

** Tondo (1991), for instance, describes a sudden remission in a severe seasonal bipolar I patient after heavy caffeine intake stopped.

*** After age 60, even one cup of coffee may trigger severe anxiety. (Boulenger)

Potential mechanisms underlying caffeine's effects on the brain

- ☐ Increases output of norepinephrine (which medicates alertness, and can foster anxiety, stress, or mania). (ROBERTSON 1978, LEVI 1967, BRUCE 1989, UHDE 1984)
- ☐ Initially increases serotonin and dopamine, which later decrease; (GREDEN 1985, MIKKELSEN 1980, CHRISTENSEN 1988, KREITSCH 1988) tyrosine and thyroid hormone similarly decrease, (PARTOLES 1984) promoting depression.
- ☐ Depletes B1, B6, other B vitamins, potassium, magnesium, calcium, zinc. (MURRAY 1995, GALTON 1979, KREITSCH 1988, BOLTON 1981, CASDORPH 1995, HEANEY 1982, HERNANDEZ-AVILA 1991, HOLLINGBERY 1985, GABY 1994)
- ☐ Promotes sugar imbalances.
- ☐ Narrows blood vessels in the brain, decreasing access to oxygen.
- ☐ Increases exposure to certain toxic metals (increases aluminum absorption* and is a major source of dietary cadmium). (CASDORPH 1995)
- ☐ Eventually, in some cases, results in cerebral allergy to caffeine.

* It can quadruple stomach acid, promoting aluminum absorption.

Withdrawal strategies (MURRAY 1995)

- ☐ B, B3, magnesium, GABA, taurine — *as needed to reduce stress.*
- ☐ Vegetable juices, salads. Fresh, uncooked whole foods. Fish.
- ☐ Outdoor light on waking (unless manic). Moderate exercise.
- ☐ Avoid sugars and foods which cause allergic reactions.
- ☐ More sleep is usually needed til the body adjusts.
- ☐ Substitutes which increase vitality and energy — ginseng, gingko, bee pollen (*if not sensitive to it*), blue green algae, wheat grass, carnitine or acetyl-L-carnitine (with antioxidants), tyrosine, cacao, etc. Keep stimulation level *lower than that previously derived from caffeine,* and *gradually* reduce further. *Be careful not to trigger mania.*)

Also see *Philpott's withdrawal strategies,* previous page.

Avoid if depressed

Because of the close association with depression (even worse when taken with sugar or sweets), Michael Murray, ND, (1995) recommends depressives avoid caffeine.

Sources

Coffee, non-herbal tea, several herb teas, colas, chocolate. Certain aspirin preparations, pain relievers, diet and alertness medications, and antihistamine-containing cold medications.

Physical effects (LEVI 1967, ROBERTSON 1978, HUGHES 1991)

Caffeine may cause nausea, stomach upset, diarrhea, muscle twitching, trembling, racing pulse, irregular heart beat, chest pain, high blood pressure (especially during stress), breathlessness, vertigo, and increased urination.

Chronic use has been associated with hypoglycemia, diabetes, arthritis, and rheumatism, and may play contribute to cancer or heart disease. (GABY 1994)

Caffeine withdrawal sedation & headaches (CASDORPH 1995, BRODY 1982)

Adenosine is a neurotransmitter which tranquilizes brain and body. It also dilates blood vessels, reducing blood pressure.

Caffeine blocks adenosine transmission, increasing energy and focus at low levels and, at higher levels, nervousness, anxiety, and panic. Chronic coffee consumption tends to produce a compensatory increase in adenosine receptors.

Subsequently, if caffeine is withdrawn, adenosine messages are temporarily magnified, producing sedation and, typically, lowering blood pressure enough to create withdrawal headaches, often severe.

Alcohol

Alcohol & biotypes (PFEIFFER 1988)

Histadelic obsession with suicide can take the form of alcoholism, which may then become particularly tenacious, thanks to histadelic compulsiveness, and also because, as a light histamine releaser, alcohol may afford temporary relief from some symptoms. Alcohol, however, incidiously undermines healing, increasing adrenaline, damaging the brain, and depleting magnesium and other nutrients critical to healing.

Histapenics experience cyclic depression and anxiety and so may engage in periodic drinking bouts. Their difficulty metabolizing alcohol makes them particularly prone to fatality if barbiturates, sleeping pills or other depressants are used concurrently.

Pyrolurics are often intolerant of alcohol due to prevalent nausea. Nonetheless, Larson (2008) finds half of all alcoholics seem to be pyroluric.

Allergy to a particular grain can manifest as an addiction to those alcoholic beverages made from that grain.

How alcoholism manifests in bipolars

Alcohol use and abuse is relatively common in bipolars. Chronic use is detrimental, as it not only promotes extensive nutritional deficiencies, but also depression, mania, psychosis and brain damage. And it has been reported to double the risk of suicide. (RUSH 2003B)

Prevalence (WHYBROW, 1997, WINOKUR 1995, 96)

Over 60% of bipolar I and almost 50% of bipolar II have a history of alcoholism or substance abuse. (DUNNER 1993) In one study, by Famularo, 7 of 10 alcohol abuse patients under age 13 were bipolar. Alcoholism also occurs more frequently in bipolar I family members.

Patterns of alcoholism in bipolars

Bipolars often drink more during mania than depression, and may stop drinking altogether when depressed. (WINOKUR 1995, 96, BRIGHAM 2001, BRADY 1992)

Bipolars with primary alcoholism tend to have fewer affective episodes, and milder illness, which may not have occured at all without the alcohol. (WHYBROW, 1997, FEINMAN 1996) In such patients, bipolar mood symptoms sometimes remit two to four weeks post-sobriety. (DUNNER 1993)

Bipolars with secondary alcoholism may use alcohol as medication and, in many cases, can stop drinking more readily than true alcoholics, especially when mood symptoms are improving. (WINOKUR 1995, FEINMAN 1996)

Potential effects

Mental symptoms

Both mania and depression can be triggered by excessive alcohol. (BROIDA 2001, DAVIDSON 1995)

Symptoms associated with both alcoholism and bipolar disorder include anxiety, hostility,inappropriate affect, altered sleep cycles, nightmares, suicidal depression, delusions, hallucinations, and unfounded physical complaints. Also, disturbed cognition, judgment, and behavior. (BRANCHEY 1984, BROIDA 2001, LARSON 1992, HAWKINS 1976)

Effects on the brain (MURRAY 1995, 98, PFEIFFER 1988, LARSON 1992)

- ☐ Impairs tryptophan transport into the brain, reducing formation of serotonin, thus promoting depression, insomnia and pellagra.
- ☐ Increases adrenal output of cortisol and adrenalin, distorting brain function.
- ☐ Can cause seizures.
- ☐ Fosters brain tissue dehydration.
- ☐ Causes neuronal damage and death, and cumulative cerebral and cerebellar degeneration.
- ☐ Creates acetaldehyde toxicity. (*See box, p. 204.*)

Also: Can interfere with antidepressants. (BROIDA 2001)

Physical effects (MURRAY 1995, PFEIFFER 1988)

Hypoglycemia. Pancreatic inflammation. Gastrointestinal complaints.

Extensive nutritional depletion: B1, B2, B6, B12, folic acid, C, zinc, etc. (BAKER 1975, SHELOCK 1984) Decreased protein synthesis.

Inflammation, scarring, and fatty degeneration of the liver. Damage may compromise the ability to derive B1, B6, folic acid, B12, A, E, and EFAs from food. (SHELOCK 1984)

Electrolyte depletion (magnesium, potassium, calcium. (SPENCER 1985)) Edema. Dehydration.

Hypertension, heart and other muscle degeneration, palpitations, angina, coagulation disorders.

Osteoporosis.

Metabolic damage to all cells.

Fetal abnormalities (even with a single drink).

Treatment (LARSON 1992, MURRAY 1998)

Treatment choices must be tailored to individual biochemical requirements. Check for biotype-related contraindications.

- ☐ Treat any contributory conditions, e.g., hypothyroidism, Candida, allergies, hypoglycemia, other adrenal disorders, etc.
- ☐ Vitamin and mineral-rich foods. Moderate portions of proteins. Avoid refined sugars and starches, allergens, fried foods, processed fat, caffeine, and depressants. (In one study, rats fed refined carbohydrates, coffee, and soda avoided water, drinking whisky instead.) (NORTON 1977, MURRAY 1995, PFEIFFER 1988, PAGE 1992, GUNTHER 1983)
- ☐ C and bioflavonoids — reduce both craving and toxicity. (MURRAY 1995, PFEIFFER 1988, WICKRAMASINGHE 1992, LARSON 1992)
- ☐ Other antioxidants (E, selenium, glutathione, etc.) — protect the liver and nervous system. (PFEIFFER 1988, BALCH 1990, TANNER 1986, LARSON 1992)
- ☐ B complex — may help restore neurological functioning. (MURRAY 1995, PAGE 1992, BALCH 1990, TANNER 1986, LARSON 1992)
- ☐ Thiamin — depleted by alcohol. Often counters alcoholic numbness, tingling, memory problems, confusion, nervousness. Prevents and treats alcohol-induced Wernicke/Korsakoff's syndrome and beriberi, both of which can lead to neurological damage, mood disorder, and psychosis. (PFEIFFER 1988, MURRAY 1998, LARSON 1992, WEINISCH 1996, PAR 1992, LARSON 1992)
- ☐ B3 — often reduces alcohol craving, lethargy, insomnia, hyperactivity, headache, apprehension. (KAHAN 1966, WILSON 1967, 68, SMITH 1974, 78, 81, KROHN 1991, HOFFER 1983, 87, 2005, LARSON 1992, CLEARY 1990, TANNER 1986, ACKERSON 1997, LARSON 1992)
- ☐ Pyridoxal-5-phosphate (P5P) — often preferable to B6, as conversion to P5P is often impaired. Supports formation of antidepressant neurotransmitters. Important to alcohol metabolism. (MURRAY 1995, PFEIFFER 1988, BAKER 1975, GLORIA 1996, LARSON 1992)
- ☐ Folic acid — may help with agitation, depression, fatigue. (TANNER 1986, GLORIA 1996, LARSON 1992)
- ☐ B12 — may help with depression, confusion, nerve damage, psychosis. (BAKER 1975, TANNER 1986, GLORIA 1996, LARSON 1992)
- ☐ Phosphatidylcholine (BALCH 1990, TANNER 1986, LIEBBER 1994) — supports nervous system repair, memory, learning capacity, liver function. Benefits cirrhosis. *May worsen bipolar depression.*
- ☐ Pantothenic acid — benefits stress, irritability, tension, adrenal exhaustion. (TANNER 1986, LARSON 1992)
- ☐ Riboflavin — addresses insomnia, trembling, lethargy. Protects liver. (DUTTA 1995, TANNER 1986, LARSON 1992)
- ☐ Zinc — a component of enzymes that detoxify alcohol. (MURRAY 1998, LARSON 1992)
- ☐ Magnesium — depleted by alcohol; low even during withdrawal. Counters mood instability, irritability, insomnia, tremor. May help with depression, liver dysfunction. (PFEIFFER 1988, MURRAY 1998, LARSON 1992)
- ☐ Calcium — may help counter depression, nervousness, insomnia. (BALCH 1990, LARSON 1992)
- ☐ Taurine — levels are lowest in psychotic alcoholics. (BALCH 1990, IKEDA 1977, LARSON 1992)
- ☐ Glutamine — effectively reduces alcohol craving and toxicity. (COUSENS, ROGERS 1956, 57B, LARSON 1992)
- ☐ Tryptophan (or 5HTP) — is often decreased, with competing aminos (tyrosine, phenylalanine, methionine, etc.) elevated. (MURRAY 1998) *May be contraindicated.*
- ☐ Acetyl-L-carnitine — supports brain energetics/activity; (CRAYHON, SACHAN 1994) *or* L-carnitine — lowers serum triglycerides, increases HDL, and helps prevent fatty liver disease. (MURRAY 1998, BERTELLI 1993) *May be contraindicated.*

Role of allergy (HAWKINS 1976, DEES 1949, PFEIFFER 1988, LARSON 2008)

Larson finds most alcoholics allergic-addicted, often with food bingeing patterns throughout the family history.

Affective symptoms emerging mainly when drinking heavily, especially if prone to one particular type of drink, suggest allergy-addiction to an ingredient in the alcohol (e.g., grain, potatoes, etc.). Treatment includes avoiding all sources of that ingredient. If the allergy is to alcohol, itself, then it must be avoided completely.

Role of blood sugar & Candida (MURRAY 1995)

Alcohol disrupts normal glucose production, and induces reactive hypoglycemia, multiplying the craving for sugar and alcohol. If indulged, hypoglycemia worsens. Alcohol and sugar also feed Candida, which, in turn, increases the cravings, and so, the hypoglycemia.

Hypoglycemia, in turn, magnifies the mental and emotional problems of alcoholism, increasing the tendency to depression, rapid cycling, (LARSON 2008) confusion, and anxiety.*

* And, headaches, tremors, rapid heart beat, increased perspiration, hunger, dizziness, visual disturbances. *See pp. 214-18.*

Severe withdrawal symptoms

Moderate symptoms usually start a few hours after withdrawal and end within 48 hours, at which point, severe symptoms may emerge. These are more likely in chronic alcoholics over 30. Murray finds that, with severe symptoms, hospitalization or comparable inpatient treatment becomes necessary. (MURRAY 1998)

Alcoholic depletion vs biotype protocols

Larson (2008b) has found long-term alcoholics can be so depleted in nutrients that some biotype restrictions may not yet apply. Thus, even with considerable pyroluria, omega 3 can be uncharacteristically low, and needed along with GLA. Similarly, she has found B vitamin depletion so pronounced, that some histadelics respond to IV B complex, despite the folic acid. Once nutrition and alcoholism improve, more typical biotype requirements and restrictions are likely to re-emerge.

Suggestions by various practitioners

HRC alcohol detox (LARSON 1992)

Larson's Health Recovery Center reports a 78% recovery rate, with patients still alcohol-free three years later. This represents an unprecedented degree of recovery.

Treatment is tailored to fit individual biochemical requirements, and distinguishes pyroluria and histamine biotypes. HRC often employs individually-tailored IV nutrients.

Larson generally emphasizes: C, B complex, glutamine, calcium, magnesium, zinc, EFAs, relevant mood-modulating neurotransmitter precursors and free-form aminos, a specially-formulated multiple, and pancreatic enzymes, *all, as relevant.*

For alcohol craving

Consider B3, glutamine, kudzu, (TANAKA 1993) zinc, B complex, C, chromium, GABA, magnesium and, perhaps, hops tea or NAC. (MURRAY 1998, LARSON 1992)

Murray's further withdrawal suggestions (MURRAY 1998)

During active consumption: P5P, riboflavin, A, zinc, milk thistle.

During withdrawal add tryptophan, and electrolyte replacement, *as indicated.*

During recovery include flax seed oil.

- ☐ SAMe, betaine, methionine — protective against fatty liver, depression. (ACKERSON 1997, MALTO 1994) *Contraindicated in histapenia.*
- ☐ Branched-chain amino acids (leucine, isoleucine, valine) — deficiency may induce cirrhosis, depression, general brain dysfunction. (MURRAY 1998)
- ☐ Free form amino acids — aminos are often deficient; in this form they are more absorbable, however, intake may need to be limited/avoided, due to cirrhosis (which is common). (PFEIFFER 1988, MURRAY 1998, LARSON 1992)
- ☐ EFAs (GLA, plus EPA or DHA) — may help support the liver and ease withdrawal. (MURRAY 1998, BALCH 1990, ERASMUS 1995, LARSON 1992)
- ☐ Spirulina or chlorella — *if not contraindicated.* (PAGE 1992)
- ☐ Milk thistle — supports the liver. (MURRAY 1998, SCHUPPAN 1995, DEAK 1990)
- ☐ Kudzu root — antioxidant, protects the liver, reduces cravings. (ACKERSON 1997, KEUNG 1993, ZIE 1992)
- ☐ Siberian ginseng — reduces stress, toxicity; supports cellular energy, oxygenation. (BALCH 1990, ACKERSON 1997) *May be contraindicated in mania.*
- ☐ Lactobacillus — to replace intestinal flora. (BALCH 1990, LARSON 1992)
- ☐ Digestive enzymes — if indicated. (BALCH 1990, LARSON 1992)
- ☐ B15 & germanium — promote oxygenation and cellular energetics. (BALCH 1990)
- ☐ Short fasts or juice diets — useful for some. Focus on freshly-made, high-mineral, low-glycemic vegetable juices. *May be contraindicated due to sugar issues, liver toxicity, unstable moods, etc.* (BALCH 1990, LARSON 1992)
- ☐ Exercise — graded, physician-approved exercise program. Helps balance mood and blood sugar; reduce stress. (MURRAY 1998)
- ☐ Psychological support — counseling, personal support, peer group support (Alcoholics Anonymous, Rational Recovery, etc.).

RECOMMENDED READING

For information on successful nutrient based, biotype-related treatment:

Larson, Joan Mathews, PhD, *Alcoholism — The Biochemical Connection,* 1992 or *7 Weeks to Sobriety,* 1997.

Larson, Joan Mathews, PhD, *7 Weeks to Emotional Healing,* 1999.

Contraindications

See contraindications listed under *Nutrients,* and *Biotype,* pp. 21-167.

Outcome with nutritional treatment (PFEIFFER 1988)

Depression and other symptoms may worsen in early treatment but then improve dramatically, (BROWN 1988, LARSON 2008) especially if the mood disorder is secondary to the alcoholism. (WHYBROW, 1997, FEINMAN 1996, DUNNER 1993) Larson finds psychological support combined with appropriate supplements (often IV) produces high rates of recovery. (LARSON 2008) Healing may be complicated by dysperceptions, drug use, hypoglycemia, alcohol-induced brain damage, or lack of individual motivation. The sooner treatment is started, the better the response, and the more likely brain and body deterioration can be corrected.* Whatever degree of moderation can be achieved should also benefit the mood disorder. (PFEIFFER 1988, LARSON 1992, 08, DUNNER 1993)

* Note: Deterioration progresses insidiously, even in people who can "hold their liquor," or who feel good the morning after. In fact, since they do not tend to seek treatment, such people are more prone to irreversible long-term damage. (Larson 2008)

Reminder: This information in this book is presented for educational purposes only. No product or service endorsements are intended. Full contraindications are not listed. Alcohol withdrawal symptoms can be severe, and in some cases, life-threatening. If you need treatment for alcoholism, affective disorder, or any other medical condition, please seek the services of a knowledgeable physician.

Substance abuse

Substance abuse or dependence is prevalent in bipolars, even as compared to other axis I diagnoses. (BRADY 1992) Rates are estimated at 21-75%, approximately 6 times the 3-13% estimated for the general population. (BRADY 1992, REGIER 1990, TOHEN 1999, MCLELLAN 1985, RUSH 2003B, SACHS, GOODWIN 1990, WHYBROW) Estimates for rates in bipolar I cluster around 60%; (BRIGHAM 2001, DUNNER 1993, FEINMAN 1996) for bipolar II, 50%. (DUNNER 1993, FEINMAN 1996)

Sample therapies (BRAVERMAN 1987, LARSON 1992, PFEIFFER 1988)

- ☐ Mood-stabilizing, and antimanic or antidepressant therapies, *as relevant.*
- ☐ Treat histadelia, or other biotypes, *as relevant.*
- ☐ Check for and address allergies/sensitivities, Candida, etc.
- ☐ Braverman suggests tyrosine [1 gm AM & PM] to reduce craving for stimulants and help repair neurotransmission.
- ☐ Larson (2008) finds you can detox from almost any drug with certain specific nutrient formulations, often IV, e.g., high-dose vitamin C, etc. (*See p. 289.*)

See also, *Withdrawal strategies* for alcohol, caffeine, and tobacco, previous pages.

Recommended reading

Gant, Charles, MD, *End Your Addiction Now,* 2002.

Considerations: Substance abuse

Why the greater rates

Street drugs may be used to medicate mood, (RUSH 2003A, STRAKOWSKI 2000, BRIGHAM 2001) or to maintain or increase mania. (WEISS 1987, NEWMAN) Or, use may reflect impaired judgment or other mood symptoms. (BRIGHAM 2001) On the other hand, common genetics or other risk factors may predispose to both drug abuse and bipolar illness. (WINOKUR 1998, BRIGHAM 2001)

Outcome (GOLD 1987, BRIGHAM 2001)

Prognosis is poor for bipolars who use substances. (BRIGHAM 2000, WEISS 1998) Repeated use (especially of stimulants and hallucinogens) worsens the illness, and can trigger it in persons who may not have otherwise become ill, or may not have become ill so soon. Drug use generally kindles more episodes, more switching, (BRIGHAM) and more mixed states, (KETTER 2001) and has been associated with twice the hospitalizations. (SONNE 1994) On the other hand, if intake is stopped, mood symptoms often improve. (DUNNER 1993, FEINMAN 1996)

Over time, such drugs deplete and replace natural brain chemicals, which may lose the ability to achieve prior levels or stop working entirely. States opposite those originally sought in the drug eventually predominate. Long-term stimulants, for example, can cause chronic apathy, depression, fatigue, anxiety, intellectual deterioration, neurological illness, and brain damage. (GOLD 1987)

Drug-induced nutrient depletion, hepatitis, AIDS, cirrhosis, TB, etc., also complicate recovery.

Stimulants (BRIGHAM 2001, COUSENS 2001, SCHEEL-KRUGER 1977, BRAVERMAN 1987)

Cocaine abuse is particularly prevalent among bipolars and associated with a several-fold increase in onset. (BRIGHAM 2001, COUSENS 1987) The drug blocks dopamine recycling, and decreases norepinephrine reuptake. The initial stimulation of catecholamines and inhibition of serotonin creates a generally hypomanic syndrome (restlessness, excitement, sleeplessness, etc.), and often, in susceptible individuals, a prolonged mania.

In many cases, the ability to process glucose also becomes compromised, creating blood sugar fluctuations in certain brain regions, further destabilizing mood.

Continual use eventually leads to melancholy. Absolute levels of dopamine and norepinephrine become depleted, and the means to create more, exhausted. Moreover, to moderate the overstimulation, receptors tend to become less sensitive. Users, craving the initial euphoria, instead find themselves needing the drug to achieve the most minimal day-to-day functioning.

Crack, a distilled cocaine, multiplies such effects.

Amphetamines decrease norepinephrine reuptake, increasing synaptic accumulation, and stimulate norepinephrine and serotonin messages. Short-term they can exacerbate or trigger mania, paranoia, or psychosis in vulnerable individuals. Gerner (1976) reports repeatedly inducing mania in a single patient (with a latency up to 34 hours), with amphetamine administration.

As with cocaine, constant use, especially when sleep is sacrificed, can produce mood symptoms, even in people with no predisposing tendencies. Eventually, with depletion of neuronal catecholamines, depression predominates, and gets more and more severe. (SCHEEL 1977, BRAVERMAN 1987, COSTA 1977)

Amphetamines, can be found in certain diet pills, and cold and cough medication, as well as "speed." Ritalin® is a type of amphetamine. Ecstasy, although primarily serotonergic, is an amphetamine.

Note: If stimulants (or other drugs) induce a first mania, whatever the genetics, the individual becomes highly prone to further affective episodes, i.e., becomes bipolar. (BRIGHAM 2001)

Marijuana (BRIGHAM 2001, GOLD 1987)

Use of marijuana and opiates is common among bipolars. Clinicians often note harmful repercussions on mood, perhaps, increased incidence of bipolar disorder. Marijuana may worsen symptoms by destabilizing blood sugar or the cholinergic/adrenergic balance. Several studies suggest it can promote depression, while abruptly stopping can trigger mania. (See *Marijuana & choline*, p. 49.)

Prescription drugs

Mark Gold, MD, (1987) cites a 1971 study which reports 3% of prescription drug-users experience psychiatric symptoms, including agitation, depression, anxiety, delusions, hallucinations, nightmares, and psychosis. Gold points out that, with polypharmacy prevalent, current rates are likely to be even higher, as drugs interact. The elderly are particularly vulnerable, due to increased difficulty metabolizing and eliminating drugs. Other especially susceptible populations include children, and medical and psychiatric patients.

A sampling of medications & potential psychiatric side effects (GOLD 1987)

Major mood stabilizers — most seem to move cycling toward depression, and, in some cases, may, over time, foster intractable manias. (FRYE, KETTER 2001).

Anticonvulsives — such as phenytoin or phenobarbitol, have similarly been associated with depression. (TRIMBLE 1996)

Lithium (and probably other stabilizers) — withdrawal greatly magnifies suicide risk over the next year.

Antidepressants — often promote mania, may increase susceptibility to depression, and frequently trigger or worsen bipolar illness. (KETTER 2001, BRIGHAM 2001)

Antipsychotics — can foster depression and increase susceptibility to psychosis and, occasionally, mania. Bipolars may have particular difficulty with rebound psychosis post withdrawal. (BRIGHAM 2001, FRYE 2000, STEINER 1990)

See *Appendix III*, pp. 285-89, for further references and more info on side effects of the above meds.

Benzodiazepines — can promote depression, suicidal thoughts, restlessness, irritability, panic, aggression, paranoia, bizarre behavior, nightmares, psychosis, incoordination, slurred speech, lethargy, confusion, amnesia. (GOLD 1987, RICHMAN 1992) Dependency is common, often with severe psychiatric reactions on withdrawal. (GOLD, 1987, GRAZIUDDIN 1990) Can interact with other psychiatric meds.

Anti-pseudo-Parkinsonism meds — can produce depression, agitation, delusions, hallucinations, attention or memory problems, confusion, insomnia, nightmares, fatigue, weakness, numbness, blurred vision, incoordination, increased risk of TD. (HAWKINS 1973, GOLD 1987, RICHMAN 1992)

Diet pills, cold and cough meds containing amphetamines or antihistamines — can alter mood and cognitive function, impair judgment, promote convulsions. (PFEIFFER) High doses of certain cough syrups may trigger mania. (MENDEZ 1992)

L-dopa — may produce depression, hypomania, confusion, agitation, hypersexuality, delusions, paranoia, or psychosis. (GOLD 1987)

Isonazid® — may produce mania, psychosis, obsessive compulsive disorder. (ALAO 1998)

Bromocriptine® — can lead to mania, hallucinations, or paranoia. (GOLD 1987)

Antabuse® (used to make alcoholics feel sick when they drink) — can induce anxiety, profound depression, mania, schizophrenia, or delirium. (GOLD 1987)

Barbiturates — can worsen depression. May increase susceptibility to anxiety, insomnia, and mania. (GOLD 1987)

Anesthesia — can lead to a month-long depression.

Birth control pills — deplete B6, alter tyrosine and tryptophan metabolism, increase copper, and are commonly associated with depression. (GOLD 1987)

Antihypertensive meds — some may cause depression, sleep problems, irritability; rarely, psychosis. (GOLD 1987)

Targamet®— an ulcer medication, may produce depression, agitation, confusion, fluctuating consciousness, and extreme paranoia, especially among the seriously ill, the elderly, and liver-damaged alcoholics. (GOLD 1987)

Chemotherapy — can produce various mental symptoms, including depression, agitation, anxiety, hallucnations, confusion, delirium, etc. (GOLD 1987)

Nonsteroidal anti-inflammatories (NSAIDS) — some occasionally cause psychiatric symptoms on the first dose. (GOLD 1987)

Similarly corticosteroids, antibiotics, and certain heart, gastrointestinal, pain, and other medications can contribute to affective and/or cognitive syndromes. (GOLD 1987)

Excitotoxicity

Neurologists John Olney and Russell Blaylock pioneered research on the excitotoxic effects of glutamate, aspartate, and certain other stimulating substances. They found that, though essential to brain function, elevated levels can overexcite brain neurons to the extent of causing severe nerve cell damage and destruction.

"Oxidative stress, poor energetics and excitotoxicity are fundamentally interrelated. The three conditions both cause and affect one another."
Woody McGinnis, MD, 2004

Excitotoxic effects on mood, cognition, & neural function (BLAYLOCK 1995, OLNEY 1989):

Excitotoxicity may play a role in the development of some cases of:

- □ Mania, moodswing, depression. (MEBANE 1984, ZARATE 2006, LEVINE 2000, MARTINI 2002)
- □ Schizophrenia. Autism. (ERB 2003)
- □ Agitation, anxiety, panic. Rage, behavior problems. (KLINGBERG 1987)
- □ Hyperactivity, learning disorders, ADD. (OLNEY 1972, ERB 2003) Disorientation, confusion, memory problems. Cognitive decline, perhaps dementias, (MARAGOS 1987, GREENAMYRE 1989) or disturbed motor function. (SPENCER 1987, PLAITAKIS 1990)
- □ Sleepiness, lethargy, insomnia.
- □ Trembling, tingling, chills, slurred speech, numbness, partial paralysis, seizures. (MARTINI 2002, MELDRUM 1983)
- □ Light-headedness, dizziness, balance problems.
- □ Brain damage, perhaps especially focusing on the hypothalamus. (OLNEY 1972, SHIMICU 1973, DAWSON 1989)
- □ Headaches, migraine. (BODNAR 1980) Exacerbations in asthma.

Glutamate sources (BRAVERMAN 1987, SLAGLE 2001))

Glutamate is abundant in food; glutamine and GABA, relatively absent. All proteins contain glutamate. Common sources include parmesan cheese, ripe tomatoes, pork, poultry, eggs, dairy, wheat germ, oats, avocados, meat, peas, mushrooms.

For the moderately sensitive individual, elimination of MSG sources (next page) is usually sufficient, though in some cases, some restriction of the above foods may be indicated.

Effects of glutamate on neural viability

Normal dietary intake of glutamate from natural sources is mediated by homeostatic mechanisms which usually keep neural exposure within healthful limits. Excess is removed from the neuron, stored (as glutamine) in glial cells, and released as needed. Greater exposure (e.g., with MSG), a weakened blood brain barrier, or conditions which reduce brain access to energy can bypass protective mechanisms. Thus:

Normal dietary exposure — Glutamate (and aspartate) receptors activate calcium (and, to some extent, zinc) channels, allowing these ions to temporarily enter the neuron, change its potential, interpret messages from other nerve cells, and intensify response.*

Greater exposure or vulnerability — Calcium channels are held open, allowing large levels of calcium to accumulate within the neuron, especially in the mitochondria. Heightened activation of calcium enzymes** stimulates profuse free radical production and depletes brain antioxidants. The nerve cell is devastated by cytoskeletal breakdown, lipid peroxidation, nucleic acid fragmentation, and a compromised ability to create ATP (its energy source). Neurons usually die within 2-18 hours, or may survive, damaged. (COYLE 1981, NAIRN 1985)

Very high levels — Excitotoxins force sodium channels open and fix them in an open position. An influx of sodium and water causes nerve cell swelling (within 15-30 minutes) and death (within 3 hours). (CHOI 1990, COYLE 1981)

* Levine (2000) poses the following model: NMDA (N-methyl-D-aspartate) receptors require glutamate or aspartate, and glycine to open the channel. A magnesium ion, bound to the channel, lets potasssium in, and keeps calcium out, moderating stimulation.
Sufficient membrane depolarization, detaches magnesium, allowing calcium in. Accumulated calcium then intensifies neural response.

** E.g., lipid peroxidase, nitric oxide synthetase, and xanthine oxidase.

Role of glutamate in the brain (BRAVERMAN 1987, PFEIFFER 88)

Glutamate is a major excitatory neurotransmitter, found throughout the body and in all brain cells, being thousands of times more abundant than norepinephrine, dopamine or serotonin. Moreover, 50% of brain neurotransmitters are made from glutamic acid, (BRAVERMAN 1987) including glutamine, glutathione,* GABA, and, possibly, histidine.

Glutamate plays an important role in learning and adaptation to external stimuli. With aspartate, it is important in sensory perception, memory, orientation, cognition and motor skills, as well as the development of cells and neural pathways in the hypothalamus. (DAWSON 1989)

Glutamate neurons connect to every major nucleus in the hypothalamus, and so affect consciousness, emotions, hunger, sleep cycles, biological clocks, autonomic activity, growth, metabolism, and glandular function.

Glutamic acid also removes ammonia and other toxic wastes from the brain, contributes to the citric acid cycle, and converts to a 6-carbon glucose which provides the brain with fuel.

* Although a metabolic defect often decreases the ability to join glutamate, cysteine and glycine to form glutathione.

See also, *GABA*, pp. 41-43, 118, & *Glutamine*, p. 201.

Major excitotoxins

Monosodium glutamate (MSG) (BLAYLOCK 1995, OLNEY 1978, 81, ERB 2003)

Acute exposure, as in "Chinese restaurant" syndrome*

Acute mental and neurological reactions to glutamate** and MSG can involve blurred vision, dizziness, flushing or burning sensations, chills, headache, or depression.***

* Many Chinese restaurants now either allow the diner to choose whether to have MSG added to their food, or no longer use it at all.

** Especially with over 3 gm.

*** Physical symptoms can include profuse perspiration, dry mouth, thirst, gums tingling, sneezing, nausea, vomiting, stomach cramps, feeling full, other GI distress, weakness, heart palpitations. (FASEB 1995)

Potential long-term effects of chronic exposure

Anxiety, learning and behavior disorders, (OLNEY 1972, KLINGBERG 1987) sleep problems, cognitive decline, (MARAGOS 1987, GREENAMYRE 1989) neurological effects, (MARTINI 2002, MELDRUM 1983) brain damage. (NAIRN 1985, CHOI 1990, COYLE 1981)

May be associated with mania, (MICHAEL 2003) perhaps depression. (ALTAMURA 1993)

Fetal exposure may alter the brain, perhaps playing a role in autism, and other childhood disorders.*(PFEIFFER 1948, GARATTINI 1979)

Note: With substantial MSG, taurates may become harmful.

* Physical symptoms can include: Addiction to MSG. Chronic gastric distress or pain, nausea, vomiting diarrhea, cramps, irritable bowel, bloating, rectal bleeding, inflammation. Obesity, changes in insulin secretion, diabetes. Hypothyroidism, decreased thyroid weight. Elevated cortisone. Growth hormone suppression. Reproductive dysfunction, prostate or vaginal swelling, vaginal spotting. With high doses, decreased pituitary, ovary or testes weight (animal studies). Extremes in blood pressure. Circulatory inflammation. Chest pain, tightness, slow or fast heartbeat, atrial fibrillation, angina. Shortness of breath, asthma. Frequent urination, noctinuria. Rash, hives, acne. Mouth lesions. Face or tongue swelling. Bags under eyes, blurred vision, difficulty focusing, pressure on eyes. With extreme intake, severe retinal lesions and degeneration.

MSG sources

Monosodium glutamate (MSG) is more readily absorbed than glutamate alone, and more damaging. Unfortunately, the FDA has considered it nontoxic, and it has been added in increasing doses to many junk and processed foods, and the meals offered by some popular fast-food restaurants. It enhances taste, but also is addictive (and causes obesity, etc.). (TANAKA 1978, DE SOUZA 2003, ERB 2003)

MSG may be present in the following: soy sauce (50% MSG), hydrolyzed vegetable protein, hydrolyzed or autolyzed yeast, other yeast, yeast extract, gelatin, bouillon, texturized protein, sodium and calcium caseinate, soy or whey protein concentrate, malt, carrageenan, vegetable gum, natural flavoring, natural chicken or turkey flavoring, modified food starch; and various unspecified spices, flavorings, enzymes, and seasonings on food labels. Canned and processed foods may contain added L-glutamate in the toxic D form to enhance flavor.

The FDA doesn't allow MSG in infant food, though it may contain other excitotoxins.

Aspartame® (MARTINI 2002, ROBERTS 2002)

Use has been associated with depression, (ZARATE 2003, SMITH 1998) bipolar disorder, suicide, panic; and memory, behavioral and neurological disorders.*(ROBERTS 2002) Research conducted by Soro, the initial manufacturer, indicates it could cause brain tumors** and seizures, destroy central nervous system tissue, and harden synovial fluids.*** Affective patients may be particularly vulnerable. (WALTON 1993)

* Also, headache, dizziness, chronic fatigue, blood sugar imbalances, eating disorders, birth defects, and vision problems; and symptoms of MS, Lou Gehrigs, lupus, or arthritis. (Roberts 2002)

** A 3-year study by Dr. Coco found aspartame breaks down into a formaldehyde-based chemical which causes leukemia, lymphoma, and malignant brain tumors. The study was confirmed by Blaylock. Even one diet cola per day was enough to increase the risk of brain tumor. (Olney)

*** Dr. Ralph Walton notes 92% of independent studies show significant negative effects; 100%, if studies by the FDA (which did not include rats who did poorly or died) and the manufacturers are excluded.

Sources (MARTINI 2002)

Used as a sweetener in some sugar substitutes, and added to many diet and other sodas, gums, and some sweet foods. Gum magnifies risk, as it facilitates access through the blood vessels under the tongue directly to the brain.

Effects of constituents (MARTINI 2002, ROBERTS 2002)

Some effects associated with Aspartame® constituents:

Phenylalanine — excess lowers seizure threshold and depletes serotonin; can worsen mania or mood instability.

Aspartate — excitotoxic; may contribute to depression; (ZARATE 2003, SMITH 1998) intensifies reactivity to chemicals, drugs and other toxins.

Methyl alcohol — a toxin, which alters the dopamine system, causing addiction.

Glutamate suppression may moderate mood

Some researchers suggest suppressing glutamate and increasing GABA as an approach to depression, mania, and mood stabilization, (BARTHOLINI 1985, BRAMBILLA 2003, KRYSTAL 2002, KENDELL 2005, ZARATE 2003) *as:*

- ☐ Glutamate may be elevated relative to GABA in mania (MICHAEL 2003), and perhaps depression. (ALTAMURA 1993)
- ☐ Antidepressants and antimanics may work by reducing glutamate activity.
- ☐ Mood stabilizers may act, in part, by increasing GABA. (KRYSTAL 2002)

Treatments (BLAYLOCK 1995)

- ☐ Don't use MSG or Aspartame® and avoid other exposures. (See *Sources,* previous page.) Limit phenylalanine.
- ☐ Avoid supplements with glutamates, and aspartates. These may be included, unlisted, in some amino acid chelates.
- ☐ Avoid toxins.

Nutrients

- ☐ Magnesium —moderates glutamate side effects, but doesn't decrease sensitivity. It limits neurotransmitter release by blocking calcium entry into the neuron. [Magnesum glycinate or -citrate]
- ☐ Zinc —blocks some excitotoxin receptors (but may enhance others).
- ☐ L-theanine (the active ingredient in green tea) — a glutamate antagonist,* which also increases GABA. *(Also see p. 55.)* (LEKH 1999, KAKUDA 2000, YAMADA 2005, DHARMANANDA 1998, KOBAYAHI 1998, MASON 2001, ESCHENAUER 2006)

* Theanine has a similar structure to glutamate and blocks the NMDA receptor. In Japan, where MSG pervades the diet, women who practice the tea ceremony show half the mortality rate.

- ☐ Taurine — increases breakdown of glutamate to GABA, and can reduce the tendency to excitotoxic convulsions.
- ☐ GABA — counteracts glutamate stimulation. (BRAMBILLA 2003, KRYSTAL 2002, KENDELL 2005)
- ☐ Antioxidants — C, E, CoQ-10, selenium, anthocyanidins, glutathione, etc.
- ☐ Resveratrol — a polyphenol derived from grape skins, and a potent antioxidant, which increases glutathione. (ZHANG 2008) Moderate intake may counter NMDA overstimulation and glutamate toxicity,*(ALMEIDA 2007) benefitting mania and mood stability.**(DASGUPTA 2007, MOYER 2008, www. resveratrol…)

* It removes glutamate, via GSH, by increasing glutamate transport proteins.

** It may also counter depression, by increasing serotonin and inhibiting MAO. (Yanez 2006)

- ☐ Support cellular energy production — Energy is required to pump excitotoxins, calcium, and sodium from the neuron. Brain infection or trauma, oxygen insufficiency, hypoglycemia, and metabolic poisons decrease energy, and compromise pump activity. Low energy levels can also foster spontaneous firing of the nerve cell, removing the magnesium blockade and allowing more calcium to enter (perhaps inducing anxiety). Consider a trial of CoQ10, carnitine, niacinamide, etc., *as relevant.*
- ☐ Support blood brain barrier integrity — with antioxidants, EFAs, *as relevant to biotype and general biochemistry.* Address hypoglycemia, oxygen deprivation, brain infection, trauma, strokes, and other neurodegenerative disorders or other conditions which reduce barrier protection.
- ☐ Glutamine instead of glutamate — for conditions in which glutamate is indicated, glutamine is usually preferable, at moderate doses, and accompanied by a generous supply of antioxidants, and other protective nutrients, as above. *For some patients, even glutamine is inadvisable.*

Populations vulnerable to excitotoxins

Protection from, and restriction of, excitotoxins becomes critical in vulnerable persons, such as the young, the elderly, and people which chronic psychiatric or medical illness. Thus:

30% of adults are susceptible to "Chinese restaurant" syndrome. (See *MSG,* box, previous page.)

Vulnerability increases with chronic physical or psychiatric illness, and other chronic stressors.

Bipolars may be especially sensitive to excitotoxins.

Children are particularly vulnerable. (KLINGBERG 1987, BODNAR 1980, SHIMICU 1973, OLNEY, 1972, 78, 88) Their brains incur damage at lower doses, since the blood brain barrier (BBB) is not fully developed until age sixteen or seventeen.

Similarly, a weakened BBB in the head-injured, and a less efficient barrier in the elderly (perhaps especially in patients with neurodegenerative diseases such as ALS, Parkinson's and Alzheimer's) increases susceptibility. (MARAGOS 1987, SPENCER 1987, PLAITAKIS 1990, GREENAMYRE 1989)

Developmental abnormalities

The diet soda or MSG habit of the pregnant or nursing mother can interfere with brain formation in the infant, and intellectual development, (KLINGBERG 1987, BODNAR1980, SHIMICU 1973, OLNEY 1978) and may play a role in the development of autism, learning and behavior disorders, etc. Large doses of MSG can damage all brain structures in infant and animal, (PFEIFFER 1948, GARATTINI 1979) especially the hypothalamus and structures near ventricles. (GARATTINI 1979)

RECOMMENDED READING

Blaylock, Russell, MD, *Excitotoxins: The Taste that Kills,* 1995.

Roberts, H J, MD, *Aspartame disease: An Ignored Epidemic,* 2002

Erb J, Erb TM, *The Slow Poisoning of America,* 2003.

Organic solvents

"[I was impressed by the] extremely violent, maniacal condition into which some of the workers, both male and female, are known to have been thrown. Some of them have been the victim of acute insanity and, in their frenzy, have precipitated themselves from the top rooms of the factory to the ground."

Thomas Oliver, 1902, reporting on his visit to the India rubber factories in London and Manchester.

"Chronic, low-level exposure to pollutants such as industrial chemicals, may be responsible for the sharp rise in childhood behavioral problems, hyperactivity, and other learning disabilities, as well as asthma and cancers... Fetal central nervous system development may be slowed, intelligence reduced."

Sandra Schwartz, director of environmental programs at the Canadian Institute of Child Health

Organic solvents are liquids used to dissolve, or reduce the viscosity of, a particular organic substance. They are also often good at dissolving the body's lipids, and at breaching the blood brain barrier and destroying myelin, glial cells, nerve cell membranes and other nervous system structures.

On exposure to air, many organic solvents become gaseous, making inhalation probable. Organic solvents are also readily absorbed through the skin. The brain is particularly vulnerable, since it is at least 50% lipid (other organs are 6-20%). Moreover, fat-soluble compounds (e.g., these solvents) are readily admitted across the blood brain barrier, but not as readily removed, since they must be made water-soluble to get back through the barrier. (PFEIFFER 1988, GOLD 1987, US OTA 1990)

Mental & neurological effects (PFEIFFER 1988, GOLD 1987, US OTA 1990, TRIEBIG 1989, SPENCER 1980, PRYOR 1978, MANCUSO 1972)

Reported symptoms include: depression, fatigue, slowed response; memory loss, decreased capacity to concentrate or learn; irritability, anxiety, sleep disturbance, psychosis, seizures; incoordination, reduced manual dexterity. Chronic exposure can produce sustained alterations in mood and personality. (GOLD 1987) Even acute exposure to glue, toluene or other such substances can lead to panic disorder and hallucinations.

Sources of exposure (PFEIFFER 1988, GOLD 1987)

At least 10 million US workers are exposed to organic solvents each day, including gas station attendants, auto mechanics, painters, and refinery workers.

Organic solvents can be found in certain glues, adhesives, cleaning fluids, degreasing agents, paints, paint removers, varnishes, dyes, print inks, floor polishes and waxes, fuels, pharmaceuticals, and plumbing supplies. Commonly used solvents include alcohol, toluene, acetone and petroleum. Exposure also occurs through contaminated water and polluted air.

Pesticides

Insecticides, rodenticides, & herbicides

The majority of the population is constantly subjected to low level exposures through treated foods, contaminated water,* or inhalation of toxic lawn and garden products. Cumulative effects have not been sufficiently investigated and most ingredients have never been tested for neurotoxic and neurobehavioral effects in humans.

Many insecticides, designed to overstimulate or otherwise destabilize the insect nervous system (ultimately causing death) can, similarly, overstimulate human nerve cells and are, in fact, used in nerve warfare.

* Runoffs often enter the water supply, but are usually permitted by US regulatory agencies, because of the dilution.

Toxic neurological, cogntiive, & mood effects (US OTA 1988, Gershon 1961, Rowntree 1950, Senakayake 1987)

- □ Depression, emotional withdrawal, other emotional problems.
- □ Agitation, tension, irritability, insomnia, nervousness, giddiness, anxiety, restlessness, hyperactivity, combativeness.
- □ Bizarre dreams, delirium, hallucinations, psychosis.
- □ Impairment of intellectual function and mental flexibility. Forgetfulness, confusion.
- □ Decreased perceptual speed and manual dexterity. Impaired judgment and coordination, increased reaction time, increased tendency to accidents and resulting fatalities.
- □ Weakness, drowsiness.

Cholinesterase inhibitors (US OTA 1988, Gershon 1961, Rowntree 1950)

Most pesticides now used in the US are cholinesterase inhibitors. This category includes *organophosphate* and *carbamate* insecticides. They promote acetylcholine accumulation, by blocking acetylcholinesterase, the enzyme which breaks it down.

Mood effects (US OTA 1988, Gershon 1961, Rowntree 1950, Sarter 1994)

Acetylcholine overstimulation can trigger depression, especially in bipolars (even more so, histadelics), who tend to be particularly sensitive to choline. Or, heightened acetylcholine may act as a psychomotor stimulant, perhaps contributing to some manias. Further research is needed to detail the effects on mood, and to determine the significance of continual low level exposure from contaminated food and water.

Other mental effects

Hayes notes persistent mental symptoms have included delirium, combativeness, and psychosis. (Hayes 1982) Several studies record irritability, anxiety, muscle twitching and seizures, and aggravation of psychosis. (Rowntree 1950, Sarter 1994, Gold, 1987, Bayer 1992) Serious mental effects are more likely in people who had experienced pronounced physical reactions.

Organophosphate effects are difficult to reverse, and besides depression, may include emotional withdrawal, lethargy, strange dreams, short-term memory loss, difficulty concentrating, confusion, irritability, tension, restlessness, giddiness, anxiety, sensory and behavioral disturbances, phosphorus psychosis (US OTA 1988, Gershon 1961, Rowntree 1950, Sarter 1994) Some studies find persistent alteration of brain function, and axonal damage. (Gold 1987)

Dietary sources

"Between 1982 and 1985, the US Food and Drug Administration (FDA) detected pesticide residues in 48% of more than two dozen frequently consumed fruits and vegetables. However, OTA recently found that FDA's analytical methods detect only about one half of the pesticides that contaminate fruits and vegetables. Use of pesticides has been so widespread that measurable levels are frequently found in human tissues."

US Office of Technology Assessment, 1988

Sources of exposure

Exposure occurs through drinking water, treated foods; home, office and yard use; and accidental poisonings. Also, agricultural, grain elevator, nursery, green house, forest, and highway applications and manufacture.

Approximately one billion pounds of pesticides are produced yearly in the United States. The EPA counts 1.3 million certified US pesticide applicator operators.

Vulnerable populations

Vulnerability increases with pyroluria, low metabolism (hypothyroids, some histapenics), MT disorders, ongoing oxidative assault, youth, age, chronic mental or physical illness, and prolonged stress.

Incidence of related illness (US OTA 1988, Pfeiffer 1988)

As of 1988, pesticide poisoning was believed to afflict somewhere between 400,000 and 2,900,000 people, worldwide, each year. Estimates of pesticide-related farm worker illness in the United States ranged from 55,000 to 300,000 people, annually.

Incidence may be much higher than suggested by such statistics, as few physicians are trained to recognize pesticide poisoning.

Acute treatment (BAYER 1992, HAYES 1991, CHEREMISINOFF 1994)

Concurrent with treatment, decontamination is essential — flushing the eyes, scrubbing the body (those assisting should wear protective gear), destruction of contaminated clothing, gastric decontamination — *as relevant.* Chelation is mainly used for mercury-type pesticides.

Treatment is often symptomatic, addressing potentially damaging or life-threatening symptoms, such as, rapid heart rate, difficulty breathing, convulsions, choking, excess bleeding, etc.

It is essential to determine the pesticide involved, as treatments which counteract one specific pesticide may be contraindicated for another. For example, supplemental oxygen, used in organophosphate and carbamate poisoning, should be avoided in paraquat toxicity, as it fuels free radical formation by paraquat. (BAYER 1992)

Appropriate treatments for all pesticide poisonings are not known, and many that are known do not reverse all effects. Persistence in body tissue creates a major obstacle to recovery.

Note: Cheremisinoff (1994) warns that phenothiazines (used for psychosis and mania) may be contraindicated when suffering from exposure to pesticides which inhibit cholinesterase.

RECOMMENDED READING

For an overview of medical treatments:

Cheremisinoff, Nicholas P, *Toxic Properties of Pesticides,* 1994.

Bayer, Marc J, MD, "Reversing the effects of pesticide poisoning," *Emergency Medicine,* 1992.

Reminder: This information is presented for educational purposes only. If you need treatment for pesticide toxicity, bipolar disorder, or any other medical condition, please seek the services of a knowledgeable physician.

Carbamates bind less readily to the neuron, so toxic effects tend to be more immediate. These may involve incoordination, anxiety, emotional instability, and severe central nervous system suppression. Reduced access to oxygen may cause a persisting brain injury.

Physical and neurological effects

Physical effects may include visual difficulties, nausea and other gastrointestinal symptoms, problems breathing, weakness, vertigo, numbness, tingling and cramps in the limbs, paralysis, convulsions, coma. Can be fatal.

Blood levels of acetylcholinesterase and plasma cholinesterase can give some indication of exposure.

Other pesticides (GOLD 1987, PFEIFFER 1988, US OTA 1988)

Organochlorine insecticides — such as DDT, are now largely banned in the US, except for limited situations, but are used other countries, and present in some imported foods.

Organochlorines are considered less acutely toxic than other pesticides, but chronic toxicity is worse. They are easily absorbed, accumulate in fatty tissue, and leave very slowly.

Acute intoxication can cause excitability, apprehension, disorientation, visual and other sensory disturbances, headaches, weakness, vertigo, incoordination, difficulty walking, tremors, convulsions and coma. Respiratory difficulties or uncontrolled seizures may damage the brain. Children have experienced behavioral and learning difficulties.

Chlorophenoxy herbicides — such as, Agent Orange, a mixture of 2,4-D and 2,4,5-T, which was used in the Vietnam War. Such herbicides are still used in forestry and weed control. They have been associated with sleep disturbances, neurological damage, and psychiatric disorders. (ROBINOWITZ 1989)

Methyl bromide — Bromides were commonly used in the early 1900's as a headache remedy, and accounted for approximately one in five psychiatric admissions. They were eventually banned. Methyl bromide, however, is one of the most widely used pesticides in the US. It is a fumigant, with a pleasant odor. Acute exposure causes visual and speech disturbances, delirium and convulsions. It can eventually produce personality changes, perceptual problems, and permanent neurological damage. (GOLD 1987, PFEIFFER 1988, ANGER 1986, US OTA 1988)

Mercury and arsenic-containing pesticides are also detrimental. See pp. 174-80; 183.

Prevention

While definitive research on the link between pesticides and affective disorder is minimal, it is probably advisable to limit exposure, to the degree possible. Prevention entails eating organic foods, drinking clean water, and supporting immune function and general health. Also, using only truly nontoxic (in most cases, natural) garden and household pesticide/herbicide products, not working in chemical pesticide industries.

IV: Health

"Mental health professionals... have a professional and a legal obligation to recognize the presence of physical disease in their patients. First, physical diseases may cause a patient's mental disorder. Second, physical disease may worsen a mental disorder, either by affecting brain function or by giving rise to a psychopathologic reaction. Third, mentally ill patients are often unable or unwilling to seek medical care and may harbor a great deal of undiscovered physical disease."

Lorrin Koran, MD, 1988

"Psychiatric symptoms are often the first and only sign of a developing illness."

Mark Gold, MD, 1987

"The diagnosis of mental disturbance is directly proportional to the degree of lack of understanding that a physician has of that patient's disease process."

Serafino Corsello, MD, 1991

"Being diagnosed with a psychiatric disorder has been correlated with a high risk of having a medical illness."

EK Koranyi, MD, 1979

"There is no longer a justification for distinguishing mental and physical illnesses... in fact mental illnesses are physical illnesses."

Michael Schachter, MD, 1999

Prevalence of undiagnosed illness in US psychiatric patients

Koranyi (1988), in a review study of Northern California psychiatric patients, found 39% with "an active, important physical disease," with nearly half such cases (47.5%) undetected by the mental health system.

In a 1981 study of 100 state mental hospital patients by Gardner and Hall, 80% were found to have a previously undiagnosed medical disorder which required treatment.* Once treated, 57% experienced marked, and often rapid, improvement of psychiatric symptoms. The most common responsive conditions were endocrine or neurological.

A 1975 study by McIntre and Roman found two-thirds of psychiatrists failed to give patients a medical exam, stating that they wouldn't know how, or that it is rarely needed. 94% of those who did conduct exams found them useful.

This situation does not seem to have changed much in four decades. Recently, Safe Harbor reported that of over 100,000 Los Angeles County Department of Mental Health outpatients, none received medical exams except during health emergencies.

* They found the SMA 34 blood test most helpful. Along with an EKG, sleep-deprived EEG, routine urine analysis, history, and complete physical and neurological exams, they concluded that 95% of confounding illnesses could be determined. (Gardner 1981) Today, tests for food allergies, toxic conditions, nutrient imbalances, biotype, etc., yield critical therapeutic information, but are even more rare, except when under the care of nutrient-oriented physicians. (Safe Harbor)

Reminder: This book is presented for educational purposes only. If in need of medical diagnosis or treatment, seek the services of a knowledgeable physician.

The reader interested in information on natural therapies for the health conditions noted in this section is encouraged to investigate the authors cited, as well as other literature on this subject.

Mood/health interactions: A vicious cycle

Comorbid illness (Ikleman 1999)

Doctors J. Hudson and H. Pope of McLean Hospital in Massachusetts find the following illnesses often comorbid with bipolar disorder, perhaps due to similar etiological factors:

Chronic fatigue.

Arthritis, fibromyalgia. Chronic pain.

Cataplexy, narcolepsy, other sleep disorders.

Irritable bowel syndrome, other chronic digestive problems

Cardiovascular disorders.

Unusual reactions to prescription medication.

Biotype influence on immunity (Pfeiffer 1987, 88, Walsh 2006)

Some examples of biotype-specific mechansims altering immunity:

Pyroluria is characterized by depleted B6 and zinc. Zinc is critical to both cellular immune function, and antibody and thymus activity. Low zinc reduces formation of T-lymphocytes, and compromises white blood cell immune function. Low B6 reduces both the quantity and effectiveness of antibodies and lymphocytes, shrinks lymphatic tissue, and compromises thymus functioning. If untreated, pyrolurics may be prone to infection and cancers.(Pfeiffer 1987, 88)

Undermethylated patients tend toward reduced resistance to cancer and other chronic illness. (Frankel 1998, Cooney 1999)

Overmethylated patients are low in histamine, which is needed for the differentiation and functioning of T and B-lymphocytes.

Influence of physical illness on mood (Koran 1988, Gold 1987, Corsello 1991, Koranyi 1979, Schachter 1999, Gardner 1981, McIntyre 1975, Brooks 2005)

Part IV explores the often profound influence of physical health on mood. Thus, treatment-resistant depression (which occurs in perhaps one-third of bipolars), can be caused or exacerbated by hypothyroidism, MS, cardiovascular disorders, cancer, or other systemic illness, and in many cases, and improves when such conditions are treated. (Levine 1986) Similarly, mania is known to occur in patients with no history of affective disorder, secondary to infection, neoplasm, epilepsy, metabolic disturbance, pharmacological effects, etc., (Krauthammer 1978) and usually then evolves into a bipolar disorder, responsive, but not reversible, with treatment of the physical illness alone.

Influence of mood on illness

Conversely, bipolar disorder and associated chemistry often compromise physical health. Some of the mechanisms:

□ **Malnutrition** — Bipolars often do not eat well enough to maintain adequate immune nutrients (e.g., C, zinc, B6, glutathione, etc.).

□ **Altered hormonal secretions** —A dysregulated hypothalamus/pituitary/endocrine axis, and otherwise altered hormonal activity, is common in bipolars, and worsens health. (Philpott 1976, Corsello 1991, Jaffe 1992, Gold 1987) (E.g., underactive thyroid increases susceptibility to illness, while overactivity promotes cardiovascular and other stress-related illness; chronic adrenal cortisol production causes an ongoing suppression of immune response; pancreatic stress acidifies the blood, facilitating opportunistic infection and degenerative illness.)

□ **Disturbed circadian rhythms** — Distortions in sleep/activity cycles, and other daily rhythms, compromise immunity. (Gold 1987)

□ **Inflammation** — Bipolar stress, allergies, autoimmunity, excess omega 6 with too little omega 3, etc., encourage inflammation. (Philpott 1976) This reduces oxygen availability, creating a fertile medium for opportunistic infection, or the development of chronic illness (and also alters signalling, perhaps leading to a severe depression). (Maes 1995, 98, Smith 1991, Connor 1998, Stoll 2002, Rudin 1987, Sterberg 1992)

□ **Weakened lymphocyte response** — Severe depression, chronic cognition-suppressing drugs, and/or reduced neural stimulation tend to suppress lymphocyte activity, increasing susceptibility to herpes and other infections, hypertension, rheumatoid arthritis, skin disorders, ulcers, possibly cancer. Immune parameters improve with mood. (Philpott 1976, Corsello 1991, Gold 1987, Torrey 1988)

□ **Uninhabited neuropeptide receptors** — Neuropeptides, which mediate the intensity of brain/body messages, decrease in depression. Viruses and neuropeptides use the same receptors to enter the cell, so the deficit affords viruses easier access. (Philpott 1976, Corsello 1991, Gold 1987, Torrey 1988)

□ **Blood brain barrier damage** — Stress promotes lipid peroxidation, damaging this barrier and increasing its permeability. Brain proteins then more readily leak into the bloodstream, and can stimulate formation of antibodies which may then launch autoimmune attacks on brain tissue. Moreover, toxins, infectious agents, allergens and reactive immune complexes gain greater access to the brain, where they can distort function, destroy tissue, and spur immune reactivity. (Philpott 1976, Corsello 1991, Jaffe 1992)

□ **Leaky gut syndrome** — Stress can similarly cause leaky gut syndrome, which permits increased levels of food particles and gut bacteria into circulation, promoting allergies, other immune reactions, and Candida. (Philpott 1976, Corsello 1991, Jaffe 1992, Gold 1987, Papez 1951, 1952ab, Trowbridge 1991)

I. Gut, Candida, Allergies, Sugar

Allergic and environmental sensitivity, Candida and general gut dysbiosis, malabsorption, and sugar imbalances occur in most bipolars, and fuel mood symptoms. Moreover, these conditions interact, cross-triggering or otherwise worsening symptoms. (Note: Low thyroid and mercury toxicity also interact with the above (but are discussed on pages 225-37 and 174-80, respectively). Oxidative stress and metal metabolism disorders (pp. 170-71), which compromise the gut barrier, can also play a significant role.)

GI integrity & function

"Any factor which impairs a person from having an adequate supply of essential nutrients can be a factor that either directly causes, or greatly contributes to, the symptoms of manic depression... a complex malabsorptive condition that affects not only the brain, but nearly every other organ... Over 60% of brain chemicals are found in the gut, including serotonin, and other mood-modulating neurochemicals." — Alan Darman, 2002

Malabsorption & nutrient deficiency (PFEIFFER 1988, JAFFE 1992, WALSH 2002, 08)

Dr. Walsh has found malabsorption primary in 10% of a 20,000 mental health patient database. Chronic malabsorption causes pervasive nutrient deficiencies, likely to distort neurotransmission and other brain activity, increase neurotoxicity and, ultimately, compromise mood and cognition. (DARMAN 1997, 2002, WALSH 1997B, 2000B, JAFFE 1992) Causes include:

- □ Stomach problems, including altered hydrochloric acid. (WALSH 2002)
- □ Incomplete digestion in the small intestine. Trouble breaking down proteins. (WALSH 2002)
- □ Problems in the intestinal villi, through which nutrients are absorbed into the blood stream. (WALSH 2002)
- □ Nutrient and enzyme deficiencies, exacerbating absorption problems. (EATON 2004, WALSH 2000B, 02, JAFFE 1992)

Leaky gut syndrome (JAFFE 1992, PHILPOTT 1976, GOLD 1987, PAPEZ 1951B, 52, TROWBRIDGE 1991, WALSH 2008)

The intestinal lining protects the blood from incompletely digested food, harmful bacteria, and toxins. This barrier can be compromised by:

- □ Toxic assault. Infection, irritation, inflammation. Chronic illness.
- □ Chronic immune overstimulation.
- □ Oxidative stress. Metal metabolism dysfunction.
- □ Overgrowth of certain bacteria, Candida, other yeast. Intestinal parasites.
- □ Stress, food allergies, autoimmune disorders.
- □ Alcohol. Certain pain meds, nonsteroidal anti-inflammatories, etc.
- □ Pancreatic insufficiency. Blood sugar imbalance.
- □ Immobility. Fluid retention.
- □ Malnutrition, prolonged fasting, starvation, parenteral nutrition, impaired digestion, malabsorption.
- □ Failure of the gut to mature properly.

If causes are not redressed, the gut is unlikely to heal, and may rapidly deteriorate, producing a host of allergic, autoimmune, and immune reactions, and allowing Candida access to internal organs. Mental symptoms may involve fatigue, confusion, stress, sleep disorders, depression, and mood instability.

Darman's list of absorption issues in bipolars

*Alan Darman, a dedicated lay researcher, has compiled a good list of absorption-related issues that can influence mood:** (DARMAN, 2008)

- □ Hidden food allergy — e.g., to glutenous grains, dairy, corn, eggs, nightshades, peanuts, citru s, etc. Often tied to mood and cognitive disorders. (ROGERS 1997)
- □ Candida — prevalent in bipolars. Can cause significant malabsorption. Also consider imbalances in other GI bacteria, and parasites. (ROGERS 1997)
- □ Low digestive enzymes or stomach acid, inadequate supportive nutrients. (ROGERS 1997)
- □ Insufficient water — required in GI function and nutrient absorption. (JENSEN 1981)
- □ Poor appetite, or poor diet. (JENSEN 1981)
- □ Stress, alcohol, sugar, caffeine, tobacco, food additives/chemicals, other toxic exposure, overwork. (ROGERS 1997)
- □ Acidosis — depletes body minerals. (ROGERS 1997, JENSEN 1981)
- □ Underfunctioning organs and glands (e.g., thyroid, pancreas, adrenals, liver) — often due to nutrient starvation. (ROGERS 1997)
- □ Other malabsorptive and biochemically depleting conditions. (ROGERS 1997, JENSEN 1981)

* And also lists more direct mood-modulating nutrients (see p. 19).

Some approaches (DARMAN, 2008)

- □ Cave man diet. Full-range multiple & free range aminos. (BALCH 1990)
- □ Avoid allergens. (ROGERS 1997)
- □ Bentonite & fiber for Candida and malabsorption.Glutamine, if helpful. Separate by several hours from bentonite/fiber intake.) (curezone.com...)

Eating habits

The atmosphere during meals should be relaxed, to promote digestion. Eat slowly and chew well to physically break down the food, mix it with carbohydrate-digesting enzymes, and stimulate digestive juices further down the digestive tract. Consider food combining (generally, don't eat fruits, desserts, etc., at the same meal as meat, poultry, fish, or vegetables). Acidosis (which is common) should respond to a mineral-rich, metabolically alkaline (vegetables, seaweeds, herbs), low immunoreactivity diet. (JAFFE 1992) Tailor diet to biochemical needs. (WALSH 2006)

Attend to metal metabolism (WALSH 2004AB, 06)

Oxidative stress from metal metabolism dysfunction can destroy key gut enzymes (including the enzyme which breaks down casein and gluten), compromising absorption and digestion, and fostering diarrhea, cramps, and food sensitivity.

Walsh finds MT therapy often makes it possible, by six to eight weeks, for patients to eat a wider variety of foods, without sensitivity reactions.

See *Lab* and *Therapy*, pp. 170-71.

Cutler's formula for gut healing

Glutamine 1-2 gm, 3-4x/day, half that much arginine, profuse liquid probiotics [25-50,000].

Approaches which may be helpful in restoring GI integrity & function

(JAFFE 1992, MURRAY 1998, BALCH 1990, SLAGLE 2001, KROHN 1991, ROGERS 1997)

Relevant IV or IM therapy may be needed to support absorption. (JAFFE 1992)

- ☐ Treat dysbiosis, digestive issues, GI irritation, allergies, nutrient deficiencies; and problems with oxidative stress and with metals.
- ☐ **B** — critical to digestion and absorption. (EATON 2004, BALCH 1990, MURRAY 1998)
- ☐ **Fiber** (in whole vegetables, fruits, grains and legumes; psyllium, pectin, guar gum, etc.) — promotes normal transit, and short-chain fatty acid production. Helps remove internal toxins. (BALCH 1990, MURRAY 1998)
- ☐ **Beneficial flora** — counterbalance detrimental bacteria, support digestion. Help ferment fiber, producing butyric and other short-chain fatty acids. Important in providing fuel to gut cells. (MITSUOKA 1990)
- ☐ **Inulin & fructooligosaccharides** (found in onions, garlic, wheat, barley, Jerusalem artichoke) — support growth of beneficial bifida bacteria, and microfloral creation of short-chain fatty acids. (HIDAKA 1986)
- ☐ **NAG** (N-acetyl-D-glucosamine) — precurses the intestine's inner mucosal layer (which selectively absorbs nutrients, and protects the gut from bacteria, enzymes, and acids); helps prevent Candida from sticking to it. Promotes growth of bifobacterium bifidum. (RHODES 1988, GLASS 1976)
- ☐ **L-glutamine** — contributes to absorption, growth, maintenance and viability of small intestines. Decreases permeability. Protects lymphoid tissue. A major fuel source for the mucosa. (FRAGA 1996, COUSENS 2001) Required in forming secretory IgA (an immune barrier). Precurses NAG. (SOUBA 1985, 90) *Can be overstimulating. Contraindicated in some manias.*
- ☐ **Phosphatidyl choline** — strengthens mucosal phospholipids. (CANTY 94)
- ☐ **Gamma-oryzanol extract** (found in rice bran oil) — antioxidant, protects mucosa, benefits various GI disorders. (MINAKUCH 1977)
- ☐ **GLA** — decreases inflammation. (TATE 1989) *Especially with pyroluria.*
- ☐ **Calcium d-glucarate** (in some vegetables and fruits) — increases toxic elimination; inhibits gut reabsorption of conjugated toxins. (DWIVEDI 90)
- ☐ **Digestive enzymes** — *as indicated.* Papain (from papaya) digests protein and, unlike pepsin, can work without hydrochloric acid. Bromelain (from pineapple) can digest 700 times its weight. Such plant enzymes are gentler on the body, but may not always get past the stomach. Pancreatic proteolytic enzymes (between meals), are sometimes indicated (though some people do not do well with them), to reduce toxic reactions and blood sugar flareups. (BALCH 1990, PHILPOTT 1978AB, 82, 87, MURRAY 1998)
- ☐ **Hydrochloric acid** issues — *low* levels are often misidentified as *over*-acidity. Low HCl compromises the ability to digest proteins, and decreases absorption of B1, B3, B5, B6 and folic acid, needed in forming HCl, creating a vicious cycle. Low HCl also means the pancreas will not be stimulated enough to create a sufficiently alkaline environment in the small intestines, for further digestion. Bitter herbs (gentian, dandelion, yellow dock, Oregon grape root, etc.), before meals, may stimulate HCl creation. Lemon may work as a mild substitute. If HCl supplements are used, sufficient protein and B3 are needed to buffer acidity. *Chronic HCl intake may suppress natural secretion.* (BALCH 1990, PHILPOTT 1987, MURRAY 1998)
  - ☐ **Bicarbonate** (as in baking soda) — *if indicated,* to prevent or reverse acidity. (PHILPOTT 1978AB, 82)
  - ☐ **Pancreatic glandulars** — *if indicated,* to nourish the pancreas. (BALCH 1990, PHILPOTT, 1978AB, 82)
  - ☐ **Limit/avoid** caffeine, alcohol, food additives, etc.

Assessments (JAFFE 1992)

Digestive disorders. MT function. Mood stability.
Difficult pregnancies. Repeated antibiotics, estrogens or steroids.
Microbial and chemical stool analysis for Candida and parasites.
Nutrient assays (including critical enzymes). Therapeutic trial.

Crohn's disease (HELZER 1984, ANDREWS 1987)

Crohn's disease involves intestinal inflammation, possibly due to immune overreactions. Stress can trigger or worsen episodes. Some researchers find high comorbidity with psychiatric illness, including depression, phobias, anxiety and OCD. Onset has been significantly correlated with that of mood syndromes.

L-Glutamine

Effects on mood

Glutamine is a mental and physical stimulant, enhances brain activity, and can be antidepresssant. (COCHIA 1976, MANNA 1988, YOUNG 1992, 93) Some of its benefit to mood may be due to normalization of gastrointestinal function and absorption.

Normal levels are rare in affective patients. Too much can trigger or worsen manias, (MEBANE 1984) and some depressions; too little can be associated with depression and fatigue. (BRAVERMAN 1987)

Support for mental function

Glutamine has been used as part of the treatment of certain cases of depression, (LEVINE 2000) schizophrenia, personality disorder, mental retardation, (ROGERS 1957B) alcoholism, (COUSENS 2001, ROGERS 1956, RAVEL 1982) and senility. It's reported to enhance memory, concentration, (MANNA 1988) alertness, mental clarity,*(ROGERS 1957) and stress tolerance (COUSENS 2001, BRAVERMAN 1987) and, perhaps, recovery from drug addictions. (LARSON 2001).

* Thus, in animals, inhibition of glutamine synthesis can produce confusion, convulsions, & dementia-like changes in brain structure. (Braverman 1987)

Brain functions

Precurses glutamic acid, a major stimulating neurotransmitter, and, to a lesser extent, GABA, a key inhibitor. (LEVINE 2000) Helps metabolize antidepressant hormones. (SLAGLE 2001)

A major brain fuel when glucose is lacking. (BRAVERMAN 1987)

Protects the brain when oxygen is low. (BRAVERMAN 1987)

Used to form niacin (which is critical to brain metabolism). (BRAVERMAN 1987)

Detoxes brain ammonia. (BRAVERMAN 1987)

Need may be suggested by

Mood and cognitive symptoms.

Intestinal irritation, ulcerative colitis, Crohn's disease, irritable bowel, leaky gut.* Ulcers. (COUSENS 2001)

Food allergies.

Sugar imbalance, cravings, hypoglycemia.**

Alcohol cravings,***(ROGERS 1956) toxicity. (RAVEL 1982, LARSON 2001)

Immune vulnerability. Major illness. (FRAGA 1996)

Injury, surgical trauma, wounds, infections,**** burns, inflammation, edema. (JAIN 1981, SLAGLE 2001)

Acidosis.*****(SLAGLE 2001)

Muscle deterioration, poor stamina. (SLAGLE 2001)

Lung susceptibility to toxic insult. (SLAGLE 2001)

* Glutamine provides energy for growth and cell division. (Fraga 1996)

** Glutamine helps metabolize sugars. When blood sugar is high, it stimulates storage as glycogen in liver and muscles; when low, insulin suppression, encouraging glycogen release and breakdown to sugar. (Fraga 1996) It also supports pancreatic growth, function, and enzyme creation. (Slagle 2001)

*** In part by stabilizing blood sugar and maintaining brain fuel. (Braverman1987, Rogers 1957b, Cousens 2001).

**** Glutamine provides energy for creating lymphocytes, macrophages, etc. Helps increase fibroblasts. Important in forming glutathione. Survival of severe infection is significantly correlated with muscle glutamine. (Slagle 2001)

***** Which can result from depression, stress, poor diet, hypoxia, fluid/electrolyte imbalance, toxicity, diabetes, trauma, etc. Glutamine helps by increasing plasma bicarbonate and detoxifying ammonia. (Slagle 2001)

Populations

Often low in chronic illness, mood and cognitive disorders. Can be low with food allergies, blood sugar imbalance, leaky gut, drug abuse. (Slagle 2001)

Nutrient interactions

Stimulates protein synthesis, inhibits degradation. Used in forming RNA and DNA. (SLAGLE 2001, BRAVERMAN 1987) Helps metabolize fats and protein. (SLAGLE 2001) Essential in forming niacin, in benzoate and arginine metabolism, and in sulfur translocation. (BRAVERMAN 1987) Supports carbon and nitrogen transport. (FRAGA 1996)

Source

Wild game, other animal protein, ricotta cheese, oats.

Supplements (COUSENS 2001, BRAVERMAN 1987, SLAGLE 2001)

Best taken as a free form amino acid. (BRAVERMAN 1987)

Take with water, not fruit juice (acidity destroys it), 1-2 hours distant from meals, not later than 3 pm.

Supportive nutrients

B6 (as *P5P**), (WALSH 2006) manganese. Choline or DMAE enhances glutamine effects. (COUSENS 2001)

Side effects, contraindications

Children, the elderly, the head-injured, and people with CNS disease, should be considered particularly susceptible to adverse reactions.

High doses can overstimulate, causing anxiety, restlessness, or insomnia. May trigger mania. (MEBANE 1984 COUSENS 2001)

If sensitive to glutamate or MSG, glutamine may produce headache, chest pain, etc., possibly, seizures (BRAVERMAN 1987)

Too much can elevate, rather than decrease ammonia.

Avoid in acute liver or kidney failure. (SLAGLE 2001)

Effect on cancer is unknown, possibly detrimental. (BRAVERMAN 1987)

See also, *Glutamate*, pp. 191-93, *GABA*, pp. 41-42, *Glutathione*, p.79.

Candida

A landmark case (TRUSS 1983)

Orion Truss, MD, had observed catatonia-like responses during premenstrual depression in some patients. In 1965, a 36 year-old woman came to Truss for treatment of allergic sinus headaches. Symptoms worsened premenstrually. She had a history of fungal infections, hormonal problems, abdominal distention, nausea, repeated sore throats and other indications of possible Candida.

She had been unsuccessfully treated for schizophrenia over the past six years with electroshock and drugs, and was about to be permanently institutionalized. She could barely speak.

Two weeks after the first injection of Candida albicans (see *Immune support*, p. 205), she became more alert. After the second injection, she was cheerful, "even able to get mad again." Stelazine® and Elavil® were discontinued at five weeks. At seven weeks, she and her husband felt she was back to normal. Ten years later, she remained well.

This case inspired further research into the link between Candida and psychiatric illness.

Overview (TRUSS 1983)

Candidiasis seems to plague most bipolars. Yeast overgrowth promotes allergies, sugar cravings, thyroid suppression, and other hormonal imbalances, all of which can lead to mood symptoms, and foster further yeast proliferation. Effective Candida therapy may help stabilize mood and implicated physical conditions.

Candida albicans is a normal inhabitant of the intestinal tract. Overgrowth, or diminished competitors (beneficial microorganisms such as lactobacilli) erode health. With breaks in the intestinal wall, Candida enters the bloodstream, and gains access to internal organs. It can also be transmitted sexually, and may enter the lungs during oral sex. Yeast colonizing tissue outside the gut become more difficult to control. In some cases, particularly if sensitivity to Candida develops, or if the brain is colonized, severe psychiatric symptoms may result.

Mental symptoms (DONSBACH 1987, MURRAY 1998, BALCH 1990, TRUSS 1978, 83, TROWBRIDGE 1986)

- ☐ Dizziness, disorientation, feelings of unreality, memory and attention problems, difficulty making decisions.
- ☐ Depression, yearning for isolation.
- ☐ Mood swings. Irritability (especially when hungry), nervousness, anxiety, agitation, hyperactivity, insomnia.
- ☐ In some cases, bipolar disorder, delusions, psychotic episodes, suicidal or violent tendencies.

Physical symptoms (DONSBACH 1987, MURRAY 98, BALCH 90, TRUSS 1978, 83, TROWBRIDGE 1986, KROHN 1991)

- ☐ Fatigue, lethargy, weakness. Headaches.
- ☐ Gastrointestinal distress (e.g., bloating, pain, heartburn, indigestion, belching, gas, diarrhea, constipation, mucus in stools, hemorrhoids)
- ☐ Craving for alcohol, sweets, chocolate, breads, pastas, other starches.
- ☐ Increasing allergic reactions to foods, often leading to environmental illness (e.g, sensitivity to perfumes, insecticides, tobacco, etc.) and, in extreme cases, universal reactor status.
- ☐ Sensitivity to dampness and molds. Cold hands and feet.
- ☐ Numb, burning, tingling, aching or weak muscles, incoordination, dizziness, paralysis, swollen or painful joints, arthritis.
- ☐ Athletes foot and other chronic fungal infections of skin or nails. Acne, rough dry skin, itchiness, ringworm, rashes.
- ☐ Vaginal burning, itching or discharge, cystitis, menstrual irregularities, PMS, endometriosis, loss of desire. Prostatitis, jock itch, impotence.
- ☐ Urinary urgency or frequency, burning upon urination, fluid retention, kidney and bladder infections.
- ☐ Recurrent infections or fluid in the ears, ear pain, deafness.
- ☐ Disturbed sense of smell and taste. Dry mouth, rash or blisters in the mouth. Bad breath. Sore or dry throat, thrush.
- ☐ Burning or tearing eyes. Erratic or failing vision.
- ☐ Chest pain or tightness. Cough. Wheezing, shortness of breath.
- ☐ Can contribute to hypothyroidism. Interferes with the thyoid, thereby promoting depression and weakening immune response.
- ☐ Can contribute to adrenal disorders, diabetes.
- ☐ Generally depresses immune function. (TRUSS 1981)
- ☐ May sometimes be important in hemolytic anemia, myasthenia gravis, MS, lupus, or other autoimmune conditions. (DONSBACH 87, VAJDANI 1996)
- ☐ IgA, IgG, or IgM antibodies may rise to 200 MONA (twice normal) or more. (LARSON 1992)

Some nutritional interactions allowing Candida to proliferate (DONSBACH 1987, MURRAY 1998, BALCH 1990, TRUSS 1978, 83, TROWBRIDGE 1986)

Decreases the magnesium and B6 available to heart and nerves, thereby increasing vulnerability to stress and futher compromising immune function and the ability to reduce Candida levels.

Produces a toxin which interferes with EFA metabolism, thus weakening membrane stability and the ability to keep allergens out. Thus, the gut and blood brain barrier become overly permeable, promoting allergies, and facilitating Candida entry into the bloodstream and brain.

Treatment (CROOK 1986, TRUSS 1980, DONSBACH 1987, TROWBRIDGE 1986)

Treatment must continue until the yeast is thoroughly controlled, which often takes a year or more.

Unfortunately, extensive die-off of Candida organisms due to treatment can induce symptom flareups (*Herxheimer reactions*), which can be life-threatening, mandating a temporary back-off on treatment intensity. (Vitamin C may moderate such reactions, to some extent.) (TRUSS 1980)

On the other hand, treatment needs to be potent enough to forestall further tissue invasion. Candida often mutates to elude therapeutic attack, frequently forming branching mycelial threads which penetrate body tissue more deeply.

Treatment is thus limited by the tolerability of the Herxheimer reaction, versus the importance of limiting Candida proliferation.

The following is an amalgam of various approaches. Treatment choices must reflect individual biochemical requirements, and careful assessment of potential contraindications. Individual patients may be intolerant to Candida therapies beneficial for most others. As improvement occurs, such intolerances may remit.

Diet, stress (DONSBACH 1987, MURRAY 1998, BALCH 1990, CROOK 1986, TRUSS 1983, TROWBRIDGE 1986)

- ☐ **General diet** — The diet should include plenty of fresh uncooked vegetables, vegetable juices, and lactobacillus sources. Fresh fish, antibiotic-free eggs and meat are usually permitted; as are non-starchy vegetables, such as artichokes, which need to be cooked (but don't overcook!) Enzyme-rich fruits, such as papaya, pineapple and mango may be helpful. Other fresh fruits, sprouted breads, and other complex carbohydrates can be consumed in moderate quantities, if they don't aggravate symptoms. Drink plenty of water.
- ☐ **Garlic, onions, & spices** (such as ginger, thyme and rosemary, especially if fresh). Also, herb teas.
- ☐ **Optimize diet, avoid refined carbohydrates, treat blood sugar imbalance** — Sugar and sugar products (candy, soda, pastry) and, often, breads and pastas, must be avoided. Refined carbohydrates feed Candida, and allow it to proliferate. Cravings for such foods tend to reflect the demand of yeast cells for fuel. Sugars also deplete B vitamins and zinc, thereby compromising immune defense, sugar and fat metabolism, and resistance to stress, and so foster Candida growth. Candida, itself, interferes with sugar metabolism, perpetuating the cycle.
- ☐ **Usually must avoid foods containing antibiotics or yeast** — Peanuts, pistachio nuts, vinegar, mushrooms, cider, soy sauce, malted products, smoked meats, cheeses, marinades, dried fruits, leftovers, and animal foods treated with antibiotics. If the candidiasis is severe enough, fresh fruit and complex carbohydrates may initially need to be avoided.
- ☐ **Avoid allergens and toxins** — Avoid foods (often gluten, dairy, etc), chemicals, or environmental substances for which there is an

Complexity (TRUSS 1980, 81)

C Orion Truss, MD, notes that 79 separate antibodies have been identified as responding to Candida antigens. (Other yeast toxins may not invoke antibodies, and so remain unidentified.) Each strain of Candida generally contains 30 to 35 out of the 79 known antigens. Thus the potential number of strains may be in the trillions.

Individual strains are also known to change their function or mutate. Furthermore, any one person may harbor more than one strain, some of which are only expressed when the yeast becomes invasive, such as after antibiotic depletion of lactobacillus and other competing organisms.

Predisposing factors (DONSBACH 1987, MURRAY 1998, BALCH 1990, TRUSS 1978, 83)

- ☐ Intake of antibiotics, especially if frequent, or consecutive for longer than one month.
- ☐ Repeated exposure, or sensitivity, to molds.
- ☐ Extended refined carbohydrate intake. Hypoglycemia, diabetes.
- ☐ Prolonged psychological or physical stress. Mood disorder.
- ☐ Repeated pregnancies. Extended use of birth control pills.
- ☐ Nutritional depletion. Leaky gut syndrome.
- ☐ Mercury toxicity.
- ☐ Metallothionein dysfunction.
- ☐ Low thyroid.
- ☐ Immune suppressive disorders (e.g., liver dysfunction, cancers, pyroluria). Use of immune-suppressing drugs (e.g. cortisone).

Immune repercussions (TRUSS 1981)

Candida is always present in the body, but usually counterbalanced by other organisms and immune system activity. However, if Candida proliferates, the immune system can become overwhelmed. An immune tolerance may develop, suppressing immune function, and increasing susceptibility to opportunistic illness, including further Candida incursions.

On the other hand, if the effectiveness of suppressor cells is compromised, immune reactions may fail to turn off. Reactions extending to body cells may promote various autoimmune conditions, including cerebral allergies and autoimmune attacks.

intolerance. Avoid alcohol, tobacco, and coffee. Avoid chemical cosmetics, chemical household cleaning products, and other common and potentially toxic or allergenic chemicals. Also, processed, preserved, chemicalized foods, and artificial colorings and flavorings.

□ **Reduce stress*** — Provide nutritive and herbal support, stress-reduction techniques, relaxation, exercise, and improvement in the psychosocial environment, *as appropriate.*

* Cortisone is secreted in response to stress or exhaustion (both common in bipolars), and enhances yeast cell activity. Yeast receptor sites are particularly keyed to cortisone, escalating Candida activity. Candida fosters stress, eliciting further cortisone, promoting further Candida activation, etc. Cortisone-type drugs are similarly detrimental.

Useful supplements

Supplements should be yeast-free.

□ **B3, B5, B6, B12, folic acid, biotin, B complex** (yeast free) — support digestive, immune and neurological function. (MURRAY 1998, BALCH 1990, GALLAND 1985)

□ **A** — helps restore intestinal walls; supports immunity. (MURRAY 1998, BALCH 1990, GALLAND 1985)

□ **Zinc, magnesium, selenium** — metabolic, immune, and neurological support. (MURRAY 1998, BALCH 1990, GALLAND 1985)

□ **CoQ-10** — stimulates immune function, energizes body cells, and increases integrity of cell membranes. (BALCH 1990)

□ **GLA, omega 3** — regulate the speed of immune reactions, help restore gut and brain-barrier integrity, increase cellular oxygenation, and enhance creation of endogenous hydrogen peroxide. (MURRAY 1998, BALCH 1990, GALLAND 1985) *Check biotype contraindications.*

□ **Probiotics** — lactobacillus and other beneficial bacteria counterbalance Candida. (DONSBACH 1987, MURRAY 1998, BALCH 1990, TRUSS 1978, 83, KROHN 1991)

□ **Fructooligosaccharides** — support growth of bifidobacteria. (MITSUOKA 1992)

□ **Iron** — *if deficient.* Not to be taken with hydrogen peroxide, germanium, CoQ10, ginkgo, or other promoters of cellular oxygenation.

□ **Lactoferrin** — antimicrobial derived from cow secretions. (BELLAMY 1993)

Acetaldehyde hypothesis (TRUSS 1984)

When intestinal oxygen becomes less available, Candida tends to convert sugar into acetaldehyde, liberating carbon dioxide (producing bloating, belching, or gas). In transporting the acetaldehyde to the liver to be detoxed, small amounts escape and become incorporated in body cells and enzymes.* Circulating blood is then repeatedly exposed, creating cumulative toxicity.

Acetaldehyde toxicity (which also occurs with alcoholism) suppresses acetyl CoA and glutathione activity, changes cell membrane permeability, and contributes to many of the important symptoms and complications associated with Candida, perhaps including chemical sensitivity.

* By binding with sulfhydryl and amine groups.

Acetaldehyde toxicity to the brain (TRUSS 1984)

Effects on the brain, altering function:

□ Impairment of synthesis or release of acetylcholine and other neurotransmitters. Formation of altered neurotransmitters (bound to acetaldehyde).
□ Metabolic disturbances in the nerve cell.
□ Changes in nerve cell membrane permeability.
□ Reductions in the availability of cerebral oxygen.
□ Free radical damage to the blood brain barrier, the neuron, neurotransmitter pathways, etc.

Effects on the body which can alter brain function:

□ Abnormalities in porphyrin metabolism. (See *Pyroluria* and *Porphyria*, pp. 147-52.)
□ Sugar metabolism abnormalities (see pp. 214-22).
□ Fatty acid imbalances (see pp. 85-94) and liver changes.
□ Increased intestinal permeability, setting the stage for allergic reactions (see pp. 199-201).
□ Increased lactate/pyruvate ratio, decreasing oxygen, and promoting anxiety and panic.

Antifungal herbs

- ☐ **Garlic** — helps prevent Candida overgrowth and conversion to mycelial form. (MURRAY 1998, KROHN 1991) *Taken separately from any homeopathics.*
- ☐ **Pau d'arco (taheebo)** — an antifungal. Murray recommends alternating with clove tea. (MURRAY 1998, KROHN 1991)
- ☐ **Oregano oil** — reputed to have strong anti-Candida activity. (INGRAM 1997) Preferred form: sublingual drops. Dosage varies with the individual.
- ☐ **Grapefruit seed extract, black walnut, Oregon grape, ginger, rosemary, thyme, German chamomile, hyssop**. (MURRAY 1998, CHRISTOPHER 1976, HUDSON 1997, ROSS 2002)

RECOMMENDED READING

Truss, Orion, MD, *The Missing Diagnosis* (1983)

Crook, William, MD, *The Yeast Connection* (1986)

Trowbridge, John, MD, *The Yeast Syndrome* (1986)

Donsbach, Kurt, ND, DC, *Candida Albicans & Systemic Candidiasis*, 1987.

Oxygen (DONSBACH 1987, MURRAY 1998, TRUSS 1983, BALCH 1990)

Yeast thrives in anaerobic environments. Oxygen deters proliferation, and supports immune action in general.

- ☐ **Vitamin E & CoQ10** — support cellular oxygenation.
- ☐ **Ginkgo** — increases brain oxygenation.
- ☐ **Organic germanium sesquioxide** — supports blood oxygenation and immunity. (BALCH 1990)
- ☐ **Daily exercise** — increases blood oxygenation.
- ☐ **Stabilized oxygen products.** (BALCH 1990)
- ☐ Donsbach (1987) gives intravenous hydrogen peroxide injections (*see box for details and contraindications*) to carry oxygen past the digestive system to other areas the yeast may have invaded.

Immune support (TRUSS 1980, 83, KROHN 1991)

- ☐ **Immune nutrients and herbs.***(THERAPIEWOCHE 1986) (*See p. 150*)
- ☐ **Thymus support.** (DONSBACH 1987, ROSS 2002)
- ☐ **Liver support** — particularly to avoid over-reaction to Candida die-off. (MURRAY 1998)
- ☐ **Treatment of other immune-suppressive conditions**.
- ☐ **Therapy for other parasites**, *if present.* (ROSS 2002)

With chronic candidiasis, the immune system tends to develop a tolerance to Candida, and loses the ability to recognize or attack it, allowing it to proliferate unchecked. To stimulate resistance, consider:

- ☐ **Oral Candida dilutions** — homeopathic drops, given orally to stimulate immune response.
- ☐ **Candida injections** — Truss employs periodic injections of uniquely tailored** Candida dilutions [the average concentration falls between 10^{-5} to 10^{-15}].
- ☐ **Mold dilutions** — Truss, similarly finds specifically calibrated** mold injections, often helpful.

* Note: Echinacea and goldenseal are often not helpful long-term.

** Patients react differently to different dilutions. The appropriate dilution and time between injections also varies with the stage of recovery. Too much worsens the illness. Too little is ineffective. Patients must also be checked for hypersensitivity to each new batch of extract. (Truss 1978, 80, 83)

Donsbach's treatments (1987)

For details, see Donsbach, 1987 (listed above).

- ☐ Food grade hydrogen peroxide, orally, on an empty stomach. (Caution: It's usually sold at 35% or 6% dilution — *EITHER ONE WILL BURN BODY TISSUE!* Donsbach dilutes this with water to a 0.5-1% concentration, then mixes in food grade aloe vera and natural flavorings.)
- ☐ Intravenous infusion of hydrogen peroxide (food grade, *appropriately DILUTED*) to oxygenate the blood and increase oxygen in body tissue.*
- ☐ Adrenal cortex and thymus extracts.
- ☐ Isoprinosine® an immune-stimulating antiviral.

After treatment:

- ☐ Healthy diet, including 5 oz plain unflavored yogurt, 3x/wk; 4 cups vegetables per day, including 2 cups raw. Avoid red meat, refined sugar and starch.
- ☐ Exercise, at least half an hour per day.
- ☐ 3 caps of one-billion count acidophilus per meal for two weeks; 2 per meal for two weeks; discontinue three weeks; then 3 per meal for one month.
- ☐ 10 one-billion-count acidophilus capsules in 4 oz warm water, injected into the rectum 3x/ week for three weeks.
- ☐ Females: a retention douche, with a specific oxygenating formulation,* 5-10 minutes, 1x/ week.
- ☐ Males wash the genital area with the commonly available 3% hydrogen peroxide before and after intercourse, and at least once per week. A weekly hydrogen peroxide bath with 16 oz of 3% hydrogen peroxide in a tub of water is also helpful.

* Developed by Donsbach.

Reminder: The information in this book is presented for educational purposes only. Full contraindications are not included. No product endorsements are intended. If you need treatment for Candida, bipolar disorder, or any other medical condition, please seek the services of a knowledgeable physician.

Medications

Eliminate or restrict: steroids, antibiotics, birth control pills, and immuno-suppressant drugs, *as medically feasible.* (DONSBACH 1987, MURRAY 1998, TRUSS 1978, 83, BALCH 1990, KROHN 1991)

Relatively mild, naturally-based medications

Caprylic acid — a contact fungicide. The enteric-coated form helps insure gradual release. (MURRAY 1998, KROHN 1991)

Sorbic and propionic acids — can selectively inhibit pathogenic forms of Candida. (TRUSS 1980)

Aramicrodin® — a tropical plant-based, broad-spectrum antimicrobial. Apparently does not interfere with normal intestinal flora. (KROHN 1991, TRUSS 1980)

Stronger drugs

Because of the importance of attacking Candida sufficiently to prevent it from mutating into treatment-resistant forms, stronger antifungals may needed for serious infestations.

James Balch, MD, (1990) warns that such drugs can weaken the immune system and encourage development of more potent strains of drug-resistant yeast, necessitating higher doses and further immune damage. He states that, for these reasons, most prescriptions are only for short-term use.

Julia Ross, MA, (2002) notes that effective treatment often involves two antifungals plus relevant nutrients, probiotics, an anti-fungal diet, and avoiding exposure to molds and reactive foods.

Some commonly prescribed drugs (KROHN 1991, DONSBACH 1987)

Nystatin® — binds to the yeast membrane, increasing permeability, especially in the intestinal tract. For oral intake, Krohn (1991) recommends the additive-free powder, taken with 1-2 gms of vitamin C (to increase stomach acidity); if nausea occurs, she suggests it be taken with meals until tolerated between meals. Donsbach (1987) warns that it can weaken the immune system, harm the liver, and occasionally provoke fatal reactions.

Nizoral® — more effective than Nystatin, enters the tissues and works on systemic yeast. In some cases, it may just suppress symptoms (as it inhibits the body's cytochrome P450 detox system), with improvement ending when intake is discontinued. Check liver enzymes monthly. (KROHN 1991)

Diflucan® — a systemic medication, which inhibits fungal cytochrome P450, compromising fungal cell survival. It also can be hard on the liver. Some people are intolerant to the dye contained in this drug. (KROHN 1991) Ross (2002) suggests testing liver enzymes monthly, and supporting the liver (e.g., with milk thistle, etc.)

Amphotericin-B® — focuses on the GI tract.

Additional contributory factors (MURRAY 1998, BALCH 1990)

Attend to contributing conditions:

- ☐ **Hypothyroidism** — thyroid helps drive immune activity. Low thyroid patients often will not recover from Candida until thyroid levels improve. (See pp. 225-37.)
- ☐ **Hypoglycemia, diabetes** — overly elevated sugar levels, and sugar surges feed Candida. (See pp. 214-22.)
- ☐ **Pyroluria** — which tends to compromise immune function, facilitating Candida overgrowth. (See pp. 147-52.)
- ☐ **Metal metabolism dysfunction** — Metallothioneins, normally abundant in gut mucosa, kill Candida and are critical to gut microflora balance. (WALSH 2006) Candida is often evident in persons with metal metabolism disorders.* Recovery, in such cases, tends to be unsustainable unless metallothionein function is supported. (WALSH 2002, 06)

* Look for elevated copper and toxic divalent metals, low plasma or serum zinc, or elevated hair zinc. Supportive nutrients include zinc, C, glutathione, etc. (See pp. 170-83.)

- ☐ **Mercury toxicity** — Alfred Zamm, MD, (1986) finds mercury can be conducive to Candida overgrowth and attendant allergies, which often improve after removal of mercury fillings.*

* Caveats: All dental fillings and adhesives carry some toxicity. Before removal, determine whether the Candida patient reacts adversely to the proposed substitute, and consider whether the increased exposure to mercury during removal, or the stress of the removal process, itself, would be prohibitive. If nonetheless indicated, maximize nutritional and other support. (See pp. 174-80.)

- ☐ **Reduced digestive secretions** — allowing parasites to flourish. Consider bitter and aromatic herbs, such as gentian, fennel, cinnamon, etc. (MURRAY 1998)
- ☐ **Leaky gut/ malabsorption** — allows Candida to more readily enter the bloodstream. Therapy may include B vitamins, fiber,* probiotics, etc. (See pp. 199-201.)

* Which counters Canddia as well as malabsorption. Water soluble fiber (e.g., guar gum, psyllium seed, pectin) decreases absorption of, binds, and promotes excretion of Candida toxins. Intestinal bacteria release fatty acids from fiber which inhibit yeast growth. Fiber also stimulates secretion of digestive enzymes.

Hygiene

- ☐ Protect throat (0.5% hydrogen peroxide gargle), and mouth (baking soda/hydrogen peroxide toothpaste). (RUSSELL-MANNING 1988)
- ☐ Jaqueline Krohn, MD, (1991) suggests thyme or tea tree oil (appropriately diluted) for topical infections, alternated with Nystatin® cream, if too drying.
- ☐ Pau d'arco (RUSSELL-MANNING 1988) or goldenseal (KROHN 1991) douche,* *when indicated.*

* Krohn's goldenseal douche: 1 Tbsp goldenseal tincture, 1 Tbsp witch hazel, 2 cups boiling water. Let sit until lukewarm (about 10 minutes). Add 1/2 tsp salt, 1/2 tsp acidophilus, 1 Tbsp yogurt. Apply slowly. (Krohn 1991)

Allergies

Allergic and environmental reactions can be critical in bipolar disorder, triggering mood changes, or worsening depression and, in some cases, mania or psychosis, (PHILPOTT 1978, LESSER 2002, LEMMO 2003) and such associated symptoms as irritability, fear, aggression, fatigue, inattention, sadness, slowed cognition, decreased activity and motivation, memory and learning difficulties. (KING 1981, STEINBERG 1997, LEMMO 2003)

Allergens (PHILPOTT 1978, HOFFER 1987, RANDOLPH 1965, 71, MANDELL 1979, HERSHEY 1996, GOLD 1987)

Any food may be suspect, but usually the allergen is a frequently eaten, favorite food, or a food which is strongly disliked. The foods to which the individual is most allergic, often become addictions, and so may interfere with willingness to cooperate with dietary treatment.

Maladaptive responses in bipolars frequently involve wheat and other glutenous grains.(WALSH 2008) Other common "allergens:" milk, eggs, beef, corn, cane sugar, chocolate, soy, peanuts, oranges, coffee, potatoes, or tomatoes. Less frequently: yeast, pork, oats, beets, carrots, apples, chicken, lettuce, green beans, other legumes, rice, salmon, oysters, salicylate-containing foods (e.g., as in the rose/apple/apricot family, *though not all members will necessarily be involved*), and sulfite-containing foods. Chemical additives, such as food dyes, preservatives, insecticides and pesticides can also cause reactions.

Potential environmental allergens: plastics, pollens, dust, mold (as in air-conditioning systems), tobacco smoke, auto exhaust, moth balls, ammonia, rubber, textiles, perfumes, air fresheners, hair sprays, cosmetics, propellants, solvents, adhesives, gas/oil fuels, refrigerants, bleach, cleaning products, combustion products, carpeting and, even, pine or cedar.

Mental symptoms (PHILPOTT 1978, PFEIFFER 1987, 88, DOHAN 1969, MANDELL,1979, KROHN 1991, FAELTEN 1983, RANDOLPH 1979, KING 1981, RIPERRE 1984, RIX 1985, HERSHEY 1996)

- ☐ Radical mood shifts related to the time and content of meals. Emotions may swing from profound depression to mania and back in a single day. (PFEIFFER)
- ☐ Often, a sullen, tense, or irritable mood.
- ☐ Erratic variation in thought processes; trouble concentrating, confusion, perhaps hyperactivity, difficulty with school or work.
- ☐ Fatigue and insomnia.
- ☐ In some cases, dysperceptions, paranoia, thought disorder.

Physical symptoms (PFEIFFER 1987, 88, MANDELL 1979, KROHN 1991, FAELTEN 1983, RANDOLPH 1979, JAFFE 1992)

- ☐ Strong food likes and dislikes. Favorite foods tend to become addictions, and induce addictive behavior. Sugar craving is common.
- ☐ Rapid pulse, especially on exposure to the allergen.
- ☐ Acidosis, digestive complaints. Tends to resolve into difficulties metabolizing carbohydrates, proteins and/or lipids.
- ☐ Possibly, rashes, eczema, hayfever, asthma, frequent rapid colds, muscle aches, convulsions, numbness, neuralgia and headaches.

Allergic stages: from adaptation & addiction to chronic illness

Philpott (1978AB, 82) uses Hans Seyles' *General Adaptation Response to Stress* (See p. 252) to describe the allergic process:

Stage 1: Acute allergic response. Initial exposure to the allergen provokes intense reactions.

"No physician in any branch of medicine can be considered as an expert in his particular field until he becomes aware of the enormous scope of medical ecology."

Marshall Mandell, MD, 1969

"I have formulated a rule that works for me: if you do not understand something, it is probably due to an allergy. Everywhere I go in the US and Canada, and it has also happened in Australia and New Zealand, the natives say, 'This is allergy valley,' or 'This is hayfever hill.'"

Lendon Smith, MD

Definitions (MANDELL 1969)

The conventional medical definition of "allergens" recognizes only those substances which cause a typical antibody-antigen immune reaction in the blood.

Foods and environmental substances which don't produce this effect on the blood, may still cause typical allergic symptoms (e.g., histamine release, edema, swelling, itching, etc.), or other reactions, not classically identified as allergic.

The field of clinical ecology developed to address this oversight. Clinical ecologists treat classical allergies, as well as unconventional ones, labelling both "maladaptive responses."

In this text, the term "allergy" is similarly used to encompass both unconventional and classical allergies.

Landmark case (RANDOLPH 1979)

In 1949, Mary Hollister was referred to Dr Theron Randolph, MD, for incapacitating headaches, extreme hyperactivity, and spells of severe depression. She ate some beets she had brought with her om his office, and two hours later was hospitalized for psychosis. Subsequently, she became depressed, amnesiac, and disoriented. Randolph tested her for milk and got no reaction, but on beets she once again became psychotic.

This case began Randolph's groundbreaking investigations into the role of allergies in mental disorders.

Increased brain immune reactions in bipolars

Young (1993) found immunoreactivity significantly elevated in the prefrontal, temporal and occipital cortex of bipolars. Thomas (2004) reports immune inflammatory reactions in the anterior cingulate cortex, a brain region researchers increasingly link to bipolar illness. (See *Structure*, pp. 280-82.)

Stage 2: Chronic adaptation. Allergies become masked with repeated exposure. A let-down occurs, perhaps hours after consuming the al-lergen, producing such symptoms as headache, depression, nasal stuffiness, insomnia, etc. These are relieved on re-exposure, obscuring the source of symptoms, and making is seem that the allergen is what makes the patient feel good. Thus, many become addicted to foods to which they are allergic, foods which steadily undermine health.

Stage 3: Chronic illness. Long-term exposure eventually overrides adaptation (2). The body becomes worn out accommodating the allergen, and strong reactions resurface; now, as chronic illness.

Predisposing factors (PFEIFFER 1987, KROHN 1991, QUILLIN 1987, LEVINE 1983, LAMKIN 1981, LAWSON 1993)

Predisposing factors include hereditary tendencies, chronic stress, digestive disorders (e.g., leaky gut syndrome, celiac sprue, malabsorption, systemic Candida (which can produce multiple allergies), etc.), nutritional deficiencies, histamine imbalances, chronic exposure to mercury or other toxins, autoimmune illness, other immune dysfunction, and disorders of the thyroid, adrenals, pancreas, or liver.

Also, see box, below, *Mechanisms*.

Role of metal metabolism disorder (WALSH 1996)

Walsh points out that oxidative stress, caused by metal metabolism dysfunction and elevated pro-oxidant metals, can destroy key gut enzymes (including one which breaks down casein and gluten), and promote multiple food sensitivities, malabsorption, and digestion dysfunction.* Sensitivities often resolve with successful treatment, allowing the patient to eat a wider variety of foods.

See pp. 170-83.

Some mechanisms underlying mood/allergy connections

(1) Blood brain barrier permeability

Drs. Jaffe and Kruesi (1992) propose the following mechanism underlying cerebral immune reactions: Especially with illness, depression, stress, or physical damage, the blood brain barrier can be compromised. Potential neurotoxins in the blood (allergens and reacting antibodies, inflammation-producing kinins, Candida, heavy metals, etc.) can then enter the brain, setting the stage for cerebral allergies, and other immune reactions. Nutrient deficiencies, especially of antioxidants, augment barrier and immune susceptibility.

Cerebral immune reactions can radically alter thought and behavior by damaging neural structures, changing neural membrane electrical potentials, causing inflammation, reducing access to nutrition and oxygen, compromising the activity of regulatory enzymes, and unbalancing neurotransmitter production.

(2) Olfactory/limbic kindling

Iris Bell, MD, (1992) suggests the following model: A chemical smell interacts with the olfactory nerve, which goes on to stimulate the amygdala, hippocampus and other limbic structures. Mood disorder, anxiety, shyness, or panic would tend to augment reactivity. (SIMON) Repeated exposures may lead to subconvulsive limbic kindling in susceptible individuals,* thus creating a chemical sensitivity. Dopamine and other excitatory pathways may be stimulated; GABA inhibitory pathways, suppressed. Such reactions may distort mood and cognitive function; increase irritability, anxiety, and social withdrawal; and create autonomic, endocrine and immune problems. Pronounced exposure may produce electrophysiological lesions which *permanently* alter neurotransmitter (and so affective and cognitive) reactions to chemical exposure.

(3) Other conditions which may kindle chemical sensitivity (MEGGS 1993, *EV HEALTH PERSPECTIVES* 1995, LANE 1997)

The following conditions, prevalent in bipolars, may help kindle chemical sensitivity (CS) and associated mood symptoms:

Depletion or damage to EFAs (as in Candida, pyroluria, bipolar disorder), compromising membrane flexibility and allergen discrimination.

Candida (prevalent in bipolars), via its toxic byproducts, acetaldehyde and ethanol. (LANE 1997)

Increased catecholamines (as in pyroluria, porphyrias, histapenia, mania), promoting kindling.

Increased corticosteroids and neuropeptides (common in bipolar disorder, headaches, fibromyalgia, asthma), fostering neural inflammation.

Allergy tests

(I) Gentler tests for hyper-reactive patients

The following types of tests are especially useful for patients who may react too severely to test meals with an allergen (e.g., patients with unstable medical conditions). Avoiding potential allergens prior to testing increases accuracy.

History — a review of clinical and dietary history (a food diary is often helpful) may give sufficient clues to determine the nature of the allergy. If not, further testing is indicated.

ELISA ACT — a lymphocyte response assay, which picks up stage 2 delayed responses. It evaluates IgA, IgG, IgM; cell-mediated reactions; and immune complexes. The test is reported to be 98% accurate, and can be used to measure reactions to foods, drugs, heavy metals, and environmental substances. (JAFFE 1992)

RAST — a blood test which measures IgE antibody-antigen response to individual allergens. (JAFFE 1992, WEINTRAUB 1995)

Electro-acupuncture techniques (EAV) — the substance to be tested is placed in a DC electrical circuit which includes the patient's hand, a specific acupuncture point, and a machine which measures galvanic skin response. This test has also been used to indicate physiological imbalances, and to give some indication of physical response to specific nutrients, herbs, homeopaths, etc. (WEINTRAUB 1995, ALI 1989, KROP 1985, 97, TSUEI 1984)

Kinesiology — decreases in muscle strength are used as a measure of allergic response. Results vary with the skill of the practitioner.

Coca pulse test — in one version, the individual fasts overnight, then is tested on a single food (small quantities) per hour. Changes in pulse rate can indicate allergic reaction. This test is not definitive, but can provide some preliminary indications of maladaptive response, and is relatively simple to administer. *Contraindicated for some.* (COCA 1994, NULL 1988)

(II) Tests which can evoke strong reactions

Warning: Extended pretest diets revert chronic allergic responses to acute reactions, like those evoked during early exposure (see p. 207). Reactions to trial meals may be too extreme for sensitive patients, though, if not contraindicated, strong reactions often underscore the importance of avoiding the allergen. Other contraindications include heart conditions, asthma, epilepsy, porphyria, diabetes, a history of severe or life-threatening mental symptoms, marked debilitated states, etc. (MANDELL 1969, 79, PFEIFFER 1987, RANDOLPH 1965)

Choice of pretest diet (PHILPOTT 1978, PFEIFFER 1987, MANDELL 1979, MESSER 1976, HOFFER 1983A)

The following choices should be made according to individual requirements and contraindications:

Fast, drinking only water.

Fast, drinking only neutral herbal teas.

Fast on non-allergenic vegetable (and perhaps fruit*) juices and water.

"Caveman" diet.

Single-food-per-meal rotation diet.**

During the pretest diet, it's helpful to avoid implicated environmental toxins and to quit smoking, if possible, as such exposures keep the individual in an allergic reactive stage, which can compromise test results.

Testing begins after four to nine days of the diet, approximately the time needed for withdrawal symptoms to subside. The pulse should be slowed and stabilized; tongue coating, cleared; and weakness, aches, chills, excess perspiration and other symptoms, abated. Psychological and musculoskeletal symptoms may be slow to clear. Paranoia or chronic depression sometimes persist.

* Not indicated if hypoglycemic, or if blood sugar is unstable.

** This diet consists of foods known to be non-allergenic for that person, or, if unknown, foods seldom eaten (e.g, perhaps, peas, rice, carrots, pears, lamb, celery, etc.). Each meal consists of a single food. If the patient reacts to it, the reaction is cleared, and the food is no longer offered. Each day, a different family of foods is presented, and then not given for at least a four-day sequence.

Choices for test procedure (MANDELL 1969, 79, PHILPOTT 1978, 79, 82, PFEIFFER 1987, 88, RANDOLPH 1965, 79, KROHN 1991, FAELTEN 1983, HOFFER 1983A)

Single test meals — meals consist of a single suspected allergen (one food/meal), three to four test meals/day, rotating food families (e.g., wheat, fish, dairy (cow), corn, dairy (goat), poultry, etc). Suspected synergistic effects (e.g., corn/beets, wheat/dairy) can also be tested, as well as reactions to cooked, raw, or non-organic foods; food additives; etc.

Serial dilutions — varying proportions of liquid dilutions of the allergen are placed under the tongue, where they are rapidly absorbed through blood capillaries into the bloodstream. Most dilutions evoke reactions, but a specific dilution (neutralizing dose) can usually be found which will block allergic response.

See *Neutralization*, next page.

Sniff test — airborne allergens, e.g., perfumes, gasoline, etc. (which were avoided, to the degree possible, during the pretest diet period) are tested, one at a time.

Intradermal tests — a liquid extract of the suspected allergen is injected sufficiently deeply into the skin to be circulated by the blood to all tissues. This test is most useful in assessing non-food allergies.

Warning: Severe reactions may occur when a restricted diet or fast is broken with allergens. The body has been made more vulnerable, and is being confronted by acute allergic stimulation. Reactions can be more intense than previously experienced. Mental and physical response must be carefully monitored by the physician. Susceptible and unstable patients require milder tests.

Clearing a reaction (PHILPOTT 1978, 79, 82, MANDELL 1979, KROHN 1991, HOFFER 1983, RIORDAN 1995)

To neutralize a strong reaction or get the patient ready for the next test, physicians may use: vitamin C powder [Philpott suggests 1-2 teaspoons, 3x/day if needed],

Allergy tests *continued*

plus (to clear the acidity) sodium bicarbonate (baking soda) and/or potassium bicarbonate [Weintraub (1995) suggests two heaping tablespoons of baking soda and one of potassium bicarbonate in two cups of water.]. To end strong histamine reactions, Hoffer suggests niacin and C.

Caution: Antihistamines, adrenalin and other relevant medical supplies should always be available to prevent anaphylactic shock. Testing should be abandoned to prevent or halt uncontrollable life or property-threatening behavior, medical flareups, or severe or prolonged reactions.

Reactions can be measured by

Behavioral and physical response (e.g., depression, headache, anxiety, diarrhea, bloating, palpitations).

Patient perceptions. A symptom diary is useful.

Pulse at 30, 60, & 90 minutes after the trial, and when symptoms occur. (COCA)

Blood immune reactions. Food antibodies include IgG (immunoglobulin G) and IgM.

Tests for complicating conditions (PFEIFFER 1987, RANDOLPH 1965, MANDELL 1979, PFEIFFER 1988, JAFFE 1992, WEINTRAUB 1995)

24-hr aminos — for metabolic and enzyme disorder.

Sugar metabolism status. Protein and lipid metabolism may also be distorted.

Hair analysis — helps identify heavy metal toxicity, mineral deficiencies, electrolyte imbalances. (Potassium and magnesium may be low; copper or sodium, high.)

Urinary and blood nutrient and enzyme assays.

Urinary pyrroles, blood histamine, basophil count.

Metal metabolism dysfunction, Candida, parasites, celiac sprue; and thyroid, adrenal, liver, digestive, and autoimmune disorders.

Extreme reactions

If not experienced in clinical ecology, patient reactions to allergic exposure may challenge credibility. Thus:

Dr. Green's patient describes his reactions to test exposures: "Peas made me very tense and I couldn't talk to people... White fish ... made my mind race and I couldn't hold on to thoughts... Pork sausage made me disorientated, insecure, lose track of who I was, and made my muscles feel rubbery... Cottage cheese made people feel miles away and I became extremely introverted." (GREEN 1985)

Dr. Theron Randolph (1965) describes a patient, D.M., who became depressed when exposed to automobile exhaust, but learned to limit exposure enough to minimize reactions. During a vacation, she slept in a recently painted room, and saw purple frogs hopping around and a lion sitting on her bed. On the bus ride home, a gorilla hugged her whenever she tried to sleep. She now maintains mental equilibrium by deliberately avoiding chemicals to which she is sensitive.

Treatment (MANDELL 1969, 79, PHILPOTT 1978, 82, 87, HOFFER 1983, 87, PFEIFFER 1987, 88, DOHAN 1969, RANDOLPH 1965, 71, KROHN 1991, COTT 1974, REES 1973, FAELTEN 1983, QUILLIN 1987, HORROBIN 1989, BALCH 1990, LEVIN 1983, MURRAY 1995, 98, LEVINE, 1983)

Choices must be tailored to individual biochemical requirements.

Dietary measures

- ☐ Adopt a four to seven day rotation diet. Food families (e.g., dairy, legume, crucifer, nightshade, mint, heath, alum, etc.) are grouped into distinct days, with no repetition til the next cycle. (ROCKWELL 1996)
- ☐ Abundant freshly-made, nonallergenic vegetable juices* can help resupply minerals and enzymes and support overall health. Tailor to individual health concerns. Rotation, as above, may be indicated.
- ☐ Decrease chemical load, (REA) and avoid fixed food allergens. (RAPP 1991) Prolonged abstinence may make it possible to eat variable allergens sparingly and infrequently, or perhaps as part of a rotation diet.
- ☐ Watch for new allergies. A food diary can help.

* Concentrate on high mineral, low sugar vegetables, such as parsley, celery, chard. Wheat or barley grass are often good choices. Cabbage family vegetables are good with overactive thyroid, or other overstimulation, but can be detrimental with low thyroid, or depression. Carrots, beets, or other sweet vegetables, should be less than half of the content and may necessitate additional water. Blue green algae, or other such supplements can help provide amino acids. Relevant herbs can be added. Be careful not to destabilize blood sugar or aggravate Candida. Do not include known or suspected allergens.

Neutralization

This approach may be especially indicated for allergens which can't be avoided or which cause severe reactions. A specific dilution is uniquely determined (*see previous page*), which does not cause the patient to react, but neutralizes response to the allergen. It's administered sublingually or, for nonfood allergens, intradermally, typically several times weekly. (WEINTRAUB 1995, WUNDERLICH,1976, RAPP 1991)

Other desensitization techniques

- ☐ Enzyme-potentiated desensitization, using beta-glucaronidase with the allergen to modify helper/suppressor T-cell ratios. (EGGER 1992)
- ☐ Acupressure or acupuncture combined with densensitization approaches.
- ☐ Psychological techniques, such as NLP, perhaps combined with other treatments.
- ☐ Philpott (1978, 79, 80, 87) suggests training out psychologically-induced allergies with injections of needed nutrients (e.g., C, B complex and adrenal cortical extract; or B6, calcium, magnesium; *as applicable*).
- ☐ Homeopathy, perhaps in conjunction with EAV (*see p. 209*).

Supplements (PHILPOTT 1978, PFEIFFER 1987, 88, QUILLIN 1987, HORROBIN 1979, HOFFER 1983, BALCH 1990, MURRAY 1992, 95, WEINTRAUB 1995, ROGERS 1997)

Treatment choices must reflect individual biochemical requirements, including biotype-based contraindications.

- □ C — antihistamine, supports immunity. [1000 mg, time-release, 2-6x/day, and to counter symptoms]
- □ Bioflavonoids — antihistamine; support immune function. (Hesperidin, quercetin and catechins, particularly, have been used to reduce allergic reactions. Bromelain supports their absorption.)
- □ B6 — aids assimilation, supports neurological function. [Typically, 50 to 200 mg; more with pyroluria and certain other conditions. (PFEIFFER 87, 88)]
- □ B1— supports metabolic and neurological functioning.
- □ B3 — antioxidant; supports circulation, sugar balance, and brain metabolism; may reduce limbic kindling. (HOFFER 1983)
- □ Pantothenic acid (B5) & potassium — support the adrenals.
- □ B complex — supports vitamin C activity, nervous and immune function, digestion and assimilation.
- □ Zinc — supports immune function and sugar metabolism.
- □ Manganese — supports use of B and C, and helps regulate blood sugar.
- □ Chromium — critical to pancreatic production of insulin.
- □ Trial of taurine, GABA, B3, tryptophan, choline, inositol, melatonin, or other inhibitors, (LEWIS, LANE 1997) *as relevant*, to reduce limbic kindling.
- □ Calcium, magnesium — decrease histamine; may reduce stress.
- □ Vitamins E, (PFEIFFER) A, carotenes — support immune activity.
- □ Omega 3 fish oil — improves food tolerance, discriminatory membrane permeability, and mood stability. Reduces anxiety, inflammation. *Take with selenium, E, other antioxidants, and B vitamins, perhaps lecithin.* (RUDIN 1981, 82, 87) *Pyrolurics often do better with an emphasis on GLA.*
- □ MSM (methylsulfonylmethane) — supplies sulfur, which is often deficient and sometimes benefits allergic symptoms. (Vitamin C supports absorption.) (WEINTRAUB 1995)
- □ Molybdenum — may similarly be helpful.
- □ Methionine or SAMe — *if* methylation is depressed (e.g., in histadelia). *Contraindicated for histapenics.*
- □ Glutamine — to support intestinal integrity, *if indicated. Can be overstimulating.*
- □ Butyric acid — to support gut regeneration, *if indicated.* (WEINTRAUB 1995)
- □ CoQ-10 — increases oxygen, energy, immunity; antioxidant.
- □ Germanium — increases oxygen availability, supports immunity.
- □ Copper and/or iron — *if deficient,* intake may provide benefit. *Use only if not contraindicated due to biotype, oxidative assault, or other factors.*
- □ Spirulina — lowers IgE and normalizes some allergic sensitivities, (WEINTRAUB 1995) *but can be overstimulating and detrimental if prone to mania or paranoia; or if copper is elevated.*
- □ Free-form aminos, especially with depression and malabsorption. *Reconsider if multi-aminos are competing with specific required aminos for absorption.*
- □ Herbs (immune, liver, kidney support) — possibilities include nettles, red clover, dandelion root, burdock root, pau d'arco (taheebo), schizandra berries, astragalus, milk thistle, cayenne, elder berries,

Turning love on & off

"Henry, seventeen years old, had been mentally ill for three years. Prior use of tranquilizers, psychotherapy, and electric shock did not succeed in helping him appreciably. He believed that people were out to kill him, and [attacked other people]. He was placed on a fast... He remained mentally ill until the fourth day, at which time his symptoms cleared... He telephoned his parents, saying, 'I love you. Please come and see me.' On the fifth day... he was fed a meal containing wheat only. Within an hour, he began to feel strange and unreal; within an hour and a half he thought people were going to kill him. He telephoned his parents again, saying, 'I hate you. You caused my illness. I don't want to ever see you again.' Further testing confirmed the fact that when specific foods were withheld, his symptoms cleared, and when given wheat again, the same paranoid reaction occurred consistently."

William Philpott, MD (1987)

Psychotic reactions to nightshades (TORREY 1980, 88, WALSH 1974, MALZBERG 1936)

Some patients are particularly sensitive to the solanaceae (nightshade) family, which includes potatoes, peppers, eggplant, tomatoes, tobacco, Jimson weed and morning glory. This family is known for its propensity to induce psychotropic effects, perhaps due to solanine or dopachrome content. Arthritic and gastrointestinal reactions are also common.

Solanine forms in potatoes exposed to light; older potatoes have greater quantities. In high enough concentrations, it has been shown to induce hallucinations and other symptoms of psychosis. Such reactions may be due to toxicity, sensitivity, or both. In one study, described by Maryellen Walsh, MD, pregnant marmosets fed blighted, discolored potatoes were observed to have offspring who could not be weaned, engaged in abnormal play patterns, and generally behaved in a manner suggestive of psychosis.

Environmental assault

"In a typical household... people wake up on synthetic foam rubber mattresses, snuggled between cotton polyester sheets and acrylic blankets... put on their drip-dry robes and acrylic slippers... brush their teeth with plastic toothbrushes, using artificially colored and flavored toothpaste. Hot water fills the air with chlorine fumes mingled with the perfumed scents of the soap, shampoo, and the plastic shower curtain. She applies some chemical dyes to her face, he 'purifies' his breath with aerosol spray.

They dress in polyester, mothproofed wool, and no-iron cotton and then sit down to breakfast. The eggs, sizzling in a Teflon pan, are full of hormones... the bacon is preserved in nitrites, the grapefruit was grown with synthetic pesticides and fertilizers; the English muffins have been processed with flavorings, extenders, and emulsifiers; and they've all been packaged in polyethylene and stored in refrigerators insulated with polyurethane and cooled by chlorofluorocarbons."

Alan Scott Levin, MD, 1983

RECOMMENDED READING

Rogers, Sherry, MD, *Depression: Cured at Last*, 1997.

Mandell, Marshall, MD, *Dr. Mandell's 5 Day Allergy Relief System*, 1979.

Philpott, William, MD, *Brain Allergies: The Psychonutrient Connection*, 1987.

Krohn, Jaqueline, MD, *The Whole Way to Allergy Relief and Prevention*, 1991.

Levin, Alan Scott, MD, *Type 1, Type 2 Allergy Relief System*, 1983.

Weintraub, Skye, ND, *Minding Your Body*, 1995.

Hunter, Beatrice T, *Gluten Intolerance*.

nettles, buchu, parsley, possibly Siberian or American ginseng, noni. *Consult herbal literature for details, and contraindications.*

- ☐ Injections of needed nutrients, *with particular attention to contraindications*, are sometimes indicated with absorption problems. (RIORDAN 1995)

Address confounding conditions

- ☐ Histamine (methylation) imbalances.
- ☐ Pyroluria or porphyria.
- ☐ Electrolyte imbalances.
- ☐ Metal metabolism dysfunction. Mercury and other metal toxicity.
- ☐ Digestive disorders: malabsorption, leaky gut syndrome,* Candida, intestinal parasites, etc.
- ☐ Mood disorders. Chronic catecholamine or neuropeptide elevation.
- ☐ Neural inflammation or certain other nervous system problems.
- ☐ Hormone imbalance. (Support adrenal balance and moderate stress. Support thyroid, spleen, liver, thymus, etc., *as relevant.* Testosterone may offer some protection from allergic sensitization *if actually depleted, and indicated.** (BELL 1992, LANE 1997) *Check the literature for contraindications, and consult with your physician.*
- ☐ Immune dysfunction, and other health issues.

* Incompletely digested protein entering the bloodstream, and treated as a foreign invaders, can initiate or aggravate allergies.

** Otherwise, it can promote mania, violence, and other extreme reactions, and should be avoided.

Lifestyle support

Supernutrition (fresh whole foods, organic, if feasible; no junk food), adequate rest, regular exercise.

Limit stressors and exposure to environmental toxins.

Clearing from food allergies and addictive reactions often increases awareness of the environment. However, vulnerability to stress may also increase, and the unfamiliarity of suddenly being well may pose problems. Friendly encouragement and support can be helpful. (HUMISTON 1979)

Antihistamines

Pfeiffer warns that though antihistamine meds may reduce insomnia and other symptoms, sustained intake tends to be counterproductive.

Outcome (MANDELL 1979, KROHN 1991, COTT 1974, HOFFER 1983, 87, PHILPOTT 1978, 82, 87)

Ninety per cent of allergies are variable. Many patients recover enough, after avoiding the offending food and taking supportive nutrients for about six months, to be able to occasionally eat small portions. Greater exposure may reactivate the allergy, and could again facilitate chronic adaptation, without the patient realizing it.

Foods which still cause reactions after six months of avoidance usually must be permanently removed from the diet.

Reminder: The information in this book is presented for educational purposes only. No product or service endorsement is intended. If you need treatment for allergies, sensitivities, celiac sprue, bipolar disorder, or any other medical condition, please seek the services of a knowledgeable physician.

Wheat & milk reactions

The majority of the world population seems to possess some sensitivity to wheat and certain other grains, and/or to dairy, especially when a mainstay of the diet. Many people react to both. The culprits are usually gluten (a mucilaginous protein contained in wheat, rye, spelt, barley) and casein (a glue-like protein found in dairy).

Mental symptoms (PFEIFFER 1987, 88, SINGH 1976, RIX 1985, DAVIES 1987)

Sensitivity is generally more pronounced, in psychiatric populations and can contribute significantly to symptoms. (PFEIFFER 1987, PHILPOTT 1974) Walsh (2008) finds gluten sensitivity is the *primary* imbalance in 5% of bipolars and, in many others, implicated to a lesser extent.

Reactions to gluten or casein can include profound depression, alienation, weeping, mania, moodswing, compulsive ritualistic behavior, anxiety, hyperactivity, problems learning to speak, introversion, and psychosis (but not usually paranoia). Such effects may be relatively constant, or occur only after eating dairy or glutenous grain. (CIACCI 1998, DOHAN 1969, 84, SINGH 1976, HUNTER 1987)

Natural approaches (gluten intolerance) (WALSH 2006, 07, MURRAY 1991)

Allergy treatments — see previous pages.

Walsh's suggestions — Look for and redress any accompanying metal metabolism dysfunction, and oxidative stress (e.g., due to mercury; or low zinc, glutathione, SOD, or NAC, etc.). Zinc is critical to small intestine enzymes which metabolize casein and gluten. Zinc, and MT support (*if indicated*) often improve sensitivities, allowing patients to eat a wider variety of food.

Murray's suggestions — Eliminate all sources of gluten, including wheat, rye, barley, and spelt, and, possibly, oats,* millet, amaranth, and buckwheat. Other sources include many processed foods, imitation cheeses, MSG, hydrolyzed vegetable protein (TVP or HVP), malt, and certain pharmaceutical products. Dairy often must also be avoided. Some must also avoid beef.

Treat associated nutrient imbalances. A good multi-vitamin/mineral and free-form aminos may be helpful, if not contraindicated.

If improvement does not occur within a month or so, search for gluten or casein still in the diet. Eventually, some patients may be able to eat small amounts of dairy (especially with added lactase), or occasional small quantites of glutenous grains (especially with papain [0.5-1.0 gm.], with meals (MESSER 1964)). Others must eliminate gluten, and perhaps dairy, permanently. (MURRAY 1998)

Common confounding disorders — Thyroid, adrenal, methylation, MT, and pyrrole disorders; Candida, blood sugar imbalances.

* Although whole oats are often acceptable, if not processed on the same equipment as wheat.

Case study: Moodswing & wheat

Davies (1987) reports on a 32-year-old female with ten years of severe mood swings, who improved markedly, within two months, on a diet restricted to fruit, vegetables, rice, meat and fish. Three days after eating wheat bread, she became severely depressed. Once she resumed the therapeutic diet, six to eight weeks passed before former improvement was reinstated.

Possible mechanisms (HORROBIN 1979, ZIOUDROU 1979, WASHBURN 1990, ASHKENAZI 1979, MYCROFT 1982, HEMMINGS 1977, RIX 1985)

The following mechanisms have been proposed to explain the gluten/casein influence on mood:

Immune reactions contribute to mania, depression, and cycling.

Malabsorption may reduce nutrient availability, compromising brain function.

Exorphins* formed in digesting casein and gluten, may compete with the body's endorphins, causing mood disturbance.**

Digestion produces an amino acid sequence which may enhance dopamine activity and create EEG changes.

Metal metabolism problems may underly both allergies and bipolar symptoms. (WALSH 2006)

* Chemicals taken in from outside the body, which, like the body's endorphins, produce morphine-like effects.

** Check for urinary opiate peptides. (William Shaw)

Reaction to meds

People with gluten/casein sensitivities do not tend to recover with conventional psychiatric treatment (which fails to address the cause). (PFEIFFER 1987, 88)

Gluten & celiac sprue (PFEIFFER 1988, JAFFE 1992, HUNTER 1987, DEAN, 1975. ASHKENAZI 1979, MURRAY 1991)

In celiac/sprue the digestive tract is irritated by gluten, and becomes smooth, with the villi flattened. Absorption of nutrients into the blood becomes severely compromised, diminishing the supply of antioxidants, precursors to various neurotransmitters, and other nourishment for the brain.

Glutenous grain often induces depression and other mood symptoms, which abate when gluten is avoided. (DEAN 1975, CIACCI 1998) The associated malnutrition can also contribute to mental symptoms.

Physical symptoms include weight loss; pale, bulky, fatty, odorous stool; and elevated serum gliadin antibodies.

Whenever the celiac eats foods with gluten, symptoms emerge, either immediately, or over a period of several weeks. Intestinal villi may appear recovered, but allow gluten to pass into the bloodstream, leaving the celiac susceptible to para-anaphylactic shock.

Sugar imbalances

"I was... suffering from severe hypoglycemia... Any degree of excitement... [caused] me to tremble, turn blue, and faint as my nervous system responded to a sudden dangerous plummet in my blood sugar level. Every step on the way down was a step by step change in my conscious awareness of my surroundings... in response to this condition, my body was releasing its own adrenalin, causing me to speed up, which I usually channeled into the [illusionary] character of Carol."

Donna Williams, 1992

Brain sugar & mood state

Blood sugar imbalances may be localized to the brain, with brain glucose levels not necessarily reflecting body blood sugar status.

Brain sugar messages may be increased in mania,* or sensitivity to insulin enhanced, with glucose burning more rapidly** in certain regions. (MOORE 1998)

Depression, on the other hand, may reflect reduced glucose messages (MOORE 1998) or relative insulin resistance. Lack of fuel during depression may sensitize neurons, perhaps contributing to over-reactivity to sugar during mania. (HENINGER 1970)

Bipolars often have a history of low brain blood sugar, (MURRAY 1995B) or altered cellular insulin metabolism. They may also be more susceptible to diabetes (chronic high blood sugar).***

* Perhaps, in part, explaining why fasting has benefitted some manias. (Cott 1974)
** Thus PET scans suggest increased glucose metabolism.
*** Neuroleptics and certain other bipolar meds have also been associated with increased diabetes.

Allergic addiction & sugar

"Any food or chemical which is frequently eaten or encountered has the potential of becoming addictive; and... any addictive substance can radically alter sugar levels. If your problems, therefore, were originally related to intake of carbohydrates, and you eliminate them in favor of eating a very-high protein diet — say, two to four eggs every day — it is very likely that within a few months or less those eggs, even though they are a superior food, loaded with many nutrients and previously caused no symptoms, will make you feel very sick again... The key points to remember are: (1) recognition of allergic specificity; (2) elimination of any incriminating substances... for two to four months; and (3) rotation of all foods."

William H Philpott, MD, 1987

Effects of too much dietary sugar & junk starch (PFEIFFER 1987, CURRIER 1979, MURRAY 1995, 98, BUCKLEY 1978, PHILPOTT 1978B, DUFY 1975)

The body is evolutionarily accustomed to handling small quantities of slowly-released glucose. Unrefined complex carbohydrates (in legumes, other vegetables, whole grains, seeds and nuts) release sugar slowly, at a pace the body should be able to handle, and also contain nutrients (B6, other B vitamins, C; zinc, chromium, manganese, potassium, magnesium, calcium, phosphorus, etc.) required in processing sugar. Thus, such foods help maintain balanced blood and brain glucose.

Refined sugars and starches (sugar, candy, soda, white breads, pastas, pastries, etc.) are absorbed too quickly, overstimulating and sensitizing the pancreas, and depleting nutrients which regulate and metabolize sugar. Very high fat or protein meals can also contribute to the sugar burden. *Eventually the following conditions may develop:*

Hypoglycemia — With extended intake of refined sugars and starches, all meals may overstimulate insulin, causing cells to absorb and use sugar too quickly. Fasting insulin rises. The adrenals become exhausted by the constant demand for insulin antagonists. Chronic high insulin, or insufficient insulin antagonists, leads to chronic low blood sugar, i.e., hypoglycemia. To feel more comfortable, the individual tends to crave more sugar, creating a vicious cycle, and perhaps, eventually leading to Type II diabetes.

Type II diabetes — Sugar also increases fasting cholesterol and triglycerides, and disturbs fat metabolism and transport, making people fat. Increased tissue fat, makes insulin less efficient, so blood sugar rises. With time, receptors lose sensitivity to insulin, resulting in chronically high blood sugar, i.e., Type II diabetes. (MURRAY 1998)

Compromised neural receptors — by altering the balance of fats available to the brain, sugar affects the composition and activity of phospholipids in neural membranes and receptors.

Candida — Sugar stimulates secretion of cortisol (SMITH 1998, CHRISTENSEN 1988) which suppresses immune response,* and allows Candida to proliferate. Candida augments the sugar craving, and further compromises mood and ability to handle stress.

Increased susceptibility to mania — A high sugar diet stimulates secretion of epinephrine (JONES 1995) and norepinephrine. This generally increases energy, pulse, (SMITH 1998, CHRISTENSEN 1988) neural activation, and suceptibility to stress and mania.**(MOORE 1998) Insulin's enhancement of serotonin availability to the brain may also elevate mood. (GOODWIN 1990)

Depression, exhaustion — As blood sugar drops, lack of brain fuel can lead to depression. With too extreme a drop, glucose may be obtained through ketosis,*** which turns proteins and keto acids into glucose, wasting muscles and otherwise depleting and weakening body tissue, promoting exhaustion.

* Sugar, cortisol, and stress suppress immune reponse, antibody production, lymphocyte effectiveness, and phagocytosis, (Smith 1998) fostering Candida proliferation.

** On the other hand, very low blood sugar (perhaps caused by low cortisol) can stimulate a profuse outflow of adrenalin to compensate, similarly fostering mania or violence.

***A process also activated during fasting and starvation.

Prevention

Move away from quick-digesting sweets

□ *Eliminate refined carbohydrates:* e.g., soda, candy, most pastries, other foods containing sugar or white flour, and alcohol.

□ *Instead, try:* honey, maple syrup, blackstrap molasses, rice syrup, canned or bottled fruit juice, dry fruit (dates, figs, raisins).

□ *And progressively move toward more optimal sweets:*
Agave. Stevia. Bee pollen *(only if not allergic).*

Modest portions of fresh whole fruits, moving toward those low on the glycemic index. Eat with seeds, nuts, yogurt, kefir, *as appropriate.*

Some substitutes for refined carbs

INSTEAD OF SODA — sparkling water with fruit juice (freshly made; the less sweet, the better), lemon water, or herb teas.

INSTEAD OF CHOCOLATE CANDY — cacao nibs, carob, tamarind, green tea. Enough magnesium, C, and protein (but small portions per meal).

SUBSTITUTIONS IN MAKING PASTRY — *instead of refined sugar, try:* cinnamon, agave, banana, other fruit, apple sauce, soaked raisins, etc.; *instead of white flour, try:* whole grains or steel cut oats, freshly ground (coffee grinders work well); *instead of oils or hydrogenated fat, try:* butter or coconut oil.

Work toward a diet which prevents insulin spikes (MURRAY 1995, BLAND, PFEIFFER 1987)

Tailor to individual biochemical requirements. Generally:

□ Whole complex carbohydrates, e.g., vegetables (squash, etc.), legumes and whole grains (presoaked before cooking). Avoid refined carbs.

□ Moderate portions of protein each meal (perhaps 5-6 small meals per day). Determine optimal balance of animal foods versus grain/legumes.

□ Plenty of fresh vegetables and salads. Low-glycemic vegetable juices. Soups (minimally cooked). Some low-glycemic fruit.

□ Modest intake of seeds, nuts, or nut butters (not roasted).

□ Most cooking herbs. Nutritional yeast. Perhaps seaweeds.

□ Water from healthful sources. Herb teas, *as relevant to individual needs.*

For further details see *Diet,* pp. 217, 222, 254-56.

Other support

Relevant supplements, sufficient sleep, moderate daily exercise, relaxation. Avoid stimulants, eliminate toxins.

"The brain does not store glucose, its major source of fuel, and so requires a continual supply, up to 25% of what's available to the body. Too much or too little alters hormone and neurotransmitter activity, and can profoundly influence mood."

Walter Lemmo, ND

Violence (PFEIFFER 1987, SCHLAUSS 1973, ADAMS 1973)

"Fighting makes one feel better."

Saying of the Quolla people

In a remote village in Peru, half the heads of household were in one way or another involved in homicide. Incidence of assault, robbery, rape, arson and divorce was high. Low blood sugar was prevalent. Their diet revolved around sporadic barley and oats, with alcohol and kola nuts.

The Quolla people of the Andes have been called the most violent people in the world. Researchers determined that the lower their blood sugar, the greater their hostility. It has been suggested that the associated adrenalin rush, which increases sugar available to blood and brain, may play a part in the violence.

Relax as you improve your diet

Being too strict* during the switch to healthier foods can be self-defeating. The most effective approach tends to be to ease into it step-by-step. Pay attention to how you feel when you support your health. Observe the effects of any lapses, without berating yourself. Over time, you will naturally prefer the healthier foods.

* Unless medically mandated.

Hypoglycemia

Contributory factors (PFEIFFER 1987, CURRIER 1979, MURRAY 1998, BUCKLEY 1978, LESSER, PHILPOTT 1978B, AIROLA 1974, TENNEY 1987)

- ☐ Prolonged stress.
- ☐ Junk food diet. Nutritional imbalances. Fasting, starvation. (PRANGE 1987)
- ☐ Poor absorption. Candida.
- ☐ Addictions and allergies, particularly fixed allergies. (E.g., sugar, alcohol, coffee, tobacco, dairy, wheat, food coloring, chlorine, etc.)
- ☐ Exhausted adrenals, insulin-secreting pancreatic tumors, enlarged pancreas.
- ☐ Insulin overload, mild diabetes (reactive hypoglycemia) after carbohydrate-rich meals. (PRANGE 1987)
- ☐ Low thyroid, pituitary, etc.
- ☐ Heavy metal toxicity (lead, cadmium, mercury, arsenic, etc.). (WALSH 2006)
- ☐ Liver damage due to toxins or enzyme defects.
- ☐ Neurosis, brain tumors, encephalitis, certain other CNS problems.
- ☐ Immune dysfunction. Asthma. Infectious disease, especially if minerals become depleted.
- ☐ Steroids, oral contraceptives, salicylates, quinine.

Chronic low blood sugar (hypoglycemia) decreases brain fuel and energy production, and undermines the brain's ability to function. Hypoglycemia thus compromises emotional balance, mental clarity, and perception, and can foster both mania and depression. Lesser (2008) finds it prevalent in bipolar disorder, especially if chronic or severe.

Walsh reports that of 20,000 psychiatric patients treated with biotype therapies, a significant percentage had chronic low blood sugar. The hypoglycemia can trigger profound mood and cognitive symptoms, usually intermittent, in relation to the timing of meals, exposure to stress, etc.

Mental symptoms (PFEIFFER 1987, CURRIER 1979, TENNEY 1987, MURRAY 1995, 98, ROSS 1989, PAGE 1993, LARSON 2001, 08, BALCH 1990, QUILLIN 1987, STEIN 1992, PRANGE 1987, GOLD 1987, CHRISTENSEN 1988)

- ☐ Late afternoon blues, uncontrollable crying spells. Lack of goals or inspiration. One in five experience a suicidal depression.
- ☐ Anxiety, fear, tension, nervous headaches, irritability, disruptive outbursts, strong temper, hostility. Hypomania. (MOORE 1998) Moodswing. Rapid cycling. (LARSON 2008)
- ☐ Confusion (especially after stress), difficulty concentrating, indecisiveness, forgetfulness, poor memory.
- ☐ Nightmares. Difficulty getting and staying asleep.
- ☐ In some, visual dysperceptions, personality changes, bizarre behavior, social withdrawal, periodic paranoid psychosis.
- ☐ Symptoms improve after meals, worsen when meals are late. (ROSS 1989)

Physical symptoms (PFEIFFER, 1987, CURRIER 1979, MURRAY 1995, 98, PAGE 1993, LESSER, BALCH 1990, QUILLIN 1987, STEIN 1992, GOLD 1987, COUSENS 2001, LARSON 2001)

- ☐ Drowsy after meals. Fatigue, exhaustion, weak spells, fainting.
- ☐ Shakiness, trembling (internal or external); in some, convulsions.
- ☐ Sugar, starch, or alcohol craving. Hunger.
- ☐ Thirst, especially after carbohydrate-rich meals, or stress.
- ☐ Low temperature. Cold hands and feet. Cold sweats. Night sweats.
- ☐ Numbness, crawling sensation under the skin.
- ☐ Muscle cramps or spasms. Unexplained aches and pains.
- ☐ Constipation, ulcers, other GI complaints. In some, enlarged liver.
- ☐ Slurred speech, unsteady gait, incoordination.
- ☐ Blurred vision, double images, sensitivity to light.

Lab (PFEIFFER 1987, ROSS 1989, PHILPOTT 1978B, 82, GOLD 1987)

Diet, symptom, and family history — may afford enough confirmation to make further testing unnecessary.

Home testing — measures sugar during a symptomatic episode. Reflects real eating conditions. (GILASSON 1991)

Glucose tolerance test — a sugar solution is given after a 12-hr fast. Blood samples are ideally taken every 30-60 min, or when symptoms occur, or on request, over the next 4-5 hrs. Beside insulin and sugar, it may be useful to monitor pulse, blood pressure, NAD, ATP, salt, symptoms, subjective impressions (e.g., a symptom diary). Sugar should rise slowly, then fall gradually to fasting level. A flat, saw tooth, or precipitously falling curve indicates hypoglycemia. *This test helps map the hypoglycemia and confirm diagnosis, but can be too stressful, and is no longer used much.*

Additional tests (PFEIFFER 1987, 88)

Allergy tests. Candida antibodies.

Endocrine tests — especially thyroid and adrenals.

Hair analysis — especially, levels of chromium, manganese, zinc;* calcium, magnesium, copper;** potassium; and lead, mercury, cadmium, arsenic.***

Blood and urinary nutrient assessments, *as relevant.*

Polyamines,**** including spermine, which is low in nutritional hypoglycemia. (PFEIFFER 1987)

Stool analysis for parasites, *if indicated.*

* Chromium, manganese and zinc are often low in hypoglycemics, and are required in sugar metabolism.

** Calcium and magnesium may elevated, and may take over in storing sugar. High copper or low magnesium can obscure test results. (Pfeiffer)

*** Lead, cadmium, mercury and arsenic can alter sugar metabolism.

**** Includes histamine, and spermidine (which indicates rapid cell growth).

- ☐ Eventually, may promote diabetes, adrenal exhaustion, or pancreatic shrinkage.
- ☐ Low blood pressure, rapid pulse, heart palpitations, feeling of a band tightening around the chest. Over time, may lead to athero- or arteriosclerosis, heart disease, or stroke.

Treatments (PFEIFFER 1987, CURRIER 1979, TENNEY 1987, MURRAY 1995, 98, ROSS 1989, AIROLA 1974, HOFFER 1983A, PAGE 1993, BALCH 1990, PHILPOTT 1978AB, 82, QUILLIN 1987, STEIN 1992, BENNETT 1974, CHERASKIN 1985)

Diet, sleep, exercise, relaxation (BALCH 90, MURRAY 95, 98, HOFFER 83, COUSENS 01)

Improved diet & lifestyle often reverses hypoglycemia: (PFEIFFER 1987)

- ☐ **Supernutrition** — Don't eat junk food! Diet is critical. Mild to moderate sugar swings can usually be controlled by switching to a diet based on high fiber (plant fiber slows sugar absorption) complex carbohydrates (emphasizing legumes, fresh vegetables and sprouts, whole grains, perhaps low-glycemic fruit), and moderate protein. *Do not eat sugar, white flour, white bread, soda, other refined food. Dry fruit and processed fruit juice should be generally avoided. Avoid allergens.* Follow a Candida diet, *as applicable.* Keep meals small, perhaps up to six or more daily, with less food later in the day.
- ☐ **Vegetable juices** — leaning toward low-glycemic veggies and herbs (e.g., more celery, parsley, ginger, etc., than carrots or beets). Freshly prepared.
- ☐ **Soups** — freshly made, not-overcooked, made of healthy proteins, vegetables, legumes, whole grains, perhaps seaweeds.
- ☐ **Proteins** — Some thrive on primarily legume/whole grain/ vegetable meals, perhaps with some meat (e.g. in burritos). For others, a focus on animal foods works better (fish, high-quality meats, free-range eggs and poultry, nonallergenic dairy (goat, buffalo, or cow, *as appropriate*)). Do not overdo rich proteins (e.g., meat) at any one meal, since excess may be turned into sugar. (With poor digestion, consider B6, papain, bromelain etc.).
- ☐ **Eat high-quality fats** — fresh fish. Seeds and nuts. Keep portions moderate. *Focus on omega 3 for histapenics and histadelics; GLA for most moderate-to-severe pyrolurics.* (WEIDERER 1992) *Avoid hydrogenated fat, fried food, peanuts, vegetable oils.*
- ☐ **Water** — from healthful sources. Also, relevant herb teas.
- ☐ **Treat allergies, Candida, low thyroid, elevated mercury,** etc., *as applicable.*
- ☐ **Exercise** — Moderate exercise moves sugar from blood to body cells, sparing insulin. Thus, blood sugar decreases, while more sugar becomes available to fuel the brain. *Do not exercise to the point of exhaustion.* (MURRAY 1995, 98, PFEIFFER 1987)
- ☐ **Get sufficient sleep & relaxation.**
- ☐ **Reduce stress** — Limit exposure to stressors. Explore stress-management techniques. Increase nutritional support when under stress.
- ☐ **Avoid allergens, caffeine, alcohol, street drugs, tobacco, aspartate, MSG, stimulants, and other toxins.**

Glucose tolerance factor (MURRAY 1998, PASSWATER 1982, PFEIFFER 1987)

Glucose tolerance factor (GTF) potentiates the effects of insulin in balancing blood sugar levels. It is critical to sugar metabolism and the prevention of diabetes, and to normal brain function.

GTF is synthesized by intestinal bacteria in the presence of sufficient chromium. Other important components include niacin and glycine.* Zinc supports its formation and use . Calcium, potassium and sodium play a secondary role.

Brewer's or nutritional yeast is perhaps the best food source of GTF, provided there's no reaction to the yeast due to Candida or sensitivity reactions.

GTF can also be taken orally.

* Each molecule of GTF contains chromium, niacin, glutamic acid, glycine and cysteine. Its structure is similar to that of B12, but with chromium (instead of cobalt) at the center. (Pfeiffer 1987)

Sugar metabolism primer (PFEIFFER 1987, CURRIER 1979, MURRAY 1998)

Sugar storage

With high enough blood sugar, the hypothalamus triggers the release of **insulin** from the beta islet cells of the pancreas. Insulin causes rapid absorption of glucose into body cells.* Any excess glucose is stored as **glycogen** in the liver and, secondarily, in muscles and other tissue.

* With one molecule of insulin, approximately one thousand molecules of glucose are absorbed.

Sugar release

When blood glucose gets too low, the hypothalamus signals the pituitary to trigger adrenal release of insulin antagonists:

Adrenalin increases cell enzyme activity, blocking glucose uptake. With adrenal **glucocorticoids**, it stimulates pancreatic alpha cells to release **glucagon**, which causes glycogen to convert back into glucose, which then reenters the blood stream.

OUTCOME: Pfeiffer finds an improved diet and lifestyle often go a long way toward resolving most hypoglycemias. Although food craving, just after sugar and allergens are eliminated, can be challenging, once dealt with, steady improvement begins. Sugar release is slowed, insulin stimulation moderated, and any underlying Candida or pyroluria is no longer fed by abundant sugars. When recovered enough, natural carbohydrates (e.g., whole grains and the less-sweet fresh fruits) can be gradually introduced, and checked for sensitivity reactions. (PFEIFFER 1987)

Herbs & superfoods (MURRAY 1995, BALCH 1990, AIROLA 1974, PHILPOTT 1982, PAGE 1992, STEIN 1992, PASSWATER 1982, CHRISTOPHER 1976)

Licorice — nourishes adrenals. *Avoid if nursing, pregnant, or hypertensive. Estrogenic, and may increase copper levels, detrimental in histapenia.* (BALCH 1990, CICERO 2004)

Bee pollen, royal jelly — rich in B5 and B6. Nourishes adrenals. *Can be overstimulating in mania.*

Nutritional or brewer's yeast — one of the best sources of GTF chromium, *if not sensitive to yeast.*

Spirulina, chlorella; alfalfa, barley or wheat grass — slow the insulin reaction, provide chlorophyll, and are highly nutritive. *But can be overstimulating in mania. Often rich in copper.**

* Which must be restricted with pyroluria, histapenia, or if MTs dysfunction; see pp. 147-51, 162-66, 170-73.

Wild yam — helps control insulin levels. *Supports progesterone formation.* (BALCH 1990)

Irish moss, bladderwrack, parsley — highly nutritive. *If needed, to support thyroid activity.*

Other useful herbs may include nettles, ginger, capsicum, suma, Siberian or american ginseng, astragalus, pau d'arco, gotu kola. (BALCH 1990, CHRISTOPHER 1976)

CONTRAINDICATIONS, DISCLAIMER: Each of these herbs has specific effects on body systems, some of which may not be beneficial for any given individual. If you are considering herbal treatment, study the relevant literature, and consult a knowledgeable physician.

RECOMMENDED READING

Dufty, William, *Sugar Blues* (1975)

Ross, Harvey, MD, *Hypoglycemia: The Disease Your Doctor Won't Treat* (1989)

Reminder to the non-clinican: The information in this book is presented for educational purposes only. If you need treatment for mood disorder, hypoglycemia, or any other medical condition, please seek the services of a knowledgeable physician.

Supplements (PFEIFFER 1987, MURRAY 98, BALCH 90, PASSWATER 1982, STEIN 1992, COUSENS 2001)

Specific supportive supplements may be indicated. Tailor choices to individual biochemical requirements, including biotype needs and contraindications.

- ☐ **Chromium** — the most important component of glucose tolerance factor (GTF). Can be antidepressant, particularly in persons with blood sugar problems.
- ☐ **B3** — important in GTF formation and carbohydrate metabolism. Has also been used for anxiety, depression, and psychosis.
- ☐ **Zinc** — supports insulin function and GTF formation. Essential to brain activity and the handling of stress.
- ☐ **Glycine** — used in forming GTF; serves as an alternate source of brain fuel; anti-anxiety.
- ☐ **B1, B6, B12, B complex** — also essential to carbohydrate metabolism.
- ☐ **B5** (pantothenic acid) — critical to adrenal function; helps convert glucose to energy.
- ☐ **Manganese** — regulates blood sugar and insulin levels, is critical to nerve/muscle interactions, needed for effective use of vitamins B and C. Important in pyroluria. *May be inadvisable if histadelic, or if prone to high blood pressure.*
- ☐ **Magnesium** — needed in energy production and carbohydrate metabolism; strengthening to the heart. Calms irritability, agitation; supports mood stability.
- ☐ **Potassium** — helps maintain glandular activity, body alkalinity, energy production; counteracts muscle spasms. *Food sources, rather than supplements.* (See *Cautions*, p. 222.)
- ☐ **Vitamin C** and bioflavonoids — essential in supporting adrenal function and carbohydrate metabolism.
- ☐ **Vitamin D3** — normalizes blood sugar, reduces sugar craving. (SULLIVAN 2000)
- ☐ **Carnitine** — burns fat, sparing glucose. (Deficiency is more likely in vegetarians, and hypothyroid patients.)
- ☐ Vitamins **B2, E, A, biotin, choline, inositol, PABA** and **folic acid** are often useful. *Folic acid is usually contraindicated in histadelia, and choline may cause symptoms; histapenics may react to inositol, especially if manic.*
- ☐ **L-glutamine** — supports GI integrity. *May be contraindicated, especially with mania, or high oxidative stress.*
- ☐ **Digestive supplements**— if needed, to support digestion and assimilation, and allow the adrenals, pancreas, and digestive system a short rest. Possibilities include bromelain, papain, betaine hydrochloride, sodium and potassium bicarbonates. Perhaps, amylase, lipase, protease, etc., though, *if taken over a prolonged period, they may suppress natural enzyme production.* (PHILPOTT 1982)
- ☐ Philpott recommends adrenal cortical extract (ACE) intramuscularly, once or twice weekly, if compromised adrenals require an occasional four to eight hour rest. (PHILPOTT 1982) Murray finds oral whole adrenal extract often preferable, starting at one-third suggested dosage and increasing to some point below that which produces any irritability, restlessness, or insomnia. Pancreatic glandulars may be useful, in some cases. (WEINTRAUB 1995) *Here, again, prolonged intake may suppress natural hormone production.*
- ☐ Injections of deficient nutrients may be temporarily indicated, in some cases, to bypass problems with absorption. (RIORDAN 1995)

Diabetes

Diabetes can trigger and exacerbate mood symptoms, particularly depression, and occasionally produces acute psychotic episodes. Associated allergies and sensitivities also influence mood. The incidence of cerebral diabetes may be relatively common in severe psychiatric disorder. Moreover, neuroleptics have been reported to increase the incidence of diabetes four to five-fold. (PFEIFFER, 1987)

Types 1 & 2 (PHILPOTT 1978B, 1982, PASSWATER,1982, MURRAY 1998)

Type 1 diabetes is characterized by insufficient insulin production. Juvenile diabetics are Type 1. Causes include heredity, autoimmune reactions, physical or chemical insult (cadmium, mercury, other environmental toxins), and viral damage.

Type 2, or insulin-resistant diabetes, is frequently endstage hypoglycemia.* 85% of diabetics are Type 2. It is typically brought on by such factors as chronic refined junk food, a general lack of exercise, and persistent allergic reactions.

* Biochemically, insulin resistance can result from a mistiming of insulin release, insufficient receptors (perhaps destroyed by chronic insulin elevation), blocked receptors or other problems with binding, or other difficulties transferring insulin's message into the cell.

Symptoms

Mental/neurological symptoms (PHILPOTT 1978AB, 1982)

Mental or neurological symptoms may be the first sign of diabetes and can include: depression, anxiety, tension, personality disorders, moodswing, mania, psychotic episodes, and/or symptoms of nerve damage.

Physical symptoms (SORENSON 1992, MURRAY 1998, GOLD 1987, BALCH, 1990, PHILPOTT 1978AB, 1982)

Intense thirst, frequent urination. Hunger or lack of appetite, weight changes. Weakness, low energy, fatigue. Frequent skin infections, itching, boils, easy bruising, slow healing of wounds, poor circulation. Vaginal fungal infections. Impotence. Blurred vision. Aches, numbness, tingling, leg cramps, transitory paralysis.

Complications (MURRAY 1998, GOLD 1987, BALCH 1990, PHILPOTT 1978AB, 82, PASSWATER 1982)

Complications are believed to result largely from a glucose deficit in the liver, fat cells or muscles; uncontrollable amounts attached to red blood cells; or excess in the brain, eyes, or kidneys. Blood sugar peaks are particularly damaging.

Fat accumulation— is common. Excess sugar which cannot be removed is turned into fat and increases cholesterol. Insulin is also fattening. (SORENSON1992) Fat, in turn, worsens insulin-resistance and creates other complications. *See box, next page.*

Allergies and sensitivities (PHILPOTT 1978AB, 1982) — insulin insufficiency and diabetic complications induce hypersensitive reactions to foods, chemicals and inhalants. Intolerances may arise to glucose, lactose, galactose, proteins, chemicals or, even, insulin. Such reactions, can go on to further compromise pancreatic function. *See box, next page.*

Candida, & other opportunistic infection — Diabetes provides fertile ground for staphylococcus, Candida, and other opportunistic infection. Candidiasis is prevalent, and contributes further to problems with refined carbohydrates, allergens, and mood.

Other complications — hardening of the arteries, high blood pressure, heart disease, gangrene, kidney disorders, blindness, increased susceptibility to tuberculosis, and a significantly decreased life expectancy.

Milk & childhood diabetes (HEAD1997)

Cow's milk may serve as a trigger to autoimmune destruction of pancreatic beta cells in genetically susceptible individuals. In a study by Karjalainen (1992), all of 142 children with newly diagnosed Type 1 diabetes, showed elevated IgG antibodies to cow serum albumin.* Concentrations in diabetics averaged sevenfold that in healthy children. The authors suggest viral exposure may stimulate the initial reaction to milk and subsequent development of diabetes. (KARJALAINEN 1992)

Other researchers have also implicated dairy and casein. (CAVALLO 1996, SAUKKONEN, 1996, VAARALA 1996, VAHASALO 1996)

A preventive approach might minimally include breast feeding for at least the first six months of infancy, and avoiding early exposure to cow's milk. (HEAD 1997, PEREZ-BRAVO 1996)

* Another study, by the same group (Levy-Marchal, 1995), found these antibodies elevated in 74.4% of newly diagnosed childhood diabetics, as compared to 5.5% of controls.

Low serotonin symptoms

The low insulin (especially in Type I) means serotonin is not preferentially transported to the brain, and often becomes depleted, typically producing such symptoms as depression, irritability, overstimulation, anxiety and carbohydrate craving.

Acidotic crisis — is brought about by a reduced availability of carbohydrates, leading to an accumulation of ketones. Early symptoms include rapid pulse, restlessness, acetone breath, excessive urination, thirst, nausea, and vomiting. Increasing apathy can evolve into a coma. Can be fatal.

Susceptible populations

The frequency of diabetes is 1%, worldwide, 5% in the US, about 30% for Naruans, Polynesians, and the Pima of Arizona. Neuroleptic antipsychotics have been reported to increase diabetes four to five-fold. Women with excess upper body fat may be particularly susceptible. Allergies and Candida also increase susceptibility. (PFEIFFER 1987, ROSS 1974)

In industrialized countries, incidence increases with age (as does chromium deficiency). One US estimate holds that 40-60% of people over age eighty are diabetic. (PASSWATER 1982)

Role of allergies in Type II diabetes (PFEIFFER 1987, PHILPOTT 1978AB, 82)

Philpott finds adult onset diabetes often results from reactions to foods and chemical inhalants, as well as, excess body fat, plasma lipids, irritants, infections, and other stressors. He suggests early and intermediate stages are usually reversible, but that without therapy, continual allergic reaction can, over time, profoundly degrade pancreatic function. Thus:

Chronic inflammation, produced by allergens and irritants, promotes a continual excess of endorphins, decreasing pancreatic ability to produce bicarbonate.

Low bicarbonate causes acidosis. (The small intestines need bicarbonate to neutralize the hydrochloric-acid-soaked food entering from the stomach.)

Acidosis inhibits production of pancreatic proteolytic enzymes, required for digestion.

Undigested food particles may then escape into the blood stream promoting further allergies.

The resulting nutrient deficiencies and pancreatic damage compromise the means for making insulin and may lead to clinical diabetes.

Low insulin inhibits transport of serotonin to the brain, fostering depression, irritability, anxiety, and carbohydrate craving. Consequent overindulgence in carbohydrates, further deteriorates pancreatic function. (MURRAY 1998)

Role of fat (SORENSON 1992, PHILPOTT 1978AB, 82)

Excess body fat often promotes insulin-resistance, since:

Plasma and tissue fat are insulin-resistant. A normal level of insulin is less effective in people with more body fat. So the demand on the pancreas increases.

Excess plasma fat irritates the circulatory system. Control of the resulting inflammation uses up additional pancreatic proteolytic enzymes.

Lipid irritation also increases hypersensitive reactions, creating further demand on the pancreas.

Therapy

Keeping a meal's fat content moderate helps prevent stimulation of insulin and supports sugar metabolism. (SORENSON 1992) However, over-restriction of healthful fats (e.g. from fish, and unprocessed seeds and nuts) can be counterproductive.

Body fat can be more effectively reduced by avoiding refined carbohydrates, and other junk food; maintaining a healthy diet in general; exercising (*diabetics should work with their physicians on an appropriate regimen*); and correction of any thyroid hypofunction, or other relevant disorders. Nutrients that may prove useful include carnitine, chromium, B3, B6, D3, CoQ10, etc. — *check first with your physician.*

Lab (MURRAY 1995, 98, PASSWATER, 1982)

HbA1$_c$ (glycosylated hemoglobin) — measures blood sugar accumulation over time, and has largely replaced the glucose tolerance test.

Home testing kits— allow patients to self-monitor.

Hair and liver chromium — levels average one-third lower than in the general population.

Allergy tests — tests involving fasts can be dangerous, particularly for Type 1 and those prone to acidotic crisis. A careful history and the less disruptive tests (e.g. ELISA ACT or EAV) are a safer choice.

Treatment (MURRAY 1998, 94, 95, HEAD 1997, BALCH 1990, PHILPOTT 1978AB, 82, PAGE 1993)

Diabetics can be extremely vulnerable, and before any changes in nutritional or herbal intake or other therapies, should consult a knowlegable physician who will tailor treatment to individual biochemical requirements (including contraindications), with special attention to ongoing blood sugar issues.

Nutrient possibilities

□ **Chromium** (GTF or picolinate) — increases insulin efficiency, and enhances its binding; and can help stabilize blood sugar swings. [200-400 mcg] (PASSWATER, 1982, VANS 1989, HEAD 1997, ROSS 1989)

□ **B3** — may slow destruction of pancreatic beta cells and support their healing. (BALCH 1990, HEAD 1997). It is an essential component of GTF. *Very high doses may be counterproductive.* (BALCH 1990)

□ **B6** — often deficient. Important to carbohydrate metabolism. Protects nerves, retina. Supports magnesium absorption. (MURRAY 1994, HEAD 1997)

□ **Vitamin D** — now known to play a critical role. (ROSS 2002) Normalizes blood sugar, reduces sugar craving, increases insulin synthesis and release. Counters glucose intolerance. (SULLIVAN 2000)

□ **Zinc** — supports insulin function and GTF formation; protects pancreatic beta cells. (MURRAY, 1994)

□ **Magnesium** — frequently low. Supports glucose metabolism. (MURRAY, 1994, HEAD 1997)

□ **Manganese** — often low. Cofactor in key glucose metabolism enzymes. (MURRAY, 1994)

□ **Thiamine** — often deficient. Helps prevent neuropathy. (HEAD 1997) *Very high doses may be counterproductive.* (BALCH 1990)

□ **Riboflavin** (*R5P*) — B2 metabolism is often abnormal. (HEAD 1997)

□ **B5** — lowers blood lipids, helps protect nerves. (HEAD 1997)

□ **Biotin** — may be low. Helps prevent neuropathy, supports liver glucose utilization. (BALCH 1990, MURRAY 1994, HEAD 1997)

□ **B12, folate** — help protect kidneys, nerves, and retina. (HEAD 1997) *Check contraindications for histadelia.*

□ **Inositol** — often deficient. Protects nerves. (HEAD 1997) *May worsen mania, particularly in histapenics.*

□ **B complex** — supports carbohydrate metabolism. (BALCH 1990, MURRAY 1998)

□ **C** — often lacking. Antioxidant; helps prevent protein glycosylation, and inhibit sorbitol accumulation (associated with complications). (MURRAY 1994, HEAD 1997) [*Moderate doses, multiple times per day, as relevant.* (BALCH 1990)]

□ **E** — often low. Antioxidant; helps prevent protein glycosylation. (HEAD 1997)

□ **CoQ-10** — often low. Antioxidant. Helps prevent diabetic neuropathy. (HEAD 1997)

□ **Selenium,** (BALCH 1990, MURRAY, 1991) **lipoic acid,** (TRITSCHIER 1995) **bioflavonoids (quercetin, hesperidin**, etc.), and other antioxidants — help prevent complications, and are often low. (HEAD 1997)

□ **Potassium** — *if indicated.* Food sources, rather than supplements. (BALCH 1990, MURRAY, 1991) (See *Cautions*, p. 222.)

□ **Omega 3, GLA, with lecithin** — normalize fat metabolism; may reduce need for insulin in Type 2 diabetes; may help prevent/reverse diabetic neuropathy. *Adjust to biotype and other contraindications.* (ERASMUS 1995, HEAD 1997)

□ **Fiber** — (guar gum, pectin, oat bran, psillium, etc.) slows sugar absorption. (BALCH 1990, MURRAY 1998)

□ **Fructooligosaccharides** — support creation of short-chain fatty acids. (CICERO 2004, HIDAKA 1986)

□ **Taurine** — often low. Decreases platelet aggregation. (HEAD 1997)

□ **Carnitine** — antioxidant. Restores inositol, nerves, retina. Brings fat to mitochondria for use as fuel. (BALCH 1990) *May be indicated with fatigue, but can be contraindicated for persons with any signs of mania.*

Herb possibilities (BALCH 1990, PAGE 1993, MURRAY, 1995, 98, CHRISTOPHER 1976, HEAD 1997)

Gymnema sylvestre — used for over 2000 years in India to treat "honey urine." Gives evidence of reducing insulin requirements and regenerating pancreatic beta cells. May help prevent sugar fluctuations. (SHANMUGASUNDARUM 1990, SRIVASTAVA 1985, MURRAY, 1995, 98, BALCH 1990)

Momordica charantia (bitter melon) — the juice has insulin-like effects and increases glucose utilization. (WILIHINDER 1982, SARKAR 1996, SHIBIB 1993)

Fenugreek — decreases fats, lowers sugar levels. (SHARMA 1990, RIBES 1986, MURRAY 1995, 98, BALCH 1990, CICERO 2004)

Salt bush — improves glucose tolerance and regulation.

Onion, garlic — lowers blood sugar. (MURRAY 95, 98, BALCH 1990, COUSENS 2001, CICERO 2004)

Blueberry leaves — reduce blood glucose, decrease triglycerides. Their anthocyanins offer protection from diabetic retinopathy. (BEVER 1979, ALLEN 1927)

Bilberry — lowers blood glucose and helps stabilize collagen. Decreases capillary permeability, thereby protecting the retina. (BONIFACE 1996, SCHARRER 1981, LAGRUE 1970, MURRAY 1995, 98, BALCH 1990, CICERO 2004)

Ginkgo — helps prevent retinopathy in animal studies. *Do not use if blood pressure is low or if medicated for hypertension.* (DROY-LEFAIX 1992, MURRAY, 1995, 98)

Siberian or Chinese ginseng — helps lower sugar, reduce acidity, control weight. *Don't use with hypertension or mania.* (BALCH 1990, MURRAY, 1995, 98)

Cedar berries — nourish the pancreas. (BALCH 1990)

Juniper berries — lower blood glucose. (BALCH 1990)

Huckleberry — helps promote insulin production. (BALCH 1990)

Dandelion root — protects the liver (which converts nutrients to glucose). Supports pancreas. *Limit with gallbladder problems.* (BALCH 1990)

Other herbs which may prove useful include burdock, prickly pear cactus; buchu, uva ursi. (BALCH 1990, MURRAY 1998, CICERO 2004)

Some cautions (BALCH 1990, MURRAY 95, 98, HEAD 97)

PABA may raise blood sugar.

Excess cysteine may break insulin bonds.

If introducing niacin to diabetics, give small doses, and increase gradually.

Excess fish oil may raise blood sugar.

Excess potassium may produce muscular fatigue, erratic heartbeat and, possibly, heart failure. Consider the balance with sodium and water. If needed, food sources of potassium are usually the best approach.

If lipoic acid is used, follow an appropriate chelation protocol. Otherwise, whatever the purpose, it will also act as a metal chelator, redistributing any mercury, etc., leading to potentially severe symptoms. (See pp. 177-78.) (CUTLER 1999, 04)

Proteolytic enzymes, in some cases, provoke adverse reactions.

Extremely high intake of thiamine may inactivate insulin. (BALCH 1990)

Diabetics must be particularly cautious in trying new treatments. The advice and care of a knowledgeable physician is essential.

For further contraindications, see Parts I & II, pp. 21-168.

Reminder

This material on diabetes is presented for educational purposes only, and does not constitute specific treatment recommendations.

Diabetics and people with unstable blood sugar are particularly susceptible to complications and must consult their physician before any change in nutritional or herbal intake. Blood sugar should be carefully monitored, especially when new therapies are introduced, or circumstances change. Improvement may necessitate a change in insulin dose.

The advice and care of a knowledgeable physician who will tailor treatment to individual requirements is essential.

□ **Vanadyl sulfate** — insulin-like activity, decreases serum glucose. (HEAD 1997) *Vanadium supplements are typically contraindicated for bipolars.*

□ **5-HTP + DL-phenylalanine** — reduce carbohydrate craving. *Avoid if premania threatens, hypomanic, manic, mixed state, a rapid cycler or histapenic.*

□ **Glutamine** — helps prevent dips in brain blood sugar, and reduce carbohydrate craving. *Contraindicated for some; can worsen manias.*

□ **Bicarbonate** — *if indicated,* to prevent/counter acidity. (PHILPOTT 1978AB, 82)

□ **Pancreatic glandulars** — *if indicated,* to nourish the pancreas. (BALCH 1990, PHILPOTT 1978AB, 82)

□ **Proteolytic or other digestive enzymes** (before meals) — *if indicated,* to reduce cytotoxic reactions and blood sugar flareups. (BALCH 1990, PHILPOTT, 1978AB, 82)

Additional support (MURRAY 1995, 98, BALCH 1990)

□ **Exercise** — reduces blood sugar, while bringing it to cells for use as fuel; increases glucose tolerance and may increase tissue chromium; increases the number of insulin receptors and sensitivity to insulin; lowers cholesterol, while increasing HDL; facilitates weight loss. *The exercise program should be graded, and approved by your physician. Special consideration is required if sugar levels tend to be unstable.* (MAIORANA 2001, MURRAY 1998)

□ **Diet** — Michael Murray, ND, (1995, 98) recommends a diet low in fat (10-15% or less) and cholesterol, low in protein (10-15%), and high in fiber and complex slow-digesting carbohydrates (75-80%). Intake of allowable carbohydrates should be steady, with abundant legumes to help normalize blood sugar levels, and five or six small meals per day, with no fasting or feasting. If animal proteins are eaten, use small portions, and choose fish and poultry over meat and dairy. Limit salt, which can raise blood sugar. *Avoid refined sugars and starches.*

□ **Foods** suggested by Balch to normalize blood sugar include brewer's yeast, dairy (if not allergic), egg yolks, fish, garlic, sauerkraut, vegetables (especially raw), spirulina, raw vegetable juices,* raw fruit, fresh berries.

* Counterbalance the sweeter vegetables (carrots, beets, etc.) with veggies lower on the glycemic index (celery, parsley, etc.), as per individual needs. Additions such as chlorophyll superfoods, nutritional yeast, and/or relevant supplements may be helpful.

□ **Weight loss**— Healthful, doctor-approved program, *if indicated.*

□ **Treat acidity, Candida, allergies, thyroid dysfunction, metal metabolism dysfunction or metal toxicity,** other contributory conditions.

□ **Avoid allergens, and addictive or other maladaptive intake.** Adopt a four to seven day rotation diet. If, after at least three months of avoidance, specific reactive substances no longer cause symptoms or blood sugar changes, occasional intake may become possible.

□ **Avoid alcohol, tobacco, other toxins.**

□ **Limit stress** — limit stressors; explore management techniques. Anger, anxiety, pain, depression, and other stress reactions increase release of adrenal glucocorticoids and adrenalin, and liver glycogen, raising blood sugar. If fight or flight cannot occur, sugar remains elevated.

□ Medical treatment, as prescribed by the physician.

Note: With plummeting blood sugar due to unstable sugar levels or too much insulin, rapidly-absorbable sugar may be temporarily needed. The eventual goal is to minimize such fluctuations.

Outcome

Philpott (1978ab) and Murray (1995, 98) find Type II (adult) diabetes, if not too advanced, often responds especially well to nutritional treatment and allergy avoidance; most Type I diabetics will always require an external source of insulin, though natural methods may reduce the quantities needed, and can help prevent complications.

2. Endocrines

"Nervous and chemical signals cannot readily be separated." — Arthur J Prange, MD, 1987

Endocrine/brain interactions

Endocrine/nervous-system interactions are crucial to mood (PRANGE 1987) Sachar points out that the major antidepressant neurotransmitters, dopamine, norepinephrine, and serotonin; and acetylcholine (an antimanic); are pivotal in regulating hormones. (MELTZER 1987) Moreover, hormones tend to localize in the tracts of mood-moderating neurotransmitters.

Thus, functional endocrine changes occur in most bipolars. (PRANGE 1987, GOLD 1987) And people with significant endocrine disorder typically experience mood dysfunction. (GOLD 1987) Imbalances of thyroid, adrenal, pituitary, pineal, pancreatic or sexual hormones can severely disrupt brain functioning. And many bipolars can be distinguished by their endocrine profile alone. (MASON 1975, 91)

Hypothalamus/pituitary interactions

Neurotransmitters involved in depression (BURCH 1983, MASON 1975, 91) and mania control the hypothalamus, which is the intermediary between the brain and the endocrine system. The hypothalamus generally targets the anterior pituitary, but can directly influence other glands. The pituitary, known as the "master gland," directly controls secretions of other endocrines.

Such symptoms as changes in appetite, sleep and libido; autonomic issues; mood variation over the day; and affective disorders can suggest hypothalamic/pituitary dysfunction. (BURCH 1983) Major mood disorders have, in fact, frequently been associated with altered hypothalamic/pituitary activity. (LASSER 1997, GOLD 1987)

Hypothalamic/pituitary/endocrine feedback dysregulation

If the hypothalamus is overactive, pituitary secretions will initially, in most cases, increase, stimulating the entire endocrine axis. Eventually, however, the pituitary can become exhausted, with diminished output profoundly impacting downstream hormonal release.

Alternately, overactive anterior pituitary secretion may be overstimulating endocrines and promoting mania; the reverse, if underactive.

On the other hand, overactive target glands sometimes initiate the dysregulation in affectives. Over time, the hypothalmus and/or pituitary become correspondingly insensitive to the hormonal feedback, and instead continue to prod already overstimulated target glands. Or, with chronically elevated hormones (particularly thyroxine and cortisol), selected peripheral tissue may become less responsive, reacting as if understimulated.

Hypothalamus
Pituitary
Thyroid
Adrenals
Sex hormones

See also *Parathyroid* p. 124, *Sugar* pp. 214-22, *Melatonin* pp. 259-62, *Endocrine rhythms*, p. 262.

Bipolar endocrine profile (MASON 1975, 91)

Bipolars tend to exhibit multiple hormone abnormalities, often due to feedback disorders. Levels of epinephrine, norepinephrine, testosterone, free thyroxine, etc., are commonly abnormal. While up to 70% of bipolars can be distinguished from schizophrenics on the basis of one of these hormones, three, taken together, distinguish 95%.

Natural therapies vs. hormone replacement

(SEE REFERENCES THROUGHOUT THIS SECTION)

When an endocrine gland is subfunctional, hormone replacement may become essential. However, especially over the long-term, hormone intake can suppress natural secretion.

So, if the situation is not critical, some natually-oriented physicians might initially prescribe a relatively short trial of supportive nutrients, health measures, and lifestyle changes (exercise, sunlight, dietary change, etc.), extended if enough improvement occurs.

At the same time, symptoms, as well as labs, are monitored, ongoing, for any need for the hormone, itself (perhaps along with the above therapies).

Overview of the interaction of the hypothalamus & pituitary with other endocrines (PRANGE 1987)

Hypothalamic hormones

Thyrotropin releasing hormone — causes the pituitary to release thyroid-stimulating hormone.
Gonadotropin releasing hormone — controls pituitary release of luteinizing and follicle-stimulating hormones.
Corticotropin-releasing hormone — controls pituitary release of ACTH.
Growth hormone releasing hormone — promotes pituitary release of growth hormone.
Growth hormone inhibiting hormone — inhibits pituitary release of growth hormone.
Prolactin releasing hormone — promotes pituitary release of prolactin.

Anterior pituitary hormones

Thyroid-stimulating hormone — stimulates creation of thyroid hormone.
Luteinizing hormone — causes ovaries to produce progesterone; testis, to produce testosterone.
Follicle-stimulating hormone — causes ovaries to produce estrogen; promotes sperm production.
Adrenocortiocotropic hormone (ACTH) — stimulates release of adrenocortical and steroid hormones.
Growth hormone — promotes muscle and bone growth, protein synthesis, use of glucose for fuel.
Prolactin — induces milk secretion, blocks ovulation & menses, reduces sexual desire. Regulates calcium, etc.
Interstitial-cell-stimulating hormone — stimulates testosterone release in men.

Posterior pituitary releases (*of hormones elaborated in the hypothalamus*)

Oxytocin — controls milk production and uterine contraction. Stimulates maternal and mating behavior.
Vasopressin — affects blood pressure, stimulates kidneys to reabsorb water, and modulates learning.

Endocrine gland secretions

Pineal — secretes melatonin (which regulates the activity/sleep cycle).
Thyroid — secretes thyroxine and triiodothyronine (T4 and T3) and other hormones (which increase metabolic rate, support growth and maturation of the nervous system and sex glands, and influence bone development.)
Parathyroid — increases blood calcium; decreases potassium.
Adrenal cortex — secretes aldosterone, androgens, estrogens, cortisol.
Adrenal medulla — secretes epinephrine, norepinephrine.
Pancreas — secretes insulin (which decreases blood sugar and increases glucose storage) and glucagon (which increases blood sugar and conversion of stored fat to glucose).
Ovaries — secrete estrogens (which govern female secondary sex characteristics, sex drive, ovulation).
Testis — secrete testosterone (which governs male secondary sex characteristics, sex drive, sperm production).

Effects of growth hormone on mood

Pituitary growth hormone increases T3 (the most active thyroid hormone) and aspartate, and promotes protein synthesis and use of glucose for fuel, suggesting antidepressant benefit. (BURMAN 1996) Acute hypersecretion, can produce euphoria, (PRANGE 1987, ANSEAU 1992) However, *chronic* oversecretion (acromegaly) is associated with reduced initiative and spontaneity, while treatment with bromocriptine can contribute to mania.*(FISHER 1999, GOLD 1987)

In many depressives, growth hormone release is blunted** (in some, even after recovery), generally suggesting a need for greater norepinephrine support,*** (while, normal GH release suggests a need for serotonin alone). (BURCH 1983, MATUSSEK 1992, DINAN 1991, ANSSEAU 1992, COUPLAND 1992)

* Acromegaly also causes enlarged face, hands, feet, and other bones, in adults; gigantism, in children.
** As measured by growth hormone response to IV clonidine.
*** Though blunting can also occur in mania, and in normals.

Effects of other pituitary disorders

Stress-induced anterior pituitary microtumors (PRANGE 1987)

Stress sometimes produces pituitary microtumors, which oversecrete prolactin, in some cases, leading to dysperceptions or psychosis.*

* Physical symptoms can include diabetes, salt/water imbalances, headaches, low libido, infertility, menstrual cycle disruption, breast secretion, and increased facial hair in women.

Hyperpituitary

Hypersecretion is most likely in the anterior lobe. The pituitary then overstimulates certain target glands, often provoking cognitive and affective symptoms.

Hypopituitary (GOLD, 1987, PFEIFFER 1988, MORGAN 1989, PRANGE 1987)

Low pituitary function can be due to burst blood vessels, tumors, tuberculosis, syphilis, steroids, surgery or other physical damage. Stimulation of downstream endocrines diminishes. 70% develop mental symptoms, e.g., apathy, confusion, depression, fatigue, low stress tolerance and, perhaps if severe, clouding of senses, paranoid delusions, auditory hallucinations, anorexia and, rarely, psychosis.*

* Physical symptoms can include impotence, amenorrhea, hypoglycemia, hypothyroidism, low blood pressure, diminished libido, reduced secondary sex characteristics, and increased susceptibility to infection.

Hyponatremia (GOLD 1987)

Oversecretion of pituitary vasopressin can cause the kidneys to reabsorb so much water as to produce hyponatremia, which can mask as psychotic depression or mania.

See *Sodium*, p. 133.

Thyroid

Overview

The thyroid gland consists of two connected lobes just below the voice box. It is crucial to production of heat and energy from food and oxygen; promotes growth and immunity; and supports heart and kidney function, bone development, and maturation of the sex glands and nervous system. (SCHACHTER 1999, GOLD 1987)

Thyroid is also critical to cognition and mood, and generally tunes in mood intensity. (GOLD 1987) Thyroid hormones are generally antidepressant, and have been used to augment antidepressants and convert nonresponders, and to treat certain rapid cycling and hypomanic patients unresponsive to other treatments (*though careful medical evaluation is essential, as thyroid may promote mania*). (GOLD 1987, LOOSEN 1987)

"Delusions and hallucinations occur in nearly half the cases, mainly where the disease is advanced... Insanity, as a complication, is noted in about the same proportion."

Clinical Society of London, 1888. They identify 16 of 45 myxedema patients as "insane," with such symptoms as, mania, melancholia, paranoid delusions, hallucinations, and slowed thought processes.

Thyroid status in bipolars

Bipolars frequently manifest thyroid abnormalities,* particularly underactivity. (LASSER 1997, PIES 1998) Moreover, two major mood stabilizers (lithium and carbamazepine) may suppress the thyroid further. (LAZARUS 1998)

In some bipolars, thyroid activity cycles with affective state, (GOLD 1987) creating transient abnormalites. (COHEN 1979, SPRATT 1982, MORLEY 1982, BOMMER 1992) Bipolars may be particularly sensitive to such fluctuations, even when within the normal range. (COLE 2002) Cognitive function, for instance seems to be significantly linked to thyroid status, rather than lithium levels. (TREMONT 1997)

Barnes (1976) warns that many patients medicated for depression, anxiety, and so forth, have undetected thyroid dysfunction, causing mood symptoms. Unfortunately, effective thyroid status is often obscured by distorted interactions of the hypothalamus/pituitary/thyroid axis, and by difficulty determining peripheral sensitivity to thyroid.**(PIES 1998)

* Even as compared to the general psychiatric populations, in which thyroid problems are common. (Gloger, 1997, Fardella 2000, Placidi 1998)

** For example, you can get high thyroxine, with an elevated pituitary TSH nonresponsive to regulatory feedback, so continuing to stimulate the thyroid further. Along with high thyroid symptoms of, for example, weight loss, rapid heart beat, etc., the patient may manifest selective insensitivity to T4 in mood-modulating neural pathways, fostering the low thyroid symptom of depression. Labs also will be contradictory: with high T4, suggesting *hyper*thyroid; high TSH, *hypo*thyroid. Thus neither effective thyroid status nor appropriate treatment will be readily apparent.

"Thyroid dysfunction is the single most important area of misdiagnosis... Failure to uncover and treat a thyroid disorder masked by mood symptoms compromises both thyroid and mood. Response to antidepressants and mood stabilizers will be suboptimal, and continued deterioration of the untreated thyroid will further erode mood."

Mark Gold, MD, 1987

"Autoimmune thyroiditis, [and] subclinical and clinical hypothyroidism may give rise to thyroxine-responsive depression."

I. S. Jackson, MD 1998

Affective symptoms in thyroid disorder patients

Thyroid dysfunction alters mood (as well as cognition and behavior), (LASSER 1997, LOOSEN 1987, PRANGE, WHYBROW 1987, TREMONT 1997) typically creates affective symptoms, (GIBSON 1962, GRAVES 1843) and is associated with increased incidence of depression, dysthymia, bipolar disorder, cyclothymia, panic disorder, phobia, and obsessive compulsive disorder. (PLACIDI 1998) Hypothyroidism characteristically creates a depressive syndrome; even subclinical hypothyroidism may be associated with mood cycling, depression, and poor or slow response to affective treatment. Autoimmune thyroiditis is often associated with depression (especially postpartum), and with rapid cycling. Hyperthyroidism creates symptoms of, and contributes to, mania. (PIES 1998)

Nonetheless, the precise impact of thyroid activity can vary from one individual to another. (LOOSEN 1987)

"Clinical observations and research suggest thyroid hormones can increase antidepressant and mood stabilizer response, especially with treatment resistance, rapid cycling, and in women."

M. Wiesel, MD, 1999

Definitions

TRH (or thyroid-releasing hormone) is secreted by the hypothalamus, and targets the pituitary and thyroid.

TSH (thyroid-stimulating hormone) is secreted by the pituitary, and targets the thyroid.

T4 (thyroxine), a 4-iodine thyroid hormone, is secreted by the thyroid, and targets peripheral tissue (i.e., outside the main thyroid axis, and including the lungs, kidneys, heart, and brain).

T3 (triiodothyronine), a 3-iodine thyroid hormone, formed from T4 in the liver, targets peripheral tissue. T3 is shorter-acting than T4, but more potent.

Effects on the brain

"The mutual influence of brain and thyroid is profound."
Arthur J Prange, MD, & Peter M Whybrow, MD, 1987

Sufficient thyroid is required for the brain to effectively create mood-modulating neurotransmitters. (ROSS 2002) Thyroid acts as a neuroregulator. (LOOSEN 1992) And thyroid hormones influence nutrition, energy, and oxygen availability to the brain. (T4, for instance, enhances general oxygen uptake and transport, and protects nerve cells when oxygen is low. (D'ALECY 1997))

Thyroid also is critical in brain development and maturation, ultimately influencing speech, coordination, movement quality, mood, thought and behavior. (LOOSEN 1992) Severe congenital hypothyroidism compromises neurological function, especially balance, coordination, fine motor movement, and language development. (BARGAGNA 2000)

Thyroid & mood-altering neurotransmitters

Stimulation of catecholamines

Thyroid metabolism interacts closely with creation and release of the antidepressant and mania-related catecholamine neurotransmitters. (K"OHRLE 1996, MANO 1998) Note the common precursor (tyrosine) to thyroid hormones, dopamine, norepinephrine, and PEA.

Elevated thyroid hormones have been associated with increased formation of the above transmitters. (SVENSON 1977, ENSTROM 1974, 75, JACOBY 1975, MANO 1998) Brain thyroid, moreover, tends to concentrate in biogenic amine tracts, and may increase receptor targets for dopamine and norepinephrine, thereby enhancing sensitivity to mood messages. (GOLD 1987, PRANGE, WHYBROW 1987, SVENSON 1974)

Furthermore, the thyroid axis may help compensate when catecholamines are low and, conversely, catecholamines may increase when thyroid activity is low (perhaps contributing to the counterintuitive irritability common in low thyroid patients). (FUKHARA 1996)

Interaction with serotonin, acetylcholine (LOOSEN, PRANGE 1984)

Thyroid hormones may increase cerebral serotonin (CLEARE 1996) (producing feelings of satisfaction and contentment), which may then feed back to the hypothalamus and suppress TSH (GOLD 1977) and T3 (CENTANNI 2000) uptake.

The thyroid may also regulate some cholinergic neurons (HAYASHI 1987) (associated with memory, nerve/muscle interaction, and the calming, parasympathetic nervous system).

Physical functions of the thyroid (LANGER 1998, GOLD 1987, BARNES 1976, SCHACHTER 1999)

The thyroid is crucial to body temperature, strength, energy, growth and vitality. Specific functions include:

Stimulates cell metabolism and other chemical reactions. Regulates creation and transfer of energy. Increases cell heat, and energy production.

Key to use and transport of oxygen and food. Increases intestinal motility and nutrient absorption. Stimulates glucose absorption and protein metabolism. Prevents organs from clogging with metabolic wastes.

Essential for efficient oxidative phosphorylation, which stores energy when oxygen burns (oxidizes) food. (Requires B1, B2, B3, B5, CoQ10, magnesium, perhaps other hormones) (GSDL 2002)

May influence action of FAD in methylation. (BELL 1992)

Key role in immunity. Protects against chronic disease. Influences autoimmune reactions.

Important to sexual function.

Supports kidney function. Influences filtration rate, fluid reabsorption, plasma flow, sodium and potassium activity. (CAPASSO 1999)

Supports muscle contraction, electrical activity, (CAPASSO 1999) and respiration. Helps regulate use of calcium in muscle contraction, and sodium/calcium exchange. (HOJO 1997)

Supports the circulatory system. Increases heart rate and strength. May directly affect alpha 1 adrenoreceptor-mediated heart activity. (ZWAVELING 1996) Influences heart mitochondrial fatty acid metabolism (involving oxygen and carnitine).

Controls growth and influences repair.

High thyroid & mania

High thyroid can interact with, trigger, or intensify mania, (GOLD 1983, NATH 2001, LOOSEN 1984, JOSEPHSON 1980, MACCRIMMON 1979, TEMPLE 1972, ESCAMILLA 2001) and can also increase switching on antidepressants. (BOTTLENDER, 2000). Even levels in the high-normal range can contribute to the development of mania. (LEE 2000, ROCA 1990)

In one study, (JOYCE 1991) over one-third of manics showed elevated thyroid (largely FT4I), and in some of the remaining two-thirds, within-patient thyroid hormones were higher in mania than depression. Lee (2000) suggests lithium's antithyroid effects may underly its benefit to mania.

Note: In some manics, however, thyroid can test low. (BRIGHAM 2001)

Thyroid/pituitary/hypothalamus interactions

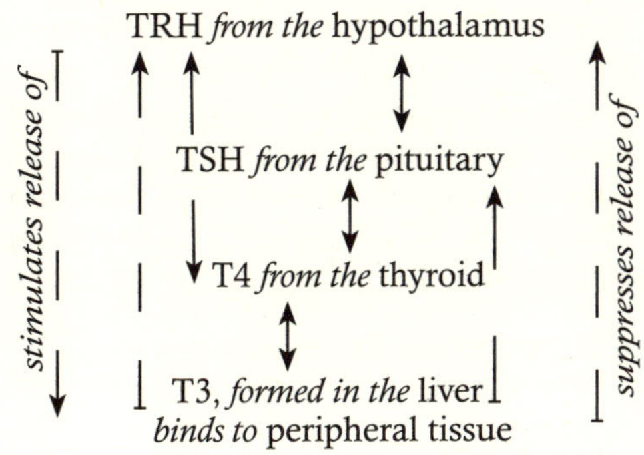

Common symptoms (GOLD 1987, MORGAN 1989, GALTON 1979, BARNES 1976, PFEIFFER 88, LANGER 1998)

Mental symptoms common to both hyperthyroid and mania include: high irritability, tension, emotional instability, explosiveness, anxiety; (WHYBROW 1969, 81, 82) exhilaration, increased motor activation, restlessness, tremors, hyperactivity, insomnia and other sleep problems; (FAN 1997, GOLD 1983, 87, NATH 2001) and, in some cases, erratic bizarre behavior, mood swings, impulsive destructive tendencies, psychosis, paranoia. (GOLD 1987, PFEIFFER 1988)

Over time, hyperthyroids may succumb to depression and social withdrawal, perhaps due to an exhaustion caused by extended thyroid overstimulation. Similarly (although usually sooner), manic overstimulation eventually gives way to depression.

Biotype vs. thyroid imbalance

Hyperthyroid and histadelia share symptoms of high metabolism; low thyroid and histapenia, those of low metabolism. Nonetheless, histadelics are more prone to depression than hyperthyroids; and histapenics, much more prone to mania than hypothyroids.

Though in many patients, histamine imbalances are not associated with thyroid disorder, in some cases, high thyroid and high histamine, co-occur; in others, low thyroid and low histamine; while in others still, they are inverse (e.g., high thyroid with low histamine). (WALSH 2000)

Distinguishing thyroid and histamine (methylation) status can be critical, as treatments are distinctive, and failure to accurately address either condition can be disastrous.

Mainstream use of thyroid for mania (LASSER 1997, PRANGE 1996, BRIGHAM 2001)

The following mainstream approaches may be instructive when considering use of nutritional and herbal thyroid therapies.

Thyroid suppression —Lithium (which is generally considered more useful in moderating mania, than in elevating depression) often suppresses thyroid function, which may be part of how it works. (LEE 2000)

Low dose* thyroid — along with medication, has benefitted certain cases of hypomania, (BRIGHAM 2001, FRYE 2001) and *occasional* manias, (PRANGE 1996) *perhaps mostly in cases where the thyroid starts off sluggish* (e.g., TSH over 2). (BRIGHAM 2001) *Warning: This approach is in developmental stages. Especially when thyroid is NOT low, intake of the hormone can pose considerable risk of aggravating mania and compounding the stress to the heart.*

* High dose T4 (a treatment sometimes used for hyperthyroids) has been tried, as a last resort, in some cases of resistant mania, to suppress thyroid overactivity. Some manics respond, others deteriorate. This is an extremely risky approach, and should be considered highly experimental.

Thyroid findings in manics (JOYCE 1991, ESCAMILLA 2001)

Thyroid may be elevated relative to levels in depression.

FT4 may correlate with the intensity of manic symptoms.

FT4I (free thyroxine index) is often elevated.

Δ TSH is often low.

Hyperthyroid

Hyperthyroidism is characterized by overproduction of thyroid hormone. Morgan (1989) cites a US incidence of 2-5 per 1,000. It's most common in women aged twenty to forty. Causes include autoimmune disease, heredity, thyroid nodules, respiratory disease, certain nutritional imbalances, and overmedication for hypothyroidism. (GOLD 1987)

Mental symptoms (WHYBROW 1969, HASKETT 1981, FAN 1997, GOLD 1983, 87, MORGAN 1989, GALTON 1979, BARNES 1976, PFEIFFER 1988, LANGER 1998)

Generalized anxiety, restlessness, irritability, emotional explosions, exhilaration, mania, insomnia and other sleep problems, mood swings, distractibility, short attention span and, especially with exhaustion, depression and social withdrawal.

In some cases, bizarre behavior, delirium, hallucinations, psychosis, impulsive destructive tendencies, feelings of persecution, or paranoid schizophrenia.

Physical symptoms (GOLD 1987, MORGAN 1989, GALTON 1979, BARNES 1976, PFEIFFER 1988, LANGER 1998)

Hunger, emaciation, heat sensitivity, excess perspiration, diarrhea, racing pulse, heart palpitations and pain, tremors, protruding eyeballs (exopthalmus), soft moist skin, hair loss, fine straight hair, scanty menses and swollen breasts in women, breast swelling in men. Eventually, may produce fatigue, and exhaustion.

Caution: Toxic metal release (KLEIN 1998)

Hyperthyroidism, as well as hyperparathyroidism, speeds bone turnover, potentially increasing the release of stored lead, strontium 90, etc.

Caution: Thyroid storm, a medical emergency

Thyroid storm results from a sudden uncontrolled release of high levels of thyroid hormone. It can be triggered by fright, physical stress (e.g. diabetic shock, surgery, toxemia), or by stopping hyperthyroid medication. Symptoms include delirium, fever, incapacitating weakness, rapid pulse, restlessness, confusion, intense emotionality, psychosis and shock. Muscles weaken, the liver often becomes swollen, and cardiovascular collapse may occur. One quarter die, even with treatment.

Thyrotoxicosis can produce symptoms of mania, (LEE 1991) delusional depression, (KRONFOL 1982) manic or depressive psychosis, (BROWNLIE 2000) and confusional states. (GREER 1968) Resolution may resolve the mental symptoms. (KRONFOL 1982, WEINBERG 1977)

Nutrients imbalances in the etiology of hyperthyroidism (BARNES 1976, PFEIFFER 1988, LANGER 1998, JENNINGS 1970)

Some studies associate low EFAs with hyperthyroid.

Thyroid hyperplasia (overgrowth) releases high levels of hormone, testing like hyperthyroid, and can be due to depleted vitamins C and E.

Excess iodine, a key component of thyroid hormones, can overstimulate and produce hyperthyroidism, especially in the elderly with autonomous nodular goiters. Some hyperthyroids improve with iodine restriction.

Alternately, hyperthyroidism is occasionally caused by a lack of iodine, especially in regions where the soil is depleted. Thus, chronic low iodine has shown some correlation with hyperthyroid and goiter. (On the other hand, mild deficiency may protect against autoimmune thyroiditis). (LAUBERG 1998, 99, AGHINI-LOMBAQRDI 1999)

WARNING: Iodine status and its effect on thyroid function can be difficult to assess. Increasing iodine in the hyperthyroid patient with already sufficient levels, may worsen hyperthyroidism, and perhaps trigger cardiovascular events, mania, or thyroid storm. (BARNES 1976, LANGER 1998, KROHN 1991)

See also, p. 235.

Drugs, medical treatment

Pfeiffer suggests that lithium, which binds and excretes iodine and slows the thyroid, might be the treatment of choice for many hyperthyroids.

See *Lithium*, p. 285, for contraindications and potential toxicity.

Standard medical treatment for hyperthyroidism usually involves suppressive drugs, radiation or, in some cases, surgery. High dose T4 has also been used, but poses substantial cardiac risk.

Low thyroid & depression (PRANGE, WHYBROW 1987)

Thyroid abnormalities, particularly low thyroid, pervade the depressed population.*(SACHAR 1975, GOLD 1981, 83, 87, FARDELLA 2000, PIES 1998, PLACIDI 1998, PRANGE 1996, MUSSELMAN 1996, FRYE 1999)

Depression is a major and consistent symptom in most low thyroid patients (WHYBROW 1981, 82) and, with lack of energy, is usually the presenting complaint. (GOLD 1983) Even mild low thyroid tends to produce depression. (JAIN 1972) And most hypothyroid symptoms are markedly like those of depression: dysphoric mood, loss of interest or pleasure, apathy, suicidal ideation, difficulty concentrating, memory problems, anergia, weakness, fatigue, anxiety, delusions, decreased libido, emotional instability, resentment, panic, mood swings, and extended sleep (more common in bipolar depressives than unipolars). (WHYBROW 1976, 81, 82, GOLD 1983, 87, JAIN 1972, SCHACHTER 1999, PLACIDI 1998, RELKIN 1969, MICHAEL 1963, LOOSEN 1984, FRYE 1999)

Low thyroid decreases cerebral glucose metabolism and blood flow, (MARANGELL 1997A) and suppresses catecholamine activity, (MANO 1998) thereby fostering depression. Such depressions are often severe and resistant to psychiatric treatment,** and complicated by additional undiagnosed medical illness. (TUNBRIDGE 1981) Thus, subclinical or clinical hypothyroidism is especially frequent in antidepressant-resistant affectives,*** (and, conversely, the greater the free thyroxine, the shorter the depressive episode tends to be).

* Even more so than the general population, where estimates (US) of low thyroid range from approximately 1% (Morgan 1989) to 40%. (Barnes 1976)

** For example, Frye (1999) notes lower mean serum FT4 is significantly associated with more affective episodes and greater depression severity during lithium treatment, and increased global severity with carbamazepine treatment.

*** Moreover, Cole (2002) found only one quarter of 65 bipolars had hormone levels in the optimal range (slightly above mid-normal) for effective antidepressant therapy.

> *"One step toward improved antidepressant efficacy is reducing the heterogeneity of depressed patients and treating fewer hypothyroid patients with antidepressants."*
> Mark Gold, MD, 1983

Myxedematous madness

Progressive hypothyroidism (myxedemia) steadily slows mental and physical functioning, compromising memory, concentration, comprehension, energy, and reflexes.

Before hormone treatment became widely available, up to half the people with progressive hypothyroidism developed an organic psychosis, "myxedematous madness."(ASHER 1949, CLIN SOC 1888).

Symptoms can include melancholia, mania, and psychosis. (GULL 1873) Also, depression, slowed thinking, dementia, morbid dreams, obsessions, frightening hallucinations, persecutory delusions, paranoia, suicidal ruminations, and physical symptoms of low metabolism. (MICHAEL 1963, PRANGE 1972, RELKIN 1969,, WHYBROW 1969, 74, 81, KLAIBER 1976, WILLIAMS 1970, GOLD 1983)

Psychiatric symptoms may precede physical, (GOLD 1983, ASHER 1949, REED 1977, BOILLET 1998) leading to misdiagnosis and incorrect treatment.

Paradoxical elevation in many depressives

On the other hand, in many depressives, the thyroid is paradoxically elevated, with regulatory feedback compromised, so it fails to turn off at usual set points. Chronic excess may, in some such cases, have selectively desensitized mood-modulating neural tracts, leading to the depressive symptoms of low thyroid, while other peripheral tissue continue to respond with classic high thyroid symptoms, e.g., insomnia, weight loss, etc. (GOLD 1987)

Adverse mood compromises thyroid

Adverse mood can compromise thyroid function. Parry (1825) first suggested fear might cause thyrotoxicosis. Studies suggest stress decreases thyroxine (T4) potency in women. (LOOSEN 1987) Wilson (1991) found stress also reduces T3, the most active thyroid hormone, and can create low thyroid symptoms, even with normal T4 (*see box, below*).

Mechanisms (LANGER 1998, MORSE 1996, KATO 1998)

Low thyroid symptoms may be due to:

- A thyroid too weak to form enough T4; or resistant to TSH or TRH.
- A pituitary too exhausted or insensitive to create enough TSH when prodded by TRH or low T4.
- A hypothalamus unable to create TRH as needed.
- Peripheral receptors which cannot bind strongly enough to thyroid hormone.
- Liver dysfunction, compromising formation of T3.
- Reverse T3 predominance, due to stress.

Wilson's syndrome (WILSON 1991)

To preserve energy during stress (e.g., fasting), the body limits peripheral conversion of T4 into T3. Blood T4 may appear adequate, but symptoms occur because T3, the more potent hormone, is low, or has been converted into reverse T3 (compromising normal T3 activity). After the stress ends, this situation should — but doesn't always — resolve.

E. Dennis Wilson, MD, has developed a protocol for reestablishing this T4 to T3 conversion. Long-acting T3 is given every 12 hours, in gradually increasing doses, determined by oral temperature. If the patient is intolerant of a specific dose, it is temporarily reduced. Once temperature is normal for approximately 3 weeks, T3 is tapered to zero. When successful, the thyroid system resets at a higher temperature, T3 increases, and hypothyroid symptoms abate. Several cycles may be required to optimize temperature. If stress again suppresses thyroid activity, treatment is repeated. Treatment often get progressively easier on the patient.

Note: This therapy may reverse the disorder, but requires discipline and commitment, and can produce difficult or harmful symptoms. Many hypothyroids, especially with adrenal or other complications, prefer a steady intake of natural desiccated thyroid. (LANGER 1998)

Hypothyroidism

Hypothyroidism is characterized by chronic underproduction of thyroid hormone. It is most common in women (especially if over 50), with the ratio of females to males about 10:1. (BARNES 1976, LANGER 1998)

Mental symptoms (GOLD 1983, SCHACHTER 1999)

Depression, suicidal ideas. Apathy.

Cognitive slowing or impairment, difficulty concentrating, memory loss.

Anxiety, fears, suspiciousness, resentment.

Emotional instability, mood swings. (SCHACHTER 1999)

May be prone to drug and alcohol abuse. (GOLD 1987, JAIN 1972, RELKIN 1969, MICHAEL 1963, WHYBROW 1969, 76, 81, LOOSEN 1984, WILLIAMS 1970)

In some cases, persecutory delusions, terrifying dreams, obsessions, auditory or visual hallucinations, paranoia, or psychosis. (GOLD 1987, SCHACHTER 1999, WHYBROW 1969, 76, 81)

Physical symptoms (MORGAN 1989, GALTON 1979, BARNES 1976, PFEIFFER 1988, LANGER 1998, CAPASSO 1999, SCHACHTER 1999, GOLD 1983)

All-consuming fatigue, especially in the morning, improving some over the day. Untreated individuals may literally sleep their lives away.

Anemia, poor circulation, cold sensitivity, hands and feet cold to the touch and intolerant to cold (and, perhaps, heat). Raynaud's Syndrome.

Weight gain, increased fat. Difficult to reverse unless thyroid activity increases. Appetite changes.

Dry, puffy, rough skin; flaky acne. Pallor, yellow tinge (due to high carotene).

Brittle, easily broken nails. Thinning, dry, brittle, hair.

Coarsened features. Fluid retention (eyebrows may be permanently raised to keep water-logged lids open).

Swelling of the ankles, and face, especially under the eyes. Missing outer third of eyebrows.

Vision problems or loss, night blindness.

Difficulty hearing. Hoarseness, slurred speech, tongue thick and swollen, difficulty swallowing.

Joint pain or stiffness, arthritis. Fatigue after minor exertion. Muscle weakness, aches, cramps. Nonathletic.

Headaches, migraines. Indigestion, gas, chronic constipation. Increased sensitivity to drugs and toxins. (SCHACHTER 1999, WHYBROW, GOLD 1987)

Often prone to allergies, Candida, hypoglycemia, or diabetes. (MACKOWIAK 1999, ROLD'AN 1999, COLEMAN 1997)

Low libido, PMS, fertility problems. Menses tend to be irregular, profuse, painful. Prone to cystic breasts or ovaries, fibroids, tumors. (GOLD 1987)

Shortness of breath, chest pain, slow pulse. Anemia. Low blood pressure initially; eventually, hypertension, elevated cholesterol, atherosclerosis, heart disease. (HAK 2000, BASTENIE 1971, FOWLER 1977)

Prone to asthma, tuberculosis, other lung disorders. (GOLD 1987, LANGER 1998)

Early history may include: high birth weight, early or late teething, late walking or talking, post-nasal drip, frequent ear, sinus, bladder, or respiratory infection. (SCHACHTER 1999, GOLD 1987)

Causes, triggers (BARNES 1976, LANGER 1998, MORSE 1996, KATO 1998)

Heredity,* iodine and other nutrient imbalances, tissue destruction,** infectious illness, toxicity,*** autoimmune reactions (e.g., Hashimoto's disease), severe stress, liver dysfunction (compromising creation of T3). (BARNES 1976, LANGER 1998) Also: fluorine (used in dental practice, or water treatment) and chlorine reduce iodine availability, impeding hormone formation. The following drugs can suppress the thyroid: lithium, certain antidepressants, sulfa drugs, certain antidiabetic drugs, thyrocyanide (a tobacco additive), corticosteroids, prednisone, estrogenergics.

* E.g., thyroid weight can vary from 8 to 50 gms. (*Prevention* 1971)
** As in hyperthyroid operations, or radioactive iodine exposure.
* Perhaps, early PCB exposure. (Langer 1998, Morse 1996, Kato 1998)

Medical treatment with synthetic hormone

Established medical treatment often consists of the prescription of synthetic hormone, usually a chemical T4; occasionally, T4 plus a *short-acting* T3.*

* If a longer-acting T3 is required, Langer (1998) suggests getting it from a compounding pharmacy, or if unobtainable, dividing the T3 into 2 or 3 doses, to take in the earlier part of the day (so as not to interfere with sleep).

Natural thyroid

Doctors Broda Barnes, MD, and Stephen Langer, MD, prefer natural dessicated thyroid,* which contains both T3 and T4. Langer also suggests concurrent B vitamins to help process the hormone and improve cell oxygen transport.

* Langer (1998) recommends starting adult hypothyroid patients on 1/4 to 1/2 grain natural thyroid daily, increasing 1/4 grain every week to ten days, up to the desired level (usually not more than 1-2 grains; occasionally, 2.5 grains or more). To achieve full therapeutic benefits, he finds it may take four to six weeks at optimal dosage (though basal temperatures may not reach normal for a year or more). If a person has recently had a heart attack, he delays treatment at least two months.

Relevance of hormone replacement in hypothyroids (BARNES 1976, LANGER 1998, AIROLA 1974, BALCH 1990, PAGE 1992, MURRAY 1998)

Depression, fatigue, low temperature, shallow breathing, poor oxygen transport, suboptimal enzyme function, high cholesterol and homocysteine, and generally compromised immunity leave inadequately treated hypothyroid patients prone to degenerative disease. (BARNES 1976, LANGER 1998)

With mild hypothyroid, iodine-deficient goiter, and euthyroid depression,* nutritional, herbal and lifestyle support for the thyroid may meet the patient's needs, though the physician should remain alert to signs of suboptimal thyroid activity.

Especially in second and third generation hypothyroids, or with severe hypofunction, nutrient therapies alone often fail to sustain mental and physical health, necessitating hormone replacement, at optimized levels. Appropriate natural therapies can be used to enhance effectiveness, and may reduce the dosage needed.

* Gold states 90% of hypothyroid depressed patients are stage 2 or 3 (see below), which is hard to detect with usual tests, so they are often given antidepressants instead of thyroid. (Gold 1981, 87)
Stage 1 — Overtly hypothyroid. Depressed, low energy, weight gain, intolerant to cold, constipated, hoarse, etc. Low T3RU or T4. High TSH and ΔTSH.
Stage 2 — Mildly hypothyroid. Dry skin, fatigued, constipated, weight gain. Normal T3 and T4. Normal to slightly elevated TSH. Elevated ΔTSH.
Stage 3 — Subclinical depression and lack of energy may be the only symptoms. ΔTSH is abnormal, but generally not T3RU, FT4 or TSH.

Mainstream use of thyroid for bipolar depression (LASSER 1997)

The following mainstream approaches (used mainly to augment meds in nonreponsive bipolar depression) may be instructive when considering use of nutritional and herbal thyroid support.

Low dose T3 augmenting antidepressants (PRANGE 1963, 96, GOODWIN 1982, LASSER 1997, JOFFE 1998, JACKSON 1998)

Depression research focuses more on T3 than T4, because of its more rapid and pronounced activity. (PRANGE 1996) A considerable database documents use of low-dose T3 in accelerating or enhancing antidepressant response, (JOFFE 1998, MUSSELMAN 1996, PRANGE 1996, JACKSON 1998) even in euthyroids, and especially in women. (PRANGE 1996) Patients who do not do well with antidepressant drugs (one-fourth to one-third of depressives, often bipolar) may be particularly responsive to thyroid; (EARLE 1970, OGURA 1974, CAVALCA 1974, BANKI 1975, 77, TSUTSUI 1979, GOODWIN 1982, LOOSEN 1992, BRIGHAM 2001, LASSER 1997, PRANGE 1996, JOFFE 1998) up to two-thirds respond.*(PRANGE 1996, JOFFE 1998, JACKSON 1998) Optimal dose and duration have not been established. (JOFFE 1998)

T3 with T4 or TSH augmenting antidepressants (WIESEL 1999)

Frye (2001) reports better response with combined hormones than with T4 alone. In some patients, the body isn't converting enough T4 into T3, so T3 alone may help, or perhaps T3 with some T4. (FRYE 2001, BUNEVICIUS 1999) Others have been previously diagnosed hypothyroid, and are already on T4, but, in many cases, experience increased stabilization or antidepressant improvement when T3 is added. (COOKE 1992, BUNEVICIUS 1999)

Loosen (1987) suggests T3 plus TSH can accelerate recovery in acute treatment-resistant depression. Whybrow (1994) has used T3 with high dose T4 for certain severe resistant depressions.

Warning 1: Excessive thyroid activity whether due to thyroid plus TSH, high-dose thyroid, even low-dose, in some cases) can trigger mania, destabilize mood (BAUER 1990, 98, RUDAS 1999, AFIELOU 1997) and pose life-threatening cardiovascular risk. High dose T4, especially, is considered a last resort approach, for extremely treatment-resistant bipolars (e.g., certain rapid cyclers, mixed state, hyperthyroid, others). If used at all, it should be accompanied by sufficient anticonvulsant mood stabilizers, and only following thorough assessment of thyroid function, complete delineation of risk, and fully informed consent. (BAUER 1991, 98, LEIBENLUFT 1996, JOFFE 1993)

TRH (hypothalamic thyroid-releasing hormone)

TRH has been found to produce temporary improvement in depression, (PRANGE 1972, KASTIN 1972) and transiently improve mood, anxiety, and cognition, (MARANGELL 1997B) as well as motivation, well being, and coping capacity in normals. (PRANGE 1979, 1978AB, 1984AB, PECKNOLD 1977) In fact, some depressed hypersecrete TRH, perhaps in an attempt by the body to reverse the depression. (POST 1996)

TRH is particularly potent. Repeated oral TRH may, in some, produce sustained thyroid activation, redressing low thyroid, (BURGER, PATEL 1977, KIELEY 1976) and thereby improving corresponding depressions, *but can also create hyperthyroidism or trigger mania (perhaps severe).*

Warning 2: TRH antidepressant therapies should be considered extreme, last resort, experimental approaches. Individualized dose and length of treatment has not been fully delineated. Mania, hyperthyroidism, or life-threatening cardiovascular complications can result. (MUSSELMAN 1996) (Warning 1, above, applies here too.)

Thyroid symptoms vs. Mood status

Hypothyroid vs. depression

Hypothyroids (unlike depressives) typically gain weight, sleep too much (though some bipolar depressives also do so), are intolerant to cold. Also, they tend toward thin, brittle hair, shortened eyebrows, thick dry skin, hoarseness, goiter, delayed reflexes, bradycardia, and constipation.

Hyperthyroid vs. mania

Generalized anxiety is more likely in hyperthyroids, euphoria less so. Increased appetite, fine tremor (though this can occur in reaction to lithium or other meds), rapid heart beat, and bulging eyes (exopthalmos) further suggest hyperthyroid. (WHYBROW 1969, 81, 82 HASKETT 1981, PRANGE 1987)

Thyroid findings in depression

*Depressives may show low or high thyroid. Findings have included:**

Low thyroid: Low T3 or T4. Abnormally elevated antithyroid antibodies. Elevated TRH or TSH (attempting to increase thyroid output). (MUSSELMAN 1996, ROCA 1990, GOLD 1983, 87, FARDELLA 2000, MARANGELL 1997A)

Cerebral hypothyroidism (with the body euthyroid): not readily detected by standard tests. (WIESEL 1999)

Normal (KIROV 1998) **or high-normal thyroid:** slightly elevated T4 (MUSSELMAN 1996, JACKSON 1998) increased FT4I (correlating with depressive severity). (ROCA 1990)

Thyroid axis dysregulation: The chronic high TRH common in bipolars, prods the pituitary, often, eventually, muting its sensitivity (and suppressing the nocturnal rise in TSH). With the downregulated TSH response, thyroxine secretion may diminish, or, the hypothalmus may directly stimulate thyroid activity, perhaps profusely (less so in bipolar II). (DEWHURST 1968, MUSSELMAN 1996, JACKSON 1998) When the depression resolves, these changes generally revert. (JACKSON 1998)

* Note: Medication can confound readings. Dilantin® and calcium channel blockers, for instance, displace T3 and T4, increasing FT3 and FT4. TSH may be more accurate, but can test deceptively low if the pituitary has become exhausted chronically trying to stimulate a poorly-responding thyroid. Tests can also be distorted by thyroid intake, or by avoiding thyroid for 24 hours. (Surks 1996)

Thyroid findings in rapid cyclers

Autoimmunity — perhaps, most common; especially, elevated thyroperoxidase antibodies (TPO-Ab). (OOMEN 1996)

Low thyroid — In some, low T4, FT4, and/or high TSH. (KILZIEH 1999, BAUER 1990, FRYE 1999)

Fluctuating thyroid levels.

Normal to high thyroid — labs suggest this is relatively common, (POST 1997) counter to some of the research. (KILZIEH 1999, BAUER 1990, FRYE 1999) However, in some such cases, perhaps a substantial number, functioning may be lower than results suggest, due to: (JOFFE 1993)

- Brain hypothyroidism — the brain may be *functionally* hypothyroid, with greater hormone requirements.
- Thyroid system inefficiency — problems creating, metabolizing, or transporting thyroid hormones; or problems with receptors.
- Pituitary exhaustion — low TSH (which usually indicates hyperthyroid) can, in the chronic hypothyroid patient, instead reflect pituitary exhaustion from long-term attempts to stimulate a nonresponsive thyroid. (POST 1997)

Rapid cycling & mixed states

Most studies find high rates of thyroid axis abnormalities in rapid cyclers, (DUNNER, FIEVE 1974, BAUER, WHYBROW 1990, CHANG 1998, COWDRY 1983) perhaps, particularly, early autoimmune thyroid disease. (KUSALIC 1992, OOMEN 1996) Some research suggests hypothyroidism is a risk factor for, and may predispose to, rapid cycling,*(KILZIEH 1999, BAUER 1990, FRYE 1999) or that oversensitivity to TRH may play a role. (BARTALENA 1990)

Mixed states also seem to involve greater thyroid axis dysfunction than found in other bipolars. (CHANG 1998)

Mainstream use of thyroid for rapid cyclers

Treatment for rapid cycling usually involves an emphasis on mood stabilizers; and discontinuing antidepressants, stimulants, bright light therapies, etc. If nonresponsive, some researchers suggest a trial of thyroid. Some of the relatively moderate approaches include:

Thyroxine — Clinical data suggests low dose T4 may be useful in refractory rapid cyclers, especially in the depressive cycle.*(KUSALIC 1992, BERNSTEIN 1992, SPOOV 1998, STANCER 1982, DZUREC 1998, WHYBROW 1990, FRYE 1999)

T3 + T4 — some clinicans find both hormones get a better response. (FRYE 1999, BUNEVICIUS 1999, AREM 1999, DARBY 2006)

* Though others (Post 1997) fail to find low thyroid. Joffe (1993) suggests considering that the brain may be functionally hypothyroid.

Autoimmune thyroid (GOLD 1987, LANGER 1998, SCHACHTER 1999)

SAT patients may appear symptomless to the endocrinologist, but not necessarily to the psychiatrist."

Mark Gold, MD

Autoimmune thyroid is becoming increasingly common, and is especially likely among women.* About half of hypothyroid patients show anti-thyroid antibodies. (SHOPSIN 1970, BASTIENIE 1967) Such antibodies seem to be most elevated in bipolar depression and mixed states, then affective disorders, then the general population. (HAGGERTY 1990)

Symptoms involve depression, often suicidal thoughts, severe fatigue and exhaustion, and weak short-term memory and concentration. Normal activity is compromised. Such symptoms may alternate or coexist with insomnia, profound anxiety and inner tension, even major panic attacks.

Physical symptoms include difficulty swallowing, allergies, gastrointestinal dysfunction, low libido, anemia, menstrual issues, headaches, ear pain, muscle and joint aches and fatigue, arthritis, irregular pulse, palpitations; often, cardiovascular complications and, perhaps, diabetes.

* Autoimmune thyroid has been associated with low thyroid volume, (Bonar 2000) or may be due to various stresses, e.g., psychosocial factors, overstimulation with iodine or certain drugs, or a viral reaction (e.g. Epstein Barr or systemic Candida). (Langer 1998)

Thyroid in other psychiatric disorders

Thyroid support has been used in treating some patients with periodic catatonia, schizophrenia, autism, and depression (LANGER 1998, PFEIFFER 1987, 88, GALTON 1979), as well as bipolar disorder, and is under investigation for some cases of PTSD, eating disorders, ADHD, behavior disorder, and borderline:

Schizophrenia — Kraepelin originally gave schizophrenics thyroid extract, and it was thought, by a number of researchers to alter the course of the disease, (BRAUCHITCH, 1961, GHESSING, 1953, WAGNER 1914) though negative studies later emerged. (HOLLISTER 1973, MICHAEL 1963) Nonetheless, a paranoid psychosis (myxedematous madness) is known to result from chronic severe, untreated low thyroid, in up to 50% of cases.

PTSD — Positive correlations have been found between FT3, T3, T4 and hyperarousal in combat PTSD. (WANG 1995)

Borderline — Garbutt (1983) found TSH blunting in 47%.

Eating disorder — Hall (1995) found eating disorder patients had double the thyroid illness of the general population.

ADHD — T4 may be needed (WEST 1996), possibly T3 for some resistant to T4 (WEISS 1997). On the other hand, in impulsive (but not inattentive) hyperactivity, thyroid may be elevated. (HAUSER 1997)

Criminality — Alm (1996) found T3 generally higher in the persistently criminal, and those with greater delinquency. Similarly, St°alenheim 1998 suggests some association of elevated T3, decreased T4 with criminality and antisocial personality disorder.

Affective drugs & thyroid

Lithium

Lithium can be cumulatively toxic to the thyroid. (WIESEL 1999) The drug concentrates in the thyroid where it inhibits iodine uptake and secretion of thyroid hormone. The resulting hypothyroidism* is often associated with autoimmunity (i.e., anti-thyroid peroxidase antibodies), and a smooth, nontender goiter in up to 60% of patients. Lithium also alters cell response to TRH and thyroglobulin structure, and inhibits coupling of iodotyrosine.**(LAZARUS 1998) Moreover, underactive thyroid decreases response to lithium. (BRIGHAM 2001).

Brigham thus suggests, *if indicated*, low dose T3, or T3 plus T4; and limiting goitrogenic foods and, where appropriate, iodine. Lazarus (1998) advises checking TSH and creatinine every three months, especially in females.

* Although lithium occasionally produces hyperthyroidism.

** Researchers are currently investigating the role of changes in hypothalamic/pituitary axis homeostasis, brain deiodinase enzymes, and hypothalamic thyroid receptor concentration in lithium's effects on mood. (Lazarus 1998, Rao 1996, Brigham 2001)

Antidepressants

As with lithium, certain level of thyroid may be needed for optimal antidepressant response, and antidepressants can decrease thyroid function. (DUVAL 1996) Some researchers suggest, *where indicated*, treating with thyroid prior to, (WHYBROW 1972, LASSER 1997, KIROV 1998, RAO 1996) and/or during antidepressant intake. (BRIGHAM 2001) Lazarus (1998) advises checking response to TRH before adding antidepressants and during treatment.

Women, children, & thyroid status

Female sensitivity to thyroid

Mixed state and rapid cycling are more common in women, as is thyroid dysfunction. (HENDRICK 1998, FARDELLA 2000, GOLD 1987) Mood-disordered women also respond better to thyroid support, even when thyroid tests normal. (HENDRICK 1998, LOOSEN 1987)

Stress may suppress T4 more in women. (PRANGE 1996) In one study by Dzurec (1998), euthyroid females experienced more substantial disruption of their lives due to fatigue and depression (as compared to males), and all women improved with low dose T4.

Maternal vulnerability

In a study by Kent (1999), one-third of pregnant women had low first-trimester FT4, and almost 12% showed thyroid dysfunction six months postpartum. The fetus uses maternal iodine and thyroid hormone; increased maternal kidney activity eliminates more iodine. Incidence of goiter increases. Hypothyroid mothers may require increased T4 intake. (KOUTRAS 2000). On the other hand, some mothers develop thyrotoxicosis.

Graves disease may cease temporarily during pregnancy, allowing reductions in antithyroid drugs. (KOUTRAS 2000) Autoimmune reactions to the thyroid may also diminish, but can rebound a few months postbirth, causing thyroiditis.

Fetal vulnerability

Maternal low thyroid reduces oxygen transport in the fetus, and stunts brain development and growth.* Poor IQ has been associated with iodine deficiency, low first trimester FT4, and positive anti-TPO antibodies in the mother. In severe cases, maternal deficit causes congenital hypothyroidism, mental retardation, or cretinism. Antithyroid antibodies readily cross the placenta and may alter the child's thyroid, (KOUTRAS 2000, DE ESCOBAR 2000) and compromise neuropsychiatric function.**(VAN WASSENAER 1998)

Maternal iodine deficiency is the greatest cause of preventable retardation and brain damage, worldwide, and generally reduces IQ 10-15 points. Severe depletion can cause cretinism (thyroid failure, neurological damage, retardation). If selenium is also low, hypothyroidism can be severe, though neurological damage may be less. (DELANGE 2000B)

Thyroid dysfunction also allows toxins to wreak greater damage on the infant nervous system.***(HAUSER 1998)

* So complete and accurate labs become important (FT3, RT3, FT4, anti-TG, anti-TPO, TSH, etc.).

** For such infants under 30 weeks, van Wassenaer (1998) suggests considering T4, perhaps also T3 replacement.

*** And may contribute to the learning, memory and attention problems associated with perinatal exposure to dioxins or PCBs. (Hauser 1998)

Warning: The medical treatments described in this chapter mandate the care of a knowledgable physician, and even so, entail varying degrees of risk, in some cases, life-threatening..

Thyroid: Lab

Include history, and physical exam. Check thyroid size, tenderness, presence of nodules or bruits. Note tremor, exopthalmos, diaphoresis, lid lag, reflex speed, blood pressure, heart rate, dysrhythmias. (Capasso 1999, Schachter 1999, Gold 1983)

Basal Temperature Test — Barnes (1976) and others find basal (underarm) temperature better reflects thyroid-controlled cell metabolism, and can pick up low thyroid status missed by other tests. (Langer 1998, Jackson 1957)

Oral glass thermometers are more accurate than digitals. Shake before retiring. On waking, before getting out of bed, place in armpit ten minutes. Record for three consecutive days. Normal is 97.8 to 98.2 F. Temperatures one to three degrees lower suggests hypothyroid, and, perhaps, a therapeutic trial of thyroid (but may be due to mercury toxicity, reactions to psych drugs, etc.). Over 98.2 suggests hyperthyroid (but can be due to infection, nervousness, or activity). During menstruation, assess only from the second through fourth day of the period, or not at all. Do not take progesterone the day before, or during these assessments.

Other tests measure blood, 24-hour urine, or salivary levels. The most common medical tests are T4 and TSH:

T4 (thyroxine) — secreted by the thyroid. Levels are usually higher in the morning. (Wilson 1992)

TSH (the pituitary's thyroid-stimulating hormone) — controls creation and release of T4, and is generally *inverse* to it.* However, after years of prodding an underactive thyroid, the pituitary can become exhausted, causing low readings for *both* TSH and T4 (common in women over 40, hypothyroid most of their lives). Physicians often mistakenly assume normal-to-overactive status and fail to prescribe thyroid.**(LoPresti 1996, Langer 1998)

* TSH increases when T4 is low to stimulate thyroid secretion. High T4 feeds back to the pituitary, reducing TSH. This feedback loop magnifies changes in T4, making this test relatively sensitive for many (but not all) patients.

** Other pituitary and hypothalamic disorders can also confound results.

Tests that may pick up some of the more subtle thyroid changes common in bipolars include T3, reverse T3 (Marangell 1999), *anti-thyroid antibodies* (Wilson 1992), *and ΔTSH.* (Gold 1987, GSDL)

T3 (liothyroxine or triiodothyronine) — the most active hormone. It's created in peripheral tissue from T4.

RT3 (reverse T3) — increases under stress, interferes with T3 functioning. (See *Wilson's Syndrome,* p. 229.)

Thyroid antibodies — anti-thyroglobulin (anti-TG), anti-thyroid peroxidase (anti-TPO), and antimicrosomal (anti-M) antibodies indicate autoimmune reactions to the thyroid. (Langer 1998, Lo Presti 1996, Gold 1987)

ΔTSH (delta TSH) — measures pituitary TSH responsiveness to hypothalamic TRH (thyroid-releasing-hormone, also called protirelin). This test is more sensitive than TSH. Very small increases in T4 and T3 decrease ΔTSH. *Caution: This test involves some risk, particularly in persons with high blood pressure, heart disease, or seizures.*

Low ΔTSH — can occur with hyperthyroid, thyroid overtreatment, depression, (Jackson 1998, Musselman 1996) and mania;* (Linkowski 1981, Extein 1980, 82, Gold 1980, Marangell 1997) and usually reflects pituitary insensitivity to chronic TRH overstimulation.

Elevated ΔTSH — occurs with early hypothyroidism, and in major (Kirkegaard 1981, Loosen 1982, Extein 1981, Frye 1999, Gold 1979, 80) and some bipolar depressions.**(Roca 1990, Gold 1983. Fardella 2000)

Abnormally high ΔTSH (equal to or greater than 20) — suggests autoimmunity. (Gold 1987, Gordin 1974)

* Also, borderline, alcoholism, (Loosen 1979, 82, 83c, 85) anorexia, aging (especially in males), Cushings, sleep problems, renal failure. Or high dopamine, growth hormone, or calcitonin; or reactions to salicylates, glucocorticoids, carbamazepine or certain other drugs.

** Also: chronic lithium or neuroleptic treatment, sleep disturbance, iodine deficiency, certain hypothalamic or pituitary disorders. (Lo Presti 1996)

Hormone ratios: Consider fT4/TSH & TT3/TT4. (Cutler)

Iodine — required to form thyroid hormone. (Gold 1987)

Tyrosine — similarly.

Lipid profiles — Low thyroid often alters lipids; hyperthyroid sometimes does. (Tsimihodimos 1999) Thyroid changes may be relatively common in lipid disorder patients.* (Bland 1997)

* Jeffrey Bland, MD, et al, suggest the following readings often corroborate low thyroid: triglycerides <200, BUN to creatinine ratio <12, cholesterol >252, total CPK >30, LDH >40, cholesterol/HDL ratio >5, and increased B2 fraction in lipoprotein electrophoresis. Yildirimkaya (1996) finds T4 intake can be corrective, decreasing cholesterol, LDL, and apolipoprotein B.

Homocysteine — can be elevated in hypothyroid patients.

Concurrent conditions — anemia, hypoglycemia, diabetes, allergies, arthritis, Candida; and respiratory, circulatory, or immune disorders may suggest thyroid dysfunction. *Note on abnormal EEGs — A lack of alpha waves or flat, low-voltage waves, suggesting brain dysfunction or a neurological disorder, may instead by due to low thyroid.* (Langer 1998, Gold 1987)

Thyroid labs can miss dysfunction (Prange 96, Lasser 97, Gold 87, Klein 98)

"Everyone has a unique FT4-TSH setpoints." — Ruz, 1999

"Thyroid labs are not conclusive. You must check symptoms." — William J Walsh, PhD, 2008

The thyroid is often mistakenly presumed normal because of the relative insensitivity of T4 and TSH; the impracticality of checking TRH, antibodies, or the status of peripheral conversion; and the influence of confounding variables (mood disorder, lithium and other meds, iodine levels, street drugs, etc.).* Thus, the thyroid assessments commonly used may not convey a complete map of function.

* Other indices, often overlooked, or hard to assess: liver dysfunction (compromising conversion), receptors resistant to T3, weak binding to the hormone, excess binding by certain proteins, poor iodide uptake, weak response in select target tissue (especially limbic), deficient transthyretin (which transfers T4 into the CSF), impaired hypothalamic response to thyroid; different brain thyroid synthesis, use and requirements from that in the rest of the body. (Langer 1998, Morse 1996, Kato 1998)

Augmentation when thyroid tests normal

So thyroid indices do not necessarily predict function, and successful augmentation of antidepressants doesn't always change thyroid data. Thus, a number of double blinds and other studies show low-dose T3 accelerating antidepressant response even without evident thyroid disorder. (Bauer 1996, Kilzieh 1999, Loosen 1987, Prange 1969, Wilson 1970, Coppen 1972b) Consequently, for *treatment-resistant* bipolar depressives with "normal" thyroid, some psychiatrists have considered: (Brigham 2001)

(1) Augmentation, whatever the thyroid labs.
(2) If TSH is over 2, treat til it's below 1.
(3) Treat until FT3 and FT4 reach high normal.
(4) Treat until FT4 is 150% of high normal.

Brigham (2001) says such approaches have "been discussed in various clinical forums and reports, and are defensible current practice."

Natural approaches

In some cases nutritional approaches, may be helpful as first line treatment; in others they can serve as an adjunct (as medically indicated) to hormone replacement or other treatment.

Suppressing thyroid overactivity (WATTS 1989. BARNES 1976, PFEIFFER 1988, LANGER 1998, JENNINGS 1970)

CONSIDER THE FOLLOWING NUTRIENTS:

□ **Lithium** — known for suppressing the thyroid. Pfeiffer suggests low doses can be preferable to radiation or surgery for hyperthyroidism.

□ **Iodine balance** — if iodine is overstimulating the thyoid, restriction can be useful. (LAUBERG 1998, 99, AGHINI-LOMBAQRDI 1999) On the other hand, overactivity is sometimes due to iodine *deficiency,* making seaweeds and other natural sources potentially helpful. (BARNES 1976, LANGER 1998)

□ **Legumes** (soy, peas, beans, peanuts), crucifers (broccoli, cabbage, etc.), rutabagas, strawberries, peaches, radish — reduce iodine availability, temporarily slowing thyroid function. (WATTS 1989)

□ **Vitamins C** and **E** — may be helpful if an enlarged thyroid is over-secreting hormone.

□ **EFAs** — support normal function (deficiency may promote hyperthyroidism). *Histamine imbalance patients tend to do best with omega 3, pyrolurics, especially if severe, with an emphasus on GLA.*

□ **B12, PABA, cobalt, calcium, sulfur, molybdenum, B17** (laetrile) — may help slow thyroid function. (Copper may, in some cases, inhibit but, most often, stimulates thyroid activity.) (WATTS 1989)

□ **Selenium** — relatively high doses may, in some cases, be helpful in reducing T3 formation. (BRATTER 1996, HOFBAUER 1997)

□ **Hormone balances** — Insulin, cortisol, and parathyroid compete with thyroid and may reduce thyroid secretions. High estrogen suppresses pituitary TSH. (WATTS 1989, LANGER 1998)

Protective nutrients:

□ **B complex** — supports neural function, protects the heart. *Check contraindications for histadelics.*

□ **B1** may protect against thyroxine toxicity. (SURE 1950)

□ **B1, B6, C, E, and calcium** — often depleted by overactive thyroid.

□ **C, zinc, magnesium, taurine, B vitamins, antioxidants** — may help calm overstimulation and protect the heart.

□ **D3** — supports calcium uptake. *But excess may overstimulate the thyroid.*

See *Nutrient contraindications,* next page.

Activating low thyroid (WATTS 1989, CRAYHON 1998, GALTON 1979, BARNES 1976, PFEIFFER 1988, AIROLA 1974, BALCH 1990, PAGE 1992, SALAMAN 1989, LANGER 1998, JENNINGS 1970)

In some patients, nutritional and herbal support alone redresses underactivity, especially when the cause is chronic insufficiency of iodine or nutrient imbalances. However, given the potentially severe complications of thyroid illness, if nutrient and herbal therapies are not completely effective, hormone replacement usually becomes essential. (BARNES 1976) *In such cases, nutrients can still help augment treatment. Many second and third generation hypothyroid patients, some first generation, require hormone replacement.*

CONSIDER THE FOLLOWING NUTRIENTS:

□ **Tyrosine** — a key component of thyroid hormones.

□ **Iodine** — critical to thyroid hormone creation. (So supports growth and development of nerve cells, general cell metabolism and energy production, and immunity.) When depleted, thyroid function is

"Any person that is suspected of bipolar disorder should without question be referred to the nearest endocrinologist for a thorough workup... lithium and other [such] drugs... destroy the thyroid. Vitamin deficiencies also are related."

Gayle Eversole, CRNP, PhD, AHG, DHom

Osteoporosis issues (LANGER 1998, GABY 1994, STARR)

Overuse of thyroid hormone (particularly high-dose T4), as well as hyperthyroidism, has been associated with increased risk of osteoporosis.

Risk can be significantly reduced by avoiding sugar, alcohol, caffeine, and stimulants; (SAFFAR 1981, HEANEY 1982, HERNANDEZ 1991, HOLLINGBERY 1985, SPENCER 1985) eating calcium-rich foods; taking supportive supplements (e.g., D3, magnesium, boron, etc.; (GABY 1994) walking and engaging in weight-bearing exercise; reducing stress; and, where appropriate, dividing the thyroid dose over the day or prescribing time-release thyroid.*

Ideally, if thyroid dose must be reduced, the patient will not have to be placed into mild hypothyroidism to protect the bones. Osteoporosis risk should be considered in the context of the risk, if thyroid is not treated sufficiently, of unresponsive bipolar depression; and an increased tendency to experience stress; use stimulants, sugar, etc., and to eschew exercise.

That said, bone density should be assessed in at-risk patients prior to treatment, measured periodically, and treatment adjusted as relevant.

See *Calcium, Magnesium,* pp. 122-26; *Vitamin D3,* pp. 119-20.

* And perhaps, considering the balance with anabolic hormones (DHEA, estrogen, progesterone, testosterone, etc.). (Brigham 2001, Gaby 1994)

Crayhon's hypothyroid support suggestions

Thyroid glandular, carnitine, CoQ10, vitamins A, B, C, E, magnesium, zinc, selenium, GLA, EPA, DHA. (CRAYHON 1998)

Nutrient cautions

Tyrosine, phenylalanine — can increase dopamine, adrenalin, noradrenalin, and thyroxine, and so exacerbate hyperthyroidism or mania. Monitor. *Contraindicated if vulnerable to melanoma.*

Iodine — though deficiency is renown for causing thyroid dysfunction, excess is, in some cases, implicated. Thus, prolonged excess sometimes leads to hypo or hyperthyroidism, thyrotoxicosis, Graves disease (especially if after chronic deficiency), (Stanbury 1998, Delange 2000a) or a worsening of the damage to follicle cells from selenium and zinc deficit. (Ruz 1999).
Too much iodine can also cause toxic rash, metallic taste, headache, difficulty breathing, free radical proliferation (Vitale 2000), and (like too much thyroid) poses cardiac risk, (Stanbury 1998) especially if intake is rapidly escalated. (Delange 2000a)

Iron — supplementation, even within a multiple, should be separated by at least 4 hours from thyroid medication, as it can interfere with absorption. (Shakir 2001)

Iron — Hypothyroid individuals are often depleted, but be wary of overcompensating, as too much creates oxidative stress. (Vitale 2000) Take only if deficient, and monitor for rising levels with thyroid corrections. Males are more prone to overload.

Copper — excess may promote anxiety, panic, mania, or psychosis in vulnerable persons. (Pfeiffer 1987)

Selenium — Excess (perhaps above 500 mcg) may depress FT3. (Br"atter 1996)

Thyroid inhibitors — Overindulgence in inhibiting substances can temporarily slow thyroid function.

Address adrenal & liver requirements

If any adrenal or liver subfunction is not addressed, reduced creation of T3 may leave the patient suffering selected low thyroid symptoms (e.g., cognitive slowing), even when treated with relatively high doses of thyroxine. The high T4 will then add a limited assortment of high thyroid symptoms (e.g., palpitations, rapid pulse, increased sweating), compounding the patient's troubles, and presenting a contradictory symptom profile to the physician.

inhibited, (Ruz 1999) and the gland enlarges, producing goiter. (Prange, Whybrow 1987)

- □ **Natural iodine sources** — seafoods (fish, kelp, dulse, other seaweeds). Modest quantities in mushrooms, garlic, onion, liver, potatoes, carrots, beef, squash, bee pollen (*avoid if allergic*), watermelon, bananas, berries. (Balch 1990, Garrison 1985, Page 1992, Lieberman 1990, Nutricircles 1996)
- □ **Selenium** — part of the deiodinase enzyme that converts T4 to T3 (the more active hormone) in peripheral tissues. (Stockdale 1996) [50-100 mcg, (Ruz 1999)] *Too much selenium can be counterproductive.* (Bratter 1996, Hofbauer 1997)
- □ **Zinc** — may help prevent thyroid atrophy and follicle degeneration; may play a role in T3 and T4 creation, (Gupt 1997) and help normalize T3 and TRH responsiveness. If T3 is low (suggested by poor response to T4 alone), 50-100 mg zinc may help maintain follicle cells. (Ruz 1999)
- □ **B6** — supports use of iodine to make thyroxine.
- □ **B12, iron, copper** — sometimes low; these nutrients help reverse any attendant anemia (which is common). (Duntas 1999) Iron and copper are also used, along with zinc and adrenal cortisol, in T4 to T3 conversion, *but may be contraindicated.*
- □ **Magnesium** — supports thyroid function. (Crayhon 1998) (Also supports mood stability, reduces stress, benefits blood pressure.)
- □ **Carnitine** — may partly spare thyroid hormone through its role in fat transport and metabolism, and enhancement of cellular energy production. (Crayhon 1998)
- □ **CoQ-10** — antioxidant, promotes stamina and cell oxygenation. Helps protect the heart. (Crayhon 1998)
- □ **B2** — supports thyroid hormone secretion. (Bell 1992)
- □ **B3** — supports respiration and metabolism, and helps control cholesterol.
- □ **A** — supports TSH formation and iodine absorption. It's often depressed in hypothyroids, due to difficulty metabolizing carotenes. Depletion compromises protein absorption.
- □ **C, bioflavonoids** — prevent bleeding of thyroid capillaries, support adrenals, help control cholesterol levels.
- □ **E** — supports creation of TSH.
- □ **Thiamine** — supports neurological function, reduces stress.
- □ **High quality protein** — moderate portions, to redress deficiencies.
- □ **Potassium** — helps reduce tissue water accumulation, due to kidney hypofunction; supports the heart. *Use food sources.*
- □ **Chromium** — supports sugar metabolism (often compromised).
- □ **Manganese** — supports joint function. Antidepressant.
- □ **Omega 3, perhaps GLA** — supports normal thyroid function, and receptor flexibility. *GLA is often preferentially needed by pyrolurics.*
- □ **Choline** — supports adrenals and thyroid hormone formation.
- □ **Barley grass, spirulina,** or other concentrated chlorophyll sources.
- □ **Liver and immune support** — the liver forms T3 from T4.
- □ **Adrenal support** — B5, B6, B, C, bee pollen or royal jelly (*if they don't provoke sensitivities*),* Siberian or American ginseng,* etc. If insufficient, consider pregnenolone,* or adrenal glandulars;* *perhaps, if required, low-dose* hydrocortisone,* (Jackson 1998, GSDL) which helps convert T4 to T3. (See *Adrenals*, pp. 238-39.)

* If not overstimulating. Contraindicated before or during mania.

- □ **Thyroid glandulars,** *if needed.* In some cases, *if required,* pituitary, adrenal, or liver glandulars. *Choose the least toxic sources. Can overstimulate.*
- □ Support for homocysteine metabolism, *if relevant* — B6, B12, folate, betaine, etc.

Note: Hypothyroid-induced deficiencies often demand immediate attention, even though they eventually tend to clear up as thyroid function is restored.

Diet (LANGER 1998, BALCH 1990, MURRAY 1998, BARNES 1976, SCHACHTER 1999)

Abundant fish (especially seafood), vegetables, seaweeds. High quality animal protein can be supportive in moderate portions. Seeds and nuts are helpful. Complex carbs and fresh fruits are okay in moderation.

Limit dried fruit and fruit juice, and avoid refined carbohydrates. Limit or avoid stimulants (coffee, colas, etc), alcohol, tobacco.
Limit thyroid-inhibiting foods (previous page); balance restriction against the need for any health benefits uniquely supplied by such foods; moderate intake of ocean fish and seaweeds may somewhat offset the depletion.

Dr Hing Hau Tsang 's herbs for hypothyroidism (TSANG 2007)

Tailor to individual biochemistry. Add cautiously, while adjusting ongoing thyroid treatment, to prevent overstimulation of the thyroid, cardiovascular complications, or aggravation of mania. (See *Reminder,* in the callout, below.)

- ☐ **Kelp** (*Ascophyllum nodosum*) — rich in iodine. Modulates hormones. (SKIBOLA 2005) Antioxidant, increases glutathione peroxidase. May help counter autoimmunity. (HOWIE 1995, SAKER 2004)
- ☐ **Bladderwrack** (*Fucus vesiculosus*) — supports iodine uptake. Counters estrogen. (SKIBOLA 2005) [Other mineral & iodine-rich choices: dulse,* other seaweeds, Irish and Iceland moss, parsley, garlic, horsetail, alfalfa.]

* Which is particularly rich in iron. See *Nutrient contraindications*, previous page.

- ☐ **Guggulu** (*Commiphora mukul*) — stimulates thyroid. (TRIPATHI 1984) Heals hypothyroidism in female mice. (PANDA 2005). Stimulates T3 production via liver enzymes and preservation of iodothyronine deiodinase activity. (PANDA 1999A, 2005, TRIPATHI 1984 Promotes peripheral receptor (retinoid X) function. (LI 2002, LEE 2005) Increases endogenous antioxidants.
- ☐ **Ashwaganda** (*Withania somnifera*) — regulates circulating thyroid hormone; increases concentration. Preserves iodothyronine deiodinase activity. (VAN DER HOOFT 2005, PANDA 1998, 99B, 2005) Promotes peripheral receptor function. (LI 2002, LEE 2005) *Can create thyrotoxicosis. Avoid excess.*
- ☐ **Coleus** (*Coleus forskohlin*) — Supports thyroglobulin production and promotes T3 and T4 secretion. (LAUBERG 1984) Mimics TSH in supporting the thyroid's iodine uptake and metabolism. (VAN SANDE 1982) Increases iodothyroinine deiodinase activity, promoting T3 creation. Supports peripheral receptor function. (LI 2002, LEE 2005)
- ☐ **Brahmi** (*Bacopa monniera*) — increases serum T4. Studies suggest support for the thyroid, (KAR 2002) memory, (ROODENRYS 2002) depression, (SAIRAM) and cognition. (STOUGH)
- ☐ **Rosemary** (*Rosmorinus officinalis*) — Preserves iodothyronine deiodinase activity. Promotes peripheral receptor function. (LI 2002, LEE 2005) Antioxidant.
- ☐ **Sage** (*Salvia officinalis*) — improves mood and cognitive performance, (TIDESLEY 2005) counters anxiety (perhaps via cholinesterase inhibition), (KENNEDY 2005) supports memory, (EIDI 2006) promotes peripheral receptor function. (LI 2002, LEE 2005) Antioxidant.
- ☐ **Hops** (*Hummulus lupulus*) — enhances iodine uptake to the thyroid. (RADOVIC 2005) Perserves iodothyronine deiodinase activity, promoting T3 creation. Decreases formation of inflammatory cytokines, perhaps helping counter autoimmunity.

Lifestyle

- ☐ **Exercise & deep breathing** — support cellular oxygenation.
- ☐ **D3, sunlight** — helps produce thyroid hormone. D3, outdoor light, or a light box stimulates the thyroid and is antidepressant. (TOMASI 1998, SHER 1999) Thyroid activity increases with increased seasonal light, decreases when light declines (winter), (TOMASI 1998, SHER 1999) which may be one means by which season influences mood. *Too much light can trigger mania.* See *Vitamin D,* p. 119-20; *Light,* p. 260.

Hormone replacement for hypothyroid

Hormone replacement is, in some cases, crucial. Natural thyroid hormones, which contain T4, some T3, and other supportive factors not in chemical thyroid, may be preferable despite minor variations in dose per tab. (Consider that thyroid secretion also varies day to day.) (LANGER 1998, JACKSON 1998)

Herb summary (TSANG 2007)

Iodine uptake: bladderwrack, kelp, hops, coleus.

Thyroid hormone secretion: coleus (T3, T4), bacopa (T4), ashwaganda.

Creation of T3 from T4: guggulu, coleus, hops, rosemary and ashwaganda.

Peripheral receptor function: Rosemary, sage, coleus, guggulu, ashwaganda.

Reducing autoimmune progression: kelp, hops, guggulsterones (which increase antioxidants), sage, rosemary, ashwaganda.

See *Reminder,* below.

RECOMMENDED READING

Barnes, Broda, MD, *Hypothyroidism: The Unsuspected Illness,* 1976.

Langer, Stephen E, MD, *Solved: The Riddle of Illness*, 1997.

Starr Mark, MD, *Hypothyroidism Type 2: The Epidemic*

Web:

brodabarnes.org
wilsonsthyroidsyndrome.com
wtsmed.org
tsangenterprise.com/news118.htm
armourthyroid.com
thyroidinfo.com

Reminder: The material in this book is presented for educational purposes only. If you need treatment for thyroid, adrenal or bipolar disorders, or any other medical condition, please seek the services of a knowledgeable physician.

Adrenals

Adrenal primer (JTI 2005, Murray 1998)

The adrenal cortex secretes:

Glucocorticoids (such as, cortisol) which, in response to stress, increase blood oxygen (by raising blood pressure) and fuel (sugar, nutrients); reduces distractions (immune and allergic response); and influences cardiovascular sodium/potassium pumps.

Corticosteroids include mineral corticoids (e.g., aldosterone, which increases kidney sodium retention and potassium excretion); and 17-ketosteroids (e.g., DHEA, testosterone, estrogen).

The adrenal medulla secretes:

Norepinephrine & epinephrine, which produce "flight or fight" reactions to stress.

Antidepressant corticosteroids (Smith 1998)

Pregnenolone* — generally elevates mood, boosts energy, and improves memory, mental performance, well-being, stress tolerance, cerebral function and sleep. It is often reduced during depression, and may be of some use for bipolar depression, (Mathis 1994) *though excess may trigger mania.*

* A precursor to DHEA and over 150 adrenal steroids including hormones critical to sexual function (progesterone, estrogens, testosterone), immune activity (cortisol), inflammation, skin health, and wound healing. Pregnenolone is made from cholesterol. Natural levels decline with age.

DHEA — enhances vitality, energy, well-being, relaxation, stress tolerance, memory and normal sleep.* It may be of particular benefit in bipolar depression, *but is more likely than pregnenolone to trigger mania.*

* It also supports immune function, and protects from the effects of excess cortisol, free radical damage, and autoimmune illness. Studies also suggest benefit to obesity, chronic fatigue, diabetes, osteoporosis, elevated cholesterol, heart conditions, lupus, Alzheimer's, and other degenerative diseases. Levels peak at age 20 and are depleted with age.

Sex hormones — see pp. 241-43.

Warning: Corticosteroids should only be used if medically indicated.

The two adrenal glands sit on the top of the kidneys, regulating reactions to stress, producing sex hormones, and influencing immune and allergic response, blood pressure, sodium retention, and carbohydrate, fat and protein metabolism.

Depressive illness, may drive the brain/adrenal system. In bipolar and major depression, the hypothalamus/pituitary/adrenal axis is often overactive and dysregulated, with increased hypothalmic stimulation, adrenal cortex hypersecretion, and/or enlarged pituitary and adrenals. (Rose 1987, Gold 1987, Reus 1987, Prange 1987) Both adrenocortical under (as in Addison's) and overactivity (as in Cushing's) have frequently been associated with mood symptoms, anxiety, behavioral lability and aggression. Adrenal function may vary with mood. (Musselman 1996)

Adrenal exhaustion (Ross 2002, Jackson 1998 Slagle 1992)

Mood disorder often exhausts the adrenals. Alternately, serious adrenal dysfunction can trigger/contribute to depression, mania, and mood instability, and may be mistaken for mood disorder. Psychiatric symptoms may emerge before physical symptoms of adrenal problems, obscuring the underlying cause, and may include:

- □ Chronic stress, irritability, tears. Sweaty hands and feet with stress. Feeling of being overwhelmed.
- □ Anxiety and depression that may improve at night, or with food.
- □ Easy startle. Fears, phobias. Paranoia.
- □ Sensitivity to light, sounds, smells. Dark circles under eyes.
- □ Trouble falling asleep. Insomnia, often with headaches or migraines.
- □ Difficulty concentrating. Confusion. Shaky, light-headed. Fainting.
- □ Dry flaky skin. Skin problems (e.g., acne, eczema, psoriasis, lupus).
- □ Small jaw, crowded uneven lower teeth. Grinds teeth at night.
- □ Sweet or salt cravings. Allergies. Heartburn. Chemical sensitivity. Intolerance to alcohol, caffeine, drugs. Weight concentrated in trunk.
- □ Fatigue. Clumsiness. Weak muscles. Feel worse after exercise.
- □ Inflammation. Chronic upper back pain. Joint or muscle pains.
- □ Heart palpitations. Low blood pressure. Low cholesterol.
- □ Indigestion, stomach pain. Alternating constipation and diarrhea.
- □ Little thirst. Infrequent urination. Low sexual vitality.
- □ Recurrent infections (change-of-season colds, Candida, etc.), perhaps severe. Breathing difficulties, especially asthma.

Weakened adrenals: Some nutritive considerations (Murray 1994, Reus 1987)

- □ C, E, other antioxidants, B5, B6, B, magnesium, potassium (*foods*), zinc.
- □ Bee pollen, royal jelly, ginseng, ginkgo, gotu kola. *Contraindicated with mania or if allergic.*
- □ Oral pregnenolone may be helpful during depression, *if deficient. Restrict or eliminate with any signs of mania, as relevant.*
- □ Address nutrient and biotype imbalance.
- □ Treat mood and eating* disorders. Avoid allergens, refined carbs.
- □ Support metal metabolism, endocrine balance, etc.
- □ Avoid chemical toxins, street drugs, alcohol,** etc.
- □ Limit exposure to stress. Employ stress reduction techniques.
- □ Get plenty of fresh, outdoor air. Walk, exercise, etc.
- □ Adrenal cortex glandulars — may be indicated in severe cases of allergy, inflammation, or stress. (Murray 1994)

* Glucocorticoids rise before and after meals. Adrenals mediate feeding, so dysfunction can be associated with anorexia, bulimia, or obesity, resolution of which may normalize adrenal axis response. (Reus 87)

** Alcohol alters cortisol release and rhythm and generally compromises adrenal function. Adrenal problems can also worsen ethanol dependence (glucocorticoids facilitate tolerance), and make withdrawal more difficult. (Reus 1987)

Glucocorticoids, stress, & mood (Reus 1987, JTI 2005)

Bipolar episodes, especially early on, seem to be triggered by mental or environmental stressors. Acute stress stimulates secretion of adrenal cortisol and other glucocorticoids, increasing fuel, oxygen, and catecholamines, (Stokes 1981, Jimerson 1983, Rubin) and decreasing distraction. The catecholamines then enhance aggression and, perhaps, memory of the event. Even with intense stressors, cortisol should return to baseline in days. In bipolars, though, ongoing stress and elevated norepinephrine may continually promote/intensify adrenal dysregulation.

"Cortisol frequently skyrockets when depressed; falls to low normal in manics."
Michael Lesser, MD, 2008

Chronic elevation in depression (& some manias) (Rose 1987, Reus 1987, Gold 1987)

In 40-60% of depressions, (Stokes 1981, 84, Stoll 1984) up to 85% of bipolar depressions, (Schlesser 1983) and some manias (often mixed), the adrenal axis becomes dysregulated, with persistently elevated glucocorticoids, unresponsive to hypothalamus or pituitary suppression. (Carroll 1976) High cortisol may persist months, even after remission.* (Rose 1987) The constant elevation often goes on to suppress receptor response and distort inhibitory feedback. Thus the pituitary may oversecrete ACTH (despite the high cortisol), (Rose 1987) the hypothalamus may oversecrete CRF targeting adrenal cortisol directly, (Gold 1987, Pfohl 1985, Halbreich 1987) or the entire HPA axis may become elevated. (Gold 1987, Sachar 1975)

Dysregulation is generally associated with greater depressive severity and greater risk of relapse or suicide.**(Ansseau 1991) With *chronic* HPA elevation, neural and physical activity decline, promoting depression. (Gold 1987, Swann 1992) Cognition and memory become impaired; and brain metabolism and access to energy and oxygen, compromised. Brain cells are damaged or die, particularly in the hippocampus, which is crucial to brain/adrenal interactions, memory, and learning. Receptors are lost; glial cells, destroyed. Impaired hippocampal flexibility and other damage can worsen depression, and may contribute to OCD, or cognitive defects. Eventual depletion of locus coeruleus norepinephrine would foster motor suppression, distraction, ambivalence, stereotypic behavior, and other depressive symptoms. Chronic high cortisol also compromises immunity, which can then further distort mood. (Reus 1987, JTI 2005)

* Cortisol may also elevate one to two weeks before relapse (especially in patients who have undergone multiple depressive episodes).

** Thus, data from the DST (a provocative challenge test which determines whether the adrenals continue to produce glucocorticoids when the pituitary stops requesting them) suggests greatest nonsuppression of adrenal secretion in suicidal, (Arana), then psychotic patients, (Mendlewicz 1992) then in pure familiar depression. (Schlesser 1983, Targum 1982, 83) Adrenals are nonresponsive in perhaps 85% of bipolar (Schlesser 1983) vs. 50% of unipolar depressives; (Stokes 1981, 84, Stoll 1984) and may normalize when depression resolves, but not necessarily in bipolars. (Watson 2004) (Nonresponse also occurs in Cushings, and in some with mixed mania, (Stokes 1981, 84, Stoll 1984, Carroll 1976) OCD, eating disorders, TLE, major illness, pregnancy, aging, uncontrolled diabetes, using/withdrawing from alcohol or narcotics, or taking CBZ, phenytoin, or barbiturates, or certain other meds.) (Ansseau 1991, Meltzer 1982)

Brain/glucocorticoid physiology

Brain NE, E --->
hypothalamic CRF --->
pituitary ACTH --->
adrenal glucocorticoids--->
NE, E *or* CRF/ACTH

□ Significant stress, depression, light/dark changes, adrenocortex feedback, and other stimuli cause the *locus coereleus* (which mediates selective attention and response) to release *norepinephrine* to the hippocampus.

□ *Hippocampal pyramid cell messages* project through neocortical sites including the hypothalamus.

□ The *paraventricular nucleus (PVN), in the hypothalamus,* releases *CRF* (corticotropin releasing factor) and other ACTH releasing factors.

□ *ACTH* stimulates adrenal secretion of: *glucocorticoids,* which increase circulating oxygen and fuel (by raising blood sugar, pressure, and pulse), and decrease distractions (suppressing feeding, etc.);

□ Acute stress, also activates *mineral corticoid receptors,* which increase catecholamine activity (perhaps, thereby, promoting aggression, and enhancing memory of the event). (Stokes 1981, Jimerson 1983, Rubin)

□ Cumulative cortisol should feed back to the hypothalamus and pituitary, *suppressing ACTH* and *CRF.*

Glucocorticoid changes & mania (Rose 1987, Reus 1987, Gold 1987)

Suppression — Chronic low cortisol reduces blood sugar, promoting hypoglycemia, perhaps with attendent depression. With lengthy or pronounced hypoglycemia, so much adrenalin may be mobilized to increase sugar that anxiety or mania, may be triggered.

See *Hypoglycemia therapies,* pp. 217-18.

Acute elevation — With acute stress, cortisol elevations may also trigger mania. And initial glucocorticoid replacement therapy can create a temporary mania, even in normals.*

* Thus, Ur (1992) reports on a depressed woman with low adrenocortical function who became manic on glucocorticoid administration, perhaps because depletion had sensitized receptors.

More on the role of adrenals in mood

Hypoglycemia, pp. 214-218.
Catecholamines, pp. 106-14.
Sex hormones, pp. 241-43.

Some basic approaches (glucocorticoid elevation) (Murray 1994, Reus 1987, Balch)

- ☐ Limit stress and employ relaxation techniques. (See pp. 252-53.)
- ☐ Mood-stabilizing nutrients, B, C, E, Mg, Zn, etc, as relevant. (21-83)
- ☐ Address biotypes (pp. 145-68), metal metabolism, blood sugar, endocrine balance, etc. (pp. 197-250)
- ☐ Avoid refined carbs (see pp. 114-22), allergens (pp. 207-13), alcohol, caffeine, street drugs, other toxins. (pp. 168-94.)

Common adrenal findings in bipolar depression

Elevated plasma or urinary cortisol often reflects depression severity. (Risch 1992)

CRF or ACTH may be elevated, unresponsive to high cortisol. (Musselman 1996) Response to ACTH and/or CRF is also often abnormal.

24 hour plasma cortisol & ACTH— secretion rhythms are often distorted,* typically with an elevated but flattened curve in the day, and high night levels, perhaps especially near midnight. Secretory episodes may also be longer and more frequent. (Pfohl 1985, Rose 1987, Ansseau 1990, Burch 1983, Krieger 1971, Sachar 1975)

Pregnenolone and/or DHEA can be low.

Pituitary or adrenal enlargement in some. (Musselman 1996)

Abdominal fat accumulation due to chronic high cortisol.

* In the general population, secretions concentrate early, peaking just before waking, and in relation to meals, followed by a steady decline, with the nadir at night. (Krieger 1971, Gallagher 1973, Gold 1987)

Adrenal disorders influencing mood

Hypoglycemia

Prevalent. See pages 214-18.

Cushing's (Gold 1987, Pfeiffer 1988, Morgan 1989, Reus1987, Prange 1987, JTI)

"Nearly all of the HPA abnormalities... in Cushing's syndrome can occur in patients with primary psychiatric disorder." — Victor I Reus, MD

Cushing's disease is characterized by *excess corticosteroids* due to elevated pituitary ACTH. In Cushing's syndrome the cause is adrenal overactivity, or prescribed hormones.

Elevated plasma cortisol can directly alter mood and cognition. Most patients exhibit psychiatric disorder, often depression, with suicidality in perhaps 10%. Psychotic symptoms, including paranoid delusions and auditory hallucinations may occur in up to 20%. Other symptoms include anxiety, euphoria, excitement, delirium, irritability, insomnia, mood elevation in some, disorientation, weak concentration, recent memory loss.*

Cushings patients may (perhaps rarely) show cyclic behavior and hormonal changes, which may suggest bipolar disorder. Early symptoms, e.g., emotional instability, nervousness and inability to cope may obscure primary Cushings, while nonetheless due to adrenal hypersecretion. Successful treatment may improve mood. (Kathol 1985)

* Physical symptoms: Some patients are only short, obese, or low in potassium, while others develop extensive symptoms, e.g., thin, easily-bruised skin; acne; puffy eyes; a flushed "moon" face; red-purple lines on abdomen, back and thighs; abdominal swelling; increased body hair; a fat neck, fat pads on the trunk and back. Complications include diabetes, Candida, high blood pressure, kidney stones, muscle and bone deterioration, menstrual irregularities, backache, impaired sexual function, poor wound healing. Cushing's is fatal if untreated.

Addison's disease (Gold 1987, Pfeiffer 1988, Morgan 1989)

Addison's disease results from a deteriorating adrenal cortex, creating *chronic reductions in adrenal hormones.** The illness comes on slowly, sometimes with temporary partial remissions. Stress can trigger an acute crisis.

Psychiatric symptoms are common, and may involve apathy, depression, low initiative, negativity, emotional instability, poverty of thought, dulled intelligence, altered cognition, insomnia, giddiness, confusion. Levels of consciousness and mental symptoms fluctuate. Acute crises can produce psychotic episodes, with clouding of senses, stupor or delirium.**(Gold 1987, Whybrow 1981, Hall)

* Thus, failure to respond to ACTH. Other causes include malignancy, tuberculosis, toxicity and inflammation. EEGs may indicate increased excitability. It's autoimmune in 90%, and relatively rare. Medical treatment may involve steroid replacement, attention to the sodium/potassium balance and causal factors. (Prange 1987)

** Physical symptoms include darkened patches of skin, spreading from areas where friction occurs; weakness, fatigue, loss of appetite, nausea, vomiting, diarrhea, weight loss, hypoglycemia, dehydration, dizziness, low blood pressure, anemia, pain, cold intolerance, immune dysfunction. Acute crises can produce severe pain in the stomach, lower back or legs and, eventually, collapse of blood vessels, kidney failure, coma. (Gold 1987, Pfeiffer 1988, Morgan 1989)

Pheochromocytoma (Gold 1987, Pfeiffer 1988, Morgan 1989, Whybrow 1981)

Pheochromocytoma, is a relatively rare condition,* in which chromaffin cell tumors, usually in the adrenal medulla, secrete *excess adrenalin and noradrenalin.*

Symptoms can be triggered by food, alcohol, physical exertion, bending, twisting, emotional stress, excitement, laughter, sneezing, gargling, sleep and pregnancy.

Mental symptoms occur mainly during attacks, and can include chronic depression, anxiety, intense apprehension, feelings of impending doom, or depressive psychosis. Panic attacks may provoke a temporary psychosis.*

* Physical symptoms can occur 20-30 times/day, and typically start with a flush at the head or neck, a sensation of heat, profuse perspiration, cold clammy skin, palpitations, wheezing, tightness in the throat, increased salivation or tears, dizziness, tingling limbs, nausea, and gastrointestinal reactions. Other symptoms can include impaired vision, fainting, chest pain, severe headaches, chronic high blood pressure. Medical treatment usually involves surgery.

Female sex hormones

Androgen, estrogen and progesterone fluctuations can profoundly influence mood and cognition (consider, the mood changes of pregnancy or menopause). (PRANGE 1987, BRIGHAM 2001) Some women may be especially sensitive to changing hormone levels. (GLICK 1987)

Estrogens: pro or anti-depressant

Estrogen promotes secondary sex characteristics, sex drive, and ovulation. It also can be antidepressant, is a MAO inhibitor, (PRANGE 1987) and has psychostimulant properties. (Thus, polycystic ovary syndrome, characterized by low estrogen, commonly produces tearful depressions (even though testosterone is elevated).*)

On the other hand, estrogen increases liver breakdown of tryptophan** to nicotinic acid, leaving less available for the brain to convert to serotonin. And high estrogen may inhibit pyridoxal phosphate (a form of B6),*** further compromising serotonin production.

Thus, estrogen tends to foster increased catecholamines and reduced serotonin, making it more likely to counter depression in patients with initially low catecholamines and relatively unexcitable temperaments, and often less than helpful in irritable patients with low serotonin and/or B6. (PRANGE 1987)

* Physical symptoms can include: profuse facial or body hair, acne, weight concentrated in the trunk, muscularity, menstrual problems, cysts or endometriosis, insulin-resistance or diabetes.

** Via tryptophan hydrogenase.

*** An estimated 80% of women taking oral contraceptives become functionally B6-deficient. (OC's can also reduce B2, folate, B12 and C, but raise A.) (Prange 1987)

Studies

A National Institute of Mental Health controlled study, of 34 women with relatively normal estrogen, found intake improved mood in 80%, relieving early-morning waking, loss of enjoyment, sadness and irritability. (SCHMIDT 2000) In another study, one-sixth of patients taking estrogen-based oral contraceptives (OCs) experienced mood elevation (and increased ability to initiate and engage in work previously avoided); one sixth, depressive symptoms; the rest, no change. (GLICK 1987)

Thus, for some patients, estrogen intake is not helpful to mood, (PRANGE 1987, SHAPIRA 1985) especially long-term. (PRANGE 1987) Ongoing use (as in OCs) can be associated with depression, fatigue, irritability, agitation, and altered libido. (PRANGE 1987)

See also *Copper overload in women*, p. 172.

Progesterone & mood moderation

Progesterone maintains pregnancy. It also has a calming, sedative influence which may help stabilize mood and moderate mania, especially if levels are low. (GLICK 1987)

Progesterone elevates synaptic MAO, (PRANGE 1987) which may explain its moderation of irritability and overexcitement. It also may increase serotonin, promoting contentment and countering some depressions.

Pfeiffer proposes: PMS tension, irritability, peeling nails,* low serotonin, and relatively high catecholamines, suggest progesterone support is more likely than estrogen to improve the depression.**

* With peeling nails, he also suggests sufficient zinc, manganese and protein.

** Similarly, such patients tend to do better with progesterone-dominant OCs. (Prange 1987, Glick 1987)

Symptoms of low sex hormones (PRANGE 1987, BRIGHAM 2001, GLICK 1987)

Low estrogen

Depressed, tearful, dazed.
Irritability, insomnia, headaches.
Infertility, low sex drive. Hot flashes, night sweats. Vaginal dryness.
Loss of hair on top of the head.

Low progesterone:

Nervousness, moodiness.
Light sleeper.
Breast pain and swelling.
Cramps, infertility.

Low testosterone

Depression, fatigue.
Low sex drive.
Reduced muscle mass.

Menstrual cycle effects (PRANGE 1987)

PMS symptoms include irritability, sadness, anxiety, insecurity, lethargy, tears, fatigue, impatience, restlessness and tension. They are usually milder than in classical depression. Nonetheless, suicide admissions increase just before, and during menses. (PRANGE 1987) Dalton finds progesterone is often low in severe/ incapacitating PMS. *Check actual hormone balances.*

Affective psychosis (and cycling in general) is sometimes tied to the menstrual cycle, and may respond to appropriate hormones (or relevant nutrients) taken with other mood-stabilizing therapy. (GLICK, STEWART, 1980)

"I am a miner. The light burns blue.
Waxy stalactites
Drip and thicken, tears.
The earthen womb
Exudes from its dead boredom."

Sylvia Plath, 1963. Plath suffered extreme moodiness and, according to Jamison, was probably bipolar II. Thompson suggests PMS may have played a key role in her mood volatility, depressions, chronic illness, and suicide. Moses (2003) suggests her literary images and content often relate to fertility, ovulation, menses, suffering, or rebirth.

Oxytocin (INSEL 1992, CARTER 1993, GETS 1996, PRANGE 1987)

Oxytocin, released through the pituitary, is known as a love and attachment hormone. It fosters social organization and, with sufficient estrogen, stimulates maternal and mating behavior. Such effects suggest some antidepessant activity.

Testosterone: Antidepressant in women (DAVIS 2000)

Known for its role in male libido, testosterone is an important mood regulator in women,* and fosters a sense of well-being.**

Androgens may also reduce allergic and sensitivity reactions, including those which produce mood symptoms.

Testosterone may drop more than 50% around menopause, up to 100% with hysterectomy or ovary removal. In some women, secretion stops independently from such factors.

Warning 1: If prescribed when not actually deficient, or if too much is given, even if indicated, testosterone can play havoc with the female reproductive system, and may promote cancer and other harmful health effects.

* Interestingly lithium initially seems to elevate testosterone (which then decreases over approximately five years). (Kusalic 1996).

** In Australia, psychiatrists often refer older depressed women, especially when postmenopausal, for testosterone replacement, at the Jean Hailes Foundation Clinic (which is studying its benefits to depression, libido, bone density and health in women).

Postpartum mood (GLICK 1987, PRANGE 1987, BRIGHAM 2001, PFEIFFER 1988)

Pregnancy elevates both estrogen and progesterone, (GLICK 1987) especially in the last month. Estrogen can double, then back down postpartum. (CONNELLY 1990) Progesterone lowers a few days pre-delivery and plumets after birth. (PRANGE 1987) Such changes repercuss on the limbic system, threatening emotional balance. (GOLD 1987) Hypothyroidism (especially, autoimmune) may develop and (perhaps along with a pervading sleep deprivation) further destabilize mood. (WEHR 1987)

Women are most vulnerable to psychiatric disorder in the first three months postpartum, (PRANGE 1987, BRIGHAM 2001) with marked estrogen drops greatly increasing risk, even more so with a personal or family history of bipolar illness. (O'HARA 1991) Mild postpartum blues occur in up to 50%, especially after a first child; 10-20% develop clinical depression. (GOLD 1987)

Postpartum symptoms often include irritability, tearfulness, fatigue, headache, insomnia, and uncharacteristic religious preoccupation, but can also involve disorientation, clouded consciousness, self-destructive tendencies, paranoia, or maternal rejection of her baby. Approximately 0.1% develop depressive psychosis (GOLD 1987), often within a week of delivery (DEAN 1981).

Just before, or by about two weeks postpartum, (MELTZER 1985) risk of mania in untreated bipolars with more than one prior episode may be over 50%. (BRIGHAM 2001)

Lab (ROSS 2002, TUTTLE 2005)

Blood estradiol, estrone, estriol, progesterone, pregnenolone, free testosterone and dihydrotestosterone, androstenedione, DHEA, insulin, glycohemoglobin, *or*

Salivary estrogens, progesterone, testosterone, cortisol, DHEA, etc.

Copper. (PFEIFFER 1988, WALSH 2004)

Natural approaches might involve (PFEIFFER 1988, WRIGHT)

- □ B6 — supports hormone balance and serotonin formation; benefits PMS.*(ADAMS 1973, 74, BRUSH 1985, BERMOND 1982, GUNN, KENDALL 1987, KLEIJNEN 1990)
- □ E, boron, EFAs, *as relevant.*
- □ Psychosocial support.
- □ If copper is elevated, restrict exposure, and support metal metabolism balance, *as relevant* (See pp. 170-73.) (WALSH 2004AB)
- □ Mood stabilizing nutrients, *as relevant.*
- □ If serotonin is low, precursors, (WYNN 1975) perhaps a complex-carbohydrate-focused diet.
- □ Appropriate herbals — may help support relevant hormone and mood balances (e.g., vitex (which is generally balancing); maca and licorice (which stimulate the adrenals to create sex hormones); other herbs which support progesterone (wild yam), estrogen (raspberry leaf, Dong Quai, liferoot, false unicorn root (an estrogen regulator), etc.), or androgen (ginsengs) levels, *as relevant to individual hormonal requirements, cancer risk, and other health factors.* (HOLISTICONLINE.COM... 2008)
- □ Hormone replacement, *only if medically indicated. Natural* hormones are preferable. Estriol may be the least risky form of estrogen. Natural progesterone is sometimes preferable to estrogen, or a combination of the two may be indicated. *Tailor to individual requirements.* (WRIGHT)

Warning 2: Hormonal birth control and hormonal replacement therapies entail substantial health risk. Estrogen, particularly, has been associated with increased risk of cancer, blood clots, stroke, and other severe conditions; chemical progesterone, with cancer, depression, fluid retention, etc. Excessive testosterone can be disastrous (see Warning 1, above). Physicians should review current literature, conduct a full assessment, coordinate or refer to OB/GYN, etc., engage in full discussion with the patient. (HOLISTIC... 2008, WRIGHT)

Male sex hormones (PRANGE 1987, GLICK 1987)

Androgens are antidepressant

Androgens (male hormones) promote secondary sex characteristics, produce sperm, and underly sex drive.

Androgens are naturally antidepressant. They increase vitality, social contact, and self-confidence. EEG profiles of high dose mesterolone, an androgen, are similar to those of stimulating antidepressants. Lowdoses produce effects similar to those of psychostimulants. (ITEL)

Deficiency in males is suppressive, possibly antimanic and, if more extreme, associated with passivity, poverty of thought, and diminished drive.

Warning: Androgen intake generally NOT indicated for males with normal levels

Though small doses of testosterone can be antidepressant in females with low levels, the larger doses needed to influence depression in males distort normal balances and tend to create prohibitive symptoms before significantly improving mood. Consider that testosterone in males is maintained in the normal adult range to advanced age. With hypogonadism, accurately-tailored hormone replacement may be corrective, but for males with generally normal levels, added androgens *can produce violence, hypersexuality, or potentially life-threatening cardiovascular disorders.* They may also contribute to mania. In one study, methyltestosterone, given with imipramine, was stimulating enough to produce florid paranoia in four of five depressed males.

Progesterone sedates males

Various studies investigate male intake of progesterone* for sedation.**

Warning: Excess can produce depression, slowed movement and reaction time, and increase temperature and heart rate variability.

* Note: The hormone, progesterone is produced by both males and females.
** Anti-androgenic chemicals (including progesterone-based formulations) have also been used to control hypersexuality associated with criminal behavior.

Effects of excess estrogen on males

Too much estrogen counters androgens, and changes male hormonal balances, posing mood, fertility, and prostate problems; even altering secondary sex characteristics. Pseudo-estrogens abound in modern industrialized countries (e.g., in many plastics, herbicides, etc.) and pose similar risk.

Important

Tampering with sexual hormones already in the normal range risks a host of severe reactions. On the other hand, when clearly deficient, and with significant symptoms of depletion, hormone replacement is sometimes indicated. *Consult with your physician*

Mania on steroid withdrawal

Venkatarangam (1988) suggests that mania, and other affective reactions to steroid withdrawal, may be more common than generally thought.

Male/female bipolar statistics

Equal numbers of men and women are bipolar. (GOODWIN1990, LAM 1999, BAUER 1996) Cumulative admissions for mania are equivalent, (SIBISI 1990), though more men experience full-blown mania, and more women are bipolar II. Initial manias tend to occur at a younger age in men. (GOLD 1987)

Women are most susceptible to mood disorder between menses and menopause, (LIEBENLUFT 1994) and are prone to premenstrual and postpartum exacerbations. (MACQUEEN)

70-90% of rapid cyclers are female. (BAUER 1994, LEIBENLUFT 1996)

Women experience more depressions than manias;* men tend toward equal occurence of both. (LEIBENLUFT 1996, ANGST 1978) Completed suicides occur about equally; women make about four times as many attempts, but men are successful four times as frequently. (GOLD 1987)

* Major depression is also more common in women, (Glick 1987) with severe symptoms in perhaps two-thirds. Women also constitute 60% of affective patients (and consume 75% of affective medications). (Gold 1987)

3. Organic brain disorders

(McCaldron 1989, Gold 1987, Davidson1983, Cohen-Cole 1987, Murray 1998, Balch 1990, Page 1992, Pfeiffer 1988, Galton 1979, Werbach 1991, 93, 94, Bagley 1971)

"All CNS disturbances... especially when chronic inflammatory and multilocal, increase the likelihood of co-occuring psychiatric symptoms." — F Engler, MD, 1991

"Neurologic etiology is generally indistinguishable from idiopathic depression." — JL Cummings MD, 1994

Certain brain disorders can trigger symptoms of, contribute to, or masquerade as mood disorder. According to Gold (1989), those most associated with bipolar disorder include partial complex seizures (see pp. 35-36), multiple sclerosis, post-concussion syndrome, and CNS tumors.

Depression occurs in 20-50% of neurological patients. Nasreddine (1997) reports lifelong prevalence of depression as: physical trauma 35%, stroke 50%, tumors 20%, MS 35%, epilepsy 30%, Parkinson's 40%, Huntington's 35%, HIV encephalopathy 30%, vascular dementia 40%, Alzheimer's 35%, Lewy body dementia 40%, and Wilson's 25%. Dysfunction or injury in depressives often involves the frontal or temporal lobes, or caudate nuclei. (Baxter 1985, Honore 1987) usually in the left hemisphere. Right hemisphere dysfunction shows greater association with mania. (See *Laterality*, pp. 283.)

Some natural therapeutic approaches are mentioned below, and on the following pages, to give the reader some sense of the relationship to nutrients used in primary bipolar disorder. This material lacks key contraindications (e.g. for lipoic acid, NAC, etc.), though some can be found in the nutrient, biotype, metals, and other sections of this book. Moreover, the following descriptions are cursory, are not intended as treatment recommendations, and are presented for educational purposes only. For more complete information, consult the relevant literature. Reminder: If you need diagnosis or treatment for mood disorder, organic brain disorders, or any other medical condition, please seek the services of a knowledgeable physician.

Conditions which can contribute to, or be misdiagnosed as, bipolar disorder

Epilepsy

Especially of the temporal lobe. See pp. 35-36.

Multiple sclerosis (MS)

Multiple sclerosis is a chronic degenerative illness caused by inflammation, deterioration, and scattering of the myelin sheath (which insulates certain nerves and accelerates nerve impulses).* Mental symptoms can include depression, euphoria, emotional upsets, intellectual deterioration and, in some cases, psychosis (usually at the onset of neurological symptoms). Temporary symptomatic remissions are typical.

MS is often mistaken for depression, sometimes, bipolar disorder (which occurs at twice the rate found in the general population). (Schiffer 1984, Horrobin 1999, Engler 1991) MS may also be more prevalent in bipolars. (Gold 1987) Depression occurs in an estimated 27-54% of MS patients. (Jaffe 1987, Minden 1990, Nasreddine 1997, Petersen 1989)

Eventually, limbs weaken, vision deteriorates, speech slurs, sensation diminishes, and seizures may occur,** suggesting the proper diagnosis.

* It may be autoimmune, (Raine 1990) or due to a virus reactivated by stress. (Johnson 1985), and is most common in women who, as children, lived in cold climates, with reduced sunlight. Symptoms usually emerge between ages 20 to 40.

** Other symptoms include transient dizziness, tingling, bladder complaints; eventually, difficulties with urination, incontinence, impotency, or vaginal numbness.

SOME NATURAL APPROACHES HAVE INCLUDED:

□ Attention to food allergies (particularly, glutenous grains and dairy), Candida, chlamydia, malabsorption. Physical therapy. (Perlmutter 2001, Murray 1998)

□ Roy Swank, MD, (1970, 77) originally suggested restricting saturated fat (to no more than 10 gm) and eating 40-55 gm of healthy, unhydrogenated, polyunsaturated oils per day. Also, whole foods, fish at least 3x/week, and limiting other animal foods, while maintaining a normal intake of total protein.

□ Michael Murray, ND, 1998, recommends flax and cod liver oils [1 Tb each], EPA [1 gm], DHA [750 mg], B12 [2-60 mg*]; selenium [200 mcg], E [600 IU], ginkgo [40-80 mg, 3x/d], a high-quality multivitamin/mineral, and pancreatin.

□ David Perlmutter, MD, generally suggests cold-water fish; nuts, seeds, dark greens, vegetarian foods; minimal dairy, no alcohol. And, hyperbaric oxygen and IM B12. Also, GLA and omega 3, magnesium, zinc, B3, B6, antioxidants (C, E, D, ginkgo, resveratrol, etc.), and brain energizers (CoQ10, NADH, phosphatidyl serine) (See *BrainRecovery.com*, 2001)

□ Researchers have also investigated bee venom therapy, which is anti-inflammatory, *but harmful if allergic.* (Hauser 2001, Fry-Welch 1996, Bellanti)

See also, *Octocosanol*, p. 245; & *Fatty acids*, pp. 85-94.

* Starting at 500 mcg, increasing gradually. Monitor; limit if causing cardiovascular reactions. (Murray 1998)

Brain trauma

Physical injury to the brain, whether due to blows to the head, toxicity, ECT, epilepsy, stroke, etc., may produce an affective syndrome, especially if the limbic system is involved. (LISHMAN 1973, GOLD 1987)

An estimated 20-50% of head trauma patients experience depression. (ROBINSON JORGE 1994, NASREDDINE 1997, SILVER 1991) One study found depression increased sevenfold (to 13.9%), panic disorder elevenfold (9%). (SHOUMITRO 1999AB) Initial symptoms relate to which part of the brain has been damaged. Anterior left hemisphere damage is associated with early major depression. Later depression or anxiety is less tied to particular brain regions. (JORGE 1993)

Studies also report manias and bipolar disorder, especially with right hemisphere damage. (POPE-HARRISON 1998, BAMRAH 1991, CLARK, DAVISON 1987, BRACKER 1987, SHUKLA 1987, YATHAM 1988)

Even mild injury can induce fatigue, absent-mindedness, irritability, anger, anxiety, depression, or prolonged elation; (GOLD 1987) or disturb concentration, attention, memory, sleep, or emotional/social interactions; and, in some cases, lead to psychosis.*(MCKENZIE 2005, WOOD 2005, GOLD 1987)

* Also, blurred or double vision, traumatic glaucoma; tinnitus, veritigo; loss of hearing, taste, or smell; head pain, drop attacks; reversal of numbers, letters, left/right; partial complex seizures; brain swelling (apraxic gait, bladder urgency, difficult cognition, etc.) or haemorrhage. (McKenzie 2005, Wood 2005, Gold 1987)

SOME NATURAL APPROACHES HAVE INCLUDED:

Note: Researchers now claim that even adults may be able to regrow some neurons. (GROSS 2000)

WITH ACUTE TRAUMA

- ☐ Hyperbaric oxygen — long enough to reduce swelling (MCKENZIE 2005, CRAYHON 1998, COLE 2005)
- ☐ C — high doses (CAMPOS 2005); or intravenous (e.g., short IV booster 2000-5000 mg, 2-3x/week; then 1000 mg time-release 3 plus x/day). (LEMMO 2005)
- ☐ Antioxidants — high intake to protect brain cells (e.g., E up to 1400 IU, selenium, resveratrol, CoQ 100mg, divided doses. Also, grape seed, milk thistle, bilberry, rosemary, green tea, zinc, etc.). (CRAYHON 1998, CAMPOS 2005)
- ☐ Magnesium — preferably injectable, otherwise as orotate. (CAMPOS 2005)
- ☐ Omega 3 and/or GLA, *as relevant,* (with B vitamins) — anti-inflammatory. (CAMPOS 2005)
- ☐ Corticosteroids, if relevant. (CAMPOS 2005)
- ☐ B1, B12 injectable. (CAMPOS 2005, EMMO 2005)
- ☐ Support blood circulation.(CAMPOS 2005)
- ☐ Avoid sugar. Limit fat. (WU 2003)
- ☐ Bach Rescue Remedy, Traumeel, Arnica (first 4 days) (ERKFRITZ 2005)

ADDRESSING CHRONIC EFFECTS

- ☐ Support circulation and tissue-building.
- ☐ Oxygenate tissue — CoQ10, gingko, etc. (CRAYHON)
- ☐ Plentiful antioxidants, including milk thistle (which is neuroptrotective), and reservatrol (which supports cellular repair). (CRAYHON 1998, HUMPHREY 2005, CAMPOS 2005)
- ☐ Magnesium. (HUMPHREY 2005, CAMPOS 2005, CRAYHON 1998)
- ☐ Symptomatic attention.
- ☐ Support brain energetics, *as relevant* — NADH, B12. Acetyl-L-carnitine with lipoic acid. (AGNELUCCI 1988, CRAYHON 98, CAMPOS, LEMMO)
- ☐ Phosphatidyl serine, (KIDD 2005, CROOK 1991) zinc — help normalize brain function. (CRAYHON 1998)
- ☐ Choline, PC, or GPC — help support memory, and perhaps, dendritic repair and growth. (MERVIS 1987, CRAYHON 1998) *May be counterproductive in some depressions*
- ☐ Essential fatty acids, *as relevant.* (HUMPHREY 2005)
- ☐ Octocosanol — a long-chain fatty acid found in wheat germ oil. May repair interneural dendrite connections, and benefit acute brain trauma.* (Dr. Andrew Ivy claims it can promote neural repair* in spastics with cerebral palsy and in post-viral encephalitic syndrome. (50% responded). Pfeiffer used 2000-4000 mcg along with zinc, B6, and C to help repair myelin, etc. Walsh also reports some success with this formula.) (CRAYHON 1998, PFEIFFER 1988)
- ☐ Green oats — used traditionally to nourish the nervous system and improve nervous debility, depression, exhaustion and, especially, stress. (KLOSS)
- ☐ Lady's slipper — thought to repair the myelin sheath. Helps allay pain and anxiety. (KLOSS)
- ☐ Chiropractic support — with spinal involvement, *if there is no bleeding and if otherwise indicated.* (WOOD 2005)
- ☐ Craniosacral work, *if indicated.* (GARY ERKFRITZ DC)

Also see, *Neuroprotective formulas*, p. 289; & *Laterality*, p. 283.

CNS tumors

Anderson (1970) and Cohen-Cole (1987) report 2-3% of purported psychiatric disorders are actually cancers. Central nervous system and hormone-secreting tumors often elicit emotional and mental symptoms, especially in early stages. (GOLD 1987) Left temporal, frontal, and limbic tumors have been associated with personality changes and a depressive syndrome. (IRLE 1994, FILEY 1995) Limbic involvement can also produce mania and a bipolar syndrome. (MCLOUGHLIN 1991)

Consider nonresponsiveness to psych meds, recent weight loss of twenty to thirty pounds or more, other suggestive symptoms, family history, and labs. (GOLD 1987)

An overview of natural approaches for CNS tumors is beyond the scope of this book.

Cerebral arterio or atherosclerosis, stroke

30 to 50% of stroke patients experience a post-stroke depression lasting a year or more. Depression has been more correlated with left frontal or left basal ganglia involvement, (STARKSTEIN ROBINSON 1989, ROBINS SZETELA 1981) and perhaps previous subcortical atrophy, (STARKSTEN 1989) than with psychosocial factors. (STARKSTEIN 1989) Serotonin (MAYBERG 1988, BYER 1992) and norepinephrine (BARRYDINAM 1990) depletion may also play a role. (NASREDDINE 1997)

Mania is rare, and strongly associated with right limbic or frontal lobe lesions, with subcortical atrophy, seizures, or genetic weakness. (STARKSTEIN 1989)

Symptoms can include hyperemotionality, exaggerated personality traits, dizziness, headaches, blackouts. At first, other areas of the brain tend to compensate for the damaged areas. Advanced illness can more permanently compromise judgment, memory, concentration, personality, and comprehension of new situations.

Stroke is more common in men, and hypertensives. Kidney circulation may indicate that of the brain.

SOME NATURAL APPROACHES HAVE INCLUDED:

- ☐ Support for cellular oxygenation: hyperbaric oxygen, (PERLMUTTER 2001) CoQ-10, germanium, ginkgo, etc. (BALCH)
- ☐ Support for cellular energetics (CoQ10, NADH, phosphatidyl serine, acetyl-L-carnitine (with lipoic acid). (PATTI 1988, PAGE 1992, PERLMUTTER 2001))
- ☐ Vinpocetine (derived from periwinkle) — enhances blood flow, prevents clots, antioxidant. (PERLMUTTER 2001)
- ☐ Address homocysteinuria, *if present.* (PERLMUTTER 2001)
- ☐ B6, niacin, B12, folic acid, B complex. (PAGE 1992, BALCH 1990, PERLMUTTER 2001)
- ☐ High doses C [buffered, 6-10 gm, divided over the day (BALCH 1990)]. Bioflavonoids, carotenes, A, E, selenium, GSH, other antioxidants. *as relevant.* (PAGE 1992, BALCH 1990)
- ☐ EPA, (BALCH 1990) and/or GLA, (PAGE 1992) *as relevant.*
- ☐ Choline *(though perhaps not with histadelia or depression).*
- ☐ Absorbable magnesium/calcium, zinc. (BALCH 1990)
- ☐ Cayenne, ginkgo, chickweed, hawthorne. (BALCH 1990) Chlorella, astragalus (for a limited time), alfalfa. (PAGE 1992)
- ☐ High-fiber diet. Limit saturated fats and animal foods. Avoid processed and refined food, alcohol, tobacco, caffeine, other stimulants. (BALCH 1990, PAGE 1992)

Common mechanisms in Parkinson's & bipolar disorder

Parkinson's is a neurogenerative disease characterized by insufficient dopamine activity, particularly in brainstem nuclei; and deteriorating and diminishing brain cells.* Serotonin and norepinephrine may also be suppressed. (MAYBERG 1990, 94, CUMMINGS 1992, 95, MCCANCE-KATZ 1992)

Early symptoms can include depression, delusions, confusion, rest tremor, rigidity, difficulty starting or stopping movements, slowed and reduced movements, stooped posture, shuffling gait, hand tremors, and a fixed, unblinking stare. Speech becomes slow, quiet, and eventually unintelligible; handwriting, illegible. Dementia eventually develops in up to one third. (MAYBERG 1990, 95, RANDRUP, CUMMINGS 1992, MCCANCE-KAT 1992)

Most Parkinson's patients have dysthymia. An estimated 40% develop depression (ROBBINS 1976, RANDRUP 1975), especially when bradykinesia and gait instability predominate. (CUMMINGS 1992)

* Contributing factors may include: distorted basal ganglia/frontal circuits trying to compensate for receptor loss; severe substantia nigra free radical damage, decreased glutathione (Jenner 1992), excitotoxicity (Blaylock 1995). Chronic neuroleptics, as well as subcortical disorders (including basal ganglia disease), can produce a Parkinsonian syndrome. (Nasreddine 1997)

Dopamine & kindling in bipolars & Parkinson's

Dopamine kindling may be a common denominator in both Parkinson's and bipolar disorders. (NAUTA 1978) Low dopamine in Parkinson's may increase receptor number and sensitivity. (CREESE 1977, 78, BUNNEY 1977) Subsequently, treatment with dopamine agonists may evoke overreaction, and in the long term, further sensitize the patient, promoting rapid dyskinesia/immobility alternations (DIMASCIO 1973, MCDOWELL 1974), as in rapid cycling bipolars, and may, in fact, lead to mood swings. L-dopa also often induces increasingly vivid dreams and waking hallucinations, and may produce mania, or paranoid or confusional psychosis. (MOSKOVITZ 1978) The difficulty Parkinson's patients have starting motor or linguistic sequences or slowing or stopping, once begun, resembles the difficulty bipolars can have getting out of a mood.

SOME NATURAL APPROACHES HAVE INCLUDED:

- ☐ IV glutathione — to counter substantia nigra oxidative stress and neural death (perhaps fostered by iron accumulation), and support mitochondrial function. (BHARATH 2002, SECHI 1996, PERLMUTTER 2001)
- ☐ Perlmutter also suggests antioxidants (C, E, D, acetyl-L-carnitine, gingko, etc); cellular energizers (CoQ10, NADH, phosphatidyl-serine); and, *if relevant,* liver detox (milk thistle, etc.).

See PERLMUTTER, *BRAINRECOVERY.COM,* 2001.

PARKINSON'S: SOME NATURAL APPROACHES (CONTINUED)

□ Balch (1990) suggests B6 (but not concurrent with L-dopa); calcium, magnesium, GABA, niacin, B; antioxidants (C, E, bioflavonoids, GSH, etc.), multivitamin-minerals, glutamine, digestive enzymes. Lecithin, brewers yeast, raw foods, seeds, nuts, and grains. Possibly, short physician-supervised fasts, chelation, or brain glandulars.

□ Amino choices — perhaps, tyrosine (which precurses dopamine), *but rule out interactions with meds, contraindications and dose restrictions.* (BALCH 1990, BRAVERMAN 1987, GELENBERG 1982) For Parkinsonian depressions, 5HTP and L-tryptophan may, in some cases, be more important than catecholamines. (MAYBERG 1990, 95, SOLOMON 1995, MCCANCE-KATZ 1992).

Reminder: With any medical condition, consult with your physician as to appropriate diagnosis and therapy.

Conditions occasionally mistaken for bipolar disorder

Huntington's chorea — a rare hereditary degenerative disorder, usually first surfacing in middle age, involving severe damage to small and intermediate-sized neurons in the basal ganglia. (MAYBERG 1992)

Symptoms may at first suggest mood disorder: indifference, depression, irritability, eccentricity, obstinacy, euphoria, paranoia, perhaps violence or psychosis. About 30% may initially be misdiagnosed with major depression,* an additional 5%, dysthymia. (CUMMINGS 1995) Some may seem to fit criteria for mania, conduct disorder, (FOLSTEIN 1989) or tardive dyskinesia.

Eventually, the deteriorating mental function, and the choreas (rapid, jerky, involuntary movements, caused by a progressive degeneration of the basal ganglia) become blatent, making the correct diagnosis more obvious. Family history also should provide some indication.

* With suicide more likely than in other neurological disorders involving depression; perhaps four to six times the rate in the general population. (Schoenfled 1984)

Dementia — a progressive deterioration of intellectual function. Many potential contributing causes can also play a role in mood disorder: chronic B12 deficiency, MT dysfunction and low zinc, (WALSH 2008) metal toxicity, (WENSTRUP 1990, CASDORPH 1995) excitotoxicity, (BLAYLOCK 1995) persistent low thyroid, recurrent severe hypoglycemia, (ROTHER1992) repeated head trauma, high fevers, multiple strokes, and medications which depress brain functioning (e.g., CCBs, neuroleptics), especially when used in combination. (GOLD 1987)

Dementias are far more likely to be initially misdiagnosed as depression than bipolar disorder. (GOLD 1987) Symptoms can include disorientation, blunted or labile emotions, inappropriate responses, deterioration of personal habits, memory loss, loss of intelligence, incoherence, delusions, and perhaps, especially in early dementias, psychosis.

Normal pressure hydrocephalus — cerebrospinal fluid is not absorbed, but suddenly seems to build up, compressing brain tissue.* (GOLD 1987)

Mental and neurological symptoms may be the most apparent, and can include delusions of persecution, depression, dementia, psychosis, incoordination, incontinence. A recent case report decribes a 22 year old male, diagnosed for two years as bipolar until an MRI revealed normal pressure hydrocephalus. Treatment resolved the manic symptoms. (REISCH 2005)

* Nonetheless, buildup may be gradual, and a prior history of brain infection or inflammation is common.

Cognitive support in neurodegenerative disorders

In MS, Parkinsons, stroke, dementias, and other neurodegenerative disorders, Paris M Kidd, PhD, 2005, generally suggests optimizing antioxidants, phospholipids, mitochondrial function, and growth factor receptors, with such nutrients (*as relevant to individual requirements*) as:

□ Glutathione, alpha lipoic acid, other antioxidants.
□ vitamins B, C, E & K
□ acetyl-L-carnitine, CoQ10, NADH.
□ phosphatidyl serine, glycerophosphocholine
□ omega 3
□ zinc, magnesium, calcium, selenium

4. Some immune & autoimmune disorders

Potentially implicated infections

Acute physical illness, anywhere from onset to many years after recovery, may trigger, or underly, chronic neurological or psychiatric disease. Alternately, a latent virus or slow infection may progressively destroy neural tissue, with symptoms only emerging decades later. Inflammatory immune chemicals add to the mix, compromising communication and function. (MAES 1995, 98, SMITH 1991, CONNOR 1998, STOLL 2002) The brain's high metabolic demands, cell specialization, lack of lymphatics, and poor ability to regenerate, enhance virulence and viral persistance. (JOHNSON 1978) Thus, infections have long been known to sometimes result in depression, delirium, psychosis, or dementia and, in some cases, have been associated with manias and bipolar syndromes. (KRISTENSSON 1986)

Influenza

Manic psychosis has been recorded following influenza. (STEINBERG 1972) The 1918 flu epidemic is infamous for the subsequent outbreak of mental illness. (TORREY 1988)

Encephalitis (GOLD 1987, KRAUTHAMMER, 1978)

Affective changes, imitating mania, depression, or psychosis, may be the only initial signs of encephalitis.* Other symptoms can include confusion, behavioral changes, memory problems, altered speech and, if severe, seizures, paralysis, or coma.

*A brain inflammation, most often occuring in the young, and usually due to a virus (e.g., herpes simplex, Epstein Barr, measles, mumps, Coxsackie virus, encephalitis lethargica, influenza). It often starts with headache and fever. Sensitivity to light or neck-ache may indicate involvement of the meninges. Mortality is high, especially in children.

Hepatitis (GOLD 1987)

Any stage of hepatitis,* even during incubation, can produce mental symptoms, including anxiety and depression. Acute delusional mania or suicide may follow physical recovery.

* Hepatitis A is incurred from contaminated food or feces; B, through the bloodstream or sex. Early physical symptoms occur 2 to 25 weeks post-infection and include loss of appetite, adversion to cigarettes, nausea, fever, malaise, aching joints, dark urine, yellowed eyes and skin.

Strep (LEMMO)

Group A streptococcus (associated with sore throats) may play a role in childhood OCD or Tourettes, can worsen anorexia, and may produce other mental symptoms.

Infectious mononucleosis (GOLD 1987)

Depression can occur at onset, during the illness, or after recovery.*

* Other symptoms can range from those of a mild cold, to swollen glands, swollen eyelids, headache, weakness, rash, sore throat, fever, liver enlargement, spleen enlargement (perhaps rupture).

Syphillis

In the early 1900s, before penicillin, syphillis* was responsible for close to a quarter of all US mental hospital placements. It is still sometimes not sufficiently screened. (GOLD 1987)

Following three to forty years of incubation, emerging symptoms can mimic almost any disease. The brain is infected in 5-15% of untreated persons, producing mental symptoms and, eventually, severe cognitive deterioration (general paresis). (GOLD 1987, PFEIFFER 1988)

Mental symptoms vary with the brain region infected. Initially, the patient may be over-talkative, restless, moody, insomniac, and headache-prone. Eventually, a relatively manic syndrome may develop (with euphoria, grandiosity, expansiveness, fabricated stories, wasted resources, rage, and, perhaps, paranoia or psychosis). Symptoms may remit for extended periods, suggesting bipolar cycles. (KRAUTHAMMER 1978, GOLD 1987)

Ultimately, judgment deteriorates, leading to moral and social mistakes. Confusion, depression, and memory lapses predominate. Alertness, ambition, abstract reasoning, even recognition of people and understanding of speech, are eventually lost. Later stages can involve dementia, seizures, paralysis, and death. (GOLD 1987)

Borna disease

Borna disease (BD)* primarily involves the limbic and olfactory systems, and the brain stem, especially its grey matter. (GOSZTONYI 1995) Bechter (1989) points out that psychiatric symptoms occur alone in some cases, perhaps with mild limbic encephalitis. (AMSTERDAM 1985, BECHTER 1987)

BD has been strongly linked to chronic fatigue, depression, and schizophrenia. (LEMMO) Mood symptoms often cycle from depression, anxiety, apathy, and passivity, to excitability, anger, and aggression, and could mimic bipolar disorder.

* An RNA virus which causes progressive immune-mediated encephalophy. (WEISMAN 1994) It is common in horses and sheep, present in most animals. Susceptibility may relate to extent of exposure. (WEISMAN 1994) Infection is latent, and triggered during brain or immune dysfunction, such as MS, HIV, or chronic malaria. (Bode 1993) Physical symptoms, such as strange gait, leg weakness, paresis, headache, etc., can fluctuate. (Bechter 1989)

Lyme disease (FALLON 1993, WWW.LYMEDISEASE... 2001)

Lyme disease* may be more prevalent in psych patients.**(HAJEK 2002) Neuropsychiatric symptoms can occur early on, leading to misdiagnosis, and may include irritability, insomnia, aggression and other manic-type symptoms; or depression. Also, incoherence, attention deficit, spatial disoridentation, memory loss, dementia, or psychosis.

In case reports by Fallon (1993), psychiatric symptoms in three Lyme patients (panic disorder, depression, and a bipolar syndrome) resolved with successful antibiotic treatment of underling Lyme disease.

* An infectious illness, usually caused by Borrelia burgdorferi (Bb), and transferred to humans from deer and furry animals (including squirrels, dogs and cats) via tick bites. Early symptoms include rash, fatigue, headache, and fever; later, numbness, tingling, seizures, muscle aches, and migrating joint pains. The tic may inject additional immune-challenging agents, besides Bb, which may further aggravate symptoms.

** In a SPECT analysis by Plutchok (1999), brain abnormalities such as hypoperfusion and poor circulation were found in 74% of 19 Lyme disease patients. Hajek (2002) found 33% of 166 psych patients with some positivity for borrelia, 19% of controls.

Miscellaneous

Herpes zoster (shingles) and rabies — attack the limbic system, creating characteristic psychotic changes, and may produce a hypomanic syndrome. (FISHER 1996)

Chronic teeth & jaw infections. (LEMMO)

Viral pneumonia — can result in depression. (GOLD 1983)

TB — produces apathy, then irritability and, in later stages, excitement, even hypomania.(GOLD 1983)

AIDS — mental symptoms occur in up to 30%.

Mad cow (Creutzfeldt-Jakob's disease) — Lendvai (1999) has reported on cases presenting as mania.

Toxoplasmosis — usually transferred to humans from cat litter, typically causes mild flu-like effects, but can produce affective syndromes.

Similarly, cytomegalovirus (a herpes virus), Epstein-Barr (which causes mononucleosis), mycoplasma pneumonia, stealth viruses, and others can have repercussions, often latent, on brain processes and affective stability.

Potentially implicated autoimmune illness

"Virtually all bipolars experience significant autoimmune issues due to the pervasive oxidative stress which alters proteins, depletes glutathione, and compromises metallothionein function."

William J Walsh, PhD, 2008

Moreover, the prevalent allergies, sensitivities, environmental illness, Candida (see pp. 202-13), etc., along with the severe psychosocial stress, challenge and dysregulate the immune system, making it more likely to start targeting body tissue. Thus, autoimmune disorders are common in bipolars: autoimmune thyroiditis (p. 232); diabetes 1 (see pp. 219-22); multiple sclerosis (p. 244); rheumatoid arthritis, narcolepsy (p. 198); some degree of celiac disease (p. 222); etc.

Autoimmune illness can also produce significant affective symptoms, for example:

Systemic lupus erythematosus (BALCH 1990, GOLD 1987, PFEIFFER, 1988, MASTERSON 1986, HOFFER 1983, ALADJEM 1972)

Systemic lupus erythematosus is thought to be largely autoimmune,* and occurs mainly in women. Central nervous system involvement can induce seizures, and symptoms of almost any mental disorder, e.g., bipolar disorder, severe depression, amnesia. Alternating immune activation and suppression may cause mood fluctuation. (STOLL 2002) Psychiatric symptoms may initially obscure diagnosis, leading to inappropriate treatment.**

* But involves specific microbes. Lupus erythematosus cells may be found in the blood and a specific antibody can be detected in 50% of patients. Blood tests often show low platelets or white blood cells, or iron-deficiency anemia. Abnormal cells may be present in the urine. Sunlight or latent viruses trigger leakage of DNA out of cell nuclei and into general circulation. The immune system forms antibodies to the leaked material, and attacks body tissue, causing relapsing tissue inflammation.**

** Physical symptoms fluctuate, and include unexplained fevers, a scaly, itchy, butterfly-shaped rash on skin exposed to the sun (typically the cheeks and bridge of the nose), inflamed blood vessels or joints, misshapen and painful joints, arthritis, kidney disease, and increased susceptibility to infection. Other symptoms include fatigue, weakness, discomfort, mouth sores, nausea, appetite and weight loss, baldness, and cardiovascular or respiratory symptoms.

Carcinoid syndrome (PRANGE 1987, GOLD 1987)

Carcinoid is an immune, possibly autoimmune illness involving hormone-secreting tumors, typically in the small intestines, stomach or appendix.* The tumors tend to profusely secrete serotonin and, in some cases, histamine, catecholamines, prostaglandins, or insulin.

Psychiatric symptoms occur in 40-75%. Depression is very common; mania less so. (KRAUTHAMMER 1978, GOLD 1982) In one series, Major (1973) found depression in 50%, anxiety in 35%, confusion in 35%. Other mental symptoms can include abrupt personality change, vagueness, memory lapses, inappropriate grinning, and psychosis (particularly with pituitary or temporal tumors).

Warning: Serotonin precursors (or serotonin-enhancing drugs) are usually contraindicated.

* Symptoms typically first become apparent when tumors spread to the lungs or liver. Food, excitement, exertion or alcohol trigger a flush (perhaps 20-30 times per day), accompanied by perspiration, heat, and perhaps tears, hyper-salivation, rapid breathing and heart beat, diarrhea, wheezing, and abdominal cramps.

Immune support. Some natural approaches have involved (BALCH 1990, MURRAY 1998, PAGE 1992, WEHRBACH 1993, 94)

Note: This outline is cursory. Actual treatment choices must be tailored to individual biochemical requirements.

- ☐ **Supernutrition** — fresh, whole foods. Avoid allergens, junk food, sugar, too much fat. Limit alcohol or caffeine. (See *Diet*, pp. 254-56.) (BALCH 1990, MURRAY 1998)
- ☐ **Antioxidants** — C, bioflavonoids, E, selenium, glutathione, resveratrol, CoQ-10, etc.
- ☐ **Carotenes, A** — antioxidant. Support thymus function. (MURRAY 1998, BEYER 1994, NICHOLS 1997, PASSWATER 1995, KIDD 1997, KETTERER 1983, KEHRER 1993)
- ☐ **B vitamins** — pantothenic acid and B6 help produce antibodies; B2, B3, and other B vitamins to counter stress, support adrenals, enhance use of C, etc. (See pp.58-72.) (MURRAY 1998, BALCH 1990, BEYER 1994, KEHRER 1993)
- ☐ **Sunlight & D3** — enhances NK and T cell production, reduces autoimmune inflammatory responses (SULLIVAN 2000)
- ☐ **Immune minerals** — zinc, magnesium, manganese, chromium (to support sugar metabolism), iron (*if deficient*). (MURRAY 1998, BALCH 1990, KEHRER 1993)
- ☐ **Omega 3** and/or **GLA** (MAES 1995, 98, SMITH 1991, CONNOR 1998, STOLL 2002), perhaps **lecithin** (KRUESI) — support oxygenation, immune function. *Take according to biotype, mood, etc.*
- ☐ **Chlorophyll sources** — dark leafy greens, barley or wheat grass, spirulina, chlorella, etc. (MURRAY 1998, 94, BALCH 1990)
- ☐ **Herbal immune builders** — pau d'arco (*taheebo*), schizandra berries, astragalus, yellow dock, burdock, Oregon grape root, milk thistle, shiitake mushrooms, cayenne, ginger, garlic, licorice,* nettles. Herbs used in acute infection (*NOT to be taken over extended periods*) include echinacea,** possibly, goldenseal.***(MURRAY 1998, BALCH 1990, CHRISTOPHER 1976, MOWREY)
- ☐ **Regular exercise** — a physician-approved program, as indicated. (MURRAY, BALCH 1990)
- ☐ **Support thymus, spleen, liver, and lymph & blood immune factors.** Glandulars, *if indicated.* (MURRAY 1998)

* If elevated estrogen or copper is NOT a factor
** Contraindicated in some autoimmune and progressive diseases.
*** Especially with mucous membrane involvement, but only with other potent immune herbs.

Liver basics (BLAND 1997)

The healthy liver effectively handles normal levels of stress, infection, and digestive byproducts. Allergies, leaky gut, chemical toxins, etc., increase the load. If detox pathways are overwhelmed, or supportive nutritients, antioxidants, conjugating agents, or critical precursors, depleted, mental and physical health can become compromised.

Phase 1: Preparation — *uses the P450 oxidase enzyme system and is supported by:* B2, B3, C, E, magnesium, molybdenum, zinc, copper, iron and various trace minerals. *Phase I normally generates free radicals and other harmful chemicals, some more potent than the original toxin. To support intracellular defense, formation of glutathione peroxidase, superoxide dismutase and catalase, may be enhanced via:* glutathione, CoQ10, A, C, E, B2, B12, carotenes, bioflavonoids (e.g, quercetin, catechins), selenium, zinc, manganese, and, *if not contraindicated,* NAC (see p. 171), or copper (pp. 171-3). (ANDERSON 1991, GUENGERICH 1984, BEUTLER 1989, MAKHTAR 1992, BLAND 1992, PERCIVAL 1996)

Phase II: Conjugation — *binds toxins and reactive intermediates from Phase I, producing conjugates, such as glucuronides, sulfates, and glutathione adducts. These are less toxic to body tissue and more easily excreted.* Glutathione and glucaronic acid *are critical. Also helpful:* glutathione precursors, sulfur-containing aminos (NAC, glycine, taurine, methionine), B5, etc. (DICKERSON 1971, GRANT 1991, QUEEN 1990, COOPER 1983, YIM 1994, LEVY 1986, KENDLER, TAHILIANI 1991)

Phase I/Phase II imbalances — may result from genetic predisposition, sustained toxic overload, chronic nutrient deficiency, or imbalanced nutrient support for both phases. *Suppressed Phase I promotes oxidative stress. Suppressed II leaves the body exposed to secondary toxins.* (BLAND 1997)

Liver support: Some natural approaches have involved

Tailor to individual requirements, including phase I/II imbalances.

Herbs — milk thistle, pau d'arco, schizandra berries, astragalus, nettles; yellow dock, burdock, dandelion, and Oregon grape roots; cayenne, ginger, garlic, licorice (*if elevated estrogen or copper is NOT a factor),* shiitake mushrooms, *as relevant.* (MURRAY 1998, BALCH 1990, CHRISTOPHER 1976, MOWREY 1986AB))

Rejuvenating diet — With the diet described on pages 254-56 as a base, emphasize specific vegetables, vegetable juices, herbs, phytonutrient-rich foods, and superfoods which address individual requirements (e.g., cabbage family foods with high thyroid; mineral rich low sugar foods with hypoglycemia, etc.). Eat vitamin C-rich food, as raw and organic as possible; freshly prepared. *Only* small portions of seeds, nuts, fats or proteins. Eat sprouted grains, beans and seeds, if possible. 1/2 to 1 gallon pure water per day. Avoid foods which may be hard to digest (dairy, glutenous grains, eggs, etc.). Get plenty of rest and sleep. Engage in a daily (physician-approved) exercise program. Take supportive supplements. (BLAND 1997)

Liver flush — *Only if indicated. On waking, juice & drink:* 1 lemon or lime, 1-2 cloves garlic, 1Tb olive oil, some ginger or cayenne, 1-3 cups water, perhaps chlorophyll. Don't eat for 2 hrs; then, have vegetable salad, and a healthy diet the rest of the day. (BALCH 1990)

RECOMMENDED READING

Bland, Jeffrey, PhD, *The 20-Day Rejuvenation Diet Program,* 1997.
Murray, Michael, ND, *Encyclopedia of Natural Medicine, 1998.*
Balch, James, MD, *Prescription for Natural Healing,* 1990.
Page, Linda, ND, PhD, *Healthy Healing,* 1992.
Pfeiffer, Carl, PhD, MD, *The Schizophrenias, Ours to Conquer,* 1998.
Werbach, Melvyn, MD, *Nutritional Influences on Mental Illness, 1991; Nutritional Influences on Illness,* 1993; *Botanical Influences on Illness, 1994.*
Salaman, Maureen, *Foods that Heal, 1989.*
Davis, Ben, *Rapid Healing Foods, 1980.*

Reminder: This information is presented for educational purposes only. This material is cursory and does not include full contraindications. The reader is referred to the abundant literature on this subject for further information. If you need treatment for physical illness, mood disorder, or any other medical condition, please seek the services of a knowledgeable physician.

V: Lifestyle

"Silence of water above a sunken tree:
The pure serenity of memory in one man—
A ripple widening from a single stone
Winding around the waters of the world."

Theodore Roethke, "The Fair Field"

A balanced lifestyle helps moderate mood, and entails

- □ Limiting exposure to psychosocial and biochemical stressors.
- □ Employing techniques to moderate stress response.
- □ Psychosocial support.
- □ Good dietary habits, optimizing nutrition.
- □ Fresh air, natural light, interaction with nature.
- □ Regular physical exercise.
- □ Breathwork, meditation, spiritual practices.
- □ Structuring daily life to match natural biological cycles.

Starting with nutrient therapies

"In our experience, best results are achieved with a two-step procedure: (1) biochemical [i.e. individualized nutritive] treatment, followed by (2) lifestyle changes, including a better diet.

We learned the hard way that most bipolars [have difficulty with] lifestyle changes until after their chemical imbalances have been corrected or at least lessened… Trying to do everything at once tends to overwhelm the patient…"

William J Walsh, PhD

1. Role of stress

"In my experience, stress is a primary cause, or an aggravating cause, of most cases of illness."

Andrew Weil, MD

"Chronic stress leads to chronic disease."

Theron Randolph, MD

Stress triggering mood episodes

Initially, bipolar illness is often triggered or worsened by identifiable stressors, either psychosocial (divorce, deaths, isolation, childhood abuse, rape, unemployment, poverty, institutional life, etc.), (WEISSMAN 1991, 96, ELICOTT 1990, HUNT 1992) or physical (e.g., seasonal change, illness, inflammation, toxic exposures, drug reactions, fatigue, sleeplessness, travel, etc).*(LEVERICH 1990, KENNEDY 1983, MALKOFF-SCHWARTZ 1998, MAES 1998, SMITH 1991, CONNOR 1998, STOLL 2002) Rush (2003) finds the length and frequency of mood episodes can increase threefold in stressed patients.*

Temperament, sensitivity, and stress interact. (ELLICOTT 1990) Mood episodes impair neural communication, reducing the capacity to interpret and cope with the psychosocial environment. Inappropriate reactions then invoke social rejection. The resulting turnmoil and hopelessness disrupt neuroendocrine homeostasis. So stress mounts, and mood is further compromised, in a vicious cycle.**(GOLD 88)

Johnson suggests negative stressors such as social rejection and blows to self-esteem are more likely to lead to bipolar depression, while stressors activating behavior, such as excess goal orientation or attainment can trigger or exacerbate mania. (JOHNSON 1999AB, 2000)

Over time, precipitating stressors become less apparent.

* Thus, a survival analyis by Ellicott (1990) finds a significant relationship between stressful life events and onset of episodes; and Hunt (1992) reports several-fold more adverse events in the month preceding an episode. (Bauer 1996)

** Also, note the similarity of symptoms of early depression to those of chronic stress, e.g., disturbed affect and motivation, disturbed "housekeeping" functions (appetite, sleep, sexual activity), and increased irritability or aggression, etc. (Gold 1988, Sachar 1973)

Hans Seyle's stress response theory (SAHLEY)

(1) Alarm, autonomic arousal, hormone response. Sudden alarm (pain, anxiety, panic, etc.) heightens limbic signals to the hypothalamus, activating fight-or-flight. Adrenaline, heart rate, and blood pressure increase, along with vigilance and tension. The pituitary stimulates cortisol and thyroxine secretion, and the liver releases sugar to the blood. Pupils dilate and limb circulation increases, while superficial blood vessels constrict. Immune stimulation should return the body to equilibrium once the threat ends.

(2) Chronic arousal/activation. The body fails to return to normal following stress, reflecting exhaustion of moderating mechanisms. Inhibitors become depleted; and the overwhelmed cortex, less rational. Vigilence and foreboding progress to anxiety and panic attacks (with intense fear, trembling, unsteady legs, profuse perspiration, difficulty breathing, disorientation, weakness, headache, diarrhea, etc.).

(3) Adaptive failure, exhaustion. Eventually, fatigue, depression, and insomnia predominate, and appetite and sexual interest diminish. Memory becomes impaired by the chronic steroid feedback. (JACOBSON 1991) Functioning of the pancreas, adrenals, heart, thyroid, or other organs is often compromised.

Post's kindling hypothesis, linking stress to mood (POST 1986)

Repeated stressors, especially those over which one has no control, might kindle anxiety, insomnia, or mania in vulnerable persons, intensifying reactions, and over time, triggering episodes with little apparent provocation, eventually leading to exhaustion/depression, and increased sensitivity to stress, with the feedback loop perhaps accelerating cycling. (See pp. 207-8.)

Psychosocial support

Although *psychotherapy* is not necessarily helpful (as memories may be distorted, promoting traumatic reactions to unreal events), *cognitive therapy* and general *psychosocial support* can be. (HUXLEY 2001B) *Consider the following goals:*

- ☐ Reduce stressors and modify reactions to stress. (OTTO 2003)
- ☐ Improve mood, with cognitive, relaxation, and mind-control techniques. (MOORE 1998)
- ☐ Encourage peer interactions and social relationships.
- ☐ Promote collaboration with family and supportive persons. (MIKLOWITZ 1997)
- ☐ Encourage work and creative achievements.
- ☐ Encourage adherence to diet, exercise, bedtimes, and other supportive lifestyle factors.
- ☐ Encourage therapeutic intake. (OTTO 2003) Provide education on benefits and side effects.
- ☐ Emphasize the importance of avoiding mania. (OTTO 2003, LAM 1997)
- ☐ Facilitate early recognition of relapse cues, and use of preventive strategies (e.g., nutritive adjustments, quiet spaces and subdued lighting for manics; morning walks for depressives, etc.). (OTTO 2003)
- ☐ Identify and address comorbid conditions which contribute to symptoms (e.g., substance abuse, (SONNE 1994) PTSD, anxiety, etc.). (OTTO 2003)

Some anti-stress techniques (Moore 1998, Lemmo)

- ☐ Support networks (family, friends, community, other social resources) (O'Connell 1985, Lam 1999, Miklowitz 1997, 98), particularly with depression. (Priebe 1989, Johnson 1999b)
- ☐ Intellectual & creative outlets. (Lemmo)
- ☐ Meditation, prayer. (Moore 1998)
- ☐ Relaxation techniques (e.g., progressive muscle relaxation and breath-work, etc. (See p. 258)) — Small controlled trials report benefit, (Broota 1990, Field 1996, Bowers 1990) comparable to tricyclics, (Murphy 1995) or cognitive therapy. (Reynolds 1986, Kahn 1990, Jorm 2002)
- ☐ Accelerated conditioning. (Moore 1998)
- ☐ Reality testing for delusions, etc. (Chadwick 1994, Kingdon 1994)
- ☐ Reciprocal, cognitive therapy (Lam 1999, Otto 2003) — Negative cognitive style, rumination, etc.,* increase the risk of depression, and can worsen and lengthen episodes. Distraction or correction improves mood, in some studies, comparably to antidepressants. (Newman 2002, Reilly-Harrington 1999, Alloy 1999, Kuehner 1999) Some manias can be addressed as defensive reactions to negative beliefs. (Newman 2002)

* Low self-worth is common in bipolars, even with positive self-report. (Winters 1985)

- ☐ Neurolinguistic programming (NLP) — generally helps facilitate subjective control over mood. (Slagle 1992, James 1999, Sutherland 2001)
- ☐ Self-hypnosis — may help prevent a manic episode, or reduce depression. (Moore 1998, Burrows 2003, Dennerstei 1980, Dryden 1986, Martin 1990, Matheson 1979)
- ☐ EEG biofeedback — a well researched-approach in epilepsy; may benefit mood. (Soc Stud Neur Reg 1995, Moore 1998, Rosenfeld 1997, 2000, Alhambra 1995)
- ☐ Emotional Freedom Technique (EFT) — involves tapping on acupuncture meridian points as part of a psychological approach to healing from negative or blocked experiences. (Lemmo) Electroacupuncture may, similarly, provide benefit. (Han 1986, Luo 1998)
- ☐ Massage — may temporarily reduce anxiety and depression in some, perhaps because it promotes relaxation and helps balance left-right frontal activation. (Field 1992, 96, 98)
- ☐ Eye Movement Desensitization & Reprocessing (EMDR) — combines counseling with specific eye exercise to alleviate & reprogram trauma. (Lemmo, Corrigan 2002, Devilly 1999)

The reader is advised to check the literature for further details.

"If the family atmosphere is good, the patient committed to taking nutrients, a tremendous amount can be done. But a family that is hostile, or a patient ambivalent to getting well (e.g., not wanting to give up addictions or drug dependence, accustomed to the illness, or just in a hurry), sabotages treatment, and the patient goes downhill."

Michael Lesser, MD, 2008

Role of stressors in mood symptoms

Parental loss

By age one, isolated orphans in group homes rarely smiled, showed little curiosity, and were often ill, as compared to children with access to mothers in prison. By age two, the latter group talked and engaged actively with others, while only 2 of 26 orphans spoke over a few words. (Spitz 1942)

In 76 major depressives, parental loss, especially permanent separation before age 9, was significantly associated with depression. In 76 bipolars early parental loss was also common. In controls, parental loss was generally associated with lower income; more physical illness, divorce, and tobacco use; and greater tendency to live alone. (Agid 1999)

Confrontation (primate study)

Suomi (1991ab) found elevated epinephrines and cortisol in adult monkeys during confrontation and fighting. The winner became the dominant monkey and his stress hormones rapidly decreased. The loser's cortisol remained high, and often rose further with additional challenges.

Most losers became withdrawn, and less inclined to explore, and eventually retreated to the edge of the troop. Epinephrines, and sex and growth hormones slowly decreased. Over time, most losers tended to sicken and die, or become prey.

Interactions of stress with brain systems

Endocrines — Chronic endocrine arousal in affectives both causes and reflects psychological pain and stress. (Sachar 1967, 73, Gold 1988) The hypothalamus and pituitary often wind up proding the thyroid, adrenals (Bauer 1988, Whybrow 1995) and other endocrines, irrespective of natural biorhythms and already elevated mood and stress hormones. (Hosboer 1995, Koob 1988, 91)

Norepinephrine — The locus coeruleus is the source of most of the brain's norepinephrine, and a key arousal center and limbic activator. Oversecretion heightens anxiety, vigilance, and vulnerability to stress and mood episodes. (Aston-Jones 1984)

Dopamine — Stress may dysregulate dopamine pathways in the behavioral activating system, fostering mania. (Gray 1990, 91, Depue 1994, 96, 97, Newman 2002) Excess dopamine contributes to manic symptoms by enhancing motivation, enthusiasm, (Depue 1994, Post 1977, 82) energy, attention, approach behavior, (Lozano 1999, Johnson 1999, Newman 2002, Depue 1998) focus on reward, and goal-directed activity at the expense of sleep and judgment. (Lozano 1999)

Limbic system — Overactivity of catecholamines and certain hormones profoundly influences the limbic system, magnifying both stress and mood instability.

2. Optimizing diet (BLAND 1997, BALCH 1990, PAGE 1992, COUSENS, HOFFER 1983, PFEIFFER 1987, LESSER 1982, MURRAY 1998, YOUNG 1993)

"Man is a food-dependent creature. If you don't feed him, he will die. If you feed him improperly, part of him will die."
— Emanuel Cheraskin, MD, DMD

"We have worked with more than 1500 bipolar patients, and found that most have an atrocious diet. I remember one young man whose only intake for the past month consisted of Pepsi and potato chips."

To the patient: On adopting a new diet

Give yourself some slack

Start wherever you are dietarily, perhaps adding just one small change at a time.

You don't have to be perfect. Try to eat as good a diet as you can at the moment. Improve your diet at your own pace. Be kind to yourself.

If you eat the "wrong" food, don't worry about it, but take advantage of this opportunity to pay attention to how you feel afterwards (over 1 to 48 hours). This helps train you to not want harmful food.

Similarly, pay attention to how you feel when you eat healthful food, and how it affects mind and body long-term. Be sure to distinguish healthy foods from those that promote mania, and from masked allergens (often, those foods you feel you can't do without. (See *Stages*, p. 207.)).

Gradually optimize your diet to what best supports your mental and physical health.

A food/ mood journal

A journal recording what you eat, what nutrients and other therapies you take, what you've been thinking about and feeling, etc., may support you in learning how food and supplements influence your mood.

Supplements may be needed first

A good diet, with regular meals, supports mental well-being and benefits the overall nutritional program. Nonetheless, Walsh (2006, 07), Hoffer (1983, 2005), and others find that some patients have to improve considerably on supplements before they feel able to improve their diets.

- ☐ Adequate but not excessive, protein per meal. Grain/legume combinations, and/or animal foods (fresh, baked or broiled, unprocessed, free range, as organic as possible). *Consider biotype requirements.*
- ☐ Soak dry legumes at least 8 hours. Then rinse and drain (you can rinse just this once, or rinse every 8 hours for another day or two). Then cook. This process cuts cooking time, and increases digestibility.
- ☐ Carbohydrates should be unrefined, whole foods (e.g, carrots, legumes, squash). Use whole grains (e.g, millet, oats, buckwheat, brown rice, amaranth, or quinoa), in preference to breads, pastas and other foods made with flour). Soak grains 8 to 10 hours, then rinse before cooking. Bread, if eaten, should be made from whole grains; preferably 100% sprouted. *Avoid sugar, white flour, refined grain.*
- ☐ Plenty of fresh raw vegetables. Multiple colors, especially deeper colors (dark greens, reds) represent a variety of antioxidants and minerals. Salads. When practical, freshly-made vegetable juice. *Some histadelics need to restrict folate foods, such as leafy greens.*
- ☐ Cooked vegetables, *as appropriate* (beans, potatoes, squash, etc.). Soups. (*Cook only as long as necessary, in descending order of cooking time.**)
- ☐ Fresh, whole fruit, with a focus on fruits lower on the glycemic index. To limit sugar reactions, fruit can be eaten three quarters of an hour before a protein meal, and taken with chromium. *Limit dry fruit. Avoid canned or bottled fruit juice.* With uncontrolled sugar imbalance, or Candida, limit fruit to lemons, limes, pomegranates, and other high vitamin C, low-sugar fruit.
- ☐ Healthy fats. Ideally, unprocessed, whole foods, such as fish (baked or broiled), seeds, and nuts (unroasted). Most people need to emphasize omega 3 fats (cold-climate fish, flax seeds, etc.). Fish provides the longer chain omega 3 needed by the brain (the nutrients or enzymes critical to converting plant sources are often insuffient, or may not function effectively). Some stores sell freshly-cooked fish in bite-size chunks (cooked shrimp, herring , sushi, etc.), making it easier to eat a little fish more often, without having to cook it. *Most moderate-to-severe pyrolurics preferentially need GLA (found in borage seed and evening primrose oil).*
- ☐ Moderate quantities of saturated fat (coconut, butter, most dairy, some meats), *as appropriate to individual biochemistry.* For cooking, use coconut oil or butter. For salad dressing, the best choice is cold-pressed virgin olive oil. *No fried food. Avoid rancid or hydrogenated fats.*

* For example: Start with beets, carrots; later add, potatoes, mushrooms; then squash, string beans, and any precooked beans, etc. Five minutes or so before completion, add garlic, onions, celery, tomatoes. Add herbs or butter (do not use oils) just before serving.)

General approach

- ☐ Eat foods as organic, fresh, and locally-grown as possible.
- ☐ Avoid allergens (e.g., wheat, dairy, soy, chocolate, eggs, etc.). Vary the diet from day to day. (See pp. 207-13.)
- ☐ Some depressives do well with a focus on raw foods (greens, sprouts, vegetables and vegetable juices, seeds, nuts) and fish; some, also with significant poultry, red meat.
- ☐ Some manics do well with animal foods, others with grain/bean meals, moderately cooked veggies.
- ☐ You can experiment with foods rich in the nutrients you most need, then observe how they influence your mood over time.

□ Chew well. Try to surround yourself with a pleasant nonstressful environment when eating. Be grateful for the food.

□ Food combining — Digestion is supported by not combining fruit (or any significant sugars) with fats, proteins or vegetables.* Do not mix melons with other foods. Limit liquids directly before, after, or with a meal; at least 30 minutes before a meal is okay.

* Though apples, peaches, berries, and other non-citrus fruit, plus yogurt is usually acceptible.

Hypoglycemic & vegetarian requirements (PFEIFFER 1987, BALCH 1990, MURRAY 1995, 98)

Hypoglycemics — usually need five to six small meals per day, with sufficient (but not excess) protein. (Ocean fish is often an excellent protein; similarly, good quality eggs or poultry. Some people do well with red meat, others with legume/grain combos; for some, meals which contain both (e.g., chilli con carne) work well.) (pp. 214-18)

Vegetarians — should make sure to take in enough protein (e.g, legume/grain combinations; and if not vegan, or allergic, dairy or eggs). Other nutrients which may have become depleted include: zinc (phytates in grains inhibit absorption), B3, B6, and B12. Carnitine (though a nonessential amino) may also be low, especially in hypothyroid vegetarians. To insure adequate calcium, vegans (especially females) should engage in weight-bearing exercise, eat calcium-rich food (sesame, carrots, cabbage family), and avoid sugar and caffeine; supplements of calcium with magnesium, boron, D3, etc. may be indicated. (pp. 124-125)

Biotype-based requirements (PFEIFFER 1987, WALSH 2006)

Pyrolurics — initially, a whole-foods, relatively vegetarian diet, as low zinc and B6 make animal protein difficult to handle. Animal protein can be increased as digestion improves. Additional B6 (and, perhaps, papain and/or bromelain) may help support digestion. Organic food helps sidestep problems processing or eliminating toxins.

Histadelia — a high protein diet with quality animal proteins (*if practical:* fish from mercury-free waters, organic meats, free-range poultry), provides methyl. The diet should also include whole foods, unrefined complex carbohydrates, fresh vegetables (*in occasional cases of already-excessive folate, leafy greens may need to be temporarily limited*), moderate portions of fresh, relatively low-glycemic fruit, and of healthy fat (emphasize omega 3).

Histapenia — plenty of fresh vegetables to supply folate. Whole foods, preferably, organic. Healthy omega-3-rich fish, etc. Meats support B3 receptors, (MILLER 2008) but may oversupply methyl, (WALSH 2008) so determine individual needs. For some, grain/legume proteins are the better choice.

In all biotypes — restrict/avoid immunoreactive foods. Avoid sugar, soda, white flour, alcohol, fried and hydrogenated fat.

Nutrient-dense & superfoods (BLAND 1997, BALCH 1990, PAGE 1992, MURRAY 1998, HOFFER 1983AB)

□ Brewers or nutritional yeast —a good source of B vitamins and chromium. May be useful in sugar metabolism imbalances.

□ Wheat, barley, kamut or other grass juices — provide magnesium, chlorophyll. May benefit anemia, fatigue, depression. *Check reactivity in patients allergic to wheat.*

□ Blue green algae, spirulina, chlorella — provides chlorophyll, A, some B12, and easily-digested amino acids. May benefit fatigue, anemia, blood sugar, depression, *but can worsen mania.*

□ Bee pollen, royal jelly — high B5, B6, some B12. Stimulating. Benefits fatigue, depression, stress. *Do not use for mania. Rule out sensitivities (more likely in patients with hayfever).*

□ Seaweed — supports the thyroid; rich in iodine & other minerals. Can be antidepressant. *For some manics, may be overstimulating.*

"The most basic intervention is [to make the diet as] organic and natural as... reasonably possible."
Andrew Cutler, PhD, 2005

Primitive nourishment (HOFFER 1983AB, 1987)

Hoffer points out that, for most of human existence, people have subsisted on a primitive diet. Our ancestors ate locally available, seasonal, whole foods. Herbicides, pesticides, chemical preservatives, and refined food didn't exist. Most food was eaten fresh and raw.

As agriculture developed over the past 10-20,000 years, many, but not all, people evolved genetically to be able to handle cooked grains.

Processed and chemicalized food have dominated our diet for only a few generations. Vitamins, minerals and enzymes are depleted, proteins and fats denatured, and toxic contaminants are rampant.

The primitive diet obviously nourished brain and body considerably better than the modern junk food counterpart.

Diet alone is usually insufficient

Some patients insist on therapy with diet alone. Unfortunately, diet usually cannot supply enough of the specific nutrients needed to redress the profound imbalances underlying bipolar disorder. Supplements are usually essential, and commonly, as a side effect, improve overall health.

Some cautions

Brewer's yeast — may cause bloating or gas (acidophilus may help). Yeast is often contraindicated in Candida.

Bee pollen — rule out allergic susceptibility, especially in patients with hayfever.

Spirulina, chlorella, other blue green algae — sometimes contain impurities. Some people are hypersensitive to certain algae. Chronic high intake can be overstimulating, triggering or worsening manias, or increasing a tendency to violence in some individuals. Research is needed to establish distinct biotype effects.

Freshly-made vegetable juices (COTT 1974, 75, BLAND 1997, MURRAY 1991, 98, WERBACH, BALCH 1990, PAGE 1992, PRITCHARD, SALAMAN, BLAUER 1989, CALBORN 1992, WALKER 1970, LEE 1982, GURSCHE 1993, SHELTON 1981)

Vegetable juices can remineralize tissue and revitalize the digestive, circulatory, immune, and other body systems, and benefit some depressions. Juices are best consumed within 20 minutes of preparation. Use ingredients that are nonallergenic, do not aggravate Candida, and are as organic as possible. Concentrate on high-mineral, low-sugar vegetables, such as parsley, celery, chard. Wheat or barley grass juices* and relevant herbs are often good additions. Choices can be tailored to what best supports individual health, e.g.: (1) Cabbage family vegetables tend to benefit overactive thyroid and overstimulation (e.g., mania), but not low thyroid and certain depressions; seaweeds add minerals and may improve low thyroid and depression; (2) Re: hypoglycemia: spirulina, chlorella, etc.,** supply aminos; nutritional yeast** adds chromium; carrots, beets, and other sweet vegetables usually should be limited.

Warning: Though individually-tailored juices often promote health and counter depression, juice fasts can be destabilizing, especially if edging toward mania.

* To avoid nausea, start with 1/4 oz, increase gradually.
** Contraindicated for some.

RECOMMENDED READING

Bland, Jeffrey, PhD, *The 20-Day Rejuvenation Diet Program,* 1998.
Cousens, Gabriel, MD, *Depression-Free for Life,* 2000.
Lesser, Michael, MD, *The Brain Chemistry Diet,* 2002.
Murray, Michael, ND, *Encyclopedia of Natural Medicine,* 1998.
Werbach, Melvyn, MD, *Nutritional Influences on Mental Illness,* 1991, *Nutritional Influences on Illness,* 1993, *Botanical Influences on Illness,* 1994.
Pfeiffer, Carl C, PhD, MD, *Nutrition and Mental Illness,* 1987.
Balch, James, MD, *Prescription for Nutritional Healing,* 1990.
Page, Linda, ND, PhD, *Healthy Healing,* 1992.
Pritchard, Paul, *Healing with Whole Foods,* 1993.
Salaman, Maureen, *Foods that Heal,* 1989
Blauer, Stephen, *The Juicing Book,* 1989.
Calborn, Cherie and Keane, Maureen, *Juicing for Life,* 1992.
Walker, Norman W, D.Sc, *Fresh Vegetable and Fruit Juices,* 1970.
Lee, William H, PhD, *The Book of Raw Fruit and Vegetable Juices and Drinks,* 1982.
Gursche, Siegfried, *Healing with Herbal Juices,* 1993.
Davis, Ben, *Rapid Healing Foods,* 1980.

- ☐ Salmon, halibut, herring, other omega 3 fish. Fish liver oils, *if from unpolluted waters.* Flax seeds (*only eat fresh*) also provide omega 3, *but are often less effective. Pyrolurics usually do better with an emphasis on primrose or borage oil.*
- ☐ Turkey — free-range; hormone-free. A good source of tryptophan.
- ☐ Deep leafy greens, parsley, salads — provide high chlorophyll, minerals, enzymes. *Occasionally, undermethylated/high-folate patients (histadelics) need to limit greens.* (PFEIFFER 1987)
- ☐ Intensely-colored vegetables. Freshly-made vegetable juices — rich in bioflavonoids and other antioxidants; high vitamin, mineral and enzyme content.
- ☐ Fresh, deeply-colored fruits — high vitamin and antioxidant content. *Patients with Candida or blood sugar susceptibilities should focus on low-glycemic-index fruits.*
- ☐ Lemon or lime — alone, or freshly squeezed into water. An excellent source of vitamin C. *Drink additional water or brush teeth within 30 minutes to reduce acid on the teeth.*
- ☐ Seeds and nuts — fresh, or as yogurts. Contain vitamin E, zinc, EFAs, and other nutrients. *Don't overdo.* Raw tahini (made from sesame seeds) is an excellent source of calcium and E.
- ☐ Sunflower, buckwheat, mung & other sprouts — nutrient and enzyme dense. (Soak seeds 8 hours. Drain. Then rinse every 6 hours for another 2 days or so, til ready to eat.)
- ☐ Acidophilus sources, e.g., yogurts or kefirs (if reactive to dairy, try goat, buffalo, or seed yogurts, *if not allergic*).
- ☐ Relevant herb teas — Including mild, nutritive herbs. If caffeine must be used, green tea is the best choice. (See pp. 53-55; 139-43.)
- ☐ Water — bathes and cleanses tissues, supports electrolyte function, removes toxins, transports nutrients, etc. Look for the cleanest, most vital sources available.

Avoid

- ☐ Refined carbohydrates (sugar, pastas, pastries, candy, sodas, alcohol). Limit breads, unless sprouted. Avoid white flour; limit other flours, and try grinding, as needed, from whole grains (coffee grinders work).
- ☐ Significant quantities of dry fruit or fruit juice. *Avoid if hypoglycemic.*
- ☐ Large meals. Too much fat and/or protein at any one meal can compromise blood sugar, and digestion.
- ☐ Hydrogenated (e.g, margarine, Crisco®), rancid or overly-processed fat. Fried food. Cooking oil (coconut or butter is okay). Limit omega 6 (meats, butter, dairy, most vegetable oils), except GLA for pyrolurics.
- ☐ Overly cooked or processed food (e.g., luncheon meat, canned food).
- ☐ Excessive salt.
- ☐ Allergens and foods causing sensitivity. *Note: Avoiding such foods may initially cause withdrawal symptoms.* If impossible to eliminate, take infrequently, in small quantities. Rotate food groups over 4 to 14 days, to reduce the development of sensitivities and allow for replenishment of digestive enzymes. (See pp 207-13.)
- ☐ Toxins. Herbicide or pesticide-treated food. MSG. Aspartate (in many diet sodas). Artificial sweeteners, food additives and preservatives. Food cooked or stored in aluminum.
- ☐ Cigarettes. Alcohol. Street drugs. Significant caffeine.
- ☐ Limit/avoid foods detrimental to biotype or health status.

3. Exercise (HOFFER 1983, PFEIFFER 1987, QUILLIN 1987)

Exercise increases the availability of glucose and oxygen, improves blood circulation to the brain, releases endorphins, and enhances the brain's ability to absorb nutrients and eliminate toxins (including elevated metals, like vanadium. (LEMMO) Exercise also decreases resting adrenaline, lowers blood fats, and transfers sugar from the liver and blood to the cells, sparing the use of insulin. (WEYERER 1994)

Exercise is reported to improve depression, anxiety, insomnia, and hyperactivity; increase alertness; and moderate psychotic symptoms.

Normalizing the reaction to stress (HOFFER 1983, PFEIFFER 1987)

When our ancestors confronted danger, fear and anger released adrenaline and glucocorticoids from the adrenals, and glycogen from the liver, which moved sugar into the blood, enhancing their ability to fight or flee. Today, constrained from either reaction, our thwarted biochemicals induce feelings of panic.

Exercise mimics the fight-or-flight response, and guides fight-or-flight biochemicals to their proper destinations.

Exercise for depression

Moreover, deep breathing and exercise increase the oxygen available to the brain, enhancing cerebral function and the ability to handle stress. Daily exercise, appropriate to health status, can be a potent antidepressant. (LEMMO, MURRAY 1995)

Note: Before exercising, take antioxidant supplements and/or foods to offset the increased production of free radicals during exercise.

Some of the studies

One study found that the rate of recovery from major depression in elderly patients who walked or jogged thirty minutes, 3x/week, for 16 weeks, was almost as high as in patients on medication (60% vs. 64%). Six months later, relapse was 8% in those who continued exercising, 38% in the group on medication alone, i.e., almost 5-fold greater in the exercise group. In patients who both exercised and took antidepressants, relapse was 31%, suggesting exercise alone may have considerably greater antidepressant benefit than exercise plus pharmaceuticals. (BLUMENTHAL 1999)

A number of randomized controlled studies report improvement in clinical depression with exercise. Pinchasov (2000) found it more effective than light therapy in patients *without* seasonal affective disorder. McNeil (1991) found benefits comparable to social contact in the elderly with moderate depression. McCann (1984) found aerobic exercise more effective than relaxation therapy. The type of exercise seemed to be less important than whether exercise occured. (DOYNE 1987, STEWART 1981, SINGH 2001, JORM 2002)

Researchers are also finding lower relapse rates than occurs with antidepressants. (BABYAK 2000, SINGH 2001, JORM 2002, BLUMENTHAL 1999)

"Alone far in the wilds and mountains I hunt,
Wandering amazed at my own lightness and glee."

Walt Whitman, in "Song of Myself"

"Physical activity of some kind has profound antidepressant properties and provides great stability to both body & mind."

Walter Lemmo, ND

"We found there was an inverse relationship between exercise and the risk of relapsing — the more one exercised, the less likely depressive symptoms [were to] return."

James Blumenthal, MD

"If mega-nutrients are not entirely effective, vigorous exercise will almost always restore the bodily equilibrium and homeostasis."

Carl C Pfeiffer, PhD, MD, 1987

Cautions

Consult your physician before engaging in an exercise program.

Exercise to the point of exhaustion reflects a transfer to anaerobic metabolism. This increases lactic acid, which can trigger panic attacks in some anxiety-prone individuals. Thus researchers suggest deep, relaxed breathing; not overexercising; and taking, as indicated, nutrients and herbs which support cellular oxygenation, and protect against free radicals.

Manics should not overdo exercise.

Consider sun exposure. Sunlight stimulates the pineal gland, is antidepressant (so should be limited in mania), and supports calcium absorption. Nonetheless, due to ozone thinning, direct U.V. exposure should be minimized, especially during midday hours, and throughout the day in some regions. Furthermore, certain neuroleptics and other meds induce sun sensitivity, as can untreated pyroluria and deficient B6.

Oxygen (HOFFER, 1983, PFEIFFER 1987, QUILLIN 1987, WILLIAMS 1956

Weil's breathwork exercises

Weil states that breathwork injects conscious control into an involuntary activity. Some of his exercises:

□ Observe your breathing.

□ Breathe slowly and deeply. Count, for example, to 10 on inhalation, hold the breath for 10, exhale for 10, repeat. Gradually increase the count.

□ Breathe in slowly. Visualize oxygen moving from your lungs to every cell in your body. Visualize your cells exchanging oxygen for carbon dioxide. Breath out slowly and visualize carbon dioxide and other cell wastes leaving your body. Repeat.

□ Breathe in through the left nostril, hold, exhale through the right. Breathe in through the right, hold, exhale through the left.

Such exercises can be done initially for a few minutes per day. Over time, such practices might extend to 15 to 30 minutes, or more. Such techniques can also be used, as needed, to reduce anger, tension, fear, stress, insomnia, etc.

The rest of the body weighs fifty times more than the brain, but the brain uses 20% of the body's oxygen. If cerebral circulation is less than optimal, access to glucose and oxygen is compromised, along with the ability to eliminate waste. Neural vitality declines, and the tendency to depression, anxiety, etc., increases.

Depressed people may breathe in six times less air. (OTT 1974) Oxygen deprivation may concentrate in areas concerned with emotion, abstract thought, and integration of experience.

Natural therapies

Cerebral access to oxygen is supported by regular exercise, deep breathing, circulatory system vitality, and nutrients and herbs which support cellular oxygenation, along with antioxidants and other protective supplements. Vitamin E and CoQ10 support the blood's ability to carry oxygen, as do vitamins C, B6, B12, folic acid,* magnesium, iron,* and copper.* Ginkgo and germanium also enhance oxygenation.

See Antioxidants, pp. 73-83.

* See *Contraindications*, pp. 66, 136, 137, respectively.

Breathwork

Andrew Weil's perspectives

To loosely quote Dr. Andrew Weil, MD (from *Breathing: The Master Key to Self-Healing)*: Breathing is a rhythmic expansion and contraction, like the oscillation of atoms and stars. The oxygen released by the green chlorophyll of plants reddens our blood and sustains our cells. The carbon dioxide waste which we breathe out sustains the plant world. The air we breathe in contains molecules from the lungs of our ancestors, of people halfway across the world, of dinosaurs, dodo birds... Einstein, Shakespeare and Eve.

Weil's patients report benefit to anxiety, panic, and insomnia (as well as high blood pressure, irregular heart beat, poor circulation, digestive problems, etc.).

Some of the studies

Several studies investigate breathwork in the treatment of depression. In a randomized comparision study, Janakiramaiah (2000) found benefit equivalent to imipramine for melancholic depression. Another study (KHUMAR 1993) reports improvement in students with multiple depressive symptoms upon 30 days of yogic breathwork.

Variations in oxygen available to the brain (WILLIAMS 1956, RIORDAN 1993, PFEIFFER 1988)

The oxygen level of the brain is relatively stable, even with the high metabolism in hyperthyroids, but is decreased in senile dementia, some cases of depression, and by high levels of carbon monoxide (which bind circulating oxygen, preventing it from reaching body tissue).* Reduced brain oxygenation can worsen depression or mania and, if extensive, cause brain damage.

The massive deforestation, and industrial pollution over the past hundred years has decreased the oxygen content of our air. The extent to which this has affected brain functioning is unclear.

* Also, during diabetic coma, or under sodium pentothal oxygen can decrease 35-40%.

4. Normalizing biorhythms

"People have been naturally programmed to sleep with the moon (or darkness) and rise with the sun. Only recently... has humanity challenged this delicate balance between the natural order of the environment and the body." — Walter Lemmo, ND

Abnormal biorhythms in bipolars

Bipolars seem to be particularly sensitive to environmental cues that interact with body rhythms. Research suggests balanced mood is supported by a repetitive daily pattern, in tune with natural environmental events, e.g., going to sleep when it gets dark, at about the same time each night, a bedtime routine to cue in sleep, getting enough sleep, waking with morning light; and eating, working and exercising regularly, at specific hours, etc.

The rationale

A genetically-controlled biological clock regulates many of our physiological and behavioral rhythms. Its timing is tied to daily, monthly and seasonal cycles in nature, (MAYEDA 1990) and altered by environmental changes, and individual choices (e.g., all-nighters, electric lights, heating, jet travel).

Bipolars tend to experience a pronounced distortion of internal daily (circadian) rhythms, (HALARIS 1987) (e.g., sleep/activity, appetite, temperature, hormone secretion, neurotransmitter release), (MAYEDA 1990, GOLD 1987, GOODWIN POST 1975) and an exaggerated response to seasonal change (e.g., with a mood episode).

Bipolars may be genetically more sensitive to changes in light, (LEWY 1980, 1985) sleep, (WEHR 1982) and the relationships of biorhythms. (KRIPKE 1978, NURNBERGER 1989) Biorhythm distortions may act as stressors, altering and aggravating mood. Originally, some researchers suggested rhythm disturbance might *cause* bipolar disorder. (WEHR 1983) In any case, seasonal changes and sleepless nights are well-known for *triggering* moodswing.

Common triggers (WEVER 1985, EHLERS 1988, 93, HEALY 1987, AMBELAS 1979, KENNEDY 1983, WEHR 1987, LIEBERMAN 1984, ANSSEAU, 1991)

Moreover, many triggers for mood episodes also disrupt natural biorhythms: changes in routine (travel across time zones; moving; a new job), emotional or social stressors (separation, loss), postpartum changes. Also, overtreatment with stimulating drugs (antidepressants, hyperactivity meds) and hormones (thyroxine); or overuse of sedative drugs (alcohol, neuroleptics, minor tranquilizers); drug abuse; and withdrawal from such drugs, especially if rapid.

"I learned not to fear infinity,
The far field, the windy cliffs of forever,
The dying of time in the white light of
tomorrow,
The wheel turning away from itself."
Theodore Roethke, from "The Fair Field"

Rhythm distortions in bipolars

Cycles out of tune with natural time cues — Day/night cues should adjust sleep/activity, temperature, REM and hormones to a 24-hr cycle, (ASCHOOF 1965, WEHR 1979) but seem to have less effect on bipolars, whose rhythms tend to increasingly focus on internal cues.

Phase changes — e.g., sleep/activity cycles typically start early (*phase-advanced*) in mania perhaps due to sensitivity to morning light; (LEWY 1985) late, in many depressives (*phase-delayed*). (WEHR 1979, CLARK 1982)

Cycle desynchronization — e.g., a 48-hr sleep/activity cycle (perhaps awake and alert 30 plus hours, sleeping 18),*(WEHR 1982, 83, WEVER 1979) may interact with a 30-hr temperature cycle, which starts too early.**(WEHR 1979)

Distorted and desynchronized biorhythms may feed on each other, and further destabilize mood. (FRANK 1994)

* Common just prior to or during the onset of mania. Thus, in a 1980 study by Wehr and Goodwin, one to four such cycles had occured in 9 of 10 manics.

** Similarly, when daily cues are absent (e.g., staying indoors in the dark), many people switch to a 25-hr cycle, (Wever 1979, Gold 1987) and biological clocks may become less responsive to external stimuli. In some, rest/activity goes to a 45-hr cycle, but temperature, REM, cortisol, etc., hover at 25 hrs, creating internal desynchronization. This sometimes leads to affective symptoms in normals. (Wehr 1982, 83)

Altered sleep architecture in bipolars

REM, is a rapid eye movement stage of sleep in which dreaming occurs.* Normally, each REM stage lasts 10 to 60 minutes, with the *shortest* REM *early* in the night, increasing toward morning. REM typically starts after 90 minutes of sleep, with approximately 90 minutes between subsequent REM stages.

As compared to normals, bipolar and unipolar depressives sleep less (though bipolars often sleep longer than major depressives (HOBSON 1988)), less deeply, fall asleep less easily, and wake more frequently and earlier. (EIBER 1999) REM occurs *sooner,* (HARTMAN 1968) and the first REM cycle may be the *longest*. REM eye movement increases, influencing dreams. Sleep levels cycle more rapidly, and less time is spent in slow-wave, deep sleep (stages III and IV). (ANSSEAU 1991, KUPFER 1988) Sleep changes may reflect limbic and brain stem arousal. (BUYSSE 1999)

In mania, the first REM stage may be *delayed*. (HARTMAN 1968) Waking occurs earlier. Sleep is reduced, without causing fatigue (especially just before the switch to mania). (BUNNEY 1977) More deep sleep may occur. Other sleep parameters are often distorted.** (EIBER 1999)

* It's also accompanied by autonomic fluctuation, slack muscles, and low voltage, desynchronized EEG.

** The sleep cycle may also be disturbed in panic disorder, OCD, anxiety, phobias, PTSD, eating disorders, borderline personality, schizophrenia and dementa, especially if the limbic system is involved.

"There's a certain Slant of light,
Winter Afternoons —
That oppresses..."

Emily Dickinson
from "There's a certain Slant of light"

Reactions to light (DOWNING, HYMAN 1990, OTT 1973, 74, DUNNE 1989)

Sensitivity to light

Lack of full spectrum (outdoor type) light has been associated with seasonal affective disorder, bipolar and other depressions, emotional instability, anxiety, irritability, vulnerability to stress, hyperactivity, fatigue, apathy, increased sleep, social withdrawal, low glandular activity,malabsorption, craving for sweets, and suppressed immunity.

Bipolars may have hypersensitive light-to-melatonin pathway receptors. (ZATZ 1979, 81, NURNBERGER 1988) Most studies find families with SAD often have a strong history of mood disorder (and perhaps alcoholism). (AVERY 1993) When light and season change, both bipolar and SAD patients experience difficulty adjusting biorhythms and regaining homeostasis. (LEWY 1981)

Altered sleep/activity rhythms influencing mood

The daily light/dark cycle is a major time cue (zeitgeber), entraining daily rhythms, such as sleep/activity, to the 24-hour cycle. (LEWY 1980, ASCHOFF 1965, MOORE 1974, SADUN 1984) Thus, a walk in the morning wakes us up, while dusk makes us sleepy.

Immediately prior to mania, sleep is markedly reduced. (BUNNEY 1972, SITAREM 1978) Continued lack of sleep accelerates mania. (WEHR 1982, STRAKOWSKI 1991) Chronic or alternate-night sleep deprivation, repeated loss of the last four hours of sleep, all-nighters (especially if accompanied by drugs), and/or irregular hours can trigger manias that last days to weeks. (WEHR 1987, 88, 91, 98, GOLD 1987) Rapid cyclers are particularly vulnerable. (WEHR 1982, 87)

Similarly, fatigue can trigger depression, which (though many depressed bipolars oversleep) often decreases sleep, eventually leading to mania, and further lack of sleep, in a vicious cycle, which may contribute to bipolar deterioration over time. (WEHR 1982)

Sensitivity to seasonal change

Among all psychiatric disorders, mood disorders show the most clear seasonality. (SUHAIL 1998) In regions with marked seasons (temperate zones), most bipolars experience seasonal mood swings, (JAIN 1992) corresponding to day length and sunlight, but not temperature. Peck (1990) suggests sunshine is strongly correlated to manic admissions one month later. Where seasons are less differentiated, episodes show less of a pattern. In a study in southern Israel (i.e., closer to the equator), mania was generally more predominant. (OSHER 2000)

Some controversy surrounds the precise association of mood with season which, in any case, varies considerably between patients. Many observational studies suggest a tendency to spring/summer mania, and fall/winter depression in temperate zones. (SUHAIL 1998, MYERS 1978, MULDER 1990, FAEDDA 1993, SAYER 1991)

Others note clusters of spring and fall peaks for suicide, major depression, and hospitalization, (FAEDDA93, GOODWIN 1990, KAMO 1993) perhaps due to more rapid changes in sun/dark ratios. Ketter (2000), therefore, suggests increased therapeutic support around late March and September.

Other patterns have been reported. (FAEDDA 1993, BAUER 1993, WEHR 1987) Male and female seasonality can also manifest differently. (SUHAIL 1998, D'MELLO 1995) Variations within patterns are common too, perhaps reflecting variable sunlight.

Seasonal affective disorder (SAD)

SAD patients become depressed as seasonal hours of daylight decrease. They have particular trouble with winter, sleeping and eating too much, and constantly fatigued, as in bipolar depression. When light increases, mood elevates. (ROSENTHAL 1984, DONNER 1993)

Susceptible populations (AVERY 1993, ROSEN 1990)

Affective patients, night-shift workers, people living closer to the poles, women,* the elderly.

* 80-90% of SAD patients are female.

Therapies for winter depression have included

□ Increased exposure to daylight, especially in the morning, e.g., outdoor walks or exercise. Light promotes shorter, more restful sleep, reduces carbohydrate craving, and elevates mood.

□ Special lamps — AM exposure to bright or blue light (20-90 minutes, *tailored to individual requirements*). (AVERY 1990, 01, TERMAN 1998, LEE 1999, WILEMAN 2001, WIRZ-JUSTICE 1996, 98, GLICKMAN 2996, LOCKLEY 2003, 06, SHILLAB 2007)

□ Dawn stimulation — either by waking slowly with sunrise, or through a gradual increase in photoelectric light in the morning. (AVERY 2001)

□ Vitamin D3 (pp. 119-20), (GLOTH 1999) tryptophan, (LAM 1997, 99, NEUMEISTER 1998) omega 3, other antidepressant nutrients, *as relevant.*

□ Rose-colored lenses in winter. (MUELLER 1984)

Too much light exposure can trigger mania. Depression may resurface when treatment is stopped, or intensity reduced. (LEWY 1980)

SES (MUELLER 1984, GOLD 1987)

SES (light sensitive energy syndrome) causes mania-like symptoms toward the summer: loss of control, violence, psychosis, acute migraine. Mueller (1984) reports epilepsy in 50% and ADD in most.*

* Also vascular problems (e.g., easy bruising) and Raynauds phenomenon (cold, painful extremities). (Mueller 1984).

Therapies have included

□ Blue green lenses. (MUELLER 1984)

□ Melatonin and mood-stabilizing nutrients.

Biorhythm therapies: Mania & mood stability

□ **Structure daily activities** — A repetitive structure of daily activity can be helpful (e.g., regular meals, work hours, bed times, etc.).

□ **Melatonin** — Melatonin, created and secreted in response to darkness, regulates the sleep/activity cycle, entraining sleep to darkness, (LERNER 1978, MARCZYNSKI 1964, REDMAN 1983) and supporting adjustment to changes in dark/light cycles (e.g., when crossing time zones). (MURAKAMI 1983) A time-release form may help maintain sleep through the night, and may, for some, be useful for mania.*(BERSANI 2000) *May be contraindicated. See box, below.*

□ **Darkness and extended bed rest** — stimulate melatonin and dampen manic cycling. (WEHR 1982, 88, 98)

□ **Avoid bright light at night, especially before bed** — even between episodes. Light suppresses melatonin, countering sleep. (LEWY 1980, 81, 84, 85, BROADWAY 1987, LAM 1990, NURNBERGER 1988)

□ **Limit exposure to electromagnetic fields** — which supress synthesis of melatonin from tryptophan, altering the sleep cycle** (perhaps more than light), worsening anxiety, stress, hypomania, and mood swing. Implicated items include fluorescent lights, older (cathode ray) TV sets and computer screens, microwave ovens, cell phones, electric blankets. Also, proximity*** to electric repeater stations and cell phone towers, even household electric wiring. (BIRDSALL 1996) (See also, p. 273.)

* In one study (Bersani 2000), melatonin intake was associated with benefits to mania, sleep duration, and daily biorhythms in 11 manics with drug-resistant insomnia.

** 24-hr exposure may shorten the sleep/activity cycle; exposure only when awake, lengthen it. (Wever 1988).

*** Exposure decreases with the square of the distance.

Approaches to insomnia

□ Morning light — morning walks; minimally, go outside for light and fresh air.

□ Exercise sufficiently during the day.

□ Dusk simulation — gradually decrease light exposure toward bedtime, or go to bed at dusk. At the least, avoid bright light at night.

□ Hot bath before bed, *if helpful.* (PFEIFFER 1987)

□ Melatonin — perhaps time-release, in the evening, 20-60 minutes before bed, optimized to what best supports sleep. (ZHDANOVA 1995) COUSENS) *Only if needed. Often not indicated for younger persons.*

□ Tryptophan, *if indicated.* (*Usually best taken early in the day, as it precurses melatonin.*) Cofactors (B6, folate) may be helpful, perhaps at a separate time. (STOCKMEIER 1997, COUSENS 2001, URSIN 1976, MELTZER 1987, HARTMAN 1974, 77, SCHNEIDER 1986)

□ Calming nutrients — B, C, zinc. Magnesium [up to 2 gm] or calcium/magnesium. GABA or taurine, *as relevant.* B3, B6, *if helpful.* Choline, *if histapenic;* inositol, *if histadelic.* Folate, *if helpful, and not histadelic.* (PFEIFFER 1987, PAGE 1992, STEIN 1992, LARSON 1992)

□ Calming herbs — Valerian, hops, passion flower, scullcap, wild lettuce, blessed thistle, catnip, nerve root, black cohosh, *as relevant.* (MOWREY 1986, CHRISTOPHER 1976, KLOSS 1973) (See *Biotypes* pp 145-68, & *Herbs* pp. 53-5 for contraindications.)

□ To prevent night waking — before bed, limit liquid and avoid sugars (even fruit); try a *small* protein snack. (HARTMAN 1974, 79, PFEIFFER 1987, BRAVERMAN 1987)

□ Support biotype, sugar, thyroid, other balances.

Melatonin: Considerations

Melatonin can be low in bipolars, (LAM 1990, BECK-FRIIS 1985) vary with mood, (LEWY 1979, 85, BRECK-FRIIS 1985, BOYCE 1985, BRANCHEY 1982, BROWN 1985, CLAUSTRAT 1984, MENDLEWICZ 1979, NAIR 1984, WETTENBERG 1983, WIRZ-JUSTICE 1979) or rhythm of secretion may be distorted. (NAIR 1984, LEWY, DAHLITZ 1991) In some, melatonin does not convert back to serotonin in the day, leading to fatigue and depression.

Depletion may be associated with:

Insomnia. Distorted biorhythms.*(MAYEDA 1990, REDMAN 1983)
Free radical toxicity.** TD. (SANDYK 1990) Aging. (BIRDSALL 1996)
Convulsive disorders. (JAN 1999, BIRDSALL 1996)
Elevated LDL, or total cholesterol.
Postmenopause osteoporosis. (BIRDSALL 1996)
SIDS, MS, heart disease, cancer. (BIRDSALL 1996)

* Melatonin influences secretion of hormone-releasing factors.

** Melatonin is a powerful free radical scavenger, and may help prevent hydroxyl injury in Alzheimer's. (Maurizi 1995)

Normal patterns of melatonin secretion

Normally,* melatonin is very low in the day, rising at night. (LEWY 1978) Levels decline as body size and age increase, (KLEIN 1984, IGUCHI 1982, SACK 1986, BIRDSALL 1996) and as luteinizing hormone increases in puberty. (WALDHAUSER 1985, 88) Magnetic fields supress melatonin synthesis from tryptophan. (BIRDSALL 1996)

* Levels and pattern are generally consistent within individuals, but vary between people, from barely detectable to abundant. (Arendt 1985)

Cautions

Manics may have high levels and not need more.
May trigger or worsen depression in some. (BRIGHAM 2001)
If taken too early, fatigue and insomnia may increase.
Contraindicated if trying to conceive, pregnant or nursing.
Extended use may suppress natural hormone production (so often inadvisable if under age 40).

Consult your physician before taking with depressive or autoimmune disorders, pregnancy, nursing, MAOIs or corticosteroids.

Light/melatonin/sleep pathways (AVERY 1982, GOLD 1987)

Light projects through the retina via acetylcholine to the SCN* and PVN.** Sufficient light stimulates norepinephrine release to the pineal,*** where it inhibits melatonin production. With darkness, the pineal secretes melatonin, promoting sleep. (PALAZIDOU 1992 MOORE 1974, SADUN 1984)

* The SCN (which lies above the chiasm where the optic nerves cross) controls melatonin production (and influences creation of vasopressin, somatostatin, serotonin, acetylcholine, substance P and other neuropeptides). (Moore, Lenn 1972, Gamlin 1982, Avery 1982, Gold 1987)

** The PVN (in the hypothalamus) regulates timing of hormonal secretions. (Avery 1982, Gold 1987)

*** The pineal gland integrates biorhythms related to light, and creates melatonin from serotonin. (Avery 1982, Gold 1987)

Biorhythm therapies: Depression

☐ **Structure daily activity** — Regular mealtimes, work, etc., in tune with natural daily rhythms.

☐ **Light therapy** — As first suggested by Wehr (1982), even when SAD is not involved, light therapy may improve bipolar depression. Thus, in a study by Delito (1991), phototherapy created significant improvement in all outcome measures in bipolar, as compared to unipolar depression, with the improvement sustained three months later. A 1998 review by Kripke also points to antidepressant benefit. Recent studies have suggested a lower intensity blue light may be even more potent, and is associated with less visual and other complaints. (GLICKMAN 2006, LOCKELY 2003, 06)

Warning: Excessive light exposure can trigger mania. (KRIPKE 1998)

More simply, researchers find that waking up to the gradually increasing light of dawn, (AVERY 2001, TERMAN 1998) or taking a daily morning walk (or at any time) frequently lifts mood. (WIRZ-JUSTICE 1996, 98, WILEMAN 2001, LEE 1999, TERMAN 1989, LEWY 1982, KRIPKE 1998)

☐ **Vitamin D3** — is antidepressant and seems to have a role in maintaining biological rhythms. Deficiency can contribute to depression in SAD and probably other depressions. (VIETH 2004, LANDSDOWNE 1998, GLOTH 1999)

See *Vitamin D3*, pp. 119-20.

☐ **Negative ions** — May promote serotonin formation. Several studies find negative ions improve winter depression. (TERMAN 1995, 98) Negative ions are produced by rain, waterfalls, ocean, and forests; and by commercial negative ion generators. (Positive ions are generally associated with smog, pollution, most electrical appliances, and pavement on hot dry days.)

A note on sleep deprivation therapy

One night's sleep deprivation is often temporarily antidepressant for both major and bipolar depression. (WEHR 1982, PFLUG 1976) Deprivation of the second (but not first) half of the night's sleep (and selective REM deprivation) can also be antidepressant. Both approaches advance wakening.*(SCHILGEN 1980)

Improvement occurs in up to 50% of depressives,** (PAREKH 1998) *however, most relapse the next day* (following recovery sleep), (WEHR 1982, 87, PFLUG 1976) *perhaps, further destabilizing mood.*

Going to sleep five or six hours earlier, and waking earlier (advancing sleep) sustains benefit, in many, for up to a week or more. (WEHR 1988, SACK 1985, 87). Antidepressants, (KASPER 1992) especially those that target serotonin, (SMERALDI 1999) may also help prevent relapse, suggesting relevant nutrients and herbs (e.g., 5HTP, B6, tyrosine, etc.) might be similarly helpful.

Care is warranted to prevent onset of mania.

* Perhaps elevating mood by correcting a sleep cycle desynchronization with other biorhythms. (Wehr 1982)

** But usually not if hypothyroid, as successful sleep deprivation therapy seems to work, in part, by stimulating the thyroid, but often fails to do so in low thyroid patients. (Kasper 1992, Kuhs 1996, Parekh 1998)

Endocrine rhythms in bipolars

Mood and endocrine rhythms appear intertwined.

Pituitary — Bipolar pituitary TSH, PRL, and pineal melatonin release may be phase advanced, or the pattern of release may be disrupted, with more secretory episodes, and secretion at abnormal hours. (WEHR 1978, 80, 82, 83) Bipolar depressives can secrete as much as fourfold normal growth hormone per day, mainly due to more secretory spikes.

Pineal melatonin — Secretion rhythm may be distorted, with peak melatonin varying with mood, typically secreted too early in mania; (LEWY 1979) too late in depression. (NAIR 1984, LEWY, DAHLITZ 1991) Melatonin entrains the biorhythms of some of the other glands.

Adrenals — Normally, plasma corticosteroids and ACTH peak before waking, followed by a steady decline, with levels minimal at night. Six to nine peaks typically cluster around early morning and meals. In many depressives, however, secretory episodes may continue through the night (often peaking near midnight), perhaps also with lengthier and more frequent episodes, and total output considerably elevated. (KRIEGER 1988, GALLAGHER 1973, SACHAR 1975, PFOHL 1985, ROSE 1987)

Acetylcholine, serotonin, and dopamine, which regulate daily ACTH and cortiocosteroid secretion, also show a circadian pattern, which may become distorted. (KRIEGER 1988)

Sex hormones — Annual sexual hormone rhythms are triggered by changes in light, probably via melatonin. (ARENDT 1985, BITTMAN 1983, BUBENIK 1986) As in herd animals, human testosterone may increase in the fall, increasing spring/early summer birth (summer in higher latitudes).*(WHYBROW 1988, LAGOGUEY 1976, COWGILL 1966)

However, estrogen (SHIBATA 1999), testosterone, and thyroid (which also supports sexual function), are among the few biochemicals that can act independently from their normal circadian rhythms, (CORFMAN) perhaps to help perpetuate the species (regardless of time of day) and support the ability to respond to physical threat. Natural sexual biorhythms in humans may currently be obscured by the effects of electric lights and a steadier food supply. (WHYBROW 1988)

Similarly, the disortion of seasonal melatonin biorhythms in the bipolar may alter sex hormone production, affecting mood. (WHYBROW 1988)

VI: Related conditions

I. Comorbid disorders

Bipolars commonly experience comorbid psychiatric disorders (Strakowski 1992, Amadeo 1992) which often complicate the illness, and may promote rapid cycling, (Bauer 1993, 94a) and mixed states, (Bauer 1994b, McElroy 1992) or mask the mood disorder.

O'Connell (1991) finds personality disorders in 58% of bipolars, especially borderline; also histrionic disorder. Personality disorders involving erratic or fearful behavior may be twice as common as those involving eccentric behavior, such as schizoid personality disorder. Panic and anxiety disorders are pervasive. (Peselow 1995)

List of comorbid disorders

J Hudson and H Pope of McLean in Massachusetts (1999) list the following conditions (best assessed during euthymia):

- □ Various depressions, including SAD.
- □ Borderline, anxiety and panic disorders. PTSD.
- □ Attention deficit and hyperactivity disorders. Autism.
- □ Obsessive compulsive disorder. Tourettes. Pathological gambling, shopping, etc. Talking too fast and too much.
- □ Body dysmorphic disorder, eating disorders.
- □ Addictions, substance abuse.
- □ Various phobias, particularly agorophobia. Hypersensitivity to light, noise, touch, crowds, etc. Social withdrawal.
- □ Pyromania, kleptomania, trichotillomania (compulsively pulling out hair), other impulse control disorders.
- □ Intermittent explosive disorder. Destructiveness, child or spousal abuse, prolonged anger. Criminality.
- □ Self-mutilation, suicide, suicide threats.
- □ Eccentric disorders.
- □ Sleep disorders, narcolepsy, cataplexy.
- □ Unusual reactions to prescription meds.
- □ Chronic pain. Severe headaches, migraines. Fibromyalgia, arthritis, chronic fatigue.
- □ Chronic digestive problems (irritable bowel syndrome, etc.).

A note on therapy

Mood stabilization plus attention to triggers and causes, tailored to individual biochemical requirements, may resolve comorbid conditions.

On the other hand, to adequately describe natural treatments currently used for the related conditions described in this book would require a library. Thus, the therapies mentioned here are necessarily incomplete, and consitute just a glimpse of what may be involved.

Reminder: This material in this book is presented for educational purposes only. If you need treatment for psychiatric disorders or any other medical condition, please seek the services of a knowledgeable physician.

See also:
Insomnia, pp. 259-62.

"The panic attacks... I can remember them prior to having language... They always have to do with death, my death...When I was about twelve... there was something about the beauty of that day, the smell, something that suddenly threw me into absolute terror that someday I would never see this again. I screamed and ran into the house with the milk bottles and dropped them on my way up the stairs. I just kept running in this frenzied way."

Patty Duke 1992

Anxiety

Panic and anxiety are prevalent in bipolars, especially during psychosis or paranoia, or perhaps replacing missed episodes. (HIMMELHOCH 1999) See *Natural anti-anxiety approaches,* in the box, below.

Panic disorder

Panic attacks typically begin with acute anxiety and intense fear, peaking within 10 minutes and ending in 20-30. Eventually, anticipatory anxiety occurs, along with avoidance behavior or agorophobia. Lifetime prevalence of panic disorder* in bipolars is over 20%, more than twice that in unipolars, and 26 times controls. (COLODNY 2000)

SOME NATURAL APPROACHES HAVE INCLUDED: (COLODNY 2000, SLAGLE 2000)
See *Anxiety therapies, below.* Optimize to individual biochemistry. GABA and serotonin support may be especially important.

Obsessive compulsive disorders (OCD)

OCD is relatively common, especially in histadelics. (PFEIFFER 1987) Some bipolars become more obsessional during mood episodes. (KETTER 2001)

SOME NATURAL APPROACHES HAVE INCLUDED:

- ☐ Mood and anxiety therapies, *as relevant*. Histadelia is common. (PFEIFFER 1987, COLODNY 2000) Serotonin support may be helpful. (YARYURAH 77, 81, FUX 96, MURPHY 89, RAMUSSEN 84, CHALEM 82, MIZUNO 75, HUWIG-POPPE 99)
- ☐ Psychological techniques, e.g., mindful attention, etc.
- ☐ Check for brain injury, which sometimes leads to OCD. (COLODNY 2000)

Natural mood-stabilizing anti-anxiety approaches have included (SLAGLE 2000)

Consult a knowledgeable physician who will rule out interactions with meds, and tailor dose, timing (taking into account daily variations in symptom intensity), and choice of nutrients to individual biochemical requirements and response.

(1) Address histapenia, histadelia, pyroluria, metallothionein dysfunction, *as relevant.* (See pp. 145-173.)

(2) Mood-stabilizing and antimanic nutrients (Consider: B1, B3, B6, and other B vitamins, magnesium glycinate, zinc, taurine, GABA, etc., *as relevant.* Lecithin (*especially if histapenic*)* or inositol (*if histadelic*).** Perhaps chromium, melatonin, nutritional doses of lithium, etc., *as relevant.* (pp. 21-75.) (ABBEY 1982, GABY 1995, KENNEDY 1980, MOHLER 1979, RUDIN 1981, WILLIAMS 1943, HOES 1981, HESEKER 1992, LEVINE 1995, REPLOGIE 1989, BUIST 1986, SEELIG 1975, DURLACH 1994, WESTON 1923, BENTON 1991, MCCLEANE 1990)

(3) Omega 3 (MILLS 1986, 89) and/or GLA. *Look at biotype requirements.* (See pp. 52, 87-94) (WALSH 2006)

(4) C, E, selenium, glutathione, other antioxidants. (73-83)

(5) Consider serotonin support (tryptophan or 5HTP, plus B6, 2-3x/day, emphasis on unrefined, whole food carbs), *but not if it worsens mania, and usually not with histapenia.* (pp. 100-5.) (SLAGLE 2000, KAHN 1987, HOES 1982, ZANG, HOYSE 1982)

(6) Kava, (SINGH 1992, LINDENBERG 1990, KINZLER 1991) scullcap, valerian, passionflower, wood betony, Bach Rescue Remedy, hops, chamomile, etc., *as relevant.* (See pp. 53-55.)

(7) Support balanced adrenals, thyroid, etc. (pp. 223-243)

(8) Treat environmental & food allergies. (*Consider favorite or frequently-eaten foods.*) (See pp. 207-13.) (KING 1981, ALVAREZ 1946)

(9) Address blood sugar, malabsorption, Candida, neurological disorders, anemias, etc. (See pp. 198-22; 244-50.)

(10) Healthy diet. Fresh whole foods, appropriate protein and vegetables, healthy fats. Avoid junk food (white sugar or flour, harmful fats, alcohol, etc.). (pp. 254-56) (SALZER 1966, RAINEY 1984, WENDEL 1973, ALBERTI 1977, VOLPI 1997, MONTEIRO 1990, BELL 1994)

(11) Limit toxins (tobacco, caffeine, other stimulants, MSG, aspartate, alcohol, street drugs, detrimental effects from meds, toxic or excess metals, etc.). (See pp. 169-96.)

(12) Balanced lifestyle. Regular hours. Relax. Nature, fresh air, light, and exercise. Psychosocial support. (251-62)

(13) If overstimulation is involved (with symptoms like tension, restlessness, trembling, racing pulse, profuse perseration), avoid caffeine, (BRUCE 1989, LEVI 1967, ROBERT 1978, SILVER 1992, HUGHES 1991, UHDE 1984) sugar, phenylalanine, street drugs, and other stimulants; limit or avoid, spirulina, bee products, ginseng (especially Korean); possibly, seaweeds, etc., *as relevant.* Rule out high thyroid. (SLAGLE 2000)

(14) If due to detrimental conditioning (anxiety triggered by stressful thoughts and fears, with minimal physical symptoms), Slagle suggests "Hypnoperipheral Processing Reprogramming" (which combines hypnosis and Neurolinguistic Programming)*** and the series "Changing Emotions" & "Feeling Better." (SLAGLE 2000)

(15) If due to low oxygen or high lactic acid, support oxygenation, e.g., with deep breathing, an appropriate exercise program,**** ginkgo, E, CoQ10; possibly carnitine or creatine. Check for low thyroid. (SLAGLE 2000)

* Note: Lecithin contains both choline and inositol with the emphasis on choline, so excess may trigger depression, especially in histadelia.

**At least one study (an 8-week double-blind crossover (Benjamin 2000), found significant decrease in panic attacks (and agoraphobia) with 12 gm per day (a high dose). Caution: Too much can trigger mania.

*** See: http://www.metamodels.com/maps/hpp.html

**** Exercise increases ability to handle stress and reduces reactivity, but if overdone, can promote lactic acid buildup and anxiety or panic attacks. So increases in exercise duration and difficulty should be gradual.

Binge eating, bulimia, anorexia (SLAGLE 2001)

Eating disorders are relatively common in bipolars. In a study by Simpson (1992), 59% of 22 eating disorder patients were bipolar II.

SOME NATURAL APPROACHES HAVE INCLUDED: (COLODNY 2000, SLAGLE 2001, NUSBAUM 1986, KAYE 1991, HOWAT 1989)

- □ Antidepressant nutrients, *if relevant.*
- □ Mood and anxiety therapies, *previous page, as relevant.*
- □ B1, B6, other B vitamins, (SLAGLE 2001), zinc; (HUMPHRIES 1989, MCCLAIN 1992, 93, PATRICK 2002) and serotonin support (evened out over the day) (WELTZIN 1991, PIJL 1995, DALVIT-MCPHILLIPS 1984) may be especially indicated.
- □ Optimize nutrient content of the diet. Avoid refined carbohydrates (DREWNOWSKI 1995) and support blood sugar balance. Small doses of chromium, 2-3x/day may be helpful, *if* timing can be adjusted so hunger does not occur between doses.
- □ Histadelia is common (consider inositol, magnesium, SAM, etc.), (PATRICK 2002) though other biotypes may be involved. (WALSH 2006)
- □ Check for thyroid, adrenal and other hormonal imbalance; allergies, Candida, malabsorption, or other contributory conditions. (SLAGLE 2001)
- □ Build the psychosocial support network.

"I am as a weed,
Flung from the rock on Ocean's foam, to sail
Where'er the surge may sweep, the tempest's breath prevail."

Lord Byron, "Child Harold's Pilgrimage," Canto 3. Byron's erratic diets, food indulgence and hard drinking, eventually compromised his kidneys.

Post traumatic stress disorder (PTSD)

PTSD involves nightmares, flashbacks and other symptoms which replay severe psychological trauma.* PTSD is common among bipolars.

SOME NATURAL APPROACHES HAVE INCLUDED: (COLODNY 2000)

- □ Mood and anxiety therapies, *as relevant.*
- □ May need to emphasize, serotonin support; and nutrients which counterbalance norepinephrine (e.g., GABA, taurine, choline), *as relevant.*
- □ Counseling, EMDR, neurolinguistic programming, acupressure, other psychological techniques, and psychosocial support. Consider the possibility of childhood abuse. (LEVIN 1999)

* PTSD typically stimulates the limbic system, and perhaps the thyroid, causing further arousal.(Wang) Activation may focus on the left frontal lobe and anterior cingulate gyrus (suggesting ability to discern threat, but not necessarily to adjust limbic arousal). (Levin 1999)

"A heap of broken images, where the sun beats,
And the dead tree gives no shelter, the cricket no relief,
And the dry stone no sound of water
There is a shadow under this red rock...
I will show you fear in a handful of dust."

TS Eliot, "The Waste Land"

Borderline personality disorder (BRIGHAM 2001, SLAGLE)

Symptoms of mixed state and rapid cycling bipolar disorder are similar to those of borderline: anger, impulsivity, stormy relationships, suicide attempts, sleep, and appetite changes.* Borderline symptoms are so common in bipolars, (POPE, BRIGHAM 2001) some researchers suggest it may be part of a bipolar spectrum. Borderlines are generally more volatile; mood can switch within hours (though changes can also be fast in atypical-mixed or rapid-cycling bipolars). Racing thoughts and adverse reactions to antidepressants are more likely in bipolars. (BRIGHAM 2001)

SOME NATURAL APPROACHES HAVE INCLUDED:

- □ Mood stabilizing and anxiety therapies, including serotonin support, *as relevant.*
- □ Counseling, EMDR, neurolinguistic programming, acupressure, etc. (SLAGLE 2000) Therapy for childhood abuse (most borderlines). (LEVIN 1999)

Note: Some practitioners consider borderline a psychiatric disorder, others suggest it represents a psychological reaction to abuse.

* Thus, in a study by Akiskal (2001), 25 of 100 borderlines met criteria for bipolar II or cyclothymia.

Behavior & conduct disorders, delinquency, violence

"Suddenly I was a famous man, and I was shot into an even higher mood state… In the end I went over the bounds of reality, or law and order. [I didn't commit any crimes] but I could easily have done so if anyone had crossed me… Should a man, friend or foe, object to anything I did or said, it was quite possible that I could poke him in the jaw."

Joshua Logan, Broadway producer, quoted in Fieve 1975

Biotypes (Walsh 1983, 91, 94, 96, 97, 2004, Pfeiffer 1988)

Doctor William J. Walsh, of Walsh Research Institute, reports the following biotypes in people prone to delinquent or violent behavior. Corresponding therapies involve correction of causal imbalances with appropriate nutritional supplements, toxic metal elimination, dietary improvements (including avoidance of coffee, alcohol, sugar and junk food), and avoidance of abused drugs. Psychosocial support can also be important.

Type A: Violence, tantrums (Walsh 1994, 96, 97, 2004)

Type A individuals are prone to violence. Boys engage in episodes of severe tantrums or fighting interspersed with excellent behavior. In girls, mood swings, oppositional behavior and nonviolent delinquency are more typical. Severe type A individuals can be extremely violent. Mild to moderate type A is characteristic of perhaps 40% of behavior-disordered children.

Biochemistry: Elevated levels of copper relative to zinc, low levels of hair sodium and potassium, and sensitivity to toxins such as lead and cadmium.

Walsh reports that adjusting these imbalances results in significant improvement within 25 days and benefits about 85% of Type A patients.

Type B: Severely antisocial, without remorse (Pihl 1990, Walsh 1983, 92, 96, 2004, Cromwell 1989)

Type B is characterized by severe antisocial activity, lack of remorse or conscience, frequent assaultive behavior, fascination with fire, cruelty to animals, extreme tendency to violence. Type B is prevalent in career criminals, serial killers and mass murderers. Perhaps 0.3% of the population is type B.

Biochemistry: Pyroluria, low hair copper, high histamine, depressed blood spermine, and elevated levels of toxic metals such as lead and cadmium.

Walsh finds prognosis is best for young Type B individuals with no involvement in drug or alcohol abuse. Response to treatment can occur within a week.

Type C: Delinquent, oppositional (Walsh 1992, 96, 2004)

Type C is characterized by irritable impulsive and oppositional behavior, and a propensity for nonviolent delinquent activity. Type C's typically underachieve in school and have difficulty keeping a job or getting a driver's license.

Biochemistry: Characteristically low in trace minerals and many amino acids; malabsorber, usually with low stomach acid, often slender.

Type D: Nonviolent delinquent behavior (Schauss 1979, 81ab, 84, 86 Reed 1983, Buckley 1979, Schoenthaler 1983, Walsh 1996, 97, 2004)

Type D individuals are prone to nonviolent, delinquent behavior.

Biochemistry: Typically hypoglycemic; deficient in manganese and chromium.

Walsh finds nutrients addressing the imbalances in types C and D are usually effective, though improvement may take one to three months to become evident.

See corresponding biotypes, health conditions, nutrients, toxins. Reminder: This information is presented for educational purposes only. If you need treatment for bipolar disorder or any other medical condition, please seek the services of a knowledgeable physician.

Pfeiffer's list of violent biochemistries (Pfeiffer 1988)

In approximately descending order of significance:

- □ Pyroluria.
- □ Low manganese, zinc and B6. (Pfeiffer 1988, Walsh 1991, 94)
- □ Hypoglycemia (especially with poor diet, low manganese). (Pfeiffer 1988, Schauss 1981, Reed 1983, Buckley 1979, Schoenthaler 1983)
- □ Histadelia, especially with addictions.
- □ Metal metabolism disorders. (Walsh 1997, 2004) Copper, aluminum, cadmium, lead, or other heavy metal toxicity. (Pfeiffer 1988, Walsh 1983, 94, 96, Pihl 1990, Schmidt 1981)
- □ Cerebral allergy (especially to milk, wheat, corn, or salicylates). (Pfeiffer 1988, Schauss 1979, 84, Moyer 1975, Rapp 1991)
- □ Psychomotor epilepsy. Head trauma. (Braverman 1993)
- □ PMS.
- □ Excess testosterone. XYY chromosome (treatment involves progesterone.)

Also: elevated catecholamines and/or suppressed tryptophan, other transmitter imbalances, (Raleigh 1987, Mawson 1978, Volavka 1990) and essential fatty acid depletion.*(Hibbeln 1996)

* Note: Forensic studies find homicide and suicide more linked to depression than mania, which is more commonly associated with benign penal infractions. (B´en´ezech 1992)

Recommended Reading

Schauss, Alexander, PhD, *Diet, Crime & Delinquency*, 1981

Reed, Barbara, PhD, *Diet, Teens, & Behavior*, 1983.

home.earthlink.net/~berniew1/violence.html

Suicide

"Remember that painting by Bosch of the end of the world? All the devils were rounding up the sinners and I pointed out one man robed like a gentleman who was rising from his table indignantly and drawing his sword. Remember? I pointed him out to you, out of all those grotesque figures, and said, see, see him there, he thinks he can handle death with a sword? And you seemed to understand so well what I was saying."

— Ernest Hemingway, shortly before his death, talking to his son, Gregory

Suicide risk in bipolars

The bipolar suicide rate is far higher than in other psychiatric illness, including major depression. (LAM 1999) Lifetime suicide rate in bipolars is 15 to 20%. Klerman (1992), reviewing twenty studies, reports a mean of 19%, with attempts in 20-56%. (GOODWIN 1990, SIMPSON 15% 1999) Accidents (perhaps related), and cardiovascular disease are also increased. (BOWDEN 1999B) Death in 15-25% results from altercations, accidents or suicide. (MARANO 2005) *Immediate therapeutic attention is critical with any signs of impending suicide.*

Mood & psychosocial risk (PFEIFFER 87, GOLD 87, TSUANGE 77, WINOKUR 75)

Suicide occurs more in bipolar depression than mania. (B'EN'EZECH 1992) Risk is greatest during early stages of recovery, (when energy may increase before mood improves), (STOLL 2002) especially in those with good insight into their condition.

Vulnerable people are commonly characterized by hopelessness, social isolation, a fall from previous achievements, and poor response to meds, combined with a relapsing course. Bipolar impulsivity, hopelessness and rigid thinking may also play a role. (BECK 1999, ELLIS 1996)

Withdrawal from lithium and probably other mood stabilizers, greatly magnifies risk, especially during the first year.

Biotype issues (PFEIFFER 1987)

Histadelics, who are often constantly obsessed with one particular form of suicide, and their tendency to discontinue treatment or succumb to addictions increases risk. Pfeiffer (1987) suggests they live with someone who provides friendly support. Pyrolurics, and other biotypes, are also at risk.

Nutritional & other risk factors (HOFFER 1967, 78, KITAHARA 1987, MILES 1977, LESTER 1990, BRANCHEY 1984, WEBB 1981)

Dr. Marie Asberg first noted a tendency to completed suicide among people with low brain serotonin. She found 20% of patients with low CSF 5HIAA (a serotonin metabolite), killed themselves within the next year. Similarly, the fluctuating serotonin status associated with chronic SSRIs or with withdrawal may contribute to suicide or violence in the young, and perhaps others (see p. 287). Markedly low cholesterol, which has been associated with decreased serotonin receptors, also increases suicide risk. (ERASMUS 1995)

Adrenal axis dysregulation, (GOLD 1987) high fat intake, (LESTER 1990) and poor uptake of C, (KITAHARA 1987) have also been associated with increased risk. In fact, risk increases with almost any significant mood-destabilizing nutrient imbalance (e.g., omega 3/6, biotype disorders, lack of B, C, magnesium, certain aminos, etc.), toxicity (e.g., alcohol, mercury, medication reaction or rebound), or implicated health conditions.

Role of orthomolecular treatment (HOFFER 1967, 1978)

"Do not go gentle into that good night/ Rage, rage against the dying of the light." — Dylan Thomas

The suicide rate in schizophrenia is reported greatly reduced by orthomolecular therapy,* especially if begun early and continued for an extended period; and may be substantially decreased, even if started later. (HOFFER 1967, 1978) Given the suspected overlap of most contributory factors, and the preliminary reports of significant effectiveness, one might project that orthomolecular methods could also help protect bipolars. Further research is needed to delineate benefit.

* Decreasing from 10%, down to appproximately 1%, about the rate found in the general population. (Hoffer)

Pfeiffer's checklist for factors underlying suicide (1987)

(Diagnostic tests are in parentheses.)

- □ Lack of nutrients to combat environmental stress.
- □ Allergies — gluten, corn, beef, dairy, etc.
- □ Histadelia. (*Basophil count, blood histamine.*)
- □ Pyroluria. (*Urinary pyrroles, serum zinc, EGOT.*)
- □ Histapenia.
- □ Vegetarian or malnourished. (*Plasma aminos, FIGLU, serum folate and B12.*)
- □ Heavy metals. (*Blood aluminum and lead, blood and serum copper, hair analysis for heavy metals.*)
- □ Paranoia (possibly histapenic) with low platelet MAO or high urinary tryptamine.
- □ Low B6, zinc, manganese, and/or tyrosine.
- □ Endocrine imbalances.
- □ Alcoholism. Substance abuse.

Pfeiffer emphasizes corresponding therapeutic nutrients, plus exercise, supportive counseling, stress reduction.

Larson's checklist

- □ Depressed, reduced well-being, self-blame, guilt.
- □ Anxiety, agitation, angry outbursts, poor self-control.
- □ Lack of support system.
- □ Drug or alcohol abuse. Sleeping pills, etc.
- □ Multiple physical ailments.

Bipolar delusions & psychosis (See corresponding chapters for further details and references)

"I would stumble into a dark narrow place between buildings, a space I could hardly squeeze myself into, and stand there, stock still for hours... I only knew the night was gone when daylight came... there were just these horrid mental images coming and going... I felt battered, pounded to a pulp... I must have stood there transfixed, like I'd looked at a Gorgon and turned to stone."

Robby Wilde, 1987

Psychotic manias* are now prevalent. (Brigham 2001) Likelihood is greatest in patients who experienced early mood disturbance, (Rosen 1983) and increases with illness severity. (Brigham 2001) Psychosis during bipolar II hypomania, redefines the episode as mania, and changes the diagnosis to bipolar I, even if other symptoms are mild. Psychosis can also occur during bipolar depression.

If antipsychotics are given long-term, bipolars are often reclassified schizoaffective. Nonetheless, Brigham (2001) contends that psychosis in bipolars may be primarily a mood symptom (more responsive to vigorous mood stabilization than antipsychotic drugs).* Similarly, for severe mixed affective states (which can look more like schizophrenia** than mania).

* This distinction becomes particularly cogent in teens presenting with a first-break psychosis.

*** E.g., with thought disorder, disorganization, or hallucinations, perhaps paranoia, and without classic manic symptoms.

Biotype distinctions

Delusional mood episodes occur mainly in histadelics, who are often diagnosed schizoaffective. The distortion is largely cognitive (i.e., delusions). Thus, typical schizoaffective characteristics can include blank mind, perhaps catatonia, lack of strong response to B3, history of high accomplishment (patient or family) and, generally, histadelic symptoms and chemistry, and responsiveness to histadelic therapies. (Walsh 2008)

See *Histadelia,* pp. 157-61.

Perceptual psychosis during mania (i.e., with sensory hallucinations and high catecholamines) is generally limited to pyroluria and histapenia, often with concurrent MT disorder and high copper (which would increase catecholamines, and so further worsen paranoia and psychosis). (Walsh 2008) Hoffer suggests bipolars with sensory psychoses might be closer to schizophrenia than bipolar disorder,* and finds they respond especially well to classic antipsychotic nutrients, particularly niacin** (perhaps with doses on the high side), and vitamin C; and attention to any pyroluria (which he finds common). (Hoffer, 2008b)

See *Histapenia,* pp. 162-6; *Hoffer's approach,* p. 17; *Niacin,* pp. 59-61; *NADH,* p. 117; *Adrenochrome,* p. 82; *Pyrrole disorder,* pp. 147-52.

* And may represent the center of a continuum between the two disorders (Hoffer, 2008b) (which seem to share some symptoms, chemistry, and genetics (Moller 2003, Rush 2003, Kidd 2004, Horrobin 1999)).

** Critical in addressing high norepinephrine, histapenia and MT dysfunction. (Walsh 2008)

Lesser's approach

Michael Lesser, MD (2008) finds acutely psychotic bipolars who agree to eat red meat every hour* often can be brought down from the psychosis within a week, even more readily if you can get them to take GABA, B3, perhaps tryptophan, etc, *as per individual requirements.* But if they can't follow the meat diet, he says meds may be a necessary evil — though usually only needed a few weeks, til ordinary reality is restored.

* Some suggestions as to why this works: The abundant meat may act through its provision of high levels of methyl (countering histadelia (Walsh 2008)), aminos (countering hypoglycemia (Lesser 2008)), B3 (countering voices & histapenia (Hoffer 2008, Lesser2008)); also: B6, B12, zinc, carnitine, or other components. Or by fostering ketone formation, thereby supporting activity of the anterior cingulate's high-affinity niacin receptors (subfunction of which may be critical in schizophrenia (Miller 2008)).

General approach (Walsh 2006)

Therapy generally involves appropriate biotype approaches, and resolution of any malnutition, malabsorption, metal metabolism disorders, and chronic oxidative stess; and of specific nutrient deficiencies, dependencies, or overloads. Also, attention to any allergies, sensitivities, blood sugar and endocrine imbalances, Candida, epilepsy and other neurological disorders, immune issues, and other implicated health conditions; and excitotoxicity, substance abuse, drug side effects, or other toxicity; and lifestyle issues, *all optimized to individual requirements.*

Recommended reading

Hoffer, Abram, MD, PhD, *Common Questions about Schizophrenia & their Answers,* 1987, and *Orthomolecular Medicine for Physicians,* 2008.

Pfeiffer, Carl C, PhD, MD, *Nutrition & Mental Illness,* 1987, and *The Schizophrenias Ours to Conquer*, 1988.

Reminder: This is a brief overview. For further information, contraindications and references, see corresponding chapters; the author's Natural Healing for Schizophrenia, and the recommended reading, above. This material is presented for educational purposes only. If you need treatment for mood disorder, or any other medical condition, please seek the services of a knowledgeable physician, who will tailor treatment to individual biochemical requirements.

2. Childhood concerns

Fifty years ago, bipolar onset clustered in the late twenties to early thirties, but now focuses on the late teens, with 20% of cases thought to emerge in childhood. (RUSH 2003, MARANO 2005, KLUGER 2002, CABF 2002)

Causes may involve: a lack of magnesium, zinc, chronium and other minerals in depleted soils and foods; profuse intake of omega 6 oils but sparse omega 3; overindulgence in sugar, sodas, caffeine, alcohol, tobacco, Aspartame®, MSG, street drugs, etc.; an epidemic of hormonal disorders; the alienation intrinsic to the modern psychosocial environment; the distortion of natural biorhythms; and widespread treatment of children with drugs for hyperactivity, depression, and with other medications that can trigger mania. (MARANO 2005)

> *"There has been an explosion in [childhood bipolar disorder] in the past five years. It represents an attempt to predict which children are headed for a bipolar type mental breakdown. [Unfortunately] the usual result is early intervention with powerful atypical antipsychotic medication."*
>
> William J Walsh, PhD, 2006

Characteristics suggesting bipolar disorder in young people

Baseline is less consistent in the young. (CARLSON 1988A) Moodiness or irritability, for instance, can suggest bipolar disorder, but be due to learning, behavior or conduct disorders, etc. (BOWDEN 1995, 96, 2001, GELLER 1995, 97, WEST 1995) On the other hand, many youth initially diagnosed with major depression, ADHD, borderline, PTSD, schizophrenia, etc., are later rediagnosed bipolar. (CABF 2002A) (Again, the role of the corresponding meds in the later development of bipolar disorder merits further investigation.) Suggested characteristics include:

- ☐ Family history of bipolar or multigeneration mood disorder. (BRIGHAM 2001)
- ☐ Very rapid cycling in children, perhaps several times per day, often with irritability, and separated by several hours of normal mood.* (CABF 2002A) *Distinguish from allergies and/or hypoglycemia.*
- ☐ Prepuberty mood symptoms, especially with anxiety disorder, (BRIGHAM 2001) (approximately 30% of children with early clinical depression later develop mania, (GELLER 1994)) perhaps, combined with early antidepressant use. *Rule out psychosocial and dietary factors; street drugs.*
- ☐ Perceptual inaccuracy, difficulty integrating information, cognitive inflexibility, adversion to complexity. (LAST 1989)
- ☐ Thought disorder, unconventionalism. (LAST 1989)
- ☐ Reduced persistence. Increased reward-dependence, harm-avoidance. (OSHER 2000, LAST 1989)
- ☐ Symptoms emerging in early puberty, or after trauma (violence, rape, etc.). (CABF 2002A) (*Often with increased risk of further trauma during mania.* (WOZNIAK 1999)) *Distinguish from PTSD.*
- ☐ Acting out of impulses (substance abuse, early promiscuity, trouble with police or school). (GOLD 1987, ZARATE 2001) *Distinguish whether due to mania, prior abuse, or both.*

* Extreme affective dysregulation syndrome — now occuring in an increasing number of children (even as young as two), (Post 2001) can involve irritability, tantrums, impulsivity, aggression, hyperactivity, attention problems. Though not quite bipolar, eventual incidence is higher, especially if moods are extreme. (Geller 1997, Kidd 2004)

> *"Rates [of depression] have increased every decade in the past century, even more so in the past 50 years, and affect increasingly younger people. 500,000 children are now on antidepressants."*
>
> GL Klerman, MM Weisman, 1989

> *"I was so depressed, I didn't care what they did. They wanted an explanation for why I do things and I didn't want to delve into my motivations. So I took what I thought was the easy way out and fed the doctor a textbook description of bipolar disorder.*
>
> *"They put me on high dose Respiridol® and Depakote.® The drugs severed a part of myself, dumbed me down, cut me off from feeling anything real. I couldn't function. I couldn't stay awake in class, and would wake up with drool all over my desk.*
>
> *"The only thing I was aware of then was the weight gain. I didn't know what the drugs were doing til after I was off them. If I had known, I would have fought it tooth and nail.*
>
> *"I was on the drugs for a year, til I weaned myself off. Now [4 years later] I am not as intelligent as I once was. I'm just a little bit slower to learn stuff. I don't read as fast, and I take just a little longer to understand what I read."*
>
> Michael, speaking of his experiences in the foster care system.

Potential benefits of early, individually-tailored nutritional therapy (PFEIFFER, 1987, HOFFER 1983B, COTT 1974, WALSH 2007)

- ☐ Opportunity to give early attention to biotype, MT imbalance, excitotoxicity, oxidative stress, hypoglycemia, and other accompanying or underlying disorders, increasing the likelihood of a more rapid and complete response.
- ☐ Decreased neuronal or other damage.
- ☐ Delayed onset of mania, or reduced number of manias, thereby slowing progression of the illness.
- ☐ Reduced risk of suicide.
- ☐ Greater ability to be vigilant about drugs which can worsen the disorder (e.g., street drugs, antidepressants, hyperactivity meds, antipsychotics).
- ☐ Less isolation. More normal psychosocial development.

"I knew from a very young age that there was something very wrong with me, but I thought it was just that I was not a good person, that I didnt try hard enough... [Starting with my first manic episode in late teens] I rode a wild roller coaster, from agitated, out-of-control heights to disabling, often suicidal lows,"

Patty Duke, in *A Brilliant Madness*,1992

Patty Duke's father was alcoholic and left when she was six. Her mother suffered major depression interspersed with explosive rage. At age 12, when Patty became a star, she was moved into the home of John and Ethel Ross, managers of child actors, who trained her rigorously. They were also heavy drinkers and eventually fed her alcohol and drugs (Thorazine,® phenobarbitol, Percodan,® and prevented her from seeing her mother, except on rare occasions. She had no friends.

Bedwetting

Pfeiffer (1987, 88) recommends niacin, B6, B complex, magnesium, vitamin E, and treatment for allergies. If this is insufficient, he suggests trying DMAE, vitamins A, B3, C, E, zinc, and manganese. Krohn (1991) finds allergies are frequently implicated, with dairy being the most frequent offender, followed by wheat, corn, egg, orange and chocolate.

Brain tissue repair (Rimland 1974, Hoffer 1983, Green 1970, Cott 1974, Gross 2000, Ivy 1993)

Brain damage (accidents, abuse, difficult deliveries, etc.) or a viral illness (Rimland) which causes brain tissue destruction might underly childhood mood symptom, in some cases, making treatment more difficult.

See *Natural approaches*, p. 245.

Therapeutic possibilities (Hoffer 1983, Rimland 1974, Green 1970, Cott 1974, Pfeiffer 1988, Fredericks 1976, Kracke 1982, Larson 1992, Reninger 1980)

Most nutrient therapies listed for adults can be used if tailored to the child's individual biochemical requirements. Doses usually must be lower, reflecting age, body weight or other concerns. Be especially careful with vitamin A. Also with herbs and aminos, many of which have not been well studied for use by children. Molybdenum is indicated only if definitely needed (check sulfite, copper, etc.), since it can inhibit growth. Consider, as relevant:

- □ **Biotype-appropriate treatment** (methylation imbalances, pyrrole disorder, metal metabolism disorder). (See pp. 145-73.)
- □ **Further mood-stabilizing nutrient therapies.**

Note: Pfeiffer advises parents to be firm enough to ensure that children take their nutrient supplements regularly.

Some key nutrients targeting mood in children (See above references and those on pp. 28-44.)

Doses are average quantities used by Hoffer, Green, Cott, or Pfeiffer. Smaller or younger children are prescribed lower doses, as appropriate. Nutrient choices and doses do not apply to all children, and must be tailored to address individual biochemical requirements.

- □ **B6** — often crucial for children and more important than B3. [100-500+ mg, *as relevant.*]
- □ **Magnesium** — key mood stabilizer. Also used for irritability, bedwetting, and sound sensitivity. Often benefits children reacting unfavorably to B6 alone, which can remove magnesium from the body. Indicated for all biotypes. (Walsh 2007) (pp. 25-28)
- □ **B3** — Improves brain respiration, metabolism, general functioning. Counters depression, anxiety, psychosis. [Non-flush, 500-1000 mg., 2-3x/day.] *Introduce gradually. Can cause flushing.*
- □ **Zinc** — helps moderate mood. Depleted with growth spurts. Benefits metal metabolism. May improve dairy sensitivity. Usually helpful for all biotypes. Critical if taking taurine (but at a separate time). (Walsh 2007) (pp. 29-31)
- □ **C** — anti-anxiety, mood-stabilizing, anti-psychotic; may increase social awareness and interaction. *Take at least twice per day.*
- □ **B1** — often helpful for insomnia, irritability, anxiety, mood stability.
- □ **B2** — supports brain metabolism and is often antidepressant.
- □ **B5** — supports adrenal function and resistance to stress (and may increase approachability).
- □ **B complex** — especially critical for children to support nervous system functioning; tends to be depleted in bipolars. *Often contraindicated in histadelia due to folate content.* (pp. 58-72)
- □ **Folic acid** (*usually contraindicated for histadelia*) & **B12** — critical to neural viability, generally antidepressant.

Lab (Gold 1987, Goldstein 1999, Green 1970, Cott 1974, Pfeiffer 1987, 88)

Family history of mood disorder or related conditions. Check for primary family or social stressors (abuse, neglect, etc.). (Gold 1987, Green 1970)

Blood, urinary, and hair nutritional analysis.

Biotype tests: Basophil count, blood histamine, methylation imbalance, urinary pyrrole.

Learning, behavior, and neurological disorders.

Metal metabolism status and metal toxicity. Hair minerals and heavy metals. Electrolyte levels.

Candida, allergies, sugar balances, malabsorption.

Thyroid, adrenal, sexual and other hormones.

Reactions to street drugs or meds (tranquilizers, sedatives, diuretics, reducing pills, amphetamines, antidepressants, hyperactivity meds), (Marano 2005) and caffeine or tobacco. (Gold 1987, Goldstein 1999)

Vision (difference in refractive power between eyes; problems with focus, convergence, binocular vision, etc.), and hearing tests. (Cott 1974)

CBC. Kidney and liver function, blood pressure, pulse, EKG, and other physical health assessments. Check for infections, autoimmune illness, cancers, anemia, other cardiovascular conditions, etc. (Gold 1987)

□ **Essential fatty acids** — support mood (especially depression); often, psychosis; and some cases of hyperactivity. *Histamine (i.e., methylation) disorder biotypes tend to do best with omega 3; moderate-to-severe pyrolurics, with a focus on GLA. If children won't take supplements, LNA or GLA can be rubbed into the skin.* (WEINTRAUB 1995) (pp. 85-94)
□ **E, bioflavonoids, selenium, other antioxidants.** (pp. 73-83)
□ **GABA, taurine, glycine, tryptophan** — calming, mood-stabilizing, anti-insomniac. *Tailor to biotype and other requirements.* (pp. 34-46)
□ **Dimethyl glycine** — may foster speech in nonverbal children. *Contraindicated in histapenia.* (KUN 1990, RIMLAND 1990, 96AB)
□ **Lecithin** — may help calm hyperactivity and mania, *but not necessarily if histadelic.* (pp. 48-51)
□ **Iron** — *only if clearly indicated* (and especially if depletion is compromising catecholamine formation, and causing depression or learning problems). (pp. 135-36)

Diet & exercise (HOFFER 1983, COTT 1969, 74, PFEIFFER 1988, WEINTRAUB 1995, PHILPOTT 1977, RENINGER 1980)

Optimize diet to individual requirements. Avoid junk food (e.g., sugar, white flour, sodas, etc.), additives (e.g., food coloring), allergens, caffeine. The diet should revolve around natural whole foods (organic, if possible), with plenty of fresh raw vegetables and fruits, unrefined slow-release carbohydrates (beans, veggies), and enough healthy proteins and fats.

Exercise (ideally, in a relatively unpolluted environment) can often provide that critical boost which leads to improvement. (PFEIFFER 1988)

Hypoglycemia (HOFFER 1983, COTT 1969, 74, PFEIFFER 1988, RAPP 1991, PHILPOTT 1977)

Hypoglycemia is often caused or aggravated by low chromium (which is vital to insulin and pancreatic action). B3 and zinc are also important. Therapy often includes eating 5-6 small nutrient-dense meals per day, with an emphasis on complex carbs and sufficient protein. Avoid sugar and junk food, alcohol, caffeine, allergens, tobacco. (pp. 214-18)

Allergies (RAPP 1991, VON HILDHEIMER 1974, WEINTRAUB 1995, PHILPOTT 1977, KROHN 1991, CLARKE 1950, BAKER 1996)

Allergens which often cause nervous system reactions in children include: wheat, dairy, corn, soy, peanuts, tomatoes, eggs, sugar, food coloring and other additives, pesticide residues, and various environmental substances. Some children react to fluorescent lights, or cathode ray TVs or computer screens (see p. 273).

Children often seem to outgrow allergies, but if exposure is resumed, a different set of reactions, less readily associated with the allergen, may emerge, e.g., depression, confusion, fatigue, irritability, anger, hyperactivity, moodswing, or psychosis. (PHILPOTT 1977)

Important natural approaches include: avoidance, rotation diet, supportive nutritients (C, bioflavonoids, zinc, B6, etc.), stress reduction, deneutralization, and relevant biotype therapies. (pp. 207-13, 271, 145-68)

Neurotoxicity (GOLD 1987, GOLDSTEIN 1999)

Children are particularly sensitive to drugs, excitotoxins, pesticides, heavy metals, and other toxins. (See pp. 169-96)

Limit or, ideally, end exposure. Check for MT disorders and toxic levels of metals. (Elevated lead, copper or sodium, with low zinc and potassium can be relatively common in underactive children. Lead may be associated with learning disorders, histadelia, or delinquency.) Attend to oxidative stress issues. (PFEIFFER 1987, 88, WALSH 2004AB, 2006) (pp. 73-83)

Illness (GOLD 1987, GOLDSTEIN 1999)

Redress thyroid, adrenal, other endocrine imbalance; malabsorption, Candida, epilepsy, infections, anemia, other cardiovascular disorders, etc. (pp. 197-250)

Repercussions of early stressors on mood (KIDD 2004)

Infant and childhood stressors may contribute to the development of bipolar disorder and/or may worsen outcome. Thus:*

□ Significant maternal stress during pregnancy can later manifest as behavior abnormalites, affective disorder, or schizophrenia. (RUSH 2003, EDWARDS 2002)

□ Obstetric complications, may also be tied to mood disorder, often early-onset and severe. (VAN OS 1997)

□ Childhood or adolescent physical or sexual abuse is associated with earlier bipolar onset,** more rapid cycling, shorter inter-episode breaks, more episodes, greater intensity of symptoms, and increased suicide attempts. (KIDD 2004, POST 2001)

* Edwards (2002) suggests overstimulated corticosteroid production may then inhibit neural formation and distort developing brain circuitry (perhaps via imbalances in growth factors, enzymes and pathways which mediate maturation and plasticity (Zing)), setting the stage for later mood disorder. (Post 2002)

** Which is associated with increased risk of substance abuse, comorbid illness, social and work difficulties, and neurophysiological dysfunction.

Psychosocial support (CABF 2002AB)

Regular counseling.
Cognitive, interpersonal, and family-focused psychotherapies.
Multi-family support groups.
Cooperation among teachers, parents and child to meet special needs.
Parent education on child relaxation techniques. Limit stress, arguments, etc.
Modify sound and light to support waking, relaxing or sleeping.
Encourage creativity.
Secure weapons, meds, etc.

Warning signs of suicide (GOLD 1987)

Threat of suicide. (At least 80% of children who threaten suicide try it.)
Preliminary stages of recovery from depression (when energy increases enough to fuel impulsivity).
Use of controlled substances. (40% of teens who use drugs or alcohol attempt suicide.)
Poor relationship with parents (reported in 90% of suicidal teens), abuse, neglect.
Other losses.
Health problems.
Adverse reactions to medication.
Family history of mood disorder.

Attention deficit & hyperactivity disorders (ADD & ADHD)

An overwhelming majority of bipolars may have comorbid attention deficit and/or hyperactivity; Wozniak (1997, 2001) claims such disorders occur in up to 90% of bipolars.

"The environment is a key determinant of children's health... Until we learn more... pollutants have to be treated as guilty until proven innocent."

Sandra Schwartz, Director, Environmental Programs, Canadian Institute of Child Health

A recent CICH profile suggests the large increase in childhood hyperactivity, learning and behavior problems may, in part, be due to chronic, low-level exposure to lead, mercury and industrial chemicals, which can reduce intelligence and slow fetal CNS development. They warn that environmental standards based on adults, can fail to reflect child vulnerability.

Hyperactivity vs. bipolar disorder

Similarities — both ADHD and bipolar disorder involve problems with impulsivity and attention. (Ketter 2001) Hyperactivity and distractibility can look like the racing thoughts and motor activation of the bipolar. (Brigham 2001)

ADHD — usually has childhood onset and involves continual problems with inattention and impulsivity. Attention is fleeting and racing, or absent. Sleep problems are ongoing, particularly difficulty getting to sleep. (Brigham 2001)

Bipolar disorder — usually emerges in adolescence or later, and involves episodic states. Bipolars can focus acutely, though attention may shift. (Ketter 2001, Brigham 2001) Bipolar hyperactivity is more goal-directed. (Brigham 2001) Sleep patterns are episodic, and typically involve phase reversal (i.e. staying up all night). (Brigham 2001)

Family history — may help diffentiate bipolar from AHDH, though, in many cases, both are found, and many bipolars, as children, were diagnosed with AHDH. (Ketter 2001)

The importance of distinguishing bipolar disorder — Ritalin®, a behavioral sensitizer, and other stimulants used for ADHD, often worsen bipolar disorder. (Brigham 2001) A large number of nonresponsive bipolars have, as children, been treated with such stimulants. (Frye 2000)

Therapeutic possibilities (Pfeiffer 1987, Cott 1974)

Choices must be tailored to individual biochemical requirements.

- ☐ Treat any methylation imbalance or pyroluria. (Walsh 2002, 06)
- ☐ Address metal metabolism dysfunction. Overloads often occur in copper, lead, mercury, or cadmium, etc. (Marlowe 1986, Thompson 1989, Walsh 2004ab)
- ☐ Provide mood-stabilizing nutrients (zinc, magnesium, B6, other B vitamins, C, choline, etc. *as relevant*). (Pfeiffer 1987)
- ☐ Supply depleted minerals. Zinc, calcium, or iron tend to be low. (Kozielec 1992) *Consider absorption issues and contraindications.*
- ☐ Optimize long-chain omega 3 (as in fish) (the means to convert shorter chain fats may be compromised; omega 6 often worsens this situation by using up desaturase enzymes). (Burgess 2000) *Take with antioxidants and B vitamins. Omega 3 is preferentially required with histamine imbalance patients; generally, GLA with significant pyrrole disorder.*
- ☐ Remit specific nutrient deficiencies or dependencies. A multiple may help address malnutrition, *but consider whether it will interfere with absorption and use of specific required nutrients, as well as biotype and other contraindications.*
- ☐ Optimize diet (Generally, plenty of fresh vegetables; and freshly-prepared beans, whole grains, soups, fish. Moderate intake of whole fruits, seeds, nuts, and good quality dairy, meat and/or poultry. *Tailor to individual requirements and contraindications.* Eliminate refined carbohydrates, detrimental fats.) (Tsang 2007)
- ☐ Reduce stressors. Support adaptive response to stress. Support adrenals (cortisol interferes with learning ability and memory).
- ☐ Look for abuse issues, and treat.

Address any:

- ☐ Sugar imbalance, malabsorption, Candida — these are common.
- ☐ Oxidative stress.* (Walsh 2007)
- ☐ Excitotoxic or other toxic exposure. (Blaylock 1995)
- ☐ Thyroid or other endocrine dysfunction.
- ☐ Other health conditions, *as relevant.*

* A full range of antioxidants is usually indicated, e.g., glutathione, E, selenium, C, bioflavonoids, grape seed extract (Tsang 2007), carotenes, A, etc.) Check for MT dysfunction, excitotoxicity and other sources of oxidative stress. (Walsh 2007)

Allergies, sensitivities

Check for allergies to gluten, dairy, soy, corn, yeast, citrus, eggs, chocolate, peanuts, etc. Reactions to salicylates or food additives are common. Ben Feingold, MD, found almost 50% of hyperactive children were sensitive to artificial flavors, colors and preservatives;* and that reactions to salicylates were also frequent.** Aspirin, apples, peaches, other rose family fruits, raspberries, and certain other foods contain salicylates. Test foods separately, as some may provoke a reaction, while others do not. (Egger 1985, Hershey 1996, Feingold 1975)

Sensitivity to fluorescent lights and ionizing radiation may also contribute to hyperactivity. (*See box, next page.*)

* Note: A 1989 National Academy of Science study reports that 73% of all food additives have never been tested for neurobehavioral effects in humans.

** Note: People with southern European ancestry are more prone to react to salicylates.

Choline & DMAE (Pfeiffer 1987, 88)

Choline or DMAE may improve learning ability and behavior. DMAE,* a precursor of acetylcholine, crosses the blood brain barrier more readily. Researchers have successfully used DMAE as a substitute for Ritalin® in many hyperactives. It has also been used for other learning disorders and certain depressions.

Adverse effects on mood: In many bipolars, *especially in histadelia,* choline may trigger depression. Occasionally, and especially as DMAE, choline can overstimulate, leading to mania.

* Commercial DMAE (dimethylaminoethanol) is usually mixed with B5 and small amounts of manganese to enhance acetylation to acetylcholine.

Other proposals

Warning: The following choices, though considerably less stimulating than hyperactivity meds, still carry some potential to contribute to mania. If indicated, keep dose modest and monitor.

□ Blue green algae —Preliminary research suggests possible benefit to some cases of hyperactivity, autism, Candida, blood sugar imbalances, and allergies. One study reports improved mental outlook and attention in school children. (Sevilla 1995) *Further research is needed. Biotype uses and contraindications have yet to be evaluated. May trigger mania.*

□ Alternatives to coffee, etc. — Hyperactives often self-medicate with coffee, chocolate candy, or other stimulants (probably unconsciously searching for Ritalin®-like effects). If so, milder alternatives like green tea or, possibly, cacao nibs, may be preferable for some.

See *Green tea,* and *Cacao,* p. 143.

Recommended Reading

Crook, William, MD, *Solving the Puzzle of Your Hard to Raise Child.64*

Rapp, Doris, MD, *Is this your child?* 1991

Rogers Sherry, MD, *Depression Cured at Last,* 1997.

von Hildheimer, George, *Allergy, Toxins, and the Learning-Disabled Child.,* 1974

Hershey, Jane, MA, *Why Can't My Child Behave,* 1996.

Reminder: This information is presented for educational purposes only. If a child needs treatment for mood disorder, hyperactivity, autism, or any other medical condition, please seek the services of a knowledgeable physician.

Fluorescent lights (Ott 1973, Gaby 2000)

Cool-white fluorescents have been associated with hyperactivity in children. Such lighting is deficient in the red and blue-violet range of the spectrum, exactly where sunlight is strongest. (Ott 1973)

In one experiment, Dr John Ott, 1973 installed full spectrum fluorescents in two of four first grade classrooms in Sarasota Florida; leaving the remaining rooms with cool white fluorescents. Within one month, behavior, performance, and academic achievement in the full-spectrum rooms improved markedly. Several extremely hyperactive, learning-disabled children calmed down and apparently overcame some learning and reading problems. In contrast, symptomatic children in other rooms did not improve.

Cathode ray TV & computer screens (Gaby 2000)

Older TVs and computer screens (cathode ray screens) emit ionizing radiation. Exposure has been associated with hyperactivity. In one study, rats placed fifteen feet from a TV screen blocked by cardboard became hyperactive and aggressive; with a lead shield, behavior normalized.

Cell phones

Cognitive and neural effects due the close proximity of cell phone radiation to the brain have not been fully explored. At least one study suggests pre and postnatal exposure may be associated with emotional and hyperactivity problems when entering school.*(Divan 2008)

Limiting the length and frequency of calls, lengthening the distance from the head (with speaker phones) and from the fetus, and restricting use in rural areas (distant from cell phone towers) offers some protection. The safest choice, of course, is to not to use them at all.

* Moreover, some preliminary research suggests greater incidence of brain tumors, increasing with extent of use, (Hardell 2007, Hours 2007) and more likely on the side of the head where the phone is held. (Hardell 2007) Given the sparcity of extensive cell phone use until relatively recently, combined with the long latency for cancer to develop (5-45 years), one might suspect a rising incidence over the next few decades.

Autism

"My mind knows... kindness will not kill me, yet my [emotions say] good feelings and gentle and loving touch can kill me or... cause me pain. When I try to ignore this message, I go into what would seem to be a state of shock, where what's coming in is either incomprehensible or has no significance. This state leads to my emotions committing suicide, leaving me without physical or emotional feeling and with a purely robotic mental response - if that...

"If I concentrated too hard, nothing would... sink in... I would drift off... Anything I tried to learn, unless it was something I sought and taught myself, closed me out and became hard to comprehend, just like any other intrusion from 'the world.' Sometimes people would have to repeat a particular sentence several times for me, as I would hear it in bits, and the way in which my mind had segmented their sentence into words left me with a strange and sometimes unintelligible message... like when someone plays around with the volume switch on the TV."

Donna Williams, 1992

Assorted nutrient proposals

- ☐ B6 & magnesium — 22 autism studies, including 13 double-blinds suggest benefit for a large percentage of autistics within days to several months. (RIMLAND 1978, 88, 96BC, PFEIFFER 1988, BARTHELEMY 1981, LELORD 1981, ELLMAN 1981, JONAS 1984).
- ☐ Zinc, B3, calcium; (RIMLAND 1988, 96, PFEIFFER 1988) perhaps B5, B complex;*(RIMLAND 1996BC, COTT 1974) possibly manganese and molybdenum.**(PFEIFFER 1988)
- ☐ Dimethyl glycine*** — may help stimulate speech and communication. (RIMLAND 1990, 96AB, KUN 1989)
- ☐ Vitamin A — suggested by Megson (2000) to reconnect retinoid receptor and G alpha proteins.
- ☐ Cutler suggests attention to toxic metals, particularly mercury. (See pp. 170-82; and Cutler 1999 and 2004.)
- ☐ Kane has proposed electrolyte solution, digestive enzymes, oxidant nutrients, and EFAs, *as relevant.*

* Not usually a good choice if overmethylated.

** Which would help address the copper elevation.

*** Though Rimland (1996a) finds it sometimes fosters hyperactivity [perhaps mainly in the few who are histapenic], in which case he suggests adding folic acid.

Autism is characterized by preoccupation with certain objects, repetitive mannerisms, fear of environmental change, and poor communication skills (problems learning to talk, and with concepts of "I," "no," and "yes;" speech often becomes high-pitched and singsong speech). Also, difficulty with emotional interactions, resistance to touch, social withdrawal, detachment, and focus on a private, self-sufficient world. (GERLACH 1992, WILLIAMS 1992) Mental retardation, vision or hearing problems, and epilepsy are common. 10% are savants, highly gifted in a particular field (e.g., music). (TORREY 1988, GERLACH 1992)

Previous estimates of frequency were close to 0.1%, but now cluster at 1 in 150 children in the US and perhaps elsewhere. (MEGSON 2000) Autism, Aspergers, or other neurodevelopmental disorders may now occur in one of six children entering school in the US. (NIH 2006)

Significance of oxidative stress

Dr. William Walsh, PhD, of Walsh Research Institute, suggests that though symptoms that look like mild autism are more prevalent in bipolars, especially males, the etiologies are distinct. Further, that autism, a developmental disorder, is not in the same spectrum as any of the other disorders described in this book. Thus, in analyzing 28,000 chemical assays on 396 brain samples of autistics and controls, Walsh (2008) has come to suspect that autism is a response to an inherited oxidative stress weakness, usually with *both** metal metabolism** and methylation*** compromised. The low metallothionein would retard brain cell development over the first three years of life. Hypodevelopment, along with the ongoing oxidative stress, probably underly the suppressed formation of dendrites and synapses seen in autistics, causing significant loss of IQ over time. (WALSH 2008)

* Thus, autistics tend to be both histadelic, and high in copper, which is unusual.

** Metallothionein is a strong antioxidant. Unregulated divalent metals form profuse free radicals.

*** Over 90% show some degree of undermethylation. The oxidative stress makes glutathione unavailable for joining B12 to methyl, a critical step in forming methionine.

Therapies

(RIMLAND 1974, 78, 88, 90, 96ABC, HOFFER 1983B, COTT 1974, PFEIFFER 1988, GERLACH 1993, HEELEY 1966, BARTHELEMY 1981, LELORD 1981, ELLMAN1981, JONAS 1984, KUN 1989, 5BAKER 1996, 97, DUKER 1996, MCDOUBLE 1996, KAPLIN 1996, SHULMAN 1994, LOVAAS 1987, MCEACHIN 1993, HARRIS 1991)

☐ **Education & training** — Intensive early behavioral intervention, emphasizing positive reinforcement provides great benefit. (RIMLAND 1996C, LOVAAS 1987, MCEACHIN 1993, HARRIS 1991) Education should be firmly structured, purposeful, and concrete. Sensory and Auditory Integration Training is often helpful. (RIMLAND 1996BC) Massage can be tailored to support implicated brain regions (brainstem, cerebellum, limbic, etc. (COURCHESNE 1997)). (BARANEK 2002) Corrective lenses may improve visual orientation. (RIMLAND 1988, SHULMAN 1994)

☐ **Reduce oxidative stress** — Walsh finds the following approaches tend to be highly effective: (WALSH 2004AB, 06, 07, 08)

— Supply a generous and wide variety of indicated antioxidants. (RIMLAND 1988, 96, PFEIFFER 1988) Avoid excitotoxins. (pp. 173-83; 191-93)

— Treat any metallothionein dysfunction (typically poorly regulated copper/zinc). (pp. 170-73.)

— Address methylation imbalance (over 90% are undermethylated) e.g., with SAMe, glutathione, methyl B12, magnesium, etc. (pp 155-61)

— Correct mitochondrial dysfunction (consider carnitine, etc.), and other causes, *as relevant.* (WALSH 2007) (pp. 115-17)

☐ **Address any gluten or dairy sensitivity** — Restrict/avoid; (ISRANGKUN 1986, SHATTOCK 1990, REICHELT 1991, KNIVSBERG 1991) consider need for zinc, MT support, etc. (WALSH 2007)

☐ **Optimize diet** — Avoid junk food, and allergens; also, MSG, Aspartame,® other food additives. (PFEIFFER 1988, RIMLAND 1996C, BAKER 1996, KANE)

- □ **Health** —Address Candida, hypoglycemia or other co-occuring illness. (PFEIFFER 1988, RIMLAND 1996C)
- □ **Meds** — The late Dr. Bernard Rimland, PhD, and founder of Autism Research Institute, contended that autism meds were often detrimental, and usually should be gradually withdrawn, corresponding to improvement with nutritive treatment. (RIMLAND 1996B)

This information is for educational purposes only. Contraindications are not included. With autism, or any medical condition, consult a knowledgeable physician who will tailor treatment to individual biochemical requirements.

RECOMMENDED READING

WIlliams, Donna, *Nobody Nowhere,* 1992, & *Somebody Somewhere.*

Baker, Sidney, M., M.D., & Pangborn, John, Ph.D., *Defeat Autism Now! Clinical Options Manual for Physicians,* 1997

Autism Research Review International. www.autism.com

Various hypotheses

Note that most of these fit into the context of a genetic oxidative-stress etiology.

Metal metabolism dysfunction (WALSH 2001AB, 2008, YAO 2006)

Pfeiffer first noted metal toxicity, especially lead, or lead in combination with copper, aluminum or cadmium, was common. Walsh reports that computer analysis of a 503 patient database has since revealed that, with only 4 exceptions, all autistics showed severe metallothionein (MT) dysfunction (pp. 171-73), much more pronounced than in behavior disorders or histapenic schizophrenia. Dr. Walsh points out that infants born with such a defect would be subject to improper neuronal development, fewer connections, and poor gut maturation. Oxidative stress could be severe; sensitivity to toxic metals, extreme; detox, difficult. The child might initially seem healthy, but vaccines,* toxic metals, illness, or other insult, overwhelming MTs and gut capacity, would allow autism to surface.

* Thus, numerous studies (recently estimated to reflect 15% of cases) report on children who develop normally til given childhood vaccinations (especially DPT, notorious for its mercury content), after which they begin to show signs of autism. (The US is reportedly phasing out the mercury in certain vaccines.) Mercury may be only in the high range of normal, but sensitivity is heightened.

Early excitotoxic exposures

Blaylock suggests exposure of the fetus or infant (through the maternal diet, or other sources) to MSG or Aspartame® (a sweetener used in some sodas, chewing gums, baby foods, etc.), flood the brain with glutamate or aspartate respectively. These neurotransmitters are critical in guiding neuronal migration and development. (BLAYLOCK 1995) Unnatural excess may so disorganize brain structure as to promote future autism, learning and behavior disorders, etc. (KLINGERG 1987, BODNAR 1980, OLNEY 1989, BLAYLOCK 1995) Large doses of MSG can damage all brain structures in animals and infants. (BLAYLOCK 1995, SHIMICU 1973, OLNEY 1978)

Gluten & dairy sensitivity (ISRANGKUN 1986, SHATTOCK 1990, REICHELT 1981, 90, 91, KNIVSBERG 1991)

Dr Reichelt initially found autism often characterized by elevated urinary peptides. Later studies pointed to combinations of increased platelet serotonin; elevated spinal fluid HVA (DA metabolite) and opioids; and excess urinary peptides and opioids. (REICHELT 1981, 91, ISRANGKUN 1986, SHATTOCK 1990)

With dairy and gluten-free diets* (avoiding milk, cheese, wheat, rye, barley, etc.) and other restrictions, Reichelt saw considerable improvement** (especially in perception, cognition and social interactions) in 90% who initially showed urinary signs. (REICHELT 1990) Seizures often decreased markedly. Improvement reversed if gluten or dairy was reintroduced.

Note: Walsh (2006) suggests dairy sensitivities can be due to the prevalent MT dysfunction, which depletes the zinc needed by gut enzymes that metabolize casein. MT treatment may thus allow the patient to handle some dairy.

* Reichelt found restricting both to be most effective. He proposed that this could be due to the marked similarity of the opioids formed in digesting both dairy and gluten. (Reichelt 1990, 91, Knivsberg 1991)

** Though, slight worsening sometimes occured in weeks 3 through 12.

Ammonia

Patricia Kane, PhD, finds autistics tend to accumulate ammonia (fogging mental function), and often show imbalanced electrolytes, fatty acid deficiencies, low oxidative tone, digestive difficulties, and gluten, dairy, and excitotoxin sensitivity. She suggests symptoms developing after infants are vaccinated with NMR or DPT may be due to interference with myelin formation.

Increased vitamin A requirements

Megson (2000) proposes that the pertussis in the DPT vaccine may cause autism when it separates brain retinoid receptors from G-alpha proteins. These receptors are critical to sensory perception, language processing, and attention (all compromised in autistics). Family histories of autistics often include a parent with a G-alpha protein defect (night blindness, pseudohypoparathyroidism, or pituitary or thyroid adenoma). Megson notes vitamin A reconnects the receptor and may help heal autism.

Other hypotheses

Dr Hugh Fudenberg, immunologist, (2001) suggests a decrease in liver enzymes, due to DPT and other vaccines, may allow undigested protein to more readily enter the bloodstream. Increased antigen-antibody complexes may then foster autism and other brain dysfunction.

Other proposed etiologies have included episodes of bleeding during pregnancy, phenylketonuria, fragile X syndrome, and viral encephalitis. (TORREY 1988)

3. Elderly concerns

Hemingway (FIEVE 1976, HEMINGWAY 1976, DONALDSON 1977)

Hemingway's life careened from violent elations (replete with rages, physical fights, hunting, car and plane crashes, feverish writing, little sleep, heavy drinking, and a sense of immortality and heroism) to deep self-doubt and depression. (FIEVE 1976)

As he aged, traumatic events, physical illness, and adverse reactions to treatment fueled depression and paranoia.

By his early sixties, his wife had died, his family had suffered financial disasters, and politics had forced him to leave his home in Cuba.

He was diabetic, his liver was deteriorating (perhaps allowing estrogen buildup), and he may have had hemochromatosis (see p. 135). He was on large doses of reserpine (see p. 50), an anti-psychotic, for high blood pressure. Side effects can include sexual dysfunction, depression (even months after the drug is stopped), and (via dopamine suppression) a dulling of inspiration, creativity, will, and *joie-de-vivre*. (HEMINGWAY 1976)

Hemingway greyed rapidly, lost both weight and zest for life, and lived in constant dread of becoming blind or impotent.

He blamed himself for his wife's death, and grew increasingly irritable and paranoid. He feared the FBI was pursuing him for tax evasion. He let no one drive his car, locked his bureau and clothes closet, and barracaded himself in his office.

His son says, "My father was never feeble in any way in his youth, either intellectually or physically, and when he became so, he refused to accept it." (HEMINGWAY 1976)

Hemingway was eventually given three courses of electric shocks. He complained of not being able to write: "What is the sense of ruining my head and erasing my memory... It was a brilliant cure, but we lost the patient."

Bipolar disorder in the elderly

As bipolars age, manic episodes usually decrease and depression predominates. Elderly onset of bipolar disorder is relatively uncommon. (GOLD 1987) If late-onset mania occurs, it's often associated with neurological* disorders. (SHULMAN 1997AB)

On the other hand, depression occurs at four times, suicide at fifteen times, the rate of the general population. 90% of suicides are completed. Attend immediately to warning signs. (GOLD 1987)

* Usually, disinhibition syndromes involving right frontal/limbic connections. (Shulman 1997)

Lab

Check heredity, family history of related disorders, biotype balances, relevant nutrients, diet, physical health. (GOLD 1987)

Gold's list of confounding factors (GOLD 1987)

Symptoms in the elderly are frequently caused or exacerbated by physical and psychosocial factors. On the other hand, mood symptoms often mask physical illness, and delay diagnosis. Look for and address the following:

- ☐ Neurological deterioration with age (dementias, strokes, etc.) Organic brain syndrome. Lesions involving frontal and limbic regions.
- ☐ Pharmaceutical interactions (polypharmacy is common) or side effects. (Adverse reactions in people over 70 are twice those in people under 50.) Educate, and reduce intake, where possible.
- ☐ Reactions to alcohol, caffeine, MSG, etc. (Again, sensitivity increases with age.)
- ☐ Hormone imbalance — thyroid disorders, diabetes, and hypoglycemia are prevalent and can profoundly alter mood. Symptoms are often denied. Laboratory hormone assessments are less indicative of actual status.*
- ☐ Other physical illness — blood pressure disorders, dizziness, emphysema, urinary or gastrointestinal disorders, dementias, brain and pancreatic cancers, rheumatoid arthritis, cardiovascular illness, etc.
- ☐ Psychosocial factors — can profoundly alter mood in the elderly.

* E.g., nonresponsive TSH, even with low thyroid, is common.

Natural therapies have included attention to (KIDD 2006, WALSH 2007)

- ☐ Biotype issues. (See pp. 145-68.)
- ☐ MT imbalance. (See pp. 170-83.) Other toxicity (pp. 184-96).
- ☐ Oxidative stress — see *Antioxidants* (pp. 73-83), *Excitotoxins* (pp. 191-93), *Metal metabolism* (pp. 170-83), and *Homocysteine* (pp. 157, 167).
- ☐ Compromised mitochondrial energy production — see *CoQ10, NADH, Acetl-L carnitine*, etc. (pp. 115-17).
- ☐ Exercise and oxygenation (pp. 257-58).
- ☐ Receptor and membrane viability — see *Glycocerophosphocholine* (GPC) (pp. 48-49), *Phosphatidyl serine* (p. 98), *Phosphatidyl inositol* (pp. 95-97), *EFAs* (pp. 85-94), etc.
- ☐ Allergy, & blood sugar (pp. 207-22).
- ☐ Nutritional depletion (poor diet (pp. 254-56), gut issues (pp. 199-206)).
- ☐ Low thyroid (pp. 225-37).
- ☐ Other health factors (pp. 244-50).
- ☐ Psychosocial support (pp. 252-53).
- ☐ Effects of medications.

Appendix I: Neurotransmission

The human brain is estimated to contain at least 100 billion nerve cells (neurons), each of which may create up to tens of thousands of communication links with other neurons. These vary though life, and together create a vastly intricate and evolving web. (CHANGEAUX 1985)

Basic neural communication mechanisms

Briefly, chemical messengers (neurotransmitters, such as serotonin, or other agonists) are conveyed from branch-like extensions on the sending (presynaptic) nerve cell across a small space (synapse) to a receiving surface (receptor(s)) on the cell membrane of another (postsynaptic) neuron. Second messengers then convey the information through the cell, changing its activity, and perhaps initiating further messages. Thus:

(1) Neurotransmitters interact with receptors of post-synaptic neurons, then return to the synapse or presynaptic cells.

(2) Transmitter/receptor interaction ⟶ second messenger cascade ⟶ a summing of inhibitory & stimulating info.

(3) If sufficiently stimulating ⟶ sodium channels open ⟶ Na/K exchange ⟶ electrical potential conveyed down the axon ⟶ calcium release ⟶ fusing of vesicles with neural membrane ⟶ neurotransmitter release

Neural communication in more detail

Neurotransmitters (NTs) are released from one or more neurons into the synapse and find their way to receptors on the membrane of the postsynaptic neuron(s). Here, neurotransmitters interact with receptors, but do not enter the cell, and return to the synapse, where they are destroyed or taken back into the presynaptic neuron(s), often via various transporters, such as VMATs.*

Second messengers convey receptor information into the body and nucleus of the postsynaptic neuron, causing a number of changes in the cell,** including a summing of various inhibitory and stimulating messages during a very short span of time:

□ *Sufficient inhibition* opens chloride channels into the neural axon, and/or potassium channels leading out, making nerve firing more difficult.

□ *Sufficient stimulation* opens the axon's sodium channels. Sodium and potassium are sequentially exchanged along the axonal membrane, conveying an electrical potential. This triggers a release of calcium, which causes a number of vesicles (sacs filled with neurotransmitter) to fuse with the membrane of small axonal branches extending from the nerve cell. On fusing, their neurotransmitter content spills into the synaptic space and links with specifically matching receptors on postsynaptic neurons, which go through a similar process.

The degree of initial stimulation at the postsynaptic receptor determines the number of electrical impulses generated,*** influencing the quantity of neurotransmitter eventually released, and the intensity of the message.

* VMATs (Vesicular Monoamine Transporters) catalyze transport of monoamines (serotonin, dopamine, norepinephrine and histamine) and storage in the vesicles at the terminal branches of the neuron. They may play a role in mood. Dr Zubieta finds euthymic bipolar males uniquely retain about 30% more VMAT2 in ventral brain stem and thalamus synaptic terminals (and show greater terminal density) than controls. He suggests cumulative overstorage (instead of use) of monoamines may suppress intellect. Overstorage also allows for more to be released when triggered (e.g., on psychostimulant intake), thereby, perhaps producing mania or other overstimulation. (Zubieta 2000, Moyer 2003)

** In gene expression, calcium movement, cyclic nucleotide function, protein and enzyme activity, receptivity, cell memory, etc.

*** But not the strength of each electric impulse, which remains constant.

Chemistry

Precursors, neurotransmitters, & thyroid

Inhibitors	
Glycine	$C_2H_5NO_2$
GABA	$C_4H_9NO_2$
Taurine	$C_2H_7NO_3S$
Acetylcholine	$C_7H_{16}NO_2$
Catecholamines, thyroid,	
Phenylalanine	$C_9H_{11}NO_2$
Tyrosine	$C_9H_{11}NO_3$
Dopamine	$C_8H_{11}NO_2$
Norepinephrine	$C_8H_{11}NO_3$
Epinephrine	$C_9H_{13}NO_3$
Thyroxine (T4)	$C_{15}H_{11}I_4NO_4$
Triiodothyronine (T3)	$C_{15}H_{12}I_3NO_4$
Other biogenic amines	
Histidine	$C_5H_9N_3O_2$
Histamine	$C_5H_9N_3$
Tryptophan	$C_{11}H_{12}N_2O_2$
Serotonin	$C_{10}H_{12}N_2O$
Melatonin	$C_{13}H_{16}N_2O_2$
More stimulating transmitters	
Carnitine	$C_7H_{15}NO_3$
ALCAR	$C_9H_{17}NO_4$
Aspartate	$C_4H_7NO_4$
Glutamate	$C_5H_9NO_4$

Nutrients supporting first messaging: Neurotransmitter precursors & cofactors

Precursor	Cofactors & supportive nutrients	Neurotransmitter
Tryptophan	B6 *(P5P)*, B3, iron, *BH4* (C, B12-folate/SAM balance*). Also, magnesium, zinc, calcium. Supported by D3, B1, complex carbs, chromium, omega 3.	**Serotonin**
Taurine, Glycine	*– These aminos are used directly as transmitters –*	**Taurine, Glycine**
Choline	B5, B6, B1, B3. Manganese supports availability.	**Acetylcholine**
Glutamate, which is the precursor, can be counterproductive, so focus on…	B6 *(P5P)*, zinc, manganese. Niacinamide (stimulates receptors). B (supports use). Inositol (but can overstimulate). C, Mg, taurine, glycine & threonine (enhance effects)	**GABA**
Histidine	B3, C, B6, B12, folic acid, zinc, manganese	**Histamine**

Catecholamine formation

Phenylalanine -----> Tyrosine ---> Dopamine ---> Norepinephrine

This process requires: *BH4* (C, B12-folate/SAM balance*), B6 *(P5P)*, iron, copper *(DBH)*.

Other supportive nutrients may include: B3 (for *NADH*, which stimulates BH4 and dopamine formation), magnesium (which seems to increase dopamine synthesis), D3, and perhaps A (increases the rate-limiting enzyme, tyrosine hydroxylase), B complex (for B1, B2, biotin). Manganese and zinc are largely regulatory.

* i.e., the appropriate folate/methyl balance. (Walsh 2007)

Enzymes which break down neurotransmitters

Enzyme	Supportive nutrients	Breaks down
MAO (monoamine oxidase)	B6, zinc, manganese copper	NE, E, Ser, DA, Glycine, Histamine
COMT (catechol-O-methyltransferase)	B3, C, folic acid, magnesium	Epinephrines

See corresponding chapters for further descriptions and references

Some nutrients influencing receptor & second messenger activity (see corresponding chapters for references)

Nutrient or health measure	Relevance
Essential fatty acids	Critical to receptor function & PI signalling
Full range of antioxidants (E, selenium, glutathione, lipoic acid, C, bioflavonoids, grape seed extract, anthocyanins, A, etc., *as relevant*	Protect membrane & receptor EFAs, NT systems, myelin, neural viability, blood brain barrier brain enzymes, metabolism, energetics.
Phospholipids (includes phosphatidyl choline, which is generally antimanic; phosphatidyl inositol, a key second messenger, generally antidepressant; and p-serine, p-carnitine, p-ethanolamine.	Incorporate EFAs into cell membranes. Protect EFAs. Critical to membrane & receptor function. and structure.
Calcium	Influences inositol cycle & key to NT release.
Magnesium	Helps regulate inositol cycle (via IMPase).
B3, B6 and other B vitamins, *as relevant to biotype.*	Support brain function, metabolism & viability.
Neurotransmitter precursors, cofactors, regulators (*above*)	Transmitter levels modulate receptor sensitivity.
Nutrients supporting methylation, *if relevant.*	Supports activation of NTs and other neurochemicals.
Support for metal metabolism, *if indicated.*	Helps prevent free radical damage to receptors & NT systems; insures mineral availability.
Nutritional support for immune, cardiovascular, respiratory, endocine, gastrointestinal systems, etc.	Suppports brain function by providing fuel, oxygen, energy; removing toxins, allergens, etc.
Sufficient protein, chromium, zinc, B6. Small meals, some complex carbs (focus on vegetables). No refined sugars.	Supports use of glucagon rather than insulin, promoting normal EFA metabolism. (Sears)
Avoid harmful fats.	Prevents displacement/damage to membrane EFAs.
Adequate exercise & stress reduction	Supports blood sugar balance, & EFA metabolism.

Second messenger signalling cascade

agonist/receptor ⟶ G protein ↗ p-inositol cycle ↘ kinases ↗ transcription factors ⟶ gene expression ↘ cell activity (including neurotransmission)
G protein ↘ ATP ⟶ cAMP ↗ kinases ↘ other messenger molecules ↗ cell activity (including neurotransmission)

(1) The neurotransmitter or other agonist interacts with neural membrane receptors, triggering a cascade of chemical reactions which transport information into the cell.

(2) G proteins,* often at the start of the pathway, modulate the incoming message. They activate second messengers, set switches on the membrane and nucleus, (AVISSAR 1989) turn ATP** into cAMP,*** and influence the phophatidylinositol cycle. *(See pp. 95-97)*

(3) cAMP and phophatidylinositols activate kinases (including PKA and PKC).

(4) Kinases activate messenger molecules down the line, including transciption factors which alter gene expression. This regulates cell memory, ion channels, receptor chemicals, and other cell chemistry and activity, including electric potential(s) down the cell axon, which cumulatively provoke neurotransmission to other cells.

* guanine nucleotide binding proteins
** adenosine triphosphate
*** 3′5′ - cyclic adenosine monophosphate, cyclic AMP

Role of second messengers in mood

Originally, researchers suspected neurotransmitter imbalances (e.g., norepinephrine/acetylcholine imbalances) as the primary culprits in bipolar disorder. A substantial body of research now indicts instability in the second messenger system. (SCHREIBER, PEREZ, 1999, 2000) In fact, most effective mood stabilizers influence signal transduction, and inhibit neural calcium mobilization (altering neurotransmitter release). Several either reduce creation of second messengers from membrane phospholipids, or inhibit kinases and G protein activity. (STOLL 1996)

Second messenger activity in bipolars

	MANIA	BOTH	DEPRESSION
G proteins	Overactive		Reduced
cAMP		Markedly disturbed in all bipolars	
Kinases:			
PKA		Elevated in all bipolars	
Rap1		Elevated in all bipolars	
PKC	Elevated		Probably reduced

Specific signalling disturbances in bipolars

G protein signalling — G proteins activate second messengers, and may be overactive in bipolars, (VAWTER 2000, FRIEDMAN 1996, YOUNG 1991) perhaps especially in mania, (AVISSAR 1989, SCHREIBER 1991B) normalizing on recovery. (SCHREIBER 2000)

Inositol cycles — disturbed, perhaps especially the conversion of phosphatidyl inositol to inositol; overactivated (as suggested by elevated PIP2). (SOARES 2001, BROWN 1993) *(See pp 95-97.)*

Adenyl-cyclase/cAMP activity — markedy disturbed. (PEREZ 1999, 2000, SCHREIBER 1991A, SPLEISS 1998, REIACH 1999) Kinases are more sensitive to cAMP in bipolars. (FIELDS 1999)

Protein kinase A (PKA) — elevated in all bipolars (SPLEISS 1998), as well as its substrate, Rap1.

PKC — PKC regulates neurotransmitter release and excitability. Frontal cortex PKC is elevated, (WANG 1996) especially in mania. (MANJI 1999B, SCHREIBER 1991A, WANG 1999, FRIEDMAN 1992, PEREZ 1999)

Calcium ion — Higher baseline (platelet) calcium in manics. Increased Ca2+ is released during both mania and depression, (DUBOVSKY 1989, 92, SOARES 1996) prevented by lithium. (DUBOVSKY 1989).

Pharmaceutical effects on signalling molecules

Moodstabilizing drugs may primarily target second messengers; (HORROBIN 1990) thus:

G proteins — Lithium and other drugs normalize G proteins. (SCHREIBER 1991AB, SPLEISS 1998)

Inositols — Lithium targets conversion of PI to I, and over three weeks, reduces PIP2 in manics. (SOARES 2000)

cAMP — influenced by antidepressants. (KNABLE 1999)

Kinases — Lithium and valproate decrease PKC activation, (MANJI 1999ABC, WANG 1989, FRIEDMAN 1993, WANG 1999, CHEN 1994) and influence kinase systems that may moderate phosphorylation. (MANJI 1999C).

Transcription factors, genes — chronic lithium (LENOX 2000, MANJI 1999ABC) or antidepressants, (KNABLE 1999) alter AP-1 transcription factors, perhaps stabilizing expression of genes involved in abnormal bipolar signaling. (LENOX 2000, PEREZ 2000)

Appendix II: Brain structures influencing mood

Neuroimaging* and other brain studies of bipolars suggest abnormalities in neural paths regulating mood,** (Buchsbaum 1986, Post 1987, Jurjus 1993ab, Strakowski 1993ab, 99: Scherk 2004) **especially** (Haldane 2004) **in the prefrontal and temporal cortex;** (Buchsbaum 1986, Kennedy 1997, Blumberg 2002, Soares 1997, Chang 2004, 2005, Davidson 1999) **in the anterior cingulate,** (Kennedy 1997, Davidson 1999, Blumberg 2002, Chang 2004, 2005, Bruno 2004) **amygdala,** (Davidson 1999, Kennedy 1997, Manj 2000, Shastry 2005 Buchsbaum 1986, Post 1987) **hippocampus,** (Harrison 2002, Rosoklija 2000, Rajkowska 2000) **hypothalamus,** (Scherk 2004, Shastry 2005) **and other limbic structures; and perhaps in the cerebellum and basal ganglia.** (Shastry 2005, Adler 2004, Chang 2005, Baxter 1985)

However, bipolar anatomy has not been definitively mapped as (1) the effect of medication on structure and function is difficult to tease out; (Monkul 2004, Chang 2005) (2) findings are not always specific to bipolars; (Chang 2005) and (3) etiological influences can be difficult to distinguish from results of the illness. (Jurjus 1993ab)

* Neuroimaging methods include: (1) MRI (structural magnetic resonance imaging, previously NMR), which surrounds patients with a cylindrical magnet which aligns hydrogen; pulses of radio waves at specific frequencies then periodically vibrate brain hydrogen protons, from which a computer maps multiple cross sections, which together yield a structural image. (2) fMRI (functional MRI) which maps brain activation (e.g., blood flow, glucose metabolism, neurotransmitter binding) as the patient performs a specific task. (3) MRS (magnetic resonance spectroscopy) which assesses biochemistry via continous radio wave frequencies which excite hydrogen in body compounds, eliciting unique frequencies of radio energy, to which the computer assigns a color. (4) PET (photon or positron emission tomography), which uses a computer to analyze the location of previously injected radioisotopes to form a video of brain biochemistry and circuitry. (Anand 2003, Chang 2005, Monkul 2004)

** These may include (Drevets, Haldane 2004, Nasralleh 1989, Strakowski 1993b): neuropsychological studies (which may suggest regional abnormalities); postmortem studies (which can measure volume of brain structures, and relative neural or glial concentrations); (Chang 2005) neuroendocrine studies; genetic analyses of subgroups; (Scherk 2004) and analysis of brain-injured patients who develop affective symptoms. (Starksen 1988)

Significant PFC regions in bipolar disorder

Dorsolateral PFC (back of sides) — *Involved in attention, working memory, sequencing of information, problem-solving, organizing and executing plans.* (Malhi 2004, Mayberg 1997, Chang 2005) Imaging suggests generally reduced activity, (Yurgelun 2000) and a role in the development of bipolar disorder. (Chang 2004, Pang 1996) Postmortems show fewer neurons and pyramid cells, and less glial density. (Rajkowska 2000, 01, Chang 2005)

Ventral PFC (underbelly) — *Governs emotions and impulses. Implicated in verbal fluency, inhibition, self-monitoring.* (Malhi 2004) *Connects directly to the amygdala, striatum, and thalamus.* (Blumberg 2004) Abnormalities on the left may be a bipolar trait. (Blumberg 2003, Haldane 2004) Bipolars show increased ventral response to emotional expressions. (Lawrence 2004) Greater activity in mania enhances verbal memory, focus and performance. (Clark 2001) Ventromedial lesions compromise decision-making, (Rubinstein 2001) and, in some, are associated with sociopathic behavior. (Price 1999)

Subgenual (under the bend of the corpus callosum; includes part of the anterior cingulate) — *Modulates visceral responses to stressful and emotionally provocative stimuli.* Studies find loss of glial cells and grey matter volume in bipolars, especially on the left. (Drevets 1998, Rajkowska 2000, Ongur 1998) Losses may disturb stress-related autonomic and endocrine response, and reward-related limbic dopamine function. (Drevets 1998)

Orbitofrontal (eyesocket basal surface) — *Associated with decision-making and risk-taking, especially where emotions are involved.* (Malhi 2004, Blumberg 2002, Chang 2005) Altered activity may be central to bipolar disorder. (Haldane 2004) Imaging suggests reduced activity in bipolar depression, perhaps reduced glial numbers and density, and changes in volume. PET scans during mania have found decreased activation during word generation and rest. (Blumberg 1999) Postmortems of affectives suggest cell atrophy. (Rajkowska 2000)

Prefrontal cortex (PFC)

The prefrontal cortex oversees most brain activity. It absorbs complex messages, relates them to previous information, and generates ideas and goal-directed behavior. It thus governs focus, attention, planning, adaptation to new situtations, creativity, imagination, cooperation, intuition, and logic.

Prefrontal cortex activity is altered with mania. (Ketter 2001, Stoll 2000; Strakowski 2000, Chang 2005)

In depression, PFC activity decreases; (Rajkowska 2000) and reduced metabolism and blood flow correlate with the symptom severity, (Ketter 2001, Soares 1997, Stoll 2000, Rajkowska 2000, Chang 2005) contributing to cognitive difficulties (even in remitted subjects). (Matsuo 2004)

Some studies suggest loss of grey or white matter, (Frey 2004 Strakowski 2002 Chang 2003a, 2005, Winsberg 2000) or of white matter bundle coherence, (Adler 2004) perhaps in specific subregions. (Bruno 2004, Lopez-Larson 2002) Such losses, however, may be effects, rather than causes of bipolar illness, (Frey 2005, Strakowski 2005, Vawter 2000) or may be due to to pharmaceuticals. (Strakowski 2005) Whatever the case, they may contribute to difficulty modulating limbic emotion. (Strakowski 2002)

Imaging also indicates loss of glial cells (Frey 2004, Vawter 2000) (which supply nutrients and growth factors to nerve cells).

Neuropsychological studies suggest relatively intact subcortical intellectual function, though some impairment may occur (Adler 2004, Malhi 2004) in executive function, learning, cognitive flexibility, (Morice 1990) memory, (Bearden 2001) or attention. (Chang 2005, Malhi 2004, Rajkowska 2000) Changes in working memory and executive control may vary with mood, (Malhi 2004) (e.g., reduced prefrontal verbal memory in acute depression, (Fossati 2004) reemerging during manic fluency. (Curtis 2001)).

Prefrontal/limbic interactions

The prefrontal cortex is intricately connected with the limbic system; some suggest it can be considered part of limbic circuitry. (SOARES 1997) Bipolar symptoms may derive especially from dorsal PFC attentional system interactions with the anterior limbic system. (STRAKOWSKI 2004, CHANG 2005)

The following interactions have been proposed:

- □ **PFC (cognitive) overactivity facilitates limbic and endocrine (emotional) extremes** — An overactivated PFC (for instance, with anxiety) heightens limbic response, (MALHI 2004) but becomes less able to modulate that response, (STRAKOWSKI 2004, 05) leading to limbic (LAWRENCE 2004) and endocrine overreactions. (CHANG 2005)
- □ **Limbic dysfunction causes PFC depletion** — Early limbic dysregulation (MALHI 2004) and hyperactivity may overstimulate the frontal cortex, eventually causing depletion. Extreme moods may thus become cumulatively toxic to prefrontal grey matter, "kindling" (POST 1992) mood dysregulation. (CHANG 2005, STRAKOWSKI 2002)
- □ **Limbic/PFC dysregulation** — Suggested by scans showing *reduced* frontal cortex blood flow and glucose metabolism in moderate to severe depressions, but *elevated* limbic (thalamus, amygdala, ventral striatum) metabolism, (KETTER 2002, MAYBERG 1997) normalizing in euthymia. (KIDD 2004)

Other cortical influences on mood

Visual cortex (in the back of the brain, in the occipital lobe) — *Mediates attention to the visual environment.* May be overactive in euthymia (STRAKOWSKI 2004) and mania, suppressed in depression. (DREVETS 1992)

Parietal cortex (at the sides; includes the sensory cortex) — *Helps support sustained attention;* (MALHI 2004) *integrates perceptions, creating a sensory map*). Plays a role in depression, and perhaps anxiety. (DAVIDSON 1999)

Mid saggital cortex — In one study involving 30 bipolars, MRI's showed manic psychosis associated with diffuse cognitive impairment and reduced midsaggital volume. (COFFMAN 1990)

"Frontostriatal loops involved in generating and modulating emotion link the anterior cingulate to the prefrontal cortex and thalamus."

Malhi 2004

Anterior cingulate

The anterior cingulate cortex acts as a gatekeeper for emotional and behavioral response to conditioned stimuli (e.g. fear), (MAMNER 1999) and processes emotions related to determining whether specific feelings, thoughts or actions will be rewarded. (TALAN 1997) Cingulate areas in the prefrontal cortex probably host emotion/cognition/drive/motor-control interactions. (DREVETS 1997) Neuroimaging and functional studies suggest a significant role in the development of, and in ongoing, bipolar symptoms. (BRUNO 2004, HALDANE 2004, MANJI 2000, CHANG 2004)

Cingulate/prefrontal role in bipolar disorder

Dr Wayne Drevets (1999) of the University of Pittsburg has proposed that anterior cingulate subfunction in bipolars might critically interfere with modulation of the amygdala, thereby distorting the processing of emotional stimuli.

Underactivity could underly the impulsive choices disregarding consequence, and the difficulty processing emotional tone in mania. ((BLUMBERG 2003, CHANG 2005, DREVETS 1999). Mayberg (1999) found hypofunction also associated with right dorsolateral prefrontal stimulation, perhaps encouraging manic focus and goal-directed activity.

On the other hand, in recurrent depression, increased left cingulate activation and circulation may contribute to depressive regret, self-chastisement, and preoccupation with consequence. An accompanying decrease in right dorsolateral prefrontal activity could underly depressive inertia and ambivalence. (DREVETS 1992, MAYBERG 1999)

"We think [compromised anterior cingulate activity] is the single most important finding in mood disorders."

WC Drevets, MD

Cingulate loss in affectives

Imaging studies have found altered, perhaps reduced blood flow and use of glucose, and decreased size in the left cingulate of severely depressed and bipolar patients. (HIRAYASU 1999, DREVETS 1988, 92, 96, MAYBERG 1999, BENES 2001, ONGUR 1998) Grey matter volume may be reduced 25-40% in familial bipolar disorder, (DREVETS 1999, HARRISON 2002) mostly due to glial loss. Pathology may also occur in neural synapses and, perhaps, dendrites. (HARRISON 2002)

Cingulate in related disorders

PTSD — The chronic activation of locus coeruleus norepinephrine may decrease anterior cingulate gating, provoking fear and other extreme reactions. (HAMNER 1999)

OCD — Frontal/limbic disturbance, especially in the cingulate gyrus, is common. (WHYBROW)

Limbic system

The limbic system is located roughly in the center of the brain, immediately above the brainstem. It generates emotions related to life-or-death survival, and initiates activity which protects and perpetuates the self (fighting, feeding, fleeing, and sexual activity). It also maintains body homeostasis (regulating temperature, blood pressure, heart rate, blood sugar), oversees endocrine response, stores life experience, and is the seat of olfactory sensation. Removal of the limbic system tames aggressive monkeys and minimizes expression of emotion. (Gyulai 2001) On the other hand, electrical stimulation (in humans), can evoke so vivid a memory of a past event, as to create a sensation of existing in two realities at once. Mood-mediating limbic structures include:

Amygdala

The amygdala is an intermediary between limbic memory and hypothalamic/endocrine response, and also has extensive connections to the prefrontal cortex. (Drevets 1999)

The amygdala is critical to primary emotion and social communication. It assigns emotional significance to experience, evaluates the emotional intent of others, (Aggleton 1981, Ladue 1992) and mediates emotional choices (e.g., partners, food, and reactions to the environment (such as fear). (Ladue 1992) It also interprets facial cues and communicates by facial expression. (Aldophs 1994) And it's crucial to childhood bonding and development. (Aggleton 1981, Ladue 1992) Animals with amygdala damage recognize favorite foods and mates, but are indifferent. Similarly, the general environment fails to evoke an emotional context, so they explore constantly, with little fear. (Ladue 1992)

In adult bipolars the amygdala, (Hurd 2002, Anand 2003) perhaps particularly the left amygdala, (Brambilla 2003) may be enlarged,*(Altshuler 1998, 2000, Strakowski 1999, Scherk 2004, Chang 2005) Imaging of the amygdala and related prefrontal regions shows activity, (Haldane 2004) circulation, (Drevets 1998) and metabolism increasing with depression severity and stress-induced cortisol elevation. Persistant amygdala activity during remission suggests a high risk of relapse. (Drevets 1998, 99)

Abnormalities in the amygdala and its prefrontal cortex connections are probably also important in mania. (Blumberg 2002)

* In contrast, pediatric volume in bipolars is low, (Blumberg 2003) and its smaller in major depression than in bipolars. (Strakowski 2002)

Prefrontal cortex/amygdala connections in bipolars

Functional neuroimaging indicates extensive orbital and medial prefrontal connections to the amygdala. (Drevets 1999) Prefrontal dysfunction interferes with the amygdala's ability to process emotional stimuli (Rubinstein 2001) (e.g., causing greater reaction to a fearful face, but reducing the ability to identify fear. (Yurgelun-Todd 2000)) Haldane suggests distorted amygdala/prefrontal interactions may be a central feature of bipolar pathology. (Haldane 2004)

Thalamus

The thalamus (literally, *center*), is located in the center of the forebrain. It has been described as a relay station; thus, it evaluates and interprets events, and projects instructions on how to react to the environment. It also helps initate consciousness.

Thalamic function may be reduced in some bipolars, compromising the ability to interpret and react to the environment. (Dasari 1999) McIntosh (2004) found anterior thalamic grey matter reduced in some bipolars, schizophrenics and relatives, perhaps marking vulnerability to psychosis.

Hippocampus

The hippocampus (literally, *sea horse*) consolidates information from the thalamus, and conveys emotionally important material to the PFC and limbic system for long-term storage. The PFC directly impacts the hippocampus. (Rajkowska 2000) Prolonged stress thus alters both PFC and hippocampal function. Dendrites shrink. and neurons die. (Yahuda 1999, Rajkowska 2000)

Rajkowska (2000) suggests hippocampal damage may be central to the development of bipolar and major depression in genetically vulnerable individuals.* MRI studies suggest reduced volume in bipolars with, perhaps, subtle synaptic or dendritic abnormalities. (Harrison 2002, Rosoklija 2000)

Hypothalamus

The hypothalamus connects the brain to the endocrine sytem. It governs "housekeeping" functions: biorhythms, temperature regulation, appetites (hunger, aggression, pleasure, sex). It's influenced by attachments, social interactions, and abstractions, such as hopes and fears.

Bipolars typically experience distorted hypothalamus/pituitary/endocrine balances, especially along the adrenal and thyroid axis.

See *Endocrines,* pp. 223-43.

Other brain regions influencing mood

Cerebellum — *mediates memory for simple learned responses, balance, position, and movement in space; deficits may be associated with cognitive impairment.* (SOARES 1997) Bipolar studies suggest reduced size, increased sulcal prominance, blood volume anomalies, and increased hyperintensities (though perhaps due to cardiac risk). (STOLL 2000, VAWTER 2000) Imaging suggests increased mood episodes are associated with greater atrophy. In treatment-resistant bipolars, cerebellar metabolism may be elevated whatever the mood. (KETTER 2000) Lauterbach (1996) suggests reduced cerebellar output to limbic, thalamic, basal ganglia, or other circuits may create the neural oscillation found in rapid-cycling or in dystonia.

Basal ganglia (located on both sides of the limbic system at the base of the cerebral hemispheres; includes the corpus striatum, subthalamic nucleus, and substantia nigra) — *regulates initiation and other aspects of movement.* Bipolar and major depression have been associated with decreased basal ganglia metabolism and circulation. (SOARES 1997) In some bipolars, the basal ganglia is enlarged. (STRAKOWSKI 2002, CHANG 2005)

Brainstem (includes midbrain, pons, medulla) — ascending projections from the brainstem may play a role in mood. (VAWTER 2000)

Laterality

The left brain controls the right side of the body; the right brain, the left. Smell doesn't cross sides. Nerves from both sides control facial muscles. Each side of the brain also governs some specialized functions.

Left side dysfunction & bipolar depression

The left half of the brain is the language hemisphere, predominantly involved in abstract, analytical thought, and sequential processing of information, and tends to be larger in women. (GEORGE 1993) The left prefrontal cortex is the depository of emotional meaning, where memories coded to feelings (by the amygdala and hippocampus) are stored. Damage can create difficulty responding emotionally to imagined emotion-laden situations. (DREVETS 1992)

Left hemisphere dysfunction has been asssociated with depression. (YAHUDA 1996) In patients who develop major depression subsequent to injury, abnormalities tend to be on the left side of the frontal, limbic temporal, or basal ganglia regions. (ROBINSON 1988, JESTED 1988) Major depression or melancholy has also been associated with stroke involving the left frontal or left basal ganglia regions. (DREVETS 1992, STARKSTEIN 1989) And PET studies show evoking of a sad mood, alters blood flow especially in the left prefrontal cortex. (GEORGE 1993, DREVETS 1992, PARDO 1993, GUR 1995, *PSYCH RES* 1994)

Right dysfunction & mania

The right hemisphere governs three-dimensional activity and perception, processes information by visual and spatial patterns, and tends to be larger in males. The right basotemporal lobe may play a major role in the modulation of mood. (STARKSTEIN 1990)

Manics tend to have right hemisphere abnormalities, (JESTED 1988) particularly in the frontotemporal region. (STARKSTEIN 1988, 89, SHYLMAN 1997) SPECT scans have shown decreased blood flow on the right. Moreover, manic trauma or stroke patients often show reduced right limbic circulation (MIGLIORELLI 1993) or exhibit right hemisphere damage, usually intwined with limbic areas. (ROBINSON 1988, STARKSTEN 1989)

Changes in laterality in rapid cyclers

Laterality can be observed to switch with mood change in rapid cyclers. (AMSTERDAM 1991, BLUMBERG 2003)

Possible nutritive adjustments

Pfeiffer suggested adjusting the copper/zinc ratio might help restore the balance between hemispheres.

A skew toward left side dysfunction

Some studies report left dysfunction in all bipolars, e.g., smaller left temporal lobe, decreased performance in the left visual field, etc. (BRUDER 1992) One explanation of this left side weakness may be a shift, induced by mood stabilizers and antimanics, toward the depressive end of the mood spectrum. (ROSSI 1991, KETTER, FRYE 2001)

Ice water treatment (AAFP 2005)

In one report, cold water* in the right ear temporarily alleviated depression; in the left, mania. The theory is that this helps reassert the normal oscillation of focus between hemispheres over the day by correcting the shift during mood episodes toward only one side of the brain.

* Cold water activates orientation pathways on the opposite side of the brain. It is also used in neurologic testing.

Laterality in other disorders (Pfeiffer 1988)

Lateral differences can also occur in schizophrenia, where compromised function in the left hemisphere,* particularly the left temporal lobe, which mediates language, may relate to the intensity of thought disorder, voices, and other hallucinations.

Epilepsy and other organic brain disorders can also cause assymetries.

Miscellaneous damage

Enlarged ventricles

Ventricle enlargement implies decreased brain size. Research conflicts, (Jeste 1988, Nasrallah 1987, Goodwin 1990, Strakowski 1993a) but enlargement may occur in some bipolars, (Botteron 1995, Strakowski 1993a) perhaps one-third, (Stoll 2000, Strakowski 1993a, Drevets 2005) and perhaps especially in the lateral ventricles. (McDonald 2004, Strakowski 1993a, Drevets 2005) Enlargement has been reported in some first-episode manias, (Strakowski 1993a) but usually correlates with age. (Botteron 1995) It may be due to affective illness; but can also be caused by medication, ECT, stress, or abuse. (Strakowski 2005)

Preliminary observations suggest adequate omega 3 may help prevent and reverse ventricle enlargement and brain shrinkage. (Horrobin)

Glial reductions

Ventricle enlargement may mainly reflect reduced glial (rather than nerve) cell numbers. Neuroimaging shows glial deficits in the posterior-lateral and posterior-medial orbital cortex, and the ventral prefrontal cortex, key regions in the processing of emotion. (Strakowski 2005)

Cortical glia are important in the homeostasis of potassium (which counters sodium cell stimulation), (Drevets 1988) and in moderating glutamate uptake (increased in acute mania). (Michael 2003) Glial reduction may reflect glutamine/GABA imbalance.

Hyperintensities

Hyperintensities are bright spots which show up on neuroimaging, indicating greater signal intensity than in nearby tissue. They suggest neural abnormalites.*(Yahuda 1996)

Over 30 MRIs or CT studies find increased hypertensities (Thomas 2004, Strakowski 2000) in some bipolars, (Chang 2005, Harrison 2002, Stoll 2000) particularly in regions bordering the ventricles, and especially in bipolar I, even in some first episode (presumably drug-naive) manics. (Botteron 1992, 95, Strakowski 1993ab) Focal subcortical hyperintensities have been associated with increased ventricle size, (Swayze 1990) more hospitalizations, decreased fluency and recall, (Dupont 1990) and late onset. (Drevets 2005)

The overall risk for hyperintensities in bipolar disorder of any age is estimated at 3-7 fold that in the general population. (Harrison 2002, Stoll 2000) However, hyperintensities do not occur in most bipolars.

Hyperintensities may contribute to symptoms, or could be caused by bipolar illness. (Strakowski 2005) Alternative explanations include extensive use of tobacco, alcohol or other substances; reactions to certain psychiatric or other medications; nutrient imbalance; and excessive stress on the cardiovascular system. (Kidd 2004)

* Hyperintensities are rare in healthy people under 30, and typically seen in cerebrovascular disorders and/or elderly patients. They can indicate myelin loss, glial inflammation, or axonal loss associated with brain ischemia and infarction. (Kidd 2004)

Enlarged ventricles in other disorders

Enlarged ventricles occur in one-third to one-half of chronic schizophrenias. (Botteron 1995, Yahuda 1996, Torrey 2005, Horrobin 2000) Larger ventricles (and a smaller corpus collosum) have also been reported in some abused children. (Yahuda 1999)

Reversing brain shrinkage (Horrobin 2000)

Steven Hirsh reports on a schizophrenic, who, at 19, had experienced violent movement disorder on antipsychotics, and then wandered London for ten years without treatment.

Eventually, he entered Horrobin's fish oil study. By the end of two months of EPA treatment, schizophrenia scores improved. At the outset, his ventricles were enlarged, presumably reflecting brain tissue loss. After six months of EPA, their size was reduced to that of the previous year. Over time, they continued to shrink (and the brain to enlarge), as his schizophrenia subsided. Four years later, he completed his first year at the university, taking only an enriched fish oil.

Concerning trials in other patients, Horrobin comments: "We are seeing EPA restore brain structure."

Appendix III: Side effects of psychiatric medications

"Prescribing tolerable drugs in tolerable dosages for each case is a psychiatric high-wire act." — H Marano, 2005

"Physicans tend toward greater suppression, patients tend toward greater stimulation." — Daniel T Moore, PhD, 1998

"Antidepressants can make you more depressed, tranquilizers more anxious, antipsychotics more psychotic... Woe to the patient whose psychiatrist thinks that the medication isn't working and prescribes more of the same." — Mark Gold, MD, 1987

"Why is the public subjected to periodic outbursts of information about how toxic vitamins are? We do not have similar outbursts against the use of drugs even though vitamins have a zero death rate, while drugs in the US alone kill 106,000 patients in hospitals annually." — Abram Hoffer, MD, PhD

"Generally [except in some cases of severe illness], use of drugs is a self-deception, which sacrifices long-term health for immediate results." — Carl C Pfeiffer, PhD, MD, 1987

CAUTION: Bipolar disorder is fatal in some 20% of patients. Medication may reduce illness severity, and provide crucial life-saving support; or pose life-threatening risks. Similarly, changes to dose or intake can save lives, or create severe consequences. This survey does not constitute advice on whether to take, reduce, or use psychiatric drugs. (*When confronting such choices, the care and advise of a knowledgeable physician is essential.*) The goal here is, rather, to provide educational information on some important side effects, especially those which involve affective and cognitive symptoms.

Major mood stabilizers (Gold 1987, Pfeiffer 1988, Psychiat News 1986, Rudra 1985, Breggin 1991, Brigham 2001)

Tolerance issues

Researchers have generally held that, short-term, approximately two-thirds of bipolars respond to lithium, (Gelenberg 1989) two-thirds to anticonvulsives (valproate or carbamazepine), gaining years of effective functioning. Over two to five years of monotherapy, however, an estimated one to two-thirds relapse. (Post 1993b, Baldessarini 1996, Gitlin 1995, Brigham 2001, Grof 1998, Coryell 1997, Frankenberg 1988) Multiple mood stabilizers, antianxiety and antipsychotic meds may eventually be prescribed but, long-term, may destabilize mood in some, as manias strengthen enough to cut through the tranquilization. Moreover, the three major stabilizers may push cycling toward depression; the newer one, lamotrigine, toward mania. (Frye, Ketter 2001, Gelenberg 1989, Gillberg 1993, Kukopulos 1995, Maj 1989, Moller 2003, O'Connell 1991, Sarantidis 1981, Swann 1997, Post 1990, 93ab, 95, 96, 99, Bowden 1999, Denicoff 1997, Leverich 1998,Weiss 1995a) Over the years, tolerance often rises with the increasing doses and number of drugs, until, for some, drugs no longer help. (Ketter, Frye 2001)

Some lithium side effects (psychiatric doses) (Gold 1987, Pfeiffer 1988, Psychiat News 1986, Rudra 1985, Breggin 1991, Brigham 2001)

Mood & cognitive

Depression, dulled emotions. (Gold 1987) Confusion, poor concentration, memory defects, suppressed cognition, blunted personality. (Millett 1990, Breggin 1991, Gold 1987, Gutton 1989, Psychiat News 1986) Progressive, irreversible intellectual deterioration may occur with chronic use. (Dawson 1970, Breggin 1991)

Withdrawal

If withdrawn, a greatly increased risk of suicide (at or above pre-treatment levels) and approximately a 50% risk of relapse within five months, especially if stopped rapidly. Resumption is often less effective, with more treatment resistance, and increased need for additional mood stabilizers. (Brigham 2001, Ketter 2001)

General

Mild symptoms — fine hand tremor, slurred speech, incoordination, sleepiness, fatigue, weakness, dry mouth, taste distortion, skin rash or acne, hair loss.

Moderate — depression, dizziness, lethargy, sedation, dull cognition, CNS effects. Nausea, diarrhea, abdominal pain, indigestion, increased appetite and thirst, excess urination, weight gain, rigidity. Often, goiter or hypothyroid; rarely, hyper-thyroid or parathyroid.

Severe — impairment of consciousness, cardiac abnormalities (20-30%), permanently increased kidney output, bedwetting, irreversible kidney scarring (Ga"sparovi'c 1990) or other damage, liver disorders,* rise in blood sugar, increased white blood cell count, blood disorders, coma. If not carefully monitored, toxic levels may accumulate*** and become lethal.***

* Although, of the major mood stabilizers, Ketter (2001) finds it the best choice for bipolars with hepatitis C.

** Whybrow suggests monitoring blood levels frequently until stabilized, then every 2-4 months, and regularly assessing liver and thyroid function, and blood cell count. Optimal dose may change due to side effects, interactions with other meds, fever, dehydration, etc. (Whybrow 1997)

*** To stop severe reactions, the physician may prescribe sudden withdrawal and substitute other mood stabilizers. For critical situations, dialysis may be indicated. In other cases, a slow taper may be indicated, accompanied by comprehensive nutritive mood stabilization. Pfeiffer (1988) recommends increasing dietary salt; Richman (1992), salt water.

Polypharmacy effects

Lithium heightens neuroleptic toxicity and can cause serious complications if given prior to ECT. It is contraindicated with high doses of neuroleptics, digitalis, diuretics; kidney or heart conditions, pregnancy, blood disorders, or a salt-free diet. (Brigham 2001)

Some side effects of anticonvulsant stabilizers

Valproate (VPA) & Carbamazepine (CBZ)

VPA and CBZ are generally used to address acute mania and, with lithium and other meds, for depression or ongoing stabilization.

Rapid administration increases side effects and can become neurotoxic. Withdrawal, especially when abrupt, can heighten anxiety, insomnia, obsessional thinking; and trigger or worsen affective episodes. Both deplete carnitine and taurine. (KIDD 2004, INTELEGEN.COM...) Interactions often occur with other pharmaceuticals. (DUNN 1998)

Long term tolerance can become substantial; and episodes, more severe. (DENICOFF 1997, LEVERICH 1998, POST 1990, 93A, 95, 96, 99, TRIMBLE 1996, WEISS 1995A) Cycling may be pushed toward depression; less often, mania. Rapid cycling or mixed states may develop; psychosis may occur or increase. (KETTER, FRYE 2001, BOWDEN 1999, TRIMBLE 1996)

Other cognitive & neurological side effects

Valproate — somnolence, drowsiness, low energy, weakness, malaise, dizziness, confusion, foggy, shaky or unsteady movement, tremor, aggressiveness, hyperactivity, constant mild headache, blurred vision.* (NASRALLAH 2003)

Carbamazepine — sedation, blurred or double vision, uncontrolled back and forth eye movement, light headedness, dizziness, incoordination, tremor, unsteady movement, headache. Elevated serum ammonia, creating fatigue, drowsiness, malaise, etc. Less commonly, behavior changes, confusion, agitation, or hostility, especially in elderly; more rarely, restless or nervous depression, trembling, uncontrolled movement, numb or tingling extremities, seizures, visual hallucinations.**(READ 2007, NASRALLAH 2003)

Some physical side effects (valproate) — Weight gain, low appetite. Increased hair growth or hair loss. Nausea, vomiting, abdominal pain, and other gastrointestinal effects. (Bowden 1997) Acne, skin rash. Swollen ankles, tissue swelling. Depletion of platelets or white blood cells; anemia, bruising, blood vessel inflammation, unusual bleeding. Jaundice, liver disorders, rarely, failure. Rarely, pancreatitis. (Stoll 1999) Neural tube defects. Irregular or absents menses. Polycystic ovaries (especially if overweight or epileptic), often fatal if untreated (note increased hairiness, acne, androgen-related infertility). Increases blood levels of lamotrigine. (Frye 2001, Ketter 2001)

Some physical side effects (carbamazepine) — Diarrhea, nausea, other gastrointestinal distress. Loss of appetite, weight gain. Muscle cramps. Hair loss. Sexual dysfunction in males. Headaches. Liver disorders, failure. Skin discoloration and hypersensitivity: hives, itching, sun sensitivity, red skin, sores, ulcers; white spots on lips or mouth, irritated or sore tongue or mouth. (Moore 1985) Skin rashes in 10-15%; may lead to exfoliative dermatitis (shedding scaly red areas), or Stevens-Johnson syndrome (a rapidly-progressing rash, which is often fatal).(Frye 2001) Low birth weight; craniofacial, (Jones 1989) neural tube (spina bifida in 1-2%), cardiac, and other birth defects. (Brigham 2001). Hyponatremia. Abnormally low white blood cells; or platelets (promoting slow coagulation, and bruising); granulocytosis (producing mucous membrane and skin ulcers); aplastic anemia (extreme depletion of red blood cells and hemoglobin). (Mehta 1994, Joffe 1985) [Monitor hematological profile, and serum electrolytes. (Birkheimer 1985)] Arrhythmia (slowed A-V conduction), tight chest, irregular pounding or slowed heartbeat. (Brigham 2001)

More rarely: Cough, hoarseness, sore throat, short breath, wheezing, chills, fever, swollen/painful glands, difficult or slurred speech; tender, swollen or weak hands and feet; lower back or side pain, bone or joint pain; blood in urine or stool, dark urine, painful or difficult urination, black tarry or pale stools; ringing or other ear sounds; pancreatitis. (Brigham 2001)

Can increase neurotoxicity of lithium, valproate, or clozapine and may contribute to the development of polycystic ovaries with VPA. Also increases elimination of numerous meds. (Brigham 2001)

Lamotrigine (NASRALLAH 2003)

Lamotrigine, a newer stabilizer, is thought to significantly improve bipolar depression, and perhaps benefit rapid cycling, but may push cycling toward mania, and can worsen irritability and insomnia. Other side effects* can include headache, dizziness, blurred or double vision, clumsiness, unsteady movement and, less commonly, anxiety, depression, confusion, slurred speech, sedation, drowsiness, uncontrollable back-and-forth eye movements, and seizures. It is not recommended for children under sixteen.

Some physical side effects: Weight gain, nausea, dry mouth, increased heart rate. Skin rash in 15%. Stevens-Johnson syndrome in 0.1%, usually in the first few months. Risk is greater if under 16, or with high or rapidly-increased dose. (Kidd 2004, Ketter 2001)

Calcium channel blockers (BRIGHAM 2001)

Calcium channel blockers often have mood stabilizing properties and are anticonvulsant. Side effects* include fatigue, depression, dizziness, numbness, or tingling, and more rarely, headache, fainting, vivid dreams.

Some physical side effects: Wheezing, coughing, shortness of breath, trouble swallowing. Stomach problems, constipation. Flushing; more rarely, rash, jaundice, fever. Edema in the legs, stomach. Bleeding, swollen or tender gums. Frequent urination (due to reduced ADH). (Dubovsky 1983) Rapid, or more often, slowed pulse (due to reduced ability of the heart to pump blood). More rarely, chest pain and severe cardiovascular effects. (Dubovsky 1983, Antman 1980) Decreased insulin secretion. Glucose intolerance. (Dubovsky 1983, Devis 1975) May compromise thyroid function. (Dubovsky 1983) May interact with lithium or CBZ.

Pregnancy & psych drugs (BRIGHAM 2001)

Lithium — increases the risk of Ebstein's disease (a heart defect) and other developmental abnormalities. Thyroid and kidneys should be monitored, particularly with altered metabolism and fluids in late pregnancy. Lithium is usually stopped two days pre-delivery (despite heightened risk of mood swing).

Carbamazepine & valproate — increased risk of spinalbifida, etc. (consider folate). Newborn withdrawal convulsions.

Diazepam — increases risk of cleft lip and palate.

Benzodiazepines — can produce major respiratory supression, floppy baby syndrome, infant withdrawal problems.

Thoridazine — may often produce limbic malformation.

Nursing & meds (LITHIUMPLUSWERKGROEP, BRIGHAM 2001, GELENBERG 1997)

Lithium — Infants are exposed to 50% of maternal intake, and are more sensitive to it, so nursing is inadvisable.

Bromocryptin-like lactation suppressors — can produce adverse psychiatric effects.

Note to the patient: Work with your physician in weighing the risks of medication to your child during pregnancy and nursing, against the risks of a mood episode.

Some side effects of antidepressant meds (BRIGHAM 2001, APA 1994, WHYBROW 1997, GOLD 1987, KETTER 2001)

"The single most effective treatment for rapid cycling is to discontinue antidepressants." — Peter M Brigham, MD

"I think that there is very clear evidence for all of the SSRI group of drugs that in addition to making people suicidal, they can make people homicidal or seriously aggressive." — Dr. David Healy, 2003

Though antidepressants can be life-saving, they are estimated to eventually trigger mania in from one-third (KETTER 2001, FRYE, KETTER 2001, MARANO 2005) to over one-half of bipolars. (POST 2003) Brigham (2001) and Ketter (2001) note that about 80% of people (whether or not bipolar) in whom antidepressants induce mania will experience another, spontaneous mania or hypomania within two years, i.e. the drug-induced mania makes them bipolar. And that antidepressant-induced manias may be the best predictor of cycle acceleration and, along with drug abuse, may underly the recent increase in rapid cycling. Vulnerability to depression may also be increased.* Use with mood stabilizers decreases, but doesn't eliminate, such risks. (*Thus, after resolution, unless depression is particularly recurrent, antidepressants are often tapered, over 2-6 months, quicker in bipolar II.* (EXPERT 2000)) (Hyperactivity meds pose similar risk.) Unfortunately, concerns over antidepressants have led to a greater use of atypical antipsychotics to suppress bipolar depression.

* Also consider the increased the risk of cardiovascular complications or fatality, (Watkins 2006) And, interactions with other meds. (Freeman 2002, Salama 1989, Sovner 1991, Gernaat 1991, Kaufman 1998, Kidd 2004)

SSRIs (WHYBROW 1997)

SSRIs block transport and reuptake of serotonin. Side-effects can take time to emerge, (KRAMER 1993) and may involve:

Altered perception (GAYFORD 1973, BRAVERMAN), drowsiness, (LARSON), grogginess (COUSENS), headache, sedation.

Bizarre dreams, acting out of nightmares, REM disorder.

Psychomotor agitation especially if taken with MAOIs. (GEYER 1976 MOURILHE 1998, KRAMER 1993)

Can trigger rapid cycling or mania on withdrawal, (DILSAVER 1984) or with ongoing intake. (DILER 1999, HOWLAND 1996) Such manias can be particularly severe and intractible, with extreme agitation and psychosis. (BRIGHAM 2001)

In some cases, profound anxiety, aggression, hostility, homicide, violence, heightened suicide risk. (BOSLEY 2004, HEALY 2003, TEICHER 1990)

Cumulatively (often rapidly) depletes tryptophan. (MOORE 1998, DELGADO 1990) Serotonin activity can also dip just before the next dose. This may lead to severe reactions *(as above)*. (HEALY 2003)

Can be detrimental in histapenia, especially if serotonin is already elevated.

Not proven effective for young people. (HEALY 2003)

Serotonin syndrome — caused by extremely elevated serotonin (e.g., when taking several SSRIs; or an SSRI plus MAOIs, tricyclics, or certain other drugs; occasionally, an SSRI plus serotonin precursors). It's usually due to interactions of pharmaceuticals that interfere with serotonin breakdown, promoting accumulation at the receptor. Symptoms may include confusion, shivering, sweating, fever, diarrhea, incoordination, impotence, muscle twitching, exaggerated reflex, severe agitation, violent muscular contractions, seizures. Can be fatal. (*NULAND 1994*)

See also *Tryptophan/5HTP side effects*, p. 105.

Some physical side effects: Dry mouth, loose stools, nausea, vomiting, other gastrointestinal effects. Excess perspiration. Impaired (or altered) sex drive, arousal, or orgasm. (Kramer 1993, Prange, Broida 2001, Whybrow 1997, Colodny). May increase blood pressure or clotting, or promote coronary artery spasm. (C, E, calcium, magnesium, fish oil, etc., may help some). (Baumel, Larson, Cousens) May contribute to deterioration of the aortic valve, or heart muscle. Contraindicated with various cardiovascular conditions. Can cause problems with pregnancy. May be associated with bronchial asthma, lupus, scleroderma. (Cousens, Whybrow 1997, Prange) Avoid in severe liver disease. (Bachmann 1983, Gilka 1975) Contraindicated with carcinoid. May interact adversely with carbidopa. (Slagle)

SSRIs, suicide, homicide (DRUGAWARENESS.ORG)

The FDA has recently warned that SSRIs double suicide risk in children under 18, and they're now evaluating the danger to adults. Use by teens is banned in the UK.

Dr. David Healy claims even healthy volunteers can become aggressive or homicidal both when taking, and when withdrawing from, an SSRI. He notes that in 2001, a US court ordered GlaxoSmith-Kline to pay $8 million to relations of a family murdered by a man the jury judged to have been reacting to an SSRI. And that many of the teens involved in the school shootings in America had been taking SSRIs, including Kip Kinkle (of Thurston), and Eric Harris (Columbine).

Tricyclics

Tricyclics focus on serotonin and norepinephrine. They are seldom given to bipolars, as they can accelerate cycling (STOLL 1994, BRIGHAM 2001) (25-30% switch on tricyclics, sometimes in a continuous cycle (APA 1994)); and can cause intense mania in depressed bipolars and worsen psychosis in schizophrenics. (GOLD 1987, BROIDA 2001, WHYBROW 1997) Other side effects include sedation, drowsiness, dizziness, confusion, insomnia. Tricyclics are not particularly effective for youth.* (BROIDA 2001, WHYBROW 1997)

Some physical side effects: Low blood pressure, rapid pulse, increased perspiration, weight gain, dry mouth and eyes, difficulty urinating, constipation. (Broida 2001, Whybrow 1997)

MAOIs

MAOIs inhibit enzymes that destroy adrenergic and serotonergic transmitters, increasing levels at the synapse, often promoting full-blown mania. Thus, they are not used much for bipolars. Other side effects include anxiety, insomnia, euphoria, depression.* (GOLD 1987, STOLL 1994, BRIGHAM 2001)

Some physical side effects: Headache, nausea, sweating. Blood pressure can dangerously increase if tyramine-rich foods are eaten (aged cheese, red wine, sausage, chocolate, preserved meat and fish, dry fruit) or with certain drugs (cold medicines, amphetamines, other antidepressants). (Broida 2001, Whybrow 1997)

Newer antidepressants (BROIDA 2001, WHYBROW 1997)

Side effects vary with the drug, and are less well explored, though seizures, sedation, sleepiness, SSRI-type reactions, changes in the efficacy of other drugs, fluid retention, weight gain, and high blood pressure have been noted.

Some side effects of antipsychotics

"For a little while you are unconscious. Then it begins. I am totally conscious, horribly awake and yet rigid, locked in the dream. There is no way out of this fate, the same dream over and over, only worse." — Kate Millett, on Prolixin®

"I was horrified to see how I deteriorated intellectually, morally and emotionally... My interest in political problems quickly disappeared, then my interest in [science], and then... in my wife and children."— Leonid Plyushch, Soviet dissident, on Haldol®

[These drugs] do not calm or sedate the nerves. They attack. They attack so deep inside you, you cannot locate the source of the pain. The drugs turn your nerves in upon yourself... The pain grinds into your fiber." — Henry Abott, on forced Prolixin®

Antipsychotics alter brain electrical activity and suppress transmission of dopamine, and sometimes norepinephrine or other transmitters. They are often used to counter mania; sometimes, as stabilizers, or antidepressants.

Mood

Researchers have reported mood-switching, increased cycling, and worsening depression with maintenance or post-manic use, (BRIGHAM 2001, FRYE 2000) perhaps promoting anhedonia (inability to feel pleasure) due to chronic dopamine exhaustion. (COHEN 1995, RICHMAN 1992)

Rebound mania or psychosis:

To compensate for dopamine suppression, receptors tend to multiply or become supersensitive. If intake is stopped, especially if abruptly, enhanced messaging may produce a supersensitivity/rebound psychosis, usually within a year. The patient may then be rediagnosed schizoaffective, with further antipsychotics reinforcing the psychosis. Similarly, mania can be triggered, and cycling accelerated, (FRYE 2000) or anxiety, insomnia, etc, intensified. (STEINER 1990, FRYE 2000)

Cognitive

Dulled thought processes, apathy; repressed creativity, consciousness, will, and personality; perhaps mutism, catatonia (especially in histadelics (PFEIFFER 1987)), or delirium. Chronic use may permanently repress intelligence, and can cause tardive dementia or psychosis. (GOLD 1987, COHEN 1995, WHYBROW 1997, BREGGIN 1991)

Neurological reactions

A high incidence of abnormal neurological signs has been reported in bipolars on long-term neuroleptics (MUKHERJEE 1984), associated with extrapyramidal,* and perhaps frontal deterioration,**(GUR 1998A) profoundly altering movement and cognition. (HOKAMA 1995, PAULESEN 1994, SACHDEV 1996)

* Including striatal changes in cell structure and the proportion and properties of synapses; (Hokama 1995) and size changes in the basal ganglia, thalamus, (Gur 1998b) or caudate. (Chakos 1994, Nielsen 1978) See *Movement disorders*, below.

** A *Lancet* letter (1998) suggests risk of atrophy increases 4-6% for each 10 gm neuroleptics.

Atypicals

Atypicals are the preferred antipsychotics in mainstream treatment of refractory bipolars. They target more neurotransmitters, and are less likely than neuroleptics to cause movement disorders, but suspected by some to be more likely to cause tardive psychosis and limbic or prefrontal damage. They promote switching and trigger mania in some patients, and can contribute to seizures, insomnia, agitation, memory problems, and oversedation. Bipolars can find withdrawal especially difficult, and are particularly prone to rebound reactions.*(FRYE, KETTER 2000, BRIGHAM 2001, REEVES 1998, POZO 1998, BREGGIN 1991, COHEN 1995, RICHMAN 1992, MCELROY 1998, GOLD 1987, GHAEMI 1997, WHYBROW 1997)

Concerns over chronic antipsychotics for bipolars (BRIGHAM 2001)

Bipolars protocols often involve a gradual taper of antipsychotics once mania and psychosis resolve (typically by 4-12 weeks). However 30-40% of patients wind up on chronic antipsychotics, usually to address repeated breakthrough manias, psychosis during taper, or psychotic depression in spite of mood stabilizers.*

Some mainstream psychiatrists are wary about giving bipolars antipsychotics. Whybrow (1997) suggests long-term use by bipolars is generally not advisable. Brigham (2001) emphasizes low doses and notes that maintenance efficacy has not been fully studied.

Also see *Manic psychosis, Medication*, p.268.

* Hopefully, further research will elucidate the extent to which such reactions are drug rebounds, made more likely by bipolar sensitivity to the status of brain stimulation.

Movement disorders (mainly associated with neuroleptics):
Akathisia —anxiety and extreme restlessness, muscles itching, inciting persistent pacing, perhaps causing blisters.

TD — involuntary muscle spasms or gimaces, perhaps severe, often triggered by stress (e.g., toxins, excitement, depression). (Sandyk 1990, Brigham 2001) Some studies link TD to cognitive impairment. (Waddington 1996, Paulsen 1994, Sachdev 1996, Chakos 1998) Affectives are at high risk. (Brigham 2001) The higher the dose, the greater the risk. One study finds for each year of use, 5% more patients develop TD. Several studies find 20 to 50% develop TD on long-term neuroleptics, particularly older people and women. (APA 1980, Sovner1986, Chouinaud 1990, Schatzberg 1986, Glaser, Cohen 1995, Saltz 1991) Symptoms are often misconstrued, and doses increased, which may temporarily suppress symptoms, while increasing deterioration. Basal ganglia free radical toxicity (Pfeiffer1987, Lohr 1995, Graham 1978) or manganese depletion (hair levels in TD are 60% that in other patients) (Kunin 1976, Hoffer 1977) may play a role. TD is rare in orthomolecular patients. (Tkacz 1984, Hoffer 1983, Hawkins 1986, 89)

Dystonias — severe, uncontrollable, painful cramps or spasms (head pulled to the side, eyes turned up in sockets; throat or pharynx spasms, interfering with breathing or swallowing).

Parkinsonism — dopamine suppression causes persistent tremors (reduced with voluntary activity and sleep), an unblinking, staring, masklike face, a stooped, shuffling gait, difficulty stopping or starting movement, slow movement, rigidity, monotonous, barely intelligible speech, mild dementia. (Gold 1987)

Other physical side effects (in various atypicals): Rampant appetite and thirst, obesity, night drooling, liver damage, blurred vision, sun sensitivity, blindness, headaches, dizziness, fever, urinary tract obstruction, impotence, grey-blue coloring to the face and heart, cardiovascular and respiratory disorders, life-threatening bone marrow suppression (Clozapine), immune impairment, sudden death. (Gold 1987, Brigham 2001, Cohen 1995, Richman 1987, 92, Breggin 1991)

Anticholinergic effects can include sedation, gastrointestinal suppression, low blood pressure, rapid pulse, stiff limbs, movement disorders. (Whybrow 1997)

Neuroleptic malignant syndrome: Occurs after chronic intake, in about 1% of patients, killing 20-30%; some, within 24 hours (due to acute kidney or respiratory failure, or cardiovascular collapse). Many survivors suffer brain damage. Acute signs include racing pulse; elevated temperature, blood pressure, and white blood cells; profuse perspiration, panting, incontinence and confusion. Deteriorates into speechlessness, rigidity, and coma. (Brigham 2001, Breggin 1991)

Neuroprotective formulas

Suggestions by Elkashef (2001) for nervous system healing & TD

Tailor to individual biochemical requirements. If swallowing is difficult, open caps, mix, and massage into skin.

- □ **Vitamin E** plus a rich assortment of **antioxidants** — to protect neurons. [2x/ day]
- □ **Distilled salmon oil** (omega 3) — provides structural support to the neural membrane; enhances neuroplasticity; optimizes function of membrane receptors, enzymes and proteins, and regulation and transport of molecules into the cell. Supports second messaging, and interactions with the sodium/potasium pump, cAMP, ATPase, etc. [2000 mg, 2x/ day]
- □ **Purified lecithin**. [1000 mg, 2x/ day; perhaps more if dopamine levels are normal to elevated.]
- □ **Phosphatidyl serine** — to support omega 3 incorporation into neural membranes. [200 mg, 2x/ day]
- □ **Flax oil** — to discourage *elongase*, etc., from converting the omega 6 in PC and PS. [2000 mg, 2x/ day]

Also see, *Brain trauma approaches*, p 245.

Suggestions by Page (1994) for nervous system healing & TD

- □ Niacin, manganese, with EFAs, B3, B6, B12, C.
- □ Lady's slipper — neural and myelin repair. Calming, relieves pain
- □ Nervines: scullcap, wood betony, kava, valerian.
- □ Rosemary — antioxidant
- □ Licorice —adrenal support, blood sugar balance.
- □ Capsicum — increases neural and glandular tone.
- □ Siberian ginseng —strengthens nervous, cardiovascular, immune systems, nourishes adrenals.

Suggestions by orthomolecular physicians for TD (Hawkins 1986, 89)

Prevention is easier than treatment. Orthomolecular researchers have found niacin and manganese* particularly helpful. (Werbach 1991, Borg 1972, Hoffer 1977, 83, Kunin 1976) Other beneficial nutrients may include choline, lecithin, (Yahr 1969, Jackson 1979, 81, Gelenberg 1979, Nasrallah 1984, Gelenberg 1990, Pfeiffer 1987, 88, Fann, Klawans) B6, (Lerner 2007, Tkacz 1969, Deveaugh-Geiss 1978) EFAs, (Vaddadi 1989, 96, Nildoon 1996) selenium, glutathione, E and other antioxidants. (Adler 1992, Lohr 1987, 88, 95, Graham 1984, Elkashef 1990, Cadet 1989) B2, B12, and tryptophan may be helpful for some. (Werbach 1991, Marshall 1983)

* Manganese can worsen histadelia, tics, and Parkinsonian stiffness. It may be unneccessary with atypicals (preferentially used for bipolars), which do not deplete it (and are not as linked to TD, anyway). (Walsh 2007)

If dose reduction or withdrawal from psychiatric medication is indicated (Richman 1992)

To avoid toxic and potentially-life threatening reactions, withdrawal or dose reductions should, in almost all cases, be gradual. Usually, practitioners start with the drug causing the most severe symptoms (e.g., antidepressants causing mania or rapid cycling; or antipsychotics causing significant depression). *Undertake only under the supervision of a knowlegeable physician.* (Richman 1992, Hoffer 2005, Pfeiffer 1987)

Withdrawal from antipsychotics frequently produces rebound mania, paranoia, or psychosis; from benzodiazepines, an excrutiating rebound anxiety; from antidepressants, severe depression or violence; etc. (Gold 1987)

Withdrawal (even reductions) of mood stabilizers is a last resort strategy, and extremely hazardous. Besides triggering severe mood episodes, lithium withdrawal has been associated with a vastly increased risk of suicide over the next year. Withdrawal from other mood stabilizers probably poses similar risk. *Note: Manics often [ill-advisedly] seek to withdraw from mood-stabilizers to feed their mania.*

In most cases where withdrawal is indicated, Walsh, Hoffer, and other orthomolecular physicians emphasize months of nutrient therapy *before* starting; then (usually focusing on one drug at a time), slow stepwise reductions, tied to nutritional improvement.* In some cases, enhanced drug effectiveness (e.g. undue suppression and fatigue associated with an antimanic med), may reflect improvement. *Unless improvement can be elicited, reductions are usually not indicated.*

David Richman, MD, suggests successive dose reductions of 10%. Each stage lasts til the patient is free of distressing withdrawal symptoms. If symptoms worsen, nutrients and other supports are enhanced. Drug dose may need to increase slightly toward the previous level (e.g, 5%), and not reduce again til enough improvement recurs. The final 10% reduction may need to be subdivided further (e.g., 1% at a time), as this stage can be particularly difficult. (Richman 1992)

Larson (2008) says you can detox from almost any drug with IVs of high-dose C. To withdraw from benzos (known to be particularly difficult), she typically gives *oral* GABA, plus IVs with C, glutathione, taurine,** perhaps some B complex, or other nutrients, *as per individual requirements.*

Ongoing support: A healthful diet, moderate physical exercise, relaxation, plenty of sleep, mental engagement, creativity, reflection, friendship and other psychosocial support, stress reduction, etc., are recommended.

Complete withdrawal is not always possible,*** though, over time, dosage can often be reduced enough to minimize side effects. (Walsh 2007)

WARNING: Bipolars are often highly sensitive to changes in drug intake. Moreover, due to the cyclic nature of the illness, their response to dose reductions can be difficult to evaluate. Withdrawal poses extreme risk, including symptom rebound with heightened intensity, even a year or more later. Violence, suicide, psychosis, or other life-threatening reactions may emerge. The care and advice of a knowledgeable physician is essential.

* Unless serious drug toxicity or other medical situations mandate a faster withdrawal.

** Before & during taurine use, optimize zinc levels relative to copper.

*** Consider that brain homeostasis may have been permanently altered by extended intake.

Appendix IV: Biochemical tests

Choice of tests is guided by signs and symptoms, individual and family history, etc. Other unlisted tests may be needed. For more complete descriptions and references, see corresponding chapters.

General exam (Gold 1987, Pfeiffer 1976, 88, Gardner 1981, Jaffe 1992)

To help pinpoint the need for specific biochemical tests.

□ Medical & psychiatric histories (individual, family): symptoms, nutrients, meds, cycling pattern, therapeutic response.

□ Personal dietary and supplement history.

□ Psychological tests.

□ Clinical observation of behavior (e.g., agitation, hyperactivity, depression, hostility, fear, general status.)

□ Physical exam: General physical condition (skin, hair, eyes, pulse, etc.). Signs of contributory illnesses, particularly nervous (especially epilepsy), endocrine (especially thyroid, adrenals, pancreas, and pituitary), and digestive (Candida, leaky gut, malabsorption, etc.). Check for abdominal pains (e.g., may indicate porphyria), head injury, headaches, joint pains (B6/ manganese deficiency, lupus), other aches and pains, immune or cardiovascular symptoms, etc.

□ Neurological exam (includes reflex, and pencil & paper tests): Suggests brain injuries, tumors, etc. EEG, *if indicated* (e.g., with episodic mood symptoms or sudden onset, genetic risk, birth complications, history of head injury, history or meningitis, encephalitis, etc.).

Pyroluria (Pfeiffer 1987, 88, Jaffe 1992, Walsh 2006)

□ Urinary pyrroles* — Normal is 4-8 mcg/dL; 20-50 is moderate pyroluria (which can be serious); over 50 is severe; below 3 suggests samples may have been handled improperly. Levels can vary over the day.

□ EGOT** — reflects B6 levels.

□ Porphyrins*** fractionated urine porphyrins (especially coproporphyrin and oroporphyrin. (Cutler)

□ Zinc — look for high or low levels in serum or hair. White spots on the nails may roughly map periods of zinc deficiency (but can be due to other causes); assume five to six months for nails to grow in.

□ Copper. Hair metals.

□ Red cell EFAs.

□ Other nutrients and corrresponding enzymes may be deficient.

□ Serum IgA may be depressed.

□ Poor health.

□ EEGs can show occasional slow waves and isolated voltage spikes.

* OHHPL (hydroxyhemopyrrolin-2-one) is the major culprit.

** Erythrocyte glutamate/oxalate transaminase.

*** Cutler advises requesting labs to put preservative in the collection vessel, rather than the sample tube.

Some key biochemical tests (Lesser 2008, Pfeiffer 1976, 88, Jaffe 1992, Braverman 1987, Walsh 2006, Werbach 1991, Gardner 1981

□ Biotype: basophils, blood histamine, urinary pyrroles, folic acid, copper, zinc, magnesium, B6, EFAs, etc.

□ Suspected imbalances in specific nutrients & related enzymes; neurotransmitters, precursors & cofactors.

□ Toxic metals, MT disorder.

□ Allergies. Absorption, Candida antibodies, etc.

□ Thyroid, adrenals, sugar metabolism, liver, etc.

□ CBC, urinalysis, neurological issues, *as relevant.*

Considerations in fine tailoring therapy (Werbach 1991, Slagle 1992, Larson 2001, Murray 1998, Walsh 2006, Pfeiffer 1988)

□ Signs, symptoms, biotype, and correspondence to a proposed nutrient's mental and physical effects.

□ Therapeutic response.

□ Nutrient blood, urine and hair analyses. Activity of key enzymes related to a suspected nutrient (depletion may occur in some, but not all enzyme systems).

□ Individualized dosage: Bipolar need for water-soluble vitamins (particularly C and B) can often be 100's of times RDA; some minerals (e.g. magnesium, often zinc), several times, while others (perhaps copper) must be kept low; dose of EFAs, aminos, etc., also vary with patient need.

□ Absorption: Are capsules/ tablets passing out of the body unabsorbed? Is the specific nutrient best utilized when taken with foods, or alone? Is another form preferable (sublingual, powdered, liquid, tincture, nasal spray, superfoods, juices, etc.)? Are health conditions causing malabsorption? *Note: With substantial malabsorption, or extreme mood, several months of IV or IM injections may be indicated.*

□ Timing: When do peak symptoms occur? Do symptoms emerge between doses? etc. Consider adjusting number of doses per day, skewing intake, changing dose or nutrient choices, using time-release forms, etc., *as relevant.*

□ Major and side effects of concurrent or prior medications. Rebound reactions, tolerance, increased symptoms as the drug wears off over the day. Nutrient/drug interactions (especially with aminos, other potent nutrients, herbs). *Adjust accordingly.*

□ Overall health profile: Allergies, hypoglycemia, caffeine, alcohol, meds, street drugs, lifestyle factors, illness.

See also, *Individualizing nutritional therapy,* p. 6.

Factors suggesting a quality supplement

Meets requirements of biotype & unique chemistry. Contains full range of nutrients supporting its function.* Organic, derived from nutrient-dense foods, wild-crafted herbs,** *as practical.* *Does not contain:* coal tar derivatives; allergens; contraindicated ingredients; mineral glutamates or aspartates;*** ferrous fumarate, magnesium oxide, calcium carbonate;**** D2.*****

* E.g, calcium supplements with magnesium, D3, boron, C, horsetail, etc.

** And, if concerned about mad cow, look for ingredients derived only from plants or fish, and vegi-based caps (or use tabs, liquids, sprays, tinctures).

*** Affectives tend to be particularly sensitive to excitotoxins.

**** Which are poorly absorbed and tend to deposit, especially if prone to malabsorption (common in bipolars) or low metabolism (some depressions).

***** Can promote calcium deposits. Look instead for D3.

Histamine/methylation imbalances (Pfeiffer 1976, 88, Jaffe 1992, Braverman 1994, Walsh 2002, 06, 07, Graham 2008)

□ Histamine — whole blood histamine is available through a limited number of labs. (Normal is 40-70ng/dL. Under 40 is low histamine; over 70, high.) Antihistamines or antigens reduce histamine, altering results. The basophil count is less sensitive, but often reflects histamine, and helps confirm histamine findings. (Normal is 30-50.)

□ Folic acid & B12 — red cell, serum or plasma folate, neutrophillic segmentation, methylmallonic acid.

□ Copper — serum, hair, ceruloplasmin saturation.

□ Zinc — serum, hair.

□ SAH/SAMe ratio — may be the best measure of methylation status, but can be hard to get. Alternately, SAH and methionine are good tests. (Walsh 2007)

□ **Undermethylation** — look for elevated histamine and folate; often low copper; low calcium, magnesium, B6, serotonin, dopamine, norepinephrine; perhaps elevated lead (especially in children). Often, respiratory allergies. *If methylation status is unclear, Walsh finds a one-to-two-week trial of SAM (cautiously!) often resolves the matter.*

□ **Overmethylation** — look for low histamine, low folate; high copper, low zinc. Metal metabolism dysfunction, heavy metals, sensitivity to metals, high mercury keeping copper high. Often, food and environmental sensitivities/allergies. Perhaps, low potassium and magnesium with metabolic acidosis. Check thyroid, estrogen, and other hormone balances, *as relevant.*

Vitamins, minerals & corresponding enzymes (Jaffe 1992, Slagle 1992, Werbach 1991, Pfeiffer Institute 2000, Watts 1990)

One to two days before testing, it's usually advisable to avoid foods (or supplements) rich in nutrients to be tested. Assays of absolute levels can fail to indicate nutrient dependencies. Readings for key related enzymes often elude this pitfall, especially if the deficient enzyme can be targeted.

□ **B1**: erythrocyte transketolase (ETK); or red cell thiamin diphosphate.

□ **B2**: erythrocyte glutathione reductase (EGR)

□ **B3**: 1NMethylnicotinamide (1NMN).

□ **B5**: not readily measured. Check for depression and stress plus high cholesterol.

□ **B6**: erythrocyte glutamate/oxalate transaminase (EGOT), kynurenic or xanthurenic acids, or red cell P5P. Test also for pyrrole disorder.

□ **Folic acid**: formiminoglutamate (FIGLU), serum folate.

□ **B12**: B12/B12 binding capacity, or serum methylmalonic acid.

□ **Biotin**: carboxylase.

□ **C**: white cell ascorbate.

□ **D**: 25(OH)D (i.e., 25-hydroxy-vitamin D).

□ **Calcium**: ionized calcium.

□ **Iron**: total iron binding capacity/% saturation, or serum ferritin.

□ **Manganese**: whole blood manganese.

□ **Potassium**: plasma potassium.

□ **Magnesium, Zinc**: plasma or red cell.

□ **Copper**: serum or plasma. Ceruloplasmin.

□ **Lithium**: serum.

Mineral loading tests — high dose copper, zinc, magnesium, manganese, or molybdenum followed, after a sufficient interval, by urinary assessment.

Electrolyte levels (24 hour urine)

Functional intracellular analysis — a blood test measuring cellular availability of key vitamins, minerals and aminos, i.e. what actually is taken to the cells. (Larson)

Amino acids, neurotransmitters (Jaffe 1992, Braverman 1987, Murray 1998, Ross 2002, Slagle 1992, Pfeiffer Inst, Gold 1987)

Typical tests: plasma aminos, 24-hour urine (reflects how the body is using aminos), serum amino chromatography (reflects tissue pools). (Slagle)

□ **Norepinephrine** — platelet, plasma or CSF NE; platelet metanephrine, or normetanephrine. Urinary MHPG, vanilmandilic acid (VMA). Check thyroid and adrenal function, and methylation.

□ **Dopamine** — Platelet DA. Urinary homovanilic acid (HVA). Thyroid, adrenals. Methylation.

□ **Serotonin** — platelet or plasma, serotonin. Urinary 5-HIAA (5-hydroxyindoleacetic acid), though concentration can change rapidly with diet, drugs, stress. (McIntyre 1984) Tryptophan loading (identifies malabsorption). Also, saliva tests for estrogen, urinary pyrroles. Methylation.

□ **Taurine** — plasma taurine, although levels can show high even when needed.

□ **GABA** — plasma GABA can be difficult to detect and may not reflect brain levels. Check for low glutamine, but elevated glutamate. Also, extremes in cortisol, or mercury toxicity, especially with high anxiety, panic, insomnia. And high progesterone (which can reduce GABA). (Braverman 1987)

□ **Glycine** — Plasma. Low serum creatinine. (Braverman)

□ **Acetylcholine** — Serum.

EFAs (See corresponding chapters for references)

□ Plasma and red cell membrane fatty acid profile. ELISA assay for measuring red cell PLA2.

□ Delta-6-desaturase.

□ Consider inflammation, cardiovascular changes, etc.

□ Response may be the most practical measure.

Toxic metals

Hair mineral/heavy metal analysis (Cutler, Jaffe 1992, Pfeiffer 1988, Pfeiffer Inst 2000, Watts 1990)

Hair analysis gives a preliminary overview of cellular mineral and heavy metal levels. It is particularly useful in evaluating tissue accumulation of heavy metals. Toxic metals plus high copper with low zinc suggest metal metabolism dysfunction. (Walsh 2006)

Readings for lead and cadmium are most accurate.

Mercury— because of its volatility, hair (as well as blood or urine) levels often yield false negatives. With amalgam illness, tin, aluminum, perhaps nickel and calcium, often test high; calcium, very high; essential elements, scattered or low; lithium, often low. (CUTLER)

Low hair chromium, manganese, vanadium, selenium etc. are often due to malabsorption. (CUTLER)

Calcium and magnesium may test high while being leached from the bones, and other minerals may similarly test high, while being depleted. This can occur with blood and urine tests as well.

Hair analysis, especially of minerals, is not definitive. It's most useful when considered along with the results of urine and blood tests, and history of exposure. Shampoos containing minerals or heavy metals, hair treatments which leach minerals, and other confounding factors should be accounted for or, ideally, avoided before testing.

Metallothionein dysfunction (WALSH 2002, 2004, 2006)

□ Elevation & increased reactivity to copper, lead, cadmium, or mercury, etc.

□ Depleted zinc and manganese.

□ Possible deficiency of B6, cysteine, and serine (which support MT activity).

□ In some cases (especially in histapenia), severe chemical and toxic metal sensitivity.

□ Milk/wheat hypersensitivity or intolerance, perhaps due to low zinc (which is required by gut enzymes that break down casein and gluten).

□ Candida overgrowth (typical in bipolars).

□ Lead: whole blood lead, upper limit erythrocyte protoporphyrin, decreased hemoglobin, hair lead. Perhaps, increased serum and whole blood copper, serum uric acid, blood spermine; decreased serum inorganic phosphate. Exposure history.

□ Mercury: whole blood,* 24 hour urine, hair mercury. CBC. History. Low T-cells, elevated white blood cells, perhaps low blood count (and B12-deficient anemia). Urine C, albumin, specific gravity and pH. Electrocardiogram. High copper which won't respond to zinc. Trial of B1, selenium, zinc, etc. (ZAMM) Plasma cysteine and sulfate (to assess sulfur needs). Plasma aminos. Urine organic acids. Elevated lactate or pyruvate.** Creatinin clearance.*** Porphyria.

* Indicates inhalation exposure.

** Can be due to interference with mitochondria, allowing carbohydrate wastes to accumulate.

*** If kidney problems are suspected.

Hormones (SEE CORRESPONDING CHAPTERS FOR REFERENCES)

□ **Thyroid** — T3, RT3, T4, TSH, TRH, and anti-thyroid (anti-TG, anti-TPO, anti-M) antibodies. Barnes basal temperature (often, the most sensitive test). Pulse. Iodine levels, lipids,* perhaps, EEG. Concurrent anemia, diabetes, allergies, arthritis, Candida; respiratory, circulatory and immune disorders. Symptoms.

□ **Adrenals** — cortisol (24-hour plasma, urinary free, peak plasma, possibly CSF). *If relevant,* 24-hr ACTH, pregnenolone, DHEA.

□ **Sex hormones** — 24-hour urine or blood tests for estradiol, estrone, estriol, progesterone, pregnenolone, free testosterone, dihydrotestosterone, androstenedione.

Other endocrine or metabolic assays, *as indicated.*

* Cholesterol over 252, triglycerides below 200, total CPK over 30, BUN/creatinine below 12, LDH over 40, cholesterol/HDL over 5, and increased B2 fraction in lipoprotein electrophoresis help corroborate low thyroid. (Bland)

Glucose metabolism (MURRAY, PFEIFFER 1988, GILASSON)

□ Dietary, symptom, medication, and family history.

□ Home testing kits can assess blood sugar when symptoms occur.

□ Glycosylated hemoglobin ($HbAl_2$) identifies hidden diabetes.

□ Glucose tolerance test — but can be too stressful

□ Blood, urine and hair analysis for relevant nutrients. Chromium, manganese and zinc may be low, compromising sugar storage, with calcium and magnesium elevated, to compensate. Also check copper, potassium, polyamines. High lead, mercury, cadmium, or arsenic can alter sugar metabolism. High copper or low magnesium may distort results.

□ Allergy tests. Candida antibodies. Other parasites, *if indicated.*

□ Adrenals, thyroid, etc., *as relevant.*

Immunity, allergies, digestive disorders (JAFFE 1992, SHAW, GRAHAM 2008, BRAVERMAN 1987)

□ Food and chemical allergies — a thorough history. ELISA ACT, RAST, EAV, ALCAT, kinesiology, or, *if advisable,* challenge tests.

□ Urinary opiates, peptides — helps detect wheat and dairy sensitivity.

□ GI profile — digestive function, intestinal permeability, parasites, bacterial overgrowth.(GRAHAM 2008, JAFFE 1992)

□ Candida antibodies — at least one of IgA, IgG, or IgM may be at 200 MONA or more.

□ Organic acids — indicates Candida, etc. (SHAW)

□ T-cell immune ratios.

□ Detox, oxidative stress, & antioxidant profiles.

□ Suspected infections (e.g., syphillis, borna, lyme disease, etc.), or autoimmune illness (e.g., lupus, fibromyalgia, MS, etc).

General health (GARDNER 1981, TAYLOR 1982, PFEIFFER 1988, JAFFE 1992, BRAVERMAN 1994)

□ Organic acids — measures amino levels (e.g., carnitine, cysteine), neurotransmitter metabolites, vitamins and minerals (including B vitamins), oxidative damage and need (including lipoic acid and CoQ10 status), detox status, mitochondrial energy production (citric acid cycle components), methylation status, dysbiosis. (GRAHAM 2008)

□ Complete blood chemistry — includes cholesterol and triglycerides, serum electrolytes, and liver, kidney, and gall bladder profiles.

□ Complete urinalysis — includes readings for glucose, albumin, ketones, acidity, hemoglobin, etc.

□ Street drugs — including amphetamines.

Diagnostic Labs

Bio Lab/ 3100 N Hillside Ave/ Witchita, KS 67219/ (316) 684-7784/ (800) 494-7785/ fax: (316) 682-2062/ www.brightspot.org/biocenter (Full service. Blood histamine, urinary pyrrole. Vitamins, minerals, lipids, toxic metals, hair analysis. Candida antibodies, parasitology. Thyroid panel. CBC. Cytotoxic food sensitivity, etc.)

Bio Health Diagnostics/ 2929 Canon St/ San Diego, CA 92106/ (800) 570-2000/ www.biodia.com (Saliva ry cortisol, DHEA, sex hormones, etc.)

Biolab Medical Unit/ The Stone House/ 9 Weymouth St/ London W1W 6DB, UK/ tel: (+44) 020 7636 5959 or 5905/ fax: (+44) 020 7580 3910/ www.biolab.co.uk/ email: info@biolab.co.uk (Vitamins (serum or red cell folate, etc.), antioxidants (GSH, etc.), minerals (ceruloplasmin, Mg loading and retention, Zn challenge, ferritin, trace minerals, etc.). Toxic metals, MT. EFAs. Pyroluria. Serum HCY. Glucose challenge, fermentation, fT4, fT3, Candida antibodies, gut permeability and function, gliadin, IgE, etc.)

Cellmate Wellness Systems (formerly Carbon Based Corporation)/ 785 Southwood Blvd, #1/ PO Box 4549/ Incline Village, NV 89451/ tel: (775) 832-8485/ website: http://www.carbonbased.com (Blood chemistry, thyroid panel, red cell membrane fatty acids, etc. Test results are matched with an extensive database of worldwide medical research.)

Diagnostechs/ 6620 South 192nd Place/ Bldg J/ Kent WA 98032/ tel: (800) 878-3787/ www.diagnostechs.com (Salivary cortisol, DHEA, thyroid. Anti-gliadin.)

Direct Healthcare Access II Laboratory/ 350 West Kensington Rd, Suite 107, Mount Prospect, IL 60056/ tel: (847) 222-9546/ www.pyroluriatesting.com (Biotype metabolic panel (includes blood histamine, urinary pyrroles, serum copper, zinc). Urine or plasma amino profile, ceruloplasmin, homocysteine, MNM, T3.)

Doctors Data/ 3755 Illinois Ave/ St Charles, IL 60174/ tel: (800) 323-2784 (US, CAN)/ tel: 0871 218 0052 (UK)/ tel: (630) 377-8139 (everywhere else)/ email: inquiries@doctorsdata.com/ www.doctorsdata.com (Toxic and essential elements in hair, red cell elements, amino acids and metabolites in blood and urine. Chemical sensitivity blood test.)

Great Plains Laboratory/ 11813 West 77th /Lenexa KS 66214/ tel: (800) 228-0383/ tel: (913) 341-8949/ fax: (912) 341-6207/ www.greatplainslaboratory.com/ email: gpl4u@aol.com (Amino acid and fatty acid metabolites. Yeast, fungal and bacterial panels. Organic acids. Opitate peptides (for dairy/gluten sensitivities), comprehensive allergies. Kreb's cycle panel. Neurotransmitter metabolites. Hair elements.) (William Shaw, PhD)

Genova Diagnostics (formerly Great Smokies Diagnostic Lab)/ 63 Zillicoa St./ Asheville, NC 28801/ tel: (828) 253-0621/ tel: (800) 522-4762/ fax: (828) 252-9303/ www.gdx.net /email: cs@gdx.net (Vitamins, minerals. Plasma aminos. Fatty acids (blood). High performance liquid chromatography. Hair elements. Allergy profile, intestinal permeability, Candida culture and antibodies; food antibodies IgG, IgE, urinary gluten, chemical sensitivity blood test, parasitology. Detox, urine toxic elements, oxidative stress and antioxidant defense profiles. Endocrine profiles.)

Meridian Valley Labs/ 801 SW 16th St #126, Renton WA 98055/ tel: (425) 271-8689/ www.meridianvalley lab.com (Comprehensive endocrine profiles. Allergies, Candida. Hair minerals, plasma EFAs, aminos, glucose, vitamins D and K.) (Associated with Tahoma Clinic.)

Metametrix Clinical Laboratory/ 3425 Corporate Way/ Duluth, GA 30096/ tel: (800) 221-4640/ fax: (770) 441-2237/ email: inquiries@metametrix.com/ www.metametrix.com (Metabolic, allergy, hormone, nutrient and toxic element panels. Fatty acids. Porphyrins. Candida antibodies. Adrenal stress. HCY. Oxidative stress. Organic acids.)

Norsom Medical Laboratories/ 497 N Hebard/ Knoxville, IL, 61448/ tel: (309) 289-2690 (Pyroluria.)

SAFE Analytical Laboratories/ PO Box 2060/ Burleigh Junction, Queensland 4220/ Australia/ tel: 61 (07) 55221919/ www.safelabs.com.au (Urinary pyrroles. Hair analysis.)

Serammune Physicians Lab/ 1890 Preston White Dr, #201/ Reston, VA 22091/ tel: (800) 553-5472/ tel: (703) 758-0610/ email: clientservices@elisaact.com (Allergies, Candida antibodies, ELISA ACT.)

Specialty Labs/ 27027 Tourney Rd/ Valencia CA 91355/ tel: (800) 421-7110 www.specialtylabs.com (SAM.)

Vitamin Diagnostics/ 2 Industrial Dr #A/ Keyport NJ 07735/ tel: (732) 583 7773. (Pyrroles, histamine. Blood platelet serotonin, catecholamines. Minerals. EFAs in red cell lining. Urinary thyroid, etc.)

No product or service endorsements or recommendations are intended. This listing is provided for informational purposes only. It is up to the reader to determine appropriate professional care.

Appendix V: Resources

No endorsements or recommendations are intended. This listing is provided for informational purposes only. It is up to the reader to determine appropriate professional care.

Orthomolecular Treatment & Research Centers

Amsterdam Kliniek, Hoogstraat 13 B/1391 BP Abcoude/ The Netherlands/ tel: 31-0-294-288-491/ fax: 31-0-294-288-492/ info@amsterdamliniek.nl/ www.amsterdamkliniek.com (Orthomolecular, environmental, cardiovascular, and life extension medicine.)

Brain Bio Centre / Institute for Optimum Nutrition/ Avalon House/ 72 Lower Mortlake Road/ Richmond TW9 2JY/ England/tel: 020 8332-9600/ www.ion.ac.uk/ foodforthebrain.org (Patrick Holford, MD)

Carl C Pfeiffer Institute/ 862 Route 518, Skillman NY 08558/ tel: (609) 924-8607/ www.suprahealth.com (Research lab. Treats allergies, sugar, osteoporosis, heart, depression, schizophrenia, autism, ADD, chronic fatigue, menopause, etc.)

Center for the Improvement of Human Functioning (formerly, Olive White Garvey Center)/ 3100 N Hillside Ave/ Wichita, KS 67219/ tel: (316) 682-3100/ fax: (316) 682-5054/ www.brightspot.org (Specializes in chronic illness and allergies/immune dysfunction. Publishes *Health Printer.* Also see, *Bio Lab,* below.)

Crayhon Research Inc/ 5355 Capital Ct #101/ Reno NV 89502/ tel: (775) 823-5333/ crayhonresearch.com

Fryer Research Center/ 30 East 40th St #608/ New York, NY 10016/ tel: (212) 808-4940 (Orthomolecular approaches for psychiatric illness, including IV and IM treatments.)

Health Recovery Center (HRC)/ 3255 Hennepin Ave South/ Minneapolis MN 55408/ tel: (612) 827-7800/ (800) 554-9155/ email: hrc@healthrecovery.com/ www.healthrecovery.com (Orthomolecular approaches for depression, anxiety, alcoholism, drug addiction.) (Joan Matthews Larson, PhD)

Institute for Optimum Nutrition (ION)/ Blades Court Deodar Road/ London, England/ SW15 2NIJ/ 0-181-877-9933. (Patrick Holford, PhD)

Linus Pauling Institute for Science and Medicine/ Oregon State University/ 571 Weniger Hall/ Corvallis, OR 97331/ tel: (541) 737-5075/ fax: (541) 737-5077/ www.lpi.oregonstate.edu (Biomedical research into the role of micronutrients, phytochemicals and other dietary constituents, in health promotion and disease prevention. *Diet & Optimum Health Conference,* May.)

Nutritional Healing Center/ Perth, Australia/ nutritional-healing.com.au (Blake Graham)

Ortho Institute/ Netherlands/ www.orthoeurope.com/intdex.htm Clinics, seminars, journals. (Dr Gert Schuitemaker)

Pfeiffer Treatment Centers / 4575 Weaver Parkway/ Warrenville, IL 60555/ tel: (630) 505-0300/ & Minnesota Pfeiffer Office/ Oakdale Square, 6230 10th Street North, Suite 310-A/ Oakdale, MN 55128/ tel: (651) 209-9282/ fax: (651) 209-9283/ www.hriptc.org (Childhood learning problems and behavior disorders; schizophrenia, depression.)

Tahoma Clinic/ 801 SW 16th St/ Suite 121/ Renton WA 98057/ tel: (425) 624-0059/fax: (425) 624-0071/ www.tahoma-clinic.com (Publishes *Nutrition & Healing.)* (Alan Gaby, MD, & Jonathan Wright, MD)

Walsh Research Institute/ 1155 South Washington St/ Naperville IL, 60540/ tel: (630) 596-5095/ www.walshinstitute.org/ email: bill.walsh@walshinstitute.org (Biotype research center. Childhood learning problems and behavior disorders. Schizophrenia, depression, bipolar disorder, etc. Physician trainings worldwide on psychiatric therapies based on extensive biochemical analysis and individualized nutritional treatments.) (William J Walsh, PhD)

Orthomolecular and Naturopathic Organizations & Conferences

American Association of Naturopathic Physicians (AANP)/ 8201 Greensboro Dr #300/ McLean, VA 22102/ tel: (703) 610-9037/ fax: (703) 610-9005/yearly conference /www.naturopathic.org

International Association of Clinical Nutrition/ 5200 Keller Springs Rd, Suite 410/ Dallas, TX 75248/ tel: (972) 250-2829/ fax: (972) 250-0233/ www.cncb.org (Referrals. Publishes *Journal of Applied Nutrition* and *Your Health.*)

International Society for Orthomolecular Medicine (ISOM) and **International Schizophrenia Foundation** (ISF)/ 16 Florence Ave/ North York, Ontario M2N 1E9/ Canada/ tel: (416) 733-2117/ fax: (416) 733-2352/ email:centre@orthomed.org/ www.orthomed.org (Publishes *Journal of Orthomolecular Medicine*, and *Nutrition and Mental Health.* Spring conference. Weblinks to international orthomolecular organizations.)

Nutrition & Vitamin Therapy Conference/ Nutritionandvitamintherapy.com/tel: (510) 845-0700/ (Michael Lesser, MD)

Orthomolecular Medical Association of Australia (OMAA)/ 13 Hilton St/ Beaumaris, Victoria 3193, Australia/ tel: 00 61 3 9589 6088/ fax: 61 3 9589 5158.

Price Pottenger Nutrition Foundation/ 7890 Broadway/ Lemon Grove, CA 91945/ tel: (800) 366-3748 or (619) 462-7600. (Supports natural, pre-industrial diet and nutritional therapies.)

Society for Orthomolecular Health Medicine/ (OHM)/ 2698 Pacific Ave/ San Francisco, CA 94115/ tel: (415) 922-6462/ fax: (415) 346-4991/ ohmsociety.com (Late winter/early spring scientific meeting.) (Dr. Richard Kunin)

Weston A Price Foundation/ PMB 106-380/ 4200 Wisconsin Ave NW/Washington DC, 20016/ tel: (202) 363- 4394/ fax: (202) 363-4396/ email: info@westonaprice.org/ www.westonaprice.org (Publishes *Wise Traditions in Foods, Farming, and the Healing Arts.*)

Educational information

Orthomolecular Vitamin Information Centre, Inc/ Suite 3a/ 2727 Quadra St/ Victoria/ BC V8T 4E5/ Canada/ tel: (250) 386-8756/ fax: (250) 386-5828/ www.orthomolecularvitamincentre.com/ email: ovicinfo@yahoo.ca/ hoffer@orthomolecularvitamincentre.com/ (Abram Hoffer, MD)

www.orthoeurope.com/ (International orthomolecular library)

Safe Harbor/ 787 West Woodbury Rd, #2/ Altadena, CA 91001/ tel: (626) 791-7868/ fax: (626) 791-7869/ email: mail@alternativementalhealth.com /www.alternativementalhealth.com (Mental health information and e-newsletter, on nutritional and medical factors affecting psychiatric function. Conference. Maintains list of practitioners.)

Townsend Letter for Doctors & Patients/ tel: (360) 385-6021/ fax: (360) 385-0699/ www.townsendletter.com (Health articles. Lists conferences.)

Newsletters: **www.cassmd.com** (Hyla Cass, MD)/ **www.doctoryourself.com** (Andrew Saul, MD)/ **www.mercola.com** (Mercola, MD)/ **www.weeksmd.com** (Bradford Weeks, MD)/ **www.thewayup.com** & **moodcure.com** (Priscilla Slagle, MD)

Support organizations

The Huxley Institute for Biosocial Researcher, 86B Dorchester Dr/ Lakewood NJ 08701 / www. schizophrenia.org (Support for the mental health consumer. Information on orthomolecular approaches.) (Elizabeth Plante)

Millennial House/ PO Box 21124/ Boulder, CO 80308/tel: (303) 641-8331/ email: drmaggie8@yahoo.com/ temporary website: www.educatebeforeyoumedicate.com (Offers othomolecular residential facilities to young people. Scheduled to open in Spring 2009.) (Maggie McClure, DC)

Well Mind Association of Greater Washington (WMAGW)/ 18606 New Hampshire Ave/ Ashton, MD 20861/ tel: (301) 774-6617/ www.ourworld.compuserve.com/homepages/WMIND (Holistic mental health clearinghouse. Newsletter, books, tapes, local talks, education, referrals.) (Alyce Ortuzar)

Well Mind Association of Minnesota/ c/o Louise Bouta/6500 Woodlake Drive/ Richfield MN 55423/ tel: (612) 823-8249/ www.wellmindminnesota.org/ info@wellmindminnesota.org (Support, orthomolecular information. Publishes *Lost Voices.*)

Well Mind Association of Seattle/ 4649 Sunnyside N/ Seattle, WA 98103/ tel: (206) 547-6167 (Newsletter, books, information, orthomolecular support group, lectures and workshops. Conference.)

Rights Protection Organizations

International Advocates for Health Freedom/ 556 Boundary Bay Road/ Point Roberts, WA 98281/ tel: (800) 333-2553 (US)/ 360 945-0352 (world)/ email: jcham@iahf.com/ www.iahf.com/ (John C Hammell, President)

National Association of Rights Protection and Advocacy (NARPA)/ PO Box 40585/ Tuscaloosa AL 35404/ tel: (205) 464-0101/ email: narpa@aol.com/ www.narpa.org (Publishes *The Rights Tenet*. Oct/Nov conference.)

National Empowerment Center/ 599 Canal St/ Lawrence, MA 01840/ tel: (800) power2u/ www.power2u.org (Peer support, drop-in centers, training to providers from consumer/survivor perspectives, referrals to statewide organizations, audio and videotapes, newsletter.)

Support Coalition International/ P.O. Box 11284/ Eugene, OR 97440/ tel: (541) 345-9106/ www.mindfreedom.org/ email: dendron@efn.org (Literature, information, support, networking. Publishes *Dendron.*)

Allergy, Clinical ecology, Toxins, Candida, Adrenals, Thyroid

Adrenal Metabolic Research Society/ 1532 Pauling Ave/ Troy, NY 12180/ (518) 272-7154. (Referrals.)

American Academy of Environmental Medicine (AAEM)/ 6505 E Central Ave #26/ Wichita KS 67206/ tel: (316) 684-5500/ fax: (316) 684-5700/ aaemonline.org/ (Directory of members, tapes, audiovisuals, referrals, books, October conference. Spring training conference.)

American Environmental Health Foundation/ 8345 Walnut Hill Lane, Suite 225/ Dallas, TX 752231/ tel: (214) 373-5132/ (800) 428-2343/ www.aehf.com (Promotes research and communication on environmental medicine.)

Broda O Barnes, MD, Research Foundation/ www.brodabarnes.org *and* **Wilsonsyndrome.com** (Thyroid info)

Candidafoundation.org

Celiac Disease Foundation/ 13251 Ventura Blvd #1/ Studio City, CA 91604/ tel: (818) 990-2354/ celiac.org// email: cdf@celiac.org/ www.celiac.org Information packet, quarterly newsletter, support.

Center for Environmental Medicine/ 10748 NE Halsey St/ Portland, OR 97220/ tel: (503) 261-0966/ fax: (503) 252-2691/ cemmed.com

Chemical Injury Info Net/ PO Box 301/ White Sulphur Springs, MT 59645/ tel: 406) 457-2255/ www.einet.net/ www.ciin.org (Support and information on chemical toxicity. Publishes *Our Toxic Times.*)

Diet Design/ PO Box 31065/ Seattle WA 98103/ tel: (206) 547-1814/ fax: (206) 547-1814. (Rotation game; self-help survival kit, referrals. Publishes a monthly newsletter, *Allergy Alert.*) (Sally Rockwell, PhD)

Electrical Sensitivity Network/ PO Box 4146/ Prescott, AZ 86302/ tel: (520) 778-4637. (Support, networking. Publishes *Electrical Sensitivity News.*)

Environmental Health Network/ PO Box 1155/ Larkspur, CA 94977/ tel: (415) 541-5075. (Support and information. Promoting public awareness of environmental sensitivities and causative factors. Publishes *The New Reactor.*)

Human Ecology Action League (HEAL)/ P.O. Box 29629/ Atlanta, GA 30359/ tel: (404) 248-1898/ fax: (404) 248-0162/ members.aol.com/HEALNatnl/ email: HEALNatnl@aol.com (Information and referrals to local chapters and support groups. Publishes *The Human Ecologist.*)

The Institute for Bio-Ecologic Medicine/ 820 NE 63rd St/ Oklahoma City, OK 73105/ tel: (405) 390-3009/ fax: (405) 840-4357. (Allergy, epilepsy, autism.) (William Philpott, MD)

Multiple Chemical Sensitivity Referral and Resources/ 2326 Pickwick Road/ Baltimore, MD 21207/ tel: (410) 448-3319/ fax: (410) 448-3317/ www.mcsrr.org (Articles, resources, support for professionals, patients.)

NO-MSG/ PO Box 367/ Santa Fe, NM 87504/ tel: (800) 232-8674 / fax: (505) 983-1733/ www.noMSG.com (Updated information, networking, newsletter.)

Northwest Center for Environmental Medicine/ 8195 166th Ave NE, #101/ Redmond WA 98052/ tel: (425) 284-1586/ drbuscher.com

Practical Allergy Research Foundation/ PO Box 60 / Buffalo NY 14223/ tel: (800) 787-8780/ (805) 356-2109/ www.drrapp.com/ www.healthychild.com. (Public awareness, research, products, teaching aids, books, audio, videotapes.) (Doris Rapp, MD)

Metals & Dental

American College for Advancement in Medicine (ACAM)//24411 Ridge Route, Ste 115/ Laguna Hills, CA 92653/ tel: (949) 309-3520/ fax (949) 309-3538/ www.acamnet.org (Spring and Fall conferences. Education on preventive and nutritional medicine. Information on metals and chelation. Referrals, reading list.)

Bio Probe/ PO Box 608010/ Orlando, FLA 32860-8010/ tel: (407) 290-9670/ (800) 282-9670/ Books, information. Publishes *Bio Probe* — for professionals.

Dental Amalgam Mercury Syndrome, Inc. (DAMS)/ P.O. Box 7249/ Minneapolis, MN 55407/ (800) 311-6265/ www.flcv.com/dams.html (Information packet. Referral list for your area.)

Environmental Dental Association/ 10160 Aviary Drive. San Diego CA 92131/ tel: (800) 388-8124 (Referrals.)

Foundation for Toxic Free Dentistry/ PO Box 608010/ Orlando, FLA 32860. (Referrals and information packet — by mail only — with SASE #10 envelope plus postage. Publishes *Dental and Health Facts.*)

Huggins Applied Healing/ 5082 List Drive/ Colorado Springs, CO 80919/ tel: (866) 948-4638/ www.hugginsappliedhealin g.com (Information and education on nontoxic dentistry.) (Hal Huggins, DDS, author, *Detoxification is Retoxification.*)

International Academy of Oral Medicine and Toxicology (IAOMT)/ 8297 Champions Gate Blvd/ Champions Gate FL 33896/ tel: (863) 420 6373/ www.iaomt.org (Professional organization limited to dentists, physicians, and researchers. Spring conference.)

www.noamalgam.com/ and **www.noamalgam.com/hairtestbook.html**/ 3006 230th Lane SE X103/ Sammamish WA 98075/ tel: (425) 557-8299/ (Andrew Hall Cutler, PhD)

Children, Autism, Hyperactivity

Autism Research Institute (ARI)/ San Diego, CA/ tel: (866) 366-3361/ www.autism.com/ (Package on autism, allergies, psychosis in children, hair mineral analysis, and violence. Publishes *Autism Research Review International.*) (Dr. Edelson)

Center for the Study of Autism/www.autism.org (Empowers parents in directing research.)

The Feingold Association of the US (FAUS)/ 554 E Main St, Suite 301/ Riverhead NY 11901/ tel: 800-321-3287/ (631) 369 9340/ fax: (631) 369-2988/ email: help@feingold.org/ www.feingold.org/ (Hyperactivity, autism, diet, monthly newsletter, *Pure Facts Food List,* literature.) (Jane Hersey, author *Why Can't My Child Behave*)

For computer links to many of these resources, visit the Borage Books website: www.boragebooks.com

Glossary

absorption — process by which the end products of food digestion pass through the epithelial cells of the gastrointestinal tract and into the circulatory system.

acetylcholine — a monoamine neurotransmitter essential to nerve/muscle communication, the initiation of short-term memory, memory storage, and parasympathetic activity.

adaptation, chronic (in allergic response) — relative decrease in sensitivity, due to prolonged or repeated exposure to an allergen. Allergies become masked. A letdown response (headache, depression, insomnia, etc.) may occur several hours after intake, but is relieved on re-exposure, fostering an addictive response to the allergen.

addiction — physical or psychological dependence causing craving and physical discomfort (withdrawal symptoms) in the absence of the addictive substance.

adrenal glands — two endocrine/exocrine glands perched on the kidneys. Secretions include cortisol, adrenalin, pregnenolone, DHEA, and sex hormones.

adrenalin — see *epinephrine.*

affect — pertaining to feelings, emotions, or mood.

agonist — a molecule that binds to certain receptors triggering receptor-specific reactions.

akathisia — a feeling of motor restlessness, typified by anxiety, extreme restlessness, and persistent pacing. In almost all cases, akathisia is produced as a side effect of antipsychotics, and can persist after withdrawal. It is also occasionally produced in Parkinson's or hysteria.

allergen — any substance, usually a protein, which causes an allergic reaction.

allergenic diet — a diet beneficial for individuals with allergies. Such diets commonly involve avoidance or limitation of foods to which the individual is allergic.

allergy — (1) an inappropriate or exaggerated immune reaction to a relatively harmless substance. Sensitization occurs when the immune system misidentifies the future allergen as a foreign antigen, and forms antibodies. On re-exposure, release of histamine, kinins, and other immune agents, create allergic reactions; (2) popularly, maladaptive response.

amino acids — the building blocks of protein. Amino acids are composed of carbon, oxygen, hydrogen, nitrogen and sometimes other elements, such as sulfur.

amino acid, essential — an amino acid indispensable to growth and life, which must be obtained from food, as it is not made by the body. Includes: threonine, leucine, isoleucine, valine, lysine, methionine, phenylalanine, tryptophan and, in infancy and sometimes childhood, histidine.

amygdala — a pair of almond-shaped regions in the temporal lobes, and an important component of the limbic system. It assigns emotional meaning to experience, and is critical to primary emotion, social communication, evaluation of emotional intent in others, and the processing and memory of emotional reactions.

anhedonia — chronic inability to experience enjoyment or pleasure.

anterior cingulate — a brain structure which acts as a gate-keeper for emotional and behavioral response to conditioned stimuli. It is critical to empathy, emotion, reward anticipation, decision-making, and creation of permanent memory. It also helps regulate heart rate, blood pressure, and other autonomic activity.

antioxidant — a substance that protects other compounds from oxidation. Antioxidants include vitamins C, E, A, bioflavonoids, carotenes, lipoic acid, glutathione, CoQ-10, pycnogenols, zinc, selenium, NAC, anthocyanins, and the enzymes: superoxide dismutase, methionine reductase, catalase, and glutathione peroxidase.

anxiety — chronic unrealistic or excessive worry, dread, or panic, typically accompanied by some sympathetic (fight-or flight) reactions.

ATP (adenosine triphosphate) — a nucleotide critical to intracellular energy transfer. It stores and releases energy for cellular activity, is used in RNA synthesis, and provides phosphorus for kinase reactions during signal transduction.

autism — a disorder, first occurring in early childhood, characterized by inability to develop social relations, preference for isolation, poverty of language, repetitive rituals, and obsessive attachment to particular objects or collections.

autoimmunity — a hypersensitivity reaction causing immune reaction to the body's own tissues. It can be caused by changes in body tissue (making it appear foreign to the immune system), or by an inability to adequately suppress lymphocytes.

autonomic nervous system — part of the peripheral nervous system which controls involuntary activities of organs, blood vessels, smooth muscles, glands, etc. It contains the *sympathetic* and *parasympathetic* nervous systems.

axon — a thin fiber which transmits neuronal impulses away from the cell body of the neuron and towards the synapse with other neurons or effectors (e.g., a gland or muscle).

basal ganglia — large nuclei at the base of the cerebral hemispheres, which control movement, particularly the initiating and stopping of movements; and also have roles in emotion, cognition, and learning. They have strong links to the cerebral cortex, thalamus and brain stem. Basal ganglia include the corpus striatum, globus pallidus, subthalamic nucleus, and substantia nigra.

basophil — a white blood cell involved in allergic reactions. Basophils are the main storage site for histamine outside the nervous system.

beriberi — a disease of the peripheral nervous system caused by thiamin deficiency. Symptoms include pain, edema, diarrhea, irritability, delirium, psychosis, and cardiovascular effects.

bioavailability — degree to which ingested nutrients are absorbed and made available to the body.

biochemical individuality — the unique individual biochemical constitution of each individual. Because people are not biochemically identical, a range exists in optimal nutrient and other requirements for maintaining health or treating any given disorder.

bioflavonoid — widely distributed water soluble pigments, present in fruits, flowers, vegetables, grains, and barks, which variously enhance the effectiveness of vitamin C; support the cardiovascular system, liver and joints; and provide anti-inflammatory and antioxidant activity. They have been used in the treatment of schizophrenia, depression, allergies, asthma, arthritis, viral infections, capillary fragility, and arteriosclerosis.

biotin — a B vitamin made by intestinal bacteria, and also found in liver, eggs, and meat. It's needed in fat, carbohydrate, and protein metabolism, and fatty acid synthesis. Deficit can cause dry skin, hair loss, nausea, glossitis, appetite loss, apathy, irritability, or depression.

biotypes, major — biochemical types often used in nutritional treatment of psychiatric illness. See *histapenia, histadelia, pyroluria.*

bipolar disorder (previously called, *manic depression*) — affective disorder in which mood swings between mania and depression.

Bipolar I — an affective disorder characterized by a history or presence of at least one manic or mixed episode (regardless of whether major depression occurs).

Bipolar II — an affective disorder characterized by a history or presence of at least one major depressive and at least one hypomanic episode, but no manic or mixed episodes.

blank mind — a mental condition characterized by periods of time in which no thought occurs.

blood brain barrier — a functional barrier which helps protect the brain from toxic substances in the blood. It can be compromised by physical brain trauma, infections affecting the central nervous system, hypertension, certain metals (e.g., lead), and increased body temperature. The barrier is weak in newborns, may not be completely developed til adulthood, and is also weak in the elderly. The hypothalamus, circumventricular organs, pineal gland, and the locus ceruleus of the brain stem do not have barrier protection.

blunted affect — an inability to express emotion and feeling in a reasonably rich and fluent manner.

brainstem — area at the base of the brain, adjacent to the spinal cord, primarily involved in life support. It controls breathing, heart rate, balance, cranial nerves, and alertness, and is important in movement. It includes the cerebellum, pons, medullar oblongata and reticular activating system.

brain waves — characteristic electrical emissions, produced by neural activity. Distinct brain wave patterns typify different stages of alertness and can reflect specific mental conditions, e.g., anxiety, depression, dementia, etc.

cAMP (3'5' - cyclic adenosine monophosphate, or cyclic AMP) — a second messenger, derived from ATP, and important in activating kinases, and regulating calcium transport through ion channels.

Candida albicans — a yeast, normally present in the gastrointestinal tract, which exists in dynamic balance with other intestinal flora.

Candidiasis — a chronic infestation of Candida albicans, commonly associated with vaginal yeast infections. Candida may also invade the mouth (*thrush*), moist skin, lungs, intestines, or other organs. Infiltration into the bloodstream can result in colonization of internal organs, including the brain.

carbohydrate — a nutrient source of fuel. Sugars, starches and cellulose are carbohydrates. *Complex carbohydrates* are found in whole grains, legumes, root vegetables, and fruits. *Refined carbohydrates*, prevalent in junk food, provide too rapid a source of fuel, without adequate nutrients to support metabolism, thus promoting blood sugar disorders and a number of degenerative diseases.

carotene— an orange-yellow pigment present in many plants and capable of being converted into vitamin A in the liver. The activity of some carotenes focus on vitamin-A type functions (e.g., supporting vision), while others are primarily antioxidant.

catatonia — a rare form of schizophrenia, also present in certain brain diseases, characterized by abnormal movement and posture, e.g., silent and immobile maintenance of odd postures for extended periods.

catecholamines — a group of neurotransmitters derived from tyrosine and phenylalanine. Catecholamines include dopamine, norepinephrine and epinephrine.

central nervous system (CNS) — brain, spinal cord and associated nerves. It produces perception, memory, thought, behavior, emotions, voluntary actions, and conscious experience.

cerebellum — two hemispheres under the occipital lobes, and attached to the brainstem. It coordinates balance, position, and motor activity, and initiates some impulses.

cerebral cortex — grey matter, about one-eighth of an inch thick, covering the surface of the cerebrum, and more densely packed with neurons than any other brain structure.

cerebrum — two hemispherical structures comprising the major part of the forebrain and the largest part of the brain. The site of most conscious and intelligent faculties and the primary coordinating center of the nervous system, governing cognitive, sensory and motor activity. It is responsible for such higher mental functions as logic, language, reason, creativity, and perception.

cheilosis — tiny lesions in the mouth, and/or cracks at the corners of the mouth. Occurs in B2 and B6 deficiency.

chelation — (1) a process in which a chelating agent, introduced into the body, binds to metals, rendering them less active and allowing for more rapid elimination; (2) a process, used in producing dietary supplements, in which minerals are made more absorbable by being bound (chelated) to amino acids and other substances.

choline — a B vitamin, and precursor of acetylcholine. It also helps maintain the myelin sheath, is a component of the neural membrane, and supports proper utilization of fats.

clinical ecology — the study and treatment of maladaptive reactions to foods and environmental agents.

coenzyme — a small molecule, often derived from a vitamin, or sometimes a mineral, required for a particular enzyme to function properly. Coenzymes combine with inactive proteins, termed *apoenzymes*, forming a complete and active enzyme, a *holoenzyme*.

coenzyme Q-10 — a coenzyme which resembles vitamin E and is an even stronger antioxidant.

cofactor — a nonprotein component, often a mineral, required for a particular enzyme to function properly. *Coenzyme* and *cofactor* are now often used interchangeably.

compulsion — a behavior an individual feels repeatedly forced to enact, often against his or her will.

COMT (catechol-O-methyl transferase) — an enzyme which breaks down catecholamines in the synapse. COMT imbalances can play a role in mood disorders.

corpus callosum — a bundle of approximately 300 million nerve fibers, which transfer information between the cerebral hemispheres.

corticosteroids — a group of hormones secreted by the adrenal cortex, including mineralocorticoids (e.g., aldosterone), 17-ketosteroids (sex hormones), and glucocorticoids (e.g., cortisol). Corticosteroids influence nutrient metabolism, sexual functioning, inflammation, immune response, and urinary excretion of salts and water.

cortisol (hydrocortisone or 17-hydroxycorticosterone) — a hormone produced by the adrenal cortex. Release is stimulated by stress, intense emotion, or injury. Cortisol suppresses inflammatory reactions to allergic and infectious agents and, somewhat, other immune activities. It also contributes to sympathetic arousal, and mediates use of fats, proteins and carbohydrates.

cortisone (11-dehydro-17-hydroxycorticosterone) — a glucocorticoid, closely allied to cortisol. Cortisone is oxidized cortisol.

cysteine — a nonessential sulfur-containing amino acid, important in providing protection from free radicals and ionizing radiation. Cysteine is a component of glutathione and glucose tolerance factor, and serves as a donor of sulfate. Isolated cysteine readily auto-oxidizes and can cause excitotoxic reactions. See *NAC*.

deficiency, nutrient — unavailability of any nutrient essential to health, either due to dietary, or secondarily, inability to effectively use, absorb, or metabolize a specific nutrient.

delusion — false beliefs, held against any argument, demonstration or other evidence to the contrary. A system of such beliefs often develops, e.g., delusions of grandeur or persecution, or involving jealousy, love, or body defects.

dementia — a progressive decline of mental ability. Dementia can result from toxicity, malnutrition, disuse, or illness.

dendrite — a treelike extension of the neuron which carries synaptic information to the nerve cell body.

dependency, nutrient — need for higher quantities of a specific nutrient than can be obtained in a good diet. Dependencies can result from genetic enzyme imbalances, or extended periods of deficiency and/or stress. They are often treatable with high levels of the nutrient, plus relevant coenzymes, precursors and activators.

depressive episode, major — an affective disorder characterized by a persistent mood of depression (despair, discouragement, apathy, irritability, self-reproach, tears, emptiness, pessimism), or loss of interest or pleasure in usual activities most of the time for at least two weeks. Plus, frequent occurrence of such symptoms as: slowed cognition, difficulty concentrating or indecisiveness, low energy, feeling of worthlessness or guilt, psychomotor agitation or retardation, sleep changes, appetite or weight changes, and recurrent thoughts of death or suicide attempts. Impairs functioning at home, school, and/or work. Not better accounted for by bereavement. Not a mixed episode and not due to medication, street drugs or a medical condition.

DHA (docosahexaenoic acid) — a long chain omega 3 fatty acid. Found in fatty fish. Important to neural membrane structure.

DMAE (dimethylaminoethanol) — a form of choline which more readily crosses the blood brain barrier and so is a more potent precursor of acetylcholine. DMAE supplements have been used in treating learning disorders, hyperactivity, and some types of depressions.

dopamine — a catecholamine neurotransmitter, and a precursor of norepinephrine. Dopamine traverses brain pathways integrating thought (frontal lobes) and emotion (limbic system). It is important to creativity, motivation, planning, judgment,concentration, learning, intelligence, activation, exploration, personality, perception of pleasure, sexual arousal, fine motor movement, and hormonal response. Excess seems to be involved in many acute psychoses.

EFA (essential fatty acid) — a fatty acid essential for normal functioning, which must be obtained from food, as it is not made in the body. Omega 3 and omega 6 are EFAs.

electron transport system — the final pathway in cellular energy production, using electrons freed by the Krebs cycle to produce energy.

endocrine glands — ductless glands, which secrete hormones directly into the blood or lymph, targeting distant organs. Endocrine glands include the thyroid, adrenals, pancreas, and pituitary.

endogenous — produced within the body.

endorphins — a group of endogenous polypeptides which produce opiate-like effects, i.e., pain suppression and a noticeably pleasurable sensation. Endorphins are stimulated by exercise, pain, and laughter. Imbalances may play a role in some depressions and psychoses.

enzyme — a complex protein, produced by living cells, which produces chemical changes in particular substrates, without itself, changing. Enzymes are often named for the substrate they act on, with the suffix *ase* attached to the end of the name (e.g., *lactase*).

EPA (eicosapentaenoic acid) — a long-chain omega 3 fatty acid, found in fatty fish (e.g. salmon, herring, cod, sardines). It counters inflammation and is critical to neural membrane function.

epilepsy — transient electrical disturbances within the brain, altering consciousness or creating convulsions.

epinephrine (also called *adrenaline*)— a brain neurotransmitter and an adrenal hormone. In response to external stress, exercise, or intense emotion (e.g., fear), it transmits sympathetic stimulation.

excitotoxins — natural or manufactured chemicals which, when present above a certain threshold, overstimulate neurons, producing nerve cell damage or death.

exorphin — an externally produced endorphin-like protein.

extrapyramidal system — a network of nerve pathways linking the cerebrum, the basal ganglia, and parts of the brain stem, and mediating voluntary movement and muscle tone.

fatty acids — the organic acids which are the building blocks of fats. They are classified as saturated or unsaturated, depending upon the number of carbon double bonds filled by hydrogen. See also, *EFA.*

folic acid — a B vitamin which supports the creation of a number of neurotransmitters, including dopamine, serotonin, and histamine. It is important in the treatment of histapenia, and some depressions.

free radicals — highly reactive molecules with at least one unpaired electron in the outer orbit. Free radicals can alter molecules of body cells, and cause extensive damage, including disruption of DNA patterns and of mitochondria; and immune, endocrine, cardiovascular, gastrointestinal, and neurological disorders.

frontal lobe — region of the cerebrum behind the forehead, which governs most brain activity. It comprehends and carries out complex actions and ideas and is critical to planning, judgment, foresight, problem-solving, decision-making, and coordinating and executing purposeful behavior. It also distinguishes similarities and differences in sensory information, and mediates attention and focus. It is important in language, cognition, personality, creativity, pleasure, drive, sexuality, adapting to new situations, and long-term memory. It is richly connected to the limbic system and RAS and thus perceives and weighs consequences of, and modifies response to, limbic emotion, suppressing unacceptable impulses, and promoting socialization.

GABA (gamma-aminobutyric acid) — an amino acid, and major inhibitory neurotransmitter. It helps the depolarized nerve recover after transmission and obstructs communication of anxiety and stress messages to motor centers.

germanium — a mineral believed to support cellular oxygenation. It is present in ginseng, garlic, aloe vera, and shiitake mushrooms.

GLA — (gamma linolenic acid) — an intermediate product in omega 6 metabolism. Found in evening primrose and black currant seed oils. As a food or supplement, it supports production of PGE1.

glial cells — "glue" cells that remove waste, provide energy, and afford other skeletal and metabolic support to the nervous system.

glossitis — inflammation of the tongue. Glossitis occurs in riboflavin, B6 and folic acid deficiency.

glucose — a simple sugar and the major source of energy for brain and body tissue. All carbohydrates are converted to glucose. Cellular metabolism of fats and protein also produces a small quantity.

glutamic acid — an amino acid and stimulatory neurotransmitter, and the source of 50% of brain neurotransmitters. It maintains and regulates cerebral tissue, helping to metabolize sugars and fats and remove ammonia and other wastes. It also converts to a 6-carbon glucose, becoming a source of brain fuel. Excess can be excitotoxic.

glutathione (GSH) — a sulfur-containing tripeptide, containing glutamate, cysteine and glycine. It is an important antioxidant, critical in methylation and liver detox. It also helps regulate cell proliferation, and supports DNA and protein synthesis, and PG metabolism.

gluten — a mixture of two proteins, glutenin and gliadin. Present in wheat, rye, oats, and barley. Some individuals are hypersensitive to gluten. See also, *celiac sprue.*

glycine — an amino acid and major inhibitory neurotransmitter, especially prevalent in the brainstem and spinal cord. It is genrally sedative, and enhances acetylcholine activity. It also stimulates glutathione peroxidase production, and benefits fats.

glycogen — a polysaccharide, the form in which glucose is stored in the liver and muscles as reserve energy.

G proteins (guanine nucleotide binding proteins)— often at the start of cell signalling pathways, modulate incoming messages and cell processes (by exchanging guanosine diphosphate for guanosine triphosphate). G proteins activate synthesis of cAMP from ATP and influence the phosphatidylinositol cycle.

gray matter — consists of nerve cell bodies, unmyelinated axons, dendrites, and glial cells. It is found chiefly on the surface of the brain, and the interior of the spinal cord.

glucose tolerance factor — a metabolic compound composed of B3, chromium, glutamate, glycine and cysteine. It works with insulin in balancing blood sugar, and is also used in lipid metabolism.

hallucination — a perception with no appropriate basis in external stimuli.

Herxheimer reaction — symptom flareups caused by toxic wastes released during extensive die-off of Candida organisms.

hippocampus (sea horse) — a temporal lobe structure which consolidates information received from the thalamus, and transfer emotionally important material to the frontal and limbic lobes for long term storage as memory.

histadelia — a condition characterized by excessive blood histamine. Histadelics typically have a rapid metabolism, and are prone to phobias, obsessions, compulsions, addictions, and severe depression. They are often labelled schizoaffective.

histamine — a polyamine and important brain neurotransmitter, mediating mood, cognition, appetite, and sleep. Histamine is also present in blood basophils and mast cells and is known for its role in allergic reactions. It also stimulates metabolism, promotes creation of hydrochloric acid, contracts smooth muscles, and plays an important role in inflammation.

histapenia — one of the five major biotypes originally found in schizophrenia. Histapenia is characterized by depressed levels of blood histamine, usually due to copper toxicity; more rarely, to allergic disruption of basophil histamine storage. Histapenics typically have a slow metabolism, food and chemical sensitivities, and such symptoms as anxiety, depression, hypomania, psychosis, paranoia.

histidine — the amino acid precursor of histamine. It is an essential amino acid in infancy and sometimes childhood. Histidine is most prevalent in animal foods.

homeostasis — a dynamic state of physiological equilibrium maintained by various body mechanisms.

homocysteine (HCY) — a chemical created in methionine and SAM metabolism. With specific enzymes and B vitamins it is metabolized into methionine or cysteine. Failing this, elevated homocysteine can alter cardiovascular, cognitive and affective function.

hormone — a secretion of an endocrine gland which enters directly into the blood or lymph and controls and regulates target substances or organs in other parts of the body.

hyperactivity — abnormally high motor activity, interfering with learning ability.

hyperparathyroid — excessive parathyroid activity. The parathyroid regulates blood calcium and phosphorus levels. Depression, delusions, hallucinations or other mental symptoms may develop.

hypersensitivity reactions — (1) inappropriate or exaggerated immune reactions to (often incorrectly) perceived threats, as in allergies; or (2) maladaptive reactions. Etiology can involve heredity, viruses, emotional stress, and/or repeated exposures.

hyperthyroidism — overactivity of the thyroid, producing such symptoms as heat sensitivity, excess perspiration, racing pulse, tremors, heart palpitations and pain, emaciation, protruding eyeballs, emotional volatility, insomnia, anxiety, and, in some cases, mania, hallucinations, delirium, or paranoia.

hypoglycemia — a condition characterized by abnormally low blood sugar, depriving the brain of fuel, often fostering mental and emotional symptoms. It can be caused by junk food, certain nutrient imbalances, glandular dysfunction, fixed allergies, toxicity, or illness.

hypomania — similar to mania, except hypomania may last only 4 days, social or occupational function is not impaired, psychotic features do not occur, and hospitalization is not required.

hyponatremia — an abnormally depressed sodium/water ratio. It can induce various mental symptoms, including psychosis. Acute hyponatremia requires medical emergency procedures.

hypothalamus — a limbic system. It coordinates the endocrine system, and regulates temperature, biological clocks, eating and drinking behavior, sleep, sex; pleasure/pain, emotion, aggression, various chemical balances, and heart rate; and also influences fat, carbohydrate and water metabolism, and the alternation of sympathetic vs parasympathetic activity. It is influenced by attachment, social interactions, and abstractions such as hope and fear.

hypothyroidism — a condition caused by thyroid underactivity and characterized by depression, slowed metabolism and mental processes, weight gain, fatigue, muscle weakness, and migraines. Severe untreated hypothyroidism may eventually produce terrifying dreams, hallucinations, paranoia, and psychosis.

inositol — a B vitamin, found in lecithin and other foods. It supports neural membrane function, is critical to signalling, and is reported to be useful in reducing anxiety and insomnia.

insomnia — chronic inability to sleep, or stay asleep.

insulin — a hormone produced by the beta cells of the pancreatic islets of Langerhans. Insulin promotes cellular absorption of glucose, and storage of glucose as glycogen.

intrinsic factor — a mucoprotein secreted by the stomach and required for B12 absorption.

isoleucine — an essential amino acid which plays a role in preventing loss of vitamin B3.

kinase — (1) enzymes which transfer phosphate from a donor (such as ADP) to a substrate molecule; (2) enzymes that catalyze conversion of a proenzyme to an active enzyme, e.g., PKA and PKC activate messenger molecules further down in the signalling cascade.

Krebs cycle (citric acid cycle) — a series of metabolic reactions, occurring in all body cells, and the major means by which the body produces energy (in the form of ATP).

lecithin — a phospholipid, found in seeds and nuts, and prevalent in the brain and nerves. Lecithin contains phosphatidyl choline, and phosphatidyl inositol.

lipids — oily fats connected to water soluble molecules

limbic system — a collection of interconnected brain structures critical to emotion (especially if related to survival); the integration of emotional with physical memory; motivation, behavior, smell, and various autonomic functions. It includes the hippocampus, amygdala, cingulate gyrus, nucleus acumbens, hypothalamus, and various other structures, and is closely linked to the cortex.

lipoic acid — a potent, sulfur-containing antioxidant, effective in both fat and water soluble tissue.

malabsorption — impaired absorption of nutrients.

maladaptive response — an inappropriate or exaggerated reaction to a food or environmental substance. Maladaptive responses include, but are not limited to, the typical antibody-antigen reactions which occur in conventionally-defined allergies.

mania — an affective disorder characterized by a persistent and abnormally elevated, expansive, or irritable mood, combined with at least three (four if only irritable) of the following symptoms: grandiosity, increased talkativeness or pressure of speech, racing thoughts or flight of ideas, distractibility, decreased need for sleep, psychomotor agitation or increased goal-directed ventures, increased indulgence in pleasurable, high-risk activities. Includes psychotic features, impaired social relationships or work, or risk of harm to self or others, significant enough to result in hospitalization. Not a mixed episode or caused by a medical condition, antidepressants or other medication, or street drugs.

manic depression — see *bipolar disorder.*

melatonin — a neurotransmitter secreted by the pineal gland in inverse response to daylight. It plays a role in Circadian rhythm, sleep, and immune function.

metabolism — (1) the absorption, assimilation, utilization and elimination of ingested food; (2) the rate of energy production and expenditure in the body.

metallothioneins (MT) — small, cysteine-rich proteins which regulate levels of divalent metals (copper, zinc, manganese, lead, cadmium), and help maintain intestinal mucosa and blood brain toxic metal barriers and counter Candida. They are also used in the development of brain cells and neural connections.

methyl — CH3 group.

methylation — transfer of methyl groups. Methylation helps produce, activate, and break down catecholamines and other neurotransmitters. It also helps maintain myelin, repair proteins, foster cell membrane fluidity, transport and eliminate fats, maintain and protect DNA, regulate gene expression, differentiate cells into body parts at conception, and control estrogen levels.

methionine — an essential, sulfur-containing amino acid, critical to methylation, and important in protecting the liver.

mitochondria — organelles which serve as cellular energy factories.

mixed episode (dysphoric mania) — criteria for both manic and depressive episodes are met nearly every day for at least one week.

molybdenum — an essential trace metal, which supports use of sulfur amino acids. It also interferes with copper absorption, making it sometimes useful for histapenia.

monoamine neurotransmitters — neurotransmitters containing one amine group, such as, dopamine, norepinephrine, serotonin.

monoamine oxidase (MAO)— a copper-containing enzyme which oxidizes and breaks down monoamine neurotransmitters and certain enzymes. Low levels may be important in mania and paranoia; elevation, in depression.

myelin sheath — the lipid and protein membrane forming a protective sheath around the axonal shafts of certain nerve cells, and increasing the efficiency of impulse conduction.

NAC (N-acetylcysteine) — an excellent source of cysteine, and a potent antioxidant. It supports formation of glutathione (which serves as a cysteine reservoir).

NAD (nicotinamide-adenine dinucleotide) — a niacinamide compound critical to cellular metabolism and respiration.

negative symptoms (schizophrenia) — include blunted affect, lack of logical connection between words or thoughts, poverty of speech, inability to initiate behavior and carry it through, anhedonia, blank mind, and attentional impairment.

nerve — bundle of neural fibers travelling to a common location.

nerve cell body — cell body of the neuron, responsible for maintenance, repair, and activity of the cell, including production of messenger substances, and energy for the creation and transmission of impulses.

nervous system (human) — a vast network of nerve cells (in the brain, spinal cord, and rest of the body) linked to sensory receptors and effector organs.

neural membrane— the structure which surrounds the nerve cell, providing insulation, promoting communication, and acting as a gatekeeper. It is composed of a double layer of lipids. Enzymes, receptors, and transport proteins, embedded in the membrane, transfer electrolytes and amino acids and send and receive signals.

neuron — the basic cellular unit of the nervous system, consisting of the nerve cell body, axon, and dendrites.

neuropeptides — simple proteins which act as neurotransmitters, mediating emotions, hunger (e.g., CCK), pain (e.g., endorphins), sleep (e.g., melatonin) and other behaviors.

neurotoxin — any substance poisonous, harmful, or destructive to nerve tissue. A substance may be beneficial or relatively harmless at one level of intake, and neurotoxic at greater levels.

neurotransmitter — small molecules, secreted at the axon terminal, which travel across the synapse to the receptors of the postsynaptic neuron (or effector organ), where they act to stimulate or inhibit neural impulses (or effector activity). *Inhibitory* neurotransmitters decrease the likelihood that the postsynaptic neuron will fire. *Excitatory* (stimulatory) neurotransmitters increase that likelihood.

neutralization — in allergy treatment, administration, over perhaps six months, of very weak dilutions of an allergen, in order to desensitize the immune system, allowing for gradual reintroduction of the allergen on an occasional basis.

niacin, niacinamide — forms of vitamin B3, a nutrient abundant in meats. It is critical to brain metabolism and respiration, mood, and cognition. See also *NAD.*

nicotinic acid, nicotinamide — older terms for *niacin, niacinamide.* Not to be confused with nicotine.

norepinephrine (also called *noradrenaline*)— a brain and sympathetic nervous system neurotransmitter, and a hormone of the adrenal medulla. It mediates intellectual performance, motivation, learning ability, arousal, pleasure, anxiety, aggression, and anger.

obsession — recurring irrational or disturbing thoughts a person cannot prevent.

obsessive compulsive disorder (OCD) — a condition, related to anxiety, involving unwanted thoughts or patterns of compulsive/ritualistic behavior that interfere with normal function.

occipital lobe — a lobe in the posterior cerebrum; it includes the visual cortex.

orthomolecular psychiatry — a practice of psychiatry, the focus of which is to restore mental health by providing optimal intake of substances normally present in the brain (e.g., vitamins), and removing substances which interfere with brain activity (e.g., toxins).

pancreas — an endocrine and exocrine gland, located behind the stomach. The pancreas supplies *bicarbonate,* which neutralizes stomach acid as food enters the small intestine; and digestive enzymes, which break down carbohydrates (*amylase*), fats (*lipase*), proteins (*chymotrypsin* and *trypsin*), and nucleic acids. Its *islets of Langerhans* secretes *insulin* and *glucagon,* which regulate blood glucose.

panic attack — a sudden rapid onset of intense psychological distress or terror (e.g., of dying or going insane) with such symptoms as trembling, sweating, dizziness, tingling, choking, shortness of breath, palpitations, heart attack symptoms, etc. It's mostly associated with a misplaced flight-or-flight response, and usually a flood of adrenaline and perhaps suppressed acetylcholine.

pantothenic acid — vitamin B5, an essential constituent of coenzyme A, acetylcholine, steroids, cortisol, hemoglobin, and antibodies. Deficit can produce fatigue, sullenness, insomnia, profound depression.

paranoia — an elaborate and fixed system of beliefs, based on a delusion that people or events carry some special significance related to oneself. It builds gradually around distorted interpretations of people's motives and actions, and the meaning of events. Typical themes include persecution, jealousy, love, or grandeur. Anger, suspicion, grandiosity, rigidity, and social isolation are common. Paranoids rarely consider themselves ill. Insomnia, drug use, or hearing loss can be triggers. Copper toxicity may often be involved.

parasympathetic nervous system — a division of the autonomic nervous system which relaxes the body, conserving energy. It primarily opposes sympathetic reactions and predominates during sleep.

parathyroids — small glands which rest on top of the two lobes of the thyroid and which control calcium and phosphorus levels.

parietal lobe — a region between the frontal and occipital lobes of the cerebrum, which receives information about touch and spatial orientation.

PEA (phenylethylamine) — formed from D-phenylalanine, may be the chemical most responsible for the feeling of "being in love." High levels can produce paranoia or psychosis. PEA may be deficient in bipolar depression, elevated in some manias.

pellagra — a nutritional disorder caused by insufficient vitamin B3 and tryptophan. Pellagra is characterized by the four Ds: dermatitis, diarrhea, dementia, and death.

phenylalanine — an essential amino acid, and precursor of tyrosine.

phobia — a deep persistent fear or dread of a certain object or situation.

phospholipids — fat/phosphorus compounds, which form the basic structural element of the cell membrane and its receptors, and are critical in conveying and activating neural response.

pineal gland — a gland at the base of the brain which governs response to light, and produces melatonin which regulates sleep.

pituitary gland (master gland) — an endocrine gland located in the limbic area of the brain, and heavily influenced by the hypothalamus. Its secretions stimulate hormone release in other glands.

porphyrin — a chemical containing a porphyrin ring, which is composed of four linked pyrrole rings. Porphyrins are found in various blood and respiratory pigments and are the basis of heme (in blood hemoglobin).

post-traumatic stress disorder (PTSD) — a disorder characterized by reliving traumatic events through nightmares, flashbacks or overreaction to triggers. Symptoms can also include irritability, angry outbursts, hypervigilence, insomnia, psychic numbing, anhedonia, depression, dissociation, memory and concentration problems, and avoiding associated people, surroundings, or feelings.

poverty of speech — scarcity of thoughts or their expression.

precursor — a substance from which another is derived.

prostaglandins (PGs) — a group of long-chain fatty acids which the body makes from EFAs. Hormones frequently stop at the cell membrane, initiating creationg of prostaglandins, which transfer their messages into the cell. PGs mediate nerve firing, immune reactions, pain perception, calcium metabolism, water retention, insulin effectiveness, muscle contractions, blood pressure, etc.

protein — the chief constituent of body tissue, composed of various amino acids, and required for growth and repair.

psychosis — loss of contact with reality, accompanied by an inability to think, perceive or judge clearly. Symptoms include hallucinations, delusions, social withdrawal.

pyridoxal-5-phosphate (P5P) — an intermediate product in B6 metabolism, especially useful when the ability to convert B6 is impaired.

pyridoxine, pyridoxal, and pyridoxamine — forms of vitamin B6, which is important to amino acid, carbohydrate and fat metabolism; hormonal balance; and neurological and immune function.

pyroluria — one of the major biotypes found in bipolar disorders and characterized by pyrrole accumulation, which depletes B6 and zinc. Symptoms include heightened susceptibility to stress, irritability (perhaps violence), nausea, immune dysfunction, anemia, joint pain.

pyrrole — unsaturated five-atom ring, containing four carbons, one nitrogen, and two carbon double bonds. A ring of four pyrroles composes the basic structure of the porphyrin molecule.

quercetin — a bioflavonoid which helps reduce inflammation and bruising; and strengthens basophil and mast cell membranes, preventing histamine loss.It's sometimes used in treating histapenia.

rapid cycling — at least 4 major depressive, manic, mixed, or hypomanic episodes per year; with partial or full remission between episodes of at least 2 months, or a switch to the opposite episode.

rebound psychosis — a psychosis which may develop when neuroleptic intake is stopped, especially with abrupt withdrawal.

receptor — specialized cells on the neural membrane and on effector organs, which receive neurochemical messages.

REM — rapid eye movement sleep, a light sleep stage in which dreaming occurs. Brain electrical activity, temperature and blood flow increases. The brain wave pattern is like that when awake.

reticular formation — densely packed neurons in the brainstem, regulating consciousness and attention.

reuptake mechanism — reabsorption of neurotransmitters from the synapse back into the presynaptic neuron.

riboflavin — vitamin B2, a yellow-green pigment, found in milk, leafy greens, and organ meats. It's important in amino acid, glucose, and fatty acid metabolism. Deficit can produce symptoms ranging from irritability and moodiness to depression and psychosis.

SAMe (S-adenysylmethionine) — a major brain and liver methylator, important in activating mood-modulating neuerotransmitters, and recently studied as an antidepressant. It also alters signalling; and supports membrane fluidity, immunity, and energy production.

schizoaffective disorders — psychotic disorder combining elements of both schizophrenia and affective disorder.

schizophrenia — (1) a group of psychotic disorders in which a number of the following symptoms occur over an extended period of time: delusions, hallucinations, disorganized speech and behavior, catatonia, negative symptoms, and deterioration in interpersonal, academic, occupational, and self-care functions; (2) dysperceptions, combined with an inability to judge whether these dysperceptions are real or not.

scurvy — a disease caused by a serious deficiency of vitamin C, disturbing normal production of collagen, and causing hemorrhages. Mental symptoms can include irritability, depression, hysteria and, in some cases, psychosis.

second messengers — chemicals which convey information from the neural membrane into the cell. Second messengers include G proteins, cAMP, cyclic GMP, IP3, phosphatidylinositols, and DAG. Second messenger instability may be critical to bipolar disorder.

serotonin — a monoamine neurotransmitter involved in mood, sleep, REM sleep, sensory perception, and body temperature. Deficiency has been associated with anxiety, depression, insomnia, and aggression. See also, *tryptophan.*

signal transduction — process by which the interaction of a neurotransmitter or other agonist with the neural receptor, activates a second messenger system, creating a cascade of biochemical events which convey information into and through the cell, reaching the nucleus and its genetic library, influencing biochemistry and activity.

stereotyped response — a repetitive and rigid response, occurring mechanically and not serving any useful purpose.

stress — imposition a stimulus to which one must adapt or adjust.

striae — subcutaneous breaks in the skin, typically on the hips. thighs, stomach, breasts or shoulders, and often accompanying significant weight gain, or extended B6 depletion.

substrate — the specific organic substance upon which a particular enzyme acts.

supersensitivity psychosis — a psychosis produced in reaction to neuroleptic suppression of dopamine. To compensate the brain may increase dopamine production, or create additional or supersensitive dopamine receptors which, in some cases, foster a psychosis, usually following reductions in drug dose, perhaps some time therafter.

sympathetic nervous system — a division of the autonomic nervous system which increases energy consumption, for fight-or-flight reactions to stress. It releases epinephrine and norepinephrine, and quickens and strengthens the pulse, widens airways, dilates blood vessels in the muscles, constricts those in the skin and abdomen, and dilates the pupils.

synapse — microscopic space between two nerve cells, across which a neurotransmitter signal may pass. One neuron may form hundreds to many tens of thousands of synapses with other neurons.

tardive dyskinesia (TD) — a chronic condition characterized by involuntary and repetitive muscle spasms, and caused almost entirely by extended intake of neuroleptics.

taurine — an amino acid and inhibitory neurotransmitter, which suppresses norepinephrine, acetylcholine and glutamic acid, and augments GABA. Taurine is reported to benefit insomnia, anxiety, hyperthyroidism, and epilepsy.

temporal lobe epilepsy (TLE) — an epilepsy involving abnormal electric discharges in the temporal lobe. Misdiagnosis as mood disorder or psychosis is not uncommon.

temporal lobes — a brain region found in the cerebral lobes near the temples, critical to mood and important in memory, perception, language, spatial tasks, and the interpretation of experience. The temporal lobes contain the auditory projection area.

thalamus — located in the center of brain, it evaluates and interprets environmental events (except smell), and sends out instructions, i.e. it ties stimuli to physical and emotional reactions. It's also critical in controlling brain wave rhythms, and helps initate consciousness, and determine stages of sleep/alertness.

thiamin — vitamin B1, used in key metabolic reactions (e.g., carbohydrate and fat metabolism) can play a role in addressing memory problems, irritability, aggression, depression, and psychosis.

thought disorder — abnormalities in the structure or content of thought, producing disorganized speech, behavior, or writing. It can involve illogical connections between thoughts (*alogia*), invention of new words (*neologisms*), thought blocking, thought insertion or withdrawal, and auditory hallucinations.

thymus — an endocrine gland located on the trachea, which mediates immune development and response, and produces T-lymphocytes.

thyroid — a horseshoe shaped endocrine gland located in the neck, and critical to metabolic function.

tolerance — physiological adaptation in which increased doses (e.g., of a drug), are required to produce the same effect as previously.

transcription factors — proteins which influence gene expression by contributing to (or blocking) transfer of genetic code via the synthesis of RNA from a DNA template. Transciption factors regulate all cell activity including cell memory, ion channels, and receptor chemicals.

tryptophan — an essential amino acid, a precursor of serotonin and B3. Deficit can be implicated in depression, anxiety, OCD, and eating disorders.

tyrosine — a nonessential amino acid, formed from phenylalanine. Tyrosine is the precursor of dopamine, norepinephrine, epinephrine, and thyroid hormones.

ultra rapid cycling — A very rapid alternation of manic and depressive symptoms (over days), often diagnosed bipolar disorder not otherwise specified.

Nutrient names

Vitamin B1 .... Thiamin
Vitamin B2 .... Riboflavin
Vitamin B3 .... Niacin, niacinamide
Vitamin B5 .... Pantothenic acid
Vitamin B6 .... Pyridoxine, pyridoxal, pyridoxamine
Vitamin C .... Ascorbic acid

References

Introduction

Altman ES, Rea NM, et al, "Prodromal symptoms and signs of bipolar relapse: A report based on prospectively collected data," *Psychiat Res*, 41(1): 1-8; 1/1992.

Angst J, Sellaro R, "Historical perspectives and natural history of bipolar disorder," *Biol Psychiat*, 48:445-7; 2000.

Bauer M, "Rapid cycling," in R Joffe, J Calabrese, eds, *Anticonvulsants in Psychiatry*, Marcel Dekker, NY, 1994; pp. 1-26.

Bellack AS, Morrison RL, et al, "Social competence in schizoaffective disorder, bipolar disorder, and negative and non-negative schizophrenia," *Schiz Res*, 2:391-401; 1989. (Poor psychosocial outcome correlated with symptoms and comparable to what occurs in schizoaffectives and positive symptom schizophrenics.)

Bowden CL, "Comparison of open versus blinded studies in bipolar disorder," in JF Goldberg, M Harrow, eds, *Bipolar disorders: Clinical course and outcome*, Am Psychiatric Press, 1999; pp 149-70.

Bratfos O, Haug JO, [The course of manic-depressive psychosis: A follow-up investigation of 215 patients], *Acta Psychiatr Neurolog Scandinavica*, 44:89-112; 1968.

Brigham PM, "The Psychopharmacology of Bipolar Disorder," updated 5-9-2001. At: http://people.ne.mediaone.net/pmbrig/BP_pharm.html

Carlson GA, Kotin J, et al, "Follow-up of 53 bipolar manic-depressive patients," *Br J Psychiat*, 124: 134-9; 1974.

Cass H, *Supplement Your Prescription, What your doctor doesn't know about nutrients*, Basic Health Publications, Laguna Beach CA, 2008.

Child & Adolescent Bipolar Foundation, "About early-onset bipolar disorder," 2002, www.bpkids.org

Compton MT, Nemeroff CB, "The treatment of bipolar depression," *J Clin Psychiat*, 61(9):57-67; 2000.

Coryell W, Keller M, et al, "Bipolar II illness: Course and outcome over a five-year period," *Psychol Med*, 19:129-41; 1989.

Coryell W, Endicott J, Keller M, "Outcome of patients with chronic affective disorder: A five-year follow-up," *Am J Psychiat*, 147:1627-1633; 1990.

Coryell W, Scheftner W, et al, "The enduring psychosocial consequences of mania and depression," *Am J Psychiatr*, 150:720-27; 1993. (Mixed affectives, 5 years later, still show educational and occupational deficits, even if recovered.)

Coryell W, Solomon D, et al, "Lithium discontinuation and subsequent effectiveness," *Am J Psychiat*, 155: 895-98; 1998.

Cott A, "From the traditional approach to biochemical treatment," *J Orthomol Psychiat*, 6(2): 178-82; 1977.

Darman A, "Natural treatment of manic depression explained," At: geocities.com/allen_dar/index.html Accessed: 3/2008.

deGroot L, Verheijden MW, et al, "Lifestyle, nutritional status, health, and mortality in elderly people across Europe: A review of the longitudinal results of the SENECA study," *J Geront Series A*, 59: 1277-84; 2004. (Healthy lifestyle delayed onset, reduced dependence and mortality, increased perception of health. Inactivity, smoking, and poor diet increased mortality.)

DeLiz A, "Large amounts of nicotinic acid and vitamin B12 in the treatment of apparently irreversible psychotic conditions found in patients with low levels of folic acid," *J Orthomol Psychiat*, 8(2): 63-5; 1979.

Denicoff KD, Smith-Jackson EE, et al, "Comparative prophylactic efficacy of lithium, carbamazepine, and the combination in bipolar disorder," *J Clin Psychiat*, 58:470-78; 1997.

Denson S, "The value of nicotinamide in the treatment of schizophrenia," *Dis Ner Sys*, 23: 167-72; 1962.

Dion G, Tohen M, et al, "Symptoms and functioning of patients with bipolar disorder six months after hospitalization," *Hosp Comm Psychiat*, 39:652-57; 1988. (80% did not have symptoms 6 months later, but only 43% worked; only 21% at prior levels.)

Fieve RR, *Moodswing*, Bantam Books, 1976.

Frye MA, Ketter TA, "Defining the Standard of Care Across the Bipolar spectrum: Q & A, Faculty: Mark A Frye MD, Terrence A Ketter MD," April 9, 2000; Bipolar Disorders Information Center, SF, at: http://www.mhsource.com/bipolar/defketter.html (Mood stabilizers may push cycling toward depression, mania, or greater severity; psychosis may emerge or worsen.)

Fugh-Berman A, Cott JM, "Dietary supplements and natural products as psychotherapeutic agents," *Psychosom Med*, 61(5):712-28; 1999.

Gelenberg AJ, Hopkins HS, "Report on efficacy of treatments for bipolar disorder," *Psychopharmacol Bull*, 29(4):447-56; 1993. (Optimal treatment adds about 10 years of major activity; 9 of health.)

Gelenberg AJ, Kane JM, et al, "Comparison of standard and low serum levels of lithium for maintenance treatment of bipolar disorder," *N Engl J Med*, 321:1489-93; 1989.

Gillberg IC, Heligren L, et al, "Psychotic disorders diagnosed in adolescence: Outcome at age 30 years," *J Child Psychol Psychiat*, 34:1173-85; 1993.

Gitlin MJ, Swendsen J, et al, "Relapse and impairment in bipolar disorder," *Am J Psychiat*, 152:1635-40; 1995.

Gold M, *The Good News About Depression*, Villard Books, NY, 1987.

Goodwin FK, Foreword, in JF Goldberg, M Harrow, eds, *Bipolar disorder: Clinical course and outcome*, American Psychiatric Press, DC, 1999; pp xii-xvii.

Green G, "Subclinical pellagra: Its diagnosis and treatment," *Schizophrenia*, 2(2-3):70-79; 1971.

Haddad P, Dursun S, [Pharmacological management of bipolar depression], *Acta Psychiatr Scand*, 105: 401-3; 2002.

Harrow M, Goldberg J, et al, "Outcome in manic disorders. a naturalistic follow-up study," *Arch Gen Psychiatr*, 47:665-71; 1990. (1.7 years postmania, 23% were continuously unemployed, 36% underemployed; significantly worse than for depressives. Social function was moderately impaired or worse in 36%. Psychotic mania was associated with profound impairment.)

Hastings D, "Follow-up results in psychiatric illness," *Am J Psychiat*, 114:1057-66; 1958 . (60% had unsatisfactory social recovery.)

D Hawkins, L Pauling, eds, *Orthomolecular Psychiat*, WH Freeman and Co, SF, 1973.

Heiden A, "Treatment of severe mania with intravenous magnesium sulphate as a supplemental therapy," *Psychiat Res*, 89(3):239-46; 1999.

Hodges RE, Hood J, "Clinical manifestations of ascorbic acid deficiency in man," *Am J Clin Nutr*, 24:432-43; 1971. (Depression is often the first symptom of clinical scurvy.)

Hoffer A, "Treatment of schizophrenia with nicotinic acid and nicotinamide," *J Clin Exp Psychopath*, 18: 131-58; 1957.

Hoffer A, "Massive niacin treatment in schizophrenia: Review of a nine-year study," *Lancet*, 1:316-20; 1962. (Double blind.)

Hoffer A, Osmond H, *How to live with Schizophrenia*, University Books, Secaucus, NJ, 1972.

Hoffer A, "Mechanism of action of nicotinic acid," in D Hawkins, L Pauling, eds, *Orthomolecular Psychiatry, Treatment of Schizophrenia*, WH Freeman and Co, SF, 1973.

Hoffer A,, "Hong Kong Veterans Study," *J Orthomol Psychiat*, 3(1):34-36; 1974.

Hoffer A, *Orthomolecular Medicine For Physicians*, Keats, New Canaan, CN, 1983.

Hoffer A, "Nutrition and behavior," in J Bland, ed, *Medical Applications of Clinical Nutrition*, Keats, New Canaan, CN, 1983.

Hoffer A, *Common Questions about Schizophrenia and their Answers*, Keats, New Canaan, CN, 1987.

Hoffer, Abram, MD, PhD, interview with author, March, 1995.

Hoffer A, "Schizophrenia: An evolutionary defense against severe stress," *Townsend Letter for Doctors & Patients*, 2-3/1996; pp 52-61.

Hoffer A, *Adventures in Psychiatry, The Scientific Memoirs of Dr Abram Hoffer*, KOS Pub, Caledon, ON, Canada, 2005.

Horrobin DF, "The role of essential fatty acids in schizophrenia," ISOM, Nutritional Medicine Today Conference, Vancouver, BC, 4/2000a.

Horrobin DF, "Phospholipid metabolism and depression: New clinical trials," *Eur Psychiat*, 17(1):76; 5/2002.

Joliffe N, "Treatment of neuropsychiatric disorders with vitamins," *JAMA*, 11/1/1941.

Kahan FH, "Out of the Quicksands," *J Orthomol Psychiat*, 6(2):87-104; 1977.

Kay DS, Naylor GJ, et al, "The therapeutic effect of ascorbic acid and EDTA in manic-depressive psychosis: Double-blind comparisons with standard treatments," *Psychol Med*, 14(3):533-9; 8/1984.

Keller, MA, "The course of manic-depressive illness," *J Clin Psychiat*, 49S:4-7; 1988.

Ketter TA, "Defining the Standard of Care Across the Bipolar Spectrum: Q & A," April 9, 2000; DC, Bipolar Disorders Information Center, at: http://www.mhsource.com/bipolar/defketter.html

Ketter TA, Kimbrell TA, et al, "Effects of mood and subtype on cerebral glucose metabolism in treatment-resistant bipolar disorder," *Biol Psychiat*, 49(2):97-109; 1/15/2001.

Kidd PM, "Bipolar disorder as cell membrane dysfunction, Progress toward integrative management," *Alt Med Rev*, 9(1):107-135; 2004.

Klerman G, Olfson M, et al, "Measuring the need for mental health care," *Health Affairs*, 11:23-33; 1992.

Klerman GL, Weissman MM, "Increasing rates of depression," *JAMA*, 261(15):2229-35; 4/1989. (Large epidemiologic and family studies. Increased post WWII, and decreased age of onset in US, Canada, Sweden, Germany, New Zealand, but NOT Korea, Puerto Rico, Mexican Americans.)

Kukopulos A, Reginaldi D, et al, "The long term prophylaxis of affective disorders," *Adv Biochem Psychopharmacol*, 49:127-47; 1995.

Larson JM, *Depression Free, Naturally*, Ballantine Wellspring, NY, 2001.

Larson, Joan M, PhD, interview with author, June 9, 2008.

Lemmo W, "Natural Treatment of Acute Mania," *International Guide to the World of Alternative Mental Health*, #30. At: www.alternativementalhealth.com/articles

Lesser M, *Nutrition & Vitamin Therapy*, Bantam Books, NY, 1983.

Lesser, Michael, MD, interview with author, 8/2008.

Lish J, Dime-Meenan S, et al, *J Affect Disord*, 31: 281-94; 1994.

Maj M, Piozzi R, Kemali D, [Long term outcome of lithium prophylaxis in patients initially classified as complete responders], *Psychopharmacol* (Berl), 98: 535-38; 1989. (Breakthrough episodes after 2 yrs in a substantial number of initially lithium-responsive and remitted patients. More, over 5 yrs.)

MacQueen GM, Young LT, et al, [A review of psychosocial outcome in patients with bipolar disorde], *Arch Psychiatr Scand*, 103:163-70; 2001.

Marano HE, "Managing bipolar disorder: A major advancement in treatment helps those who suffer," *Psychol Today*, 6/30/2005.

Masters JC, "When lithium does not help: The use of anticonvulsants and calcium channel blockers in the treatment of bipolar disorder in the older person," *Geriatr Nurs*, 17(2):75-8; 3-4/96. (Each manic episode increases the risk of progressively more severe episodes, more closely spaced.)

Mental Health Today at: http:www.mental-health-

today.com/bp/dep.htm
Meyers S, "Use of neurotransmitter precursors for treatment of depression," *Altern Med Rev,* 5: 64-71; 2000.
Mintz J, Mintz LI, et al, "Treatment of depression and the functional capacity to work," *Arch Gen Psychiat,* 49:761-68; 1992.
Moller HJ, Nasrallah HA, "Treatment of bipolar disorder," *J Clin Psychiat,* 64:9-17; 2003.
Murray MT, Pizzorno J, *Encyclopedia of Natural Medicine,* Prima, Rocklin, CA, 1998.
O'Connell RA, Mayo JA, et al, "Outcome of bipolar disorder on long-term treatment with lithium," *Br J Psychiat,* 159:123-29; 1991.
Owens MJ, "Molecular and cellular mechanisms of antidepressant drugs," *Depress Anxiety,* 4:153-59; 1996.
Pauling L, "Orthomolecular Psychiatry," *Science;* 4/19/1968; p 268.
Perry A, Tarrier N, "Randomized controlled trial of efficacy of teaching patients with bipolar disorder to identify early symptoms of relapse and brain treatment," *BMJ,* 318(7177):149-53; 1/16/1999.
Pfeiffer CC, *Nutrition and Mental Illness*, Healing Arts Press, Rochester, VT, 1987.
Pfeiffer CC, *The Schizophrenias, Ours To Conquer*, Bio-Communications Press, Wichita, KS, 1988.
Plumlee AA, "Biological rhythms and affective illness," *J Psychosoc Nurs,* 24:12-17; 1986. (92% report finishing high school; 60%, further education.)
Popper CW, "Do vitamins or minerals (apart from lithium) have mood-stabilizing effects?" *J Clin Psychiat*, 62:933-5; 2001.
Popper, Simmons, "Nutritional approach to bipolar disorder," *J Clin Psychiat,* 64; 2003.
Post RM, Leverich GS, et al, "Carbamazepine prophylaxis in refractory affective disorders: A focus on long-term follow-up, *J Clin Psychopharmacol,* 10:318-27; 1990.
Post RM, "Transduction of psychosocial stress into the neurobiology of recurrent affective disorder," *Am J Psychiat,* 149:999-1010; 1992.
Post RM, Ketter TA, et al, "Assessment of anticonvulsant drugs in patients with bipolar affective illness," in I Hindmarch, PD Stonier, eds, *Human Psychopharmacology Methods and Measures,* V4, Wiley, Chichester, England, 1993a; pp 71-84.
Post RM, Leverich GS, et al, "Lithium tolerance and discontinuation as pathways to refractoriness," in NJ Birch, C Padgham, MS Hughes, eds, *Lithium in Medicine and Biology,* Marius Press, Lancashire, England, UK, 1993b; pp 72-84. (34.8% of 66 patients developed tolerance over long term prophylaxis.)
Post RM, Weiss SRB, "The neurobiology of treatment-resistant mood disorders," in FE Bloom, DJ Kupger, eds, *Psychopharmacology: The Fourth Generation of Progress,* Raven Press, NY, 1995; pp 1155-1170.
Post RM, Denicoff KD, et al, "Long-term outcome of anticonvulsants in affective disorders," in JE Goldberg, M Harrow eds, *Bipolar Disorders: Clinical Course and Outcome,* Am Psychiatric Press, Inc, DC, 1999.
Post RM, Leverich GS, "A re-evaluation of the role of antidepressants in the treatment of bipolar depression: Data from the Stanley Foundation Bipolar Network," *Bipolar Disorders,* 5(6):396; 12/2003. (Antidepressant augmentation created modest response over 2 months, though 35% relapsed by a year and 18% switched to hypomania or mania.)
Quillin P, *Healing Nutrients,* Contemporary Books, Chicago, 1987.
Quiroz JA, Singh J, et al, "Emerging experimental therapeutics for bipolar disorder: Clues from the molecular pathophysiology," *Molec Psychiat,* 9: 756-76; 2004.
Richman DL, *Dr Caligari's Psychiatric Drugs,* Network Against Psychiatric Assault, Berkeley, 1992.
Sarantidis D, Waters B, "Predictors of lithium prophylaxis effectiveness," *Prog Neuropsychopharmacol,* 5:507-10; 1981.
Slagle P, *The Way Up from Down,* St. Martin's Paperbacks, NY, 1992.
Spies T, "The mental symptoms of pellagra; their relief and nicotinic acid," *Am J Med Sci,* 196:461; 1938.
Stoll AL, Sachs GS, et al, "Choline in the treatment of rapid-cycling bipolar disorder: Clinical and neurochemical findings in lithium-treated patients," *Biol Psychiat,* 40(5):382-8; 1996.
Stoll AL, Severus WE, "Mood stabilizers: Shared mechanisms of action at postsynaptic signal-transduction and kindling processes," *Harv Rev Psychiat,* 4(2):77-89; 7-8; 1996.
Stoll AL, Severus WE, et al, "Omega 3 fatty acids in bipolar disorder: A preliminary double-blind placebo-controlled trial," *Arch Gen Psychiat,* 56: 380-81; 1999.
Stork C, Renshaw PF, "Mitochondrial dysfunction in bipolar disorder: Evidence from magnetic resonance spectroscopy research," *Mol Psychiat,* 10:900-19; 2005. (Impaired oxidative phosphorylation, shift to glycolysis for energy, decreased energy or substrate availability, altered phospholipid metabolism.)
Stone I, *The Healing Factor: Vitamin C against Disease,* 1974.
Swann AC, Bowden CL, et al, "Mania: Clinical and biological predictors of outcome," *ACNP Scientific Abstracts;* 1997; p 252. (The greater the illness, and the more prior episodes, the less likely the response to lithium.)
Tohen M, Waternaux C, et al, "Outcome in mania. A 4-year prospective follow-up of 75 patients utilizing survival analysis," *Arch Gen Psychiat,* 47(12):1106-11; 12/1990. (Poor outcome post recovery in 77 manics correlated with: history of alcoholism, more episodes, poor prior occupational status, depression or psychotic features during index mania, affective symptoms at 6 mo follow-up, male.)
Tohen M, Strakowski SM, et al, "The McLean-Harvard first-episode project: 6-month symptomatic and functional outcome in affective and nonaffective psychosis," *Biol Psychiat,* 48(6):467-76; 2000a. (257 first-hospitalization patients. Syndromal recovery in half by 3 mo. In 2/3 of these, functional recovery did not occur by 6 mo. Functional recovery was significantly associated with syndromal recovery, diagnosis, older onset, shorter hospitalizations.)
Tohen M, Hennen J, et al, "Two year syndromal and functional recovery in 219 cases of first episode major affective disorder with psychotic features," *Am J Psychiat,* 157(2):220-8; 2000b.
Trimble MR, "Anticonvulsant-induced psychiatric disorders. The role of forced normalization," *Drug Saf,* 15(3):159-66; 9/1996.
Walsh WJ, "Biochemical treatment of mental illness and behavior disorders," at: www.hriptc.org/BioTreatment.html Accessed: 11/17/1997.
Walsh, WJ, PhD, "Commentary on nutritional treatment of mental disorders, *International Guide to the World of Alternative Mental Health,* at: www.alternativementalhealth.com/articles.walshMP.htm#Py Accessed:10/08/2006
Weiss SRB, Clark M, et al, "Contingent tolerance to the anticonvulsant effects of carbamazepine: Relationship to loss of endogenous adaptive mechanisms," *Brain Res Rev,* 20:305-325; 1995a. (Tolerance in animals was associated with failure of seizure-related adaptions (e.g., increased GABA receptors.)
Werry JS, McClellan JM, Chard L, "Childhood and adolescent schizophrenic, bipolar, and schizoaffective disorders: A clinical and outcome study," *J Am Acad Child Adolesc Psychiat,* 30:457-65; 1991.
Whybrow PC, *A Mood Apart, Depression, Mania, and Other Afflictions of the Self,* Basic Books, HarperCollins, NY, 1997.
Williams R, *Biochemical Individuality,* John Wiley & Sons, Texas, 1956.
R Williams, D Kalita, eds, *A Physician's Handbook on Orthomolecular Medicine,* Keats, New Canaan, CN, 1979.
Winokur G, Clayton PJ, et al, *Manic Depressive Illness,* Mosby, St Louis, MO; 1969.
Wittenborn JR, Weber, Brown, et al, "Niacin in the long term treatment of schizophrenia," *Arch Gen Psychiat,* 28:308-15, 1973. (Negative.)
Wittenborn JR, "A search for responders to niacin supplementation," *Arch Gen Psychiat,* 31:547-52, 1974. (Double blind. A subgroup in Wittenborn, 1973, had responded.)
Wolpert EA, Goldberg JF, et al, "Rapid cycling in unipolar and bipolar affective disorders," *Am J Psychiat,* 147(6):725-78; 6/1990.
Wozniak J, Biederman J, "Diagnostic and therapeutic dilemnas in the management of pediatric-onset bipolar disorder," *J Clin Psychiat,* 62; 2001
Wozniak J, Biederman J, "Childhood mania: Insights into diagnostic and treatment issues," *J Assoc Acad Minor Phys*, 8(4):78-84; 1997. (Childhood bipolar commonly presents with atypical symptoms (e.g., irritability, chronicity, mixed state) and ADHD.)
Young, SN, "The use of diet and dietary components in the study of factors controlling affect in humans: A review," *J Psychiat Neurosci,* 18(5):235-44; 1993.
Zarate, Bipolar Disorders Information Center At: http://www.mhsource.com/bipolar/defzarate.html Accessed: 6/11/2001

Definition, Gifts & Trials

Akiskal KK, Savino M, Akiskal HS, "Temperament profiles in physicians, lawyers, managers, industrialists, architects, journalists, and artists: A study in psychiatric outpatients," *J Affect Disord,* 85(1-2):201-6; 3/2005. (Artists and architects may benefit from cyclothymia. Lawyers and physicians tended to dysthmia and OCD; managers and industrialists to hyperthymia.)
Amadeo S, Abbar M, et al., "Clinical study of five families with bipolar disorder," *Encephale,* 18S(1): 78-82; 1/92. (Each family line, had at least one bipolar with panic disorder, borderline, retardation with dysmorphia, anorexia-bulimia, etc.)
Anderson N, Pfohl B, "Linguistic analysis of speech in affective disorders," *Arch Gen Psychiat,* 33: 1361-7; 1976.
Andreason N, Glick I, "Bipolar affective disorder and creativity," *Compr Psychiat,* 1988.
Andreason N, "Genius and Insanity Revisited: Psychiatric symptoms and family history in creative writers," *Studies in Life History Research,* V3; 1987
Angst J, Sellaro R, "Historical perspectives and natural history of bipolar disorder," *Biol Psychiat,* 48:445-7; 2000.
Atre-Vaidya N, Taylor MA, "Differences in the prevalence of psychosensory features among schizophrenic, schizoaffective, and manic patients," *Compr Psychiat,* 38(2):88-92; 3-4/1997. (Greatest in schizoaffective manics.)
Bauer M, McBride L, *Structured Group Psychotherapy for Bipolar Disorder,* Springer, NY, 1996.
Berlioz H, *Memoirs.*
bipolar.about.com/cs/celebs/a/virginiawoolf.htm Accessed: 6/2/2005.
bipolarsurvivor.com/famous.html Accessed: 6/2/2005.
Brigham PM, "The Psychopharmacology of Bipolar Disorder," updated 5-9-2001. At: http://people.ne.mediaone.net/pmbrig/BP_pharm.html
Dax EC, *Experimental Studies in Psychotic Art,* London, Faber & Faber, 1953.
Dickens C, *A Tale of Two Cities,* 1859.
DSMIIIR & DSM IV
Eby D, "Depression, Women, and Creativity," Gifted Women Forum, AOL, Online Psych, 12/1996, at: DouglasEby@aol.com,
Enachescu C, "Aspects of pictorial creation in manic-depressive psychosis," *Confinia Psychiatrica,* 14:133-42, 1971.
Fieve RR, *Moodswing,* Bantam Books, 1976.
Freeman MP, Freeman SA, et al, "The comorbiditiy of bipolar and anxiety disorders: Prevalence, psychobiology, and treatment issues," *J Affect Disord,* 68:1-23; 2002.
Ghaemi SM, Bauer M, et al, "A summary of the International Society for Bipolar Disorder Guidelines Task Force report, *Bipolar Disord,* 10(1pt2):117-8; 2/2008.
Hirschfeld RM, Calabrese JR, et al, "Screening for bipolar disorder in the community," *J Clin Psychiat,* 64:53-9; 2003
Hudson J, Pope H, of McLean in Massachusetts, in Inkleman, 1999: www.frii.com/~parrot/tree.html
Jamison K, "Mood disorders and patterns of creativity in British writers and artist," *Psychiat,* 52(3):125-34; 5/1989.

Jamisons K, *Moods & Music,* Kennedy Center, DC
Jamison KR, *Touched with Fire, Manic Depressive Illness and the Artistic Temperament,* Free Press, Macmillan, NY, 1993.
Jamison KR, *An Unquiet Mind, A Memoir of Moods and Madness,* Knopf, NY, 1995.
Kaplan A, "Experts reach 'extraordinary' consensus on bipolar disorder," *Psychiatric Times,* 2000.
Kidd, PM, "Bipolar disorder as cell membrane dysfunction. Progress toward Integrative management," *Alt Med Rev,* 9(2)107-35; 2004.
Kraepelin E, *Manic depressive insanity and paranoia,* Livingston, Edinburgh, 1921.
Kubie LS, *Neurotic Distortion of the Creative Process,* Noonday Press, 1961.
Lange Jessica, Interview, *LA Times,* 3/1995.
Gustav Mahler, quoted in Jamison, 1995
Lemmo W, "Mental health care: Under the microscope" At: www.lemmo.com/mental.html#microscope Accessed: 2003.
Lesser, Michael, MD, interview with author, 8/2008.
Ludwig AM, "Mental illness within the professions," in *The Price of Greatness: Resolving the Creativity and Madness Controversy,* Guilford Press, 1995.
Marano HE, "Managing bipolar disorder: A major advancement in treatment helps those who suffer," *Psychol Today,* 6/30/2005.
Mather JH, "How Healthy was Churchill," at: winstonchurchill.org./i4a/pages/index.cfm?pageid=78 Accessed: 2006. (Unwilling to accept sick role; devised therapies, e.g., painting).
McElroy S, Keck P, et al, "Clinical and research implications of the diagnosis of dysphoric or mixed mania or hypomania," *Am J Psychiat,* 149: 1633-44; 1992.
Mental Health Today, at: http:www.mental-health-today.com/bp/dep.htm
mentaljokes.com/famous_manic.html Accessed: 6/2/2005.
themoodynews.com/inspiration.htm Accessed: 6/2/2005.
Moran L, *Winston Churchill: The Struggle for Survival: 1940-1965,* Houghton Mifflin, Boston, 1966.
Nettle D, *Strong imagination: Madness, creativity and human nature,* Oxford University Press, 2002.
Nowakowska C, Strong CM, "Temperamental commonalities and differences in euthymic mood disorder patients, creative controls, and healthy controls," *J Affect Disord,* 85(1-2):207-15; 3/2005.
O'Connell RA, Mayo JA, et al, "PDQ-R personality disorders in bipolar patients," *J Affect Disord,* 23(4)-217-21; 12/1991. (In 58% of 50 bipolars. Borderline was especially. Histrionic was also common.)
Osher Y, Cloninger CR, Belmaker RH, "TPQ in euthymic manic-depressive patients," *J Psychiatr Res,* 30(6);353-7; 2000. (Persistence significantly reduced; harm avoidance, reward dependence, increased.)
ourworld.compuserve.com/homepages.malcolmi/creativity.htm
parrot@frii.com
Pearson J, *The private lives of Winston Churchill,* Simon & Schuster, NY, 1991.
Peselow E, Sanfilipo M, et al, "Relationship between hypomania and personality disorders before and after successful treatment," *Am J Psychiat,* 152: 232-238; 1995.
Reitman F, *Psychotic art,* Routledge & Kegal, London, 1950.
Roeper, Annemarie, quoted in Eby 1996.
Rowse AL, *The Early Churchills,* Macmillan, London, 1956.
Rush AJ, "Bipolar disorder: Origin, recognition, and treatment," *J Clin Psychiat,* 64:3; 2003.
Anne Sexton, *Self;* 6/1958.
Slagle: healthrecovery.com/HRC_2006/Depression_06/D_sadness_inside_you.htm#bipolar
Storr A, *Churchills Black Dog and Kafka's Mice,* Ballantine Books, NY 1990.
Strakowski SM, Tohen M, Stoll AL, et al, "Comorbidity in mania at first hospitalization," *Am J Psychiatr,* 149:554-56; 1992. (May be greater in females, perhaps contributing to rapid cycling.)
Wadeson HS, Carpenter WT, "A comparative study of art expression of schizophrenic, unipolar depressive, and bipolar manic depressive patients," *J Nerv Ment Dis,* 162:334-44; 1976.
Weissman MM, Livingston BM, et al, "Affective disorders," in *Psychiatric Disorders in America,* Free Press, 1991.
Wolpert EA, Goldberg JF, et al, "Rapid cycling in unipolar and bipolar affective disorders," *Am J Psychiat,* 147(6):725-78; 6/1990.
Woolf V: "On writing & mood," in Leonard Woolf, *An Autobiography,* U Press, Oxford 1980.
Zimmerman J, Garfinkle L, "Preliminary study of the art productions of the adult psychotic," *Psychiat Quart,* 16:313-8, 1942.

Genetics

Bertelsen, A, Harvald B, et al, "A Danish twin study of manic-depressive disorders," *Br J Psychiat,* 130: 330-51; 1977.
Child and Adolescent Bipolar Foundation, "About early-onset bipolar disorder," 2002. At: wwwbpkids.org
Coryell W, Endicott J, et al, "Bipolar affective disorder and high achievement: A familial association," *Am J Psychiatr,* 146:983-8; 1989. (Type II often highly successful and higher socioeconomic status.)
De Paolo JR, Simpson SG, et al, "The new genetics of bipolar affective disorder: Clinical implications," *Clin Chem,* 35(7): B28-32; 1989.
DePaulo JR, Simpson SG, et al., "Bipolar II disorder in six sisters," *J Affect Disord,* 19(4):259-64; 9/90. (Less responsive, more comorbidity & family incidence.)
Gershon ES, Hamovit J, et al, "A family study of schizoaffective, bipolar I, bipolar II, unipolar, and normal control probands," *Arch Gen Psychiat,* 39: 1157-67; 1982.
Gershon ES, Hamovit JH, et al, "Birth cohort changes in manic and depressive disorders in relatives of bipolar and schizoaffective patients," *Arch Gen Psychiat,* 33:214-19; 1987.
Gold, MS, *The Good News About Depression,* Villard Books, NY, 1987.
Goodwin FK, Jamison KR, *Manic -depressive Illness,* Oxford U Press, NY;1990.
Goodwin GM, et al, "New international consensus statement on bipolar depression at the 21st European Neuropsychopharmacological Congress, Barcelona, based on discussion of 60 bipolar experts," European *Neuropsychopharmacol,* 7/2007.
Gurling H, Smyth C, et al, "Linkage findings in bipolar disorder," *Nat Genet,* 10:8-9; 1995.
Hirschfeld RM, Calabrese JR, et al, "Screening for bipolar disorder in the community," *J Clin Psychiat,* 64:53-9; 2003.
Horrobin DF, Bennett CN, "New gene targets related to schizophrenia and other psychiatric disorders: Enzymes, binding proteins and transport proteins involved in phospholipid and fatty acid metabolism," *Prosta Leukot Essent Fatty Acids,* 60: 141-67; 1999.
Horrobin DF, "The role of essential fatty acids in schizophrenia," ISOM, Nutritional Medicine Today Conference, Vancouver, BC, 4/2000.
Kidd, PM, "Bipolar disorder as cell membrane dysfunction. Progress toward integrative management," *Alt Med Rev,* 9(2)107-35; 2004.
Kluger J, Song S, "Young and bipolar," *Time,* 163: 38-46, 51; 2002
Lasch K, Weissman M, et al, "Birth-cohort changes in the rates of mania," *Psychiat Res,* 33(1):31-7; 7/90. (17,827 respondents. The risk of mania increased in those born after 1935.)
Lenzi A, Lazzerini F, et al, "Social class and mood disorders: Clinical features," *Social Psychiatr Epid,* 28:56-59; 1993.
Maier W, Rietschel M, et al, "Family and genetic studies on the relationship of schizophrenia to affective disorders," *Eur Arch Psychiat Clin Neurosci,* 249(4S):57-61; 1999.
McInnis MG, McMahon FJ, et al, "Anticipation in bipolar affective disorder," *Am J Hum Genetics,* 53: 385-90; 1993.
Moller HJ, "Bipolar disorder and schizophrenia: Distinct illnesses or a continuum?" *J Clin Psychiatr, 64:23-27; 2003.*
Moore DT, "A Holistic Approach for Treating Manic Depressive Disorders," 1998. At: familyclinic.simplenet.com/bipolar/bipaper.html
Robbins L, Helzer Z, et al, "Lifetime prevalence of specific psychiatric disorders in three sites," *Arch Gen Psychiat,* 41:949-958; 1984.
Rush AJ, Bipolar disorder: Origin, recognition, and treatment," *J Clin Psychiat,* 64:3; 2003a.
Rush AJ, "Toward an understanding of bipolar disorder and its origin," *J Clin Psychiat,* 64:4-8; 2003b.
Sklar P, Smoller JW, "Whole-genome association study of bipolar disorder," *Mol Psychiat,* 13(6):558-69; 6/2008. (Pooled intrnl data: 4,387 bipolars, 6000 controls. The most robust associations were to an axonal gene, ANK3, which helps decides whether the neuron will fire, and to a calcium channel gene.)
Slagle: healthrecovery.com/HRC_2006/Depression_06/D_sadness_inside_you.htm#bipolar
Strakowski SM, Woods BT, et al, "MRI subcortical signal hyperintensities in mania at first hospitalization," *Biol Psychiat,* 33:204-06; 1993.
Strober M, "Relevance of early age-of-onset in genetic studies of bipolar affective disorder," *J Am Acad Child Adolesc Psychiat,* 31(4):606-10; 7/92. (Early onset may predict higher familial loading.)
Torrey EF, *Schizophrenia and Manic Depressive Disorder, The Biological Roots of Mental Illness as Revvealed by the Landmark Study of Identical Twins,* Basic Books, HarperCollins, NY, 1994.
Tsuang M, Winokur G, Crowe R, "Psychiatric disorders among relatives or surgical controls," *J Clin Psychiat,* 45:420-2; 1984.
Walsh WJ, "Commentary on nutritional treatment of mental disorders, *International Guide to the World of Alternative Mental Health,* at: www.alternativementalhealth.com/articles.walshMP.htm#Py Accessed: 10/08/2006
Weissman MM, Bland RC, et al, "Cross-national epidemiology of major depression and bipolar disorder," *JAMA,* 276:293-99; 1996. (Lifetime rates of depression: 1.5% in Taiwan, 19% in Beirut. Bipolar: 0.3 in Taiwan to 1.5% in New Zealand.)
Winokur G, Tsuang M, Crowe R, "The Iowa 500: Affective disorder in relatives of manic and depressed patients," *Am J Psychiatr,* 139:209-212; 1982.
Winokur G, Wesner R, [From unipolar depression to bipolar illness: 29 who changed], *Acta Psychiatrica Scandinavica,* 76:59-63; 1987.
Yatham LN, Srisurapanont M, et al, "Comparative studies of the biological distinction between unipolar and bipolar depressions," *Life Sci,* 61: 1445; 1997.
Young RC, Klerman GL, "Mania in late life: Focus on age at onset," *Am J Psychiat,* 149(7):867-76; 7/1992. (Late onset associated with certain diseases, drug use, and low familial mood disorder.)

Approaches

Ascherio A, Rimm EB, et al, "Dietary intake of marine omega-3 fatty acids, fish intake, and the risk of coronary disease among men," *NEJM,* 332: 977-82; 1995.
Bibus DM, Holman RT, Walsh WJ, "Fatty acid profiles of schizophrenic phenotypes," *Abst, 91ST Annual Mtg, AOCS,* San Diego, 4/25-28; 2000.
Boullin DJ, Orr MW, "Blood platelets as a model for the action of psychotropic drugs on central serotoninergic neurones," *Proc 7th Intl Cong,* 1979.
Bowden CL, "Comparison of open versus blinded studies in bipolar disorder," in JF Goldberg, M Harrow, eds, *Bipolar disorders: Clinical course and outcome,* Am Psychiatric Press; 1999; pp 149-70.
Brigham PM, "The Psychopharmacology of Bipolar Disorder," updated 5-9-2001. At: http://people.ne.mediaone.net/pmbrig/BP_pharm.html
Broida M, *New Hope for People with Depression,* Prima Publishing, Roseville CA, NY, 2001
Connor TJ, Leonard BE, "Depression, stress and immunological activation: the role of cytokines in depressive disorders," *Life Sci* 1998; 62:583-606.
Cooney, Craig PhD, "Methyl Magic and the Mind," in *Methyl Magic,* Andrews McMeel Pub, Kansas City, 1999; pp 154-66.

Darman A, personal communication, Sept 2000, CCS conference. (Inhibitors) and, Sept 2007.

Darman A, "Natural treatment of manic depression explained." At: geocities.com/allen_dar/index.html (Malabsorption, etc.) Accessed: 3/2008.

Dilsaver SC, Greden JF, "Antidepressant withdrawal-induced activation (hypomania and mania): Mechanism and theoretical significance," *Brain Res*, 319(1):29-48; 3/1984.

Eby G, "Magnesium & stress: Rapid recovery from severe, treatment-resistant depression using magnesium," At: george-eby-research.com/html/depression-anxiety.html epub Mar 20 2006

Patty E Fleener MSW. At: mental-health-today.com/bp/selfcare3.htm, Accessed 2005

gojibook.com/ BRO9.html

Gold MS, *The Good News About Depression*, Villard Books, NY, 1987.

Hoffer A. At: orthomolecular vitamincentre.com/mooddisorders.php Accessed: 3/2008

Holian O, Nelson R, "Action of long-chain fatty acids on protein kinase C activity: Comparison of omega-6 and omega-3 fatty acids," *Anticancer Res*, 12:975-80; 1992.

Horrobin DF, Bennett CN, "Depression and bipolar disorder: Relationships to impaired fatty acid and phospholipid metabolism and to diabetes, cardiovascular disease, immunological abnormalities, cancer, aging and osteoporosis. Possible candidate genes," *Prostaglandins, Leukot, Essent Fatty Acids*, 60(4):217-34; 4/1999.

Kaplan BJ, Simpson JS, et al, "Effective mood stabilization with a chelated mineral supplement: An open-label trial in bipolar disorder," *J Clin Psychiat*, 62:936-44; 2001. (Case series. Depression, mania and general psychiatric rating scales improved significantly in 7/11 who completed the trial. Meds were more than half reduced, in 2, eliminated.)

Ketter TA, "Defining the Standard of Care Across the Bipolar Spectrum: Q & A," April 9,2000; DC, Bipolar Disorders Information Center. At: http://www.mhsource.com/bipolar/defzarate.html

Kidder M, "The role of amino acids in bipolar disorder and mental health," *International guide to the world of alternative mental health*, Safe Harbor; 3/2008. At: alternativementalhealth.com/articles/aminobipolar.htm

Larson JM, *Depression Free, Naturally*, Ballantine Wellspring, NY, 2001

Leonard DE, Song C, "Stress and the immune system in the etiology of anxiety and depression," *Pharmacol Biochem Behav*, 54:299-303; 1996.

Lesser, Michael, MD, interview with author, August 2008.

Logan J, *Movie stars, real people and me*, Delacorte Press, NY; 1978; pp 342-50.

Machado-Viera R, Kapczinski F, "Perspectives for the development of animal models of bipolar disorder," *Prog Neuro Psychopharmacol Biol Psychiat*, 28(2): 209-224; 2004.

Maes M, et al, "Interleukin-2 and interleukin-6 in schizophrenia and mania: Effects of neuroleptics and mood stabilizers," *J Psychiatr Res*, 29:141-52; 1995.

Maes M, Smith RS, "Fatty acids, cytokines, and major depression," *Biol Psychiat*, 43:313-4; 1998.

McEnany GW, "Psychobiological indices of bipolar mood disorder: Future trends in nursing care," *Arch Psychiatr Nurs*, 4(1):29-38; 1990.

McGinnis W, "Pyroluria: Hidden cause of schizophrenia, bipolar, depression, and anxiety symptoms," Orlando FL, 5/21/2004. At: alternativemental health.com/articles/pyroluria.htm

Murray MT, Pizzorno J, *Encyclopedia of Natural Medicine*, Prima, 1998.

Murck H, Song C, Horrobin D, et al, "Ethyl-eicosapentaenoate and dexamethasone resistance in therapy-refractory depression," *Intl J Neuropsychopharm*, 7(3):341-9; 9/2004.

Pfeiffer CC, *Nutrition and Mental Illness*, Healing Arts Press, Rochester, VT, 1987.

Pfeiffer CC, *The Schizophrenias Ours to Conquer*, Bio-Communications Press, Wichita, KS, 1988.

Philpott WH, "Selective substance reactivity in pancreatic insufficiency," *J Orthomol Psychiat*, 7(3):179-89; 1978a.

Philpott W, "Methods of reversing the stimuli-evoked pancreatic insufficiencies of chronic degenerative diseases," *J Orthomol Psychiat*, 7(3):190-201; 1978b.

Philpott W, Philpott K, "Principles of bio-ecologic medicine," *J Orthomol Psychiat*, 11(3):204-7; 1982.

Philpott W, Kalita D, *Brain Allergies: The Psychonutrient Connection*, Keats, New Canaan, CN, 1987.

Popper CW, "Do vitamins or minerals (apart from lithium) have mood-stabilizing effects?" *J Clin Psychiat*, 62:933-35; 2001. (Improvement in 20/23. 11/15 were able to stop meds, and remained stable 6-9 mo. later.)

Rogers S, *Depression, Cured at Last*, SK Pub, Sarasota FL, 1997.

Sachs G, Printz DJ, et al, "Expert Consensus Guideline Series: Medication Treatment of Bipolar Disorder, 2000." At: www.psychguides.com

Scherk H, Reith W, et al, [Changes in brain structure in bipolar affective disorders], *Nervenarzt*, 75(9): 861-72; 9/2004.

Seung Kim HF, Weeber EJ, et al, "Inhibitory effects of omega-3 fatty acids on protein kinase C activity in vitro," *Mol Psychiat*, 6(2):246-8; 2001. (EPA, DHA and combo inhibit PKC.)

Simmons M, "Nutritional approaches to bipolar disorder," *J Clin Psychiat*, 642:338; 2003. (12/19 improved markedly, 3 moderately, 1 mildly. 13 mo. later 11 remained on formula, without meds.)

Quiroz JA, Singh J, Manji, et al, "Emerging experimental therapeutics for bipolar disorder: Clues from the molecular pathophysiology," *Molecular Psychiat*, 8(8):756-76; 8/2004. (Impaired cell plasticity and resilience in key neuronal circuits.)

Slagle P, *The Way Up from Down*, St. Martin's Paperbacks, NY, 1992.

Smith RS, "The macrophage theory of depression," *Med Hypotheses*, 35:298-306; 1991.

Stoll AL, Severus WE, "Mood stabilizers: Shared mechanisms of action at postsynaptic signal-transduction and kindling processes," *Harv Rev Psychiat*, 4(2):77-89; 1996.

Stoll AL, Severus WE, et al, "Omega 3 fatty acids in bipolar disorder: A preliminary double-blind, placebo-controlled trial," *Arch Gen Psychiat*, 56(5): 407-12; 5/1999.

Stoll, AL, *The Omega-3 Connection*, Simon & Schuster, NY, 2002.

Stork C, Renshaw PF, "Mitochondrial dysfunction in bipolar disorder: Evidence from magnetic resonancy spectroscopy", *Mol Psychiat*, 20:900-19; 2005.

Truss CO, "Tissue injury induced by Candida albicans, mental and neurological manifestations," *J Orthomol Psychiat*, 7(1):17-37; 1978.

Truss CO, "Restoration of immunologic competence to Candida albicans," *J Orthomol Psychiat*, 9(4):287-301; 1980.

Truss CO, "The role of Candida albicans in human illness," *J Orthomol Psychiat*, 10(4):228-38; 1981.

Truss CO, *The Missing Diagnosis*, Orian Truss, Birmingham, Alabama, 1983.

Truss CO, "Metabolic abnormalities in patients with chronic candidiasis: The acetylaldehyde hypothesis," *J Orthomol Psychiat*, 13(2):66-93; 1984.

Trowbridge J, Walker M, *The Yeast Syndrome*, Bantam Books, NY, 1986.

Walsh WJ, "Biochemical treatment of mental illness and behavior disorders." At: www.hriptc.org/BioTreatment.html Accessed: 11/17/1997b

Walsh WJ, "Biochemical individuality and nutrition" 2000. At: www.hriptc.org/biochemical_individuality.html

Walsh WJ, "A biological basis for neurologic disorders: autism, hyperactivity, attention deficit disorder, depression, obsessive-compulsive disorder, Tourette's syndrome, and violence, An interview with William Walsh PhD," *Latitudes*, 5(2)1-8; 2002. At: www.Latitudes.org

Walsh, WJ, PhD, "Commentary on nutritional treatment of mental disorders," *International Guide to the World of Alternative Mental Health*. At: www.alternativementalhealth.com/articles.walshMP.htm#Py Accessed:10/08/2006

Whybrow, Peter C, MD, *A Mood Apart, Depression, Mania, and Other Afflictions of the Self*, Basic Books, HarperCollins, NY, 1997.

Yurgelun-Todd DA, Gruber SA, et al, "fMRI during affect discrimination in bipolar affective disorder," *Bipolar Disord*, 2(3 Pt 2):237-48; 9/2000.

Minerals; Magnesium

Abraham GE, "Magnesium deficiency in premenstrual tension," *Magnesium Bull*, 1:68-73; 1982.

Altura BM, "Calcium antagonist properties of magnesium: implications for anti-migraine actions," *Magnesium*, 4:169-175; 1985.

Amari L, Layden B, et al, "Competition between Li+ and Mg2+ in neuroblastoma SH-SY5Y cells: a fluorescence and 31P NMR study," *Biophys J*, 76(6): 2934-42; 6/99. (Increased free intracellular Mg2+ following Li+ incubation. Li and Mg have similar properties; competition may displace Mg.)

Ananth J, Yassa R, "Magnesium in mental illness," *Comprehensive Psychiatry*, 20:475-82; 9-10/1979.

Balch JF, Balch P, *Prescription for Nutritional Healing*, Avery, Garden City Park, NY, 1990.

Banki CM, et al, "Aminergic studies and cerebrospinal fluid cations in suicide," *Ann NY Acad Sci*, 487:221-30; 1986. (CSF magnesium significantly lower in suicidal depressives.)

Tenney L, Stress, Woodland Health Books, 1987.

Baumel S, *Dealing with Depression Naturally*, Keats, New Canaan, CN, 1995.

Blasbicher T, Heiden A, et al, "Magnesium sulfate IV as an adjunction to treatment of severe mania," *Eur Neuropsychopharmacol*, 7(2):285; 9/1997.

Blaylock, Russell, MD, *Excitotoxins: The Taste that Kills*, Health Press, Santa Fe, NM, 1995.

Bosc M, Roche M, et al, "Magnesium and vitamin B6 intake reduces central nervous system hyperexcitability in children," *J Am Coll Nutr*, 23(5): 5455-85; 10/2004.

Chouinard G, Beauclair L, et al, "A pilot study of magnesium aspartate hydrochloride (Magnesiocard) as a mood stabilizer for rapid cycling bipolar affective disorder patients," *Prog Neuropsychopharma Biol Psychiat*, 14(2):171-80; 1990. (Small open label trial. 40mEq/day was at least as effective as lithium in 50% of severe rapid-cyclers.)

Clague JE, et al, "Intravenous magnesium loading in chronic fatigue syndorme," *Lancet*, 340:124-125; 7/11/1992.

Colodny L, Hoffman RL, "Inositol: Clinical Applications for exogenous use," *Alt Med Rev*, 3(6):4323-447, 1998.

Cousens G, *Depression free for Life*, Quill, HarperCollins, NY, 2001.

Cox IM, et al, "Red blood cell magnesium and chronic fatigue syndrome," *Lancet*, 337:757-60; 3/30/1991.

Dishashi T, Iwaoka T, et al, "Magnesium metabolism in hyperthyroidism," *Endocr J*, 43:397-402; 1996.

Dunner DL, Meltzer HL et al, "Plasma and erythrocyte magnesium levels in patients with primary affective disorders during chronic lithium treatment," *Acta Psychiat Scand*, 51:104-9; 1975.

Durlach, "Diverse Applications of Magnesium Therapy" in *Handbook of Metal-Ligand Interactions in Biological Fluids — Bioinorganic Medicine*, V2, Marcel Dekker, Inc, New York, 1995.

Durlach, "Chronic fatigue syndrome and chronic primary magnesium deficiency," *Magnesium Res*, 5:68; 3/1992.

Ebel H, Gunther T, "Magnesium metabolism: A review," *J Clin Chem Bio-chem*, 257-70; 1980.

Eby G, "Magnesium & stress: Rapid recovery from severe, treatment-resistant depression using magnesium," Austin, Texas, last revision: 12/09/01.

Friedman E, Wang HY, "Receptor-mediated activation of G proteins is increased in postmortem brains of bipolar affective disorder subjects," *J Neurochem*, 67(3):1145-52; 1996. (Suggesting increased transmembane signaling.)

Garrison RH, Somer E, *The Nutrition Desk Reference*, Keats, New Canaan, CN, 1985.

Giannini AJ, Nakoneezie AM, et al, "Magnesium oxide augmentation of verapamil maintenance therapy in mania," *Psychiat Res,* 93(1):83-7; 2/14/2000. (Significantly more effective than the drug alone.)

Gold MS, *The Good New About Depression,* Bantam Book, NY, 1995

Hall RCW, Joffe JR, "Hypomagnesemia: physical and psychiatric symptoms," *JAMA,* 224(13):1749-51; 1973.

Heiden A, Frey R, et al, "Treatment of severe mania with intravenous magnesium sulphate as a supplemental therapy," *Psychiat Res,* 89(3): 239-46; 1999. (Open study. Up to 23 days of the magnesium treatment allowed significant reductions in neuroleptics and benzodiazepines. 7/10 improved markedly.)

Henrotte JG, "Type A behavior and magnesium metabolism," *Magnesium,* 5:201-10; 1986.

Herzberg L, Herzberg B, "Mood changes and magnesium. A possible interaction between magnesium and lithium," *J Nervment Dis,* 165: 423-26; 1977.

Hoschl C, "Do calcium antagonists have a place in the treatment of mood disorders?" *Drugs,* 42(5): 721-29; 1991.

Iseri LT, French JH, "Magnesium: Nature's physiologic calcium blocker," *Am Heart J,* 108: 188-93; 1984.

Jaffe R, Kruesi OR, "The biochemical immunology window: A molecular view of psychiatric case management," *J App Nutr,* 44(2); 1992.

Kirov GK, Tsachev KN, "Magnesium, schizophrenia, and manic-depressive disease," *Neuropsychobiol,* 23:79-81; 1990.

Larson JM, *Depression Free, Naturally,* Ballantine Wellspring, NY, 2001.

Larson, Joan M, PhD, interview with author, June 2008.

Layden B, Diven C, et al, "Li+/Mg+ competition at therapeutic intracellular Li+ levels in human neuroblastoma SY5Y cells," *Bipolar Disord,* 2(3 Pt 1):200-4; 2000.

Lesser M, *Nutrition & Vitamin Therapy,* Bantam Books, NY, 1983.

Levine J, Stein D, et al, "High serum and cerebrospinal fluid Ca/Mg ratio in recently hospitalized acutely depressed patients," *Neuropsychobiol,* 39(2):63-70; 1999. (Ca/Mg ratios were elevated in acute bipolar and unipolar depression vs controls.)

Lieberman S, Bruning N, *The Real Vitamin & Mineral Book,* Avery, Garden City Park, NY, 1990.

Marlowe M, et al, "Decreased magnesium in the hair of autistic children," *J Orthomol Psychiat,* 13: 117-22; 1984. (Calcium and magnesium were low. B6 without magnesium can worsen symptoms.)

McCarty MF, "Complementary vascular-protective actions of magnesium and taurine: A rationale for magnesium taurate," *Med Hypotheses,* 46(2): 89-100, 1996.

McGuire R, "Type A stress: A drain on magnesium," *Med Tribune,* 5/15/1984.

Mousain-Bosc M, Roche M, et al, "Improvement of neurobehavioral disorders in children supplemented with magnesium-vitamin B6. I. Attention deficit hyperactivity disorders," *Magnes Res,* 19(1):46-52; 2006.

Muller P, Address at *First International Symposium on Magnesium Deficit in Human Pathology*; 1971.

Murray MT, *Encyclopedia of Nutritional Supplements,* Prima, Rocklin, CA, 1996.

Lininger SW, Gaby A, et al, The Natural Pharmacy, HealthNotes, Roseville CA, 1999.

Neguib MA, "Effect of magnesium on the thyroid," *Lancet,* 1:1405; 1963.

Nizankowska-Blaz T, Korczowski R, et al, [Level of magnesium in blood serum in children from the province of Rzesz'ow], *Wiad Lek,* 46(3-4):120-2; 2/1993. (Low in 24/247 children.)

NutriCircles®, Strickland Computer Consulting, Version 3.25, April 29, 1996.

Page LR, *Healthy Healing,* Healthy Healing, CA, 1992.

Pavlinac D, et al, "Magnesium in affective disorders," *Biol Psychiat,* 14(4):657-61; 1979.

Pfeiffer CC, *Mental and Elemental Nutrients,* Keats, New Canaan, CN, 1975.

Pfeiffer CC, *The Schizophrenias Ours to Conquer,* Bio-Communications Press, Wichita, KS, 1988.

Plenge P, Rafaelsen OJ, "Lithium effects on calcium, magnesium and phosphate in man. Effects on balance, mineral content, faecal and urinary excretion," *Acta Psychiatr Scand,* 66(5):361-73; 1982. (Decreased urinary excretion of calcium and phosphorus, and, over time, increased magnesium loss, and decreased bone mineral content.)

Quillin P, *Healing Nutrients,* Contemporary Books, Chicago, 1987.

Rajkowska G, "Postmortem studies in mood disorders indicate altered numbers of neurons and glial cells," *Biol Psychiat,* 48(8):766-77; 10/15/2000. (Prolonged stress damages PFC and hippocampal function.)

Robinet ML, *Bulletin of the Academy of Medicine,* France, 1934. (Magnesium content of soil strikingly relates to suicide.)

Rogers S, *Depression, Cured at Last,* SK Publishing, Sarasota FL, 1997.

Simontacchi C, *Crazy Makers - How the Food Industry is Destroying Our Brains and Harming Our Children,* Jeremy P Tarcher, Putnam, NY, 2000.

Slagle P, "Magnificent Magnesium," *The Way Up Newletter Archives,* #30; 1995 At: thewayup.com/newletters/newsarch.htm

Smith L, *Feed Yourself Right,* 1983.

Srinivasan C, Minadeo N, et al, "Competition between Li+, and Mg+ for red blood cell membrane phospholipids: Nuclear magnetic resonance study," *Lipids,* 34(11):1211-21; 1999.

Standley CA, Mason BA, et al, "Differential regulation of seizure activity in the hippocampus of male and female rats," *Am J Obstet Gynecol,* 173(4):1160-5; 1995. (Magnesium sulfate (often used to prevent eclampsia seizures) reduced seizure duration in female rats; duration and number in males. NMDA seizures were more severe in males.)

Starabrat-Hermelin B [The effects of magnesium supplementation on hyperactivity in children with attention deficit hyperactivity disorder (AHDH)], *Magnes-Res,* 10(2):149-56; 1997.

Starabrat-Hermelin B, [The effect of deficiency of selected bioelements on hyperactivity in children with certain specified mental disorders] *Ann Acad Med Stn,* 44:297-314; 1998. (Low magnesium in 116 hyperactive children as compared to controls.)

Stoll AL, Severus WE, "Mood stabilizers: Shared mechanisms of action at postsynaptic signal-transduction and kindling processes," *Harv Rev Psychiat,* 4(2):77-89; 7-8; 1996.

Tenney L, *Stress,* Woodland Health Books, 1987.

Wallach JD, Lan M, *Rare Earths, Forbidden Cures,* Double Happiness Pub Co, Bonita, CA, 1994.

Weintraub S, *Minding Your Body,* Complementary Medicine Pub, Portland, OR, 1995.

Werbach, MT, *Nutritional Influences on Mental Illness,* Third Line Press, Tarzana, CA, 1991.

Wessely S, "Magnesium and chronic fatigue syndrome," *Lancet,* 337:1094-5; 5/4/1991.

Weston PG, "Magnesium as a sedative," *Am J Psychiat,* 1:637-8; 1921-2. (IV magnesium sulfate led to relaxation and 4-6 hrs sleep in 50 manic, agitated depression, or agitation patients. Calcium chloride reversed side effects.)

Young LT, Robb JC, et al, "Serum Mg2+ and Ca2+/Mg2+ ratio in major depressive disorder," *Neuropsychobiology,* 34(1)):26-28; 1996. (Serum Mg2+ implicated in depressive severity.)

CCBs

Aldenhoff JB, Schlegel, et al, "Antimanic effects of the calcium antagonist D-600: A double-blind placebo controlled study," *Clin Neuropharmacol,* 9:553-55;1986. (4/5 acute manics on 8 days D-600 improved marginally compared to placebo, mainly with reduced psychomotor activity.)

Auby P, Olivier F, et al, "Calcium channel blockers and dysthymic disorders. Recent data," *Encephale,* 18(S1):67-9, 1992. (Inconsistant in hypomania; preventive alone or with lithium.)

Barton BM, Gitlin MJ, "Verapamil in treatment-resistant mania: An open trial," *J Clin Psychopharmacol,* 7:101-3; 1987.

Brotman AW, Farhadi AM, Gelenberg AJ, "Verapamil treatment of acute mania," *J Clin Psychiat,* 47:136-8; 1986. (6 acute manics (4 psychotic), lithium intolerant, or nonresponders rapidly improved by 3 wks. 3 patients relapsed within 3 wks of stopping.)

Brunet G, Cerlich B, et al, "Open trial of a calcium antagonist nimodipine in acute mania," *Clin Neuropharmacol,* 13:224-28; 6/1990. (Significant improvement by 1 wk in all 6 mild, acute manics. Mood and speech benefitted most, sleep least.)

Caillard V, "Treatment of mania using a calcium antagonist: Preliminary trial," *Neuropsychol,* 14:23-26;1985. (Significant improvement in 5/7 manics by 2 wks. Nonresponders had organic mood disorder.)

Currier MD, Goodnick PJ, "Calcium antagonists and newer anticonvulsants," in PJ Goodnick, ed, *Mania: Clinical and Research Perspectives,* Am Psychiatric Press, DC, 1998; pp 337-62.

de Falco FA, Bartiromo U, et al, "Calcium antagonist nimodipine in intractable epilepsy," *Epilepsia,* 33: 343-45; 1992.

Dinan TG, Silverstone T, et al, "Cortisol, prolactin, and growth hormone levels with clinical ratings in manic patients treated with verapamil," *Int Clin Psychopharmacol,* 3:151-6; 1988 (High doses led to signifcant improvement in 5/6 acute manics. The sixth withdrew due to severe mania.)

Dose M, Emrich HM, et al, "Use of calcium antagonists in mania," *Psychoneuroendocrinol,* 11:241-43; 1986. (Significant improvement in 7 of 8 manic or schizoaffective manics.)

Dubovsky SL, Franks RD, et al, "Effectiveness of verapamil in the treatment of a manic patient," *Am J Psychiat,* 139:502-4; 1982.

Dubvosky SL, Franks RD, "Intracellular calcium ions in affective disorders: A review and an hypothesis," *Biol Psychiat,* 18:781-97; 1983.

Dubovsky SL, "Calcium antagonists: A new class of psychiatric drugs?" *Psychiatric Annals,* 16:724-28; 1986.

Dubovsky SL, Franks RD, et al, "Calcium antagonists in mania: A double-blind study of verapamil," *Psychiat Res,* 18:309-20;1986

Dubovsky SL, "Calcium channel antagonists as novel agents for manic-depressive disorder, in AF Schatzberg, CB Nemeroff, eds, *Textbook of Psychopharmacology,* Psychiatric Press, DC, 1995; pp 377-88.

Dunn RT, Frye MS, et al, "The efficacy and use of anticonvulsants in mood disorders," *Clin Neuropharmacol,* 21(4):215-35; 7-8/1998.

Garzo-Trevino ES, Overall JE, et al, "Verapamil versus lithium in acute mania," *Am J Psychiat,* 149: 121-22; 1992. (Equivalent improvement.)

Giannini AJ, Houser WL, et al, "Antimanic effects of verapamil," *Am J Psychiat,* 141:1602-1603; 1984. (Response equivalent to lithium.)

Giannini AJ, Loiselle RH, et al, "Comparison of antimanic efficacy of clonidine and verapamil," *J Clin Pharmacol,* 25:3307-8; 1985 (Verapamil was significantly more effective and preferred by 60%.)

Goldstein JA, "Calcium channel blockers in the treatment of panic disorder," *J Clin Psychiat,* 46: 546; 1985.

Goodnick PJ, "Nimodipine treatment of rapid cycling bipolar disorder letter," *J Clin Psychiat,* 56: 330; 1995.

Goodnick PJ, "Treatment of mania; relationship between response to verpamil and changes in plasma calcium and magnesium levels," *South Med J,* 89:225-26; 1996.

Hoschl C, Kozeny J, "Verpramil in affective disorders: A controlled, double blind study," *Biol Psychiat,* 25: 128-40;1989.

Manna V, "Bipolar affective disorders and role of intraneuronal calcium. Therapeutic effects of the treatment with lithium salts and/or calcium antagonists in patients with rapid polar inversion," *Minerva Med,* 82(11):757-63; 11/1991.

Masters JC, "When lithium does not help: The use of anticonvulsants and calcium channel blockers in the treatment of bipolar disorder in the older person,"

Geriatr Nurs, 17(2):75-8; 3-4/1996. (Depression improves in 25-30%; mania, in even more.)
McDermut W, Pazzaglia PJ, et al, "Use of single case analysis in off-on-off trials in affective illness: A demonstration of the efficacy of nimodipine," *Depression,* 2:259-71; 1995.
Pazzaglia PJ, Post RM, et al, "Preliminary controlled trial of nimodipine in ultra-rapid cycling affective dysregulation," *Psychiat Res,* 49:257-72; 1993.
Post RM, Ketter TA, et al, "The place of anticonvulsant therapy in bipolar illness," *Psychopharmacol (Berl),* 128(2):115-29; 11/1996.
Post RM, Denicoff KD, et al, "Long-term outcome of anticonvulsants in affective disorders," in Joseph E Goldberg, M Harrow, eds, *Bipolar Disorders: Clinical Course and Outcomes,* Am Psychiatric Press Inc, DC, 1999; pp 95-96.
Post RM, Kramlinger KG, et al, "Treatment of rapid cycling bipolar illness," *Psychopharmacol Bull,* 26(1):37-47; 1990.

Zinc

Balch F, Balch P, *Prescription for Nutritional Healing,* Avery, Garden City Park, NY, 1990.
Baumel S, *Dealing with Depression Naturally,* Keats, New Canaan, CN, 1995.
Blaylock R, *Excitotoxins: The Taste that Kills,* Health Press, Santa Fe, NM, 1995.
Braverman E, Pfeiffer CC, *The Healing Nutrients Within,* Keats, New Canaan, CN 1987.
Bryce-Smith D, Simpson RID, "Anorexia, depression and zinc deficiency," *Lancet,* 1162; 11/17/1984.
Edwards N, "Mental disturbances related to metals," in RCW Hall, ed, *Psychiatric Presentations of Medical Illness,* Spectrum Publications, Jamaica, NY, 1980; 283-308.
Ferbabdez-Madrif F, Prasad AS, et al "Effect of zinc deficiency on nucleic acids, collagen and non-collagenous protein of the connective tissue," *J Lab Clin Med,* 82:951-61; 1973.
Garbarg M, Babbin G, et al, "Histaminergic pathway in rat brain evidenced by lesions of the medial forebrain bundle," *Sci,* 186:833-35; 1974.
Garrison RH, Somer E, *The Nutrition Desk Reference,* Keats, New Canaan, CN, 1985.
Harrison FM, et al, "Timm's sulfide-silver reaction for zinc during experimental anterograde degeneration of hippocampal mossy fibers," *J Compar Neurol,* 142:23-31; 1971a.
Harrison FM et al, "Depletion of metal in the rat hippocampal mossy fiber system by intravital chelation with dithizone," *Histochemie,* 28:211-19; 1971b.
Hoffer A, in *Orthomolecular Medicine for Physicians,* Keats, New Canaan, CN, 1983a.
Hoffer A, "Nutrition and behavior," in J Bland, ed, *Medical Applications of Clinical Nutrition,* Keats, New Canaan, CN, 1983b.
Humphries L, et al, "Zinc deficiency and eating disorders," *J Clin Psychiat,* 50:456-59; 12/1989.
Ibata Y, Otsuka N, "Electron microscopic demonstration of zinc in hippocampus formation using Timm's sulfide-silver technique," *J Histochem Cytochem,* 17:171-75; 1969. (Zinc concentrated in hippocampal neuron terminal vesicles.)
Irvine D, Bayne W, Miyashita H, *Nature,* 224(81); 1969. (Urinary kryptopyrrole in psychosis.)
Jaffe R, Kruesi OR, "The biochemical-immunology window: A biomolecular view of psychiatric case management," *J App Nutr,* 44(2); 1992.
Kimura, I, Kimura, J, "Preliminary reports on the metabolism of trace elements in neuropsychiatric diseases, I: Zinc in schizophrenias," *Proc Japan Acad Sci,* 1965; p 943. (Postmortem schizophrenics had 50% less frontal, occipital, and hippocampal zinc.)
Krohn J, *The Whole Way to Allergy Relief & Prevention,* Hartley & Marks, Pt Roberts, WA, 1991.
Kruesi, Oscar Rogers, MD, interview with author, February, 1996.
Larson JM, *Depression Free, Naturally,* Ballantine Wellspring, NY, 2001
Lesser M, *Nutrition & Vitamin Therapy,* Bantam Books, NY, 1983.
Lieberman S, Bruning N, *The Real Vitamin & Mineral Book,* Avery, Garden City Park, NY, 1990.
Little KY, Castellanos X, et al, "Altered zinc metabolism in mood disorder patients," *Biol Psychiat,* 26(6):646-8; 10/1989.
McGinnis W, "Pyroluria: Hidden cause of schizophrenia, bipolar, depression, and anxiety symptoms," Orlando, 5/21/2004. *At:* alternativementalhealth.com/articles/pyroluria.htm
McLardy T, "Hippocampal zinc and structural deficit in brain from schizophrenics and chronic alcoholics," Presented at the*Trace Elements and Brain Function Symposium,* Princeton, NJ, 1973. (Reduced. May play a role in histamine storage in mossy fiber terminal vesicles.)
McLoughlin IJ, Hodge JS, [Zinc in depressive disorder], *Acta Psychiatr Scand,* 82:451-53; 12/1990.
Moyer D, *Nutrients to Quiet the Unquiet Brain,* Nu-tune Press, Penn Valley, CA, 2003.
Moynahan EJ, "Zinc deficiency and disturbance of mood and visual behavior," 1(7950):91; 1/1976.
Murray MT, *Encyclopedia of Nutritional Supplements,* Prima CA, 1996.
Murphy JV, "Intoxication following ingestion of elemental zinc," *JAMA,* 212:2119-20; 1970.
Nichols J, Morgan J, et al "Postnatal depression and zinc status- a preliminary report," *J Nut Med,* 3:1, 35-42; 1992.
Niklowitz WJ, "Interference of Pb and Mg with essential brain tissue Cu, Fe and Zn as main determinant in experimental metal encephalopathy," Presented at the *Trace Elements and Brain Function Symposium,* Princeton, NJ, 1973.
Page LR, *Healthy Healing,* Healthy Healing, CA, 1992.
Pfeiffer CC, Iliev V, "A study of zinc deficiency and copper excess in the schizophrenias," *Int Ref Neurobiol,* 1S:141-65; 1972. (Mn can triple Cu excretion. Effectiveness is enhanced by Zn. Estrogens raise ceruloplasmin and serum Cu, lower Zn.)
Pfeiffer CC, Jenney EH, "Fingernail white spots: Possible zinc deficiency," *JAMA,* 228:157; 1974.
Pfeiffer, CC, *Mental and Elemental Nutrients,* Keats, New Canaan, CN, 1975.
Pfeiffer, CC, *Nutrition and Mental Illness,* Healing Arts Press, Rochester, VT 1987.
Pfeiffer CC, Audette L, "Pyroluria, zinc and B6 deficiencies," *Intl Clin Nutr Rev,* 8(3):107-110; 1988b.
Prasad, A.S, et al. "Experimental zinc deficiency in humans," *Ann Intern Med,* 89:483; 1978. (Irritability, depression, amnesia, apathy, paranoia, lethargy, retardation. slow learning.)
Quillin P, *Healing Nutrients,* Contemporary Books, Chicago, 1987.
Reuven S, "Zinc deficiency and cerebellar disease," *Intnl J Neurosci,* 60:21-26; 1991.
Rogers S, *Depression, Cured at Last,* SK Publishing, Sarasota FL, 1997.
Rosenberg IH, "Importance of zinc for hormone binding and signal transduction: Limiting mechanisms in zinc deficiency?" *Nutr Rev,* 49:12: 369-70; 1991.
Slagle P, *The Way Up from Down,* St. Martin's, NY, 1992.
Toren, et al, "Zinc deficiency in attention deficit hyperactivity disorder," *Biol Psychiat,* 40:1308-10; 1996. (Significantly lower than in controls.)
Wallwork J, Sandstead H, "Effect of zinc deficiency on brain catecholamine concentration," *Fed Proc,* 40:939; 1981. (Catecholamines elevated.)
Walsh, William J, PhD, "Biochemical treatment: Medicines for the next century," *NOHA News,* 16(3); 1991.
Walsh, William J, PhD, "Zinc deficiency, metal metabolism, and behavior disorders," A Report of the Health Research Institute, Naperville, IL, March, 1996.
Walsh WJ, "Biochemical treatment of mental illness and behavior disorders." At: www.hriptc.org/BioTreatment.html Accessed: 11/17/1997.
Walsh, WJ, "Biochemical individuality and nutrition," *NOHA News,* XXV(2):6-8; 2000. At: www.hriptc.org/biochemical_individuality.html
Walsh, WJ, "A biological basis for neurologic disorders: autism, hyperactivity, attention deficit disorder,depression, obsessive-compulsive disorder, Tourette's syndrome, and violence, An interview with William Walsh PhD." At: www.Latitudes.org 5(2):1-8; 2002.
Walsh WJ, "Zinc deficiency, metal metabolism, and behavior disorders.," At: hriptc.org/zinc_deficiency.html 12/6/2004.
Walsh, WJ, PhD, "Commentary on nutritional treatment of mental disorders, *International Guide to the World of Alternative Mental Health.* At: www.alternativementalhealth.com/articles.walshMP.htm#Py Accessed:10/08/2006.
Walsh WJ, PhD, interview with author, Nov. 2007.
Werbach M, *Nutritional Influences on Mental Illness,* Third Line Press, Tarzana, CA, 1991.

Lithium

Abou Saleh MT, Copen AJ, "Prediction of lithium treatment outcome of mood disorder on prophylactic lithium," *Lithium,* 1:27-35; 1990.
Ahrens B, Mueller-Oerlinghausen D, et al, "Cardiovascular and suicide mortality of affective disorders may be reduced by lithium prophylaxis," *J Affect Dis,* 33:67-75; 1995.
Dr. Manfred Anke of Karl Marx School, Leipzig Germany, as reported in Hoffer, 1983.
Baldessarini RJ, Tondo L, "Does lithium treatment still work? Evidence of stable responses over three decades," *Arch Gen Psychiat,* 57(2):187-90; 2000.
Baraban JM, Worley PF, Snyder SH, "The second messenger systems and psychoactive drug action: Focus on the phosphoinositide system and lithium," *Am J Psychiat,* 146:1251-60; 1989.
Beliles RP, "Lithium," in GD Clayton, FE Clayton, eds, *Patty's Industrial Hygiene and Toxicology,* 4th ed, V: IIC, John Wiley & Sons, Inc, NY, 1994.
Brigham PM, "The Psychopharmacology of Bipolar Disorder," updated 5-9-2001. At: http://people.ne.mediaone.net/pmbrig/BP_pharm.html
Cade J, "The story of lithium," in Ayd FJ, B Blackwell, eds, *Discoveries in Biological Psychiatry,* JB Lippincott, Phil, PA, 1970; pp 218-29.
Cade JFJ, "Lithium salts and the treatment of psychotic excitement," *Med J Australia,* 1:195-8; 1949.
Compton MT, Nemeroff CB, "The treatment of bipolar depression," *J Clin Psychiat,* 61(9):57-67; 2000. (Relatively understudied. Lithium is the "gold standard and most appropriate initial treatment.")
Coppen A, et al, "Plasma folate and affective morbidity during long-term lithium therapy," *Biol Psychiat,* 141:87-89; 1982. (Of 107 lithium-treated patients, those with lower folate (which may reduce serotonin) showed greater affective morbidity.)
Coppen A, et al, "Depression and tetrahydrobiopterin: The folate connection," *J Affect Disord,* 16(2-3):103-07; 1989. (BH4 is reduced in lithium patients.)
Dawson E, in *Diseases of the Nervous System,* 1970.
Dean, Ward, MD, "Lithium orotate the unique safe mineral with multiple uses," 2006 (Orotate increases lithium utilization and effectiveness many-fold; transports it to mitochondria, lysosomes and glial membranes; stabilizes lysosome membranes.)
Gelenberg AJ, Kane JM, et al, "Comparison of standard and low serum levels of lithium for maintenance treatment of bipolar disorder," *N Engl J Med,* 321:1489-93; 1989.
Gold MS, *The Good News About Depression,* Villard Books, NY, 1987.
Grof P, Alda M, et al, "The challenge of predicting response to stabilizing lithium treatment. The importance of patient selection," *Br J Psychiat,* 9/21/1993.
Grof P, "Has the efficacy of lithium changed? Impact of a variety of lithium's effects," *Neuropsychopharmacol,* 19(5)183-8; 9/1998.
Hoffer A, *Orthomolecular Medicine for Physicians,* Keats, New Canaan, CN, 1983.
Horrobin DF, "The role of essential fatty acids in schizophrenia," ISOM, Nutritional Medicine Today Conference, Vancouver, BC, 4/2000.
Ketter TA, "Defining the Standard of Care Across the Bipolar spectrum: Q & A, April 9,2000; DC,

Faculty: Terrence A Ketter MD," Bipolar Disorders Information Center. At: http://www.mhsource.com/bipolar/defketter.html

Kleindienst N, Grell W, "Lithium in longterm treatment of bipolar disorder," *Eur Arch Psychiatr Clin Neurosis*, 253(3):120-5; 6/ 2003.

Kruesi, Oscar Rogers, MD, interview with author, February, 1996.

Kukopulos A, Reginaldi D, et al, "The long term prophylaxis of affective disorders," *Adv Biochem Psychopharmacol,* 49:127-47; 1995.

Larson JM, *Depression Free, Naturally,* Ballantine Wellspring, NY, 2001

Larson, Joan M, PhD, interview with author, June 9, 2008.

Maj M, Pirozzi R, Kemali D, "Long-term outcome of lithium prophylaxis in patients initially classified as complete responders," *Psychopharmacol,* 98:535-38; 1989.

Markar HR, Mander AJ, "Effectiveness of lithium prophylaxis in clinical practice," *Br J Psychiat,* 156: 146-7; 1990. (41 bipolars with 2 -3 admissions in 5 years, showed only modest benefit.)

Mueller-Oerlinghausen D, Ahrens B, et al, "Reduced mortality of manic-depressive patients in long-term lithium treatment. An international collaborative study by IGSLI," *Psychiat Res,* 36:329-333; 1991.

Mueller-Oerlinghausen D, Mueser-Causemam B, et al, "Suicides and parasuicides in a high risk patient group on and off lithium long-term medication," *J Affect Dis,* 25:261-70; 1992.

Nieper HA, [The clinical applications of lithium orotate], *Agressologie,* 14(6):407-11; 1973.

Page, Linda, PhD, *Healthy Healing,* Healthy Healing Pub, CA, 1992. (Up to 5 plus mg/day, though occasionally at mainstream levels.)

Pfeiffer CC, *The Schizophrenias Ours to Conquer,* Bio-Communications Press, Wichita, KS, 1988.

Post RM, Leverich GS, et al, "Lithium tolerance and discontinuation as pathways to refractoriness," in NJ Birch, C Padgham, MS Hughes, eds, *Lithium in Medicine and Biology,* Marius Press, Lancashire, England, 1993b; pp 71-84. (23/66 long-term patients developed tolerance.)

Prakash R et al, "A case of megaloblastic anemia secondary to lithium, *Am J Psychiat,* 138:849; 1981. (A 40-year old developed anemia after 5 mo lithium, but improved steadily over 6 mo when whole blood and folate were added. Lithium alone for 9 mo again led to anemia til very high dose folate was added.)

Rosenblatt S, *Beyond Valium,* G.P. Putnam's Sons, NY, 1981.

Sartori HE, "Lithium orotate in the treatment of alcoholism and related condtions," *Alcohol,* 3(2): 97-100; 3/1986.

Schou, M, "Mortality-lowering effect of prophylactic lithium treatment. A look at the evidence," *Pharmacopsychiat,* 28:1; 1995.

Smith DF, Schou M, "Kidney function and lithium concentrations of rats given an injection of lithium orotate," *Pharm Pharmacol,* 31(3):161-3; 1979.

Snyder, *Biological Aspects of Mental Disorder,* Oxford U. Press, NY, 1980.

Whybrow PC, *A Mood Apart, Depression, Mania, and Other Afflictions of the Self,* Basic Books, HarperCollins, NY, 1997.

Werry JS, McClellan JM, et al, "Childhood and adolescent schizophrenic, bipolar, and schizoaffective disorders: A clinical and outcome study," *J Am Acad Child Adolesc Psychiat,* 30: 457-65; 1991.

Wright JV, Lithium, "Part I: Protect and renew your brain," *Townsend Letter,* 2-3/2004, pp 78-81.

Young AM, Newham JI, "Lithium in maintenance therapy for bipolar disorder," *J Psychopharmacol,* 20(2)S17-22 2006. (New episodes increase if stopped.)

Kindling, Epilepsy

Balch JF, Balch PA,*Prescription for Nutritional Healing,* Avery, Garden City Park, NY, 1990.

Bell I, Miller C, et al, "An olfactory-limbic model of multiple chemical sensitivity — Possible relationships to affective spectrum disorders and to kindling," *Biol Psychiatr,* 32:218; 1992.

Blumer D, "The illness of Vincent van Gogh," *Am J Psychiat,* 159(4):519-26; 4/2002.

Braverman E, Pfeiffer CC, *The Healing Nutrients Within,* Keats, New Canaan, CN, 1987.

Charlie Foundation to Help Cure Pediatric Epilepsy: An Introduction to the Ketogenic Diet," Santa Monica, CA, 1997. (Samuel Livingston, MD, of John Hopkins, (1954) reported 43% of 304 pediatric patients completely controlled seizures on this diet; with marked improvement in another 34%. His later work suggests seizures stop completely in one third, are significantly reduced in another third.)

Davidson, K, "Schizophrenia-like psychosis associated with organic cerebral disorders: A review," *Psych Dev,* 1; 1983. (In 17%.)

Denicoff KD, Smith-Jackson EE, et al, "Comparative prophylactic efficacy of lithium, carbamazepine, and the combination in bipolar disorder," *J Clin Psychiat,* 1997.

Destaing F, [Le soleil et l'orage ou la maladie de Van Gogh], *La nouvelle Presse Medicale,* 1(46); 12/23/1972.

Dilsaver SC, Swann AC, et al, "Treatment of bipolar depression with carbamazepine: Results of an open study," *Biol Psychiat,* 40:935-37; 1996.

Emrich HM, Von Zerssen D, et al, "Effect of sodium valproate in mania; the GABA hypothesis of affective disorders," *Arch Psychiatr Neurol Sci,* 229:1-16; 1980.

Fieve RR, *Moodswing,* Bantam Books, 1976.

Galton L, *You May Not Need A Psychiatrist,* Simon & Schuster, NY, 1979.

Geschwind N, Penfield H, *Epilepsy and the functional anatomy of the human brain,* Little Brown, Boston, 1954.

Ghaemi SN, Boiman EE, Goodwin FK, "Kindling and second messengers: An approach to the neurobiology of recurrence in bipolar disorder," *Bipolar P,* 45:137-44; 1999.

Gold MS, *The Good News About Depression,* Villard Books, NY, 1987.

Hoffer A, *Orthomolecular Medicine for Physicians,* Keats, New Canaan, CN, 1983.

Hoffer A, At: orthomolecular vitamincentre.com/mooddisorders.php Accessed: 3/2008

Kessler AJ, Barklage NE, et al, "Mood disorders in the psychoneurology borderland. Three cases of responsiveness to carbamezepine," *Am J Psychiat,* 146:81-83; 1989.

Ketter TA, "Defining the Standard of Care Across the Bipolar spectrum: Q & A," April 9,2000; DC, Bipolar Disorders Information Center. At: http://www.mhsource.com/bipolar/defketter.html

Kidder M, "The role of amino acids in bipolar disorder and mental health," *International guide to the world of alternative mental health,* Safe Harbor; 3/2008. At: alternativementalhealth.com/articles/aminobipolar.htm

John Kuehne, MD, quoted in LaPlante 1993.

Tom Lane, communication with author, 5/1997.

LaPlante E, *Seized,* HarperCollins, NY, 1993.

Larson JM, *Depression Free, Naturally,* Ballantine Wellspring, NY, 2001.

Lewis A, Clowatre D, *Melatonin and the Body Clock,* Keats (Stabilizes CNS electrical activity; May help some cases of seizures, depression, panic, schizophrenia.)

Lewis DO, Feldman M, et al, "Psychomotor epileptic symptom in six patients with bipolar mood disorders," *Am J Psychiat,* 141:1583-6; 1984. (6/12 consecutive bipolars each had five or more symptoms, including olfactory hallucinations, multiple deja vu or mystical experiences.)

Maclean P, "The temporal lobe and limbic system," *J Nerv Ment Dis,* 186(11):728-30; 11/1998.

Mazza M, Nicola M, et al, "Bipolar disorder and epilepsy: A bidirectional relation? Neurobiological underpinnings, current hypotheses, and future research directions," *Neuroscientist,* 13(4):392-404, 2007.

Mendez MF, Cummings JL, "Depression in epilepsy. Signs and phenomenology," *Arch Neurol,* 1986

Moore, Daniel T, PhD, "A Holistic Approach for Treating Manic Depressive Disorders," 1998. At: familyclinic.simplenet.com/bipolar/bipaper.html (Seizure theory: Acute bipolar episodes can be only mildly related to life events. Sleep-deprived EEGs help confirm diagnosis. Anticonvulsant meds show comparable benefit to lithium.)

Nagera H, "Vincent Van Gogh: A Psychological Study," International Press, NY, 1967.

Negash A, Kebede D, et al, "Neurological soft signs in bipolar I disorder patients," *J Affect Disord,* 80(2-3): 221-30, 2003. (Treatment-naive bipolar I patients showed a number of significant deficits (NES), particularly in sequencing complex motor activity.)

Pfeiffer CC, *The Schizophrenias Ours to Conquer,* rev ed, Bio-Communications Press, Wichita, KS, 1988. (Pyrolurics especially vulnerable.)

Post RM, Uhde TW, et al, "Antidepressant effects of carbamazepine," *Am J Psychiat,* 143:29-34; 1986.

Rogers S, *Depression, Cured at Last,* SK Publishing, Sarasota FL, 1997.

Ross J, The Mood Cure, Viking Penguin, NY, 2002.

SC Schacter, O Devinsky, eds, *Behavioral Neurology and the Legacy of Norman Geschwind,* Lippincott-Raven, NY, 1997.

Slagle P, "Anxiety & taurine," *The Way Up Newletter,* 16; 1/15/2000.

Dr. Paul Spiers, quoted in La Plante.

Stoll AL, Severus WE, "Mood stabilizers: Shared mechanisms of action at postsynaptic signal-transduction and kindling processes," *Harv Rev Psychiat,* 4(2):77-89; 7-8; 1996.

Victoroff J, "DSM IIIR psychiatric diagnosis in candidates for epileptic surgery, Lifetime prevalence," *Neuropsychiat Neuropsychol Behav Neurol,* 1994.

Walsh WJ, "Biochemical treatment of mental illness and behavior disorders," www.hriptc.org/BioTreatment.html Accessed: 11/17/1997

Walsh, WJ, PhD, "Commentary on nutritional treatment of mental disorders, *International Guide to the World of Alternative Mental Health* At: www.alternativementalhealth.com/articles.walshMP.htm#Py Accessed:10/08/06

Walsh, William J, PhD, interview with author, November 2007.

Walsh, William J, PhD, interview with author, July 2008.

Waxman SG, Geschwind N, "Hypergraphia in TLE," *Epileptic Behavior,* 6(2) 282-91, 3/2005.

Anticonvulsants

Bowden CL, Swann AC, Calabrese JR, et al, "Maintenance clinical trials in bipolar disorder: Design implications of the divalproex-lithium-placebo study," *Psychopharmacol Bull,* 33(4): 693-699; 1997.

Brigham PM, "The Psychopharmacology of Bipolar Disorder," updated 5-9-2001. At: http://people.ne.mediaone.net/pmbrig/BP_pharm.html

Calabrese JR, Delucchi GA, "Spectrum of efficacy of valproate in 55 patients with rapid-cycling bipolar disorder," *Am J Psychiat,* 147(4):431-434; 1990.

Calabrese JR, Bowden CL, et al, "A double blind placebo conrolled study of lamotrigine monotherapy in outpatients with bipolar I. Lamictal 602 Study Group," *J Clin Psychiat,* 60(2):79-88; 2/1989.

Coxhead N, Silverstone T, et al, "Carbamazepine versus lithium in the prophylaxis of bipolar affective disorder," *Acta Psychiatr Scand,* 85:114-18; 1992.

Cullen M, Mitchell P, et al, "Carbamazepime for treatment-resistant melancholia," *J Clin Psychiat,* 52:4742-76;1991.

Freeman TW, Clothier JL, et al, "A double-blind comparison of valproate and lithium in the treatment of acute mania," *Am J Psychiat,* 149: 108-11; 1992.

Frye MA, "Defining the Standard of Care Across the Bipolar spectrum: Q & A, April 30,2000; DC, Faculty: Mark A Frye MD," Bipolar Disorders Information Center. At: http://www.mhsource.com/bipolar/deffryewa.html

Frye MA, "Defining the Standard of Care Across the Bipolar spectrum: Q & A, April 9,2000, SF, Faculty: Mark A Frye MD, Terrence A Ketter MD,"

Bipolar Disorders Information Center. At: http://www.mhsource.com/bipolar/defzarate.html

Ghaemi SN, Boiman EE, Goodwin FK, "Kindling and second messengers: An approach to the neurobiology of recurrence in bipolar disorder," *Bipolar P,* 45:137-44; 1999.

Greil W, Ludwig-Mayerhofer W, et al, "Lithium vs carbamazepine in the maintenance treatment of bipolar disorders — A randomized study," *J Affect Disord,* 43:151-61; 1997b.

Lambert PA, Venaud G, "Comparative study of valpromide vs lithium in treatment of affective disorders," *Nervure,* 5(2):57-65;1992.

Marano, HE, "Managing bipolar disorder: A major advancement in treatment helps those who suffer," *Psychology Today,* 6/30/2005.

McElroy SL, Suppres T, et al, "Open-label adjunctive topiramate in the treatment of bipolar disorders," *Biol Psychiat,* 47(12):1025-33; 6/15/2000.

Pope HG, McElroy SL, et al, "Valproate in the treatment of acute mania," *Arch Gen Psychiat,* 48: 62-68; 1991.

Post RM, Uhde TW, et al, "Kindling and carbamazepine in affective illness," *J Nerv Ment Dis,* 170(12):717-31; 12/1982.

Post RM, Uhde TW, et al, "Antidepressant effects of carbamazepine," *Am J Psychiat,* 143:29-34; 1986.

Post RM, Weiss SR, "Sensitization, kindling and anticonvulsants in mania," *J Clin Psych,* 50S:23-30, 45-47; Dec 1989.

Post RM, Weiss SRB, "Endogenous biochemical abnormalities in affective illness: Therapeutic versus pathogenic," *Biol Psychiat,* 32:469-84; 1992.

Post RM, Weiss SRB, et al, "Mechanisms of action of carbamazepine in seizure and affective disorders," in RT Joffe, JR Calabrese, eds, *Anticonvulsants in Mood Disorders,* Marcel Dekker, NY, 1994b; pp 43-92.

Post RM, Ketter TA, et al, "The place of anticonvulsant therapy in bipolar illness," *Psychopharmacol (Berl),* 128(2):115-29; 11/1996a. (Especially if multiple episodes, rapid cycler, dysphoric mania, dual diagnosis, medical factors, no close bipolar relatives.)

Post RM, Ketter TA, et al, "Rational polypharmacy in the bipolar affective disorders," *Epilepsy Res,* 11S: 153-80; 1996b.

Post RM, Weiss SRB, "The neurobiology of treatment-resistant mood disorders," in FE Bloom, DJ Kupger, eds, *Psychopharmacology: The Fourth Generation of Progress,* Raven Press, NY, 1995; pp 1155-1170.

Post RM, Mark AF, et al, "Anticonvulsants in the long-term prophylaxis of affective disorders," in A Honig, HM van Praag, eds, *Depression: Neurobiological, Psychopathological and Therapeutic Advances,* John Wiley & Sons Ltd, 1997; pp 487-493.

Post RM, Denicoff KD, et al, *Long-Term Outcome of Anticonvulsants in Bipolar Disorders: Clinical Course and Outcome, JE Goldberg,* M Harrow eds, Am Psychiatric Press, Inc, DC, 1999.

Post RM, Weiss SR, et al, "Sensitization and kindling-like phenomenon in bipolar disorder: Implications for psychopharmacology," *Clin Neurosci Res,* 1(1): 69-81; 1/2001.

Stoll AL, Banov M, et al, "Neurologic factors predict a favorable valproate response in bipolar and schizoaffective disorders", *J Clin Psychopharmacol,* 14(5):311-3; 1994. (E.g., history of seizures, head injury and abnormal EEG. 44% with a neurological abnormality responded vs. 24%, without.)

Walden J, Normann C, "Differential treatment of bipolar disorder with old and new antiepileptic drugs," *Neuropsychobiology,* 38(3):181-4; 10/98.

Weiss SRB, Clark M, et al, "Contingent tolerance to the anticonvulsant effects of carbamazepine: Relationship to loss of endogenous adaptive mechanisms," *Brain Res Rev,* 20:305-325; 1995a.

Whybrow, PC, *A Mood Apart, Depression, Mania, and Other Afflictions of the Self,* Basic Books, HarperCollins, NY, 1997.

Yang YY, Deng HC, Wang BH, "The increasing use of anticonvulsants in prophylactic treatment of bipolar disorder," *Psychiat Clin Neurosci,* 52(4): 429-31; 8/1998.

Inhibitors

Braverman E, Pfeiffer CC, *The Healing Nutrients Within,* Keats, New Canaan, CN 1987.

Hoffer A, *Orthomolecular Medicine for Physicians,* Keats, New Canaan, CN, 1983.

Larson JM, *Depression Free, Naturally,* Ballantine Wellspring, NY, 2001

Rogers S, *Depression, Cured at Last,* SK Publishing, Sarasota FL, 1997.

Ros J, The Mood Cure, Viking Penguin, NY, 2002.

Slagle P, "Anxiety &, taurine," *The Way Up Newletter,* 16; 1/15/2000.

Walsh WJ, "Biochemical treatment of mental illness and behavior disorders." At:www.hriptc.org/BioTreatment.html Accessed: 11/17/1997

Walsh WJ, PhD, "Commentary on nutritional treatment of mental disorders, *International Guide to the World of Alternative Mental Health* At: www.alternativementalhealth.com/articles.walshMP.htm#Py Accessed:10/08/06

Walsh William J, interview with author, November 2007.

Taurine

Azuma J, Sawamura A, et al, "Double blind randomized crossover trial of treatment in congestive heart failure," *Curr Ther Res,* 34(4):543-57; 1983.

Balch, JF, Balch PA, *Prescription for Natural Healing,* Avery, Garden City Park, NY, 1990.

Birdsall TC, "Therapeutic applications of taurine," *Alt Med Rev,* 3(2):128-36; 1998.

Bonhause DW, Huxtable RJ, "Seizure susceptibility and decreased taurine transport in the genetically epileptic rat," *Neurochem Intl,* 6(3):365-68;1984. (Seizure-susceptible had half the taurine uptake.)

Braverman E, Pfeiffer CC, *The Healing Nutrients Within,* Keats, New Canaan, CN 1987.

Feekes, D, Pepplinkhuizen L, et al, "Plasma levels of serine, methionine and taurine in transient acute polymorphic psychosis," *Psych Res,* 51(1):11-18; 1994. (Bipolars show significantly lower plasma serine as compared to other aminos.)

Feuer L, Fekete M, et al, [Effect of intraventricular administration of glutathione on norepinephrine, dopamine, and serotonin turnover in different brain regions in rats] *Acta Physiol Hungarica,* 61(3):163-67; 1983.

Feuer L, Nagy SU, et al, [Effect of glutathione (gamma-L-glutamyl-taurine) on the serum glucocorticoid and estriol level in rats] *Endokrinologie,* 79(3):437-38; 1982.

Hayes KC, "Taurine requirements in primates," *Nutr Rev,* 43(3):65-70; 1985.

Kendell SF, Krystal JH, et al, "GABA and glutamate systems as therapeutic targets in depression and mood disorders," *Expert Opinon on Therapeutic Targets,* 9(1):153-68; 2/2005.

Krystal JH, Sanacora G, et al, "Glutamate and GABA systems as targets for novel antidepressant and mood-stabilizing treatments," *Mol Psychiat,* 7S(1): 71-80; 2002. (Mood stabilizers and antidepressants may target GABA and glutamate. Antidepressants may reduce NMDA glutamate receptor function. Anti glutamatergics may also be antimanic. MRS suggests unipolar (but not bipolar) depression is associated with low cortical GABA. Mood stabilization raises GABA and repletes deficits.)

Lampson WG, Kramer JH, et al, "Potentiation of the actions of insulin by taurine," *Can J Physiol Pharmacol,* 61:457-63; 1983.

Larson JM, *Depression-free, Naturally,* Ballantine Wellspring, NY, 2001.

Larson, Joan M, PhD, interview with author, June 9, 2008.

Machado-Viera R, Viale CJ et al, "Mania associated with an energy drink: The possible role of caffeine, taurine and inositol," *Can J Psychiat,* 46(5):454-5; 2001.

Martin WG, Truex RC, et al, "The synthesis of taurine from sulfate, A constitutive enzyme in mammals," *Proc Soc Exp Bio Med,* 147(2):563-5; 1974.

Martin WG, Truex RC, et al, "The synthesis of taurine from sulfate; Vitamin B6 deficiency and taurine synthesis in the rat," *Proc Soc Exp Bio Med,* 147(3):835-8; 1974.

Michael N, Erfurth A, et al, "Acute mania is accompanied by elevated glutamate/glutamine levels within the left dorsolateral prefrontal cortex," *Psychopharmacol,* 168, 3; 2003. (Proton MRS found elevated glutamate/glutamine in mania.)

Murphy BL, Stoll A, "Taurine as an anti-manic agent: A double-blind, placebo-controlled study." (Slated for completion in 2007.)

Murray MT, Pizzorno J, *Encyclopedia of Natural Medicine,* Prima, Rocklin, CA, 1998.

Page LR, *Healthy Healing,* Healthy Healing Pub, CA, 1992.

Pfeiffer CC, *Mental and Elemental Nutrients,* Keats, New Canaan, CN, 1975.

Pfeiffer CC, *Nutrition and Mental Illness,* Healing Arts Press, Rochester, VT, 1987.

Pfeiffer CC, *The Schizophrenias, Ours To Conquer,* Bio-Communications Press, Wichita, KS, 1988.

Rogers S, *Depression, Cured at Last,* SK Publishing, Sarasota FL, 1997.

Ross J, *The Mood Cure,* Viking Penguin, NY, 2002.

Schaffer S, Takahashi K, et al, "Role of osmoregulation in the actions of taurine," *Amino Acids,* 19(3-4): 527-46; 2000.

Sebring LA, Huxtable RI, "Cardiovascular actions of sulfur amino acids, Introduction," *Prog Clin Biol Res,* 125:3-4; 1983.

Seidl R, Peyrl A, "A taurine and caffeine-containing drink stimulates cognitive performance and well being," *Amino acids,* 19(3-4):635-42; 2000. (Contains caffeine, taurine, glucaronolactone. Claimed to improve mental performance and mood. May act via caffeine's effects on adenosine receptors and taurine's receptor modulation.)

Shimada M, Shimono R, et, "Distribution of 35S-taurine in rat neonates and adults. A whole-body autoradiographic study," *Chem Cell Biol,* 80(3):225-30; 1984. (Taurine can be reduced by as much as half in patients prone to seizures.)

Slagle P, "Anxiety & Taurine," *The Way Up Newletter Archives,* #16; 2000 At: thewayup.com/newletters/newsarch.htm

Stoll A, et al, "Taurine as an anti-manic agent: A double-blind controlled study in adolescents with bipolar disorder." (Slated for completion in 2007.)

Sturman JA, Cohen PA, "Cystine metabolism in vitamin B6 deficiency: Evidence of multiple taurine pools," *Biochem Med,* 5(3):245-68; 1971.

Sturman JA, Cohen PA, "Taurine in nutrition," *Comp Thera,* III:59-65; 1977.

Sturman JA, Cohen PA, "Taurine in developing rat brain: Changes in blood-brain barrier," *J Neurochem,* 32:811-816; 1979.

Tachiki KH, Hendrie HC, et al, "A rapid column chromatographic procedure for the routine measurement of taurine in plasma of normals and depressive patients," *Clin Chimm Acta,* 75(3): 455-65; 1977.

Urquhart N, Perry TL, et al, "Passage of taurine into adult mammalian brain," *J Neurochem,* 22: 871-72; 1974.

Voaden MJ, Hussain IP, et al., "Studies on retinitis pigmentosa in man. Inositol, taurine and blood platelets," *Br J Opthamol,* 66:771-5; 1982.

Walsh WJ, "Biochemical treatment of mental illness and behavior disorders," At: www.hriptc.org/BioTreatment.html Accessed: 11/17/1997.

Walsh WJ, "Biochemical individuality and nutrition." At: www.hriptc.org/biochemical_individuality.html Accessed: 2000.

Walsh WJ, "A biological basis for neurologic disorders: autism, hyperactivity, attention deficit disorder, depression, obsessive-compulsive disorder, Tourette's syndrome, and violence, An interview with William Walsh PhD," *Latitudes,* 5(2)1-8, 2002. At: www.Latitudes.org

Walsh, WJ, "Commentary on nutritional treatment of mental disorders," *International Guide to the World of Alternative Mental Health.* At: www.alternativementalhealth.com/articles.walshMP.htm#Py Accessed: 2006.

Walsh, William J, PhD, interview with author, November, 2007, & July, 2008

Warburton DM, Bersellini E, "An evaluation of a caffeinated taurine drink on mood, memory and information processing in healthy volunteers without caffeine abstinence," *Psychopharmacol,* 158(3): 322-28; 2001. (Improved information processing, attention, verbal reasoning.)

Yamori Y, Wang H, et al, "The role of sulfur amino acids in the prevention and regression of cardiovascular disorders," *Prog Clin Biol Res,* 125: 103-15; 1983.

GABA

Akasu T, "5-hydroxytryptamine facilitates GABA-induced depolarization in bullfrog primary afferent neurons," *Neursci Lett,* 92(3):270-4; 10/17/1988.

Antonaccio, MJ, "Central GABA receptor stimulants as potential novel antihypertensive agents," *Drug Devl Res,* 4(3):315-329; 1984.

Balch JF, Balch PA, *Prescription for Natural Healing,* Avery, Garden City Park, NY, 1990.

Bartholini G, "GABA receptor agonists: Pharmacological spectrum and therapeutic agents," *Med Res Rev,* 5(1):55-75; 1-3/1985.

Baloyannis SJ, Karakatsamis K, et al, "Effects of GABA, glycine, and sodium barbiturate on dendritic growth in vitro," *Acta Neuropathol,* 59(3):171-82; 1983. (GABA or glycine (relative to sodium barbiturate) enhanced dendritic growth and arborization in cerebellar and cerebral dendrites.)

Berrettini WH, Nurnberger JI, et al, "Plasma and CSF GABA in affective illness," *Br J Psychiat,* 141:483-87;1982. (Lithium increases plasma GABA.)

Berrettini WH, Post RM, *Neurobiology of Mood Disorders,* Williams & Baltimore, 1984.

Bird ED, Iversen I, "Huntington's chorea — postmortem measurement of glutamic acid decarboxylase choline acetyltransferase and dopamine in basal ganglia," *Brain,* 97:457; 1974. (Low GAD (which synthesizes GABA).)

Bohlen P, Huot S, et al, "The relationship between GABA concentrations and cerebrospinal fluid," *Brain Res,* 167(2):297-305; 5/11/1979.

Brambilla P, Perez J, et al, "GABAergic dysfunction in mood disorders," *Molecular Psychiat,* 8(8):721-3; 2003. (Levels have been low in animal models of depression and in affectives. Drugs which increase its activity can act as antidepressants or stabilizers. GABA support may benefit a subset of bipolars.)

Braverman E, Pfeiffer CC, *The Healing Nutrients Within,* Keats, New Canaan, CN 1987.

Braverman E, *Path Wellness Manual,* Publications for Achieving Total Health, NJ, 1994.

Christensen AV, Svendsen O, et al, "Pharmacodynamic effects and possible therapeutic uses of THIP, a specific GABA-agonist," *Pharm Weekbi [Sci],* 4(5):145-53; 10/22/82. (Parkinsons and Huntingtons brains have shown low basal ganglia GABA and GAD. GABA may be helpful in epilepsy, dementia, pain, perhaps mania, depression.)

Chouinard, G, et al, "A controlled clinical trial of L-tryptophan in acute mania," *Biol Psychiat,* 20:546-57; 1985. (Double blind. Significant improvement.)

Chouinard G, Young SN, et al, "Tryptophan-nicotinamide combination in depression," *Lancet,* 1(8005):249; 1/1977.

Chouinard G, Young SN, et al, "Tryptophan-nicotinamide combination in the treatment of newly admitted depressed patients," *Commun in Psych,* 2:311-18; 1978.

Coryell W, Winokur G, et al, "Alcoholism and primary major depression: A family study approach to co-existing disorders," *J Affect Disord,* 24:93-99; 1992.

Cousens G, *Depression free for Life,* Quill, HarperCollins, NY, 2000.

Darman A, personal communication with author, September, 2000.

Emrich HM, Zerssen DV, et al, [Effect of sodium valproate on mania: The GABA-hypothesis of affective disorders], *Archiv fur Psychiatrie und Nervenkrakheiten,* 229:1-16; 1980.

Emrich HM, von Zerssen D, et al, "On a possible role of GABA in mania. Therapeutic efficacy of sodium valproate," *Adv Biochem, PsychoPharmamacol,* 26: 287–96; 1981.

Ferkany JW, Smith LA, "Measurement of gamma-aminobutyric acid (GABA) in blood," *Life Sci,* 22(23): 2121-8; 1978.

Francois-Bellan AM, Hery M, "Analysis of the inhibitory of effect of oestradiol on functional GABA/5HT relationship in the rat brain," *J Neuroendocrinol,* 1989.

Gerner RH, Fairbanks L, "CSF neurochemistry in depressed, manic and schizophrenic patients compared with that of normal controls," *Am J Psychiat,* 141:1533-40; 1984.

Gillis RA, Yamada KA, et al, "Central gamma-aminobutyric acid involvement in blood pressure control," *Fed Proc,* 43(1):32-8; 1/1984.

Gray JA, Green AR, "GABA-B-receptor mediated inhibiton of potassium-evoked release of endogenous 5-hydroxytryptamine from mouse frontal cortex," *Br J Pharmacol,* 91(2):517-22; 7/1987.

Jaffe R, Kruesi OR, "The biochemical-immunology window: A molecular view of psychiatric case management," *J App Nutr,* 44(2); 1992.

Kendell SF, Krystal JH, et al, "GABA and glutamate systems as therapeutic targets in depression and mood disorders," *Expert Opinon on Therapeutic Targets,* 9(1):153-68; 2/2005.

Krystal JH, Sanacora G, et al, "Glutamate and GABA systems as targets for novel antidepressant and mood-stabilizing treatments," *Mol Psychiat,* 7S(1):71-80; 2002. (Mood stabilization raises and repletes GABA. MRS suggest an association of major depression with low cortical GABA. Clinical data suggest NMDA/glutamate receptor suppression can be antidepressant. Anti-glutamatergics may be antimanic.)

Larson JM, *Depression Free, Naturally,* Ballantine Wellspring, NY, 2001

Larson, Joan M, PhD, interview with author, June 9, 2008.

DeMontis G, et al, "Neurochemical and neuropharmacologial indications for the involvement of GABA and glycine receptors in neuropsychiatric disorders," Adv Biochem Psychopharmacol, 37:137-48; 1983. (GABA agonists in dyskinesias, epilepsy, depression, animal models. GABA concentrates in the forebrain and upper brain stem; glycine in the lower brain stem and spinal cord; both are found in the substantia nigra.)

Lloyd KG, et al, "The GABAergic hypothesis of depression," *Prog Neuropsychopharmacol Biol Psychiat,* 133(3-4):341-51; 1989.

Lloyd KG, Morselli PL, et al, "The potential use of GABA agonists in psychiatric disorders: Evidence from studies with progabide in animal models and clinical trial," *Pharmacol Biochem Behav,* 18(6): 957-66; 6/1983. (Improves mood.)

Loscher W, Schmidt D, "Plasma GABA levels in neurological patients under treatment with valproic acid," *Life Sci,* 28:2383-88; 1981.

Loscher W, Nau H, "Valproic acid: Metabolite concentrations in plasma and brain, anticonvulsant activity, and effects on GABA metabolism during subacute treatment in mice," *Arch Int Pharmacodyn Ther,* 257(1):20-31; 5/1982.

Loscher W, Siemes H, "Cerebrospinal fluid gamma-aminobutyric acid levels in children with different types of epilepsy: Effect of anticonvulsant treatment," *Epilepsia,* 26(4):314-9; 7-8/1985.

Michael N, Erfurth A, et al, "Acute mania is accompanied by elevated glutamate/glutamine levels within the left DLPFC," *Psychopharmacol,* 168:3; 2003.

Moss HB, Yao JK, Burns M, et al, "Plasma GABA-like activity in response to ethanol challenge in men at high risk for alcoholism," *Biol Psychiat,* 27(6): 617-25; 3/15/1990.

Motohashi N, "GABA receptor alterations after chronic lithium administration: Comparison with carbamazepine and sodium valproate," *Neuropsychopharmacol Biol Psychiat,* 16:571-9; 1992. (All increase GABA-B hippocampal receptor density.)

Page LR, *Healthy Healing,* Healthy Healing Publications, CA, 1992.

Petty F, Sherman AD, "GABAergic modulation of learned helplessness," *Pharmacol Biochem Behav,* 156:567-570; 1981. (Pharmacologic and animal data strongly suggest low plasma GABA is a trait marker in a subset of depressives.)

Petty F, Kramer GL, et al, "Low plasma gamma-aminobutyric acid levels in male patients with depression," *Biol Psychiat,* 32:334-63; 1992.

Petty F, Kramer GL, Hendricks W, "GABA and Depression," in *Biology of Depressive Disorders PART A, A Systems Perspective,* J Mann, DJ Kupfer, eds, Plenum Press, NY, 1993a; pp 82-99.

Petty F, Kramer GL, et al, "Low plasma GABA is a trait-like marker for bipolar illness," *Neuropsychopharmacol,* 9(2):125-32; 9/1993b. (30-40% of bipolars are low, even if manic.)

Petty F, "Plasma concentrations of gamma-amminobutyric acid (GABA) and mood disorders: A blood test for manic depressive disease?" *Clin Chem,* 40:296-302; 1994. (Plasma (which reflects brain levels) is significantly lower in manic and depressed bipolars vs controls. Low levels persist after depressive recovery and are a familial marker in some affectives.)

Petty F, "GABA and mood disorders: A brief review and hypothesis," *J Affect Disord,* 34(4): 275-81; 9/18/1995. (GABA agonists, and upregulation of GABA-B receptors benefit mood. Clinical data show reduced plasma GABA and GABA activity during episodes.)

Petty F, Rush A, "Plasma GABA predicts acute response to divalproex in mania," *Biol Psychiat,* 39(4):278-84; 1996.

Petty F, Kramer GL, Davis LL, "Gamma-Aminobutyric Acid," in P Goodnick, ed, *Mania: Clinical and research perspectives,* Am Psychiatric Press, DC, 1998; pp 164-66.

Pfeiffer CC, *Mental and Elemental Nutrients,* Keats, New Canaan, CN, 1975.

Pfeiffer CC, *The Schizophrenias Ours to Conquer,* Bio-Communications Press, Wichita, KS, 1988.

Post R, Denicoff KD, Frye M, et al "Long term outcome of anticonvulsants," in JE Goldberg, M Harrow, eds, *Bipolar Disorders: Clinical Course and Outcome,* Am Psychiatr Press Inc, DC, 1999.

Priestley CM, Williamson EM, et al, "Thymol, a constituent of thyme essential oil, is a positive allosteric modulator of human GABA-A receptors and a homo-oligomeric GABA receptors from Drosophila melanogaster," *Br J Pharmacol,* 140: 1363-72; 2003. (It potentiates GABA-A receptors.)

Ring HA, Crellin R,et al, "Vigabatrin and depression", *J Neurol Neurosurg Psychiatr,* 56:925-28; 8/1993.

Roberts, "GABA in nervous system function", Raven Press, TN, 1976.

Ross J, *The Mood Cure,* Viking Penguin, NY, 2002.

Sahley BJ, *Healing with Amino Acids,* Pain & Stress Center Pub., TX, 1995.

Schlicker E, "GABA B receptor-mediated inhibition of serotonin release in the rat brain," *Arch Pharmacol,* 326(2):6/1984.

Shiah IS, Yatham LN, "GABA function in mood disorders: An update and critical review," *Life Sci,* 63(15):1289-303; 1998. (GABA inhibits NE, Ser.)

Silverstone T, "Dopamine in manic depressive illness. A pharmacological synthesis," *J Affect Disord,* 8(3):225-31; 5-6/1985. (DA/choline/GABA pathways link in limbic and vental tegmental regions influencing bipolar illness.)

Slagle P, *The Way Up Newletter Archives,* At: thewayup.com/newletters/newsarch.htm #0285

Strahlendorf JC, Lee M, "Modulatory role of serotonin on GABA-elicited inhibition of cerebellar Purkinje cells," *Neurosci,* 30(1):117-25; 1989.

Suzdak PD, Gianutsos G, "GABA-noradrenergic interaction: Evidence for differential sites of action for GABA-A and GABA-B receptors," *J Neural Transmission,* 64(3-4):163-72; 1985.

Suzdak PD Gianutsos G, "Effect of chronic imipramine or baclofen on GABA-B binding and cyclic AMP production in cerebral cortex," *Eur J Pharmacol,* 131(1):129-33; 11/12/1986.

Taylor M, Bhagwagar Z, et al, "GABA and mood disorders," *Psychol Med,* 33:387-93l 2003.

Tews JK, Rogers QR, et al, "Effect of dietary protein and GABA on food intake, growth and tissue amino

acids," *Physiol Behav,* 32(2):301-8; 2/1984.
van Kammen DP, "Gamma-aminobutyric acid (GABA) and the dopamine hypothesis of schizophrenia," *Am J Psychiat,* 134:138-43; 1977.
Wehrbach MR, *Nutritional Influences on Mental Illness,* Third Line Press, Tarzana CA, 1991.

Glycine

Balch JF, Balch PA, *Prescription for Natural Healing,* Avery, Garden City Park, NY, 1990.
Baloyannis SJ, Karakatsamis K, et al, "Effects of GABA, glycine, and sodium barbiturate on dendritic growth in vitro," *Acta Neuropathol,* 59(3):171-82; 1983. (GABA or glycine-enriched medium enhanced in vitro dendritic growth and arborization.)
Braverman, Pfeiffer CC, *The Healing Nutrients Within,* Keats, New Canaan CN, 1987
Deutsch SI, Peselow ED, et al, "Effect of lithium on glycine levels in patients with affective disorders," *Am J Psychiat,* 138:683-4; 1981. (Lithium increases RBC glycine, whatever the mood.)
Deutsch SI, "Erythrocyte glycine in depressed, hypomanic and euthymic bipolar patients treated with lithium carbonate," *Psychopharmacol,* 78(4):314-16; 1982. (In 27 bipolars on lithium at least 8 mo, serum levels strongly correlated with RBC glycine, for all moods, and varied significantly from controls.)
Deutsch SI, Stanley M, et al, "Glycine: A possible role in lithium's action and affective illness," *Neuropsychobiol,* 9(4):215-18; 1983. (Some bipolars show elevated RBC glycine. Chronic lithium elevates brain and RBC glycine.)
Eby G. At: george-eby-research.com/html/magnesium-for-depression.pdf
Hendler S, *The Oxygen Breakthrough,* NY, William Morrough, 1989.
Heresco-Levy U, Javitt DC, et al, "Double-blind, placebo-controlled, crossover trial of glycine adjuvant therapy for treatment-resistant schizophrenia," *Br J Psychiat,* 169:610-17; 1996. (Glycine may improve negative symptoms, depression, cognitive symptoms, especially if low at baseline.)
Jaffe R, Kruesi OR, "The biochemical-immunology window: A molecular view of psychiatric case management," *J App Nutr,* 44(2); 1992.
Kasai K, Suzuki H, et al, "Glycine stimulates growth hormone release in man," *Acta Endocrin,* 93:283-6; 1980.
Page LR, *Healthy Healing,* Healthy Healing Pub, CA, 1992.
Pearson D, Shaw S, *Life Extension Companion,* Warner Books, NY, 1983.
Pfeiffer CC, *The Schizophrenias Ours to Conquer,* rev ed, Bio-Communications Press, Wichita, KS, 1988.
Rosenblatt S, Gaull GE, et al, "Amino acids in bipolar affective disorders: Increased glycine levels in erythrocytes," *Am J Psychiat,* 136(5):672-74; 5/1979. (RBC, but not plasma, glycine was generally elevated in female bipolars, whatever the mood.)
Rosenblatt S, Leighton WP, et al, "Elevation of erythrocyte glycine levels during lithium treatment of affective disorders," *Psychiat Res,* 6(2):203-14; 4/1982. (RBC glycine was increased (up to 90%) in a group of lithium-treated bipolars, peaking after about 100 days, and decreasing toward normal after three plus years. If lithium was stopped abruptly, RBC glycine increased dramatically and paradoxically, and remained elevated about 100 days.)
Ross J, *The Mood Cure,* Viking Penguin, NY, 2002.
Slagle P, *The Way Up Newletter Archives,* At: thewayup.com/newletters/newsarch.htm #0193
Smythies JR, "The role of one-carbon cycle in neuropsychiatric disease," *Biol Psychiat,* 19(5):755-58; 5/1984. (Carboxymethlation transmethylation reactions are important in coupling receptors to adenylate cyclase, and in neurotransmitter release. In some schizophrenics and depressives, the Vmax of MAT (methionine adenosine transferase) is decreased, and in some manics increased. MAT produces SAM, a key methylator; often an effective antidepressant.)
Tomaszewski A, Kleinrok A, et al, "The influence of strychnine and glycine on the metabolism of acetylcholine in the rat striatum and hippocampus," *Pol J Pharmacol Pharma,* 35(4):27; 1983.
Walsh WJ, PhD, "Commentary on nutritional treatment of mental disorders, *International Guide to the World of Alternative Mental Health.* At: www.alternativementalhealth.com/articles.walshMP.htm#Py Accessed:10/08/2006.
Yamamoto HA, McCain HW, et al, "Effects of amino acids, especially taurine and gamma-amminobutyric acid (GABA) on analgesia and calcium depletion induced by morphine in mice," *Euro J Pharma,* 71: 177-84; 1981.

Threonine

Baumel Syd, *Dealing with Depression Naturally,* Keats, New Canaan, CN, 1995
Blin O, "A double-blind placebo controlled trial of L-threonine in amyotrophic lateral sclerosis," *La Presse Medicale,* 18(30):1469-70; 9/1989.
Braverman E, Pfeiffer CC, *The Healing Nutrients Within,* Keats, New Canaan, CN 1987.
Doolittle TH, Hauser SL, et al, "Antispasticity effect of threonine in multiple sclerosis," *Arch Neurol,* 49: 923-6; 9/1992. (May also benefit depression.)
Fukuda N, Hidaka T, et al, "Altered hepatic metabolism of free fatty acid in rats fed a threonine-imbalanced diet," *J Nutr Sci Vitaminol,* 36(5):467-74; 10/1990.
Haas EM, *Staying healthy with nutrition: The complete guide to diet and nutritional medicine,* Celestial Arts, 2006.
Hendler S, *The Oxygen Breakthrough,* NY, William Morrough, 1989. (Can be low in depression.)
Honda T, "Amino acid metabolism in the brain with convulsive disorders. Part 2. The effects of anticonvulsants on convulsions and free amino acid patterns in the brain of E1 mouse," *Brain Dev,* 6(1):22-6; 1984.
Larson, Joan M, PhD, interview with author, June 9, 2008.
Lotan R, et al, "The effect of lysine and threonine supplementation on the immune response of growing rats fed wheat gluten diets," *Nutr Reports Intl,* 22(3):313-8; 1980.
Maes M, Verkerk R, et al, [Serum levels of excitatory amino acids, serine, glycine, histidine, threonine, taurine, alanine, and arginine in treatment-resistant depression: Modulation by treatment with antidepressants and prediction of clinical responsivity], *Acta Psychiatr Scand,* 97(4):302-8; 4/1998. (Over 5 wks, antidepressant nonresponders had significantly lower serum aspartate, asparagine, serine, threonine and taurine — which may predict response. Treatment reduced aspartate, glutamate and taurine; increased glutamine. Antidepressants may modulate excitatory aminos and taurine.)
Pfeiffer CC, *The Schizophrenias Ours to Conquer,* Bio-Communications Press, Wichita, KS, 1988.
Rogers QR, Tichenal CA, et al, "Threonine imbalance, deficiency and neurologic dysfunction in the kitten," *J Nutr,* 110(12):2444-59, 12/1980. (A food mix lacking threonine led to neurologic dysfunction in 14/17, and lameness, corrected via threonine.)

Serotonin

Annitto W, Shopsin B, "Neuropharmacology of Mania," in B Shopsin, ed, *Manic Illness,* Raven Press, NY 1979; pp 141-49. (Bipolars may underutilize serotonin.)
Baumel Syd, *Dealing with Depression Naturally,* Keats, New Canaan, CN, 1995.
Benkelfat C, et al, "Mood lowering effect of tryptophan depletion: Enhanced susceptibility in a young man at genetic risk for major affective disorders," *Arch Gen Psychiat,* 51:687-97; 1994.
Brewerton TD, et al, "Lithium carbonate and L-tryptophan in the treatment of bipolar and schizoaffective disorders," *Am J Psychiat,* 140:757-60; 1983. (3 gm L-tryptophan 3x/d with lithium created significantly greater improvement vs. lithium alone.)
Brigham PM, "The Psychopharmacology of Bipolar Disorder," updated 5-9-2001. At: http://people.ne.mediaone.net/pmbrig/BP_pharm.html
Chouinard G, Young SN, et al, "Tryptophan-nicotinamide combination in the treatment of newly admitted depressed patients," *Commun in Psych, Psychopharmacol,* 2(4):311-7; 1978.
Chouinard, G, et al, "A controlled clinical trial of L-tryptophan in acute mania," *Biol Psychiat,* 20:546-57; 1985. (Double blind. 24 manics were given 12 gm/d tryptophan for 1 wk; then 1/2 were given placebo. In wk 1, manic scores decreased significantly. In wk 2, scores worsened only in controls.)
Chouinard G, et al, "Tryptophan in the treatment of depression and mania," *Adv Biol Psychiat,* 10:47: 411-18; 1990. (Double blind. Some antidepressants may depend on serotonin availability.)
Coppen A, Prange AJ, et al, "Abnormalities of indoleamines in affective disorders," *Arch Gen Psychiatr,* 26:474-78; 1972.
Coppen AJ, Doogan DP, "Serotonin and its place in the pathogenesis of depression," *J Clin Psychiat,* 49S:4-11; 8/1988.
Coppen A, Shaw DM, et al, "Tryptamine metabolism in depression," *Br J Psychiat,* 111(479):993-8; 1965.
Coppen A, Prange AJ Jr, et al, "Abnormalities of indoleamines in affective disorders," *Arch Gen Psychiatr,* 26:474-78; 1972.
Copper A, Wood K, "Tryptophan and depressive illness" *Psychol Med,* 8:49-57; 1978.
Gayford JJ, Parker AL, et al, "Whole blood 5-hydroxytryptamine during treatment for endogenous depressive illness," *Br J Psychiat,* 122(570):597-8; 1973. (Caused hypomania in 2 depressives. Perhaps more likely if serotonin is elevated to start.)
Gelenberg AJ, et al, "Neurotransmitter precursors for the treatment of depression," *Psychopharmacol Bull,* 18(1):7-18; 1982. (Negative.)
JE Goldberg, M Harrow, eds, *Bipolar Disorders: Clinical Course and Outcome,* Am Psychiatric Press Inc, DC, 1999.
Landry P, Chouinard G, "Lithium-tryptophan combination in the maintenance treatment of bipolar affective illness," *Lithium,* 2:135-40; 1991. (Double blind. Drug resistant bipolars).
Maes M, et al, "The decreased availability of L-tryptophan in depressed females: Clinical and biological correlates," *Neuro Psychopharm Biol Psychiat,* 14:903-13; 1990.
Malone K, "Serotonin and major depression," in JJ Mann, DJ Kupfer, eds, *Biology of Depressive Disorders Part A,* Plenum Press, NY 1993.
Marazziti D, Lenzi A, "Decreased platelet serotonin uptake in bipolar I patients," *Int Clin Psychopharmacol,* 6(1):25-30; Spring/1991a. (The Vmax for uptake of 14C-5HT was significantly lower in 12 bipolars, indicating a transport problem.)
Marazziti D, Lenzi A, et al, "Serotinergic dysfunction in bipolar disorder," *Pharmacopsychiat,* 24(5):164-67; 9/1991b.
Murphy DL, et al, "L-tryptophan in affective disorders: Indoleamine changes and differential clinical effects," *Psychopharmacologia,* 34:11-20; 1974. (36% of 44 patients responded.)
Post RM, "Biochemical Theories of Mania," in R Belmaker, HM van Praag, eds, *Mania: An Evolving Concept,* Spectrum Pub, Jamaica NY, 1980; pp 233-35.
Prange AJ, et al, "L-tryptophan in mania," *Arch Gen Psychiat,* 30:56-62; 1974. (Double blind crossover. Tryptophan benefits acute mania, as well as, or better than, chlopromazine.)
Rogers S, *Depression, Cured at Last,* SK Publishing, Sarasota FL, 1997.
Ross J, *The Mood Cure,* Viking Penguin, NY, 2002.
Sachs GS, "Adjuncts and alternatives to lithium therapy for bipolar affective disorder," *J Clin Psychiat,* 50S:31-39; 12/1989. (Tryptophan antimanic for some at very high doses.)
Swann AC, Secunda S, et al, "CSF monoamine metabolites in mania," *Am J Psychiat,* 140:396-400; 1983.
Takahashi S, Kondo H, et al, "Effect of L-5-hydroxytryptophan on brain monoamine metabolism and evaluation of its clinical effect in depressed patients," *J Psychiat Res,* 12:177-87; 1975.
van Praag HM, "Indoleamines in depression," *Neuroregulators and Psychiatric Disorders,* 1977a.
van Praag HM, [Neuro-endocrine disorders in depression: Their importance for the study of the pathogenesis of depression] *Ned Tijdschr Geneeskd,* 121(50):2002-9; 1977b. (Serotonin, protirelin,

catecholamines, L-dopa, and peptides.)

Intro & Choline

Alarcon RD, et al, "One carbon metabolism disturbances in affective disorders, a preliminary report," *J Affect Dis,* 9:297-301; 1985.

Barabeau A, Growden JH, Wurtman RH, eds, "Choline and lecithin in brain disorders," in *Nutrition and the Brain,* V5, Raven Press, 1979.

Bartholini G, "GABA receptor agonists: Pharmacological spectrum and therapeutic agents," *Med Res Rev,* 5(1):55-75; 1-3/1985.

Beckman, H, "DL-phenylalanine in affective disorders," *Adv Biol Psychiat,* 10:137-47; 1983.

Benedito MA, Camarini R, "Rapid eye movement sleep deprivation induces an increase in acetylcholinesterase activity in discrete rat brain regions," *Braz J Med Biol Res,* 34(1):103-9; 1/2001.

Blusztajn JK, Wurtman RJ, "Choline and cholinergic neurons," *Science,* 221:614-619; 9/1983.

Braverman ER, Pfeiffer CC, *The Healing Nutrients Within,* Keats, New Canaan, CN, 1987.

Braverman ER, *Path Wellness Manual,* Publications for Achieving Total Health, NJ, 1994.

Braverman ER, "Brain mapping: A short guide to interpretation and philosophy," *J Orthomol Med,* 5(4):196-7; 1990.

Carroll PT, Buterbaugh GG, et al, "High affinity choline uptake by guinea pig brain: Effect of norepinephrine," *J Neurochem,* 24(5):917-24; 1975.

Casey DE, "Deanol in the mangement of involuntary movement disorders: A review," *Dis Nerv Syst,* 38: 7-15; 1977.

Charles HC, Lazeyras F, et al, "Brain choline in depression: In vivo detection of potential pharmacodynamic effects of antidepressant therapy using hydrogen localized spectroscopy," *Prog Neuropsychopharmacol Biol Psychiat,* 18(7): 1121-7; 11/1994. (Supports Ach hypothesis.)

Cohen BM, Miller AL, et al, "Lecithin in mania: A preliminary report," *Am J Psychiat,* 137:242-3; 1980. (4 manics responded markedly to 15-30 gm/day augmenting medication. After stopped, symptoms re-emerged in 3/4.)

Cohen BM, Lipinski JF, et al, "Lecithin in the treatment of mania: Double-blind, placebo-controlled trials," *Am J Psychiat,* 139(9):1162-4, 1982. (Lecithin significantly better than placebo in 5/6 manics, even when anticholinergics are used.)

Cooney C, *Methyl Magic,* Andrews McNeel Publishing, Kansas City, 1999; pp 154-66.

Cousens G, *Depression Free for Life,* Quill, HarperCollins, NY, 2000.

Crook TH, Thinklenberg J, et al, "Effects of phosphatidylserine in age-associated memory impairment," *Neurology,* 41:644-49; 1991.

D'Aldessariani RJ, "Dopamine and the patho-physiology of dyskinesias induced by anti-psychotic drugs," *Ann Rev Neuro Sci,* 3:23-41; 1980.

Davis JM, "Critique of single amine theories: Evidence of a cholinergic influence in the major mental illnesses," *Re Publ Assoc Re Ment Dis,* 54: 333-546; 1975.

Davis KL, et al, "Choline for tardive dyskinesia," *NEJM,* 293:152; 1976.

Davis KL, Berger PA, "Pharmacolgocial investigations of the cholinergic imbalance hypotheses of movement disorders and psychosis," *Biol Psychiat,* 13(1):23-49; 1978a.

Davis RE, Midalia ND, et al, "Illegal drugs and nutrition in undergraduate students," *Med J Aust,* 1(11):617-20; 1978b. (Perhaps low B6 or folate.)

Davis KL, Hollister LE, et al, "Cholinergic inhibition of methylphenidate-induced sterotype: Oxotremorine," *Psychopharmacol,* 56(1); Jan/1978c.

DeMet EM, Sodolski KN, "Sodium valproate increases pupillary responsiveness to a cholinergic agonist in responders with mania," *Biol Psychiat,* 46(3):432-6; 8/1999.

Dilsaver SC, Greden JF, "Antidepressant withdrawal-induced activation (hypomania and mania): Mechanism and theoretical significance," *Brain Res,* 319(1):29-48; 3/1984.

Dilsaver SC, "Pharmacologic induction of cholinergic system upregulation and supersensitivity in affective disorders research," *J Clin Psychopharmacol,* 6(2): 65-74; 4/1986.

Domino EF, Sharp RR, "NMR chemistry analysis of red blood cell contents in normal subjects and lithium-treated psychiatric patients," *Biol Psychiat,* 20(12):1277-83; 12/1985.

Duncan GE, Dagirmanjian R, et al, "Delta 9 tetrahydrocannabinol sensitization of the rat brain to direct cholinergic stimulation," *Psychopharmacol,* 60(3); 1/1979.

Egorov AV, Gloveli T, et al, "Muscarinic control of dendritic excitability and Ca2+ signaling in CA1 pyramidal neurons in rat hippocampal slice," *J Neurophysiol,* 82(4):1909-15; 10/1999.

Elkashef AM, Ruskin PE, et al, At: http://www.ncbi.nlm.nih.gov/entrez/query.fcgi?cmd=Retrieve&db=pubmed&dopt=Abstract&list_uids=1987837

El-Yousef MK, Janowsky DS, et al, "Induction of severe depression by physostigmine marijuana intoxicated individuals," *Br J Addict Alcohol Other Drugs,* 68(4):321-5; 12/1973.

Finney JW, et al, "Deanol and Tourette's syndrome," *Lancet,* 989; 10/31/1981.

Gelenberg Alan J, et al, "Choline and lecithin in the treatments of tardive dyskinesia: Preliminary results from a pilot study," *Am J Psychiat,* 136(6): 772-6; 1979.

Gelenberg AJ, et al, "A crossover study of lecithin treatment of tardive dyskinesia," *J Clin Psychiat,* 51(4):149-53, 1990. (Double blind crossover. Minimal, but definite benefit.)

Gershon, S, Shaw, F.H, "Psychiatric sequelae of chronic exposure to organophosphate insecticides," *Lancet,* (1):1371; 1961.

Gross CG, "Neurogenesis in the adult brain: Death of a dogma," *Nature Rev, Neurosci,* 1(2):67-73; 2000.

Groth DP, Bain JA, Pfeiffer CC, "The comparative distribution of C14-labeled 2-dimethylaminoethanol and choline in the mouse," *J Pharmacol Exp Ther,* 124(4):290-5; 1958. (DMAE is a stimulant.)

Growdon JH, "Use of phosphatidylcholine in brain diseases: An overview," in I Hanin, GB Ansell, eds, *Lecithin,* Plenum Publ, 1987.

Growden JH, Wurtman RJ, "Lecithin treatment of neuroleptic-induced tardive dyskinesia," in G Hemmings, ed, *Biological Aspects of Schizophrenia and Addiction,* Wiley, London, 1982; 129-38.

Growdon J, Cohen EL, Wurtman RJ, "Treatment of brain diseases with dietary precursors of a neurotransmitter," *Ann Intern Med,* 86:337-39; 1977.

Gundermann KF, Chapter 19, in G Cerv, F Paltauf, eds, *Phospholipids: Characterization, Metabolism And Novel Biological Applications,* AOCS Press, Champaign, IL, 1995; pp 209-227.

Hamakawa H, Kato T, "Quantitative proton magnetic resonance spectroscopy of the bilateral frontal lobes in patients with bipolar disorder," *Psycholog Med,* 29:639-44; 1999.

Hamakawa H Kato T, et al, "Quantitative proton magnetic resonance spectroscopy of the basal ganglia in patients with affective disorders," *Eur Arch Psychiat Clin Neurosci,* 248:53-8; 1998.

Haudrich R, Wang FLP, et al, "Increase in rat acetylcholine induced by choline or deanol," *Life Sci,* 17:975; 1975.

Hirata F, "Enzymatic methylation of phosphatidyl ethanolamine increased erythrocyte membrane fluidity," *Nature,* 275:219-20; 1978.

Hitzemann R, Mintzer MC, et al, "Characteristics of phospholipid methylation in human erythrocyte ghosts: Relationship(s) to the psychoses and affective disorders," *Biol Psychiat,* 20:397-407; 1985.

Hoffer A, "Mega amino acid therapy," *J Orthomol Psychiat,* 9(1):2-5; 1980.

Horrobin DF, "The role of essential fatty acids in schizophrenia," ISOM, Nutritional Medicine Today Conference, Vancouver, BC, 4/2000a.

Horrobin DF, "Essential fatty acids and mental health," *10th Winter schizophrenia workshop,* Davos, Switzerland, 2/5-12/2000." At: www.mhnj.com 10/15/2000b.

Jackson IV, et al, "Treatment of tardive dyskinesia with lecithin," *Am J Psychiat,* 136(11):1458-60, 1979. (Double blind crossover. All 6 improved.)

Jackson IV, et al "Lecithin administration in tardive dyskinesia: Clinical and medical correlates," *Biol Psychiat,* 16:85, 1981. (Double blind crossover.)

Jaffe R, Kruesi OR, "The biochemical-immunology window: A molecular view of psychiatric case management," *J App Nutr,* 44(2); 1992.

Janowsky DS, El-Yousef MK, et al, "Cholinergic reversal of manic symptoms," *Lancet,* 1:1236-37; 1972a.

Janowsky DS, el-Yousef MK, "A cholinergic-adrenergic hypothesis of mania and depression," *Lancet,* 2(7778):632-5; 9/1972b.

Janowsky DS, El-Yousef, et al, "Parasympathetic suppression of manic symptoms by physostigmine", *Arch Gen Psychiatr,* 28:542-47; 1973. (While low acetylcholine enhances catecholamine activity.)

Janowsky DS, Overstreet DH, et al, "Is cholinergic sensitivity a genetic marker for the affective disorders?" *Am J Med Genetics,* 54(4):335-44; 1994.

Jope RS, Jenden DJ, et al, "Erythrocyte choline concentrations are elevated in manic patients," *PNAS,* 77(10); 10/1/1980.

Kato T, Hamakawa H, et al, "Choline-containing compounds detected by proton magnetic resonance spectroscopy in the basal ganglia in bipolar disorder," *J Psychiatr Neurosci,* 21(4):248-54; 7/1996. (The choline to creatine and phosphocreatine peak ratio was higher in 19 euthymic bipolars (whether or not lithium-treated) than controls. Results suggest possible basal ganglia membrane breakdown.)

Kato T, Inubushi T, et al, "Magnetic resonance spectroscopy in affective disorders," *J Neuropsychiat Clin Neurosci,* 10(2):133-47; Spring, 1998. (MRS suggests abnormal metabolism of phosphate and membrane phospholipids, and abnormal intracellular pH. Lithium increases brain phosphomonoester peak (perhaps inositol-1-phosphate), but not the peak for choline-containing substances.)

Kidd, Paris M, "Phosphatidyl choline: A superior protectant against liver damage," *Alt Med Rev,* 1(4): 258-74; 1996. (PC protects membranes and is their most abundant constituent. It's safer than choline, 90% bioavailable, and enhances bioavailability of other nutrients.)

Kidd PM, "Phosphatidyl serine; membrane nutrient for memory. A Clinical and mechanistic assessment," *Alt Med Rev,* 1(2):70-84; 1996.

Krasnoperova MG, et al, "Use of cholinomimetics in the treatment of endogenous autism in children," *Zhurnal nevrologii i psikhiatrii,* 6:35; 2004.

Kuchel PW, Hunt GE, et al, "Lithium, red blood cell choline and clinical status: A prospective study in manic-depressive patients," *J Affect Disord,* 6(1): 83-94; 2/1985. (Lithium fostered RBC choline accumulation.)

Leiva DB, "The neurochemistry of mania: A hypothesis of etiology and rationale for treatment," *Prog Neuropsychopharmacol Biol Psychiatr,* 14(3): 423-9; 1990. (10 manics experienced permanent remission, supporting the cholinergic lack, adrenergic dominance hypothesis.)

Lewis JA, Young R, "Deanol in learning disorders," *J Clin Pharmacol Ther,* 15:210; 1974.

Lewis JA, Young RA, "A double-blind comparison of deanol and methylphenidate in children with learning disorders," unpubd data, Riker Laboratories, 1973.

Liscovitch M, Ben-Av P, et al, "Phospholipase D-mediated hydrolysis of phosphatidylcholine: Role in cell signalling," *J Lipid Mediat,* 8(3):177-82; 11/1993. (PLD, PLC and PLA2 signalling cascades are used by virtually all calcium-mobilizing agents.)

Mallinger AG, Kopp U, et al, "Erythrocyte choline transport in drug-free and lithium-treated individuals," *J Psychiatr Res,* 18(2):107-17; 1984.

Mandell AJ, Knapp S, "The effects of chronic administration of some cholinergic and adrenergic drugs on the activity of choline acetyltransferase in the optic lobes of the chick brain," *Neuropharmacol,* 10(4):513-6; 7/1971.

JJ Mann, ed, *The Biology of Depressive Disorders,* 1993.

Mervis RF, Parker KL, et al, "Chronic dietary choline and phosphatidylcholine induces dendritic growth in pyramidal cells of aging mouse neocortex," in Wurtman RJ, et al, ed, *Alzheimer's Disease: Advances in Basic Research and Therapies: Proceedings of the Fourth Meeting of the International Study Group on the Pharmacology of Memory Disorders Associated with Aging,* Zurich, Switzerland; 1987.

Miller E, "Deanol in the treatment of levodopa-induced dyskinesias," *Neurology,* 24:116-19; 1974.

Mitterauer B, "Imbalance of glial-neuronal interaction in synapses: A possible mechanism of pathophysiology of bipolar disorder," *The Neuroscientist,* 10(3):199-206; 2004. (Glial binding protein, by reducing free acetylcholine and other transmitters, may promote depression; if underexpressed, mania.)

Modestin J, Hunger J, et al, [Depressive effects of physostigmine], *Arch Psychiatr Nervenkr,* 218(1): 67-77; 11/1973.

Moore CM, Breeze JL, et al, "Choline, myo-inositol and mood in bipolar disorder: A proton-magnetic resonance spectroscopic imaging study of the anterior cingulate cortex," *Bipolar Disorders,* 2(3), 207-16; 8/2000. (PC metabolites and other choline compounds are altered.)

Morand, C, et al, "Clinical response of aggressive schizophrenics to oral tryptophan," *Biol Psych,* 18(5):575-78; 1983. (Double blind. Aggressive patients improved with tryptophan; nonaggressive patients worsened.)

Murray MT, Pizzorno J, *Encyclopedia of Natural Medicine,* Prima, Rocklin, CA, 1998.

Nakamura S, "Phosphatidyl choline hydrolysis and protein kinase C activation for intracellular signaling network," *J Lipid Mediat Cell Signal,* 14(1-3):197-202; 9/1996. (DAG transfers signals into the cell via PKC. Phospholipid degradation products can activate distinct PKCs, perhaps with distinct signal transduction roles, to control specific activity. Agonists may hydrolyze phosphotidyl choline via PLA2 and PLD, causing cell proliferation, differentiation, etc.)

NutriCircles®, Strickland Consulting, 1996.

Pace-Schott EF, Hobson JA, "The neurobiology of sleep: Genetics, cellular physiology, and subcortical networks," *Nat Rev Neurosci,* 3:591-605; 2002.

Pfeiffer CC, *Mental and Elemental Nutrients,* Keats, New Canaan, CN, 1975.

Pfeiffer CC, *Nutrition and Mental Illness,* Healing Arts Press, Rochester, VT, 1987.

Pfeiffer CC, *The Schizophrenias Ours to Conquer,* Bio-Communications Press, Wichita, KS, 1988.

Risch SC, Janowsky DS, "Cholinergic-adrenergic balance in affective illness," in RM Post, JC Ballenger, eds, *Neurobiology of Mood Disorders,* Williams & Wilkkins, Baltimore, 1984; pp 652-63.

Roe CM, Anderson MJ, Use of anticholinergic medications by older adults with dementia, *J Am Ger Soc,* 50(5):836-42; 2002.

Rogers S, *Depression, Cured at Last,* SK Publishing, Sarasota FL, 1997.

Rosenblatt JE, Janowsky DS, et al, "The augmentation of physostigmine toxicity in the rat by 9 tetrahydrocannabinol," *Res Commun Chem Pathol Pharmacol,* 3(3):479-82; 5/1972.

Ross J, *The Mood Cure,* Viking Penguin, NY, 2002.

Rowntree DW, Nevin S, Wilson A, "The effects of diis opropylfluorophosphate in schizophrenia and manic depressive psychoses," *J Neurol Neurosurg Psychiat,* 13:47; 1950. (Racing thoughts, hypomania.)

Samples JR, Janowsky DS, "Lethal effects of physostigme plus lithium in rats," *Psychopharmacol,* 52(3); 1/1977. (Physostigme increased lithium's toxicity. Reversed by scopolamine.)

Schreier HA, "Mania responsive to lecithin in a 13-year-old girl," *Am J Psychiat,* 139:108-10; 1982.

Senakayake, N, et al, "Neurotoxic effects of organophosphates," *NEJM,* 316:761; 1987.

Shopsin B, Janowsky D, et al, "Rebound phenomena in manic patients following physostigmine. Preliminary observations," *Neuropsychobiol,* 1(3): 180-7; 1975.

Sitaram N, Weingartner H, et al, "Human serial learning: Enhancement with arecholine and choline impairment with scopalamine," *Science,* 201(4352): 274-6; 7/21/1978.

Slagle P, "5-hydroxy-tryptophan (5HTP) and L-tryptophan," *The Way Up Newletter Archives,* #13 At: thewayup.com/newletters/newsarch.htm

Soares JC, Krishnan KR, et al, "Nuclear magnetic resonance spectroscopy: New insights into the pathophysiology of mood disorders," *Depression,* 4(1):14-30; 1996. (Increased basal ganglia choline resonance, and phospholipid and energy metabolism abnormalities in bipolars.)

Solana-Figueroa R, Prado-Alcala RA, "Retrograde amnesia produced by intrastriatal atropine and its reversal," *Life Sci,* 46(10):679-86; 1990.

Stadler H, Lloyd KG, et al, "Dopaminergic inhibition of striatal cholinergic neurons: Synergistic blocking action of gamma butyrolactone and neuroleptic drugs," *Arch Pharmacol,* 283(2); 6/1974.

Stoll AL, Cohen BM, et al, "Erythrocyte choline concentration in bipolar disorder: A predictor of clinical course and medication response," *Biol Psychiatr,* 29(12):1171-80; 6/15/1991.

Stoll AL, Sachs GS, et al, "Choline in the treatment of rapid-cycling bipolar diorder: Clinical and neurochemical findings in lithium-treated patients," *Biol Psychiat,* 40(5):382-88; 9/1/1996. (Choline bitartrate augmentation of lithium reduced manic symptoms substantially in 5/6 consecutive rapid-cyclers; all mood symptoms in 4.)

Stoll, AL, *The Omega-3 Connection,* Simon & Schuster, NY, 2002.

Sulser S, Bickel MH, et al, "Action of desmethyl-imipramine in counteracting sedation and cholinergic effects of reserpine-like drugs," *J Pharmacol Exp Ther,* 144(3):321-331, 1964.

Swann AC, "Biology of bipolar disorder," in JJ Mann, ed, *The Biology of Depresssive Disorders,* 1993. (Exaggerated response to choline.)

Tune LE, Anticholinergic effects of medication in elderly patients, *J Clin Psychiat,* 62(21):11-4; 2001

Uney JB, Duggan C, et al, "A pilot study of erythrocyte choline flux and content in affective disorders," *Psychol Med,* 16(2):337-41; 5/1986. (Choline did not increase with age unless taking lithium.)

Uney JB, Marchbanks RM, et al, "Lithium prophylaxis inhibits choline transport in post-mortem brain", *Lancet,* 2(8504):458; 8/23/1986.

Walsh WJ, "Biochemical individuality and nutrition," at: *NOHA News,* XXV(2):6-8; 2000.

Walsh WJ, "Commentary on nutritional treatment of mental disorders," *International Guide to the World of Alternative Mental Health.* At: www.alte rnativementalhealth.com/articles.walshMP.htm#Py Accessed:10/08/06.

Walsh, William J, PhD, interview with author, November, 2007.

Wehr TA, Goodwin FK, *Arch Gen Psychiat,* 36(5); 1979. (Rapid cycling induced by tricyclic.)

Williams CL, Meck WH, et al, "Hypertrophy of basal forebrain neurons and enhanced visuospatial memory in pernatally choline-supplemented rats," *Brain Res,* 794(2):225-38; 6/1998.

Wurtman RJ, "Effects of dietary amino acids, carbohydrates, and choline on neurotransmitter synthesis," *Mount Sinai J Med,* 55(1):75-86; 1988.

Wurtman RJ, et al, "Lecithin consumption raises serum-free choline levels," *Lancet,* 2:68-69; 1977.

Counterbalancing inositol

Agam G, Shamir A, et, "Myo-inositol-1-phosphate (MIP) synthase: A possible new target for antibipolar drugs," *Bipolar Disord,* 4(s1)15; 9/2002.

Bersudsky Y, Einat H, et al, "Epi-inositol and inositol depletion: Two new treatment approaches in affective disorder," *Curr Psychiat Reports,* 1:141-7; 1999. (Inositol restriction may benefit mania and augment lithium.)

Brown A, Mallinger A, et al, "Elevated platelet membrane phosphatidylinositol-4, 5-bisphosphate in bipolar mania," *Am J Psychiatr,* 150:1252-554; 1993.

Dubovsky SL, Murphy J, et al, "The calcium second messenger system in bipolar disorders: Data supporting new research directions," *J Neuropsychiatr Clin Neurosci,* 4(1):3-14, Winter/1992. (In bipolars and mania phosphotidylinositol and calcium signaling mechanisms are hyperactive. Lithium and other stabilizers normalize these systems.)

Kato T, Shioiri T, et al, "Measurement of brain phosphoinositide metabolism in bipolar patients using in vivo 31P-MRS," *J Affect Disord,* 22(4): 185-90; 1991.

Kato T, Inubushi T, et al, "Magnetic resonance spectroscopy in affective disorders," *J Neuropsychiat Clin Neurosci,* 10(2):133-47; 1998. (MRS suggests abnormal intracellular pH, and phosphate and membrane phospholipid metabolism. Lithium increases the phosphomonoester peak (perhaps inositol-1-phosphate), but not for choline-containing substances.)

Kim H, McGrath BM, et al, "A review of the possible relevance of inositol and the phosphatidylinositol second messenger system (PI-cycle) to psychiatric disorders — focus on magnetic resonance spectroscopy (MRS) studies," *Hum Psychopharmacol,* 20(5):309-26; 7/2005. (Particularly relevant to bipolars.)

Soares JC, Mallinger AG, "Abnormal phosphatidylinositol (PI)-signalling in bipolar disorder," *Biol Psychiat,* 39:461-4; 1996.

Shaldubina A, Ziva S, et al, "Inositol deficiency diet and lithium effects," *Bipolar Disord,* 8(2):152; 4/2006. (Major improvement, even in acute nonresponsive mania and rapid cycling, by 2 wks.)

Steen VM, "Does inositol signalling have a role in disease susceptibility and drug treatment of bipolar disorder?" *Bipolar Disord,* 4(S1):53-5; 2002.

Walsh, William J, PhD, interview with author, 11/2007

Wolfson M, Bersudsky Y, et al, "Chronic treatment of human astrocytoma cells with lithium, carbamazepine or valproic acid decreases inositol uptake at high inositol concentration but increases it at low inositol concentrations," *Brain Res,* 855(1):158-61; 2/7/2000. (May explain conflicting studies.)

EFAs

Buydens-Branchey L, Branchey M, "Omega-3 polyunsaturated fatty acids decrease anxiety feelings in a population of substance abusers," *J Clin Psychopharmacol,* 26(6):661-5; 2006. (Randomized double blind. Over 3 mo, 13 patients received 3 gm DHA and EPA. Anxiety decreased progressively and significantly. Over 3 post-treatment months, anxiety remained low in the 6 experimental subjects.)

Chiu CC, Huang SY, et al, "Omega-3 fatty acids are more beneficial in the depressive phase than in the manic in patients with bipolar I disorder," *J Clin Psychiat,* 66(12):1613-4; 12/2005.

Chiu CC, Huang SY, et al, "Polyunsaturated fatty acid deficit in patients with bipolar mania," *Eur Neuropsychopharmacol,* 13(2):99-103; 3/2003. (Red cell AA and DHA were significantly reduced over 20 manics, though total omega 3 and 6 were unchanged. Future studies should rule out the effect of meds, immune status, diet, smoking, etc, and check post remission PUFAs.)

Connor TJ, Leonard BE, "Depression, stress and immunological activation: The role of cytokines in depressive disorders," *Life Sci,* 62:583-606; 1998.

Hirashima F, Parow AM, Stoll AL, et al, "Omega-3 fatty acid treatment and T2 whole brain relaxation times in bipolar disorder," *Am J Psychiat,* 161:1922-24; 10/2004. (Omega 3 increased membrane fluidity in a dose-dependent manner.)

Horrobin DF, Bennett CN, "Depression and bipolar disorder: Relationships to impaired fatty acid and phospholipid metabolism and to diabetes, cardiovascular disease, immunological abnormalities, cancer, aging and osteoporosis. Possible candidate genes," *Prostaglandins Leukot Essent Fatty Acids,* 60(4):217-34; 4/1999. (

Kidd, PM, "Bipolar disorder as cell membrane dysfunction. Progress toward integrative management," *Alt Med Rev,* 9(2):107-35; 2004.

Maes M, "Interleukin-2 and interleukin-6 in schizophrenia and mania: Effects of neuroleptics and mood stabilizers," *J Psychiatr Res,* 29:141-52; 1995.

Maes M, Smith RS, "Fatty acids, cytokines, and major depression," *Biol Psychiat,* 43:313-4; 1998.

Rudin, Donald O, MD, et al, *The Omega-3 Phenomenon,* Rawson Assn, NY, 1987.

Seung Kim HF, Weeber EJ, et al, "Inhibitory effects of omega-3 fatty acids on protein kinase C activity in vitro," *Mol Psychiat,* 6(2):246-8; 2001. (Preliminary data suggest omega 3 is an effective mood stabilizer. Here, EPA, DHA, and the combo inhibited PKC, as do lithium and valproic acid. AA had no effect.)

Smith RS, "The macrophage theory of depression," *Med Hypotheses,* 35:298-306; 1991.

Sperling RI, Benincaso AI, et al, "Dietary omega-3 polyunsaturated fatty acids inhibit phosphoinositide formation chemotaxis in neutrophils," *J Clin Invest,* 91(2):651-60; 1999. (Omega 3 suppressed PI signal transduction pathways.)

Andrew Stoll MD, quoted in Kaplan, A, "Omega 3 fatty acids evaluated for bipolar disorder," *Psychiatric Times,* 16(12); 12/1999. At: psychiatrictimes.com/p991211.htm

Stoll AL, Severus WE, et al., "Omega 3 fatty acids in bipolar disorder: A preliminary double-blind, placebo-controlled trial," *Arch Gen Psychiat,* 56(5): 407-12; 5/1999.

Stoll AL, *The Omega-3 Connection,* Simon & Schuster, NY, 2002.

Su KP, Shen WW, et al, "Are omega 3 fatty acids beneficial in depression but not mania?" *Arch Gen Psychiat,* 57(7):716-7; 2000.

Sublette ME, Bosetti F, et al, "Plasma free polyunsaturated fatty acid levels are associated with symptom severity in acute mania," *Bipolar Disord,* 9(7):759-65; 2007. (Preliminary results suggest low EPA vs AA related to manic severity.)

Herbs

Akhondzadeh S, Naghavi HR, et al, "Passionflower in the treatment of generalized anxiety: A pilot double-blind randomized controlled trial with oxazepam," *J Clin Pharm Ther,* 26(5):363; 10/2001. (Equivalent effectiveness. Drug had more rapid onset but significantly more side effects.)

Almeida JC, Grimsley EW, "Coma from the health food store: Interaction between kava and alprazolam," *Annals Int Med,* 125(11):940-1; 12/1996. (May act on the same receptor and regions as benzos. One case of coma.)

Ambuehi, H, [Anatomical and chemical investigations on passiflora coerula L and passiflora incarnata L], *Dis Nr,* 3830, ETH Zurich; 1966.

Ayd FJ, "Evaluating interactions between herbal and psychoactive medications," *Psychiatric Times,* XVII (12); 12/2000. At: http://www.mhsource.cm/pt/p001245.html

Balch JF, Balch P, *Prescription for Natural Healing,* Avery, Garden City Park, NY, 1990.

Boeters U, "Treatment of autonomic dysregulation with valepotriates (Valmane)," *Muenchener Medizinische Wochenschrift,* 37:1873-6; 1969.

Cass H, healthy.net, nove 2002 (Most cases were taking alcohol or some other drug known to hurt the liver, consider effect of benzos on the body.)

Christopher JR, *School of Natural Healing,* Provo, UT, 1976.

Cropley M, Cave Z, et al, "Effect of kava and valerian on human physiological and psychological responses to mental stress assessed under laboratory condtions," *Phytother Res,* 16(1):23-7; 2002 (May reduce physiological reactivity under stress.)

Dressing H, Riemann D, et al, [Insomnia: Are valerian/melissa combinations of equal value to benzodiazepine?], *Therapiewoche,* 42:726-36; 1992.

Fugh-Berman A, Cott JM, "Dietary supplements and natural products as psychotherapeutic agents," *Psychosom Med,* 61(5):712-28; 9-10 1999. (Significant evidence supports St Johnswort for depression; ginkgo, dementia; kava, anxiety; valerian, insomnia; SAM, depression.)

Gammerman and ID Yourkevitch, eds, *Wild Medical Plants,* AF Bello-Russ Pubs, Acad Sci, Inst Exp Botanics Microbiology, Minsk, Bello-Russia, 1965.

Herberg KW, et al, [Effect of kava-special extract WS 1490 combined with ethyl alcohol on safety-relevant performance parameters], *Blutalkohol,* 30(2):96-105; 3/1993. (Concentration significantly improved in the group on kava alone, without alcohol.)

Hoenk, E, [Concerning psychic vegetative effects of a supposed antihistamineic], *Nervenarzt,* 37: 448-53; 1952.

Hoffman D, *The New Holistic Herbal,* Element Books, GB, 1990

Jussofie A, Schmiz A, et al, "Kavapyrone enriched extract from Piper methysticum as modulator of GABA binding site in different regins of rat brain," *Psychopharmacol (Berlin),* 116:469-75; 1994.

Kilch R, Gladbach B, [Childhood behavior disorders and their treatment], *Medizinische Welt,* 26(25): 1251-4; 1975.

Kinzle E, Kromer J, Lehmann E, [Clinical efficacy of a kava extract in patients with anxiety syndrome], *Arzheim-Forsch,* 41:584-8; 1991.

Kloss J, *Back to Eden,* Lifeline Bks, Riverside CA 1973.

Larson JM, *Depression Free — Naturally,* Ballantine Pub Gp, NY, 1999.

Larson JM, *Alcoholism — The Biochemical Connection,* Villard Books, NY, 1992.

Leathwood, PD, et al, "Aqueous extract of valerian root improves sleep quality in man," *Pharmacol Biochem Behav,* 17(1):65-71; 1982. (Double blind, 128 subjects. Sleep quality improved; latency decreased.)

Lesser M, *Nutrition & Vitamin Therapy,* Bantam Books, NY, 1983.

Lindahl O, "Double blind study of a valerian preparation", *Pharmacol Biochem Behav,* 32(4): 1065-66; 1989. (Improvement in 89%; perfect sleep in 49%.)

Lindenberg D, Pitule-Schodel HD, [L-kavain in comparison with oxazepam in anxiety disorders], *Forscht Med,* 108:49-50, 53-4; 1990.

Lutomski J, Alkaloidy, [Passiflora incarnata L], *Dissertation, Institut for Medicinal Plant Res,* Poznan, 1960.

Lutomski J, Segiet E, et al, [The meaning of passion flower in the healing arts], *Pharmazie in Unserer Zeit,* 10(2):45-9; 1981.

Malsch U, Kieser M, "Efficacy of kava-kava in the treatment of non-psychotic anxiety, following pre-treatment with benzodiazepines," *Psychopharmacol,* 157(3):277-83; 9/2001. (Benefits anxiety. Increases improvement after switching from benzos.)

Matthews JD, et al, "Effects of heavy usage of kava on physical health: Summary of a pilot survey in an aboriginal community," *Med J Aust,* 148:548-55; 1988.

Mowrey DB, *The Scientific Validation of Herbal Medicine,* Keats, New Canaan, CN, 1986a.

Mowrey DB, *Proven Herbal Blends,* Keats, New Canaan, CN, 1986b.

Murray MT, *Stress Anxiety and Insomnia,* Prima, Rocklin, CA, 1995.

Page LR, *Healthy Healing,* Healthy Healing Pub, CA, 1992.

Pfeiffer CC, Murphree HB, "Effect of kava in normal subjects and patients," *Psychopharmacol Bull,* 4(3): 12; 12/1967.

Pittler MH, Ernst E, "Kava extract for treating anxiety," Cochrane Database Syst Rev, CD003383; 2001, 02, 03: (Literature review. Superior to placebo.)

Ross J, *The Mood Cure,* Viking Penguin, NY, 2002.

Slagle P, *The Way Up from Down,* St Martin's Paperbacks, NY, 1992.

Spinella M, *The Psychopharmacology of Herbal Medicine: Plant drugs That Alter Mind, Brain, and Behavior,* MIT Press

Stein D, *The Natural Remedy Book for Women,* Crossing Press, Freedom, CA, 1992

Stevinson C, Huntley A, et al, "A systematic review of the safety of kava extract in the treatment of anxiety disorder," *Drug Saf,* 25(4):251-61; 2002. (Side effects mostly mild, can include skin and neurological reactions, and liver damage. Doesn't impair cognitive performance or vigilance. May interact with benzos.)

Walsh, William J, PhD, interview with author, April, 1995.

Werbach M, Murray MT, *Botanical Influences on Illness,* Third Line Press, Tarzana, CA, 1994.

Zinchernko TV, Feter IM, [Investigation of glycosides from betonica officinalis], *Armatsevt Shurnal,* 17(3): 35-8; 1962.

Theanine

Dharmananda S, *Biosci, Biotech, Biochem,* 1998, (Rats produced 26% more tryptophan and showed less anxiety.)

Eschenauer G, Sweet BV, "Pharmacology and therapeutic uses of theanine," *Am J Health Syst Pharm,* 63(1):26-30; 2006. (Dose dependent increase in alpha waves 40 minutes post ingestion.)

Kakuda T, "Inhibiting effect of theanine on caffeine stimulation evaluated by EEG in the rat," *Biosci, Biotech, Biochem,* 64:287-93; 2000.

Kobayahi K, Nagato Y, et al, "Effects of L-theanine on the release of alpha-brain waves in human volunteers," *Nippon Nogei Kagakukaishi,* 72(2): 153-7; 1998. (Counters caffeine stimulation. In 8 females with anxiety, 200 mg produced alpha waves in occiptal and parietal regions, more so with greater anxiety.)

Lekh RJ, et al, "L-theanine — A unique amino acid of green tea and its relaxation effect in humans," *Fooc Sci Tech,* 10(6-7):199-204; 1999.

Mason R, "L-theanine boosts alpha waves, promotes alert relaxation," *Alt Complementary Ther,* 7(2):91-95; 4/2001.

Yamada T, Terashima T, et al, "Effects of theanine, r-glutamylethylamide, on neurotransmitter release and its relationship with glutamic acid neurotransmission," *Nutr Neurosci,* 8(4):219-26; 8/2005. (Animal study. Theanine may inhibit excitatory, and promote inhibitory messages, especially glycine.)

Acute strategies

Cocchi P, et al, *J Orthomol Med,* 4(2):96-7; 1989. (Patients responded to IV ascorbic acid.)

Gaby A, "Intravenous vitamin and mineral therapy" presented at: *Nutritional Therapy in Medical Practice Conference,* Seattle, 1998.

Gaby AR, Intravenous nutrient therapy: "The Myers Cocktail," *Alt Med Rev,* 7(5):389-403; 2002.

Lemmo W, "Natural Treatment of Acute Mania," *International Guide to the World of Alternative Mental Health,* #30. At: www.alternativementalhealth.com/articles

Rebec GB, et al., "Ascorbic acid and the behavioral response to haldoperidol: Implications for the action of antipsychotic drugs," *Science,* 227:438-40; 1985. (Ascorbic acid blocks amphetamine response in rats.)

Saleeby, JP, MD, "Nutrient Cocktail for Schizophrenia and Bipolar Disorder: At: www.alternativementalhealth.com/articles/cocktail.htm 9/6/2005 (Drs. Alan Gaby and Harry Adelson pilot study at Naturopathic Medical Center at UI Bridgeport, and Saleeby in Savannah.)

Tolbert LC, et al., "Ascorbate affects conversion of tyrosine to dopamine in mouse brain," Abst., *Trans Am Soc Neurochem,* 1979a.

Tolbert LC, et al., "Effect of ascorbic acid on neurochemical, behavioral, and physiological symptoms mediated by catecholamines," *Life Sci,* 25:2189-95; 1979b. (Injections block amphetamine-induced stereotyped behavior in mice.)

B vitamins

General bibliography for all B vitamins:

Balch JF, Balch P, *Prescription for Nutritional Healing,* Avery, Garden City Park, NY, 1990.

Baumel S, *Dealing with Depression Naturally,* Keats, New Canaan, CN, 1995.

Braverman E, Pfeiffer CC, *The Healing Nutrients Within,* Keats, New Canaan, CN 1987.

Broida, Marian, RN, *New Hope for People with Depression,* Prima Publishing, Roseville CA, 2001.

Cousens G, *Depression free for Life,* Quill, HarperCollins, NY, 2001.

Garrison RH, Somer E, *The Nutrition Desk Reference,* Keats, New Canaan, CN, 1985.

Gold MS, *The Good News About Depression,* Villard Books, NY, 1987.
Hoffer A, *Common Questions on Schizophrenia and their Answers,* Keats, New Canaan, CN 1987.
Krohn J, *The Whole Way to Allergy Relief & Prevention,* Hartley & Marks, Pt Roberts, WA, 1991.
Larson JM, *Depression Free, Naturally,* Ballantine Wellspring, NY, 2001
Lesser M, *Nutrition & Vitamin Therapy,* Bantam Books, NY, 1983.
Lieberman S, Bruning N, *The Real Vitamin & Mineral Book,* Avery, Garden City Park, NY, 1990.
Murray MT, Pizzorno J, *Encyclopedia of Natural Medicine,* Prima, Rocklin, CA, 1998.
Murray MT, *Encyclopedia of Nutritional Supplements,* Prima, 1996.
Newbold HL, *Mega-nutrients for Your Nerves,* Berkeley Books, NY, 1975.
NutriCircles®, Strickland Computer Consulting, Version 3.25, April 29, 1996.
Pfeiffer CC, *Mental and Elemental Nutrients,* Keats, New Canaan, CN, 1975.
Pfeiffer CC, Nutrition and Mental Illness, Healing Arts Press, Rochester, VT, 1987.
Pfeiffer CC, *The Schizophrenias Ours to Conquer,* rev ed, Bio-Communications Press, Wichita, KS, 1988.
Quillin P, *Healing Nutrients,* Contemporary Books, Chicago, 1987.
Rogers S, MD, *Depression, Cured at Last,* SK Publishing, Sarasota FL, 1997.
Ross J, *The Mood Cure,* Viking Penguin, NY, 2002.
Slagle P, *The Way Up from Down,* St. Martin's Paperbacks, NY, 1992. Newsletters at: thewayup.com/newsletters/
Tenney L, *Stress,* Woodland Health Books, 1987.
Werbach MT, *Nutritional Influences on Mental Illness,* Third Line Press, Tarzana, CA, 1991.

Niacin, niacinamide (B3)

Ananth IV, et al, "Potentiation of therapeutic effects of nicotinic acid by pyridoxine in chronic schizophrenics," *Can Psychiatr Assoc J,* 18:377-83; 1973.
Birkmayer W, Birkmayer JG, "Nicotinamide adenine dinucleotide (NADH): The new approach in the therapy of Parkinsons disease," *Ann Clin Lab Sci,* 19(1):38-43; 1989a.
Birkmayer JG, Birkmayer W, [Stimulation of endogenous L-dopa biosynthesis — a new principle for the therapy of Parkinson's disease: The clinical effect of nicotinamide adenine dinucleotide (NADH) and nicotinamide adenine dinucleotidephosphate (NADPH)], *Acta Neurol Scand,* 126S:183-87; 1989b.
Birkmayer W, et al, "The coenzyme nicotinamide adenine dinucleotide (NADH) improves the disability of Parkinsonian patients," *J Neural Transm Park Dis Dement Sect,* 1(4):297-302; 1989c.
Birkmayer W, Birkmayer JG, "Coenzyme nicotinamide adenine dinucleotide (NADH) as a biological antidepressive agent. Experience with 205 patients," *New Trends Clin Neuropharmacol,* 5:19-25; 1991; 6:1-7; 1992 (Open label trial. 205 depressives, treated with NADH orally, IM or IV, over 5 to 310 days. 93% improved.)
Birkmayer JG, et al, [Nicotinamide adenine dinucleotide (NADH): A new therapeutic approach to Parkinson's disease: Comparison of oral and parenteral application], *Acta Neurol Scand,* 87(S146):32-35; 1993.
Birkmayer JG, "Coenzyme nicotinamide adenine dinucleotide: New therapeutic approach for improving dementia of the Alzheimer's type," *Ann Clin Lab Sci,* 26(1):1-9; 1996a.
Birkmayer JG, Vank P, "Reduced coenzyme 1 (NADH) improves psychomotoric and physical performance in athletes," *White Paper Report,* NY, Menuco Corp; 1996b.
Chaturvedi SK, Upadhyaya M, "Secondary mania in a patient receiving isonicotinic acid hydrazide and pyridoxine: Case report," letter, *Can J Psychiat,* 33(7):675-76; 10/1988.
Chouinard G, Young SN, et al, [Tryptophan-nicotinamide, imipramine and their combination in depression], *Acta Psychiatr Scand,* 59:395-414; 1979. (Double blind. Nutrient response was significantly correlated with plasma tryptophan elevation, but not in the group which also took the antidepressant (perhaps serotonin became too high). Study suggests appropriate doses are comparable to imipramine in major depression, and that lower doses augment medication. Bipolars may require more tryptophan.)
Cleary, JP, "The NAD deficiency diseases," *J Orthomol Med,* 1(3):149-57; 1986.
Curr Ther Res, 41:1017-1021; 1987. (With IV B3, benzodiazepine withdrawal symptoms decreased significantly.)
Glen AI, Cooper SJ, et al, "Membrane fatty acids, niacin flushing and clinical parameters," *Prostaglandins Leukot Essent Fatty Acids,* 55(1-2):9-15; 7-8/1996. (In negative symptom schizophrenia, flushing was associated with red cell AA and DHA, and increased affective symptoms.)
Green A, et al, "Metabolism of an oral tryptophan load: Effect of pretreatment with the putative tryptophan pyrrolase inhibitors nicotinamide or allopurinol," *Br J Clin Pharmacol,* 10:611-5; 1980.
Green GR, "Subclinical pellagra: Its diagnosis and treatment," *Schizophrenia,* 2(2-3):70-79; 1971.
Head KA, "Inositol hexaniacinate: A safer alternative to niacin," *Alt Med Rev,* 1(3):176-184; 1996. (Numerous trials suggest virtual absence of the flushing, pruritus, and altered glucose tolerance or liver enzymes that can occur with niacin. Extensive research indicates benefit to hyperlipidemia, intermittent claudication, Raynaud's disease. Benefit has been suggested in hypertension, diabetes, alcoholism, dysmennorrhea.)
Hoffer A, et al, "Treatment of schizophrenia with nicotinic acid and nicotinamide," *J Clin Exp Psychopath,* 18:131-58, 1957.
Hoffer A, *Niacin Therapy in Schizophrenia,* Charles C Thomas, Springfield IL 1962.
Hoffer A, Osmond H, "Treatment of schizophrenia with nicotinic acid: A ten-year follow-up," *Acta Psychiatr Scand,* 40:171-89; 1964.
Hoffer A, "The effect of nicotinic acid on the frequency and duration of rehospitalization of schizophrenic patients; A controlled comparison study," *Int J Neuro Psych,* 2:234-240; 1966.
Hoffer A, "Treatment of schizophrenia with a therapeutic program based upon nicotinic acid as the main variable," in O Wallaas, ed, *Molecular Basis of Some Aspects of Mental Activity,* V3, Academic Press, NY, 1967.
Hoffer A, "Mega vitamin B3 therapy for schizophrenia," *Cana Psych Assoc,* 16:499-504; 1971.
Hoffer A, "Mechanism of action of nicotinic acid and nicotinamide in the treatment of schizophrenia," in D Hawkins, L Pauling, eds, *Orthomolecular Psychiatry,* W H Freeman and Co, San Francisco, 1973.
Hoffer A, Walker, *Nutrients to Age without Senility,* Keats, New Cannaan, CN, 1980.
Hoffer A, "Nutrition and behavior," in J Bland, ed., *Medical Applications of Clinical Nutrition,* Keats, New Canaan, CN, 1983.
Hoffer A, Walker M, *A Guide to Nutrients that can Prevent and Reverse Senility,* Avery, Garden City Park, NY, 1994.
Hoffer A, "Another anecdote of schizophrenia, Psychological activity of nicotinamide adenine dinucleotide (NAD)," *J Orthomol Med,* 10:68-9; 1995.
Hoffer A, *Adventures in Psychiatry, The Scientific Memoirs of Dr Abram Hoffer,* KOS Pub, Caledon, ON, Canada, 2005.
Hoffer A, "Vitamin B3, niacin and its amide." At: Doctoryourself.com/hoffer_niacin.html Accessed 4/2007.
Horrobin DF, "The role of essential fatty acids in schizophrenia," *ISOM, Nutritional Medicine Today Conference,* Vancouver, BC, 4/2000a
Horrobin DF, "Essential fatty acids and mental health," *10th Winter Schizophrenia Workshop,* Davos, Switzerland, 2/5-12/2000. At: www.mhnj.com Accessed: 10-15-2000b.
Jaffe R, Kruesi OR, "The biochemical immunology window: A molecular view of psychiatric case management, *J App Nutr,* 44(2); 1992.
Joliffe, Norman, MD, 1939.
Kahan F, Hoffer A, Osmond H, *New Hope for Alcoholics,* University Books, NY, 1966.
Kuhn W, "Parenteral application of NADH in Parkinson's disease: Clinical improvement partially due to stimulation of endogenous levodopa biosynthesis," *J Neural Transm,* 103(1):1187-93; 1996.
McGinnis W, "Pyroluria: Hidden cause of schizophrenia, bipolar, depression, and anxiety symptoms," Orlando, 5/21/2004. *At:* alternativem entalhealth.com/articles/pyroluria.htm
Miller CL, Dulay JR, "The high affinity niacin receptor HM74A is decreased in the anterior cingulate cortex of individuals with schizophrenia," *Brain Res Bull,* 77(1):33-41; 9/2008.
Mohler H, et al, "Nicotinamide is a brain constituent with benzodiazepine-like actions," *Nature,* 278: 563-65; 1979.
Newbold HL, *Mega-nutrients for Your Nerves,* Berkeley Books, NY, 1975.
Osmond H, Hoffer A, "Massive niacin treatment in schizophrenia: Review of a nine year study," *Lancet,* 1:316-20; 1962. (Decreased long-term suicide rate.)
Osmond H, Hoffer A, "Naturally occurring endogenous major and minor tranquilizers," *J Orthomol Psychiat,* 9(3):198-205; 1980.
Patrie WM, "The use of nicotinic acid and pyridoxine in the treatment of schizophrenia," *Int Pharmacopsychiat,* 16(4):245-50; 1981. (B3 and B6 groups showed significant improvement. In B3 + B6 group, average phenothiazine dose decreased.)
Patton, Alva R, "Nutrient pioneers," *J Orthomol Psychiat,* 13(3):193-6; 1984.
Pfeiffer CC, *Mental and Elemental Nutrients,* Keats, New Canaan, CN, 1975.
Pfeiffer CC, *Nutrition and Mental Illness,* Healing Arts Press, Rochester, VT, 1987.
Pfeiffer CC, *The Schizophrenias Ours to Conquer,* Bio-Communications Press, Wichita, KS, 1988.
Prousky J, Seely D, "The treatment of migraines and tension-type headaches with intravenous and oral niacin (nicotinic acid): Systematic review of the literature," *Nutr J,* 4:3; 2005. (Vasodilation and improved brain energetics suggest benefit.)
Rudin DO, "The three pellagras," *J Orthomol Psychiat,* 12(2):91-110; 1983.
Smith RF, "A five year field trial of massive nicotinic acid therapy of alcoholics in Michigan," *J Orthomol Psychiat,* 3:327-32; 1974.
Smith RF, "Status report concerning the use of megadose nicotinic acid in alcoholics," *J Orthomol Psychiat,* 7:52-5; 1978.
Smith, Russell, *Drug and Cosmetic Industry,* 129(4): 68-69, 104-5; 1981. (B3 helped normalize blood sugar in hypoglycemic alcoholics.)
Spies T, "The treatment of subclinical and classical pellagra," *JAMA,* 111:584; 8/1938.
Spies T, "The mental symptoms of pellagra; their relief and nicotinic acid, *Am J Med Sci,* 196:461; 1938.
Strohle A, "The neuroendocrinology of stress and the pathophysiology and therapy of depression and anxiety," 74(3):279-92, Nervenarzt 3/2003a.
Strohle A, Holsboer F, "Stress responsive neurohormones in depression and anxiety," 36(3):207-14, *Pharmacopsychiat,* 36(3S):207-14; 12/2003b.
Sydenstricker VP, Cleckley HM, "The effect of nicotinic acid in stupor, lethargy and various other psychiatric disorders," *Am J Psychiat,* 98: 83-92; 1941.
Tonge, WL, "Nicotinic acid in the treatment of depression," *Ann Intern Med,* 38:551-3; 1953.
Velling DA, Dodick DW, et al, "Sustained-release niacin for prevention of migraine headache," *Mayo Clin Proc,* 2003.
Vrecko K, et al, [NADH stimulates endogenous dopamine biosynthesis by enhancing the recycling of tetrahydrobiopterin in rat phaeochromocytoma cells], *Biochim, Biophys Acta,* 361(1):59-65; 1997.
Walsh WJ, "Biochemical individuality and nutrition," *NOHA News,* XXV(2):6-8; 2000.
Washburne AC, "Nicotinic acid in the treatment of certain depressed states: A preliminary report,"

Ann Int Med, 32:261-69; 2/1950. (14/15 withdrawn, retarded depressives improved in days, many dramatically, on megadoses. 11 responded again when depression recurred.)

Wilson B, "The vitamin B3 therapy: The first communication to AA's Physicians," 1967; & "A Second Communication to AA's Physicians," 1968.

Wittenborn JR, "A Search for responders to niacin supplementation," *Arch Gen Psychiatr,* 31:547-552; 1974.

Pyridoxine (B6)

Adams PW, Wynn V, et al, "Vitamin B6, depression, and oral contraception," letter, *Lancet II,* 1974; pp 516-7.

Adams PW, Wynn V, et al, "Effect of pyridoxine hydrochloride upon depression associated with oral contraception," *Lancet,* ii:899-904; 1973. Postive double blind.)

Ananth IV, et al, "Potentiation of therapeutic effects of nicotinic acid by pyridoxine in chronic schizophrenics," *Can Psychiatr Assoc J,* 18:377-83; 1973.

Benton D, Hallert J, et al, "Vitamin supplementation for 1 year improves mood," *Neuropsychobiol,* 32(2): 98-105; 1995. (Mood improvement in females was associated with increased B6 status.)

Bernstein AL, "Vitamin B6 in clinical neurology," *Ann NY Acad of Sci,* 585:250-60; 1990. (Some studies suggest B6 improves depression, pain, headache, hyperactivity, and aggression. Support for serotonin formation may play a role.)

Bermond P, "Therapy of side effects of oral contraceptive agents with vitamin B6," *Acta Vitaminol Enzymol,* 4(1-2):45-54; 1982. (Poor B6 and tryptophan metabolism due to OCs can lead to depression, anxiety, poor glucose tolerance, and low libido. 40 mg B6/day relieved symptoms in low B6-women on OCs.)

Brenner A, "The effects of megadoses of selected B complex vitamins on children with hyperkinesis: controlled studies with long-term follow-up," *J Learn Disabil,* 15(5):258-64; 1982.

Brooks SC, et al, "An unusual schizophrenic illness responsive to pyridoxine HCl subsequent to phenothiazine butyrophenone toxicities," *Biol Psychiat,* 18(11):1321-8; 1983. (500 mg B6 was effective in 2 nonresponsive catotonics.)

Buist RA, "Anxiety neurosis: The lactate connection," *Int Clin Nutr Rev,* 5:1-4; 1984.

Brush MG, Perry M, "Pyridoxine and the premenstrual syndrome," *Lancet,* 1399; 5/15/1985.

Bukreev VI, [Effect of pyridoxine on the psychopathology and pathochemistry of involutional depressions], *Zh Nevropatol Psikhiatr,* 78(3):402-08; 1978. (B6 is a cofactor of DOPA decarboxylase, so promotes creation of catecholamines. Intake by 31 involutional melancholics and 17 late-onset bipolars improved mood, increased NE excretion.)

Carney MWP, et al, "Thiamin, riboflavin and pyridoxine deficiency in psychiatric in-patients," *Br J Psychiat,* 141:271-72; 1982. (Affectives tended to be low in both B2 and B6.)

Chaturvedi SK, Upadhyaya M, "Secondary mania in a patient receiving isonicotinic acid hydrazide and pyridoxine: Case report," letter, *Can J Psychiat,* 33(7):675-76; 10/1988.

Dakshinamurti K, "Neurobiology of Pyridoxine," in HH Draper, ed, *Adv Nutr Res,* Vol 4, Plenum, NY, 1982; pp143-79.

Deijen JB, et al," Vitamin B6 supplementation in elderly men. Effects on mood, memory, performance and mental effort," *Psychopharmacol,* 109(4):489-96; 1992.

Doll H, "Pyridoxine (vitamin B6) and the premenstrual syndrome: A randomized crossover trial," *J Royal Coll Gen Practitioners,* 39:364-368; 9/1989.

Green AR, Aronson JK, "The pharmacokinetics of oral L-tryptophan: Effects of dose and concommitant pyridoxine, allopurinol or nicotinamide administration," *Adv Biol Psychiat,* 10:67-81; 1983. (A high dose and lengthier tryptophan therapy may be needed, unless B6 is also used to help degrade kynurenine.)

Gunn ADG, "Vitamin B6 and premenstrual syndrome (PMS)," *Int J Vitam Nutr Res,* 27S:213-24 [review]. (Helps with PMS depression.)

Hallert C, Astrom J, et al, [Reversal of psychopathology in adult coeliac disease with the aid of pyridoxine], *Scand J Gastroenterol,* 18(2):299-304; 1983. (In 12 consecutive celiac depressives, 1 yr post gluten withdrawal, mood remained low, despite GI improvement. After 1.5 more yrs, 6 mo. of 80 mg B6 reduced MMPI depression scale ratings from an average 70 to 56. B6 may influence CNS mood-regulating mechanisms.)

Hoes MJ, "L-tryptophan in depression and strain," *J Orthomol Psychiat,* 11(4):2231-42; 1982. (B6, zinc and tryptophan.)

Hoffer A, "Nutrition and behavior," in J Bland ed, *Medical Applications of Clinical Nutrition,* Keats, New Canaan, CN, 1983.

Hoffer A, *Orthomolecular Medicine For Physicians,* Keats, New Canaan, CN, 1983.

Jaffe, R, Kruesi OR, "The biochemical—immunology window: A molecular view of psychiatric case management," *J App Nutr,* 44(2); 1992.

Joshi, Vasant MB, et al, "Vitamins B1, B6, and B12 in the adjunctive treatment of schizophrenia — further studies to examine the effect of reduction of chlorpromazine dosage," *J Orthomol Psychiat,* 11(1):45-9; 1982.

Kakuma S, et al, "Enhanced acetaldehyde hepatotoxicity in vitamin B6 deficiency," *Gastroenterology,* 71:914; 1976.

Kendall KE, Schnurr PP, "The effects of vitamin B6 supplementation on premenstrual syndrome," *Ob Gyn,* 70:145-49; 1987.

Kleijnen J, Knipschild P, "Niacin and vitamin B6 in mental functioning: A review of controlled trials in humans," *Biol Psychiat,* 29(9):931-41; 1991.

Martineau J, et al, "Vitamin B6, magnesium, and combined B6-magnesium: Therapeutic effects in childhood autism," *Biol Psychiat,* 20(5):467-78; 5/1985. (Double blind involving 60 autistics. B6 and magnesium led to significant improvement.)

McGinnis W, "Pyroluria: Hidden cause of schizophrenia, bipolar, depression, and anxiety symptoms," Orlando, 5/21/2004. *At:* alternativementalhealth.com/articles/pyroluria.htm

Nobbs BT, "Pyridoxal phosphate status in clinical depression," letter, *Lancet,* i:405-406; 3/9/1974.

NutriCircles®, Strickland Computer Consulting, Version 3.25, April 29, 1996.

Patrie WM, "The use of nicotinic acid and pyridoxine in the treatment of schizophrenia," *Int Pharmacopsychiat,* 16(4):245-50; 1981.

Pfeiffer CC, Sohler A, et al, "Treatment of pyroluric schizophrenia (malvaria) with large doses of pyridoxine and a dietary supplement of zinc," *J Orthomol Psychiat,* 3(4):292-3; 1974.

Pfeiffer CC, Bacchi D, "Copper, zinc, manganese, niacin and pyridoxine in the schizophrenias," *J Appl Nutr,* 27:9-39, 1975b.

Pfeiffer CC, "Pyroluria, zinc, and B6 deficiencies," *Intl Clin Nutr Rev,* 8(3):107-110; 1988b.

Russ CS, et al, "Vitamin B6 status of depressed and obsessive-compulsive patients," *Nutr Rep Intl,* 27(4): 867-73; 1983. (Plasma pyridoxal phosphate was almost 50% lower in 7 depressives compared to controls. B6 enzymes were low in all depressed; no controls.)

Schaumberg HH, et al, "Sensory neuropathy from pyridoxine abuse: A new megavitamin syndrome," *NEJM,* 309:445-48; 1983.

Shiloh R, Weizman A, et al, [Antidepressive effect of pyridoxine (vitamin B6) in neuroleptic-treated schizophrenic patients with comorbid minor depression — preliminary open-label trial], *Harefuah,* 140(5):359-73; 5/2001. (2/9, with greater pre-trial HAM-D and SANS, lengthier illness, older, showed marked symptomatic improvement (about 25% lower HAM-D and SANS).)

ME Shils, VR Young, eds, *Modern Nutrition in Health and Disease,* Leo & Febiger, Philadelphia, PA, 1988. (Volunteers on a low B6 diet, and given a B6 antagonist, became irritable and depressed.)

Stewart TW, Harrison W, et al, "Low B6 levels in depressed outpatients," *Biol Psychiat,* 19(4):613-6; 1984. (Levels were low in 21/101 depressives without confounding disorders. 14/21 showed neurological symptoms.)

Tohoku, *J Experimental Med,* 140:45-51; 1983.

Wyatt KM, Dimmock PW, et al, "Efficacy of vitamin B-6 in the treatment of premenstrual syndrome: Systematic review," *BMJ,* 318:1375-81; 1999. (Meta analysis, 10 studies, suggests improvement.)

Wynn V, et al, "Tryptophan, depression and steroidal contraception," *J Steroid Biochem,* 6:965-70; 1975. (Placebo controlled. B6 was highly effective in severely-depressed, low-B6 women on OCs.)

Walsh WJ, "Biochemical individuality and nutrition," *NOHA News,* XXV(2):6-8; 2000.

Choline, Inositol

Cohen M, Miller AL, et al, "Lecithin in mania: A preliminary report," *Am J Psychiat,* 137:242-3; 1980. (4 manics responded markedly to 15-30 gm/day p-choline with ongoing meds. After discontinuing lecithin, manic symptoms re-emerged in 3/4.)

Cohen BM, Lipinski JF, et al, "Lecithin in the treatment of mania: Double-blind, placebo-controlled trials," *Am J Psychiat,* 139(9):1162-4, 1982. (Lecithin was significantly better than placebo in 5/6 patients, even when anticholinergics were used.)

Janowsky DS, El-Yousef MK, "Cholinergic reversal of manic symptoms," *Lancet,* 1:1236-37; 1972.

Janowsky DS, El-Yousef, et al, "Parasympathetic suppression of manic symptoms by physostigmine," *Arch Gen Psychiatr,* 28:542-47; 1973b. (Low acetylcholine enhances catecholamine potency.)

Leiva DB, "The neurochemistry of mania: A hypothesis of etiology and rationale for treatment," *Prog Neuropsychopharmacol Biol Psychiatr,* 14(3): 423-9; 1990. (Permanent remission of mania in 10 subjects. Support for cholinergic insufficiency, adrenergic dominance hypothesis of mania.)

Risch SC, Janowsky DS, "Cholinergic-adrenergic balance in affective illness," in RM Post, JC Ballenger, eds, *Neurobiology of Mood Disorders,* Williams & Wilkkins, Baltimore, 1984; pp 652-63.

Stoll AL, Sachs GS, et al, "Choline in the treatment of rapid-cycling bipolar disorder: Clinical and neurochemical findings in lithium-treated patients," *Biol Psychiat,* 40(5):382-88; 9/1/96.(Choline bitartrate augmentation of lithium substantially reduced manic symptoms in 5/6 consecutive rapid-cyclers; all mood symptoms, in 4. Basal ganglia choline compounds increased considerably in responders.)

Walsh, William J, PhD, interview with author, November 2007.

B12, folic acid

Abalan F, et al, [Frequency of deficiencies of vitamin B12 and folic acid in patients admitted to a geriatric-psychiatry unit], *Encephale,*10:9-12; 1984.

Abou-Saleh MT, Coppen A, "The biology of folate in depression: Implications for nutritional hypotheses of the psychoses," *J Psychiatric Res,* 20(2):91-101; 1986.

Abou-Saleh MT, Coppen A, [Serum and red blood cell folate in depression], *Acta Psychiatr Scand,* 80(1):78-82; 1989. (Associated with severity.)

Acta Med Scand, Vitamin B12 hypovitaminosis in mental disease, 1965. (About 30x greater deficit in hospitalized mental patients vs general population.)

Alpert JE, Fava M, "Nutrition and depression: The role of folate," *Nutr Rev,* 55:145-9; 1997.

Alpert JE, Mischoulon D, et al, "Nutrition and depression: Focus on folate," *Nutr,* 16(7-8):544-6; 2000.

Alpert M, Silva RR, et al, "Prediction of treatment response in geriatric depression from baseline folate levels," *J Clin Psychpharmacol,* 23:3; 6/2003.

Bagnelie DV, et al., *Am J Clin Nutr,* 531:659; 1991. (Enlarged RBCs in second generation vegans failed to improve with nori, but fish was beneficial.)

Bell IR, Edman JS, "Relationship of normal serum vitamin B12 and folate levels to cognitive test performance in subtypes of geriatric major depression," *J Geriatr Psychiat Neurol,* 3(2): 98-105; 4-6/1990. (In psychotic depressives (vs. nonpsychotic, bipolars and dementia) B12 significantly correlated with IQ, verbal and visual memory, and other cognitive measures.)

Bell IR, Edman JS, et al, "Vitamin B12 and folate status in acute geropsychiatric inpatients: Affective and cognitive characteristics of a vitamin nondeficient population," *Biol Psychiatr,* 27(2):125-37; 1/15/1990. (Below median B12 and folate were associated with more severe symptoms. Low folate was associated with lengthier hospitalizations and late-onset depression. Low B12 was more common with organic psychoses and no family psychiatric history.)

Bell IR, et al, "B-complex vitamin patterns in geriatric and young adult inpatients with major depression," *J Am Ger Soc,* 39(3):252-57; 3/1991.

Bendich, A., "Safety issues regarding the use of vitamin supplements," *Ann NY Acad Sci,* 669: 300-10; 1992.

Bjelland I, Ueland PM, et al, "Folate and depression," *Psychother Psychosom,* 2003.

Botez MI, Fontaine F, et al, "Folate-responsive neurological and mental disorders: Report of 16 cases," *Eur Neurol,* 16(1-6):230-46; 1977.

Botez MI, et al, "Relapsing neuropathy, cerebral atrophy, and folate deficiency. A close association," *Appl Neurophysiol,* 42(3):171-83; 1979.

Bottiglieri R, Crellin RF, "Folate and neuropsychiatry," in *Folate in Health and Disease,* Marcel Dekker, NY 1995.

Bottiglieri T, Lanundry M, et al, "Homocysteine, folate, methylation, and monoamine metabolism in depression," *J Neurol, Neurosurg Psychiat,* 2000.

Br J Psychiat, 153:266-7; 8/1988. (B12 deficit may predispose to psychotic symptoms during depression.)

Carney MW, "Serum folate in 423 psychiatric patients," *Br Med J,* iii:512-8; 1967.

Carney MW, Sheffield BF, "Associations of subnormal serum folate and vitamin B12 and effects of replacement therapy," *J Nerv Ment Dis,* 150:404-12; 1970.

Carney MW, Sheffield BF, "Serum folic acid and B12 in 272 psychiatric in-patients," *Psychol Med,* 8:139-44; 1978.

Carney MW, "Psychiatric aspects of folate deficiency," in MI Botex, EH Reynolds, eds, *Folic Acid in Neurology, Psychiat, and Internal Medicine,* Raven Press, NY, 1979.

Carney MW, Chary TK, et al, "Red cell folate concentrations in psychiatric patients", *J Affect Disord,* 19(3):207-13; 7/1990. (Low in depressives.)

Coppen A, Chaudhry S, "Folic acid enhances lithium prophylaxis," *J Affect Disord,* 10(1):9-13; 1986.

Coppen A, Bolander-Gouaille, "Treatment of depression: Time to consider folic acid and vitamin B12," *J Psychopharmacol,* 2005.

Coppen A, et al, "Plasma folate and affective morbidity during long-term lithium therapy," *Br J Psychiat,* 141:87-89; 1982. (Affective morbidity was greater in those with lower folate. Animal studies indicate an association with low serotonin.)

Coppen A, Bailey J, "Enhancement of the antidepressant action of fluoxetine by folic acid: A randomized, placebo-controlled trial," *J Affect Disord,* 60:121-30; 2000.

Coppen A, Swade C, "Depression and tetrahydrobiopterin: The folate connection," *J Affect Disord,* 16(2-3):103-7; 1989.

Crellin R, Bottiglieri T, et al, "Folates and psychiatric disorders: Clinical Potential," *Drugs,* 45:623-36; 1993.

Curtis H, Muldner H, Niederwieser, "Tetrahydro-biopterin: Efficacy in endogenous depression and Parkinson's disease," *J Neural Trans,* 55:301-8; 1982.

Curtis H, et al, "Successful treatment of depression with tetrahydrobiopterin," *Lancet,* 657-8; 1983.

DeLiz AJ, "Large amounts of nicotinic acid and vitamin B12 in the treatment of apparently irreversible psychotic conditions found in patients with low levels of folic acid," *J Orthomol Psychiat,* 8(2):63-5; 1979.

Di Palma C, Urani R, et al, "Is methylfolate effective in relieving major depression in chronic alcoholics? A hypothesis of treatment," *Curr Ther Res,* 55:559-67; 1994. (Large intake of methylfolate was beneficial.)

Dommisse J, "Subtle vitamin B12 deficiency and psychiatry: A largely unnoticed but devastating relationship?" *Med Hypotheses,* 34:131-40; 1991.

Duthie SJ, Whalley LJ, et al, "Homocysteine, B vitamin status, and cognitive function in the elderly," *Am J Clin Nutr,* 2002.

Eastley R, Wilcock GK, et al, "Vitamin B12 deficiency in dementia and cognitive impairment," *Intl J Geriatric Psychiat,* 2000.

Edwin E, et al, "Vitamin B12 hypovitaminosis in mental disease," *Acta Med Scand,* 177:689-99; 1965.

Ellis FR, Nasser S, "A pilot study of vitamin B12 in the treatment of tiredness," *Br J Nutr,* 30:277-83; 1973. (Double blind. B12 injections enhanced energy and mood in chronically fatigued patients, even without obvious deficiency.)

Engelborghs S, Vloeberghs E, et al, "Correlations between cognitive, behavioral and psychological findings and levels of vitamin B12," *Intl J Geriatr Psychiat,* 19L:365-70; 2004.

Engstrom G, Traskman-Bendz L, "Blood folate, vitamin B12, and their relationships with cerebrospinal fluid monoamine metabolites," *Nordic J Psychiat,* 1999.

Fava M, "Folate, vitamin B12, and homocysteine in major depressive disorder," *Am J Psychiat.* At: ajp.psychiatryonline.org 1997.

Gaby AR, "The story of vitamin B12: Is vitamin B12 a panacea or placebo?" *Nutrition & Healing,* 2(7); 7/1995.

Geagea K, Ananth J, "Response of a psychiatric patient to vitamin B12 therapy," *Dis Nerv Sys,* 36: 323-344; 6/1975.

Ghadirian AM, Ananth J, et al, "Folic acid deficiency and depression," *Psychosom,* 21(11):926-29; 1980. (Folate inversely correlated with severity.)

Godfrey PSA, et al, "Enhancement of recovery from psychiatric illness by methyl folate," *Lancet,* 336:392-95; 8/18/1990. (Double blind. Major depressives and schizophrenics with low red cell folate improved significantly over 6 mo. with high dose methylfolate.)

Goggans FC, "A case of mania secondary to vitamin B12 deficiency," *Am J Psychiatr,* 141(2): 300-301; 1984. (A mania, presenting without other symptoms of pernicious anemia, resolved in 6 mo. with monthly B12 shots.)

Guaraldi GP, Fava M, et al, "An open trial of methyltetrahydrofolate in elderly depressed patients," *Ann Clin Psychiat,* 5(2):101-5; 1993.

Hasannah CI, et al, "Reduced red-cell folate in mania," J Affect Disord, 46(2):95-99; 11/1997. (Especially with neurological symptoms.)

Hashimoto R, Ozaki N, et al, "The plasma tetrahydrobiopterin levels in patients with affective disorders," *Biol Psychiat,* 28:526-8; 1990.

Hector M, Burton JR, "What are the psychiatric manifestations of vitamin B12 deficiency?" *J Am Geriatr Soc,* 36(12):1105-12; 12/1998. (Confusion, cognitive slowing, memory problems, delirium, depression, delusions, hallucinations, acute psychosis. Less commonly, reversible mania.)

Hermest H, Weizman A, [Vitamin B12 and folic acid serum levels in obsessive compulsive disorder], *Acta Psychiatr Scand,* 78(1):8-10; 1988.

Heseker H, Kubler W, et al, "Psychological disorders as early symptoms of a mild to moderate vitamin deficiency," *Ann NY Acad Sci,* 669:352-7; 1992.

Hilsson Ehle, H, "Age-related changes in cobalamin handling, Implications for therapy," *Drugs Aging,* 1998.

Hintikka J, Tolmunen T, et al, "High vitamin B12 levels and good treatment outcome may be associated in major depressive disorder," *Bio Med Central Psychiat,* 2003. (Mood can improve dramatically with repletion.)

Hoffer A, "Nutrition and behavior," in Jeffrey Bland, ed, *Medical Applications of Clinical Nutrition,* Keats, New Canaan, CN, 1983.

Hoffer A , Walker M, *Orthomolecular Nutrition,* Keats, New Canaan, CN, 1978.

Hommes OR, Hollinger JL et al, "Convulsant properties of folate compounds: Some considerations and speculations," in MI Botez, EN Reynolds, eds, *Folic Acid in Neurology, Psychiatry and Internal Medicine,* Raven Press, 1979.

Holmes JM, "Cerebal manifestations of vitamin B12 deficiency," *Br Med J,* ii:1394-8; 1956.

Howard JS, "Folate deficiency in psychiatric practice," *Psychosomatics,* 16:112-15; 1975. (May be associated with depression, weakness, spasticity, numbness, stiffness, muscular atrophy.)

Hunter, R, "Serum B12 and folate concentration in mental patients," *Br J Psych,* 113:1291-95; 1967. (About 25% of hospitalized patients are deficient.)

Hutto BR, "Folate and cobalamin in psychiatric illness," *Compr Psychiat,* 38(6):1; 1997.

Jaffe R, Kruesi OR, "The biochemical immunology window: A molecular view of psychiatric case management," *J App Nutr,* 44(2); 1992.

Joshi, Vasant MB, et al, "Vitamins B1, B6, and B12 in the adjunctive treatment of schizophrenia — further studies to examine the effect of reduction of chlorpromazine dosage," *J Orthomol Psychiat,* 11(1):45-9; 1982.

J Nutr Med, 2:89-90; 1991. (Depression can occur even without anemia.)

Kallstrom B, et al, [Vitamin B12 and folate concentrations in mental patients], *Acta Psychiat Scand,* 45:137-52; 1969.

Karnase DS, Carmel R, "Neurologic and evoked potential abnormalities in subtle cobalamin deficiency states, including deficiency without anemia and with normal absorption of free cobalamin," *Arch Neurol,* 47(9):1008:12; 1990.

Kivela SL, Pahkala, et al, "Depression in the aged: Relation to folate and vitamins C and B12," *Biol Psychiat,* 26: 209-13; 1989.

Lancet, V. II, 7/28/1984, pp 196-8. (Folic acid benefitted depressed patients, and helped those who didn't respond well to medications.).

Larner AJ, Janssen JC, "Cognitive profile in dementia associated with vitamin B12 deficiency due to pernicious anaemia," *J Neurol,* 1999.

Lee S, Chow CC, et al, "Folate concentration in Chinese psychiatric outpatients on long-term lithium treatment," *J Affect Disord,* 24(4):265-70; 4/1992. (Folate deficiency is uncommon in China, though relatively higher blood folate was associated with better response to lithium.)

Lee S, Wing YK, et al, "A controlled study of folate levels in Chinese inpatients with major depression in Hong Kong," *J Affect Disord,* 49(1):73-7; 4/1998.

Leeming R, et al, "Tetrahydrofolate and hydroxycobalamin in the management of dihydropteridine reductase deficiency," *J Ment Def Res,* 26:21-5; 1982.

Levitt AJ, Joffe RT, "Folate, B12, and thyroid function in depression," *Biol Psychiat,* 33:52-3; 1993.

Levitt AJ, Joffe RT, "Folate, B12 and life course of depressive illness," *Biol Psychiat,* 25(7):867-72; 1989. (Low folate & lengthier depressions.)

Levitt AJ, Wesson VA, et al, "Impact of suppression of thyroxine on folate status during acute antidepressant therapy," *Psychiat Res,* 79(2):123-9; 6/15/98. (Antidepressant response has been linked to red cell folate and reduced T4. 4-wk double blind. Improvement occured in 14/25 and was associated with increased folate.)

Lindenbaum J, Healton EB, et al, "Neuropsychiatric disorders caused by cobalamin deficiency in the absence of anemia or macrocytosis," *N Engl J Med,* 318:1720-28; 1988. (Deficiency affects mood, which improves with supplementation.)

Mesulam MM, Moran MA, "Cholinesterase within neurofibrillary tangles related to age and Alzheimer's patients," *Nature,* 1985.

Morris MS, "Folate, homocysteine, and neurological function," *Nutr Clin Care,* 5(3):124; 2002.

Morris MS, Fava M, "Depression and folate status in the US population," *Psychother Psychosom,* 2003.

Newbold HL, MD, "The use of vitamin B12b in psychiatric practice, *J Orthomol Psychiat,* 1(1): 27-36; 1972.

Newbold HL, "Vitamin B12: Placebo or neglected therapeutic tool," *Med Hypotheses,* 28:155-164; 1989.

Ohta T, et al, "Daily activity and persistent sleep-wake

schedule disorders," *Prog Neuro-Psychopharmacol Biol Psychiat,* 16:529-37; 7/1992.

Papakostas GI, Petersen T, "Serum folate, vitamin B12, and homocysteine in major depressive disorder, Part I," *J Clin Psychiat,* 2004.

Passeri M, Cucinotta G, et al, "Oral 5-methyltetrahydrofolic acid in senile organic mental disorders with depression: Results of a double-blind multicentre study," *Aging Clin Expt Res,* 51:63-71; 1993. (At least equivalent to the pharmaceutical.)

Paul RTP, McDonnell AP, "Folic acid: Neurochemistry, metabolism and relationship to depression," *Hum Psychopharmacol Clin Exp,* 2004.

Penninx BWJ, Guralnik JM, "Vitamin B12 deficiency and depression in physically disabled older women: Epidemiological evidence," *Am J Psychiat,* 157:715-721; 2000. (Serum B12 was significantly lower in 122 severely depressed vs 478 nondepressed. Deficit was 2x as likely with severe depression.)

Pfeiffer CC, Braverman ER, "Folic acid and vitamin B12 therapy for the low histamine, high copper biotype of schizophrenia," in MI Botez, EN Reynolds, eds, *Folic Acid in Neurology, Psychiatry and Internal Medicine,* Raven Press, NY; 1979; pp 483-87.

Prakash R, Sethi N, et al, "A case of megaloblastic anemia secondary to lithium," *Am J Psychiat,* 138(6): 849; 6/1981. (Reversed by high-dose folate.)

Procter A, "Enhancement of recovery from psychiatric illness by methylfolate," *Br J Psychiat,* 1991.

Reading CM, "Latent pernicious anaemia: A preliminary report," *Med J Aust,* 1:91-4; 1975.

Reutens S, Sachdev P, "Homocysteine in neuropsychiatric disorders of the elderly," *Intl J Geriatric Psychiat,* 17:859-64; 2002.

Reynolds EH, Carney MW, Toone BK, "Methylation and mood," *Lancet,* 2(8396):196-8; 7/1984. (Folic acid benefitted depressives including those non responsive to medication.)

Reynolds E, Stramentinoli G, "Folic acid, S-adenosylmethionine and affective disorder," *Psychol Med,* 13:705-10; 1983.

Reynolds EH, "Folic acid, aging, depression, and dementia," *Br Med J,* 2002.

Reynolds E, et al, "Folate deficiency in depressive illness," *Br J Psychiat,* 117:287-92; 1970. (Low in a large number of depressives.)

Rita M, Paola T, et al, "Vitamin B12 and folate depletion in cognition: A review," *Neurology (India),* 2004.

Rosche J, [Depression and folic acid in patients with epilepsy], *Nervenheilkunde,* 2002.

Schilling RF, Morris FK, "Is vitamin B12 a tonic?" *Wis Med J,* 70(5):143-4; 1971.

Shorvon SD, Carney MWP, et al, "The neuropsychiatry of megaloblastic anaemia," *Br Med J,* 281:1036-43; 1980.

Slagle P, "Vitamn B12, Folic Acid/ Homocysteine," *The Way Up Newletter Archives,* #33 At: thewayup.com/newletters/newsarch.htm

Tiemeier H, van Tuijl HR, et al, "Vitamin B12, folate and homocysteine in depression: The Rotterdam study," *Am J Psychiat,* 159:2099-2101; 12/2002. (112 depressives vs controls. Depression related to low B12. Also, homocysteinemia and low folate, but less so after adjusting for disability and heart disease.)

Taylor MJ, Carney SM, Goodwin GM, et al, "Folate for depressive disorders: Systematic review and meta-analysis of randomized controlled trials," *J Psychopharm,* 2004.

Thornton WE, Thornton BP, "Geriatric mental function and folic acid: A review and survey," *Southern Med J,* 70:919-22; 1977.

Tolmunen T, Voutilainen S, et al, "Dietary folate and depressive symptoms are associated in middle-aged Finnish men;" 2003. At: hn.nutrition.org

Tolmunen T, Hintikka J, "Association between depressive symptoms and serum concentrations of homocysteine," *Am J Clin Nutr,* 2004.

van Tiggelen CJM, Peperkamp JPC, et al, "Vitamin B12 levels of cerebrospinal fluid in patients with organic mental disorder," *J Orthomol Psychiat,* 12(4): 305-11; 1983.

Walsh WJ, "Commentary on nutritional treatment of mental disorders, *International Guide to the World of Alternative Mental Health.* At: www.alternativementalhealth.com/articles.walshMP.htm#Py Accessed: 10/08/2006.

Walsh William J, PhD, interview with author, November 2007.

Whyte EM, Mulsant BH, "Cognitive and behavioral correlates of low vitamin B12 levels in elderly patients with progressive dementia?" *Am J Geriatr Psychiat,* 10:321-7; 6/2002.

Wolfersdorf M, Knoig F, "Serum folic acid and vitamin B12 in depressed inpatients. A study of serum folic acid with radioimmunoassay in 121 depressed inpatients," *Psychiatr Prax,* 22(42):162-64; 1995.

Zhang X, Fan C, "Study on serum folic acid and vitamin B12 levels of patients with depression," *J Clin Psychological Med,* 2006.

Zucker DK, et al, "B12 deficiency and psychiatric disorders: Case report and literature review," *Biol Psychiat,* 16:197-205; 1981.

Thiamin (B1)

Bell IR, Edman JS, et al, "Vitamin B1, B2 and B6 augmentation of tricyclic antidepressant treatment in geriatric depression with cognitive dysfunction," *J Am Coll Nutr,* 11:159-63; 4/1992. (Randomized controlled double blind. Modest doses of B1, B2, and B6 enhanced antidepressant response.)

Benton D, Hallert J, et al, "Vitamin supplementation for 1 year improves mood," *Neuropsychobiol,* 32(2): 98-105; 1995. (In the 90 female students, low baseline B1 was associated with low POMS on several measures of mood. Increased B1 over 3 mo. was associated with improved mood. By 1 yr, sleep improved.)

Benton D, Donohoe RT, "The effects of nutrients on mood," *Public Health Nutr,* 2:403-9; 1999. (Double blind, placebo-controlled. B1 improves mood in the general population.)

Benton D, Griffiths R, et al, "Thiamin supplement-ation, mood and cognitive function," *Psychopharmacol,* 129(1):66-71; 1997. (Even with adequate initial levels, 50 mg per day given to 120 young adult females, increased clarity, composure, and energy.)

Bowman KM, Goodhart R, Joliffe N, "Observations on the role of vitamin B1 in the aetiology and treatment of Korsakoff's psychosis," *J Nerv Mental Disease,* 1939.

Brozek J, "Psychologic effects of thiamine restriction and deprivation in normal young men," *Am J Clin Nutr,* 5(2):109-20; 1957. (5/9 developed marked depression and irritability on a low B1 diet.)

Carney MWP, et al, "Thiamin, riboflavin and pyridoxine deficiency in psychiatric in-patients," *Br J Psychiat,* 141:271-72; 1982. (53% were low B1 (especially schizophrenics), B2, and/or B6.)

Carney MWP, Williams DG, et al, "Thiamin and pyridoxine lack in newly admitted psychiatric patients," *Br J Psychiat,* 135:249-54; 1979.

Clin Neuropharmacol, 8:286-93; 7-9/1985. (30% of 172 psychiatric patients were deficient in B1, though only one showed clinical symptoms.)

Connor DJ, "Thiamin intake and monoamine oxidase activity," *Biol Psychiat,* 16:869-72; 9/1981. (Double blind. 3 days of 400 mg B1 (divided doses) significantly inhibited MAO in 21 male students.)

Fattal-Valevski A, Kesler A, et al, "Outbreak of life-threatening thiamine deficiency in infants in Israel caused by a defective soy-based formula," *Pediatrics,* 115(2); 2/2005. (Physicians reported irritability, lethargy, anorexia, and developmental delay, in 156 infants inadvertently fed B1-deficient formula. Irreversible brain damage can occur.)

Heseker H, Kubler W, et al, "Psychological disorders as early symptoms of a mild to moderate vitamin deficiency," *Ann NY Acad Sci,* 669 352-7; 1992. (Of 1081 healthy males, those with chronic B1 deficiency showed significantly more depression.)

Jaffe R, Kruesi OR, "The biochemical immunology window: A molecular view of psychiatric case management," *J App Nutr,* 44(2); 1992.

Lonsdale D, "Thiamine," *J Orthomol Psychiat,* 13(3): 197-209; 1984.

Lonsdale D, Shamberger RJ, "Red cell transketolase as an indicator of nutritional deficiency," *Am J Clin Nutr,* 33:205-11; 2/1980.

McConachie, Haskew A, "Thiamine status after major trauma," *Intensive Care Medicine,* 14(6); 10/1988. (Sedative effects. Prospective study of patient with severe injury found severe deficiency (low transketolase) though feeding included B1.)

McConachie I, Haskew A, Lereboullet J, Pluvinage R, et al, "Sedative action of a thiazole derivative of thiamine in delirium tremens," *Bull Mem Soc Med Hop,* 72(28-9):693-6; 1958.

Osterman E, Bellander-Lofvenberg S, et al, "SCTZ, a new sedative and hypnotic related to thiamine," *Acta Psychiatr Scand,* 34(136S):56-61; 1959.

Sacks W, et al, "Acetzolamide and thiamine: A preliminary report on an ancilliary therapy for chronic mental illness," *J Clin Psychopharmaco,l* 8:70; 1988.

Smidt IJ, Cremin FM, et al, "Influence of thiamin supplementation on the health and general well-being of an elderly Irish population with marginal thiamine deficiency, *J Gerontol,* 46(1): M16-22; 1991. (Double blind. B1, given to 80 marginally-deficient women, improved appetite, energy, low weight, well-being, activity, fatigue, sleep patterns.)

Thiessen, Imgard, PhD, "The role of thiamine in research with animals and in humans," *J Orthomol Psychiat,* 7(2):107-13; 1978.

Williams RD et al, "Induced thiamin (B1) deficiency in man: Relation of depletion of thiamine to development of biochemical defect and of polyneuropathy," *Arch Inter Med,* 71:38-53; 1943.

Riboflavin (B2)

Bell IR, et al, "Complex vitamin patterns in geriatric and young adult inpatients with major depression, *J Am Geriatr Sci,* 39(3):252-7; 3/1991. (28% of 20 elderly and 16 young adult unipolars were low in B2, B6 or B12.)

Bell IR, Morrow FD, et al, [Low thyroxine levels in female psychiatric patients with riboflavin deficiency: Implications for folate-dependent methylation], *Acta Psychiatr Scand,* 85(5):360-3; 5/1992b. (Methylation can include a step dependent on FAD, a B2-dependent enzyme. 9/52 acute inpatients were B2 deficient; all female, relatively young, with low baseline thyroxine, and a nonsignificant tendency to depression, but not schizophrenia or bipolar disorder. Only one also had another B deficiency. B2 deficit may mark thyroxine status in some females, and may indicate methylation defects.)

Carney MWP, et al, "Thiamin, riboflavin and pyridoxine deficiency in psychiatric in-patients," *Br J Psychiat,* 141:271-72; 1982. (B2 was deficient in up to 29% of 172 sucessive admissions, especially depressives, schizophrenics and alcoholics.)

Easlove M, et al, "Severe riboflavin deficiency: A previously undescribed side-effect of phenothiazines," *J Orthomol Psychiat,* 12(2):113-5; 1983.

Heseker 1992, ibid. (Of 1081 healthy males, those with chronic B2 deficiency showed significantly more depression on the Adjective Check List.)

Jaffe R, Kruesi OR, 1992, ibid.

Miyake Y, Sasaki S, et al, "Dietary folate and vitamins B1, B2, B6 and B2 intake and the risk of postparum depression in Japan: The Osaka maternal and child health study," *J Affect Disord,* 96(1-2):133-38; 2006. (Third trimester B2 may decrease risk of postpartum depression.)

Pinto J, et al, "Inhibition of riboflavin metabolism in rat tissues by chlorpromazine, imipramine and amitriptyline," *J Clin Invest,* 67(5):1500-06; 1981.

Sterner RT, Price WR, "Restricted riboflavin: Within-subject behavioral effects in humans," *Am J Clin Nutr,* 26:150-60; 1973. (56 days of severe B2 restriction in 6 male COs, produced symptoms of hypomania, hysteria, psychopathy, depression, shallow emotions, or hypochondriasis, reflected in MMPI scores. 2 wks repletion did not readily reverse scores. Deficiency may also lead to physical complaints, hypersensitivity, weakness, lethargy.)

Pantothenic acid (B5)

Adams PW, Rose DO, et al, "Effect of pyridoxine hydrochloride (vitamin B6) upon depression associated with oral contraception," *Lancet*, 1:899-904; 1973. (Better than placebo in depressed women low in B6 and taking birth control pills.)

Amrich L, Hurley LS, et al, "Response to stress by riboflavin-deficient and pantothenic acid-deficient dogs," *Am J Physiol*, 184(3):515-20; 1956.

Baker H, et al, "Inability of chronic alcoholics with liver disease to use food as a source of folates, thiamin and vitamin B6," *Am J Clin Nutr*, 28, 1377-80; 1975.

Brenner A, "The effects of megadoses of selected B complex vitamins on children with hyperkinesis: controlled studies with long-term follow-up," *J Learn Disabil*, 15(5):258-64; 1982. (Double blind. ADD children, often also emotional unstable, most on stimulants, were consecutively given 3 days of: B1 (100 mg, 4x/day), lactose placebo, calcium pantothenate (110 mg, 2x/day), B6 (100 mg, 3x/day). With improvement, a 2nd wk of that vitamin was assigned, plus 1 wk placebo; with dramatic improvement, a long-term trial, with dose periodically reduced or discontinued. Initially, 4 improved on B5, vs. 2 on methylphenidate.)

Casentini S, [Relations between pantothenic acid and cold stress], *Boll Soc Ital Biol Sper*, 32(12): 1419-22; 12/1956.

Early RG, Carlson BR, [Water-soluble vitamin therapy in the delay of fatigue from physical activity in hot climatic conditions], *Int Z Angew Physiol*, 27: 43-50; 1969. (B5 is critical to CoA which helps B6 and fatty acids enter the TCA cycle. Depletion may result from increased metabolism or perspiration. Energy production might then focus on glycolysis. Fat metabolism may also be compromised.)

Fry PC, et al, "Metabolic response to a pantothenic acid deficient diet in humans," *J Nutr Sci Vitaminol*, 22:239-46; 1976. (Half of 10 males on a low B5 diet were given 10 mg, daily. By 63 days, the remaining half seemed listless, and complained of fatigue.)

Gensini GF, Prisco D, et al, "Changes in fatty acid composition of the single platelet phospholipids induced by pantethine treatment," *Int J Clin Pharmacol Res*, 5:309-18; 1985. (Double blind crossover. 20 dislipidaemics. B5 increased HDL, phospholipids, selectively increased omega 3; decreased AA (omega 6), cholesterol, triglycerides, saturated and monounsaturated fats.)

Hodges RE, Ohlson MA, et al, "Pantothenic acid deficiency in man," *J Clin Invest*, 1958.

NutriCircles®, Strickland Computer Consulting, Version 3.25, April 29, 1996.

Thornton GHM, et al, *J Clin Invest*, 34:1073; 1955. (A B5-deficient diet, left subjects easily upset, and prone to anger. Other reactions: extreme fatigue, sleep problems, dizziness, reduced blood pressure, rapid pulse on exertion, muscle weakness, GI issues, chronic upper respiratory infections. Progressively reduced adrenal hormones, and sharply reduced digestive and gastric secretion and motility.)

Tohoku J Experimental Med, 140:45-51; 1983. (B5 used clinically in epilepsy, postencephalitis syndrome, retardation, childhood disorders.)

Vecsci L, Widerlov E, "Preclinical and clinical studies with cysteamine and pantethine related to the central nervous system," *Prog Neuropsychopharmacol, Biol Psychiat*, 14:835-862; 1990. (B5 is metabolized into CoA, which degrades into cysteamine. Cystaeamine (and, somewhat, B5) deplete somatostatin, prolactin and NE. Cystamine influences avoidance, kindled seizures, and pain perception.)

Biotin

Firestone, "Growth-promoting effects of biotin and biotin derivatives for the oral yeast Candida albicans," 1959.

Haneke E, [Biotin as a therapeutic hair and nail substance], *Med Monatsschr Pharm*, 17(6):187; 6/1994.

Levinson JL, "Biotin-responsive depression during hyperalimentation," *J Parenteral Enteral Nutr*, 7(2): 181-3; 1983. (General parenteral intake, if overdone, can create severe depression, delirium, paresthesia, anorexia, headaches, nausea, pallor, dermatitis. Biotin improved symptoms.)

Mock DM, Mock NI, et al, "Disturbances in biotin metabolism in children undergoing long-term anticonvulsant therapy," *J Pediatr Gastroenterol Nutr*, 1998. (Can be due to chronic antibiotics or antiseizure meds.)

Pawlowski A, Kostanecki W, [Effect of biotin on hair roots and sebum excretion in women with diffuse alopecia], *Pol Med J*, 5(2):447-52; 1966.

Shirayama Y, Andrew CH, et al, "Brain-derived neurotrophic factor produces antidepressant effects in behavioral model of depression," *J Neurosci*, 22(8):3251-61; 4/2002. (Benefit equivalent to antidepressants (as indicated by forced swim test and learned helplessness) emerging as early as 3 days after a single infusion, and lasting 10 or more days.)

Yamaguchi H, [Mycelial development and chemical alteration of Candida albicans from biotin insufficiency], *Sabouraudia*, 12(3):320-8; 11/1974.

Antioxidants

Abdalla DS, Manteiro HP, et al, "Activities of superoxide dismutase and glutathione peroxidase in schizophrenic and manic depressive patients," *Clin Chem*, 32:805-7; 1986.

Agen V, Serbinova E, "Antioxidant effects of unbiquinones in microsomes and mitochondria are mediated by tocopherol recycling," *Biochem Biophys Res Commun*, 169:851-57; 1990.

Akbaraly NT, Hininger-Faveir I, et al, "Plasma selenium over time and cognitive decline in the elderly," *Epidemiology* 18(1):52-8; 2007. (The greater the decrease in plasma selenium in 1389 elderly, the greater the cognitive decline.)

Aleksandrovskii P, Neznamov GG, et al, [Lipid peroxidation in emotional stress and neurotic disorders], *Zh Nevropatol Psikhiatr Im SS Korsakova*, 88(11):95-101;1988. (Membrane lipid peroxidation correlated with emotional stress severity. Neurotic disorders were inverse to alpha tocoperol.)

Altenkirch H, et al, "Effects of lipoic acid in hexacarbon-induced neuropathy," *Neurotoxicol Teratology*, 12(6):619-22; 11-12/1990.

Altschule MD, Siegel EP, et al, "Blood glutathione level in mental disease before and after treatment," *Arch Psychiat*, 71:69-74; 1955. (Affirms early case reports of low glutathione in bipolars.)

Altschule MD, Goncz RM, et al, "Carbohydrate metabolism in brain disease. VII. The effect of glutathione on carbohydrate intermediary metabolism in schizophrenic and manic-depressive psychoses," *AMA Arch Intern Med*, 99(1):22-7; 1/1957.

Anderson R, "The immunostimulatory, anti-inflammatory, and anti-allergic properties of ascorbate", in Harold H Draper ed, *Advances in Nutritional Research*, Vol 6, Plenum, NY, 1984; pp. 19-45. (Deficiency increases likelihood of drug-induced delirium or sensitivity, addictions , alcoholic psychosis, toxic metal accumulation.)

Anonymous patient quoted at: *www.alternativementalhealth.com/testimonials/bipolar5.htm*

Balch JF, Balch PA, *Prescription for Nutritional Healing*, Avery, Garden City Park, NY, 1990.

Barak Y, Swartz M, et al, "Vitamin E (alpha-tocopherol) in the treatment of tardive dyskinesia: A statistical meta-analysis," *Ann Clin Psychiat*, 10(3); 9/1998. (In 12 double blinds over 223 patients given 400-1600 IU/day, 28.3% showed improvement. Side effects were rare and not significant.)

Baumel S, *Dealing with Depression Naturally*, Keats, New Canaan, CN, 1995.

Beauclair L, et al," An adjunctive role for ascorbic acid in the treament of schizophrenia," *J Clin Psychopharmacol*, 7:282-3; 1987. (Symptoms in 10/13 neuroleptic-treated patients improved on up to 8 gm C /day for 8 wks.)

Bendich A, Machlin LJ, "The safety of oral intake of vitamin E: Data from clinical studies from 1986 to 1991," in L Packer, J Fuchs, eds, *Vitamin E in Health and Disease*, Marcel Dekker, NY, 1993.

Bendich, A, "Safety issues regarding the use of vitamin supplements," *Ann NY Acad Sci*, 669: 300-10; 1992.

Benton D, Cook R, "Selenium supplementation improves mood in a double blind crossover trial," *Psychopharmacol*, 102(4); 12, 1990. (50 subjects. Substantial improvement at 2.5 and 5 weeks with 100 mcg/day vs. placebo.)

Benton D, Cook R, "The impact of selenium supplementation on mood," *Biol Psychiat*, 29(11): 1092-98; 1/1/1991. (The greater the deficit, the more the improvement in anxiety, depression, and fatigue after 5 wks of selenium.)

Benton D, "Selenium intake, mood and other aspects of psychological functioning," *Nutritional Neurosci*, 5(6):363-74; 2002. (5 studies associate low intake with poor mood. Brain retention increases with deficiency. Selenium, as an antioxidant role may benefit Alzheimer's, Parkinson's, schizophrenia, TD.)

Berry IT, "Negative symptoms, glutathione peroxidase and dopamine receptors," *J Orthomol Med*, 7(1):24-30; 1992.

Berry IT, "Selenium deficiency and clinical findings in schizophrenia: A common thread," *J Orthomol Med*, 8(1):21-4; 1993.

Berson EL, Rosner B, "A randomized trial of vitamin A and vitamin E: Supplementation for retinitis pigmentosa," *Arch Opthamol*, 111:7661-72; 1993.

Beyer R, "The role of ascorbate in antioxidant protection of biomembranes: Interaction with vitamin E and coenzyme Q," *J Bioenerget*, 26(4): 349-58; 1994.

Biol Trace El Res, 7:161-8; 4-5/1985. (Double blind. Se and E helped older patients reduce fatigue, anorexia, depression, anxiety, mood swing, hostility; improved well-being, alertness, motivation, initiative, self-care, interest in the environment.)

Bland J, *Bioflavonoids*, Keats, New Canaan, CN, 1984.

Bland J, *The 20-Day Rejuvenation Diet Program*, Keats, New Canaan, CN, 1997.

Braverman ER, Pfeffer CC, *The Healing Nutrients Within*, Keats, New Canaan, CT, 1987.

Buckman TD, Kling AS, et al, "Glutathione peroxidase and CT scan abnormalities in schizophrenica," *Biol Psychiatr*, 22:349-356; 1987.

Buckman TD, Kling AS, et al, "Platelet glutathione peroxidase and monoamine oxidase activity in schizophrenics with CT scan abnormalities: Relation to psychosocial variables," *Psychiatr Res*, 31:1-14; 1990.

Can J Neuro Sci, 11:561-4; 11/1984. (Childhood neurological disorders related to fat absorption respond to vitamin E.)

Capel ID, "Factors affecting antioxidant defense potential," in CK Chow, ed, *Cellular Antioxidant Defense Mechanism*, CRC Press, Boca Raton, 1988; pp 191-215.

Casey-Smith, JR, "Benzopyrones in the treatment of schizophrenia," letter, 1:4211; 1983.

Casey-Smith JR, et al, "Benzopyrones in the treatment of chronic schizophrenic diseases," *Psychiat Res*, 18(3):267-73; 1986. (Mean improvement of 27% in 8/16 chronic patients taking benzopyrone, a hydroxyethylrutinoside.)

Cheraskin E, *The Vitamin C Connection*, Harper & Row, NY, 1983.

Cicero AFG, Derosa G, et al, "What do herbalists suggest to diabetic patients in order to improve glycemic control? Evaluation of scientific evidence and potental risks," *Acta Diabetologica*, 41(3); 9/2004.

Cocchi P, et al, *J Orthomol Med*, 4(2):96-7; 1989. (Patients responded to IV ascorbic acid.)

Cohen G, "Oxy-radical toxicity in catecholamine neurons," *Neurotoxicology*, 5:77-82; 1984.

Cousens G, *Depression free for Life*, Quill, HarperCollins, NY, 2001.

Crayhon R, *The Carnitine Miracle*, M Evans & Co, 1998

Cutler A, "Amalgam Illness: Diagnosis and Treatment of Mercury Poisoning," 2000. Also at: home.earthlink.net/~moriam/ANDY_INDEX.html And: onibasu.com/archives/am/552.html and 520.html Accessed: 2007

Dager SR, "Brain metabolic alterations in medication-free bipolar patients", *Arch Gen Psychiat*, 61:450-8;

5/2004. (Mitochondria showed increased oxidative stress, a shift from oxidative phosphorylation to glycolysis, and decreased expression (perhaps due to fewer synapses (where mitochondria concentrate), possibly associated with psychosis).)

De Leve LD, Kaplowitz N, "Glutathione metabolism and its role in hepatotoxicity," *Pharmac Ther,* 52: 287-305; 1991.

DeLiz, AJ, MD, PhD, "Administration of massive doses of vitamin E to diabetic schizophrenic patients," *J Orthomol Psychiat,* 4(1): 85-7, 1975.

DeVos N, Pioli R, et al, "Lower serum E concentrations in major depression," *J Affect Disord,* 1995.

De Vos N, Pioli R, et al, "Lower serum vitamin E concentrations in major depression. Another marker of lowered antioxidant," *J Affect Dis,* 2000.

Dhalla RN, et al, "Measurement of adrenolutin as an oxidative product of catecholamines in plasma," *Molec Cell Biochem,* 87:85-97; 1989.

Eikasbef AM, et al, "The effect of coenzyme Q10 on the cognitive functions in patients with schizophrenia," *Institute for Biomedical Research,* University of Texas at Austin, 1994.

Emerit J, Claudiere J, "Free radicals and lipid peroxidation in cell pathology," in J Miquel, A Quintanilha, H Weber, eds, *Biomedicine,* Vol 1, CRC Press, Boca Raton, 1989; pp 177-85.

Engin A, Atlan N, et al, "Erythrocyte glutathione levels in lithium-induced hypothyroidism," *Drugs in R & D,* 6(1):35-40; 2005. (Eventually lithium may elevate TSH, often reducing RBC glutathione 40%, and leaving SOD unchanged, increasing vulnerability to oxidative stress.)

Ernster I, "Lipid peroxidation in biological membranes: Mechanisms and implications," in K Yagi, ed, *Active Oxygens, Lipid Peroxides and Antioxidants,* CRC Press, Japan, 1991; pp 1-38.

Folkers K, Simonsen R, "Two successful double-blind trials with coenzyme Q10 on muscular dystrophies and neurogenic atrophies," *Biochim Biophys Acta,* 1271(1):281-86; 5/24/1995.

Foster HD, Hoffer A, "Schizophrenia and cancer: The adreochrome balanced morphism, *Med Hypotheses,* 62:415-19; 2004a.

Foster HD, Hoffer A, "The two faces of L-dopa: Benefits and adverse side effects in the treatment of encephalitis lethargica, Parkinsons disease, multiple sclerosis, and amyotrophic lateral sclerosis, *Med Hypotheses,* 62:177-81; 2004b.

Free Radical Biol Med, 6:189-207; 1989. (Neurological dysfunction and degeneration in older patients helped with E.)

Gaby AR, "The role of coenzyme Q10 in clinical medicine: Part I," *Alt Med Rev,* 1:11-17; 1996. (Effective in peridontal disease. May support immunity and physical performance.)

Gal, E.M, "Reversal of selective toxicity of (-)-alpha-lipoic acid by thiamine in thiamine-deficient rats," *Nature,* 207:535; 1965.

Gant, C, "Vitamin E in the treatment of tardive dyskinesia," *Am J Psychiat,* 148(2):279; 2/1991.

Gardner R, Gasnier BCH, et al, "Selenium supplementation in patients with autoimmune thyroiditis decreases thyroid peroxidase antiobodies concentration," *J Clin Endocrin & Metabolism,* 87(4): 1687-91; 2002. (Se may benefit inflammation in autoimmune thyroiditis, especially if extreme.)

Garrison RH, Somer E, *The Nutrition Desk Reference,* Keats, New Canaan, CN, 1985.

Gold, MS, *The Good News About Depression,* Villard Books, NY, 1987.

Gotz ME, et al, "Influence of N-methyl-4-phenyl-1, 2, 3, 6-tetrahydropyridine, lipoic acid and L-deprenyl on the interplay between cellular redox systems," *J Neural Transm,* 43S:145-62; 1994.

Graham, DG, "Oxidative pathways for catecholamines in the genesis of neuromelanin and cytotoxic quinones," *Mol Pharmacol,* 14: 633-43; 1978.

Grunert RR, "The effect of DL alpha lipoic acid on heavy-metal intoxication in mice and dogs," *Arch Biochem Biophys,* 86:190-94; 1960.

Hadjimarkos DM, "Selenium in relation to dental carries," *Fd Cosmet Toxicol,* 11:1083-95; 1973.

Harr JR, Muth OH, "Selenium poisoning in domestic animals and its relationship to man," *Clin Toxicol,* 5(2):175-86; 1972.

Hodges RE, Hood J, "Clinical manifestations of ascorbic acid deficiency in man," *Am J Clin Nutr,* 24:432-43; 1971.

Hoffer A, Osmond H, Smythies J, "Schizophrenia: A new approach II. Results of a year's research," J Ment Sci, 100:29-54; 1954.

Hoffer A, "Mechanism of action of nicotinic acid and nicotinamide in the treatment of schizophrenia," in D Hawkins, L Pauling, eds, *Orthomolecular Psychiat,* WH Freeman and Co, SF, 1973.

Hoffer A, Walker M, *Orthomolecular Nutrition,* Keats, New Canaan, CT, 1978. (Critical in schizophrenia.)

Hoffer, Abram, *Orthomolecular Medicine for Physicians,* Keats, New Canaan, CN, 1983.

Hoffer A, "Nutrition and behavior," in J Bland, ed, *Medical Applications of Clinical Nutrition,* Keats, New Canaan, CN, 1983b

Hoffer A, Osmond H, "The adrenochrome hypothesis and psychiatry," *J Orthomol Med,* 5: 32-45; 1990.

Hoffer A, *Adventures in Psychiatry, The Scientific Memoirs of Dr Abram Hoffer,* KOS Pub, Caledon, ON, Canada, 2005.

Hoffer A, "Bipolar disorder and antioxidants," *Townsend Letter,* 2008, submitted.

Holloway DE, Peterson FJ, "Ascorbic acid in drug metabolism," in DA Roe, TC Campbell, eds, *Drugs and Nutrients,* Marcel Dekker, NY, 1984, pp 225-95.

Horrobin DF, Bennett CN, "Depression and bipolar disorder: Relationships to impaired fatty acid and phospholipid metabolism and to diabetes, cardiovascular disease, immunological abnormalities, cancer, aging and osteoporosis. Possible candidate genes," *Prostaglandins, Leukot, Essent Fatty Acids,* 60(4):217-34; 4/1999.

Horrobin DF, "The role of essential fatty acids in schizophrenia," *ISOM, Nutritional Medicine Today Conference,* Vancouver, BC, 4/2000a.

Jaffe R, Kruesi OR, 1992, ibid.

Kalaiselvi T, "Effect of L-carnitine on the status of lipid peroxidation and antioxidants in aging rats," *J Nutr Biochem,* 9(1):575-81; 1998.

Kanofsky JD, et al, "Ascorbate: An adjunctive treatment for schizophrenia," *J Am Coll Nutr,* 8(5): 425, 1989. (Sustained benefits of up to 6 gm in 6/21 neuroleptic-refractory patients.)

Kato T, Kato N, "Mitochondrial dysfunction in bipolar disorder," *Bipolar Disord,* 2:180-90; 2000. (The initial proposal that mitochondrial dysregulation altering energy metabolism and calcium uptake could underly bipolar.)

Kay DS, Naylor GJ, et al, "The therapeutic effect of ascorbic acid and EDTA in manic-depressive psychoses: Double blind comparisons with standard treatments," *Psychol Med,* 14:533-9; 1984. (C plus EDTA was comparable to the antidepressant. Manics responded better to lithium.)

Kehrer, JP, "Free radicals as mediators of tissue injury and disease," *Crit Rev Toxicol,* 23(1):21-48; 1993.

Ketterer B, Coles B, et al, "The role of glutathione in detoxication," *Environ Health Perspectives,* 49: 59-69; 1983.

Kidd PM, "Glutathione: Systemic protectant against oxidative and free radical damage," *Alt Med Rev,* 2(3):155-76; 1997. At: thorne.com/altmedrev/fulltext/glut.html

Konradi C, et al, "Molecular evidence for mitochondrial dysfunction in bipolar disorder," *Arch Gen Psychiatr,* 61:300-8; 2004. (Marked reduction in mitochondrial energy metabolism gene expression in postmortem bipolar brains.)

Krohn J, *The Whole Way to Allergy Relief & Prevention,* Hartley & Marks, Point Roberts, WA, 1991.

Ku H, Brunk UT, et al, "Relationship between mitochondrial superoxide and hydrogen peroxide production and longevity of mammalian species," *Free Radical Biol Med,* 15:621-27; 1993.

Kuloglu M, Ustundag B, et al, "Lipid peroxidation and antioxidant enzyme level in patients with schizophrenia and bipolar disorder," *Cell Biochem Funct,* 20:171-5; 2002.

Kut'ko I, Frolov VM, et al, [Antioxidants in the treatment of schizophrenia (the correction of lipid peroxidation processes)], *Zh Nevropatol Psikhiatr Im SS Korsakova,* 96:32-34; 1996. (185 patients. During relapse, lipid peroxidation intensified. Antioxidants improved mental status.)

Larson Joan M, PhD, interview with author, June 2008.

Leitner ZA, Church IC, "Nutritional studies in a mental hospital," *Lancet,* 1:565-647; 1956. (Over 10% of 465 psychiatric patients showed delayed ascorbic acid saturation — to a degree similar to that of borderline or clinical scurvy.)

Leng GC, Lee AJ, et al, "Impact of antioxidant therapy on symptoms of anxiety and depression. A randomized controlled trial in patients with peripheral arterial disease," *J Nutr Environ Med,* 8(4):321-8; 12/1998. (After 2 yrs beta carotene, C, pyridoxine, zinc sulphate, and sodium selenite, depression was significantly less than in controls.)

Leo MA, Lieber CS, "Alcohol, vitamin A, and beta-carotene: Adverse interactions, including hepatoxicity and carcinogenicity," *Am J Clin Nutr,* 69:1071-1085; 1999. (Alcohol isoenzymmes convert retinol and ethanol to aldehydes, which are toxic to the liver. Prolonged use of certain drugs or alcohol stimulates enzymes which break down retinol. Ethanol and retioic acid precursors compete, depleting A. Beta carotene also interacts with ethanol, obstructing conversion to retinol, and perhaps creating liver toxicity. In smokers who drink, it may promote lung cancer or cardiovascular effects.)

Levy TR, *Vitamin C, Infectious Diseases, & Toxins: Curing the Incurable,* Xlibris Corp, Phil, PA, 2002.

Levy DI, Sucher NJ, et al, "Glutathione prevents N-methyl-D-aspartate receptor-mediated neuro-toxicity," *Neuroreport,* 2(6):345-47; 1991.

Lieberman S, Bruning N, *The Real Vitamin & Mineral Book,* Avery, Garden City Park, NY, 1990.

Lorano RM, et al, "Thioredoxin-linked reductive inactivation of venom neurotoxins," *Arch Biochem Biophys,* 309(2):356-62; 3/1994.

Maas JW, *Arch Gen Psychiat,* 4:109; 1961. (C breakdown increases with anxiety or excitement.)

Mahadik SP, Scheffer RE, "Oxidative injury and potential use of antioxidants in schizophrenia," *Prostaglandins Leukot Essent Fatty Acids,* 55(1-2): 45-54; July, August/1996.

Makhtar, H, Wamg Z.Y, et al, "Tea components: Antimutagenic and anticarcinogenic effects," *Prev Med,* 21:351-60; 1992. (Catechins protect the liver from oxidative stress.)

Marlowe M, Errera J, et al, "Hair selenium levels and children's classroom behavior, *J Orthomol Med,* 1(2):91-96; 1986.

Masoro EJ, "A critical review: Nutrition and aging — A current assessment," *J Nutr,* 115:842-48; 1984.

Mathews SB, et al, "The adrenochrome pathway: The major route for adrenaline catabolism by polymorphonuclear leucocytes," *J Molec Cell Cardiol,* 17:339-46; 1985.

Milner G, "Ascorbic acid in chronic psychiatric patients: A controlled trial," *Br J Psychiat,* 109:294-9; 1963. (Chronic psych patients may have borderline scurvy. Double blind. 40 patients, 4 bipolars. 1 gm C/day over four weeks. Significant improvement for depression, paranoia, and bipolar.)

Mohler, H, et al, "Nicotinamide is a brain constituent with benzodiazepine-like actions," *Nature,* 278: 563-65; 1979.

Morishita S, Sonohara M, et al, "Vitamin E treatment of prolonged depression: A report of nine cases," *Int Med J,* 7:33-6; 2000. (E augmentation created significant improvement in 6/9 depressives.)

Muller DP, "Vitamin E — its role in neurological function," *Postgrad Med J,* 62:107-12; 1986. (Deficit associated with impaired neurological function.)

Muller L, Menzel H, "Studies on the efficacy of lipoate and dihydroilipoate in the alteration of cadmium toxicity in isolate hepatocytes," *Biochem Biophys Acta,* 1052:386-91; 1990.

Murray MT, *Encyclopedia of Nutritional Supplements,* Prima, 1996.

Murray MT, Pizzorno J, *Encyclopedia of Natural Medicine*, Prima, Rocklin, CA, 1998.

Naylor GJ, Smith AH, "Vanadium: A possible aetiological factor in manic depressive illness," *Psychol Med*, 11:249-56; 57-63; 1981ab. ((1) Over 2 days, manic and depressive patients reported significant improvement by 3-4 hrs; (2) Double blind placebo controlled crossover. 11 manic and 12 depressed bipolars were given 3 gm C or placebo on day 1; the opposite, on day 2. Severity decreased more rapidly with C, especially at 3-5 hrs; (3) An 82-yr-old woman with severe, medication-resistant bipolar illness became mildly hypomanic after 2 wks EDTA, high C, and a low vanadium diet, and showed no mood swings for 8 wks. 5 days postwithdrawal she fell into severe depression, resolving when C was resumed; (4) C enabled a 28-yr-old treatment-resistant bipolar woman, ill 15 yrs, to avoid a depressive cycle, though mania did not remit.)

Naylor GJ, "Vanadium and manic-depressive psychosis," *Nutrition and Health*, 3:79; 1984.

Naylor GJ, Smith AH, et al, "Trace elements in manic depressive psychosis," *J Affect Disord*, 8(2):131-6; 1985. (Analysis of hair, blood, serum and urine. Molybdenum was the only element that showed a significant change in more than one tissue.)

Newbold HL, *Vitamin C Against Cancer*, Stein & Day, NY, 1979.

Nichols TW, "Alpha-lipoic acid: Biological effects and clinical implications," *Alt Med Rev*, 2(3):177-83; 1997.

NutriCircles®, Strickland Computer Consulting, Version 3.25, April 29, 1996.

Nutr Rev, "Vanadium, vitamin C and depression," 40(10):293-95; 1981. (C reduces vanadate (+5) to vanadyl (+4), a less potent NA+K+ATPase inhibitor, perhaps thereby benefitting bipolars.)

Ohlenschlager, G, Treusch, G, "Reduced glutathione and anthocyanins: Redox cycling and redox recycling in living systems," *Praxis Telegramm*, 6: 1-20; 12/1996.

Oliveira CR, Agostino P, et al, "Reactive oxygen species and GABA release," *Ann NY Acad Sci*, 738: 130-40; 1994.

Owen AJ, Batterham MJ, "Low plasma vitamin E levels in major depression: Diet or disease?" *Eur J Clin Nutr*, 59:304-6; 2005. (Low alpha tocoperol related inversely to Beck Depression Inventory.)

Packer L, et al, "A-lipoic acid: A metabolic antioxidant and potential redox modulator of transcription, Antioxidants in disease mechanisms and therapy," in H Sies, ed, *Advances in Pharmacology*, Acad Press, 1997.

Page LR, *Healthy Healing*, Healthy Healing, CA, 1992.

Pal SN, Dandiya PC, "Glutathione as a cerebral substrate in depressive behavior," *Pharmacol Biochem Behav*, 48(4):845-51; 8/1994. (Appreciable reduction in cortical GSH. GSH and various antidepressants prevented or reversed shock-induced behavioral depression.)

Panneerselvam SR, Govindasamy S, "Effect of sodium molybdate on the status of lipids, lipid peroxidation and antioxidant systems in all oxan-induced diabetic rats," *Clinicas Chimica Acta*, 345: 1-2:93-8; 7/2004. (Prevents lipid oxidation, protects antioxidant systems.)

Papaioannou R, Pfeiffer CC, "Sulfite sensitivity — Unrecognized threat. Is molybdenum deficiency the cause?," *J Orthomol Psychiat*, 13(2):105-10; 1984.

Passwater RA, *Lipoic acid: The metabolic antioxidant*, Keats, New Canaan, CT, 1995; pp 1-47.

Pauling L, "L Pauling before Congress," *Healthline*, 1(2). (Supports immunity, heart, connective tissue. Animal equivalent dose for adult humans is 2-19 gm /day.)

Pfeiffer CC, *Mental and Elemental Nutrients*, Keats, New Canaan, CN, 1975.

Pfeiffer CC, *Nutrition and Mental Illness*, Healing Arts Press, Rochester, VT, 1987.

Pfeiffer CC, *The Schizophrenias Ours to Conquer*, rev ed, Bio-Communications Press, Wichita, KS, 1988.

Podda M, et al, "Alpha-lipoic acid supplementation prevents symptoms of vitamin deficiency," *Biochem Biophys Res Comm*, 204:98-104; 1994.

Prabakaran S, et al, "Mitochondrial dysfunction in schizophrenia: Evidence for compromised brain metabolism and oxidative stress," *Mol Psychiatr*, 4/2004.

Quillin P, *Healing Nutrients*, Contemporary Books, Chicago, 1987.

Quiroz JA, Singh J, Manji, et al, "Emerging experimental therapeutics for bipolar disorder: Clues from the molecular pathophysiology," *Molec Psychiat*, 8(8):756-76; 8/2004. (Impaired cell plasticity and resilience in critical neuronal circuits.)

Rafalowska U, Liu J, et al,"Peroxidation induced changes in synaptosomal transport of dopamine and aminobutyric acid," *Free Radical Biol Medicine*, 6: 485-92; 1989.

Ranjekar P, "Decreased antioxidant enzymes and membrane essential polyunsaturated fatty acids in schizophrenic and bipolar mood disorder patients," *Psychiat Res*, 121(2):109-22, 2003.

Rebec GB, et al, "Ascorbic acid and the behavioral response to haldoperidol: Implications for the action of antipsychotic drugs," *Science*, 227:438-40; 1985. (Ascorbic acid blocks amphetamine response in rats.)

Reddy R, et al, "Enzymes of the antioxidant defense system in chronic schizophrenic patients," *Biol Psychiatr*, 30:409-12; 1991.

Reddy R, Kelkar H, et al, "Abnormal erythrocyte catalase activity in schizophrenic patients," *Schizophr Res*, 9:227; 1993.

Reddy RD, Yao, J, "Free radical pathology in schizophrenia: A review," *Prostaglandins Leukot Essent Fatty Acids*, 55(1 & 2):33-44; 7-8/1996.

Rogers S, *Depression, Cured at Last*, SK Publishing, Sarasota FL, 1997.

Rudin DO, et al, *The Omega-3 Phenomenon*, Rawson Assn, NY, 1987.

Saez G, Thornalley PJ, et al, "The production of free radicals during the autoxidation of cysteine and their effects on isolated rat hepatocytes," *Biochim Biophys Act*, 719:24-31; 1982.

Salazar MR, "Alpha lipoic acid: A novel treatment for depression," *Med Hypotheses*, 2000.

Schorah CG, et al, "Plasma vitamin C concentration in patients in a psychiatric hospital," *Hum Nutr Clin Nutr*, 37C:447-52; 1983. (In 885 patients, average plasma C /1000 ml was .51mg (vs .87mg in controls). In about a third, readings were below .35mg (a level associated with immune and behavioral changes).

Schwartz RD, Skolnick P, et al, "Regulation of gamma butyric acid/barbiturate receptor grated chloride ion flux in brain vesicles by phospholipase A2: Possible role of oxygen radicals," *J Neurochem*, 50: 565-71; 1988.

Schweitzer AN, "Pegging pathology on mitochondrial dysfunction. Studies strengthen suspicions about brain disorder pathophysiology," *The Scientist*, 18(10):28; 5/2004.

Sher L, "Role of thyroid hormones in the effects of selenium on mood, behavior, and cognitive function, *Med Hypothesis*, 57(4):480-3; 10/2001. (Consider deficiency, especially if depressed, low thyroid, experiencing viral infection, or if soil is depleted.)

Sher L, "Role of selenium depletion in the effects of dialysis on mood and behavior," *Med Hypotheses*, 59(1):89-91; 7/2002a.

Sher L, "Role of selenium depletion in the etiopathogenesis of depression in patient with alcoholism," *Med Hypotheses*, 59(3):330-3; 9/2002b.

Smythies J, "Oxidative reactions and schizophrenia: A review-discussion," *Schiz Res*, 24:357-64; 1997.

Smythies J, "Recent advances in the neurobiology of schizophrenia," *Ger J Psychiat*, 1:24-40; 1998.

Smythies J, Galzigna L, "The oxidative metabolism of catecholamines in the brain: A review," *Biochim Biophys Acta*, 1380:159-62; 1998.

Smythies J, "The adrenochrome hypothesis of schizophrenia revisited," *Neurotox Res*, 4:147-50; 2002.

Sohal RS, Sohal BH, et al, "Relationship between antioxidant defenses and longevity in different mammalian species," *Mech Aging Dev*, 53:217-27; 1990.

Sohal R, Ku H, et al, "Oxidative damage, mitochondrial oxidant generation, and antioxidant defenses during aging and in response to food restriction in the mouse," *Mech Aging Dev*, 74: 121-33; 1994.

Stoklasova, Zapletalek M, et al, [Glutathione peroxidase activity of blood in chronic schizophrenics] *Shorniku Bedeckych Praci Lekarske Fakulty UK v Hradci Kralove*, 291-2:103-108; 1986.

Stoklasova A, Ranjekar P, "Decreased antioxidant enzymes and membrane essential polyunsaturated fatty acids in schizophrenic and bipolar mood disorder patients," *Psychiat Res*, 121(2):109-22, 1990.

Stoklasova A, Petrakova K, et al, [Activities of blood glutatione peroxidase in schizophrenic and depressive patients], *Sb Ved Pr Lek Fak Karlovy Univerzity Hradci Kralove*, 33(5):495-500; 1990. (GSH activity may be reduced in depressives.)

Stoll S, et al, "The potent free radical scavenger alpha-lipoic acid improves memory in aged mice: Putative relationship to NMDA receptor deficits," *Pharmacol, Biochem Behav*, 16(1):799-805; 12/1993.

Stone I, *The Healing Factor: Vitamin C against Disease*, 1974.

Stone I, "Eight decades of scurvy. The case history of a misleading dietary hypothesis," *J Orthomol Psychiat*, 8(2):58-63; 1979. (Humans need high-dose C to achieve normal mammalian levels.)

Stork C, Renshaw PF, "Mitochondrial dysfunction in bipolar disorder: Evidence from magnetic resonance spectroscopy research," *Mol Psychiatr*, 10:900-19; 2005. (Impaired oxidative phosphorylation; shift to glycolysis; decrease in total energy or substrate availability; altered phospholipid metabolism.)

Stram RJ, Binkova B, et al, "Antioxidant effects on alcohol, drugs, and aging," in ML Medelsohn, RJ Albertini, eds, *Mutation and the Environment*, Wiley-Lioss, NY, 1990; pp 327-37.

Suboticanec K, et al, "Vitamin C and schizophrenia," *Acta Med Iugosl*, 38(5):299-308, 1984. (Hospitalized schizophrenics retain less C than neurotics.)

Suboticanec K, "Vitamin C status in schizophrenia," *Bibl Nutr Dieta*, 38:173-81, 1986.

Suboticanec K, et al, "Plasma levels and urinary C excretion in schizophrenic patients," *Hum Nutr Clin Nutr*, 40C:421-28, 1986.

Sumathi R, Baskaran G, et al, "Relationship between glutathione and DL alpha-lipoic acid against cadmium-induced hepatotoxicity," *Jpn J Med Sci Biol*, 49:39-48; 1996.

Sumathi R, Devi VK, et al, "DL alpha-lipoic acid protection against cadmium-induced tissue lipid peroxidation," *Med Sci Res*, 22:23-25; 1994.

Suzuki YJ, Tsuchiya M, et al, "Thioctic acid and dihydrolipoic acid are novel antioxidants which interact with reactive oxygen species," *Free Rad Res Comm*, 15(5):255-63; 1991.

Szabo L, Lajko K, et al, "Effects of neuroleptics on lipid peroxidation and peroxide metabolism enzyme activities in various discrete areas of the rat brain," *Chem Pharmacol*, 14:537-539; 1983.

Tateishi N, Higashi T, et al, "Relative contribution of sulfur atoms of dietary cysteine and methionine to rat liver glutathione and proteins," *J Biochem*, 90: 1603-10; 1981.

Tatum LR, "Selenium supplementation as a treatment for mild to moderate depression in the elderly," Texas Tech University, thesis/dissertation, 2004.

Tenney L, *Stress*, Woodland Health Bks, 1987.

Tolbert LC, et al, "Effect of ascorbic acid on neurochemical, behavioral, and physiological symptoms mediated by catecholamines," *Life Sci*, 25:2189-95; 1979. (C injections in mice blocked amphetamine-induced stereotyped behavior.)

Tolbert LC, et al, "Ascorbate affects conversion of tyrosine to dopamine in mouse brain," Abst, *Trans Am Soc Neurochem*, 1979.

Tritschier HJ, et al, "Thioctic (lipoic) acid: A therapeutic metal-chelating antioxidant?" *Biochem Pharmacol*, 1:123-26; 1995.

VanderKamp H, "A biochemical abnormality in schizophrenics involving ascorbic acid," *Intl J*

Neuropsychiat, 2(3):204-6, 1966. (Schizophrenics required about 40 gm/day (10x controls) before C was excreted. Socialization & well-being improved.)

van Zandwijk, "N, N-acetylcysteine (NAC) and glutathione (GSH): Antioxidant and chemopreventive properties, with special reference to lung cancer," *J Cell Biochem,* 22:24-32; 1995.

von Hilsheimer G, Philpott W, "Ascorbic acid metabolism in a population of adolescent psychiatric patients," *J Orthomol Psychiat,* 5(1):35-42; 1976. (Unusually high tolerance for C.)

Walsh WJ, Rehman F, "Methylation syndromes in mental illness," *Neurosci Soc,* Abst, New Orleans, 11/1997.

Walsh, WJ, "Biochemical individuality and nutrition," *NOHA News,* XXV(2):6-8; 2000.

Walsh, William J, PhD, interview with author, November, 2000.

Walsh WJ, "A biological basis for neurologic disorders: autism, hyperactivity, attention deficit disorder, depression, obsessive-compulsive disorder, Tourette's syndrome, and violence, An interview with William Walsh PhD," Latitudes, 5(2)1-8; 2002. At: www.Latitudes.org

Walsh WJ, "Metal metabolism and human function." At: www.hriptc.org/metal_metabolism.html Accessed 12/6/2004a

Walsh WJ, "Zinc deficiency, metal metabolism, and behavior disorders." At: hriptc.org/zinc_deficiency.html Accessed 12/6/2004b.

Walsh, WJ, PhD, "Commentary on nutritional treatment of mental disorders, *International Guide to the World of Alternative Mental Health.* At: www.alternativementalhealth.com/articles.walshMP.htm#Py Accessed: 2006.

Walsh, William J, PhD, interview with author, July 2008.

Werbach, MT, *Nutritional Influences on Mental Illness,* Third Line Press, Tarzana, CA, 1991.

Essential Fatty Acids

Abdalla DSP, Manteiro HP, et al, "Activities of superoxide dismutase and glutathione peroxidase in schizophrenic and manic depressive patients," *Clin Chem,* 32:805-7; 1986.

Abdulla YH, Hamadah K, "Effect of ADP on PGE1 formation in blood platelets from patients with depression, mania and schizophrenia," *Br J Psychiat,* 127:591-95; 1975. (PGE1 increased in mania, decreased in depression. Schizophrenic platelets did not make PGE1 normally.)

Adams PB, Lawson S, et al, "Arachidonic acid to eicosapentaenoic acid ratio in blood correlates positiviely with clinical symptoms of depression," *Lipids,* 31:S157-61; 1996.

Aruoma OI, Halliwell B, "Superoxide-dependent and ascorbate-dependent formation of hydroxyl radicals from hydrogen peroxide in the presence of iron," *Biochem J,* 241:273-78; 1987.

Ascherio A, Rimm EB, et al, "Dietary intake of marine omega-3 fatty acids, fish intake, and the risk of coronary disease among men, *NEJM,* 332: 977-82; 1995.

Axelrod, J, "Receptor-mediated activation of phospholipase A2 and arachidonic acid release in signal transduction," *Biochem Soc Trans,* 19: 503-7; 1990.

Ayton AK, Azaz A, Horrobin DF, "A pilot open case series of ethyl-EPA supplementation in the treatment of anorexia nervosa," *Prostaglandins Leukot, Essent Fatty Acids,* 71(4):205-9; 10/2004. (By three months, on 1 gm/day EPA plus standard treatment, 3/7 anorexics recovered, the other 4 improved.)

Barefoot JC, Schroll M, "Symptoms of depression, acute myocardial infarction, and total mortality in a community sample," *Circulation,* 93:1976-80, 1996.

Bates PR, Hawkins A, et al, "Heat stress lipids and schizophrenia," *Prostaglandins Leukot Essent Fatty Acids,* 55(1 & 2):1901-8; 7-8/1996.

Barton PG, Gunstone FD, "Hydrocarbon chain packing and molecular motion in phospholipid bilayers formed from unsaturated lecithins. Synthesis and properties of sixteen positional isomers of 1, 2-dioctadecenolyl-sn-glycero-3-phosphorylcholine," *J Biol Chem,* 250(12):4470-76; 1975.

Berridge MJ, Downes CO, et al, "Lithium amplifies agonist dependent phosphatidylinositol response in brain and salivary glands," *Biochem J,* 206(3): 587-95; 1982.

Bibus DM, Holman RT, Walsh WJ, "Fatty acid profiles of schizophrenic phenotypes," *Abst, 91ST Annual Mtg, AOCS,* San Diego, 4/25-28; 2000.

Buckman TD, Kling AS, et al, "Glutathione peroxidase and CT scan abnormalities in schizophrenia," *Biol Psychiatr,* 22:349-356; 1987.

Buckman TD, Kling AS, et al, "Platelet glutathione peroxidase and monoamine oxidase activity in schizophrenics with CT scan abnormalities: Relation to psychosocial variables," *Psychiat Res,* 31:1-14; 1990.

Capel ID, "Factors affecting antioxidant defense potential," in CK Chow, ed, *Cellular Antioxidant Defense Mechanism,* CRC Press, Boca Raton, FL, 1988; pp 191-215.

Carney RM, et al, "Major depressive disorder predicts cardiac events in patients with coronary artery disease," *Psychosom Med,* 50(6):627-33; 1988.

Carney RM, Freedland KE, et al, "Depression, the autonomic nervous system, and coronary heart disease," *Psychosom Med,* 67S:29-33; 2005.

Chen G, Manji HK, et al, "Chronic valproate selectively decreases protein kinase C alpha and epsilon in vitro," *J Neurochem,* 63(6):2361-4; 1994.

Chiu CC, Huang SY, et al, "Polyunsaturated fatty acid deficit in patients with bipolar mania," *Eur Neuropsychopharmacol,* 13(2):99-103; 2003. (Significantly reduced red cell AA and DHA in 20 manics vs. controls. No difference in total n-3 and n-6. Future studies should control for meds, immunity, diet, smoking, and remissions.)

Chiu CC, Huang SY, et al "Omega-3 fatty acids are more beneficial in the depressive phase than in the manic in patients with bipolar I disorder," *J Clin Psychiat,* 66(12):1613-4; 12/2005.

Connor TJ, Leonard BE, "Depression, stress and immunological activation: the role of cytokines in depressive disorders," *Life Sci,* 1998; 62:583-606.

Cooney Craig, Lawren Bill, et al, *Methyl Magic: Maxium Health Through Methylation,* 1999.

Cott J, NIH Workshop on Omega 3 EFAs & Psychiatric Disorders, Bethesda, MD, 9/1998.

Davis D, "Omega 3 fatty acids in clinical practice," *J Adv Med,* 8(1):5-35; 1995.

Davis, Donald R, PhD, interview with author, February, 1996.

Dennis EA, Rhee SG, et al, "Role of phospholipase in generating lipid second messenger signal transduction, *FASEB J,* 5:2068-77; 1991.

Dunbar LM, Bailey JM, *J Biol Chem,* 250:1152-1154; 1975.

Edwards R, Peet M, et al, "Omega-3 polyunsaturated fatty acid levels in the diet and in red blood cell membranes of depressed patients," *J Affect Disord,* 48:149-55; 1998.

Elkashef AM, Ruskin PE, et al. At: http://www.ncbi.nlm.nih.gov/entrez/query.fcgi?cmd=Retrieve&db=pubmed&dopt=Abstract&list_uids=1987837

Emerit J, Claudiere J, "Free radicals and lipid peroxidation in cell pathology," in J Miquel, A Quintanilha, H Weber, eds, *Biomedicine,* V1, CRC Press, Boca Raton, 1989; pp 177-85.

Erasmus U, PhD, *Fats that Heal, Fats that Kill,* Alive Books, Burnaby, Canada, rev ed, 1995.

Ernster I, "Lipid peroxidation in biological membranes: Mechanisms and implications," in K Yagi, ed, *Active Oxygens, Lipid Peroxides and Antioxidants,* CRC Press, Japan, 1991; pp 1-38.

Farooqui AA, Hirashima Y, et al, "Brain phospholipases and their role in signal transduction," in NG Bazan, B Toffano, DF Horrobin, eds, *Neurobiology of Essential Fatty Acids,* Plenum Press, NY, 1992; pp 11-25.

Fleischman AI, Philpott H, et al, "Lipid chemistry and the psychiatric patient," *J Orthomol Psychiat,* 4(2):168-73; 1975.

Frasure-Smith, Lesperance F, et al, "Depression following myocardial infarction. Impact on survival," *JAMA,* 270(15); 10/1993.

Fugh-Berman A, Cott JM, "Dietary supplements and natural products as psychotherapeutic agents," *Psychosom Med,* 61(5):712-28; 1999.

Gattaz WF, Schmitt, A, et al, "Increased platelet phospholipase A2 in schizophrenia," *Schizophr Research,* 16:1-6; 1995.

Gattaz, W.F, Brunner, J, "Phospholipase A2 and the hypofrontality hypothesis of schizophrenia," *Prostaglandins Leukot Essent Fatty Acids,* 55(1 & 2):109-14; July, August/1996.

Gattaz, W.F, Hubner C, et al, "Increased serum PLA2 in schizophrenia: A replication study, *Bio Psychiatr,* 28:495-501; 1990. (Increased PLA2 removes AA, DHA, DGLA and EPA from the Sn 2 position.)

Glen AIM, Glen EMT, Horrobin DF, et al, "A red cell membrane abnormality in a subgroup of schizophrenic patients: Evidence for two diseases," *Schizophr Res,* 12:53-61; 1994.

Glen AI, Cooper SJ, et al, "Membrane fatty acids, niacin flushing and clinical parameters," *Prostaglandins Leukot Essent Fatty Acids,* 55(1-2): 9-15; 8/1996. (6 mo. multicenter. Failure to flush was tied to reduced AA & DHA, affective symptoms. May play a role in schizophrenia and bipolar flareups.)

Gundermann KF, Chapter 19, in G Cerv, F Paltauf, eds, *Phospholipids: Characterization, Metabolism And Novel Biological Applications,* AOCS Press, Champaign, IL, 1995; pp 209-227.

Haglund O, Hamfelt A, et al, "Effects of fish oil supplementation with pyridoxine and folic acid on homocysteine, atherogenic index, fibrinogen and plasminogen activator inhibitor-1 in man," *Nutr Res,* 13:1351-65; 1993.

Heron D, Hershkowitz, et al, "The lipid fluidity of synaptic membranes and the binding of serotonin and opiate ligands," in UZ Littauer, Y Dudai, I Silman, V Teichbergy, Z Vogel, eds, *Neurotransmitters and their Receptors,* John Wiley, 1980; pp 125-38.

Heron D, Shinitzky M, et al, "Lipid fluidity markedly modulates the bindings of serotonin to mouse brain membrane," *Proc Natl Aca Sci,* USA, 77:7463-67; 1980.

Hibbeln JR, Palmer JW, et al, "Are disturbances in lipid-protein interactions by phospholipase-A2 a predisposing factor in affective illness?" *Biol Psychiat,* 25:945-61; 1989.

Hibbein JR, Saleni N, "Dietary polyunsaturated fatty acids and depression when cholesterol does not satisfy," *Am J Clin Nutr,* 62:1-9; 1995.

Hibbeln JR, Umhau JC, et al, "Do plasma polyunsaturates predict hostility and depression," *World Rev Nutr Diet,* 82:175-86; 1997. (Low omega 3 strongly associated with depression. Intake helpful.)

Hibbein JR, "Fish consumption and major depression," *Lancet,* 351:1213; 1998a. (More depression in countries with diets low in fish.)

Hibbeln JR, "Essential fatty acid status and markers of serotonin neurotransmission in alcoholism and suicide," presented at *NIH Workshop, Omega 3 and Psychiatric Disorders,* Sept/2-3/1998b.

Hippisley Cox J, Fielding K, Pringle M, "Depression as a risk factor for ischaemic heart disease in men: Population based case-control study," *Br Med J,* 316: 1714-9; 1998.

Hirashima F, Parow AM, Stoll AL, et al, "Omega-3 fatty acid treatment and T2 whole brain relaxation times in bipolar disorder," *Am J Psychiat,* 161: 1922-24; 10/2004. (4-wk study. Omega 3 increased membrane fluidity in a dose dependent manner.)

Hirata F, Axelrod, J, "Phospholipid methylation and biological signal transmission," *Science,* 209: 1082-1090; 1980.

Holian O, Nelson R, "Action of long-chain fatty acids on protein kinase C activity: Comparison of omega-6 and omega-3 fatty acids," *Anticancer Res,* 12:975-80; 1992.

Horrobin DF, "Prostaglandin deficiency and endorphin excess in schizophrenia," *J Orthomol Psychiat,* 8(1):13-19; 1979.

Horrobin DF, Manku MS, "Possible role of prostaglandin E1 in the affective disorders and in alcoholism," *Br Med J,* 280(6228):1363-66; 6/7/1980. (Platelet production of PGE1 is elevated in mania; reduced in depression. Drinking increases PGE1, though when stopped, it declines sharply (precursors may be reduced), perhaps worsening depression. Lithium decreases PGE1 synthesis.)

Horrobin, DF, *Med Hypotheses,* 5:969-985; 1979. 6: 469-486, 785-800; 1980. 10:329-36; 1983.

Horrobin DF, "EFAs in plasma phospholipids in schizophrenia," *Biol Psychiat,* 25(5):562-68; 1989.

DF Horrobin, ed, *Neurobiology of Essential Fatty Acids,* Plenum Press, NY, 1992; pp 11-25.

Horrobin DF, Glen AIM, Vaddadi KS, "The membrane hypothesis of schizophrenia," *Schiz Res,* 13:195-207; 1994.

Horrobin DF, "Schizophrenia as a membrane lipid disorder which is expressed throughout the body," *Prostaglandins Leukot Essent Fatty Acids,* 55(1 & 2): 3-7; 7-8/1996.

Horrobin DF, "The membrane phospholipid hypothesis as a biochemical basis for the neurodevelopmental concept of schizophrenia," *Schiz Res,* 30:193-208; 1998.

Horrobin DF, Bennett CN, "New gene targets related to schizophrenia and other psychiatric disorders: Enzymes, binding proteins and transport proteins involved in phospholipid and fatty acid metabolism," *Prostaglandins Leukot Essent Fatty Acids,* 60(3):141-67; 3/1999. (Role of PLA2 and PLC in signal transduction.)

Horrobin DF, Bennett CN, "Depression and bipolar disorder: Relationships to impaired fatty acid and phospholipid metabolism and to diabetes, cardiovascular disease, immunological abnormalities, cancer, aging and osteoporosis. Possible candidate genes," *Prostaglandins, Leukot, Essent Fatty Acids,* 60(4):217-34; 4/1999. (Bipolar depression is especially resistant to meds. Concurrent conditions (diabetes, immune or cardiovascular disorders, MS, cancer, osteoporosis, aging) often worsen outcome, and have been associated with impaired phospholipid metabolism and signal transduction, which may also underly depression.)

Horrobin DF, "The role of essential fatty acids in schizophrenia," *ISOM, Nutritional Medicine Today Conference,* Vancouver, BC, 4/2000a.

Horrobin DF, "Essential fatty acids and mental health," *10th Winter Schizophrenia Workshop,* Davos, Switzerland, 2/5-12/2000. At: www.mhnj.com 10-15-2000b.

Horrobin DF, "Phospholipid metabolism and depression: New clinical trials," *Eur Psychiat,* 17(1):76; 5/2002.

Horrocks LA, Yeo YK, "Health benefits of docosahexaenoic acid (DHA)," *Pharmacol Res,* 40(3):211-25; 1999.

Hrelia, et al, "Kinetic analysis of delta-6-desaturation in liver microsomes: Influences of GLA dietary supplementation to young and old rats," *Prostaglandins Leukot Essent Fatty Acids,* 44: 191-94; 1991.

Hudson CJ, Lin A, Horrobin DF, "Phospholipases: In search of a genetic base of schizophrenia," *Prostaglandins Leukot Essent Fatty Acids,* 55(1 & 2): 119-122; 7-8/1996.

Kaiya, H, "Prostaglandin E1 treatment of schizophrenia," *Biol Psychiat,* 19(3):457-63; 1984. (Clinical improvement in acute, unmedicated patients given IV PGE1, related to initial low PG.)

Kaplan A, "Omega 3 fatty acids evaluated for bipolar disorder," *Psychiatric Times,* 16(12); 12/1999. At: psychiatrictimes.com/p991211.html

Kidd PM, "Bipolar disorder as cell membrane dysfunction. Progress toward integrated management," *Alt Med Rev,* 9(2):107-35; 2004.

Klerman GL, Weisman MM, "Increasing rates of depression," *JAMA,* 261:2229-35; 1989.

Kolata G, "Which comes first: Depression or heart disease?" *NY Times,* 1/14/1997.

Kruesi, Oscar Rogers, MD, interview with author, February, 1996.

Ku H, Brunk UT, et al, "Relationship between mitochondrial superoxide and hydrogen peroxide production and longevity of mammalian species," *Free Radical Biol Med,* 15:621-27; 1993.

Kut'ko I, Frolov VM, et al, [Antioxidants in the treatment of schizophrenia (the correction of lipid peroxidation processes)], *Zh Nevropatol Psikhiatr Im SS Korsakova,* 96:32-34; 1996. (During relapse, lipid peroxidation intensified in the 185 patients examined. Antioxidants improved mental state.)

Laugharne JD, Mellor JE, Peet M, "Fatty acids and schizophrenia," *Lipids,* 31:S163-5; 3/1996. (Schizophrenic red cells showed substantial depletion, with AA and DHA particularly low. Another study found adequate intake, but symptomatic improvement with greater dietary omega 3. 10 gm MaxEPA/day created significant improvement, related to increased red cell membrane omega 3.)

Lemmo W, "Mental health care: Under the microscope" At: www.lemmo.com/mental.html#microscope Accessed: 2003.

Leonard DE, Song C, "Stress and the immune system in the etiology of anxiety and depression," *Pharmacol Biochem Behav,* 54:299-303; 1996.

Levin EY, Kaufman S, *J Biol Chem,* 236:2043-48; 1961.

L'Hirondel M, Cheramy A, et al, "Effects of arachidonic acid on dopamine synthesis, spontaneous release, and uptake in striatal synaptosomes from the rat," *J Neurochem,* 64: 1406-9; 1995.

Lieb J, Karmali R, Horrobin D, "Elevated levels of prostaglandin E2 and thromboxane B2 in depression," *Prostaglandins, Leukot Med,* 10(4): 361-7; 4/1983. (In all 30 depressives, thromboxane B2 was increased. MAOIs inhibit synthesis, and tricyclics may antagonize PG activity.)

Maes M, "Interleukin-2 and interleukin-6 in schizophrenia and mania: Effects of neuroleptics and mood stabilizers," *J Psychiatr Res,* 29:141-52; 1995.

Maes M, Smith R, eta l, "Fatty acid composition in major depression: Decreased omega 3 fractions in cholesteryl esters and increased c20:4 omega 6/c20:5 omega 3 ratio in cholesteryl esters and phospholipids," *J Affect Disord,* 38:35-46; 1996.

Maes M, Smith RS, "Fatty acids, cytokines, and major depression," *Biol Psychiat,* 43:313-4; 1998.

Maes M, Christophe A, et al, "Lowered omega 3 polyunsaturated fatty acids in serum phopholipids and cholesteryl esters of depressed patients," *Psychiat Res,* 85(3):275-91; 1999.

Mahadik SP, Mukherjee S, "Elevated levels of lipid peroxidation products in plasma from drug-naive patient at the onset of psychosis," *Schizophr Res,* 15:66; 1995.

Mahadik SP, Scheffer RE, "Oxidative injury and potential use of antioxidants in schizophrenia," *Prostaglandins Leukot Essent Fatty Acids,* 55(1 & 2):45-54; 7-8/1996.

Maidment ID, "Are fish oils an effective therapy in mental illness — An analysis of the data?" *Acta Psychiatr Scand,* 102:3-11; 1990. (Plasma or red cellatty acids may be reduced during depression. Omega 3 may be effective in bipolars.)

Mandell AJ, "Non-equilibrium behavior of some brain enzyme and receptor systems," *Annu Rev Pharmacol Toxicol,* 24:237-74; 1984.

Manji HK, Bersudsky Y, et al, "Modulation of protein kinase C isozymes and substrates by lithium: The role of myo-inositol," *Neuropsychopharmacol,* 15(4).

Martinez M, Mougan I, "Fatty acid composition of human brain phospholipids during normal development," *J Neurochem,* 71:2538-33; 1998.

Masoro EJ, "A critical review: Nutrition and aging — A current assessment," *J Nutr,* 115:842-48; 1984.

Mathe AA, "Combined prostaglandin 1 decrease with PGE2 increase found in schizophrenics," *Clin Psychiat News;* 1981.

Medini L, Colli S, "Diets rich in n-9, n-6 and n-3 fatty acids differentially affect the generation of inositol phosphates and of thromboxane by stimulated platelets in the rabbit," *Biochem Pharmacol,* 39(1): 129-33; 1990.

Mellor JE, Peet M, "Double blind placebo-controlled trial of omega-3 fatty acids as an adjunct to the treatment of schizophrenia," *Winter Schizophrenia Workshop;* Davos, Switzerland: 2/7-13/1998. www.mhnj.com

Miyakawa T, Sumiyoshi S, et al, [Electron microscopic study on schizophrenia. Mechanism of pathological changes], *Acta Neuropathologica,* 20:647-77; 1972.

Mozaffarian D, Rimm EB, *JAMA,* 296:1885-99; 10/2006. (Health benefits of fish usually outweigh the risk of mercury contamination.)

Mukherjee S, Mahadik SP, Horrobin DF, "Membrane fatty acid composition of fibroblasts from schizophrenic patients," *Biol Psychiat,* 35: 700; 1994.

Murck H, Song C, Horrobin D, et al, "Ethyl-eicosapentaenoate and dexamethasone resistance in therapy-refractory depression," *Intl J Neuropsychopharm,* 7(3):341-9; 9/2004.

Murray MT, Pizzorno J, *Encyclopedia of Natural Medicine,* Prima, Rocklin, CA, 1998.

Nemets B, Stahl Z, et al, "Addition of omega-3 fatty acid to maintenance medication treatment for recurrent unipolar depressive disorder," *Am J Psychiat,* 159(3):477-9; 2002. (Double blind. EPA augmentation of antidepressants created highly significant improvement by wk 3.)

Oliveira CR, Agostino, P, et al, "Reactive oxygen species and GABA release," *Ann NY Acad Sci,* 738: 130-40; 1994.

Osher Y, Bersudsky Y, et al, "Omega-3 eicosa-pentaenoic acid in bipolar depression: Report on a small open-label study," *J Clin Psychiat,* 66(6):726-9; 2005. (8/10 bipolar I depressed on 1.5-2 gm EPA, up to 6 mo, showed 50% or more reduction in HamD, without significant side effects or hypomania.)

Pall HS, Williams AC, et al, "Evidence of enhanced lipid peroxidation in cerebrospinal fluid of patients taking phenothiazines," *Lancet,* ii:596-99; 1987.

Passwater, Richard, PhD, *Evening Primrose Oil,* Keats, New Canaan, CN, 1981.

Passwater, Richard, *Fish Oils Update,* Keats, New Canaan, CN, 1987.

Peet M, Laugharne J, et al, "Tardive dyskinesia, lipid peroxidation, and sustained amelioration with vitamin E treatment," *Int Clin Psychopharmacol,* 8: 151-53; 1993.

Peet M, Horrobin DF, et al, "Arachidonic acid, a common link in the biology of schizophrenia," *Arch Gen Psychiatr,* 5:665-666; 1994.

Peet M, Laugharne JDE, "Depleted red cell membrane essential fatty acids in drug-treated schizophrenic patients," *J Psychiatr Res,* 29:227-32; 1995.

Peet, M, Laugharne JDE, et al, "Essential fatty acid deficiency in erythrocyte membranes from chronic schizophrenic patients, and the clinical effects of dietary supplementation," *Prostaglandins Leukot Essent Fatty Acids,* 55(1 & 2):71-76; 7- 8/1996.

Peet M, Edwards RW, "Lipids, depression and physical diseases," *Curr Opinion Psychiat,* 10: 477-80; 1997b.

Peet M, et al, "Fatty acid supplementation in schizophrenic patients," *Schiz Res,* 24:255; 1997a. Abst. Presented at Fatty Acids & Psychiatric Disorders, NIMH conference, Sept, 1998. (12-wk placebo-controlled, blinded trial. 9% improved on DHA; 23%, EPA; vs controls, 11%.)

Peet M, Murphy B, Shay J, Horrobin D, "Depletion of omega-3 fatty acid levels in red blood cell membranes of depressive patients," *Biol Psychiat,* 43:315-9; 1998.

Peet M, Mellor J.E, "Double blind placebo controlled trial of n-3 polyunsaturated fatty acids as an adjunct to neuroleptics," *Schizophr Res,* 29:160; 1998.

Peet M, Horrobin DF, *Phospholipid Spectrum Disorder in Psychiatry,* Marius Press, London, 1999.

Peet M, Horrobin DF, *Phospholipid Spectrum Disorder in Psychiatry,* Marius Press, London, 1999.

Peet M, Horrobin DF, "A multicenter trial of ethyl-eicosapentaenoate in schizophrenia," *Schizophr Res,* 41:225; 2000.

Peet M, Horrobin DF, "A dose-ranging study of the effects of ethyl-eicosapentaenoate in patients with ongoing depression despite apparently adequate treatment with standard drugs," *Arch Gen Psychiat,* 59:913-9; 2002. (Double blind. Over 12 wks, 70 treatment-resistant depressives were given 1, 2 or

4 gm EPA/day, or placebo, plus medication. Results suggest 1 gm is optimal.)

Pellegrew JW, Keshavan MS, et al, "NMR spectroscopy, neurodevelopment and schizophrenia," *Schiz Bull*, 19:35-53; 1993. (Phospholipid breakdown.)

Potter WZ, Rudorfer MV, et al, "Biological findings in bipolar disorders," in RE Hales, AJ Frances, eds, *APA Annual Rev*, V. 6, DC, 1987.

Pratt LA, Ford DE, Eaton WW, et al, "Depression, psychotropic medication, and risk of myocardial infarction," *Circulation*, 94:3123-9; 1996.

Prostaglandins Leukot Essent Fatty Acids, 55(1 & 2); July, August/1996. Pearson Professional Ltd.

Puri BK, Richardson AJ, "Sustained remission of positive and negative symptoms of schizophenia following treatment with eicosapentaenoic acid," *Arch Gen Psychiat*, 55: 188-189; 1998.

Puri BK, Richardson AJ, Horrobin DF, et al, "Eicosapentaenoic acid treatment in schizophrenia associated with symptom remission, normalization of blood fatty acids, reduced neuronal membrane phospholipid turnover and structural brain changes," *Int J Clin Pract*, 54(1):57-63; 1-2/2000a. (A drug-naive patient improved dramatically on 6 mo EPA. Red cell membrane n-3 and n-6 normalized, membrane phospholipid turnover decreased, the previous year's ventricle enlargement and cerebral atrophy reversed.)

Puri BK, Richardson AJ, Easton T, et al, "Reduced neuronal membrane phospholipid turnover and normalization of blood fatty acids associated with symptom remission in a patient with schizophrenia treated solely with eicosapentanoic acid," *Schizophr Res*, 41:243; 2000b.

Puri BK, Counsell SJ, et al, "Eicosapentaenoic acid in treatment-resistant depression associated with significant remission, structural brain changes, and reduced neuronal phospholipid turnover," *Int J Clin Pract*, 55(8):560-3; 2001. (Severely suicidal male, with 7 yrs unremitting depression. One mo adjunctive EPA created sustained improvement in suicidal ideation, social phobia, etc., and niacin response. Lateral ventricular volume decreased (increasing brain size).)

Puri BK, Counsell SJ, et al, "Eicosapentaenoic acid in treatment-resistant depression," *Arch Gen Psychiat*, 59(1):91-2; 1/2002.

Rafalowska U, Liu J, et al, "Peroxidation induced changes in synaptosomal transport of dopamine and aminobutyric acid," *Free Radical Biol Medicine*, 6: 485-92; 1989.

Reddy R, Kelkar H, et al, "Abnormal erythrocyte catalase activity in schizophrenic patients," *Schizophr Res*, 9:227; 1993.

Reddy R, et al, "Enzymes of the antioxidant defense system in chronic schizophrenic patients," *Biol Psychiatr*, 30:409-12; 1991.

Reddy RD, Yao JK, "Free radical pathology in schizophrenia: A review," *Prostaglandins Leukot Essent Fatty Acids*, 55(1 & 2):33-44; 7-8/1996.

Rintala J, Seenabb R, et al, "85 kDA cytosolic phospholipase A2 is a target for chronic lithium in rat brain," *Molec Neurosci Neuroreport*, 10(18): 3887-3890; 12/1999.

Ross BM, Turenne S, et al, "Differential alteration of phospholipase A2 activities in brain of patients with schizophrenia," *Brain Res*, 821(2):407-13; 3/13/1999. (In contrast to Horrobin, Ross suggests brain PLA2 activity is normal in bipolars. In schizophrenics, he finds temporal, prefrontal, and putamen calcium-stimulated PLA2 suppressed (perhaps due to high dopamine), but not temporal calcium-independent PLA2.)

Rudin, Donald O, "The major psychoses and neuroses as omega 3 essential fatty acid deficiency syndrome: Substrate pellagra," *Biol Psychiat*, 16(9): 837-50; 1981. (3 patients with dry skin, fatigue, tinnitus, autonomic symptoms, improved on flax.)

Rudin, DO, "The dominant diseases of modernized societies are omega-3 essential fatty acid deficiency syndrome: Substrate beriberi," *Med Hypoth*, 8:17-47; 1982.

Rudin DO, *The Omega-3 Phenomenon*, Rawson Assn, NY, 1987.

Rudin DO, "The modernization disease syndrome as substrate pellagra-beriberi," *J Orthomol Med*, 2(1): 3-14; 1987.

Rudin DO, Felix C, *Omega-3 Oils: To improve mental health, fight degenerative diseases, and extend your life*, Avery, NY, 1996.

Schwartz RD, Skolnick P, et al, "Regulation of gamma butyric acid/barbiturate receptor grated chloride ion flux in brain vesicles by phospholipase A2: Possible role of oxygen radicals," *J Neurochem*, 50: 565-71; 1988.

Sohal RS, Sohal BH, et al, "Relationship between antioxidant defenses and longevity in different mammalian species," *Mech Aging Dev*, 53:217-27; 1990.

Sohal R S, Ku H, et al, "Oxidative damage, mitochondrial oxidant generation, and antioxidant defenses during aging and in response to food restriction in the mouse," *Mech Aging Dev*, 74: 121-33; 1994.

Stoklasova A, Zapletalek M, et al, [Glutathione peroxidase acivity of blood in chronic schizophrenics], *Shorniku Bedeckych Praci Lekarske Fakulty UK v Hradci Kralove*, 291-2:103-108; 1986.

Seko C, [Relationship between fatty acid composition in blood and depressive symptoms in the elderly], *Jpn J Hyg*, 52:539; 1997.

Seung Kim HF, Weeber EJ, et al, "Inhibitory effects of omega-3 fatty acids on protein kinase C activity in vitro," *Mol Psychiat*, 6(2):246-8; 2001. (EPA, DHA and both inhibit PKC (as do lithium and valproic acid).)

Slater SJ, et al, "The modulation of protein kinase C activity by membrane lipid bilayer structure," *J Biol Chem*, 269:4866-71; 1994.

Smith RS, "The macrophage theory of depression," *Med Hypotheses*, 35:298-306; 1991.

Sperling RI, et al, "Dietary omega-3 polyunsaturated fatty acids inhibit phosphoinositide formation and chemotaxis in neutrophils," *J Clin Invest*, 91:651-60; 1999.

Stevens LJ, Zentall SZ, et al, "Essential fatty acid metabolism in boys with attention-deficit hyperactivity disorder," *Am J Clin Nutr*, 62:761-8; 1995.

Stevens LJ, Zentall SS, et al, "Omega-3 fatty acids in boys with behavior, learning, and health problems," *Physiol Behav*, 59:915-20; 1996.

Stoll AL, Severus E, "Mood stabilizers: Shared mechanisms of action at postsynaptic signal transduction and kindling processes," *Harvard Rev Psychiat*, 4:77-89; 1996.

Stoll AL, Severus WE, et al, "Omega 3 fatty acids in bipolar disorder: A preliminary double-blind, placebo-controlled trial," *Arch Gen Psychiat*, 56(5): 407-12; 5/1999a.

Stoll AL, Locke CA, et al, "Omega-3 fatty acids and bipolar disorder: A review," *Prostaglandins, Leukot, Essent Fatty Acids*, 60:329-37; 1999b.

Stoll AL, Marangell, "Commentary: fish oils and bipolar disorder: A promising but untested treatment, in reply," *Arch Gen Psychiat*, 56:415-16; 1999c.

Stoll, AL, *The Omega-3 Connection*, Simon & Schuster, NY, 2002.

Stram RJ, Binkova B, et al, "Antioxidant effects on alcohol, drugs, and aging," in ML Mendelsohn, RJ Albertini, eds, *Mutation and the Environment*, Wiley-Lioss, NY, 1990; pp 327-37.

Su KP, Shen WW, et al, "Are omega 3 fatty acids beneficial in depression but not mania?" *Arch Gen Psychiat*, 57:716-7; 2000.

Sublette ME, Bosetti F, et al, "Plasma free polyunsaturated fatty acid levels are associated with symptom severity in acute mania," *Bipolar Disord*, 9(7):759-65; 2007. (Preliminary results suggest low EPA vs AA related to manic severity.)

Szabo,L, Lajko K, et al, "Effects of neuroleptics on lipid peroxidation and peroxide metabolism enzyme activities in various discrete areas of the rat brain," *Chem Pharmacol*, 14:537-539; 1983.

Timonen M, Horrobin D, et al, "Fish consumption and depression: The Northern Finland 1966 birth cohort study," *J Affect Disord*, 82(3):447-52; 11/2004. (2986 females, up through age 31. Adjusting for cholesterol, body mass, and socioeconomics, those who rarely ate fish ran 2.6x the risk of depression.)

Trowbridge JP, Walker M, *The Yeast Syndrome*, Bantam Books, 1986.

Truss CO, "Tissue injury induced by Candida Albicans: Mental and neurologic manifestations," *J Orthomol Psychiat*, 1978.

Truss CO, "Restoration of immunological competence to Candida albicans," *J Orthomol Psychiat*, 1980.

Truss CO, "The role of Candida albicans in human illness," *J Orthomol Psychiat*, 1981.

Truss CO, "Metabolic abnormalities in patients with chronic candidiasis: The acetylaldehyde hypothesis," *J Orthomol Psychiat*, 13(2):66-93; 1984.

Vaddadi KS, Horrobin DF, *J Med Sci*, 7:52; 1979.

Vaddadi KS, Courtney P, et al, "A double blind trial of essential fatty acid supplementation in patients with tardive dyskinesia," *Psychiatr Res*, 27(3):313-23, 1989. (RBC membrane ALA, EPA, and DHA correlated inversely with TD severity.)

van Kammen D, Uao JG, et al, "Polyunsaturated fatty acids, prostaglandins, and schizophrenia," *Ann NY Acad Sci*, 559:411-23; 1989.

Walsh, William J, PhD, interview with author, November, 2000.

Walsh, WJ, PhD, "Commentary on nutritional treatment of mental disorders, *International Guide to the World of Alternative Mental Health*. At: www.alternativementalhealth.com/articles.walshMP.htm#Py Accessed:10/08/2006.

Williamson PC, Brauer M, et al, "^{31}P magnetic resonance spectroscopy studies in schizophrenia," *Prostaglandins Leukot Essent Fatty Acids*, 55(1 & 2): 115-18; 7-8/1996.

Yao JK, van Kammen DP, et al, "Red blood cell membrane dynamics in schizophrenia. II. Fatty acid composition," *Schizophr Res*, 13:217-26; 1994.

Inositol

Agam G, Shamir A, et al, "Myo-inositol-1-phosphate (MIP) synthase: A possible new target for antibipolar drugs," *Bipolar Disord*, 4(S1):15; 9/2002.

Atack JR, "Inositol monophosphatase, the putative therapeutic target for lithium," *Brain Res Rev*, 22(2): 183-90; 1996. (Lithium may work by attenuating phosphatidyl inositol cell signaling pathways (by inhibiting inositol, and reducing PI synthesis).

Aukema HM, Holub BJ, "Inositol and pyrroloquinoline quinone," in E Shills, JA Olson, M Shike, eds, *Modern Nutrition in Health and Disease*, 8th ed, Lea & Febiger, Philadelphia, PA, 1994; pp 466-73.

Banks RE, Aiton JF, et al, "Incorporation of inositol into the phosphoinositides of lymphoblastoid cell lines established from bipolar manic-depressive patients," *J Affect Disord*, 19(1):1-8; 5/1990. (50-60% less than in controls.)

Barak Y, Levine J, et al, "Inositol treatment of Alzheimer's disease: A double blind, cross-over placebo-controlled trial," *Prog Neuropsychopharmacol Biol Psychiat*, 20(4):729-35; 5/1996a.

Barkai IA, Dunner DL, et al, "Reduced myo-inositol levels in cerebrospinal fluid from patients with affective disorder," *Biol Psychiat*, 13:65-72;1978.

Belmaker RH, Bersudsky Y, et al, "How does lithium work on manic depression? Clinical and psychological correlates to inositol theory," *Annu Rev Med*, 47(1):47-56; 1996.

Belmaker RH, Agam G, et al, "Behavioral reversal of lithium effects by four inositol isomers correlates perfectly with biochemical effects on the PI cycle: Depletion by chronic lithium of brain inositol is specific to hypothalamus, and inositol levels may be abnormal in postmortem brain from bipolar patients," *Neuropsychopharmacol*, 19:220-32; 1998.

Berridge MG, Irvine RF, "Inositol phosphates and cell signalling," *Nature*, 341, 197, 9/1989.

Berridge MJ, Downes CP, et al, "Lithium amplified agonist-dependent phosphatidylinositol responses in brain and salivary glands," *Biochem J*, 206(3): 587-95; 9/1982.

Bersudsky Y, Einat H, et al, "Epi-inositol and inositol depletion: Two new treatment approaches in affective disorder," *Curr Psychiat Rep*, 1:141-71 1999. (Inositol restriction benefits mania, augments lithium.)

Brown A, Mallinger A, et al, "Elevated platelet membrane phosphatidylinositol-4, 5-bisphosphate in bipolar mania," *Am J Psychiatr,* 150:1252-54; 1993.

Casebolt TL, Jope RS, "Chronic lithium treatment reduces norepinephrine-stimulated inositol hydrolysis in rat cortex," *Eur J Pharmacol,* 140(2): 245-6; 1987.

Chengappa KN, Levine J, et al, "Inositol as an add-on treatment for bipolar depression," *Bipolar Disord,* 2(1):47-55; 2000. (6/12 given 12 gm/day inositol, showed 50% or greater reduction in HAM-D, and much to very-much improvement on the CGI scale, versus only 3/10 controls. 67% of the experimental group also showed a 50% reduction in MADRS vs 33% of controls. Inositol was highly tolerated.)

Colodny L, Hoffman RL, "Inositol — Clinical applications for exogenous use," *Alt Med Rev,* 3(6): 432-47; 1998.

Colodny L, Hoffman RL, "Inositol treatment of obsessive compulsive disorder, *Am J Psychiat,* 153:1219-21; 1996.

Cooney, C, *Methyl Magic,* Andrews McNeel Publishing, Kansas City, 1999; pp 154-66.

Cousens G, *Depression Free for Life,* Quill, Harper Collins, NY, 2001.

Crayhon, R, *The Carnitine Miracle,* M Evans & Co, 1998.

Drummond AH, Raeburn CA, "The interaction of lithium with thyrotropin-releasing hormone-stimulated lipid metabolism of GH3 pituitary tumour cells. Enhancement of stimulated 1,2 diacylglycerol formation," *Biochem,* 224:129-36; 1984.

Drummond AH, "Inositol lipid metabolism and signal transduction in clonal pituitary cells," *J Exp Biol,* 124(1):337-58: 1986 (Inositol/calcium/PKD effects.)

Drummond AH, "Inositol Lipids in Cell Signalling," in Alan H Drummond, C Peter Downes, et al, *Inositol,* 1989.

Dubovsky SL, Christiano J, et al, "Increased platelet-intracellular calcium concentration in patients with bipolar affective disorders," *Arch Gen Psychiat,* 46: 632-8; 1989.

Dubovsky SL, Murphy J, et al, "The calcium second messenger system in bipolar disorders: Data supporting new research directions," *J Neuropsychiatr & Clin Neurosci,* 4(1):3-14; Winter 1992. (Lithium and other therapies may act by normalizing hyperactive phosphotidylinositol and calcium second messaging.)

Eden EA, Demopulos C, et al, "Inositol augmentation of lithium or valproate for bipolar depression," *Bipolar Disord,* 8(2):168-74 2006. (Over 6 wks, HRSD reduced 50% in 4/9 on inositol (none in placebo), but increased 50% in 2 (who, at baseline showed significantly greater irritability, disruptive/ aggressive behavior, unkempt appearance.)

Einat H, Kofman O, et al, "Augmentation of lithium's behavioral effect by inositol uptake inhibitors", *J Neural Transmission,* 105(1):31-38; 3/1998.

Einat H, Belmaker RH, "The effects of inositol treatment in animal models of psychiatric disorders," *J Affect Disord,* 62(1-2):113-21; 1/2001. (Positive benefits in animals.)

Einat H, Karbovski H, et al, "Inositol reduces depressive-like behaviors in two different animal models of depression," *Psychopharmacol,* 144(2): 158-62; 5/1999.

Einat H, Belmaker RH, "Chronic inositol treatment reduces depression-like immobility of Flinders Sensitive Line rats in the forced swim test," *Depress Anxiety,* 15(3):148-51; 2002.

el-Mallakh R, et al, "Is Na(+)-K(+)-ATPase the link between phosphoinositide metabolism and bipolar disorder?" *J Neuropsychiatr Clin Neurosci,* 5(4): 361-68; 1993.

Fisher SK, Heacock AM, et al, "Inositol lipid and signal transduction in the nervous system: An update," *J Neurochem,* 58(1):18-38; 1992.

Greil W, Steber R, et al, "The agonist-stimulated accumulation of inositol phosphatides is attenuated in neutrophils from male patients under chronic lithium therapy," *Biol Psychiat,* 30(5):442-51; 1991.

Hardan A, Vagnucci A, et al, "Inositol as an add-on treatment for bipolar depression," *Bipolar Disorders,* 2(1):47-55; 2000.

Honchar MP, Vogler GP, et al, "Evidence that phosphoinositide metabolism in rat cerebral cortex stimulated by pilocarpine, physotigmine and pargyline is changed by chronic lithium treatment," *J Neurochem,* 55(5):1521-5; 11/1990.

Jaffe R, Kruesi OR, "The biochemical-immunology window: A molecular view of psychiatric case management," *J App Nutr,* 44(2); 1992.

Jenkinson S, Nahorski SR, et al, "Disruption by lithium of phosphatidylinositol-4,5-bisphosphate supply and inositol-1,4,5-trisphosphate generation in Chinese hamster ovary cells expressing human recombinant m1 muscarinic receptors," *Molec Pharmacol,* 46(6):1138-48; 1994.

Jope RS, Song L, et al, "The phosphoinositide signal transduction system is impaired in bipolar affective disorder brain," *J Neurochem,* 66(6):2402-09; 6/1996. (Hydrolysis on stimulation in postmortem brains, suggests bipolars may experience reduced phosphoinositide signaling in the occipital cortex and certain other regions.)

Kato T, Shioiri T, et al, "Measurement of brain phosphoinositide metabolism in bipolar patients using in vivo 31P-MRS," *J Affect Disord,* 22(4): 185-90; 1991.

Kato T, Inubushi T, et al, "Magnetic resonance spectroscopy in affective disorders," *J Neuropsychiat Clin Neurosci,* 10(2):133-47; Spring, 1998. (Suggests abnormal intracellular pH and metabolism of phosphate and membrane phospholipids. Lithium increases phosphomonoester peaks (perhaps inositol-1-phosphate), but not peaks for choline.)

Kim H, McGrath BM, et al, "A review of the possible relevance of inositol and the phosphatidylinositol second messenger system (PI-cycle) to psychiatric disorders — focus on magnetic resonance spectroscopy (MRS) studies," *Hum Psychopharmacol,* 20(5):309-26; 7/2005.

Larson JM, *Depression Free, Naturally,* Ballantine Wellspring, NY, 2001.

Lenox R, Watson D, "Lithium and the brain: A psychopharmacological strategy to a molecular basis for manic depressive illness," *Clin Chem,* 40(2):L309-314; 1994. (Inositol may influence mood indirectly via the Na/K pump and cell osmosis.)

Levine J, Double blind controlled trial of inositol, *Am J Psychiat,* 137(5):622-23; 1980.

Levine J, Rapaport A, et al, "Lithium raises CSF inositol levels," *Brain Res,* 627:168-70; 1993. (6 gm did not produce signficant improvement, perhaps because urinary loss can be 7-8 gm/day; some may require large doses to insure CNS absorption.)

Levine J, Barak Y, et al, "Double-bind, controlled trial of inositol treatment of depression, *Am J Psychiat,* 152(5):792-4; 1995a. (On 12 gm/day (10x average intake) for 4 wks, 11/13, improved significantly (HAM-D) by wk 4; controls remained the same or deteriorated. Side effects were mild: nausea, flatus.)

Levine J, Barak Y, et al, "Follow up and relapse analysis of an inositol study of depression," *Isr J Psychiat Relat Sci,* 32(1):14-21; 1995b. (Half of prior responders relapsed rapidly after stopping. A yr later, HAM-D showed little difference among responders, nonresponders, placebo.)

Levine J, Kurtzman L, et al, "CSF inositol does not predict antidepressant response to inositol," *J Neural Transm,* 103(12):1457-62; 1996.

Levine J, "Controlled trials of inositol in psychiatry," *Eur Neuropsychopharmacol,* 7(2):147-55; 1997.

Lieberman S, Bruning N, *The Real Vitamin & Mineral Book,* Avery, Garden City Park, NY, 1990.

Manji HK, McNamara R, et al, "Signalling pathways in the brain: Cellular transduction of mood stabilization in the treatment of manic-depressive illness," *Aust NZJ Psychiat,* 33S:65-83; 12/1999.

Moore GJ, Bebchuk JM, et al, "Temporal dissociation between lithium-induced changes in frontal lobe myo-inositol and clinical response in manic-depressive illness," *Am J Psychiat,* 156(12):1902-8; 12/1999. (12 depressed bipolars. Lithium, after 2+ wks washout. MRS then found right frontal myoinositol reduced about 30%, through wks 3-4. Depressive severity decreased, but not in wk 1 (perhaps awaiting signaling and gene expression changes).

Murray MT, *Encyclopedia of Nutritional Supplements,* Prima, 1996.

Murray MT, Pizzorno J, *Encyclopedia of Natural Medicine,* Prima, Rocklin, CA, 1998.

Nemanov L, Ebstein RP, et al, "Effect of bipolar disorder on lymphocyte inositol monophosphatase mRNA levels," *Int J Neuropsychopharmacol,* 2(1): 25-29; 1999.

Palatnik A, Frolov K, et al, *J Clin Psychopharmacology,* 21(3):335-8; 6/2001. (Double blind crossover trial of inositol vs. fluovoxamine for panic.)

Pfeiffer CC, *Mental and Elemental Nutrients,* Keats, New Canaan, CN, 1975.

Pfeiffer CC, *Nutrition and Mental Illness,* Healing Arts Press, Rochester, VT, 1987.

Pfeiffer CC, *The Schizophrenias Ours to Conquer,* Bio-Communications Press, Wichita, KS, 1988.

JW Putney, ed, *Inositol Phosphates and Calcium Signalling,* 1992.

Ragan C, "The effect of lithium on inositol phosphate metabolism," in *Lithium and Cell Physiology,* Springer, NY, 1990.

Rogers S, *Depression, Cured at Last,* SK Publishing, Sarasota FL, 1997.

Schreiber G, Avissar S, "Lithium sensitive hyperfunction: A dynamic model for the pathogenesis of bipolar affective disorder," *Med Hypotheses,* 35(3): 237-43; 7/1991. (Lithium may work by attenuating G protein function, thus altering PI & cAMP, and so, PKA (which is cAMP-dependent) & PKC. These may influence phosphorylation, thereby mood.)

Shaldubina A, Ziva S, et al, "Inositol deficiency diet and lithium effects," *Bipolar Disord,* 8(2):152; 4/2006. (Major decrease in severity by 1-2 wks, even in nonreponsive manics and rapid cyclers.)

Shears S, *Signalling by Inositides: A practical approach,* 1997.

Sherman WR, Leavitt AL, "Evidence that lithium alters phosphoinositide metabolism: Chronic administration elevates primarily D-myo-inositol-L-phosphate in cerebral cortex of the rat," *J Neurochem,* 36:1947-51; 1981.

Shimon H, Agam G, Belmaker RH, et al, "Reduced frontal cortex inositol levels in postmortem brain of suicide victims and patients with bipolar disorder," *Am J Psychiat,* 154(8):1148-50; 1997.

Soares JC, Mallinger AG, "Platelet membrane phospholipids in euthymic bipolar disorder patients: Are they affected by lithium treatment?" *Biol Psychiat,* 45(4):435-7; 2/15/1999.

Soares JC, Mallinger AG, "Abnormal phosphatidylinositol (PI)-signalling in bipolar disorder," *Biol Psychiat,* 39:461-4; 1996.

Soares JC, Mallinger AG, et al, "Effects of lithium on platelet membrane phosphoinositides in bipolar disorder patients: A pilot study," *Psychopharmacol (Berl),* 149:12-6; 2000.

Steen VM, "Does inositol signalling have a role in disease susceptibility and drug treatment of bipolar disorder?" *Bipolar Disord,* 4(S1):53-5; 2002.

Wang HY, Markowitz P, et al, "Increased membrane-associated protein kinase C activity and translocation in blood platelets from bipolar affective disorder patients," *J Psychiatr Res,* 33(2):171-79; 3-4/1999. (Suggests increased PKC signal transduction in mania (n=44); reduced in depression & schizophrenia.)

Walsh WJ, "Biochemical individuality and nutrition," at: www.hriptc.org/biochemical_individuality.html Accessed: 2000.

Walsh WJ, "A biological basis for neurologic disorders: autism, hyperactivity, attention deficit disorder, depression, obsessive-compulsive disorder, Tourette's syndrome, and violence, An interview with William Walsh PhD," *Latitudes,* 5(2)1-8, 2002. At: www.Latitudes.org

Walsh, WJ, PhD, "Commentary on nutritional treatment of mental disorders," *International Guide to the World of Alternative Mental Health.* At: www.alternativementalhealth.com/articles.walshMP.htm#Py Accessed:10/08/2006

Walsh, William J, PhD, interview with author, November, 2007.

Wolfson M, Einat H, "Nordidemnin potentially inhibits inositol uptake in cultured astrocytes and dose-dependently aguments lithium's proconvulsant effect in vivo," *J Neurosci Res,* 60(1):116-21; 1992.

Wolfson M, Bersudsky Y, et al, "Chronic treatment of human astrocytoma cells with lithium, carbamazepine or valproic acid decreases inositol uptake at high inositol concentration but increases it at low inositol concentrations," *Brain Res,* 855(1): 158-61; 2/7/2000. (Which may explain conflicting studies on the effect of lithium on inositol.)

Phosphatidyl serine

Balch JF, Balch PA, *Prescription for Natural Healing,* Avery, Garden City Park, NY, 1990.

Brambilla F, et al, "Beta-endorphine concentation in peripheral blood mononuclear cells of elderly depressed patients — effects of phosphatidylserine therapy," *Neuropsychobiol,* 34:18-21; 1996.

Broida, Marian, RN, *New Hope for People with Depression,* Prima Publishing, Roseville CA, 2001.

Crayhon R, *The Carnitine Miracle,* M Evans & Co, 1998.

Crook TH, "Effects of PS in age-associated memory impairment," *Neurology,* 41:644; 1991.

Elkashef AM, Ruskin PE, et al. At: http://www.ncbi.nlm.nih.gov/entrez/query.fcgi?cmd=Retrieve&db=pubmed&dopt=Abstract&list_uids=1987837 Accessed 2001.

Jaffe R, Kruesi OR, "The biochemical-immunology window: A molecular view of psychiatric case management," *J App Nutr,* 44(2); 1992.

Kidd PM, "Phosphatidylserine; membrane nutrient for memory. A clinical and mechanistic assessment," *Alt Med Rev,* 1(2):70-84, 1996.

Kidd PM, *Phosphatidyl serine, Nature's brain Booster,* Total Health Communications, St George UT, 2005.

Maggioni M, et al, [Effects of phosphatidyl serine therapy in geriatric patient with depressive disorders], *Acta Psychiatr Scand,* 81:265-270; 1990.

Page LR, *Healthy Healing,* Healthy Healing Pub, CA, 1992.

Pfeiffer CC, *The Schizophrenias Ours to Conquer,* Bio-Communications Press, Wichita, KS, 1988.

Wilcox, J, et al, *Biol Psychiat,* 1985; p 49. (Serine absorption may be less efficient among psychotics.)

Wsaziri, "Plasma serine to cysteine ratio as a biological marker for psychosis," *Br J Psych,* 143:69-73; 1983. (Degree of psychosis showed a correspondence to serine and serine/cysteine levels.)

Aminos

Balch JF, Balch P, *Prescription for Nutritional Healing,* Avery, Garden City Park, NY, 1990.

Beckman H, "DL-phenylalanine in affective disorders," *Adv Biol Psychiat,* 10:137-47; 1983.

Beckman H, et al, "DL-phenylalanine versus impramine: A double-blind controlled study," *Arch Psychiat Nervenkr,* 227:49-58; 1979.

Bell KM, et al, "S-adenosylmethionine treatment of depression: A controlled clinical trial," *Am J Psychiatr,* 145(9):1110-14; 1988. (Benefit over imipramine.)

Branchey L, et al, "Depression, suicide and aggression in alcoholics and their relationship to plasma amino acids," *Psychiat Res,* 12(3):219-26; 1984. (Tryptophan was low relative to competing aminos in alcoholics with a history of both aggression and depression.)

Braverman ER, "Brain mapping: A short guide to interpretation and philosophy," *J Orthomol Med,* 5(4):196-7; 1990.

Buist R, "The therapeutic predictability of tryptophan and tyrosine in the treatment of depression," *Int J Clin Nutr Rev,* 3:1-3; 1983.

Carney MWP, "Rapid antidepressant response with SAMe. A double-blind study," *Ala J Med Sci,* 25(3): 16; 1988.

Chouinard G, et al, "Tryptophan in the treatment of depression and mania," *Adv Biol Psychiat,* 10:47-66; 1983. (Enhances MAOIs. Adding niacinamide is not always helpful. Chlorpromazine and nitrazepam can obscure the benefit of tryptophan.)

Delgado PD, Chouinard G, et al, "Serotonin function and the mechanism of antidepressant action. Reversal of antidepressant-induced remission by rapid depletion of plasma tryptophan," *Arch Gen Psychiat,* 47(5):411-18; 1990. (Double blind. Some antidepressants may require tryptophan availability.)

Galton L, *You May Not Need A Psychiatrist: How Your Body May Control Your Mind,* Simon & Schuster, NY, 1979.

Geracioti T, Loosen P, et al, "Uncoupling of serotonergic and noradrenergic systems in depression: Preliminary evidence from continuous cerebrospinal fluid sampling," *Depress Anxiety,* 6(3): 89-94; 1997. (5HIAA (serotonin metabolite) and MHPG (NE) are significantly inverse in normals, but not depressives.)

Gibson CJ, Gelenberg, A, "Tyrosine for the treatment of depression," *Biol Psychiat,* 10:148-59; 1983. (Double blind.)

Hoffer, "Mega amino acid therapy," *J Orthomol Psychiat,* 9(1):2-5; 1980.

Jaffe R, Kruesi OR, "The biochemical—immunology window: A molecular view of psychiatric case management," *J App Nutr,* 44(2); 1992.

King DS, "Can allergic exposure provoke psychological symptoms? A double blind test," *Biol Psychiat,* 16(1):3-19, 1981.

Lesser M, *Nutrition & Vitamin Therapy,* Bantam Books, NY, 1983.

McGrath RE, et al, "The effect of L-tryptophan on seasonal affective disorder," *J Clin Psychiat,* 51(4); 162-63; 1990. (Double blind. Tryptophan/B6/C was more effective than placebo, and comparable to light therapy.)

Mongeau R, Blier P, et al, "The serotonergic and noradrenergic systems of the hippocampus: Their interactions and the effects of antidepressant treatments," *Brain Res Rev,* 23:145-95; 1997.

Murray MT, Pizzorno J, *Encyclopedia of Natural Medicine,* Prima, Rocklin, CA, 1998.

Morand C, et al, "Clinical response of aggressive schizophrenics to oral tryptophan," *Biol Psych,* 18(5):575-78; 1983. (Double blind. Aggressive patients improved, others did not.)

Pfeiffer CC, *The Schizophrenias Ours to Conquer,* Bio-Communications Press, Wichita, KS, 1988.

Pope HG, et al, "Toxic reactions to the combination of monoamine oxidase inhibitors and tryptophan," *Am J Psychiat,* 142(4):491-92; 1985.

Raleigh MJ, "Differential behavioral effects of tryptophan and 5-hydroxytryptophan on vervet monkeys: Influence of catecholamine systems, *Psychopharmacol (Berlin),* 93(1):44-50; 1987.

Ross J, *The Mood Cure,* Viking Penguin, NY, 2002.

Sabelli HC, et al, "Clinical studies on the phenylethylamine hypothesis of affective disorder: Urine and blood phenylacetic acid and phenylalanine dietary supplements," *J Clin Psychiat,* 47(2):66-70; 1986. (May benefit bipolar depression. Side effects include anxiety, insomnia, constipation, transient nausea, headaches.)

Slagle P, *The Way Up from Down,* St Martin's Paperbacks, NY, 1992.

Slagle P, "5-hydroxy-tryptophan (5HTP) and L-tryptophan," *The Way Up Newletter Archives,* #13 At: thewayup.com/newletters/newsarch.htm

Walsh, WJ, PhD, "Commentary on nutritional treatment of mental disorders, *International Guide to the World of Alternative Mental Health.* At: www.alternativementalhealth.com/articles.walshMP.htm#Py Accessed: 10/08/2006.

Werbach MR, *Nutritional Influences on Mental Illness,* Third Line Press, Tarzana, CA, 1991.

Young SN, Teff KL, "Tryptophan availability, 5HT synthesis and 5HT function," *Prog Neuropsychopharmacol Biol Psychiat,* 13(3-4):373-79; 1989 (Tryptophan firing increased with arousal, perhaps underlying effectiveness in aggressive patients, but not normals, even during aggression.)

Zmilacher K, et al, "L-5-hydroxytryptophan in combination with a peripheral decarboxylase inhibitor in the treatment of depression," *Neuropsychobiol,* 20(2):205-12; 1987. (Equivalent to traditional antidepressant drugs.)

Serotonin

Agren H, "Symptom patterns in unipolar and bipolar depression correlating with monoamine metabolites in the cerebrospinal fluid, I. General patterns," *Psychiat Research,* 3:211-23; 1980.

Agren H, et al, [Low brain uptake of L-(11C)5-hydroxytryptophan in major depression: A positron emission tomography study on patients and healthy volunteers], *Acta Psychiatr Scand,* 83: 449-55; 1991.

Alino JJ, et al, "5-hydroxytryptophan (5-HTP) and a MAOI (nialamide) in the treatment of depression. A double-blind controlled study," *Int Pharmaco Psychiat,* 11(1):9-15; 1976.

Anst J, et al, "The treatment of depression with L-5-hydroxytryptophan versus imipramine: Results of two open and one double-blind study," *Arch Psychiatr Nervenkr,* 224:175-86; 1977.

Asberg M, Thoren P, et al, "Serotonin depression: A biochemical subgroup within affective disorders," *Science,* 191:478-80; 1976a. (CSF 5HIAA is low in many patients with depression or suicidality.)

Asberg M, Traskman L, et al, "5-HIAA in the cerebrospinal fluid. A biochemical suicide predictor?" *Arch Gen Psychiat,* 33:1193-97; 1976b.

Asberg M, Bertelson L, et al, [CSF monoamine metabolites in melancholia], *Acta Psychiatr Scand,* 69(3):201-19; 3/1984.

Ashcroft GW, Sharman DF, "5-hydroxyindoles in human CSF," *Nature,* 186:1050-51, 1960.

Asheychick R, et al, "The efficacy of L-tryptophan in the reduction of sleep disturbance and depressive state in alcoholic patients," *J Studies Alcohol,* 50: 525-32; 11/1989.

Ballenger J, Wheadon D, et al, "Double-blind, fixed-dose, placebo-controlled study of paroxetine in the treatment of panic disorder," *Am J Psychiat,* 155:36-42; 1998.

Baumel Syd, *Dealing with Depression Naturally,* Keats, New Canaan, CN, 1995.

Beitman BD, Dunner DL, "L-tryptophan in the maintenance treatment of bipolar II manic-depressive illness," *Am J Psychiat,* 139:1598-99; 1982.

Belongia EA, et al, "An investigation of the cause of the eosinophilia-myalgia syndrome associated with tryptophan use," *NEJM,* 323:357-65; 1990.

Benjamin J, Ebstein RP, Belmaker RH, "Personality genetics," *Isr J Psychiat Relat Sci,* 34(4):270-80; 1997. (The dopamine D4 receptor gene related to novelty-seeking among 1224 Israelis, 215 Americans. In Israelis, an interaction emerged between reward dependence and the serotonin 2C receptor gene.)

Benkelfat C, et al, "Mood lowering effect of tryptophan depletion: Enhanced susceptibility in a young man at genetic risk for major affective disorders," *Arch Gen Psychiat,* 51(9):687-97; 1994.

Bernstein AL, "Vitamin B6 in clinical neurology," *Ann NY Acad Sci,* 585:250-60; 1990. (Some studies find B6 helpful in depression, chronic pain, headache; perhaps hyperactivity, aggressive behavior.)

Bhatti T, et al, "Effects of a tryptophan-free amino acid drink challenge normal human sleep electroencephalogram and mood," *Biol Psychiat,* 43(1):52-59; 1998.

Blauvelt A, Falanga V, "Idiopathic and L-trytophan-associated eosinophilic fascitis before and after L-tryptophan contamination," *Arch Derm,* 127: 1159-66; 8/1991.

Blundell JE, "Serotonin and appetite," *Neuropharmacol,* 23(12B):1537-51; 12/1984.

Boman B, "L-tryptophan: A rational antidepressant and a natural hypnotic?" *Aust NZ J Psychiat,* 22(1): 83-97; 1988. (Review. May benefit mild depression and resistant bipolar depression. May be involved in sleep chemistry.)

Botez MI, et al, "Relapsing neuropathy, cerebral atrophy and folate deficiency. A close association," *Appl Neurophysiol,* 42(3):171-83; 1979. (Folate deficiency may interfere with serotonin synthesis.)

Braverman ER, Pfeiffer CC, *The Healing Nutrients Within,* Keats, New Canaan, CN, 1987.

Bridges PK, Bartlett JR, et al, "Precursors and

metabolites of 5-hydroxytryptamine and dopamine in the ventricular cerebrospinal fluid of psychiatric patients," *Psycholog Med,* 6:399-405; 1976.

Brigham PM, "The Psychopharmacology of Bipolar Disorder," updated 5-9-2001. At: http: //people.ne.mediaone.net/pmbrig/BP_pharm.html

Brewerton TD, Reus, et al, "Lithium carbonate and L-tryptophan in the treatment of bipolar and schizoaffective disorders," *Am J Psychiat,* 140: 757-60; 1983.

Broida, *New Hope for Depression,* Prima Publishing, Roseville CA, NY, 2001.

Brown, Ebert et al, "Aggression, suicide, and serotonin: relationships to CSF amine metabolites," *Am J Psychiat,* 139:741-46; 1982a. (Aggression and suicide were associated with low 5HIAA in various psychiatric patients and some XYY violent and aggressive criminals.)

Brown GL, Goodwin FK, et al, "Human aggression and suicide: Their relationship to neuropsychiatric diagnoses and serotonin metabolism," *Adv Biochem Psychopharmacol,* 34:287-307; 1982b.

Brown L, Rosellini RA, "Evidence for a serotonergic mechanism of the learned helplessness phenomenon," *Pharmacol Biochem Behav,* 17(5): 877-83; 11/1983.

Buydens-Branchey L, et al, "Age of alcoholism onset. II. Relationship to susceptibility to serotonin precursor availability," *Arch Gen Psychiat,* 6:231-6; 3/1989.

Buydens-Branchey L, Branchey M, et al, "Craving for cocaine in addicted users. Role of serotonergic mechanisms," *Am J Addict,* 6(1):65-73; 1997. (Suggests serotonin modulates cravings.)

Byerley WF, Judd LL, et al, "5-hydroxytryptophan: A review of its antidepressant efficacy and adverse effects," *J Clin Psychopharmacol,* 7:127-37; 1987.

Cangiano C, Ceri F, et al, "Eating behavior and adherence to dietary prescriptions in obese subjects treated with 5-hydroxytryptophan," *Am J Clin Nut,* 56:863-68; 1992.

Cannell JJ, "Vitamin D and Your Health," At: vitamindcouncil.com/depression.shtml

Caruso I, Sarzi Puttini P, "Double blind study of 5-hydroxytryptophan versus placebo in the treatment of primary fibromyalgia syndrome," *J Int Med Res,* 18:201-9; 1990.

Cass H, *Supplement Your Prescription,* Basic Health Press, Laguna Beach CA, 2007.

Catterall WE, "Tryptophan and bladder cancer," *Bio Psychiat,* 24:733-34; letter, 10/1988.

Chouinard G, Young SN, et al, "Tryptophan-nicotinamide combination in depression," *Lancet,* 1(8005):249; 1/1977.

Chouinard G, Young SN, et al, "Tryptophan-nicotinamide combination in the treatment of newly admitted depressed patients," *Commun in Psych,* 2:311-18; 1978.

Chouinard G, Young SN, et al, [Tryptophan-nicotinamide, imipramine and their combination in depression, A controlled study], *Acta Psychiatr Scand,* 59(4):395-414; 4/1979a. (These nutrients were as effective as imipramine, but not at excessive doses (though bipolars may need high levels.)

Chouinard G, Jones BD, et al, "Potentiation of lithium by tryptophan in a patient with bipolar illness," *Am J Psychiat,* 136(5):719-20; 5/1979b.

Chouinard, G, et al, "A controlled clinical trial of L-tryptophan in acute mania," *Biol Psychiat,* 20:546-57; 1985. (Double blind. Significant improvement.)

Cleare AJ, McGregor A, et al, "Thyroxine replacement increases central 5-hydroxytryptamine activity and reduces depressive symptoms in hypothyroidism," *Neuroendocrinology,* 64(1):65-69; 7/1996. (In 7 hypothyroids, T4 significantly increased 5-HT-mediated cortisol response. TSH correlated with depressive symptoms; cortisol, inversely.)

Cleare AJ, et al, "Effects of alterations in plasma tryptophan levels on aggressive feelings," *Arch Gen Psych,* 51:1004-5; 12/1994.

Cohen BM, et al, "Lecithin in the treatment of mania," *Am J Psychiat,* 139:1162-64; 1982. (Double blind. Significantly better than placebo.)

Collins D, Davis C, et al, "Tryptophan depletion and aggressive responding in healthy males," *Psychopharmacology,* 126:97-103; 1996.

Comings DE, "Blood serotonin and tryptophan in Tourette's syndrome," *Am J Med Genetics,* 36: 418-30; 8/1990.

Conlay LA, et al, "Effect of running the Boston marathon on plasma concentrations of large neutral amino acids," *J Neural Transmission,* 76: 65-71; 1989.

Coppen AJ, Doogan DP, "Serotonin and its place in the pathogenesis of depression," *J Clin Psychiat,* 49S:4-11; 8/1988.

Coppen A, Prange AJ, et al, "Abnormalities of indoleamines in affective disorders," *Arch Gen Psychiat,* 26:474-78; 1972.

Coppen A, Brooksbank BW, "Tryptophan metabolism in depressive illness," *Psychol Med,* 4(2):164-73; 5/1974.

Coppen A, et al, "Plasma folate and affective morbidity during long-term lithium therapy," *Br J Psychiat,* 141:87-89; 1982. (Morbidity in 107 long-term lithium patients was greater when folate was lower (perhaps due to reduced serotonin creation.)

Coppen A, Brooksbank BW, "Tryptophan metabolism in depressive illness," *Psychol Med,* 4(2):164-73; 5/1974.

Copper A, Wood K, "Tryptophan and depressive illness," *Psychol Med,* 8(1):49-57; 2/1978. (Reduced plasma free tryptophan in major depression.)

Cousens G, *Depression Free for Life,* Quill, HarperCollins, NY, 2000.

Deakin JF, "The role of serotonin in panic, anxiety, and depression," *Intl Clin Psychopharmacol,* 13(4S): 1-5; 4/1998.

De Benedittis G, Massei R, "5-HT precursors in migraine prophylaxis: A double-blind crossover study with L-5-hydroxytryptophan versus placebo," *Clin J Pain,* 3:123-29; 1986.

Delgado PL, Price LH, et al, "Serotonin and the neurobiology of depression: Effects of tryptophan depletion in drug-free depressed patients," *Arch Gen Psychiat,* 51(11):865-74; 11/1994. (Some improved comparably to antidepressants.)

Drevets W, "Pet imaging of serotonin 1A receptor binding in depression," *Biol Psychiat,* 46(10):1375-87; 1999.

Dyer W, at: www. healthtimesonoma.com/ spring04.wayne.html Accessed 3/2004.

Evans GW, "Normal and abnormal zinc absorption in man and animals: The tryptophan connection," *Nutr Rev,* 38:137-41; 1980.

Farinelli S, Marianai A, et al, "Eosinophilia-myalgia syndrome associated with 5-OH-tryptophan. Description of a case," *Recenti Prog Med,* 82: 381-84; 1991.

Farkas T, Dunner DL, Fieve RR, "L-tryptophan in depression," *Biol Psych,* 11(3); 1976. (More effective in bipolars.)

Ferrier IN, et al, "Relapse in chronic depressives on withdrawal of L-tryptohan," *Lancet,* 336:380-81; 8/11/1990.

Gelenberg AJ, Gibson CJ, et al, "Neurotransmitter precursors for the treatment of depression," *Psychopharmacol Bull,* 18(1):7-18; 1982.

Gilka L, [Schizophrenia, a disorder of tryptophan metabolism], *Acta Psychiatr Scand,* 258S:1-83; 1975. (Tryptophan may benefit confusion, dementia.)

Gilka L, "Relationship of dietary tryptophan and niacin to tryptophan metabolism in schizophrenics and nonschizophrenics," *Am J Clin Nutr,* 27:565-71; 1974.

Glickman G, Byrne B, "Light therapy for seasonal affective disorders with blue narrow-band ligh-emitting diocides (LEDs)," *Biol Psychiatr,* 59(6): 502-7; 2006.

Gold MS, *The Good News About Depression,* Villard Books, NY, 1987.

JE Goldberg, M Harrow, eds, *Bipolar Disorders: Clinical Course and Outcome,* Am Psychiat Press Inc, DC, 1999.

Golden RN, Gilmore JH, et al, "The effects of age, gender and season on serotonergic function in healthy subjects," *Prog Neuropsychopharmacol Biol Psychiat,* 20(8):1315-23; 11/1996. (Age may be the strongest influence.)

Goldenberg D, Mayskiy M, et al, "A randomized, double-blind crossover trial of fluoxetine and amitriptyline in the treatment of fibromyalgia," *Arthritis Rheum,* 39:1852-59; 1996.

Goodnick PJ, Sandoval R, "Psychotropic treatment of chronic fatigue syndrome and related disorders," *J Clin Psychiat,* 54:13-20; 1/1993.

Goodwin FK, Jamison KR, *Manic-depressive illness,* Oxford University Press,1990.

Gorman J, "The use of newer antidepressants for panic disorder," *J Clin Psychiat,* 58(14S):54-58.

Green AR, Aronson JK, et al, "Metabolism of an oral tryptophan load. I. Effects of dose and pretreatment with tryptophan; II. Effect of pretreatment with the putative tryptophan pyrrolase inhibitors nicotinamide or allopyrinol; III. Effect of a pyridoxine supplement," *Br J Clin Pharmacol,* 10(6):603-19; 12/ 1980abc. (As dose and length of treatment increase, the kynurenine pathway can become relatively saturated, perhaps due to depleted B6 (critical to metabolic enzymes). 7 days of B6 with tryptophan decreased basal plasma kynurenine 50%.)

Gronier B, Axorin JM, et al, "Evidence for a defective platelet L-tryptophan transport in depressed patients," *Intl Clin Psychopharmaco,* 8(2):87-93; 1993.

Halbreich U, Tworek H, "Altered serotonergic activity in women with dysphoric premenstrual syndromes," *Internat J Psychiat Med,* 23(1):1-27; 1993.

Hartmann E, Spinweber CL, "Sleep induced by L-typtophan. Effect of dosages within normal dietary intake," *J Nerv Ment Dis,* 167(8):497-9; 1979.

Hartmann E, Cravens J, et al, "Hypnotic effects of L-tryptophan," *Arch Gen Psychiat,* 31(3):394-7; 9/1974.

Hartmann E, "L-tryptophan: A rational hypnotic with clinical potential," *Am J Psychiat,* 134:366-70; 1977. (Review of 9 studies. Tryptophan, unlike hypnotics, doesn't distort sleep physiology.)

Hauri P, Chernik D, Hawkins D, "Sleep of depressed patients in remission," *Arch Gen Psychiat,* 31:386-91; 1974. (Stage 4 (probably Ser-dependent), slow-wave sleep disturbance remains after remission.)

Heeley AG, Roberts GE, "A study of tryptophan metabolism in psychotic children," *Developmental Medicine and Child Neurology,* 3:708-718; 1966.

Heninger GR, Delgado PL, et al, "Tryptophan-deficient diet and amino acid drink deplete plasma tryptophan and induce a relapse of depression in susceptible patients," *J Chem Neuroanat,* 5(4):347-8; 7-8/1992.

Howard JS, "Folate deficiency in psychiatric practice," *Psychosomatics,* 16:112-15; 1975.

Huether G, et al, "Effects of tryptophan administration on circulating melatonin levels in chicks and rats: Evidence for stimulation of melatonin synthesis and release in the gastrointestinal tract," *Life Sci,* 51:945-53; 1992.

Jouvet M, "Biogenic amines and the states of sleep," *Sci,* 163:32-41; 1969.

Kahn R, Westenberg H, et al, "Effect of a serotonin precursor and uptake inhibitor in anxiety disorders: A double-blind comparison of 5-hydroxtryptophan, clomipramine and placebo," *Intl Clin Psychopharmacol,* 2:45; 1987.

Kahn R, Westenberg H, "L-5-hydroxytryptophan in the treatment of anxiety disorders, " *J Affect Disord,* 8:197-200; 1985.

Khazali H, Parhiskar A, et al, "Effect of serotonin infusions on the mean plasma concentrations of growth hormone, thyroid hormone, and the amount and constituents of milk in the Sanan goat," *African J Biotech,* 5(1):31-34; 1/2006. (Serotonin may increase thyroid and growth hormone secretion.)

Kirstein L, Bowers MB, et al, "CSF amine metabolites, clinical symptoms, and body movement in psychiatric patients," *Biol Psychiat,* 11(4):421-34; 8/1976.

Kitahara M, "Dietary tryptophan ratio and suicide in the United Kingdom, Ireland, the United States, Canada, Australia, and New Zealand," *Omega: Journal of Death and Dying,* 18(1):71-6; 1987.

Knutson B, Wolkowitz OM, et al, "Selective

alteration of personality and social behavior by serotonergic intervention," *Am J Psychiat,* 155: 373-9; 1998.

Lam RW, et al, "L-tryptophan augmentation of light therapy in patients with seasonal affective disorder," *Can J Psychiat,* 42(3):303-6; 1997.

Lambert GW, Reid C, "Effect of sunlight and season on serotonin turnover in the brain," *Lancet,* 360(9348):1840-2; 12/2002.

Lampert A, Joly P, et al, "Scleroderma-like syndrome with bulbous morphea during treatment with 5-hydroxytryptophan, carbidopa and flunitrazepam," *Ann Dermatol Venereol,* 119:209-11; 1992. (In case 3, 5HTP may not have been involved.)

Landry P, Chouinard G, "Lithium-tryptophan combination in the maintenance treatment of bipolar affective illness," *Lithium,* 2:135-40; 1991 (Double blind. Drug resistant bipolars).

Larson JM, *Depression Free, Naturally,* Ballantine Wellspring, NY, 2001.

Lidberg L, Tuck JR, et al, [Homicide, suicide and CSF5-HIAA], *Acta Psychiatr Scand,* 71(3):230-6; 3/1985. (Violence and emotional turmoil were associated with lower CSF serotonin.)

Linnoila VM, Virkkunen M, "Aggression, suicidality and serotonin," *J Clin Psychiat,* 53S:46-51; 10/1992.

Lloyd K, Farley L, et al, "Serotonin and 5-hydroxyindoleacetic acid in discrete areas of the brainstem of suicide victims and control patients," *Adv Biochem Psychopharm,* 11:387-98; 1974.

Lopez-Ibor JJ, "Serotonin and psychiatric disorders," *Intl Clin Psychopharmacol,* 7(2): 5-11; 10/1992.

Lindberg D, Ahlfors UG, [Symptom reduction in depression after treatment with L-tryptophan or imipramine. Item analysis of Hamilton rating scale for depression], *Acta Psychiatr Scand,* 60(3):287-94; 9/1979.

Loew D, [L tryptophan. An essential amino acid for structural and functional metabolism], *Fortschr Med,* 115:40-42; 1997.

Lucca A, et al, "Plasma tryptophan levels and plasma tryptophan/neutral amino acids ratio in patients with mood disorder, patients with obsessive-compulsive disorder, and normal subjects," *Psychiat Res,* 44(2): 85-91; 1992.

Maes M, et al, "The decreased availability of L-tryptophan in depressed females: Clinical and biological correlates," *Neuro Psychopharm Biol Psychiat,* 14:903-13; 1990.

Maes M, et al, "Symptom profiles of biological markers in depression: A multivariate study, *Psychoneuroendocrinol,* 15(1):29-37; 1990.

Maes M, et al, "Disturbance in dexamethasone suppression test and lower availability of L-tryptophan and tyrosine in early puerperium and in women under contraceptive therapy," *J Psychosom Res,* 36:191-97; 9/1992.

Maes M, Meltzer H Y, et al, "Relationships between lower plasma L-tryptophan levels and immune-inflammatory variables in depression," *Psychiat Res,* 49(2):151-65; 11/1993.

Maes M, et al, "Stimulatory effects of L-5-hydroxytryptophan on postdexamethasone beta-endorphin levels in major depression," *Neuropsychopharmacol,* 15:340-48; 1996.

Malison R, et al, "Reduced brain serotonin transporter availability in major depression as measured by [123I]-2-carbomethoxy-3-(4-iodophenyl)tropane and single photon emission computed tomography," *Biol Psychiat,* 44(11):1090-98; 1998.

Malone K, "Serotonin and major depression, in JJ Mann, DJ Kupfer, eds, *Biology of Depressive Disorders Part A,* Plenum Press, NY 1993.

Mann JJ, Yates PO, "Neurotransmitter deficits in Alzheimer's disease and in other dementing disorders," *Hum Neurobiol,* 5(3):147-58; 1986.

Mann JJ, Marzuk PM, et al, "Neurochemical studies of violent and nonviolent suicide," *Psychopharmacol Bull,* 25(3):407-13; 1989.

Mann JJ, Arango V, et al, "Evidence for the 5-HT hypothesis of suicide. A review of post-mortem studies," *Br J Psychiatr,* (8S): 7-14; 12/1989.

Mann JJ, Arango V, et al, "Serotonin and suicidal behavior," *Ann NY Acad Sci,* 600(1):476-84; 1990.

Mann JJ "Role of the serotinergic system in the pathogenesis of major depression and suicidal behavior," *Neuropsychopharmacol,* 21(2S):99-105; 1999.

Marazziti D, Lenzi A, "Decreased platelet serotonin uptake in bipolar 1 patients," *Intl Clin Psychopharmacol,* 6(1):25-30; Spring/1991a. (The Vmax for uptake of 14C-5HT (important in serotonin transport) was significantly lower in 12 bipolars vs controls, suggesting a 5HT transport problem.)

Marazziti D, Lenzi A, et al, "Serotinergic dysfunction in bipolar disorder," *Pharmacopsychiatr,* 24(5):164-67; 9/1991b.

Mc Grath RE, et al , The effect of L-tryptophan on seasonal affective disorder, *J Clin Psychiat,* 51: 162-63; 4/1990.

McIntyre IM, Stanley M, "Postmortem and regional changes of serotonin, 5-hydroxyindoleacetic acid and tryptophan in brain," *J Neurochem,* 42(6): 1588-92; 1984.

Brigham PM, "The Psychopharmacology of Bipolar Disorder," updated 5-9-2001. At: http: //people.ne.mediaone.net/pmbrig/BP_pharm.html

Meltzer CC, et al, "Serotonin in aging, late-life depression, and Alzheimer's disease: The emerging role of functional imaging," *Neuropsychopharmacol,* 18(6):407-30; 1998.

Miller HL, "Acute tryptophan depletion: A method of studying antidepressant action," *J Clin Psychiat,* 53S:28-35; 10/1992. (Tryptophan deprivation can make most people depressed within hours.)

Moldofsky H, Warsh H, "Plasma tryptophan and musculoskeletal pain in non-articular rheumatism," *Pain,* 5:65-71; 1978.

Moldofsky H, Lue F, "The relationship of alpha and delta EEG frequencies to pain and mood in fibrositis patients treated with chlorpromazine and L-tryptophan," *Electroencephalogr Clin Neurophysiol,* 50:71-80; 1980.

Moller S, et al, "Tryptophan availability in endogenous depression: Relation to efficacy of L-tryptophan treatment," *Adv Biol Psychiat,* 10: 30-46; 1983.

Moore P, et al, "Rapid tryptophan depletion, sleep electroencephalogram, and mood in men with remitted depression on serotonin reuptake inhibitors," *Arch Gen Psychiat,* 55(6):534-39; 1998.

Mundo E, Bianchi L, et al, "Efficacy of fluvoxamine, paroxetine, and citalopram in the treatment of obsessive-compulsive disorder: A single-blind study," *J Clin Psychopharmacl,* 17:267-71; 1997.

Murphy DL et al, "L-tryptophan in affective disorders: Indoleamine changes and differential clinical effects," *Psychopharmacologia,* 34:11-20; 1974. (36% of 44 patients responded.)

Murray MT, *Encyclopedia of Nutritional Supplements,* Prima, Rocklin, CA, 1996.

Murray MT, Pizzorno J, *Encyclopedia of Natural Medicine,* Prima, Rocklin, CA, 1998.

Nardini M, et al, "Treatment of depression with L- 5-hydroxytryptophan combined with chlorimipramine: A double blind study," *J Clin Pharmacolog Res,* 3: 239-50; 1983.

Neumeister A, et al, "Effects of tryptophan depletion on drug-free patients with seasonal affective disorder during a stable response to bright light therapy," *Arch Gen Psychiat,* 54:133-38; 1997.

Nishizawa S, Benkelfat C, et al, "Differences between males and females in rates of serotonin synthesis in human brain," *Proc Natl Acad Sci US,* 94:5308-13; 1997. (52% higher in males.)

Persson T, Roos B, "5-hydroxytryptophan for depression," *Lancet,* ii:987; 1967.

Nolen WA, et al, [Treatment strategy in depression. II. MAO inhibitors in depression resistant to cyclic antidepressants: Two controlled crossover studies with tranylcypromine versus L-5-hydroxy-tryptophan and nomifensine], *Acta Psychiat Scand,* 78(5):676-83; 1988.

Panzer A, "Depression or cancer: The choice between serotonin or melatonin," *Med Hypotheses,* 50(5):385-87; 1998.

Gayford JJ, Parker AL, et al, "Whole blood 5-hydroxytryptamine during treatment for endogenous depressive illness," *Br J Psychiat,* 122(570):597-8; 1973.

Poldinger W, Calanchini B, et al, "A functional-dimensional approach to depression: Serotonin deficiency as a target syndrome in a comparison of 5-hydroxytryptophan and fluvoxamine," *Psychopathol,* 24(2):535-81; 1991. (Double blind. Both 5HTP and drug groups improved significantly at 2, 4, and 6 wks (reports and HAM-D). Depression scores reduced 50% by 6 wks. Side effects in both gps included early GI symptoms. Drug groups experienced 4x as many treatment failures, and more side effects.)

Poldinger W, Macke S, [Progress toward functional diagnosis in psychiatry. The serotonin deficiency syndrome], *Ther Umsch,* 53(3):225-7; 3/1996.

Poldinger W, [Impulse control disorders and other serotonin function disorders], *Schweiz Rundsch Med Prax,* 87(41):1348-55; 10/1998. (Especially if episodic.)

Pollock Robert L, et al, *The Pain-Free Tryptophan Diet,* Warner Books, NY, 1986.

Prange AJ, Jr, Wilson IC, et al, "L-tryptophan in mania. Contribution to a permissive hypothesis of affective disorders," *Arch Gen Psychiat,* 30:56-62; 1974. (Double blind crossover. Tryptophan as good or better than chlopromazine.)

Price LH, Malison RT, et al, "The neurobiology of tryptophan depletion in depression: Effects of intravenous tryptophan infusion," *Biol Psychiat,* 43(5):339-47; 1998.

Puttini P, Caruso I, "Primary fibromyalgia syndrome and 5-hydroxy-L-tryptophan: A 90-day open study," *J Int Med Res,* 20:182-89; 1992.

Quadbeck H, Lehmann E, et al, "Comparison of the antidepressant action of tryptophan, tryptophan/5-hydroxytryptophan combination and nomifensine," *Neuropsychol,* 11(2):111-15; 1984.

Reilly J, Mc Tavish S, et al, "Rapid depletion of plasma tryptophan: A review of studies and experimental methodology," *J Psychopharmacol,* 11:381-92; 1997.

Reuven S, "L-tryptophan in neuropsychiatric disorders: A review," *Intl J Neurosci,* 67:127-44; 1992.

Rogers S, *Depression, Cured at Last,* SK Publishing, Sarasota FL, 1997.

Ross J, *The Mood Cure,* Viking Penguin, NY, 2002.

Russell I, Michalek J, et al, "Serum amino acids in fibrositis/fibromyalgia syndrome," *J Rheumatol,* 16(19S):158-63; 1989.

Sachs GS, "Adjuncts and alternatives to lithium therapy for bipolar affective disorder," *J Clin Psychiat* 50S:31-39; 12/1989.

Salomon RM, Miller HL, et al, "The use of tryptophan depletion to evaluate central serotonin function in depression and other neuropsychiatric disorders," *Inter Clin Psychopharmacol,* 8S(2):41-46; 11/1993.

Sano I, ["Precursor-therapy" with active amines. Part I: Treatment of depression by L-5-HTP (L-5-hydroxytryptophan)], *Psychiatr Neurol Japn,* 73: 809; 1971.

Sano I, [L-5-hyroxytryptophan (L-5-HTP) therapy], *Folia Psychiat Neurol Japn,* 26:7; 1972.

Soulairac A, Lambinet H, "Action of 5-hydroxytryptophane, precursor of serotonin, on sleep disorder," *Ann Med Psychol,* 135:792-98; 1977.

Schneider-Helmet, D, et al, "Evaluation of L-tryptophan for treatment of insomnia: A review," *Psychopharmacol,* 89(1):1-7; 1986.

Schweiger U, et al, "Macronutrient intake, plasma large neutral amino acids and mood during weight-reducing diets," *J Neural Transm,* 67(1-2): 77-86; 1986.

Shaw K, Turner J, "Tryptophan and 5-hydroxytryptophan for depression," *The Cochrane Database of Systematic Review,* Issue 3; 2006.

Slagle P, "5HTP" *The Way Up Newsletter,* V#13; 10/15/1999. At: http://www.thewayup.com

Slutsker L, et al, "Eosinophilia-myalgia syndrome associated with exposure to tryptophan from a single manufacturer," *JAMA,* 264:213-17; 1990.

Brigham PM, "The Psychopharmacology of Bipolar Disorder," updated 5-9-2001. At: http: //people.ne.mediaone.net/pmbrig/BP_pharm.html

Smith KA, Fairburn CG, "Relapse of depression

after rapid depletion of tryptophan," *Lancet,* 349: 915-9; 1997.

Steiger H, Eating disorders and the serotonin connection: State, trait and developmental effects, *J Psychiat Neurosci,* 2004.

Sternberg E, Van Woert M, et al, "Development of a scleroderma-like illness during therapy with L-5-hydroxytryptophan and carbidopa," *NEJM,* 1980.

Stockmeier C, Shapiro LA, et al, "Increase in serotonin 1-A autoreceptors in the midbrain of suicide victims with major depression — Postmortem evidence for decreased serotonin activity," *J Neurosci,* 18(18): 7394-7401; 9/1998.

Stockmeier CA, "Neurobiology of serotonin in depression and suicide," *Ann NY Acad Sci,* 836: 220-32; 1997.

Strosznaider J, Samochocki M, "Serotonin, a potent modulator of arachidonic acid turnover, interaction with glutaminergic receptor in brain cortex," *Neurochem Int,* 25:193-99; 1994.

Swann AC, Secunda S, et al, "CSF monoamine metabolites in mania," *Am J Psychiatr,* 140:396-400, 1983.

Takahashi S, Kondo H, et al, "Effect of L-5-hydroxytryptophan on brain monoamine metabolism and evaluation of its clinical effect in depressed patients," *J Psychiat Res,* 12:177-87; 1975.

Thomas DE, et al, "Tryptophan and nutritional status of patients with senile dementia," *Psychol Med,* 16: 297-303; 5/1986.

Thomson J, et al, "The treatment of depression in general practice: A comparison of L-tryptophan, amitriptyline, and a combination of L-tryptophan and amitriptyline with placebo," *Psychol Med,* 12: 741-51; 11/1982.

Titus F, Davaolos A, et al, "5-hyroxytryptophan versus methysergide in the prophlaxis of migraine. A randomized clinical trial," *Eur Neurol,* 25:327-29; 1986.

Ursin R, "The effect of 5-hydroxytryptophan and L-tryptophan on wakefulness and sleep patterns in the cat," *Brain Res,* 106:106-15; 1976.

van Hiele LJ, "L-5 hydroxytryptophan in depression: The first substitution therapy in psychiatry," *Neuropsychol,* 6:230-40; 1980.

van Praag H, de Haan S, "Depression vulnerability and 5-hydroxytryptophan prophylaxis," *Psych Res,* 3:75-83; 1980.

van Praag HM, "Management of depression with serotonin precursors," *Biol Psychiat,* 16:291-310; 1981.

van Praag HM, Westenberg HG, "The treatment of depressions with L-5-hydroxytryptophan. Theoretical backgrounds and practical application," *Adv Biol Psychiat,* 10:94-128; 1983.

van Praag HM, "Studies on the mechanism of action of serotonin precursors in depression," *Psychopharm Bull,* 20:599-602; 1984.

van Praag H, "Biological suicide research: Outcome and limitations," *Biol Psychiat,* 21:1305-23; 1986.

van Praag HM, Lemus C, "Monoamine precursors in the treatment of psychiatric disorders," in RJ Wurtman, JJ Wurtman, eds, *Nutrition and the Brain,* Raven Press, NY, V7; 1986.

van Praag H, Kahn R, "L-5-hydroxytryptophan in depression and anxiety," *Schweiz Rundschau Med,* 77:40-46; 1988. (5HTP and SSRIs sometimes increase anxiety or depression in first few weeks, before improvement occurs. Benzos decrease Ser activity.)

Widner, B, Laich A, et al, "Biopterin production, tryptophan degradation and mental depression — what is the link?" *Brain, Behav, Immun,* 16: 590-95; 2002.

Wood K, "Total and non-bound plasma tryptophan in depressive illness," *Lancet,* 1977.

Wurtman J, "Carbohydrate craving, mood changes, and obesity," *J Clin Psychiat,* 49S:37-39; 1988.

Wurtman RJ, Wurtman JJ, "Carbohydrates and depression," *Sci Am,* 68-75; 1/1989.

Yaryura-Tobias J, Bhagavan H, "L-tryptophan in obsessive-compulsive disorders," *Am J Psychiat,* 134:1298-99; 1977a.

Yarura-Tobias JA, Neziroglu F, "Tryptophan and perceptual schizophrenias," *J Orthomol Psychiat,* 6(2):193-94; 1977b.

Young SN, Sourkes TL, "Antidepressant action of tryptophan," *Lancet,* 2(7885):897-8; 10/1974. (Niacinamide may help limit tryptophan breakdown in the liver.)

Young SN, Chouinard G, et al, "Tryptophan in the treatment of depression," *Adv Exp Med Biol,* 133: 727-37; 1981.

Young SN, Smith SE, et al, "Tryptophan depletion causes a rapid lowering of mood in normal males," *Psychopharmacol,* 87(2):173-7; 1985.

Young SJ, "The clinical psychopharmacology of tryptophan," in RJ Wurtman, JJ Wurtman, eds, *Nutrition and the Brain,* Raven Press, NY, V7: 49-88; 1986.

Young, "Use of tryptophan in combination with other antidepressant treatments: A review," *J Psychiat Neurosci,* 16(5):241-6; 1991.

Zmilacher K, et al, "L- 5-hydroxytryptophan alone and in combination with a peripheral decarboxylse inhibitor in the treatment for depression," *Neuropsychobiol,* 20:28-35; 1988.

Dopamine, Norepinephrine

Adler LE, Gerhardt GA, et al, "Sensory physiology and catecholamines in schizophrenia and mania," *Psychiat Res,* 31(3):297-309; 3/90. (Manics may have a transient deficit in sensory gating via NE. Schizophrenics have a fixed familial deficit, unchanged by meds; sensitivity increases during acute illness, probably via DA.)

Akiskal HS, McKinney WT, "Depressive disorders: Toward a unified hypothesis," *Science,* 182:20-29; 1973.

Akiskal HS, McKinney WT, "Overview of recent research in depression. Integration of ten conceptual models into a comprehensive clinical frame," *Arch Gen Psychiat,* 32:285-305, 1975.

Andrews J, Ninan PT, et al, "Venlafaxine: A novel antidepressant that has a dual mechanism of action," *Depression,* 4:48-56; 1996.

Ansseau M, "Biological markers of depression," Proc Intl Congress Biol Markers Depression: State of the Art, Liege, Belgium, 6/13-15, 1990, in M Ansseau, R Von Frenckell, G Franck, eds, *Elsevier Sci Pubs, Excerpta Medica,* NY, 1991; pp 4-9.

Arango V, Underwood MD, "Fewer pigmented locus coeruleus neurons in suicide victims: Preliminary results," *Biol Psychiat,* 39:112-20; 1996.

Arborelius L, Owens MJ, et al, "The role of corticotropic-releasing factor (CRF) in depression and anxiety disorders," *J Endocrinol,* 160:1-12; 1999.

Ashcroft GW, Glen AIM, "Mood and neuronal functions: A modified amine hypothesis for the etiology of affective illness," *Adv Biochem Psychopharmacol,* 11, 335-39; 1974.

Ashcroft GW, Blackburn IM, et al, "Changes on recovery in the concentration of tryptophan and the biogenic amine metabolites in the CSF of patients with affective illness," *Psychol Med,* 3: 319-325; 1973.

Aston-Jones G, Chiang C, et al, "Discharge of noradrenergic locus coeruleus neurons in behaving rats and monkeys suggests a role in vigilance," *Prog Brain Res,* 88:501-20; 1991a.

Axelrod J, Whitby L, et al, "Effect of psychotropic drugs on the uptake of ^{3}H-norepinephrine by tissues," *Science,* 133:383-4; 1961

Baron B, Ogden A, et al, "Rapid down-regulation of B-adrenoreceptors by co-administration of desipramine and fluoxetine," *Eur J Pharmacol,* 154: 125-34; 1998.

Banki CM, "Correlation between cerebrospinal fluid amine metabolites and psychomotor activity in affective disorders," *J Neurochem,* 28, 225-57; 1977

Baumel S, *Dealing with Depression Naturally,* Keats, New Canaan, CN, 1995.

Beaulieu JM, Sotnikova TD, et al, "An Akt/beta-arrestin 2/PP2A signaling complex mediates dopaminergic neurotransmission and behavior," *Cell,* 122(2):153-5; 7/2005.

Beckman H, et al, "DL-phenylalanine versus impramine: A double-blind controlled study," *Arch Psychiat Nervenkr,* 227:49-58; 1979.

Belmaker R, Ebbesen K, et al, "Electrophoresis of platelet monoamine oxidase in schizophrenia and manic-depressive illness," *Br J Psychiat,* 129:227-32; 1976. (Platelet MAO may be higher in manics than schizophrenics or normals, though effects of lithium need to be controlled for.)

Belmaker RH, "Receptors, adenylate cyclase, depression, and lithium," *Biol Psychiat,* 16(4):333-50; 4/1981. (Beta adrenergic receptor sensitivity may be a better indicator of antidepressant effectiveness than NE turnover. Lithium reduces beta adrenergic adenylate cyclase and partially inhibits plasma cyclic GMP (balancing) response to epinephrine.)

Benkert O, Grunder G, et al, "Dopamine autoreceptor agonists in the treatment of schizophrenia and major depression," *Pharmacopsychiat,* 25(6):254-60; 11/1992.

Benjamin J, Ebstein RP, Belmaker RH, "Personality genetics," *Isr J Psychiat Relat Sci,* 34(4):270-80; 1997. (DA receptor gene may relate to novelty seeking, and may interact with the serotonin 2C receptor gene, and reward dependence.)

Berman R, Krystal J, et al, "Mechanism of action of antidepessants: Monoamine hypotheses and beyond," in S Watson, ed, *Biology of Schizophrenia and Affective Disease,* Am Psychiatric Press Inc, DC; 1996; pp 395-46.

Biegon A, Fieldust S, "Reduced tyrosine hydroxylase immunoreactivity in locus coeruleus of suicide victims," *Synapse,* 10:79-82; 1992.

Biegon A, Israeli M, "Regionally selective increases in beta-adrenergic receptor density in the brains of suicide victims," *Brain Res,* 442(1):199-203; 2/1988.

Blomberg P, Kopin I, et al, "Conversion of MHPG to vanillylmandelic acid," *Arch Gen Psychiat,* 37: 1095-8; 1980.

Blum K, Braverman ER, et al, "Association of polymorphisms of dopamine D2 receptor (DAD2), and dopamine transporter (DAT1) genes with schizoid/avoidant behaviors (SAB)," *Mol Psychiat,* 2(3):239-46; 5/1997.

Bond PA, Jenner FA, et al, "Daily variation of urine content of MHPG in two manic-depressive patients," *Psychol Med,* 2:81; 1972. (Increased preceding and during mania.)

Bowden C, et al, "Reduced dopamine turnover in the basal ganglia of depressed suicides," *Brain Res,* 769(1):135-40; 1997.

Bowers MD, JR, "Acute psychosis induced by psychomimetic drug abuse II. Neurochemical findings," *Arch Gen Psychiat,* 27:440-42; 1972.

Bowers MB, "CSF acid monoamine metabolites as a possible reflection of central MAO activity in chronic schizophrenia," *Biol Psychiat,* 11, 245-49; 1976. (Greater HVA in manics vs depressives.)

Braverman ER, Pfeiffer CC, *The Healing Nutrients Within,* Keats, New Canaan, CN, 1987.

Braverman ER, *Path Wellness Manual,* Publications for Achieving Total Health, NJ, 1994.

Breggin PR, MD, *Toxic Psychiatry,* St. Martin's Press, NY, 1991.

Bunney WE, Davis JM, Norepinephrine in depressive reactions: A review," *Arch Gen Psychiat,* 13:483-94; 1965.

Bunney WE, Murphy D, et al, "The 'switch process' in manic-depressive illness. I. A systematic study of sequential behavior change," *Arch Gen Psychiatr,* 27:195-302; 1972a; "II: Relationship to catecholamines, REM sleep, and drugs," 27: 304-09; 1972b; "III: Theoretical implications," 27: 312-17; 1972c.

Bunney WE Jr, "Psychopharmacology of the switch process in affective illness, in MA Lipton, A DiMascio, KF Killam, eds, *Psychopharmacology: A Generation of Progress,* Raven, NY, 1978, pp 1249-59.

Cabib S, Puglisi-Allegra S, "Stress, depression and the mesolimbic dopamine system," *Psychopharmacol,* 128(4):331-42; 1996.

Casper RC, Davis JM, et al, "Neuroendocrine and amine studies in affective illness," *Psychoneuroendocinol,* 2:105-13; 1977.

Chan-Palay V, Asan E, "Quantitation of catecholamine neurons in the locus coeruleus in human brains of normal young and older adults and in depression," *J Comp Neurol,* 287:357-72; 1989.

Charney D, "Monoamine dysfunction and the pathophysiology and treatment of depression," *J Clin Psychiat,* 59(14S):11-14; 1998.

Charney D, Heninger G, et al, "Presynaptic adrenergic receptor senstiivity in depression: The effect of long-term desipramine treatment," *Arch Gen Psychiat,* 38:1334-40; 1981. (Postmortem studies show increased alpha2R density.)

Checkley SA, Wiecke A, et al, "Hormones, genes and the triggering of bipolar illness in the puerperium," in SA Montgomery, TH Corn, eds, *Psychopharmacology of Depression,* Oxford U Press, Oxford, 1994; pp 57-65.

Cleare A, Murray R, et al, "Do noradrenergic reuptake inhibitors affect serotonergic function in depression?" *Psychopharmacology,* 134:406-10; 1997. (Intricate connections.)

Cohen D, Cailloux-Cohen, S, l'AGIDD-SMQ, [*Guide Critique des Medicaments de l'Ame*], Les Editions de l'Homme, Quebec, 1995.

Cole B, Robbins T, "Forebrain norepinephrine: role in controlled information processing in the rat," *Neuropsychopharmacol,* 7:129-41; 1992.

Cools AR, "Basic considerations on the role of concertedly working dopaminergic, GABAergic, cholinergic, and serotonergic mechanisms within the neostriatum and nucleus accumbens in locomotor activity, sterotyped gnawing, turning, and dyskinetic activities," in EH Ellinwood and NM Kilbey, eds, *Cocaine and Other Stimulants, Advances in Behavioral Biology,* V21, Plenum, NY, 1977; pp 97-142.

Costall B, Naylor R, "Mesolimbic and extrapyramidal sites for the mediation of sterotyped behavior patterns and hyperactivity by amphetamine and apomorphine in the rat," in EH Ellinwood and MM Kilbey eds, *Cocaine and Other Stimulants, Advances in Behavioral Biology,* V21, Plenum, NY, 1977; pp 47-76.

Cousens G, *Depression Free for Life,* Quill, HarperCollins, NY, 2000.

Crow T, Deakin J, "Affective change and the mechanisms of reward and punishment: A neurochemical hypothesis," in C Perris, G Struwe, B Jansson, eds, *Biol Psychiat,* Elsevier, Amsterdam, 1981; pp 536-41.

Curzon G, Goodwin-Austin RB, et al, "The CSF HVA concentration in patients with Parkinsonism treated with L-dopa," *J Neurol Neurosurg Psychiat,* 33:1-6; 1970.

Davis JM, et al, "A behavioral-biochemical study of lithium treatment," *Am J Psychiat,* 125:499; 1968.

deBoer T, "The pharmacologic profile of mirtazepine," *J Clin Psychiat,* 57(4S):19-25; 1996.

DeLeon-Jones F, Maas JW, et al, "Urinary catecholamine metabolites during behavioral changes in a patient with manic-depressive cycles," *Science,* 179:300-2; 1973.

De Parmentier F, Cheetham S, et al, "Brain beta-adreno-receptor binding sites in antidepressant-free depressed suicide victims," *Brain Res,* 525:71-7; 1990.

Diehl DJ, Gershon S, "The role of dopamine in mood disorders," *Compr Psychiat,* 33(2):115-20; 1992.

Drevets W, "Functional neuroimaging studies of depression: The anatomy of melancholia," *Ann Rev Med,* 49:341-61; 1998.

Durman R, Heninger G, et al, "A molecular and cellular theory of depression," *Arch Gen Psychiat,* 54:597-606; 1997. (Depression may occur when stress alters neurotrophic factors (which protect neural viability).)

Duval F, Mokrani MC, et al, "Dopamine function in men with bipolar depression," *Biol Psychiat,* 47(8S):73; 2000.

Fischer E, "Biogenic amines in schizophrenia" in D Hawkins, L Pauling, eds, *Orthomolecular Psychiatry,* WH Freeman and Co, SF, 1973.

Foote S, Aston-Jones G, "Pharmacology and physiology of central noradrenergic systems," in F Bloom, D Kupfer, eds, *Psychopharmacology: The Fourth Generation of Progress,* Raven Press Ltd, NY, 335-45; 1995.

Freis E, "Mental depression in hypertensives treated for long periods with large doses of reserpine," *NEJM,* 241:1006-8; 12/1954. (Depletes catecholamines and can cause severe depression, reversible when discontinued or opposed by l-DOPA.)

Geracioti T, Loosen P, et al, "Uncoupling of serotonergic and noradrenergic systems in depression: Preliminary evidence from continuous cerebrospinal fluid sampling," *Depress Anxiety,* 6(3): 89-94; 1997. (Depressives don't tend to significant inverse relation between 5HIAA and MHPG (Ser/NE metabolites).)

Gerner RH, Post RM, Bunney WE, "A dopaminergic mechanism in mania, *Am J Psychiat,* 133, 1177-80; 1976. (Case report. Amphetamine or a DA agonist consistently triggered mania.)

Glowinski J, Axelrod J, "Inhibition of uptake of noradrenaline in the intact rat brain by imipramine structurally related compounds," *Naturek,* 204: 1318-9; 1964.

Gold MS, *The Good News About Depression,* Villard Books, NY, 1987.

Goldberg IK, "L-tyrosine in depression," *Lancet,* 8/1980.

Goodwin F, Bunney WE, "Depression following reserpine: A re-evaluation," *Seminars in Psychiatry,* 3:435-48; 1971.

Goodwin FK, Post RM, et al, "Cerebrospinal fluid amine metabolites in affective illness: The probenecid technique," *Am J Psychiatr,* 130, 73-9; 1973.

Goodwin FK, Sack RL, "Behavioral effects of a new dopamine-beta-hydroxylase inhibitor (dusaric acid) in man," *J Psychiatr Res,* 11:211-217; 1974.

Goodwin FK, Post RM, "Studies of amine metabolites in affective illness and in schizophrenia: A comparative analysis," in D Freedman, ed, *The Biology of the Major Psychoses,* Raven NY 1975; pp 299-332.

Gordon EK, Oliver J, [3-Methoxy-4-hydroxy-phenylethylene glycol in human cerebrospinal fluid], *Clin Chim Acta,* 35, 145-50; 1971. (CSF MHPG lowest in depressed patients.)

Greenhoff J, Nisell M, "Noradrenergic modulation of midbrain dopamine cell firing elicited by stimulation of the locus coeruleus in the rat," *J Neural Trans,* 93:11-25; 1993.

Greenspan K, Schildkraut J, et al, "Catecholamine metabolism in affective disorders, MHPG and other catecholamine metabolites in patients treated with lithium carbonate," *J Psychiatr Res,* 7:171-184; 1970. (NE and NM greater during hypomania.)

Grunder G, Wetzel H, et al, "Roxindole, a dopamine autoreceptor agonist, in the treatment of major depression," *Psychopharmacol,* 111(1); 4/1993. (A powerful selective DA receptor agonist showed potent antidepressant activity. 4/12 responded by week one, 3 more by two, 1 by four.)

Guldberg HC, Yates CM, "Some studies of the effect of chlorpromazine, reserpine and dihydroxyphenylalanine on the concentrations of homovanillic acid, 3,4-dihydroxyphenylacetic acid and 5-hydroxyindole-3-acetic acid in ventricular cerebrospinal fluid of the dog using the technique of serial sampling of the cerebrospinal fluid," *Br J Pharmacol,* 33:457-71; 1968.

Halper MJ, Brown RP, et al, "Blunted beta-adrenergic responsivity of peripheral blood mononuclear cells in endogenous depression. Isoproterenol dose-response studies," *Arch Gen Psychiat,* 45(3): 3/1988.

Hamner MB, Lorberbaum JP, et al, "Potential role of the anterior cingulate cortex in PTSD: Review and hypothesis," *Depress Anxiety,* 9(1):1-14; 1999. (Chronic LC NE transmissions may decrease cingulate grating, facilitating over-response, such as in PTSD.)

Hansson L, Hunyor SN, et al, "Blood pressure crisis following withdrawal of clonidine, with special reference to arterial and urinary catecholamine levels, and suggestions for acute management," *Am Heart J,* 85:605; 1973.

Heninger G, Delgado P, et al, "The revised monoamine theory of depression: A modulatory role for monoamines, based on new findings from monoamine depletion experiments in humans," *Pharmacopsychiat,* 29:2-11; 1996.

Hoffer A, "Nutrition and behavior" in J Bland, ed, *Medical Applications of Clinical Nutrition,* Keats, New Canaan, CN, 1983.

Jaffe R, Kruesi OR,"The biochemical-immunology window: A molecular view of psychiatric case management," *J App Nutr,* 44(2); 1992.

Janowsky DS, Golden RN, et al, "Neurochemistry of Depression and Mania," in A Georgotas, R Cancho, eds, *Depression and Mania,* Elsevier Sci Pub Co, Inc, NY, 1988; pp 244-259.

Janssen PAG, Leysen JE, et al, "Does phenylethylamine act as an endogenous amphetamine in some patients," *Intl J Neuropsychopharmacol,* 2:249-40; 1999. (Not stored, rapidly degraded. Low levels have been tied to ADD, & depression; elevation to schizophrenia.)

Kapur S, Mann JJ, "Role of the dopaminergic system in depression," *Bio Psychiat,* 32:1-17; 1992.

Karege F, Bovier P, et al, "Platelet membrane alpha-2-adrenergic receptors in depression," *Psychiat Res,* 43:243-52; 1992.

Karege F, Bovier P, et al, "Plasma MHPG and AMDP depression relations, evolution and drug effect in a follow up study of depressed patients," *Hum Psychopharmacol,* 6:11-17; 1991.

Karki NT, [The urinary excretion of noradrenalin and adrenaline in different age groups, its clinical variation and the effect of muscular work on it], *Acta Physiol Scand,* 132(39S):1-96; 1956.

Kasamatsu T, Itakura T, et al, "Neuronal plasticity in cat visual cortex: A proposed role for the central noradrenaline system," in L Discarries, T Read, H Jasper, eds, *Monoamine Innervation of Cerebral Cortex,* Alan R Liss Inc, NY, 1984; pp 9-40.

Kitayama I, Yaga T, et al, "Long-term stress degenerates, but imipramine regenerates, noradrenergic axons in the rat cerebral cortex," *Biol Psychiat,* 42:687-96;1997.

Klimek V, Stockmeier C, et al, reduced levels of norepinephrine transporters in the locus coeruleus in major depression, *J Neurosci,* 17(21):8451-8; 1997.

Krauthammer C, Klerman GL, "Secondary mania: Manic syndromes associated with antecedent physical illness or drugs," *Arch Gen Psychiat,* 35: 133-1339; 1978.

Leonard BE, "Noradrenaline in basic models of depression," *Eur Neuropsychopharmacol,* 7(1S): 11-16, 71-73; 1997a. (Review.)

Leonard BE, "The role of noradrenaline in depression: A review," *J Psychopharmacol,* 11(4S): 39-47; 1997b.

Levitt P, Rakic P, et al, "Comparative assessment of monoamine afferents in mammalian cerebral cortex," in L Descarries, T Read, H Jasper, eds, *Monoamine innervation of Cerebral Cortex,* Alan R Liss Inc, NY, 1984.

Lindvall O, Bjorkland A, "General organization of cortical monoamine systems," in L Descarries, T Read, H Jasper, eds, *Monoamine innervation of Cerebral Cortex,* Alan R Liss Inc, NY, 1984.

Lewander T, [Neuroleptics and the neurolpeptic-induced deficit syndrome], *Acta Psychiatrica Scandinavica,* 89:8-13; 1994. (Can be similar to lobotomy.)

Maas J, Fawcett J, et al, "Catecholamine metabolism, depressive illness and drug response," *Arch Gen Psychiat,* 26:252-62; 1972.

Mann JJ, Stanley M, et al, "Increased serotonin2 and beta-adrenergic receptor binding in the frontal cortices of suicide victims," *Arch Gen Psychiat,* 43(10); 10/1986.

Mann JJ, Brown RP, et al, "Reduced sensitivity of lymphocyte beta-adrenergic receptors in patients with endogenous depression and psychomotor agitation," *NEJM,* 313:715; 9/1985.

Mann J, Peselow ED, et al, "D-phenylalanine in endogenous depression," *Am J Psychiatr,* 137(12): 12; 1980.

Matussek N, Ackenheil M, et al, "Effects of clonidine

on growth hormone release in psychiatric patients and controls," *Psychiat Res,* 2:25-36; 1980.

Meana J, Barturen F, et al, "2-adrenoceptors in the brains of suicide victims: Increased receptor density associated with major depression," *Biol Psychiat,* 31: 471-90; 1992.

Melia KR, Nestler EJ, et al, "Chronic imipramine treatment normalizes levels of tyrosine hydroxylase in the locus coeruleus of chronically stressed rats," *Psychopharmacol,* 108:23-6; 1992.

Messiha FS, Agallianos D, et al, "Dopamine excretion in affective states and following lithium carbonate therapy," *Nature,* 225:868-69; 1970.

Meyers S, "Use of neurotransmitter precursors for treatment of depression," *Alt Med Rev,* 2000.

Mongeau R, Blier P, et al, "The serotonergic and noradrenergic systems of the hippocampus: Their interactions and the effects of antidepressant treatments," *Brain Res Rev,* 23:145-95; 1997.

Moore KE, Kelly PH, "Biochemical pharmacology of mesolimbic and mesocortical dopaminergic neurons," in MA Lipton, A DiMascio, KF Killam, eds, *Psychopharmacology: A Generation of Progress,* Raven, NY, 1978; pp 221-34.

Muscat R, et al, "Antidepressant-like effects of dopamine agonists in animal model of depression," *Biol Psychiat,* 31(9):937-46; 1992.

Muscettola G, Potter W, et al, "Urinary 3-methoxy-4-hydroxyphenylglycol and major affective disorders: A replication and new findings," *Arch Gen Psychiat,* 41: 337-42; 1984. (Bipolar I depressives generally have lower NE and urinary MHPG, increased in mania.)

Muller J, Pryer W, et al, "Depression anxiety occuring during Rauwolfia therapy," *JAMA,* 159: 836-9; 1955.

Muth E, Haskins J, et al, "Antidepressant biochemical profile of the novel bicyclic compound WY-45,030, an ethyl-cyclohexanol derivative," *Biochem Pharmacol,* 35:4493-7; 1986.

Nathan K, Musselman D, "Biology of mood disorders," in A Schatzberg, C Nemeroff, eds, *Textbook of Psychopharmacology,* Am Psychiatric Press Inc, DC, 1995; pp 439-77.

Nathanson JA, Greengard P, "'Second messengers' in the brain," *Sci Am,* 237, 108-19; 1977. (Transynaptic induction of new protein involves receptor, adenylate cyclase, PK activation, phosphorylated protein translocation to the nucleus, RNA changes, synthesis of the protein, and a change in enzyme or receptor activity.)

Nestler E, McMahon A, et al, "Chronic antidepressant administration decreases the expression of tyrosine hydroxylase in the rat locus coeruleus," *Proc Natl Acad Sci,* US, 87:7522-26; 1990.

Nierenberg AA, Dougherty D, et al, "Dopaminergic agents and stimulants as antidepressant augmentation strategies," *J Clin Psychiat,* 59 (S5):60-3; 1998.

Nibuya M, Nestler E, et al, "Chronic antidepressant administration increases the expression of cAMP response element-binding protein (CREB) in rat hippocampus," *J Neurosci,* 16:2365-72; 1996.

Nutt DJ, "Noradrenaline in depression: Half a century of progress," *J Psychopharmacol,* 11(4S):3; 1997.

Ordway GA, Smith KS, et al, "Elevated tyrosine hydroxylase in the locus coeruleus of suicide victims," *J Neurochem,* 62:680-5; 1994a.

Ordway GA Widowson PS, et al, "Agonist binding to alpha2 adrenoceptors is elevated in the locus coeruleus from victims of suicide," *J Neurochem,* 63:617-24; 1994b.

Owens MJ, Morgan WN, et al, "Neurotransmitter receptor and transporter binding profile of antidepressants and their metabolites," *J Pharmacol Exp Ther,* 283:1305-22; 1997.

Owens MJ, Ieni Jr, et al, "The serotonergic antidepressant nefazadone inhibits the serotonin transporter: In vivo and ex vivo studies," *Life Sci,* 57:373-80; 1995.

Pandey GN, Dysken MW, "Beta-adrenergic receptor function in affective illness," *Am J Psychiat,* 136:675-78; 1979. (Significantly less NE-stimulated cAMP in depressives, suggesting reduced beta adrenergic receptor sensitivity.)

Park SK, Nguyen MD, et al, "Par-4 links dopamine signaling and depression," *Cell,* 122(2):275-87; 7/2005. (Par-4 interacts with the D2 receptor via calmodulin binding. Dysfunction alters cAMP and DA signalling promoting depression without anxiety.)

Perugi G, Toni C, et al, "Adjunctive dopamine agonists in treatment-resistant bipolar II depression: An open case theory. Dopamine agonists may be useful as an adjunct to meds in drug resistant bipolar II depression: An open case series," *Pharmacopsychiat,* 34(4):137-41; 7/2001.

Plaznik A, Kowtowski W, "The involvement of serotonin and noradrenaline in the psychopathological processes of stress and depression: Animal models and the effect of antidepressant drugs," *Pol J Pharmacol Pharm,* 43(4):301-22; 1991.

Pfeiffer CC, *Mental and Elemental Nutrients,* Keats, New Canaan, CN, 1975.

Pfeiffer CC, *Nutrition and Mental Illness,* Healing Arts Press, Rochester, VT, 1987.

Pfeiffer CC, *The Schizophrenias Ours to Conquer,* Bio-Communications Press, Wichita, KS, 1988.

Piletz J, Halaris A, "Involvement of I_1-imidazoline receptors in mood disorders," *Ann NY Acad Sci,* 763:510-9; 1995.

Plotsky P, Owens M, et al, "Psychoneuroendocrinology of depression," *Psychoneuroendocrinol,* 21:293-307; 1998. (LC important in coordinating CRF/NE stress response.)

Pollack A, "Coactivation of D1 and D2 dopamine receptors: In marriage, a case of his, hers and theirs," *Sci STKE,* 255:50; 10/2004. (D1 and D2 are slow G protein-coupled dopamine receptors. D1 activates adenyl cyclase, D2 uncouples or suppresses it. Activation of both does neither, and leads to PLC mediated calcium mobilization.)

Post RM, Gordon EK, et al, "Central norepinephrine metabolism in affective illness: 3 methoxy-4-hydroxyphenylethylene glycol in the cerebrospinal fluid," *Science,* 179:1002-3; 1973. (Higher MHPG in mania than depression, but not greater than normals and neurological controls.)

Post RM, Stoddard FJ, et al, "Slow and rapid alterations in motor activity, sleep, and biochemistry in a cycling manic-depressive patient," *Arch Gen Psychiat,* 34, 470-7; 1977.

Post RM, Lake CR, et al, "Cerebrospinal fluid norepinephrine in affective illness," *Am J Psychiat,* 135, 907-12; 1978. (NE increased in mania.)

Post RM, Jimerson DC, "Dopamine and mania: Behavioral and biochemical effects of the dopamine receptor blocker pimozide," *Psychopharmacol,* 67(3); 3/1980.

Post RM, "Biochemical Theories of Mania," in R Belmaker, HM van Praag, eds, *Mania: An Evolving Concept,* Spectrum, NY, 1980; pp 216-65.

Potter W, Muscettola G, et al, "Sources of variance in clinical studies in MHPG," in J Maas, ed, *MHPG: Basic Mechanisms and Psychopathology,* Academic Press, NY, 1983.

Prange A, "The pharmacology and biochemistry of depression," *Dis Nerv Syst,* 25:217-21; 1964.

Potter WZ, Grossman F, et al, "Noradrenergic function," in J Mann, DJ Kupfer eds, *Biology of Depressive Disorders, Part A, A Systems Perspective,* Plenum, NY, 1993; 1-27.

Randrup A, Munkvad I, et al, "Mania, depression, and brain dopamine," *Curr Dev Psychopharmacol,* 2:205-248; 1975.

Redmond AM, Leonard BE, "An evaluation of the noradrenergic system in the neurobiology of depression: A review," *Hum Psychopharmacol Clin Exp,* 12(5):407-30; 12/1998. (Inconsistent results with metabolites and receptor binding. Antidepressants commonly downregulate, suggesting they act on gene expression. CRF may regulate thyroid release. Glutamate and sigma receptors may also play a role.)

Ressler KJ, Nemeroff CB, "Role of norepinephrine in the pathophysiology and treatment of mood disorders," *Bio Psychiat,* 46(9):1219-33; 1999.

Richman DL, *Dr. Caligari's Psychiatric Drugs,* Network Against Psychiatric Assault, Berkeley, 1987; 1992.

Robbins T, Everitt B, "Central norepinephrine neurons and behavior," in F Bloom, D Kupfer, eds, *Psychopharmacology: The Fourth Generation of Progress,* Raven Press Ltd, NY, 363-72; 1995.

Robinson DS, Nies A, "Aging, monoamines, and monoamine oxidase levels," *Lancet,* 2:290-291; 1972. (Studies indicate MAO increases with age.)

Roos BE, Sjostrom R, "5-Hydroxyindoleacetic acid (and homovanillic acid) levels in the CSF after probenecid application in patients with manic-depressive psychosis," *Pharmacol Clin,* 1: 153-55; 1969.

Ross J, *The Mood Cure,* Viking Penguin, NY, 2002.

Roy A, et al, "Marked reduction in indexes of dopamine metabolism among patients with depression who attempt suicide", *Arch Gen Psychiat,* 49(6):447-50; 1992.

Roy A, Nielsen D, et al, "Genetics of suicide in depression, *J Clin Psychiat,* 60(2S):12-17; 1999.

Sabelli HC, et al, "Clinical studies on the phenylethylamine hypothesis of affective disorder: Urine and blood phenylacetic acid and phenylalanine dietary supplements," *J Clin Psychiat,* 47(2):66-70; 1986. (PA can be effective in bipolar depression. Side effects: anxiety, insomnia, constipation, transient nausea, headaches.)

Sabelli HC, "Phenylethylamine modulation of affect: Therapeutic and diagnostic implications," *J Neuropsychiat,* 7:6-14; 1995. (PEA modulates aminergic synapses, and can promote energy, elevate mood, foster aggression. Phenylacetic acid, its major metabolite, is decreased in depressives, increased in schizoaffectives.)

Sabelli J, Fink P, "Sustained antidepressant effect of PEA replacement," *J Neuropsychiat Clin Neurosci,* 8:168-71; 1996. (PEA increases animal attention and activity, and may revert 60% of human depressions. 12/14 responded rapidly to 10-60 mg/d (with selegiline to prevent deterioration), including some nonresponsive to meds. Response continued 20-50 wks later without side effects or tolerance.)

Sack RL, Goodwin FK, "Inhibition of dopamine beta hydroxylase in manic patients," *Arch Gen Psychiat,* 31, 649-54; 1974. (Inhibition of *DBH* (which converts DA to NE) did not improve mania, and worsened psychosis.)

Schatzberg A, Schildkraut J, "Recent studies on norepinephrine systems in mood disorders," in F Blom, D Kupfer, eds, *Psychopharmacology: The Fourth Generation of Progress,* Raven Press Ltd, NY, 1995; pp 911-20.

Schatzberg A, "Noradrenergic vs serotonergic antidepressants: Predictors of treatment response," *J Clin Psychiat,* 59(14S):15-18; 1998.

Schatzberg A, Samson J, et al, "Toward a biochemical classification of depressive disorders, Urinary catecholamines, their metabolities, and D-type scores in subgroups of depressive disorders," *Arch Gen Psychiat,* 46:260-8; 1989.

Schildkraut JJ, "The catecholamine hypothesis of affective disorders: A review of supporting evidence," *Am J Psychiat,* 122:509-22; 1965.

Schildkraut JJ, Kety SS, "Biogenic amines and emotion," *Science,* 156:21-30; 1967.

Schildkraut J, Orsulakk P, et al, "Toward a biochemical classification of depressive disorders. II. Application of multivariate discriminant function analysis to data on urinary catecholamines and metabolites," *Arch Gen Psychiat,* 35:1436-9; 1978.

Schweizer E, Feighner J, "Comparison of venlafaxine and imipramine in the acute treatment of major depression in outpatients," *J Clin Psychiat,* 55: 104-8; 1994.

Sci STKE, "Disecting dopamine's behavioral effects," 295:277; 8/2005. (Reduced D2 receptors are associated with mood disorder, schizophrenia, and addiction.)

Shinfuku N, Michio O, Masao K, [Catecholamine excretion in manic depressive psychosis], *Yonago Acta Med,* 5:109-14; 1961.

Shopsin B, Gershon S, "Pharmacology-toxicology of the lithium ion," in S Gershon, B Shopsin, eds, *Lithium: Its Role in Psychiatric Research and Treatment,* Plenum, NY, 1973.

Siever L, Trestman R, et al, "The growth hormone

response to clonidine in acute and remitted depressed male patients," *Neuropsychopharmacol,* 6:165-77; 1992.

Sjostrom RB, [Steady-state levels of probenecid and their relation to acid monamine metabolites in human cerebrospinal fluid], *Psychopharmacologia (Berlin),* 25:96-100; 1972.

Slagle P, *The Way Up from Down,* St. Martin's Paperbacks, NY, 1992.

Sloane RB, Hughes W, et al, "Catecholamine excretion in manic depressive and schizophrenic psychosis and its relationship to symptomatology," *Can Psychiatr Assoc J,* 11, 6-19; 1966. (Increased DA excretion in mania.)

Snyder, Solomon MD, *Madness and the Brain,* McGraw Hill, NY, 1974.

Spector S, Sjoerdsma A, et al, "Blockade of endogenous norepinephrine synthesis by a-methyl-tyrosine, an inhibitor of tyrosine hydroxylase," *J Pharmacol Exp Ther,* 147:86-95; 1965.

Spyraki C, Fibiger H, "Functional evidence for subsensitivity of noradrenergic alpha2 receptors after chronic desipramine treatment," *Life Sci,* 27: 186-7; 1980.

Strom-Olsen R, Weil-Malherbe H, "Humoral changes in manic depressive psychosis with particular reference to the excretion of catecholamines in urine," *J Ment Sci,* 104, 696-704; 1958.

Sulser F, Bickel M, et al, "The action of desmethylimipramine in counteracting sedation and cholinergic effects of reserpine-like drugs," *J Pharmacol Exp Ther,* 144:321-30; 1964.

Svensson TH, "Central alpha adrenoceptors and affective symptoms and disorders," in *Depressive Disorders Symposium, Rome, May 9-11, 1977,* FK Schattauer Verlag, NY; pp 248-53.

Szabo A, Billett E, et al, "Phenylethylamine, a possible link to the antidepressant effects of exercise," *Br J Sports Med,* 35:342-3; 2001. (In 20 healthy males, mean 24-hr urinary PEA excretion increased 77% 0.5 hr after treadmill exercise at 70% max heart rate.)

Valentino R, Aston-Jones G, "Physiological and anatomical determinants of locus coeruleus discharge," in F Bloom, D Kupfer, eds, *Psychopharmacology: The Fourth Generation of Progress,* Raven Press Ltd, NY, 1995; pp 373-85.

Walsh TJ, Schulz DW, et al, "Acute exposure to triethyl lead enhances the behavioral effects of dopaminergic agonists: Involvement of brain dopamine in organolead neurotoxicity," *Brain Res,* 363(2):222-29; 1/22/1986. (Rats exposed to lead 1 wk prior to testing showed increased motor stimulation/hyperactivity on exposure to D-amphetamine and apomorphine, and stereotypy in response to apomorphine.)

Wang P, Kitayama I, et al, "Tyrosine hydroxylase gene expression in the locus coeruleus of depression-model rats and rats exposed to short-term and long-term forced walking stress," *Life Sci,* 62(23):2083-2092; 1998.

Waterhouse B, Sessler F, et al, "New evidence for a gating action of norepinephrine in central neuronal circuits of mammalian brain," *Brain Res Bull,* 21: 425-32; 1988.

Whybrow, "The Emerging Neurobiology of Mood Disorder," in PC Whybrow, HP, Akiskal, WT McKinney, eds, *Mood Disorders: Toward a New Psychobiology,* Plenum, NY, 1984; pp 119-50.

Wolf ME, Mosnaim AD, "Phenylaethylamine in neuropsychiatric disorders," *Gen Pharmacol,* 14(4): 385-90; 1983.

Yehuda R, et al, "Plasma norepinephrine and 3-methoxy-4-hydroxyphenylglycol concentrations and severity of depression in combat post-traumatic stress disorder and major depressive disorder," *Biol Psychiat,* 44(1):56-63; 1998. (Depression severity related to low plasma NE and MHPG.)

Phenylalanine, Tyrosine

Axorin JM, Bovier P, et al, "L-tyrosine and L-tryptophan membrane transport in eryythrocytes and antidepressant drug choice," *Biol Psychiat,* 27: 723-4; 1990.

Banderet LE, et al, "Treatment with tyrosine, a neurotransmitter precursor, reduces environmental stress in humans," *Brain Res Bull,* 22:759-62; 1989.

Baumel S, *Dealing with Depression Naturally,* Keats, New Canaan, CN, 1995.

Beckmann H, Strauss MA, "DL-phenylalanine in depressed patients: An open study," *J Neural Trans,* 41:123-34; 1977.

Beckmann H, Ludolph E, [DL-phenylalanine as an antidepressant: Open study], *Arzneimittelforschung,* 28:1283-84; 1978.

Beckmann H, et al, [DL-phenylalanine versus imipramine: A double-blind controlled study], *Archiv fur Psychiatrie und Nervenkrankheiten,* 227(1):49-58; 3/1979. (Double blind. 40 depressives received 150-200 mg DLPA/day or imipramine for 1 mo. Improvement (HamD and a questionaire) with DLPA was statistically equivalent to the drug. Imipramine took longer to achieve optimal benefit.)

Beckman H, Goodwin FK, "Urinary MHPG in subgroups of depressed patients and normal controls," *Neuropsychopharmacol,* 6:91-100; 1980. (Low MHPG excreters responded better to antidepressants.)

Beckman H, "DL-phenylalanine in affective disorders," *Adv Biol Psychiat,* 10:137-47; 1983a. (DLPA equal or better than low dose imipramine.)

Beckmann H, Schmauss M, "Clinical investigations into antidepressive mechanisms. I. Antihistaminic and cholinolytic effects: amitriptyline versus promethazine," *Arch Psychiatr Nervenkr,* 223(1): 59-70; 1983b.

Benkert O, et al, "Blood-brain movements of tryptophan and tyrosine in manic-depressive illness and schizophrenia," *J Neural Transm,* 15S: 189-96; 1979.

Bessman SP, "The justification theory: The essential nature of non-essential amino acids," *Nutr Rev;* 37: 209-20; 1979.

Birkmayer W, et al, "L-deprenyl plus L-phenylalanine in the treatment of depression," *J Neural Transmission,* 59:81-87; 1/1984. (69% of 155 unresponsive depressives recovered with low dose LPA, another 15% improved.)

Braverman E, Pfeiffer CC, *The Healing Nutrients Within,* Keats, New Canaan, CN 1987.

Broida M, *New Hope for People with Depression,* Prima Publishing, Roseville CA, NY, 2001.

Budd K, "Use of D-phenylalanine, an enkephalinase inhibitor, in the treatment of intractable pain," *Adv Pain Res Ther,* 5:305-8; 1983.

Bukreev VI, [Effect of pyridoxine on the psychopathology and pathochemistry of involutional depressions], *Zh Nevropatol Psikhiatr,* 78(3):402-08; 1978. (B6 is a cofactor of *dopadecarboxylase,* a critical enzyme in forming catecholamines. B6 improved symptoms and increased NE excretion, and relatively decreased E excretion in 31 involutional melancholics and 17 late onset bipolars.)

Buist R, "The therapeutic predictability of tryptophan and tyrosine in the treatment of depression," *Intl J Clin Nutr Rev,* 3:1-3; 1983.

Cousens G, *Depression Free for Life,* Quill, HarperCollins, NY, 2000.

Da Diehl DJ, Gershon S, "The role of dopamine in mood disorders," *Compr Psychiat,* 33(2):115-20; 1992.

Darby P, "Causes and natural treatments for bipolar disorder." At: www.alternativementalhealth.com/articles/bipolartreatment.htm, 2/12/2006 (Claims PA (up to 4000 mg/day) alleviates approximately 75% of bipolar depressions, but can trigger mania.)

Fischer E, Heller B, et al, [Therapy of depression by phenylalanine. Preliminary note], *Arneimittelforschung,* 25(1):143; 1975. (17/23 depressives, unreponsive to MAOIs or imipramine type drugs, recovered on 50-100 mg PA over 15 days, without important side effects.)

Fox A, Fox B, *DLPA to end chronic pain and depression,* Pocket Books, NY 1985. (Even in severe cases.)

Gelenberg AJ, Wojcik JD, et al, "Tyrosine for the treatment of depression," *Am J Psychiat,* 137: 622-23; 1980.

Gelenberg AJ, et al, "Tyrosine for Depression," *J Psychiatric Res,* 17(2):175-80; 1982. (Double blind followup. 4/6 treated with tyrosine recovered in 4 wks compared to 3/8 on placebo. 3/5 unimproved placebo patients responded to followup tyrosine.)

Gelenberg AJ, Wojcik JD, et al, "Tyrosine for depression: A double-blind trial," *J Affect Disord,* 19:125-32; 1990. (In 65 depressives, over 4 wks, the difference in effectiveness between tyrosine and imipramine was only 5%, while tyrosine produced less clinical deterioration or other side effects.)

Giannini AJ, Sternberg DE, et al, "Prevention of late luteal phase dysphoric disorder symptoms with DL-phenylalanine in women with abrupt beta-endorphin decline: A pilot study," *Ann Clin Psychiat,* 1:259-63; 1989.

Gibson CJ, Gelenberg A, "Tyrosine for the treatment of depression," *Biol Psychiat,* 10:148-59; 1983. (Double blind.)

Gold MS, *The Good News About Depression,* Villard Books, NY, 1987.

Goldberg IK, "L-tyrosine in depression," *Lancet,* 2: 364-5; 1980.

Growdon JH, "Neurotransmitter precursors in the diet: Their use in the treatment of brain diseases," *in* RJ Wurtman, JJ Wurtman, eds, *Nutrition and the Brain,* V3:117-81, Raven, NY, 1979.

Hale AS, Sandler M, et al, "Tyramine conjugation test distinguishes unipolar from bipolar depressed patients and controls," *J Psychiatr Res,* 25(4):185-90; 1991. (24 unipolars showed significantly impaired tyramine sulphate conjugation as compared to 24 bipolars.)

Halpern LM, Dong WK, "D-phenylalanine: A putative enkephalinase inhibitor studied in a primate acute pain model," *Pain,* 24(2):223-37; 1986.

Hashimoto H, et al, [Metabolism of D-phenylalanine and its effects on concentrations of brain monoamines and amino acids in rats — a basic study of possibility of clinical use of D-phenylalanine as an antidepressant], *Folia Psychiatr Neurl Jpn,* 37(2): 137-44; 1983.

Hendler LC, Hendler S, *The Oxygen Breakthrough,* William Morrow, NY, 1989.

Holford, P, "Depression: The nutrition connection," *Primary Care Mental Health,* 1(1):9-16; 3/2003.

Kravitz HM, et al, "Dietary supplements of phenylalanine and other amino acid precursors of brain neuroamines in the treatment of depressive disorders," *J Am Osteopathic Org,* 84S:119-23; 9/1984. (11 refractory depressives recovered and 20 improved with large doses of LPA.)

Larson JM, *Depression Free, Naturally,* Ballantine Wellspring, NY, 2001.

Maes M, Claes M, et al, "Disturbances in dexamethasone suppression test and lower availability of L-tryptophan and tyrosine in early puerperium in women under contraceptive therapy," *J Psychosom Res,* 36(2):191-7; 2/1992.

Mandell AJ, Knapp S, "Adaptive regulation in central biogenic amine neurons," MA Lipton, A DiMascio, KF Killam, eds, *Psychopharmacology: A Generation of Progress,* Raven, NY, 1978; pp 205-16.

Mann J, Peselow E, et al, "D-phenylalanine in endogenous depression," *Am J Psychiat,* 137: 1611-12; 1980. (Negative trial.)

Meyers S, "Use of neurotransmitter precursors for treatment of depression," *Altern Med Rev,* 5:64-71; 2000. (Catecholamine precursors may be needed if DA, NE or endorphin activity is reduced.)

Pfeiffer CC, *Mental and Elemental Nutrients,* Keats, New Canaan, CN, 1975.

Pfeiffer CC, *Nutrition and Mental Illness,* Healing Arts Press, Rochester, VT, 1987.

Pfeiffer CC, *The Schizophrenias Ours to Conquer,* rev ed, Bio-Communications Press, Wichita, KS, 1988.

Puchacz E, Stumpf WE, et al, "Vitamin D increases expression of the tyrosine hydroxylase gene in adrenal medullary cells," *Brain Res Mol brain Res,* 36(1):193-6; 2/1996. (Rapidly creates 3-fold increase in expression of tyrosine hydroxylase, the rate-limiting enzyme in creating catecholamines.)

Reeves PG, O'Dell BL, "The effect of dietary tyrosine levels on food intake in zinc-deficient rats," *J Nutr,* 114(4):761-7; 4/1984.

Reinstein DK, Lehnert H, et al, "Dietary tyrosine suppresses plasma corticosterone following acute stress in rats," *Life Sci,* 37(23):2157-63; 1985. (Low tyrosine may then lead to depression.)

Rogers S, *Depression, Cured at Last,* SK Publishing, Sarasota FL, 1997.

Ross J, *The Mood Cure,* Viking Penguin, NY, 2002.

Sabelli HC, et al, "Antidepressant effects of L-phenylalanine," *Paper presented at Second World Conference of Clinical Pharmacology and Therapeutics,* DC, 8/1983.

Sabelli HC, "Clinical studies on the phenylethylamine hypothesis of affective disorder: Urine and blood phenylacetic acid and phenylalanine dietary supplements," *J Clin Psychiat,* 47(2):66-70; 1986. (31/40 depressives responded to up to 14 gm/day.)

Sabelli H, "Rapid treatment of depression with selegiline-phenylalanine combination," letter, *J Clin Psychiat,* 52:137; 3/1991.

Salter CA, "Dietary tyrosine as an aid to stress resistance among troops," *Military Med,* 154:144-46; 3/1989.

Serretti A, et al, "Tyrosine hydroxylase gene associated with depressive symptomatology in mood disorder," *Am J Med Genet,* 81(2):127-30; 1998.

Simonson M, "L-phenylalanine," letter, *J Clin Psychiat,* 46:355, 8/1985. (50% of depressed bipolars recovered rapidly with low dose LPA.)

Slagle P, "Low moods/ Light therapy/ L-tyrosine," *The Way Up Newletter Archives,* #3 At: thewayup.com/newletters/newsarch.htm

Spatz H, et al, "Effects of D-phenylalanine on clinical picture and phenylethylaminuria in depression," *Biol Psychiat,* 10:235; 1975.

Steiner W, Fontaine R, "Toxic reaction following the combined administration of fluoxetine and L-tryptophan: five case reports," *Biol Psychiat,* 21: 1067-1071; 1986.

Takahashi R, Utena H, et al, "Tyrosine metabolism in manic depressive illness," *Life Sci,* 7(22):1219-31; 11/15/1968.

van Praag HM, "In search of the mode of action of antidepressants: 5-HTP/tyrosine mixtures in depression," *Adv Biochem Psychopharmacol,* 39: 301-14; 1984.

van Praag HM, Lemus C, "Monoamine precursors in the treatment of psychiatric disorder," in RJ Wurtman, JJ Wurtman, eds, *Nutrition and the Brain,* 7:89-138; Raven, NY, 1986.

Wojcik JD, Gibson DJ, Wurtman RJ, "Tyrosine for depression," *J Psychiat Res,* 17(2):175-80; 1983.

Wurtman RJ, et al, Brain catechole synthesis: Control by brain tyrosine concentration, *Sci,* 185: 183-84; 1974.

Wurtman RJ, "Effects of dietary amino acids, carbohydrates, and choline on neurotransmitter synthesis," *Mt Sinai Med,* 55:75-76; 1/1988.

Yaryura-Tobias JA, et al, "Phenylalanine for endogeous depression," *J Orthomol Psychiat,* 3(2): 80-81; 1974. (The majority recover within 2 wks, most within 2 mo.)

Yaryura-Tobias JA, Neziroglu F, "Phenylethylamine and glucose in true depression," *J Orthomol Psychiat,* 5(3):199-202; 1976.

Young SN, "Behavioral effects of dietary neurotransmitter precursors: Basic and clinical aspects," *Neurosci Biobehav Rev,* 20:313-23; 1996.

Energetics: Carnitine, Creatinine, etc.

Agnelucci L, et al, "Nerve growth factor bind in aged rat CNS: Effect of acetyl-L-carnitine, *J Neurosci Res,* 20:491; 1988.

Amenta F, et al, "Reduced lipofuscin accumulation in senescent rat brain by long-term acetyl-L-carnitine treatment," *Arch Gerontol Geriatr,* 9(2): 147-53; 1989.

Aureli T, et al, "Aging brain: Effect of acetyl-L-carnitine treatment on rat brain energy and phospholipid metabolism. A study by 31P and 1H NMR spectroscopy," *Brain Res,* 526(1):108-12; 1990.

Bella R, Biondi R, et al, "Effect of acetyl-L-carnitine on geriatric patients suffering from dysthymic disorders," *Intl J Clin Pharmacol Res,* 10(6):355-60; 1990.

Bodis-Wollner I, "Physiological effects of acetyl-levo-carnitine in the central nervous system," *Intl J Clin Pharm Res,* X(1/2):109-14; 1990.

Brooks JO et al, "Acetyl-L-carnitine shows decline in younger patients with Alzheimer's disease," *Intl J Clin Pharmacol Res,* 10:101; 1990.

Calvani M, et al, "Action of acetyl-L-carnitine in neurodegeneration and Alzheimer's disease," *Ann NY Acad Sci,* 663:483-86; 1992.

Calvallini G, Caracciolo S, et al, "Carnitine versus androgen administration in the treatment of sexual dysfunction, depressed mood and fatigue associated with male aging," *Urology,* 641-6; 2004. (20 patients on testosterone; 45, carnitine. Depression, fatigue, and ED significantly improved in both vs placebo.)

Cook EH Jr, Lindgren V, et al,"Relative carnitine deficiency in autism," *J Autism Dev Disord,* 34: 615-23; 2004.

Crayhon, R, *The Carnitine Miracle,* M Evans, 1998.

Corredor C, Mansbach C, et al, "Carnitine depletion in the choline-deficient state," *Biochim Biophys Acta,* 144(2):366-74; 1967.

Dager SR, "Brain metabolic alterations in medication-free bipolar patients," *Arch Gen Psychiatr,* 61:450-8; 5/2004. (Mitochondria showed reduced expression, increased oxidative stress, and a shift from oxidative phosphorylation to glycolysis.)

Di Giulo AM, Gorio A, et al, "Acetyl-L-carnitine prevents substance P loss in the sciatic nerve and lumbar spinal cord of diabetic animals," *Int J Clin Pharmacol Res,* 12:5-6:243-46; 1992.

Drevets WC, Bogers W, et al, "Functional anatomical correlates of antidepressant drug treatment assessed using PET measures of regional glucose metabolism," *Eur Neuropsychopharmacol,* 12(6): 527-44; 12/2002.

Furlong, JH, "Acetyl-L carnitine: metabolism and applications in clinical practice," *Alt Med Rev,* 1(2):85-93; 1996.

Gadaleta MN, et al, "Reduced transcription of mitochondrial DNA in the senescent rat. Tissue dependence and effect of L-carnitine," *Eur J Biochem,* 187(3):501-6; 1990.

Garzya G, Corallo D, et al, "Evaluation of the effects of L-acetylcarnitine on senile patients suffering from depression," *Drugs Exp Clin Res,* 16(2):101-6; 1990.

Gecele M, Francesetti G, et al, "Acetyl-L-carnitine in aged subjects with major depression: Clinical efficacy and effects in the circadian rhythm of cortisol," *Dementia,* 2:333-37; 1994.

Hirata F, Azelrod J, "Phospholipid methylation and biological signal transmission," *Science,* 209: 1082-90; 1980.

Kato T, Takahashi S, et al, "Brain phosphorus metabolism in depressive disorders detected by phosphorus-31 magnetic resonance spectroscopy," *J Affect Disord,* 16(4):223-30; 1992.

Kato T, Kato N, "Mitochondrial dysfunction in bipolar disorder," *Bipolar Disord,* 2:180-90; 2000. (First proposed mitochondrial dysregulation altering energy metabolism and calcium uptake could underly bipolar. Phosphocreatine, which acts as a cellular energy reservoir for ATP, is decreased.)

Kidd PM, "Bipolar disorder as cell membrane dysfunction. Progress toward integrative management," *Alt Med Rev,* 9(2):107-35; 2004.

Kohjimoto Y, et al, "Effects of acetyl-L-carnitine on the brain lipofuscin content and emotional behavior in aged rats," *Jpn J Pharmacol,* 48(3):365-71; 1988

Konradi C, et al, "Molecular evidence for mitochondrial dysfunction in bipolar disorder," *Arch Gen Psychiatr,* 61:300-8; 2004. (Marked reduction in mitochondrial energy metabolism and gene expression in postmortem bipolar brains.)

McGinnis W, "Pyroluria: Hidden cause of schizophrenia, bipolar, depression, and anxiety symptoms," Orlando, 5/21/2004. At: alternativementalhealth.com/articles/pyroluria.htm

Modica-Napolitano JS, Renshaw PF, "Ethaloamine and phosphoethanolamine inhibit mitochondrial function in vitro: Implications for mitochondrial dysfunction hypothesis in depression and bipolar disorder," *Biol Psychiat,* 55:273-7; 2004. (Lactate and glutamate/glutamine increased. pH reduced.)

Mayberg HS, "Frontal lobe dysfunction in secondary depression," *J Neuropsychiat Clin Neurosci,* 6:428-42; 1994.

Patacchioli FR, Amenta F, et al, "Acetyl-L carnitine reduces the age-dependent loss of glucocorticoid receptors in the rat hippocampus: An autoradiographic study," *J Neurosci Res,* 23:462-66; 1989.

Persky AM, Brazeau GA, "Clinical pharmacology of the dietary supplement creatine monohydrate," *Pharm Rev,* 53:161-76; 2001.

Pettegrew JW, Levine J, et al, "31P-MRS study of acetyl-L-carnitine treatment in geriatric depression: Preliminary results," *Bipolar Disord,* 4(1):61-6; 2/2002. (Increased prefrontal phosphomonoesters, correlating with improved HAM-D.)

Pettegrew JW, Levine J, et al, "Acetyl-L-carnitine physical-chemical, metabolic and therapeutic properties: Relevance for its mode of action in Alzheimer's disease and geriatric depression," *Mol Psychiat,* 5(6):616-32; 11/2000.

Prabakaran S, et al, "Mitochondrial dysfunction in schizophrenia: Evidence for compromised brain metabolism and oxidative stress," *Mol Psychiatr,* in press, 4/2004.

Quiroz JA, Singh J, Manji, et al, "Emerging experimental therapeutics for bipolar disorder: Clues from the molecular pathophysiology," *Molec Psychiat,* 8(8):756-76; 8/2004. (Impaired cell plasticity and resilience in key neuronal circuits.)

Rampello L, et al, [Trophic action of acetyl-L-carnitine in neuronal cultures], *Acta Neurol (Napoli),* 14(1):15-21; 1992. (Increases levels of, and enhances hippocampal, etc., response to NGF (which preserves neurons, especially Ach neurons, but declines with age.)

Rogers S, *Depression, Cured at Last,* SK Publishing, Sarasota FL, 1997.

Salvioli G, et al, "L-acetyl carnitine treatment of mental decline in the elderly," *Drugs Exptl Clin Res,* 20(4):169-76; 1994.

Shapira B, Levine J, "A double-blind, parallel, randomized, add-on clinical trial of creatine versus placebo added to antidepressant treatment of patients with major depressive episode," 2007.

Schweitzer AN, "Pegging pathology on mitochondrial dysfunction. Studies strengthen suspicions about brain disorder pathophysiology," *Scientist,* 18(10):28; 5/2004.

Silveri MM, Parow AM, et al, "S-adenosyl-L-methionine: Effects on brain bioenergetic status and transverse relaxation time in health subjects," *Biol Psychiat,* 54(8):833-9; 2003.

Stork C, Renshaw PF, "Mitochondrial dysfunction in bipolar disorder: Evidence from magnetic resonance spectroscopy research," *Mol Psychiat,* 10:900-19; 2005. (Impaired oxidative phosphorylation, shift to glycolysis for energy, decreased energy or substrate availability, altered phospholipid metabolism.)

Temesta E, et al, "L-acetylcarnitine in depressed elderly subjects, A cross-over study vs placebo," *Drugs Exp Clin Res,* 13:417-23; 1987.

Tommaso A, Micheli A, et al, "Aging brain: Effect of acetyl-L-carnitine treatment on rat brain energy and phospholipid metabolism, A study by 31H NMR," *Brain Res,* 526; 106-12; 1990.

Walsh, WJ, PhD, "Commentary on nutritional treatment of mental disorders, *International Guide to the World of Alternative Mental Health.* At: www.alternativementalhealth.com/articles.walshMP.htm#Py Accessed:10/08/2006.

White HL, Scates PW, "Acetyl-L-carnitine as a precursor of acetylcholine," *Neurochem Res,* 15: 6, 597-601; 1990.

Wyss M, Kaddurah-Daouk R, "Creatine and creatinine metabolism," *Physiol Rev,* 80:1107-213; 2000.

NAD

Birkmayer W, Birkmayer JG, "Nicotinamide adenine dinucleotide (NADH): The new approach in the therapy of Parkinsons disease," *Ann Clin Lab Sci,* 19(1):38-43; 1989a.

Birkmayer JG, Birkmayer W, [Stimulation of endogenous L-dopa biosynthesis — a new principle for the therapy of Parkinson's disease: The clinical effect of nicotinamide adenine dinucleotide (NADH) and nicotinamide adenine dinucleotidephosphate (NADPH)] *Acta Neurol Scand,* 126S:183-87; 1989b.

Birkmayer W, et al, "The coenzyme nicotinamide adenine dinucleotide (NADH) improves the disability of Parkinsonian patients," *J Neural Transm Park Dis Dement Sect,* 1(4):297-302; 1989c.

Birkmayer W, Birkmayer JG, "Coenzyme nicotinamide adenine dinucleotide (NADH) as a biological antidepressive agent. Experience with 205 patients," *New Trends Clin Neuropharmacol,* 5:19-25; 1991. (Open label trial. Clinical improvement in 93% of 205 depressives, treated orally, IM or IV, over 5-310 days.)

Birkmayer JG, et al, [Nicotinamide adenine dinucleotide (NADH): A new therapeutic approach to Parkinson's disease: Comparison of oral and parenteral application], *Acta Neurol Scand,* 87(S146):32-35; 1993.

Birkmayer JG, "Coenzyme nicotinamide adenine dinucleotide: New therapeutic approach for improving dementia of the Alzheimer's type," *Ann Clin Lab Sci,* 26(1):1-9; 1996a.

Birkmayer JG, Vank P, "Reduced coenzyme 1 (NADH) improves psychomotoric and physical performance in athletes," *White Paper Report,* NY, Menuco Corp; 1996b.

Cleary JP, "The NAD deficiency diseases," *J Orthomol Med,* 1(3):149-57; 1986.

Cousen G, *Depression Free for Life,* Quill, HarperCollins, NY, 2000.

Hoffer A, MD, PhD, "Mechanism of action of nicotinic acid and nicotinamide in the treatment of schizophrenia," in D Hawkins, L Pauling, eds, *Orthomolecular Psychiatry,* WH Freeman and Co, San Francisco, 1973.

Hoffer A, "Nutrition and behavior," in J Bland, ed, *Medical Applications of Clinical Nutrition,* Keats, New Canaan, CN, 1983.

Hoffer A, "Another anecdote of schizophrenia, Psychological activity of nicotinamide adenine dinucleotide (NAD)," *J Orthomol Med,* 10:68-9; 1995.

Hoffer A, *Adventures in Psychiatry, The Scientific Memoirs of Dr Abram Hoffer,* KOS Pub, Caledon, ON, Canada, 2005.

Kuhn W, "Parenteral application of NADH in Parkinson's disease: Clinical improvement partially due to stimulation of endogenous levodopa biosynthesis," *J Neural Transm,* 103(1):1187-93; 1996.

Vrecko K, et al, [NADH stimulates endogenous dopamine biosynthesis by enhancing the recycling of tetrahydrobiopterin in rat phaeochromocytoma cells], *Biochim, Biophys Acta,* 361(1):59-65; 1997.

Co Q-10

Balch JF, Balch P, *Prescription for Natural Healing,* Avery, Garden City Park, NY, 1990.

Beyer R, "The role of ascorbate in antioxidant protection of biomembranes: Interaction with vitamin E and coenzyme Q," *J Bioenerget,* 26(4):349-58; 1994.

Eikasbef AM, et al, "The effect of coenzyme Q10 on the cognitive functions in patients with schizophrenia," Institute for Biomedical Research, University of Texas at Austin, 1994.

Garrison RH, Somer E, *The Nutrition Desk Reference,* Keats, New Canaan, CN, 1985.

Kagen V, Serbinova E, "Antioxidant effects of unbiquinones in microsomes and mitochondria are mediated by tocopherol recycling," *Biochem Biophys Res Commun,* 169:851-57; 1990.

Krohn J, *The Whole Way to Allergy Relief & Prevention,* Hartley & Marks, Point Roberts, WA, 1991.

Lieberman S, Bruning N, *The Real Vitamin & Mineral Book,* Avery, Garden City Park, NY, 1990.

Inhibitors

Balch JF, Balch P, *Prescription for Natural Healing,* Avery, Garden City Park, NY, 1990.

Bartholini G, "GABA receptor agonists: Pharmacological spectrum and therapeutic agents," *Med Res Rev,* 5(1):55-75; 1-3/1985.

Baumel S, *Dealing with Depression Naturally,* Keats, New Canaan, CN, 1995

Baloyannis SJ, Karakatsamis K, et al, [Effects of GABA, glycine, and sodium barbiturate on dendritic growth in vitro], *Acta Neuropathol,* 59(3):171-82; 1983. (GABA or glycine-enriched medium enhanced in vitro dendritic growth and arborization cf sodium barbiturate.)

Birdsall TC, " Therapeutic applications of taurine," *Alt Med Rev,* 3(2):128-36; 1998.

Braverman E, Pfeiffer CC, *The Healing Nutrients Within,* Keats, New Canaan, CN, 1987.

Cousens G, *Depression Free for Life,* Quill, HarperCollins, NY, 2000.

Haas EM, *Staying healthy with nutrition: The complete guide to diet and nutritional medicine,* Celestial Arts, 2006.

Hendler S, *The Oxygen Breakthrough,* NY, William Morrough, 1989. (Threonine can be low in depression.)

Heresco-Levy U, Javitt DC, et al, "Double-blind, placebo-controlled, crossover trial of glycine adjuvant therapy for treatment-resistant schizophrenia," *Br J Psychiat,* 169:610-17; 1996. (Glycine (especially if baseline is low) may improve negative and cognitive symptoms and depression.)

Kendell SF, Krystal JH, et al, "GABA and glutamate systems as therapeutic targets in depression and mood disorders," *Expert Opinon on Therapeutic Targets,* 9(1):153-68; 2/2005.

Krystal JH, Sanacora G, et al, "Glutamate and GABA systems as targets for novel antidepressant and mood-stabilizing treatments," *Mol Psychiat,* 7S(1):71-80; 2002. (Mood stabilizers and antidepressants may target GABA and glutamate. Clinical data suggest suppressing NMDA/glutamate receptor activity can be antidepressant. Anti-glutamatergic drugs may be antimanic. MRS suggests unipolar, but not bipolar, depression is associated with low cortical GABA. Stabilization raises and repletes GABA.)

Larson JM, *Depression Free, Naturally,* Ballantine Wellspring, NY, 2001

Lloyd KG, et al, "The GABAergic hypothesis of depression," *Prog Neuropsychopharmacol Biol Psychiat,* 133(3-4):341-51; 1989.

Machado-Viera R, Viale CJ et al, "Mania associated with an energy drink: The possible role of caffeine, taurine and inositol," *Can J Psychiat,* 46(5):454-5; 2001.

Maes M, Verkerk R, et al, [Serum levels of excitatory amino acids, serine, glycine, histidine, threonine, taurine, alanine, and arginine in treatment-resistant depression: Modulation by treatment with antidepressants and prediction of clinical responsivity], *Acta Psychiatr Scand,* 97(4):302-8; 4/1998. (5 wks treatment reduced aspartate, glutamate and taurine; increased glutamine. Nonresponders had significantly lower serum aspartate, asparagine, serine, threonine, taurine. Antidepressants may modulate excitatory aminos and taurine.)

Petty F, Kramer GL, Hendricks W, "GABA and Depression," in J Mann, DJ Kupfer, eds, *Biology of Depressive Disorders PART A, A Systems Perspective,* Plenum Press, NY, 1993a.

Petty F, Kramer GL, et al, "Low plasma GABA is a trait-like marker for bipolar illness," *Neuropsychopharmacol,* 9(2):125-32; 9/1993b. (Low in 30-40% of bipolars.)

Petty F, "GABA and mood disorders: A brief review and hypothesis," *J Affect Disord,* 34(4): 9/18/1995. (Depressed animals show regional Baseline GABA deficits where GABA agonists are antidepressant. Upregulation of GABA-B receptors benefits mood. Clinical data shows reduced plasma GABA and supressed GABA activity during episodes. Agonists benefit mood, without normalizing GABA levels.)

Petty F, Kramer GL, Davis LL, "Gamma-Aminobutyric Acid," in Paul Goodnick, ed., *Mania: Clinical and Research Perspectives,* Am Psychiatric Press, DC, 1998; pp 164-66.

Pfeiffer CC, *Mental and Elemental Nutrients,* Keats, New Canaan, CN, 1975.

Pfeiffer CC, *Nutrition and Mental Illness,* Healing Arts Press, Rochester, VT, 1987.

Pfeiffer CC, *The Schizophrenias Ours to Conquer,* Bio-Communications Press, Wichita, KS, 1988.

Ring HA, Crellin R, et al, "Vigabatrin and depression," *J Neurol,* 56 925-8; 1993.

Sahley BJ, *Healing with Amino Acids,* Pain & Stress Ctr Pub, TX, 1995.

Seidl R, Peyrl A, "A taurine and caffeine-containing drink stimulates cognitive performance and well being," *Amino acids,* 19(3-4):635-42; 2000. (Contains caffeine, taurine and glucaronolactone. Improves mental performance and mood. May act via caffeine's effects on adenosine receptors and taurine's receptor modulation.)

Slagle P, *The Way Up from Down,* St. Martin's Paperbacks, NY, 1992.

Smythies JR, "The role of one-carbon cycle in neuropsychiatric disease," *Biol Psychiat,* 19(5):755-58; 5/1984. (In some schizophrenics and depressives, the Vmax of MAT is decreased; in some manics, increased. MAT produces SAM, an important methylator, and potent antidepressant.)

Sturman JA, Cohen PA, "Cystine metabolism in vitamin B6 deficiency: Evidence of multiple taurine pools," *Biochem Med,* 5(3):245-68; 1971.

Sturman JA, Cohen PA, "Taurine in nutrition," *Comp Thera,* III:59-65; 1977.

Suzdak PD Gianutsos G, "Effect of chronic imipramine or baclofen on GABA B binding and cyclic AMP production in cerebral cortex," *Eur J Pharmacol,* 131(1)129-33; 11/12/1986.

Tomaszewski A, Kleinrok A, et al, "The influence of strychnine and glycine on the metabolism of acetylcholine in the rat striatum and hippocampus," *Pol J Pharmacol Pharma,* 35(4):27; 1983.

Warburton DM, Bersellini E, "An evaluation of a caffeinated taurine drink on mood, memory and information processing in healthy volunteers without caffeine abstinence," *Psychopharmacol,* 158(3):322-28; 2001. (Improved info processing, attention, and verbal reasoning.)

Vitamin D

Bettica P, Bevilacqua M, et al, "High prevalence of hypovitaminosis D among free-living postmenopausal women referred to an osteoporosis outpatient clinic in northern Italy for initial screening," *Osteoporos Int,* 9:226-9; 1999.

Cannell JJ, Vieth R, "Epidemic influenza and vitamin D," *Epid Infect,* 134(6):1129-40; 2006.

Cannell JJ, "Vitamin D and Your Health." At: vitamindcouncil.com/depression.shtml (Increases brain Ser. Receptors for D in the nucleus of neurons and glial cells. Brain cells contain genes which encode enzymes that metabolize D. It may support brain detox, in that it helps make neurotrophic factors, increases GSH, and inhibits formation of nitric oxide synthase. Antioxidant. SAD studies do not provide enough sun, light, or D3 to move levels to at least 35ng/mL. 400 IU is inadequate. Ergocalciferol (D2) is significantly less potent than cholecalciferol (D3).)

Cantorna MT, "Vitamin D and autoimmunity: Is vitamin D status an environmental factor affecting autoimmune disease prevalence?" *Proc Soc Exp Biol Med,* 223:230-3; 2000.

Cousens G, *Depression Free for Life,* Quill, HarperCollins, NY, 2000.

Dawson-Hughes B, Heaney R, et al, "Vitamin D round table," *Nutritonal Aspects of Osteoporosis,* B Dawson-Hughes, R Heaney, P Burckhardt, eds, Academic Press, NY, 2004. (1000 IU per day.)

Eyles D, Brown J, et al, "Vitamin D3 and brain development," *Neurosci,* 118:641-53; 2003.

Garcion E, Wion-Barbot N, "New clues about vitamin D functions in the nervous system," *Trends Endocrinol Metab,* 13(3):100-5; 4/2002 (May help brain detox: Inhibits formation of nitric oxide synthase; increases GSH.)

Garland CF, et al, "Calcium and vitamin D. Their potential roles in colon and breast cancer prevention," *Ann NY Acad Sci,* 889:107-19; 1999.

Garland CF, Gorham ED, et al, "Vitamin D and prevention of breast cancer: pooled analysis," *J Steroid Biochem Mol Biol,* 103(3-5):708-11; 2007.

Garrison RH, Somer E, *The Nutrition Desk*

Reference, Keats, New Canaan, CN, 1985.

Glerup H, Mikkelsen K, et al, "Commonly recommended daily intake of vitamin D is not sufficient if sunlight exposure is limited," *J Intern Med,* 247:260-8; 2000.

Gloth FM III, Alam W, Hollis B, "Vitamin D vs broad spectrum phototherapy in the treatment of seasonal affective disorder," *Nutr Health Aging,* 3(1):5-7; 1999. (Supplement doubled D as compared to light. Only D patients improved on all 3 depression scales)

Kenny AM, Biskup B, et al, "Effect of vitamin D supplementation on strength, physical function, and health perception in older, community-dwelling men," *J Am Geriatr Soc,* 51(12):1762-7; 12/2003. (25(OH)D correlated directly with mental health scores in highly functional older adults.)

Kozielec T, Starobrat-Hermelin B, et al, [Deficiency of certain trace elements in children with hyperactivity], *Psychiatr Pol,* 28:345-53; 1994.

Krohn J, *The Whole Way to Allergy Relief & Prevention,* Hartley & Marks, Point Roberts, WA, 1991.

Kleibeuker JH, et al, "Calcium and vitamin D: Possible protective agents against colorectal cancer? *Eur J Cancer,* 31A:1081-4; 1995.

Lambert GW, Reid C, "Effect of sunlight and season on serotonin turnover in the brain," *Lancet,* 360(9348):1840-2; 12/2002. (Summer sun doubles winter increase in serotonin).

Landsdowne AT, Provost SC, "Vitamin D3 enhances mood in healthy subjects during winter," *Psychopharmacol, Berl,* 135(4):319-23; 2. 1998.(5 day trial, 44 subjects. 400 or 800 IU or placebo.)

Lappe JM, Travers-Gustafson D, "Vitamin D and calcium supplementation reduces cancer risk: Results of a randomized trial," *Am J Clin Nutr,* 85(6):1586-91; 2007.

Lieberman S, Bruning N, *The Real Vitamin & Mineral Book,* Avery, Garden City Park, NY, 1990.

Mariani E, Ravaglia G, et al, "Vitamin D, thyroid hormones and muscle mass influence natural killer (NK) innate immunity in healthy nonagenarians and centenarians," *Clin Exp Immunol,* 117(1):206; 1999.

Michelson C, Stratakis L, et al, "Bone mineral density in women with depression," *NEJM,* 335: 1176-1181; 1996.

Miller GJ, "Vitamin D and prostate cancer: Biologic interactions and clinical potential," *Cancer Metastasis Rev,* 17:353-60; 1998

Pfeiffer CC, *Nutrition and Mental Illness,* Healing Arts Press, Rochester, VT, 1987.

Puchacz E, Stumpf WE, et al, "Vitamin D increases expression of the tyrosine hydroxylase gene in adrenal medullary cells," *Brain Res Mol Brain Res,* 36(1):193-6; 2/1996. (Rapidly creates 3x increase in genetic expression of tyrosine hydroxylase.)

Quillin P, *Healing Nutrients,* Contemporary Books, Chicago, 1987.

Sardar S, Chakraborty A, et al, "Comparative effectiveness of vitamin D3 and dietary vitamin E peroxidation of lipids and enzymes of the hepatic antioxidant system in Sprague-Dawley rats," *Int J Vitam Nutr Res,* 66:39-45; 1996.

Saul AW, "Vitamin D: Deficiency, diversity and dosage," *J Orthomol Med,* 18(3-4):194-204; 2003. (No deaths from D.)

Schneider B, Weber B, Frensch A, et al, "Vitamin D in schizophrenia, major depression, and alcoholism," *J Neural Transm,* 107(7):839-42; 2000. (Depressed averaged 37 ng/mL; healthy, 46.)

Starobrat-Hermelin B [The effect of deficiency of selected bioelements on hyperactivity in children with certain specified mental disorders], *Ann Acad Med Stetin,* 44:297-314; 1998.

Sullivan, Krispin, CN, "The miracle of vitamin D," *Wise Traditions in Food, Farming and the Healing Arts,* Weston A Price Foundation, fall 2000. At: www.westonaprice.org/basicnutrition/ vitamindmiracle.html

Trang H, Cole DE, et al, "Evidence that vitamin D3 increases serum 25-hydroxyvitamin D more efficiently than does vitamin D2," *Am J Clin Nutr,* 68:854-8; 1998.

Vieth R, "Vitamin D may ease depression," Inst Med Nutr, 2004b. At:webmd.com/depression/news/ 20040803/vitamin-d-ease-depression (Low blood D may be linked to a cause of depression.)

Vieth R, Kimball S, et al, "Randomized comparison of the effects of the vitamin D3 adequate intake versus 100 mcg (4000 IU) per day on biochemical responses and the wellbeing of patients," *Nutr J,* 3(8); 7/2004a. (130 adults with normal D (24 ng/mL in summer; about 16 in winter. Those most likely to develop depression were given 600 or 4000 IU summer through winter. Both reached at least 40 ng/mL Mood improved with increasing D. Instead of worsening, they felt better in winter. The 4000 IU group benefitted most.)

Vogelsang H, Ferenci P, et al, "Bone disease in vitamin D-deficient patients with Crohn's disease," *Dig Dis Sci,* 34:1094-9; 1989.

Watson KE, Abrolat ML, et al, "Active serum vitamin D levels are inversely correlated with coronary calcification," *Circulation,* 96:1755-60; 1997. www.westonaprice.org/basicnutrition/ vitamindmiracle.html

Wiseman H, "Vitamin D is a membrane antioxidant. Ability to inhibit iron-dependent lipid peroxidation in liposomes compared to cholesterol, ergosterol and tamoxifen and relevance to anticancer action," *FEBS Lett,* 326(1-3):285-8; 7/1993.

Zitterman A, "Vitamin D in preventive medicine: Are we ignoring the evidence?" *Br J Nutr,* 89(5): 552-72; 5/2003.

Calcium

Abdullah H, Bliss R, "Pathology and outcome of surgical treatment for lithium-associated hyperparathyroidism," *Br J Surg,* 86(1):91-93; 1/ 1999. (Lithium can cause parathyroid hyperplasia or adenoma. Retrospective review of 11 bipolars who had surgery for hyperparathyroidism due to chronic lithium. Multigland involvement was common.)

Alarcon RD, Franceschine JA, "Hyperparathyroidism and paranoid psychosis: Case report and review of the literature," *Br J Psychiat,* 145:477; 1984.

Alvir JM, Thys-Jacobs S, "Premenstrual and menstrual symptom clusters and response to calcium treatment," *Psychopharmacol Bull,* 27(2): 145-48; 1991.

Baastrup PC, Christiansen C, et al, [Calcium metabolism in lithium-treated patients: Relation to uni/bipolar dichotomy], *Acta Psychiatrica Scandinavica,* 57(2):124-28; 2/1978. (83 bipolars on chronic lithium had lower bone mineral content than unipolars, and 88% lower than controls. Both uni and bipolar serum calcium, magnesium, proteins, were consistent with hyperparathyroidism.)

Balch JF, Balch PA, *Prescription for Nutritional Healing,* Avery, Garden City Park, NY, 1990.

Baumel S, *Dealing with Depression Naturally,* Keats, New Canaan, CN, 1995.

Berk M, Bodemer W, et al, "Dopamine increases platelet intracellular calcium in bipolar affective disorder and controls," *Int Clin Psychopharmacol,* 9(4):291-3; 1994.

Birdsall TC, " Therapeutic applications of taurine," *Alt Med Rev,* 3(2):128-36; 1998.

Blaylock R, *Excitotoxins: The Taste that Kills,* Health Press, Santa Fe, NM, 1995.

Bowden CL, Huang LG, et al, "Calcium function in affective disorders and healthy controls," *Biol Psychiatr,* 23(4):367-76; 2/15/88. (Unipolar, manic, and bipolar depressives all show abnormal calcium activity, but differently. Plasma calcium was lower in 11 manics than in controls.)

Broida M, *New Hope for People with Depression,* Prima Publishing, Roseville CA, 2001.

Carman JS, et al, "Calcium and calcitonin in bipolar affective disorder," in RM Post, JC Ballenger, eds, *Neurobiology of Mood Disorders,* Williams & Wilkins, Baltimore, 1984; pp 340-355.

Carman JS, Post RM, et al, "Increased serum calcium and phosphorous with the 'switch' into manic or excited psychotic state," *Br J Psychiat,* 135:55-61; 1979.

Carroll BJ, et al, "Neuroendocrine regulation in depression. II. Discrimination of depressed from nondepressed patients," *Arch Gen Psychiat,* 33: 1051-58; 1976.

Colodny L, Hoffman RL, "Inositol: Clinical Applications for exogenous use," *Alt Med Rev,* 3(6):432-447, 1998.

Currier MD, Goodnick PJ, "Calcium antagonists and Newer Anticonvulsants," in PJ Goodnick, ed, *Mania: Clinical and Research Perspectives,* Am Psychiatric Press, DC, 1998; pp 337-62.

Dubovsky SL, Franks RD, "Intracellular calcium ions in affective disorders: A review and an hypothesis," *Biol Psychiat,* 18:781-97; 1983.

Dubovsky SL, Franks RD, et al, "Calcium antagonists in mania: A double-blind study of verapamil," *Psychiat Res,* 18:309-20;1986.

Dubovsky SL, Christiano J, et al, "Increased platelet intracellular calcium ion concentration in patients with affective disorders," *Arch Gen Psychiat,* 46:632-38; 1989. (Baseline, and agonist-stimulated increases were greatest in untreated manics, then untreated bipolar depressed, untreated unipolars, controls.)

Dubovsky, SL, Lee, C, et al, "Elevated platelet intracellular calcium concentrations in bipolar depression," *Biol Psychiatr,* 29(5):441-50; 1990. (Greatest in untreated bipolar depressed, then unipolar depressed, then controls.)

Dubovsky SL, Lee C, et al, "Lithium decreases platelet intracellular calcium ion concentrations in bipolar patients," *Lithium,* 2:167-74; 1991 (Baseline platelet and lymphocyte intracellular calcium is significantly elevated in bipolars.)

Dubovsky SL, Murphy J, et al, "Abnormal intracellular calcium ion concentration in platelets and lymphocytes of bipolar patients," *J Am J Psychiatr,* 149(1):118-20; 1/92a. (Mean intracellular calcium ion concentration higher in bipolars and manics. Mechanisms regulating calcium homeostasis may be disturbed.)

Dubovsky, SL, Murphy J, Christiano J, Lee C, "The calcium second messenger system in bipolar disorders: Data supporting new research directions," *J Neuropschiatr Clin Neurosci,* 4(1):3-14, Winter 1992b. (In bipolar episodes, PI and Ca signaling mechanisms are hyperactive. Li and other stabilizers may act via these second messenger systems.)

Dubovsky SL, "Calcium antagonists in manic-depressive illness," *Neuropsychobiol,* 27(3): 184-92; 1993. (Free intracellular blood platelet calcium (which, though less than 0.1% of total, may be more sensitive, and more important to excitability) is elevated in acute bipolars. Lithium alters calcium dynamics and lowers platelet levels in actively ill patients, but not controls. CCBs modulate hyperactive calcium, have been used for mania, and are most effective in lithium responders.)

Dubovsky SL, Sarfati Y, Spadone C, et al, "Calcium antagonists and lithium in preventive treatment of manic depressive disorder," *Encephale,* 22(2): 149-53; 1996. (Calcium-regulated activity may play a role in bipolar etiology. Lithium may act via calcium-dependent processes.)

Edwards N, "Mental disturbances related to metals," in RCW Hall, ed, *Psychiatric Presentations of Medical Illness,* Spectrum Pub, Jamaica NY, 1980; pp 283-308.

El Mallakh RS, Jaziri WA, "Calcium channel blockers in affective illness: Role of sodium-calcium exchange," *J Clin Psychopharmacol,* 10: 203-06; 1990.

Emamghoreishi M, Schlichter L, et al, "High intracellular calcium concentrations in transformed lymphoblasts from subjects with bipolar I disorder," *Am J Psychiatr,* 154(7):976-82; 7/1997. (Bipolars show elevated basal intracellular calcium ion in lymphocytes and platelets. Here, basal Ca2 was significantly greatest in bipolar I (especially males), then bipolar II, depressed, other psychiatric patients, normals.)

Ericsson Y, Angmar-Mansson B, et al, "Urinary mineral ion loss after sugar ingestion," *Bone Miner,* 9(3):233-7; 6/1990.

Felberg W, Sherwood SL, "Effects of calcium and potassium injected into the cerebral ventricles of the cat," *J Physiol,* 139(3):408-16; 12/1957.

Fitzpatrick L, Heaney RP, "Got soda?" *J Bone Miner Res,* 18:1570-2; 9/2003.

Flach FF, "Calcium metabolism in states of

depression," Br J Psychiat, 110:588-93; 1964.

Flach FF, Faragalla F, "The effects of imipramine and electroconvulsive therapy on the excretion of various minerals in depressed patients," *Brit J Psychiat,* 116:437-38; 1970.

Gaby AR, *Preventing and Reversing Osteoporosis,* Prima, Rocklin CA, 1994.

Garrison RH, Somer E, *The Nutrition Desk Reference,* Keats, New Canaan, CN, 1985.

Gold MS, *The Good News About Depression,* Villard Books, NY, 1987.

Groat RD, MacKenzie TB, "The appearance of mania following intravenous calcium replacement," *J Nerv Ment Dis,* 168(9):562-3; 1980. (A 35-year-old depressive, character-disordered woman, with low magnesium and calcium, given rapid IV calcium, developed sleeplessness, racing thoughts, pressure of speech, psychomotor hyperactivity, euphoria, exaggerated feelings of power and other manic symptoms. Symptoms resolved after 6 days.)

Haden ST, Brown EM, et al, "The effect of lithium on calcium-induced changes in adrenocorticotrophin levels," *J Clin Endocrinol Metab,* 84(1):198-200; 1/1999. (Chronic lithium alters calcium sensing, shifting the parathyroid set-point. Calcium citrate infusions given to 7 lithium-treated bipolars, increased inonic calcium, stimulating ACTH increases.)

Heaney RP, "Effects of nitrogen, phosphorus and caffeine on calcium balance in women," *J Lab Clin Med,* 99:46-55; 1982.

Heaney RP, Recker RR, et al, "Calcium absorption in women: Relationships to calcium intake, estrogen status, and age," *J Bone Miner Res,* 4(4): 469-75; 8/1989. (In 189 middle-aged women at self-selected calcium intake, absorption was inversely proportional to intake. (Mean absorption fraction was 0.45 at 200 mg per day; one third that at over 2000 mg.) Absorption efficiency decreased about .002/year, with a one-time .02 loss at menopause.)

Hernandez-Avila M, et al, "Caffeine, moderate alcohol intake, and risk of fractures of the hip and forearm in middle-aged women," *Am J Clin Nutr,* 54:157-63; 1991.

Himmelhoch JM, Garfinkle ME, "Sources of lithium resistance in mixed mania," *Psychopharmacol Bull,* 22:613-20; 1986.

Hojo Y, Ikeda U, et al, "Thyroid hormone stimulates NA(+)-Ca2+ exchanger expression in rat cardiac myoctes," *J Cardiovasc Pharmacol,* 29(1):75-80; 1/1997. (Thyroid and sodium may act through distinct pathways in regulating expression of the Na(+)-Ca2+ exchanger gene.)

Hollingbery PW, et al, "Effect of dietary caffeine and aspirin on urinary calcium and hydroxyproline excretion in pre and postmenopausal women," *Fed Proc,* 44:1149; 1985.

Hoschl C, Kozeny J, "Verpramil in affective disorders: A controlled, double blind study," *Biol Psychiat,* 25:128-40;1989. (12 acute manics were given verapamil 35 days; 24, neuroleptics; 11, low-dose neuroleptic plus lithium. Results were equivalent.)

Hoschl C, "Do calcium antagonists have a place in the treatment of mood disorders?" *Drugs,* 42:721-29; 1991. (Review.)

Hu JF, et al, "Dietary calcium and bone density among middle aged and elderly women in China," *Am J Clin Nutr,* 58:219; 1993. (Previous studies suggested that in populations with relatively physically strenuous lives, those who do not eat dairy, but eat other calcium-rich food (e.g., greens), have considerably less osteoporosis. This study finds that within such populations, those who eat dairy show greater bone density.)

Jaffe R, Kruesi OR,"The biochemical immunology window: A molecular view of psychiatric case management," *J App Nutr,* 44(2); 1992.

Jimerson DC, et al, "CSF calcium: Clinical correlates in affective illness and schizophrenia," *Biol Psychiat,* 14(1):37-51; 1979. (CSF calcium correlated with depressive severity, and tended to decrease with improvement. In 4 rapid cyclers, CSF calcium increased with depression (though absolute levels did not differ significantly from controls).)

Joborn C, et al, "Psychiatric symptomatology in patients with primary hyperparathyroidism," *Ups J Med Sci,* 91(1)77-87; 1986. (23% of 441, especially older patients, had psychiatric symptoms; most frequently, depression and anxiety.)

Johnson FN, Birch NJ, et al, "Mechanisms of lithium action," *Rev Contemp Pharmacother,* 4: 287-318; 1993.

Johnson RK, Frary C, "Choose beverages and foods to moderate your intake of sugars: The 2000 dietary guidelines for Americans — What's all the fuss about," *J Nutr,* 131S:2766-71; 2001 (Diets high in added sugars have been associated with bone loss and fractures. Sodas are the greatest source and constitute one third of total sugar.)

Klein M, Barb'e F, et al, "Lead poisoning secondary to hyperthyroidism: Report of two cases," *Eur J Endocrinol,* 138(2):185-8; 2/98. (Hyperthyroidism, as well as hyperparathyroidism, increased bone turnover, potentially releasing stored lead.)

Konig P, "Psychopathological alterations in cases of symmetrical basal ganglia sclerosis," *Biol Psychiat,* 25(4):459-68; 2/15/89. (35 basal ganglia sclerosis patients (due to parathyroid dysfunction, thyroidectomy, etc.). Presenting symptoms were psychiatric in 40%; neurological, in 50%. Almost all chronic patients showed intellectual impairment. Organic affective syndromes occured in 21% of acute and 65% of chronic patients; 37% were depressive, 20% bipolar, 11% manic. Thyroidectomy was associated with parathyroid deficiency and extensive calcification leading to more severe mental deterioration.)

Krohn J, *The Whole Way to Allergy Relief & Prevention,* Hartley & Marks, Point Roberts, WA, 1991.

Kusumi I, Koyama, et al, "Thrombin-induced platelet calcium mobilization is enhanced in bipolar disorders," *Biol Psychiat,* 32(8):731-4; 1992.

Larson JM, *Depression Free, Naturally,* Ballantine Wellspring, NY, 2001

Levine J, Stein D, "High serum and cerebrospinal fluid Ca/Mg ratio in recently hospitalized acutely depressed patients," *Neuropsychobiology,* 39(2):63-70; 1999. (Increased CSF and serum Ca/Mg ratio in unipolar and, especially, bipolar depression.)

Lieberman S, Bruning N, *The Real Vitamin & Mineral Book,* Avery, Garden City Park, NY, 1990.

Linnoila M, MacDonald E, et al, "RBC membrane adenosine triphosphatase activities in patients with major affective disorders," *Arch Gen Psychiat,* 40(9): 1021-26; 9/1983. (8 affectives, 12 controls. Mean RBC Ca2+ATPase activity was greatest in mania, then depression, then controls, though mood did not correlate in all patients. Na, K, Mg, and Ca ATPase activity fluctuated more in affectives than controls but did not reflect Li or Va levels. Authors suggest mood changes may be due to extreme sensitivity to, or elevated levels of, a pump regulator.)

Manna V, "Bipolar affective disorders and role of intraneuronal calcium. Therapeutic effects of the treatment with lithium salts and/or calcium antagonist in patients with rapid polar inversion," *Minerva Med,* 82(11):757-63; 11/1991. (In 12 rapid-cyclers, a CCB plus lithium was more effective than either alone. Calcium ionic disorders may play a role in bipolar disorder. Some studies suggest lithium may act as a calcium antagonist.)

Marlowe, Mike, PhD, et al, "Decreased magnesium in the hair of autistic children," *J Orthomol Psychiat,* 13:117-22; 1984. (Ca and Mg are low. B6 without magnesium can worsen symptoms.)

Mattarello MJ, Benedini S, et al, "Effect of licorice on PTH levels in healthy women," *Steroids,* 71(5): 403-8; 2006. (Has aldosterone and estrogen-like activity; counters androgens. PTH and urinary calcium increased after only 2 months.)

Meltzer HL, "Lithium mechanisms in bipolar illness and altered intracellular calcium functions," *Biol Psychiatr,* 21(5-6):492-510; 5/1986. (Lithium may alter many calcium-dependent processes.)

Meltzer HE, Caesar S, et al, "Calmodulin-activated calcium ATPase in bipolar illness," *Neuropsychobiol,* 20:169-73; 1988.

Morgan B, Morgan R, *Hormones,* Price, Stern, Sloan, LA, 1989.

Murphy HJ, et al, *J Neuropsychiat Clin Neurosci,* 4(1):3-14; 1992. (Importance of Ca signalling dysfunction. Lithium influences Ca hyperactivity.)

Nieves JW, Komar L, et al, "Calcium potentiates the effect of estrogen and calcitonin on bone mass: Review and analysis," *Am J Clin Nutr,* 67: 18-24; 1998.

NutriCircles®, Strickland Computer Consulting, Version 3.25, April 29, 1996.

Okamoto Y, Kagaya A, et al, "Serotonin-induced platelet calcium mobilization is enhanced in mania," *Life Sci,* 56(5):327-32; 95. (Ser induces intracellular platelet Ca mobilization with a rapid peak within 10 seconds, then a prolonged plateau. Reports suggest increased peak amplitude in affectives. This study found an enhanced plateau phase in untreated bipolars, reversed with treatment.)

Page LR, *Healthy Healing,* Healthy Healing, CA, 1992.

Pappenheimer JR, Held D, et al, "Bulk flow and diffusion in the cerebrospinal system of the goat," *Am J Physiol,* 203:775-8; 1962.

Pang P, et al, "Parathyroid hypertensive factor and intracellular calcium regulation," *J Hypertension,* 14:1053-60; 1996.

Pavlinac D, et al, "Magnesium in affective disorders," *Biol Psychiat,* 14(4):657-61; 1979.

Pfeiffer CC, *Mental and Elemental Nutrients,* Keats, New Canaan, CN, 1975.

Pfeiffer CC, *The Schizophrenias Ours to Conquer,* Bio-Communications Press, Wichita, KS, 1988.

Pollack MH, Rosenbaum JF, "Calcium channel blockers in psychiatry," *Psychosomatics,* 28:356-69; 1987.

Post RM, Denicoff KD, et al, "Long-term outcome of anticonvulsants in affective disorders," in Joseph E Goldberg MD, Martin Harrow PhD, *Bipolar Disorders: Clinical Course and Outcomes,* Am Psychiatric Press Inc, DC, 1999; pp 95-96.

Post RM, :Biochemical theories," in RH Belmaker, HM van Praag, eds, *Mania: An evolving concept,* Spectrum Publications, Jamaica NY, 1980.

Prange A, Whybrow P, Loosen PT, "Depression and Other Mental Symtoms in Endocrine Disorders: An Overview," in U Halbreich, ed, *Hormones and Depression,* Raven Press, NY, 1987, pp 313-324.

Quillin P, *Healing Nutrients,* Contemporary Books, Chicago, 1987.

Rogers S, *Depression, Cured at Last,* SK Publishing, Sarasota FL, 1997.

Sklar P, Smoller JW, "Whole-genome association study of bipolar disorder," *Mol Psychiat,* 13(6):558-69; 6/2008. (Pooled international data on 4,387 bipolars, over 6000 controls. The second most robust association was to a calcium channel gene.)

Slagle P, "Cancer/ Osteoporosis/ Stress" *The Way Up Newletter Archives,* #1 At: thewayup.com/newletters/newsarch.htm

Smigan L, [Long term lithium treatment. Some clinical, psychological and biological aspects], *Acta Psychiatrica Scandinavica,* 71(2):160-70; 2/1985. (In responsive patients, blood calcium elevated during the first 4 months.)

Spencer H, et al, "Alcohol osteoporosis," *Am J Clin Nutr,* 41:847; 1985.

Sullivan, Krispin, CN, "The miracle of vitamin D," Wise Traditions in Food, Farming and the Healing Arts, Weston A Price Foundation, Fall 2000

Swartz CM, "Albumin decrement in depression and cholesterol decrement in mania," *J Affect Disord,* 19(3);173-6; 7/90. (Over 4 yrs, serum calcium/protein was 2.2% higher in manics than other psychiatric admissions.)

Thakar JH, et al, "Erythrocyte membrane sodium-potassium and magnesium ATPase in primary affective disorder," *Biol Psychiat,* 20:734-40; 7/1985.

Veal WL, Myers RD, "Emotional behavior arousal and sleep produced by sodium and calcium ions, perfused within the hypothalamus of the cat," *Physiol Behav,* 7(4):601-7; 10/1971.

Walsh WJ, "Biochemical individuality and nutrition," NOHA News, XXV(2):6-8; 2000.

Walsh WJ, "Biochemical individuality and nutrition," 2000. At: www.hriptc.org/biochemical_individuality.html

Walsh WJ, "A biological basis for neurologic disorders: autism, hyperactivity, attention deficit disorder, depression, obsessive-compulsive disorder, Tourette's syndrome, and violence, An interview with William Walsh PhD, Latitudes, 5(2)1-8, 2002. At: www.Latitudes.org

Walsh, William J, PhD, interview with author, November, 2007.

Watts DL, "The nutritional relationships of calcium," *J Orthomol Med,* 5(2):61-6; 1990.

Weintraub S, *Minding Your Body,* Complementary Medicine Pub Co, Portland, OR, 1995.

Werbach MT, *Nutritional Influences on Mental Illness,* Third Line Press, Tarzana, CA, 1991.

Weston PG, Howard MQ, "The determination of sodium, potassium, calcium and magnesium in the blood and spinal fluid of patients suffering from manic depressive insanity," *Arch Neurol Psychiat,* 8:179-83; 1922.

Winter A, Winter R, *Eat Right, Be Bright,* St Martin's Press, NY, 1988.

Wood K, "The neurochemistry of mania: The effect of lithium on catecholamines, indoleamines, and calcium mobilization," *J Affect Disord,* 8:215-223; 1985.

Wyshak G, "Teenaged girls, carbonated beverage consumption, and bone fractures," *Arch Pediatr Adolesc Med,* 154:620-13; 6/2000. (Associated with bone fracture, particularly cola beverages.)

Yudkin J, *Sweet and Dangerous,* Bantam, NY, 1973.

Magnesium

Ananth J, Yassa R, "Magnesium in Mental illness," *Comp Psychiat,* 20:475-82; 9/10/1979.

Balch JF, Balch P, *Prescription for Nutritional Healing,* Avery, Garden City Park, NY, 1990.

Banki, C.M, et al, "Aminergic studies and cerebrospinal fluid cations in suicide," *Ann NY Acad Sci,* 487:221-30; 1986. (CSF magnesium significantly lower in suicidal depressives.)

Berube B, "Depression, Virus link," *Medical Post,* 23:1-2l; 6/2/1992.

Biol Psychiat, 19:871-6; 6/1984. (Boys with schizophrenia, depression or sleep disorders had significantly lower blood Mg than controls.)

Biol Psychiat, 20:163-71; 2/1985. (Suicidal psychiatric patients had low magnesium.)

Bjorum, N, [Electrolytes in blood in endogenous depression], *Acta Psychiatr Scand,* 48:59-68; 1972. (Higher plasma Mg in depressed patients.)

Blaylock R, *Excitotoxins, The Taste that Kills,* Health Press, Santa Fe, NM, 1995.

Bosc M, Roche M, et al, "Magnesium and vitamin B6 intake reduces central nervous system hyperexcitability in children," *J Am Coll Nutr,* 23(5): 5455-85; 10/2004.

Cousens G, *Depression free for Life,* Quill, HarperCollins, NY, 2000.

Davis, W, et al, Presentation at The 2nd Intl Symposium on Magnesium, Montreal, 1976. (99% of 200 subjects experienced improved sleep.)

Dubovsky SLm Franks RD, et al, "Effectiveness of verpamil in the treatment of a manic patient," Am J Psychiat, 139:502-4; 1982.

Dubovsky SL, "Calcium channel antagonists as novel agents for manic-depressive disorder," in AF Schatzberg, CB Nemeroff, eds, *Textbook of Psychopharmacology,* Am Psychiatric Press, DC, 1995; pp377-88.

Dubovsky SL, Buzan RD, "Novel alternatives and supplements to lithium and anticonvulsants for bipolar affective disorder," *J Clin Psychiatr,* 58(5): 224-42; 5/1997. (Review: Includes thyroid, CCBs, benzos, etc.)

Eby KL, "Rapid recovery from major depression using magnesium treatment," *Med Hypotheses,* 2006.

Eby G, At: coldcure.com/html/dep.html (Serum Mg was low in suicidally and severely depressed.)

george-eby-research.com/html/magnesium-for-depression.pdf

Frazer A, Ramsey TA, et al, "Plasma and erythrocyte electrolytes in affective disorders," *J Affect Disord,* 5(2):103-13; 1983. (Depressives and manics showed greater plasma Mg than controls; depressives, also, greater red cell Mg.)

Frizel D, Coppen A, et al, "Plasma magnesium and calcium in depression," *Br J Psychiat,* 115: 1375; 1969.

Garrison RH, Somer E, *The Nutrition Desk Reference,* Keats, New Canaan, CN, 1985.

Garza-Trevino ES, Overall JE, et al, "Verpamil versus lithium in acute mania," *Am J Psychiat,* 149: 121-22; 1992.

Gold MS, *The Good News About Depression,* Villard Books, NY, 1987.

Hashizume N, Mri M, "An analysis of hypermagnesemia and hypomagnesemia," *Jap J Med,* 29(4):368-472; 7-8, 1990. (Personality changes and depression improved when Mg increased.)

Jaffe R, Kruesi OR,"The biochemical immunology window: A molecular view of psychiatric case management," *J App Nutr,* 44(2); 1992.

Kirov GK, Tsachev KN, "Magnesium, schizophrenia and manic-depressive disease," *Neuropsychobiol,* 23(2):79-81; 1990. (Plasma magnesium was low in 15 schizophrenias and 10 depressions, but not manias or Alzheimer's. Levels increased with improvement in schizophrenia. Stress may marginally decrease magnesium, worsening anxiety, hallucinations, weakness, body complaints, etc.)

Langley WF, Mann D, "Central nervous system magnesium deficiency," *Arch Intern Med,* 593-96; 1991.

Levine J, Stein D, "High serum and cerebrospinal fluid Ca/Mg ratio in recently hospitalized acutely depressed patients," *Neuropsychobiol,* 39(2):63-70; 1999.

Lieberman S, Bruning N, *The Real Vitamin & Mineral Book,* Avery, Garden City Park, NY, 1990.

Linder J, et al, [Calcium and magnesium concentrations in affective disorder: Difference between plasma and serum in relation to symptoms], *Acta Psychiatr Scand,* 80:527-37; 1989. (Depressive symptoms correlated with high serum magnesium.)

Marlowe M, "Decreased magnesium in the hair of autistic children," *J Orthomol Psychiat,* 13:117-22; 1984.

Mousain-Bosc M, Roche M, et al, "Improvement of neurobehavioral disorders in children supplemented with magnesium-vitamin B6. I. Attention deficit hyperactivity disorders," *Magnes Res,* 19(1):46-52; 2006.

Murray M, *Glandular Extracts,* Keats, New Canaan, CN, 1994.

Nizankowska-Blaz T, Korczowski R, et al, [Level of magnesium in blood serum in children from the province of Rzesz'ow], *Wiad Lek,* 46(3-4):120-2; 2/1993.

NutriCircles®, Strickland Computer Consulting, Version 3.25, April 29, 1996.

Page LR, *Healthy Healing,* Healthy Healing, CA, 1992.

Pavlinac D, et al, "Magnesium in affective disorders," *Biol Psychiat,* 14(4):657-61; 1979.

Penland J, "Effects of trace element nutrition on sleep patterns in adult women," *Fed Am Soc Exp Biol J,* 2: A434, 1988. (High-magnesium, low-aluminum diet associated with better quality sleep.)

Pfeiffer CC, *Mental and Elemental Nutrients,* Keats, New Canaan, CN, 1975.

Rasmussen HH, "Depression and magnesium deficiency," *Int J Psychiat Med,* 19(1):57-63; 1989. (Check serum, loading, urine, symptoms, health.)

Starabrat-Hermelin B, [The effects of magnesium supplementation on hyperactivity in children with attention deficit hyperactivity disorder (AHDH)], *Magnes-Res,* 10(2):149-56; 1997.

Starabrat-Hermelin B [The effect of deficiency of selected bioelements on hyperactivity in children with certain specified mental disorders], *Ann Acad Med Stetin,* 44:297-314; 1998.

Quillin P, *Healing Nutrients,* Contemporary Books, Chicago, 1987.

Robinet ML, *Bull Acad Med (France),* 1934 (Soil Mg strikingly relates to suicide.)

Sahley BJ, *Healing with Amino Acids,* Pain & Stress Center Pub., TX, 1995.

Tenney L, *Stress,* Woodland Health Books, 1987.

Thase M, "Bipolar depression: Pharmacotherapy and related therapeutic strategies," *Biol Psychiatr,* 48(6):559-72.

Ubell, E, science ed, *Herald Tribune,* 5/1966, reporting on, *Am Soc Exp Biol,* Meeting, 5/1966. (One study found rapid rise urinary adrenal breakdown products before successful suicide. Adrenalin depletes magnesium.)

Watts DL, "The nutritional relationships of magnesium," *J Orthomol Med,* 3(4):197-201; 1988.

Werbach, MT, *Nutritional Influences on Mental Illness,* Third Line Press, Tarzana, CA, 1991.

Widmer J, "Evolution of blood magnesium, sodium and potassium in depressed patients followed for three months," *Neuropsychobiol,* 26(4):173-79; 1992.

Chromium

Attenburrow J, Odontiadis BJ, et al, "Chromium treatment decreases the sensitivity of 5-HT2A receptors," *Psychopharmacol,* 159:432-6; 2002. (Chromium may moderate endocrine response to mood dysregulation.)

Balch JF, Balch PA,*Prescription for Nutritional Healing,* Avery, Garden City Park, NY, 1990.

Bennett JB, "Physiological and biochemical changes in impaired sugar metabolism," *J Orthomol Psychiat,* 3(4):246-53, 1974.

Buckley RE, "Hypoglycemic kindling of limbic system disorder," *J Orthomol Psychiat;* 1978, pp 118-21.

Christensen, L, "Psychological distress and diet — effects of sucrose and caffeine," *J Appl Nutr,* 40(1):44-50; 1988. (Double blind.)

Cohen D, "Dementia, depression, and nutritional status," *Primary Care Clinics in Office Practice,* 21(1): 107-19; 3/1994.

Cousens G, *Depression Free for Life,* Quill, HarperCollins, NY, 2001.

Currier, William, et al, "Hypoglycemia: The end of your sweet life," in R Williams, D Kalita, eds, *A Physician's Handbook on Orthomolecular Medicine,* Keats, New Canaan, CN, 1979.

Docherty JP, Sack DA, et al, "A double-blind, placebo-controlled, exploratory trial of chromium picolinate in atypical depression: Effect of carbohydrate craving," *J Psychiatric Practice,* 11(5): 302-14; 9/2005. (8 wk double blind multicenter replication study. 113 outpatients with dysthymia, major depression, or depression NOS. 600 mcg/d led to significant improvement in appetite and craving regulation on HAM-D, especially in atypical depressives with severe carbohydrate craving.)

Dufy W, *Sugar Blues,* Warner Books, NY, 1975.

Garetz, "Breaking the dangerous cycle of depression and faulty nutrition," *Geriatrics,* 31(6):73-75; 6/1976

Gold MS, et al, *The Good News About Depression,* Villard Books, NY, 1987.

Jonathan RT, Davidson MD, et al, "Effectiveness of chromium in atypical depression: A placebo-controlled trial," *Biol Psychiat,* 53(3):261-4; 2003. (Randomized 8-wk clinical trial. 7/10 major depressives with weight gain, fatigue, and carbohdrate cravings given 400-600 mcg Cr improved significantly. Symptoms reduced over 66%; no side effects; and no need for additional meds. Controls did not improve.)

Larson, JM, *Depression Free Naturally,* Ballantine, Wellspring, NY, 2001.

Lesser M, *Nutrition & Vitamin Therapy,* Bantam Books, NY, 1983.

Lieberman S, Bruning N, *The Real Vitamin & Mineral Book,* Avery, Garden City Park, NY, 1990.

Malcolm N, McLeod MN, et al, "Chromium potentiation of antidepressant pharmacotherapy for dysthymic disorder in 5 patients," *J Clin Psychiat,* 60(4):237-40; 1999. (In 5 chronic dysthymic depressives, augmentation, especially with chromium picolinate, produced a rapid response.)

Malcolm N, McLeod MN, Golden RN, "Chromium treatment of depression," *Intrntl J Neuropsychiat,* 3:311-14; 2000. (Case series. Chromium intake by 8 chronic refractory affectives (including bipolar II) led to remission and productive functioning. Self-described improvements were dramatic. For most, decreased carbohydrate craving and excessive appetite. Side effects were rare or mild (e.g., enhanced dreaming, mild psychomotor activation). Improved insulin use. Increasing Ser availability or NE release, may contribute to benefit.)

McCarty MF, "Enhancing central and peripheral insulin activity as a strategy for the treatment of endogenous depression — an adjuvant role for chromium picolinate?" *Med Hypotheses,* 43(4): 247-52; 10/1994. (Cr enhances insulin sensitivity. The insulin resistance often found in depressives may be due to elevated cortisol. Brain insulin receptors are widespread, and concentrated in catecholamine terminals. Insulin also increases tryptophan uptake. A low fat diet and aerobic exercise may also help.)

Moore, Daniel T, PhD, "A Holistic Approach for Treating Manic Depressive Disorders," 1998. At: familyclinic.simplenet.com/bipolar/bipaper.html (Clients report sugar and caffeine can start a mild mania; similarly, junk or chemicalized food)

Murray MT, *Stress, Anxiety & Insomnia,* Prima, Rocklin CA, 1995.

Murray MT, *Encyclopedia of Nutritional Supplements,* Prima, Rocklin, CA, 1996.

Nutricircles®, Strickland Computer Consulting Version 3.25 April 29, 1996.

Page LR, *Healthy Healing,* Healthy Healing Pub, CA, 1992.

Pfeiffer CC, *Mental and Elemental Nutrients,* Keats, New Canaan, CN, 1975

Pfeiffer CC, *Nutrition and Mental Illness,* Healing Arts Press, Rochester, VT, 1987.

Philpott W, Kalita D, *Brain Allergies: The Psychonutrient Connection,* Keats, New Canaan, CN, 1987.

Prange A, Whybrow PC, Loosen PT, "Depression and other mental symtoms in endocrine disorders: An overview," in U Halbreich, ed, *Hormones and Depression,* Raven Press, NY, 1987, pp 313-324.

Rogers S, *Depression, Cured at Last,* SK Publishing, Sarasota FL, 1997

Ross H, et al, *Hypoglycemia, The Disease Your Doctor Won't Treat,* Pinnacle Books, 1989.

Ross H, "Hypoglycemia," *J Orthomol Psychiat,* 3(4): 240-5; 1974.

Schrauser GN, Shrestha KP, et al, "Somato-psychological effects of chromium supplementation," *J Nutr Med,* 3:1, 43-48; 1992.

Weintraub S, *Minding Your Body,* Complementary Medicine Pub Co, Portland, OR, 1995.

Manganese

Ali MM, Murphy RC, "Effect of low protein diet on manganese neurotoxicity. III. Brain neurotransmitter levels," *Neurobehav Toxicol Teratol,* 7(5):427-31; 1985. (Significant increase in DA and NE.)

Balch JF, Balch P, *Prescription for Nutritional Healing,* Avery, Garden City Park, NY, 1990.

Baly DL, et al, "Effects of manganese deficiency on pyruvate carboxylase and phosphoenolpyruvate carboxykinase activity and carbohydrate homeostasis in adult rats," *Biol Trace Elem Res,* 11: 201-212; 1986.

Barceloux DG, "Manganese," *J Toxicol Clin Toxicol,* 37(2):293-307; 1999. (Industrial toxicity has been associated with compulsivity, lability, hallucinations, a Parkinson's syndrome.)

Buthieau AM, Autissier N, "Effects of manganese ions on thyroid function in rat," *Arch Toxicol,* 54(3): 243-6; 1983.

Carl EG, Keen BB, et al, "Association of low blood manganese concentrations with epilepsy," *Neurol,* 336:1584-7; 1986.

Casdorph HR, Walker M, *Toxic Metal Syndrome: How Metal Poisoning Can Affect Your Brain,* Avery, Garden City Park, NY, 1995.

Colipp PJ, et al, "Manganese in infant formulas and learning disability," *Ann Nutr Metab,* 26(6): 488-94; 1983.

Cook DG et al, "Chronic manganese intoxication," *Arch Neurol,* 30:59, 1/1974.

Crawte J, "Accounts of a mystery illness. The Groote Eylandt Syndrome," *Aust New Zealand J Psychiat,* 18:179-87; 1984.

Donaldson J, Labella FS, et al, "Enhanced autoxidation of dopamine as a possible basis of manganese neurotoxicity," *Neutotoxicol,* 2:53-64; 1981.

Donaldson J, McGregor D, et al, "Manganese neurotoxicity: A model for free radical medicated neurodegeneration," *Can J Physiol Pharmacol,* 60: 1398-1405; 1982.

Dupont CL, Tanaka Y, "Blood manganese levels in children with convulsive disorder," *Biochem Med,* 33:246-55; 1985.

Eder K, Kralik A, et al, "The effect of manganese supply on thyroid hormone metabolism in the offspring of manganese-depleted dams," *Biol Trace Elem Res,* 55(1-2):137-45; 1996. (Mn supports thyroid function, but too much can reduce serum T3. Too little impairs growth and food conversion and alters serum Ca and Mg.)

English WM, "Report on the treatment with manganese chloride of 181 cases of schizophrenia, 33 of manic depression and 16 other defects or psychoses at the Ontario Hospital, Brockville, ON, 11/1929," *Amer J Psychiat,* 9:569; 1964.

Garrison RJ, Somer E, *The Nutrition Desk Reference,* Keats, New Canaan, CN, 1985.

Gold MS, et al, *The Good News About Depression,* Villard Books, NY, 1987.

Gottschalk LA, Rebello T, et al, "Abnormalities in hair trace elements as indicators of aberrant behavior," *Compr Psychiat,* 32(3):229-37; 1991. (High manganese.)

Hawkins D, "Successful prevention of tardive dyskinesia," *J Orthomol Med,* 4(1):35-36, 1989.

Hoffer A, "A tardive dyskinesia treated with manganese," letter, *Can Med Assn J,* 117(8):859, 1977. (In a Vancouver nursing home in which gives patients manganese and other nutrients, TD is no longer a problem.)

Hoskin RG, "The manganese treatment of schizophrenic disorders," *J Nerv Ment Dis,* 79: 59; 1934.

Hurley LS, Wooley DE, et al, "Influence of manganese on susceptibility of rats to convulsions," *Am J Physiol,* 204:493-6; 1963.

Jaffe R, Kruesi OR,"The biochemical immunology window: A molecular view of psychiatric case management," *J App Nutr,* 44(2); 1992.

Kawada J, Nishada M, et al, "Manganese ion as a goitrogen in the female mouse," *Endocrinol Jpn,* 32(5):635-43; 1985.

Kimura M, Yagi N, et al, "Effect of subacute manganese feeding on serotonin metabolism in the rat," *J Toxicol Environ Health,* 4(5-6):701-7; 1978. (By 3+ wks, Ser decreased.)

Kunin RA, "Manganese and niacin in the treatment of drug induced dyskinesias," *J Orthomol Psychiat,* 5(1):4-27, 1976. (14/15 TD patients responded to Mn alone or Mn plus niacin, often with striking improvement.)

Kontur PJ, Flechter LD, "Brain regional manganese levels and monoamine metabolism in manganese-treated neonatal rats," *Neurotoxicol Teratol,* 10(4): 295-303; 1988. (25 or 50 mg manganous chloride/ day for 2 or 3 wks did not decrease monoamines and metabolites.)

Krohn J, et al, *The Whole Way to Allergy Relief & Prevention,* Hartley & Marks, Point Roberts, WA, 1991.

Larson JM, *Depression Free, Naturally,* Ballantine Wellspring, NY, 2001.

Lieberman S, Bruning N, *The Real Vitamin & Mineral Book,* Avery, Garden City Park, NY, 1990.

Misiewicz A, Radwan K, et al, "Effect of occupational environment containing manganese on thyroid function," *Endokrynol Pol,* 44(1):57-63; 1993. (Low T3 and T4, elevated TSH. Environment also had iron chromates.)

Montes S, Alcaraz-Zubeldia M, et al, "Striatal manganese accumulation incudes changes in metabolism in the cirrhotic rat," *Brain Res,* 891(1-2):123-9; 2001.

Murray MT, Pizzorno J, *Encyclopedia of Natural Medicine,* Prima, Rocklin, CA, 1998.

Neff NH, et al, "Selective depletion of caudate nucleus dopamine and serotonin during chronic manganese dioxide administration," *Experimentia,* 25:1140-41; 1969.

Norris JP, Sams R, letter, *Am J Psychiat,* 134(12): 1448, 1977.

Nutr Rev, "Manganese and glucose tolerance," 26: 207-10; 1968.

NutriCircles®, Strickland Computer Consulting, Version 3.25, April 29, 1996.

Page LR, *Healthy Healing,* Healthy Healing, CA, 1992.

Papavasiliou P, et al, "Seizure disorders and trace minerals: Manganese in epileptics," *Neurology,* 29: 1466-73; 1979.

Patterson KY, Holbrook JT, et al, "Zinc, copper, and manganese intake and balance for adults consuming self-selected diets," *Am J Clin Nutr,* 40: 1397, 1403; 1984.

Penalver R, "Manganese poisoning, *Ind Med Surge,* 24:107; 1955.

Pfeiffer CC, Iliev V, "A study of zinc deficiency and copper excess in the schizophrenias," *Intl Rev Neurobiol,* 1972; p 141. (Mn can triple Cu excretion, especially when used with Zn.)

Pfeiffer CC, *Mental and Elemental Nutrients,* Keats, New Canaan, CN, 1975a.

Pfeiffer CC, Bacchi D, "Copper, zinc, manganese, niacin and pyridoxine in the schizophrenias, *J Appl Nutr,* 27:9-39, 1975b.

Pfeiffer CC, LaMola S," Zinc and manganese in the schizophrenias," *J Orthomol Psychiat,* 12:215-34; 1983. (Cu may increase 1-3 months before falling. This can be prevented by including Mn, B6 and, if unavoidable, D-penicillamine.)

Pfeiffer CC, *Nutrition and Mental Illness,* Healing Arts Press, Rochester, VT 1987.

Pfeiffer CC, *The Schizophrenias Ours to Conquer,* Bio-Communications Press, Wichita, KS, 1988.

Quillin P, *Healing Nutrients,* Contemporary Books, Chicago, 1987.

Rico H, Gomez-Raso N, "Effects on bone loss of manganese alone or with copper supplement in ovariectomized rats. A morphometric and densitometric study," *Eur J Obstet Gynecol Reprod Biol,* 90(1):97-101; 2000.

Rogers S, *Depression, Cured at Last,* SK Publishing, Sarasota FL, 1997.

Ross J, *The Mood Cure,* Viking Penguin, NY, 2002.

Rubinstein AH, Levin NW, et al, "Manganese-induced hypoglycemia," *Lancet,* 2:1348-51; 1962.

Saltman PD, Staruse LG, "The role of trace minerals in osteoporosis," *J Am Coll Nutr,* 12(4): 384-9; 1993.

Sampson P, "Low manganese level may trigger epilepsy," *JAMA,* 238:1805; 1977.

Shirani Ranasinghe JG, Ming-Chjeh L, et al, "Manganese administration induces the increased production of dopamine sulfate and depletion of dopamine in Sprague-Dawley rats," *J Biochem,* 128: 477-80; 2000. (Stimulates production of dopamine sulfates, depleting dopamine.)

Slagle, Phyllis, MD, *The Way Up from Down,* St. Martin's Paperbacks, NY, 1992.

Sohler A, Pfeiffer CC, "A direct method for the determination of manganese in whole blood: Patients with seizure activity have low blood levels," *J Orthomol Psychiat,* 8:275-80; 1979.

Stauber JL, Florence TM, "Manganese in scalp hair: Problems of exogenous manganese: Implications for manganese monitoring in Groote Eylandt Syndrome Aborigines," *Sci Total Environ,* 83(1-2): 85-98; 1989.

Subhash MN, Padmashree TS, "Effect of manganese on biogenic amine metabolism in regions of the rat brain," *Food Chem Toxicol,* 29(8):579-82; 1991. (Variable.)

Tkacz C, "A preventive measure for tardive dyskinesia," *J Intl Acad Preventive Med,* 8(5):5-8, 1984. (Not one case in 10,000 outpatients and 1,000 inpatients receiving nutrient-based treatments.)

Walsh, William J, PhD, "Biochemical treatment: Medicines for the next century," *NOHA News,*

16(3); 1991.

Walsh, William J, PhD, "Zinc deficiency, metal metabolism, and behavior disorders," *A Report of the Health Research Institute,* Naperville, IL, 3/1996.

Walsh WJ, "Biochemical individuality and nutrition,"*NOHA News,* XXV(2):6-8; 2000.

Watts, David L, PhD, "The nutritional relationships of manganese," *J Orthomol Med,* 5(4):219-22; 1990.

Werbach, MT, *Nutritional Influences on Mental Illness,* Third Line Press, Tarzana, CA, 1991.

Windhurst JM, Manchester KL, "Comparison of ability of Mg and Mn to activate the key enzymes of glycolysis," FEBS Letters, 27:321-6; 1972.

Zinc

Am J Clin Nutr, 42:1229-39; 1985. (Monkeys deprived of zinc were less active, and engaged in fewer types of activities.)

Jeffrey Bland, ed, *Medical Applications of Clinical Nutrition,* Keats, New Canaan, CN, 1983.

Blaylock R, *Excitotoxins, The Taste that Kills,* Health Press, Santa Fe NM, 1995.

Br Med J, 289:273-6; 8/1984.

Constantinidis J, "The hypothesis of zinc deficiency in the pathogenesis of neurofibrillary tangles," *Med Hypoth,* 35:319-23; 1991.

Crawford LL, "Zinc and hippocampal function," *J Orthomol Psychiat,* 4(1):39-52;1974.

Garrison RH, Somer E, *The Nutrition Desk Reference,* Keats, New Canaan, CN, 1985.

Hansen CR, Malecha M, "Copper and zinc deficiencies in association with depression and neurological findings," *Biol Psychiat,* 18(3):395-401; 1983.

Hoffer, Abram, *Orthomolecular Medicine for Physicians,* Keats, New Canaan, CN, 1983.

Jaffe R, Kruesi OR,"The biochemical immunology window: A molecular view of psychiatric case management," *J App Nutr,* 44(2); 1992.

Khan W, et al, "Trace element studies on Karachi population, Part IV: Blood copper, zinc, magnesium and lead levels in psychiatric patients with depression, mental retardation and seizure disorders," *J Pak Med Assn,* 39(10):269-74; 10/1989. (Depressives had significantly lower zinc than normals; significantly higher lead. Similarly, in seizure patients. At least one metal abnormality was found in 21/31 depressives; 6/7 seizure patients.)

Kimura I, Kimura J, "Preliminary reports on the metabolism of trace elements in neuropsychiatric diseases, I. Zinc in schizophrenia," *Proc Japanese Acad Sci,* 1965; p 943. (50% less zinc in frontal, occipital, and hippocampal regions.)

Kroczka B, Branski P, et al, "Antidepressant-like properties of zinc in rodent forced swim test," *Brain Res Bull,* 55:297-300; 2001.

Kroczka B, Zieba A, et al, [Zinc exhibits an antidepressant-like effect in the forced swim test in mice], *Pol J Pharmacol,* 52:403-6; 2000.

Little KY, Castellanos X, "Altered zinc metabolism in mood disorder patients," *Biol Psychiat,* 26(6): 646-8; 1989.

Maes M, D'Haese PC, et al, "Hypozincemia in depression," *J Affect Disorders,* 31:135-40; 1994.

Maes M, Vandoolaeghe H, et al, "Lower serum zinc in major depression is a sensitive marker of treatment resistance and of the immune/inflammatory response in that illness," *Biol Psychiat,* 42(5):349-58; 9/1997. (Intake is effective, though improvement can take 6 wks to emerge.)

Markovits PM, Sankey AW, "Zinc taste test and postnatal depression," *Br J Psychiat,* 156:451-2; 3/1990. (Plasma copper was significantly higher during depression. Zinc increased in recovered patients.)

McLoughlkin IJ, Hodge JS, [Zinc in depressive disorder], *Acta Psychiat Scand,* 82 421-53; 1990.

Murray MT, *Encyclopedia of Nutritional Supplements,* Prima, 1996.

Murray MT, Pizzorno J, *Encyclopedia of Natural Medicine,* Prima, Rocklin, CA, 1998.

Narang RL, Gupta KR, et al, "Levels of copper and zinc in depression," *Indian J Physiol Pharmacol,* 35(4):272-4; 10/1991.

Nichols J, Morgan J, "Postnatal depression and zinc status — A preliminary study," *J Nutr Med,* 3(1): 35-42; 1992.

Nowak G, Siwek M, et al, "Effect of zinc supplementation on antidepressant therapy in unipolar depression: A preliminary placebo-controlled study," *Polish J Pharmacol,* 55:1143-7; 2003.

Nowak G, et al, "Serum trace elements in animal models and human depression, Part I, Zinc," *Hum Psychopharmacol Clin Exp,* 14(2):83-6; 3/1999. (Low serum zinc in 19 unipolars, 16 controls. Confirms prior findings. Chronic severe stress in rats.)

Ossowska G, Lenk-Majewska B, et al, "Antidepressant-like effect of zinc hydroaspartate in a chronic unpredictable stress model of depression," in H Lach, AP Wud Nauk, eds, *Molecular and Physiological Aspects of Regulatory Processes of the Organism,* Krakow, 2003; pp 288-9.

Pfeiffer, CC, Iliev V, "A study of zinc deficiency and copper excess in the schizophrenias," *Intl Rev Neurobiol;* 1972, p 141. (Manganese can triple copper excretion. Effectiveness is enhanced by zinc.)

Pfeiffer CC, "Observations on trace and toxic elements in hair and serum," *J Orthomol Psychiat,* 3(4):259-64; 1974.

Pfeiffer CC, *Mental and Elemental Nutrients,* Keats, New Canaan, CN, 1975.

Pfeiffer CC, LaMola S, "Zinc and manganese in the schizophrenias," *J Orthomol Psychiat,* 12: 215-34; 1983.

Pfeiffer CC, Audette L, "Pyroluria, zinc and B6 deficiencies," *Intl Clin Nutr Rev,* 8(3):107-110; 1988.

Prasad AS, et al, "Experimental zinc deficiency in humans," *Ann Intern Med,* 89:483; 1978. (Associated with lethargy, amnesia, apathy, retardation, irritiability, depression, paranoia.)

Prasad AS, "Clinical biochemical and nutritional spectrum of zinc deficiency in human subjects: An update," *Nutr Rev,* 41;197-208; 1983.

Rogers S, *Depression, Cured at Last,* SK Publishing, Sarasota FL, 1997.

Schlegel-Zawadzka M, et al, "Effect of depression and of antidepressant therapy on serum zinc levels — a preliminary clinical study," in Kluwer, ed, *Trace Elements in Man and Animals,* Academic Plenum Press, 2000; pp 607-10.

Szewczyk B, Branski P, et al, [Interaction of zinc with antidepressant in the forced swimming test in mice], *Pol J Pharmacol,* 54:681-5; 2002.

Tenney L, *Stress,* Woodland Health Bks, 1987.

Walsh WJ, "Zinc deficiency, metal metabolism, and behavior disorders," *A report of the Health Research Institute,* Naperville IL, March 1996.

Watts DL, "The nutritional relationships of zinc," *J Orthomol Med,* 3(2):62-7; 1988.

Werbach, MT, *Nutritional Influences on Mental Illness,* Third Line Press, Tarzana, CA, 1991.

Sodium/Potassium

Balch JF, Balch P, *Prescription for Nutritional Healing,* Avery, Garden City Park, NY, 1990.

Bartoszewicz S, Rybakowski J, [Sodium, potassium and water in affective psychoses], *Psychiatr Pol,* 7(5):577-81; 1973.

Baumel S, *Dealing with Depression Naturally,* Keats, New Canaan, CN, 1995.

Beard TC, et al, "Randomized controlled trial of no-added-sodium diet for mild hypertension," *Lancet,* 455-58; 8/28/1982.

Birdsall TC, "Therapeutic applications of taurine," *Alt Med Rev,* 3(2):128-36; 1998.

Blum A, "The possible role of tobacco cigarette smoking in hyponatremia of long-term psychiatric patients," *JAMA,* 252(20):2864-5; 1984a.

Blum A, "Smoking and hyponatremia in psychiatric patients," *J Clin Psychiat,* 45(8):360-1, 1984b.

Cater, RE, "The use of sodium and potassium to reduce toxicity and toxic side effects from lithium," *Med Hypotheses,* 20(4):359-83; 9/86.

Cox JR, et al, "Changes in sodium, potassium and fluid spaces in depression and dementia," *Gerontol Clin,* 13:232-245; 1971. (Depressed patients may retain more intracellular sodium.)

Demers RG, Heninger GR, "Sodium intake and lithium treatment in mania," *Am J Psychiat,* 128: 199-204; 7/1971. (Increases manic symptoms, reduces lithium side effects.)

Dick DA et al, "Plasma vanadium concentrations in manic- depressive illness," *J Physiol,* 310:27; 1981. (Plasma vanadium correlated negatively with the NA+K+ATPase/ magnesium ratio in 72 bipolars, but not controls.)

Dick DA, Naylor GJ, et al, "Plasma vanadium concentration in manic depressive illness," *Psychol Med,* 12(3):533-37; 8/1982. (Vanadium may alter Na-K-Mg-ATPase activity.)

Ebel H, Gunther T, "Magnesium metabolism: A review," *J Clin Chem Biochem,* 257-70; 1980.

Garrison RH, Somer E, *The Nutrition Desk Reference,* Keats, New Canaan, CN, 1985.

Goggans FC, "Acute hyperkalemia during lithium treatment of manic illness," *Am J Psychiat,* 137(7): 860-1; 1980

Gold MS, *The Good News About Depression,* Villard Books, NY, 1987.

Harland BF, Harden-Williams BA, "Is vanadium of human nutritional importance yet?" *J Am Diet Assoc,* 94:891-4; 1994.

Hiyama T, Yoshimuta N, et al, "Lithium-potassium cotransport across the erythrocyte membrane in affective disorders," *FEBS Letters,* 5(3):265 9/1995.

Hiyama T, [Red cell lithium-potassium cotransport in affective disorders and its clinical significance], *Tokyo Jikeikai Medical J,* 2002.

Jaffe R, Kruesi OR,"The biochemical immunology window: A molecular view of psychiatric case management," *J App Nutr,* 44(2); 1992.

Jandhyala BS, Hom GJ, "Minireview: Physiological and pharmacological properties of vanadium," *Life Sci,* 33(14):1325-40; 10/3/1983.

Joffe RT, Blank DW, et al, "Erythrocyte sodium and potassium in affective illness," 73(4):416-9; 1986. (Sodium was significantly lower, potassium, significantly higher, in 24 depressed and euthymic patients vs. controls.)

Jose CJ, Barton JL, "Hyponatremic seizures in psychiatric patients," 14(5):839-43; 1979. (Review of 34 cases.)

Tom Lane, communication with author, 5/1997.

Larson JM, *Depression Free, Naturally,* Ballantine Wellspring, NY, 2001.

Lesser M, *Nutrition & Vitamin Therapy,* Bantam Books, NY, 1983.

Lieberman S, Bruning N, *The Real Vitamin & Mineral Book,* Avery, Garden City Park, NY, 1990.

Linnoila M, MacDonald E, et al, "RBC membrane adenosine triphosphatase activities in patients with major affective disorders," *Arch Gen Psychiat,* 40(9): 1021-26; 9/1983. (Mean Ca2+ATPase activity was greatest in mania, then depression, then controls, but not in all patients. ATPase activity fluctuated more in affectives and did not reflect Li or Va levels.)

Murray MT, *Encyclopedia of Nutritional Supplements,* Prima, 1996.

Murray MT, Pizzorno J, *Encyclopedia of Natural Medicine,* Prima, Rocklin, CA, 1998.

Naylor, GJ, Corrigan, FM, et al, "Further studies of vanadium in depressive psychosis," *Br J Psychiat,* 150:656-61; 5/87. (In 58 patients, red cell Na/K pump activity showed strong negative correlation with serum vanadium.)

Naylor GJ, Dick DA, et al, "Possible explanation for therapeutic action of lithium, and a possible substitute (methylene-blue)," *Lancet,* 2(8256): 1175-76; 11/21/1981a.

Naylor GJ, Smith AH, "Defective genetic control of sodium pump density in manic depressive psychosis," *Psychol Med,* 11:257-63; 1981b. (Bipolar lymphocytes showed less ability to create new Na pumps upon challenge. Response to Li is accompanied by increased pump activity.)

Naylor GJ, "Reversal of vanadate-induced inhibition of NA-K-ATPase, A possible explanation of the therapeutic effect of carbamazepine in affective illness," *J Affect Disorder,* 8(1):91-93; 1-2/1985.

NutriCircles®, Strickland Computer Consulting, Version 3.25, April 29, 1996.

Ohsawa H, Kishimoto T, et al, [An epidemiological study on hyponatremia in psychiatric patients in mental hospitals in Nara Prefecture], *Jpn J Psychiat Neurol,* 46(4):883-9; 1992. (Retrospective survey found hyponatremia in 10.5% of 1114 schizophrenia, epilepsy, and other psych patients. They tended to early onset, chronic duration, perhaps, nonresponse.)

Page LR, *Healthy Healing,* Healthy Healing, CA, 1992.

Pfeiffer CC, *Mental and Elemental Nutrients,* Keats, New Canaan, CN, 1975.

Pfeiffer CC, *The Schizophrenias Ours to Conquer,* rev ed, Bio-Communications Press, Wichita, KS, 1988.

Quillin P, *Healing Nutrients,* Contemporary Books, Chicago, 1987.

Rayssiguier Y, "Magnesium and lipid interrelationships in the pathogenesis of vascular diseases," *Magnesium Bull,* 3:165; 1981a.

Rayssiguier Y, Gueux E, et al, "Effect of magnesium deficiency on lipid metabolism in rats fed a high carbohdrate diet," *J Nutr,* 111:1876-83; 1981b.

Rayssiguier Y, "Role of magnesium and potassium in the pathology of arteriosclerosis," *Magnesium Bull,* 3:226-38; 1984.

Reddy PL, Khanna S, et al, "Erythrocyte membrane — sodium/potassium adenosine triphosphatase activity in affective disorders," *J Neural Transmission,* 89(3):183-218; 10/1992. (In drug-naive subjects, response to lithium was associated with significantly increased NaK-ATPase activity.)

Rose, JDR, "Disturbed hypothalamic control of Na, K-ATPase: A cause of somatic symptoms of depression," *Med Hypotheses,* 19:179-83; 1986.

Rybakowski J, Potok E, et al, "The activity of the lithium-sodium countertransport system in erythrocytes in depression and mania," *J Affect Disord,* 1981. (Mean countertransport lowest in mania, then bipolar depression, remitted bipolars, controls. Major depressives had higher levels than bipolars.)

Rybakowski J, Potok E, et al, [Decreased activity of ouabain-dependent sodium and potassium fluxes in erythrocytes during depression and mania], *Acta Nerv Super (Praha),* 25(1):72-4; 3/1983.

Rybakowski J, Lehman W, "The activity of erythrocyte sodium-potassium ATPase in affective patients treated with lithium," *Lithium,* Edinburgh, 1993.

Rybakowski J, Strzyzewski W, et al, "Evaluation of the water-electrolyte balance (erythrocyte model) in the course of endogenous depression," *Psychiatr Pol,* 15(3):243-49; 2000.

Tandon R, Channabasavanna SM, et al, [CSF biochemical correlates of mixed affective states], *Acta Psychiatr Scand,* 78(3):289-97; 1988. (Manics showed significantly higher CSF HVA, 5HIAA and sodium.)

Tenney L, *Stress,* Woodland Health Books, 1987.

Thakar JH, Lapierre YD, et al, "Erythrocyte membrane sodium-potassium and magnesium ATPase in primary affective disorder," *Biol Psychiat,* 20:734-40; 7/1985. (Mg-ATPase activity is elevated in well members of affective families. NaK-ATPase was similar for all groups. Lithium didn't change magnesium or sodium pump activity.)

Tollefson GD, Zander J, et al, "Prediction of postdexamethasone cortisol levels by serum sodium levels in patients with major depression," *Am J Psychiat,* 143:81-84; 1986. (Serum sodium was significantly correlated with DST nonsuppression.)

Webb WL, Gehi, M, "Electrolyte and fluid imbalance: Neuropsychiatric manifestation," *Psychosomatics,* 22(3):199-203; 1981. (Low potassium is frequently associated with weakness, fatigue, depression, perhaps, organic brain syndrome. Depressed patients tend to low intracellular potassium. Suicides often show low cerebral potassium.)

Widmer J, et al, "Evolution of blood magnesium, sodium and potassium in depressed patients followed for three months," *Neuropsychobiol,* 26(4):173-79; 4/1992.

Xie X, Hagan RM, "Cellular and molecular actions of lamotrigine: Possible mechanisms of efficacy in bipolar disorder," *Neuropsychobiol,* 38(3): 119-30; 10/1998. (This stabilizer inhibits neuron hyperexcitability, and controls synapse plasticity by inhibiting voltage activated sodium, and perhaps calcium, channels. Presumably, this could modify limbic intra and intercellular signalling.)

Vanadium

Balch JF, Balch PA, *Prescription for Nutritional Healing,* Avery, Garden City Park, NY, 1990.

Bencherif M, Lukas RJ, "Vanadate amplifies receptor-mediated accumulation of inositol trisphosphates and inhibits inositol tris- and tetrakis-phosphatase activities," *Neurosci Lett,* 134(2):157-60; 1/6/1992.

Brichard SM, Henquin JC, "The role of vanadium in the management of diabetes," *Trends Pharmamacol Sci,* 16:265-70; 1995.

Cohen N, et al, "Oral vanadyl sulfate improves hepatic and peripheral insulin-sensitivity in patients with non-insulin-dependent diabetes mellitus," *J Clin Invest,* 95:2501-9; 1995.

Dick DA, et al, "Plasma vanadium concentrations in manic-depressive illness, *J Physiol,* 310:27; 1981. (Plasma vanadium was negatively correlated with Na+K+ATPase/magnesium ratio in 72 bipolars, but not in controls.)

Dick DA, Naylor GJ, et al, "Plasma vanadium concentration in manic depressive illness," *Psychol Med,* 12(3):533-37; 8/1982. (8 bipolars, 9 controls. Mean plasma vanadium was highest in manics, then depressed, then euthymics, then normals. Vanadium may alter sodium pump and Na-K-Mg-ATPase activity in bipolars.)

Dick DA, Naylor GJ, et al, "Plasma vanadium concentration in manic-depressive illness," *Med Hypotheses,* 12(3):253-68; 1983.

Harland BF, Harden-Williams BA, "Is vanadium of human nutritional importance yet?" *J Am Diet Assoc,* 94:891-4; 1994.

Harvey NS, Jarratt J, et al, "Trace elements and the electroencephalogram during long-term lithium treatment," *Br J Psychiat,* 160:654-58; 5/1992. (In 12 patients, irregular cortical activity (EEG) was associated with elevated Br, Va, and Li.

Jandhyala BS, Hom GJ, "Minireview: Physiological and pharmacological properties of vanadium," *Life Sci,* 33(14):1325-40; 10/3/1983. (Vanadium was first noted as an inhibitor of the membrane sodium/potassium pump. It may also influence certain intracellular enzymes, homeostatic mechanisms, and neurological and cardiovascular status.)

Kay DS, Naylor GJ, et al, "The therapeutic effect of ascorbic acid and EDTA in manic depressive psychosis: Double-blind comparisons with standard treatments," *Psychol Med,* 14(3):533-39; 9/1984. (Depressed patients responded to C plus EDTA, and to amitriptyline. Manics responded better to lithium. Vanadium may play a role in depressive psychosis, but not mania.)

Larson JM, *Depression Free, Naturally,* Ballantine Wellspring, NY, 2001

Murray MT, Pizzorno J, *Encyclopedia of Natural Medicine,* Prima, Rocklin, CA, 1998.

Naylor GJ, Smith AH, et al, "Elevated vanadium content of hair and mania," *Biol Psychiat,* 19(5): 759-64; 5/1984a. (Significantly greater than in recovered manics or controls.)

Naylor GJ, Smith AH, "Tissue vanadium levels in manic-depressive psychosis," *Psychol Med,* 14(4): 767-72; 11/1984b. (Elevated whole blood and serum vanadium in depression, decreased with recovery. High hair levels in mania. Serum and blood vanadium strongly correlated; hair levels were unrelated.)

Naylor GJ, Dick DA, et al, "Possible explanation for therapeutic action of lithium, and a possible substitute (methylene-blue)," *Lancet,* 2(8256):1175-76; 11/21/1981a.

Naylor GJ, Smith AH, "Vanadium: A possible aetiological factor in manic depressive illness," *Psychological Med,* 11:249-63; 1981b.

Naylor GJ, Smith AH, et al, "Catalysis of the reduction of vanadate by psychotropic drugs," *Neuropharmacol,* 22(5):653-56; 5/1983. (Methylene blue was the most effective. Phenothiazines and MAOIs catalyze vanadate reduction by NADH. Tricyclics and benzodiazepines do not.)

Naylor GJ, "Reversal of vanadate-induced inhibition of NA-K-ATPase. A possible explanation of the therapeutic effect of carbamazepine in affective illness", *J Affect Disord,* 8(1):91-93; 1-2/1985. (CBZ largely reverses inhibition of Na-K ATPase in vitro.)

Naylor, GJ, Corrigan, FM, et al, "Further studies of vanadium in depressive psychosis," *Br J Psychiatr,* 150:656-61; 5/1987. (Hair, blood and serum levels decreased with recovery in 13 depressive psychosis patients (perhaps underlying Na transport changes). In another study of 31 patients, mean renal vanadium clearance was supressed and mean serum concentration elevated in depression vs. controls. In a third study, red cell Na-K ATPase activity was strongly negatively correlated to serum vanadium.

Pfeiffer CC, *The Schizophrenias Ours to Conquer,* rev ed, Bio-Communications Press, Wichita, KS, 1988.

Witkowska D, Brzyinski J, [Alteration of brain noradrenaline, dopamine and 5-hydroxytryptamine levels during vanadium poisoning], *Pol J Pharmacol Pharm,* 31:393-98; 1979.

Yung CY, "A synopsis on metals in medicine and psychiatry," *Pharmacol Biochem Behav,* 21(S1): 41-47; 1984. (Review. Excess vanadium may contribute to bipolar symptoms.)

Iron

Arthur JR, Beckett GJ, "Thyroid function," 55(3):658-668; 11/1999. (Too much or too little Fe, Zn, and Cu adversely alter thyroid hormone metabolism.)

Balch JF, Balch PA, *Prescription for Nutritional Healing,* Avery, Garden City Park, NY, 1990.

Beard J, Tobin B, et al, "Evidence for thyroid hormone deficiency in iron-deficient anemic rats," *J Nutr,* 119(5):772-8; 5/1989. (May underly poor response to cold in iron-deficient anemia.)

Beard JL, Borel MJ, et al, "Impaired thermoregulation and thyroid function in iron-deficiency anemia," *Am J Clin Nutr,* 52:813-99; 1990. (Sufficient iron to correct anemia improved temperature and partially corrected plasma thyroid.)

Beard JL, Brigham DE, et al, "Plasma thyroid hormone kinetics are altered in iron-deficient rats," *J Nutr,* 12/1997.

Beard JL, Erikson KM, et al, "Neurobehavioral analysis of developmental iron deficiency in rats," *Behav Brain Res,* 134(1-2):517-24; 2002. (Anxiety behaviors increased; activity and exploration decreased, in weaned rats on a 6 wk, Fe-deficient diet. Low corpus striatum, PFC, and midbrain iron was associated with reduced DA receptors and transporters. Anxiety related to reduced D1 receptor density, and reduced PFC DA transporter density.)

Bocchetta A, Severino G, et al, "Associations between heterozygous beta-thalasemia, glucose-6-phosphate dehydrogenase deficiency, and affective disorders of the bipolar spectrum," *It J Psychiat Behav Sci,* 3:107-10; 1993.

Bocchetta A, Del Zompo M, "Bipolar affective disorder and heterozygous beta-thalasemia," *Am J Psychiat,* 147(8):1094; 1990.

Brodie, BB, "Heterozygous beta-thalassemia as a susceptibility factor in mood disorders: Excessive prevalence in bipolar patients," *Clin Prac Epid Ment Health,* 1(6):1745-9; 2005. (In an estimated 16% of 732 bipolars; 10% of 282 other psych patients.)

Casdorph HR, Walker M, *Toxic Metal Syndrome:* Avery, Garden City Park, NY, 1995.

Cousens G, *Depression Free for Life,* Quill, HarperCollins, NY, 2001.

Cutler P, "Iron overload in psychiatric illness," *Am J Geriat,* 148:147-48; 1/1991.

Eseh R, Zimmerberg B, "Age-dependent effects of gestational and lactational iron deficiency on anxiety behavior in rats," *Behav Brain Res,* 164(2):214-21; 11/2005. (Worsened by maternal deficiency, somewhat reversed with repletion, though some effects continue through adulthood.)

Garrison RH, Somer E, *The Nutrition Desk Reference,* Keats, New Canaan, CN, 1985.

Gold MS, *The Good News About Depression,* Villard Books, NY, 1987.

Heath AL, Skeaff CM, "The treatment of mild iron deficiency by iron supplementation and diet and its impact on mood," *New Zealand Nutrition Society Conference,* Auckland, New Zealand, 1999.

Heath AL, Penland JG, et al, "Cognitive effects of non-anaemic iron deficiency in adult women," *Ann Nutr Metab,* 45:510; 2001.

Heath AL, Fairweather-Tait SJ, "Health implications of iron overload: The role of diet and genotype," *Nutr Rev,* 61:45-62; 2003.

Hoffer A, *Orthomolecular Medicine for Physicians,* Keats, New Canaan, CN, 1983.

Jaffe R, Kruesi OR,"The biochemical immunology window: A molecular view of psychiatric case management," *J App Nutr,* 44(2); 1992.

Konofal E, Lecendreux M, "Iron deficiency in children with attention-deficit/hyperactivity disorder," *Arch Pediatr Adolesc Med,* 158:113-5; 2004. (Controlled comparison study. Serum ferritin was abnormal in 84% of 53 ADHD children and some children with behavior disorders, retardation, mood, or anxiety disorders. Low levels correlated with more severe symptoms.)

Leedman PJ, Stein AR, et al, "Thyroid hormone modulates the interaction between iron regulatory proteins and the ferritin mRNA iron-responsive element," *J Biol Chem,* 271(20):12017-23; 5/1996. (T3 can thus upregulate liver ferritin expression, increasing serum ferritin. Elevation is seen in hyperthyroids.)

Lieberman S, Bruning N, *The Real Vitamin & Mineral Book,* Avery, Garden City Park, NY, 1990.

Maes M, Van de Vyvere J, "Alterations in iron metabolism and the erythron in major depression: Further evidence for a chronic inflammatory process," *J Affect Disord,* 40(1-2):23-33; 1996. (38 depressives showed significantly reduced serum iron and red cells, related to inflammatory markers.

NutriCircles®, Strickland Computer Consulting, Version 3.25, April 29, 1996.

Nutr Rev, "Do diets high in iron impair manganese status?," 51(3):86-88; 1993.

Page LR, *Healthy Healing,* Healthy Healing, CA, 1992.

Parker, SD, "Depression and nutrition: Anemia and glucose imbalances," *Anabolism;* 1-2/1984.

Pfeiffer CC, *Mental and Elemental Nutrients,* Keats, New Canaan, CN, 1975.

Pfeiffer CC, *Nutrition and Mental Illness,* Healing Arts Press, Rochester, VT, 1987.

Pfeiffer CC, *The Schizophrenias Ours to Conquer,* rev ed, Bio-Communications Press, Wichita, KS, 1988.

Politt E, "Iron deficiency and cognitive function," *Ann Rev Nutr,* 13:521-37; 7/1993.

Politt E, "Developmental sequel from early nutritional deficiencies: Conclusive and probability judgments," *Am Soc Nutr Sci,* 130:350-3S; 2000.

Quillin P, *Healing Nutrients,* Contemporary Books, Chicago, 1987.

Richardson JS, Subbarao KV, et al, "On the possible role of iron-induced free radical peroxidation in neural degeneration in Alzheimer's disease," *Ann NY Acad Sci,* 648:326-27; 1992.

Rogers S, *Depression, Cured at Last,* SK Publishing, Sarasota FL, 1997.

Slagle P, "Iron deficiency/ Iron excess/ hemochromatosis," *The Way Up Newletter Archives,* #37 At: thewayup.com/newletters/newsarch.htm

Swain J, Penland J, "Energy, mood and attention did not consistently improve with iron status in non-anemic women with moderate to low iron stores," *Fed Am Soc, Experimental Biology Conference,* 3/2006. (Randomized, blind. 52 premenopausal low-iron women given heme, electrolytic iron, reduced iron, FeSO4, or placebo. Fatigue improved only with heme or FeSO4. Attention improved most at the outset. Improvements in mood and attention were subtle.)

Tucker DM, et al, "Iron status and brain function," *Am J Clin Nutr,* 39:105-13; 1984.

Walsh, WJ, PhD, "Commentary on nutritional treatment of mental disorders, *International Guide to the World of Alternative Mental Health* at: www.alternativementalhealth.com/articles.walshMP.htm#Py Accessed:10/08/2006.

Werbach, MT, *Nutritional Influences on Mental Illness,* Third Line Press, Tarzana, CA, 1991.

Youdim MB, Ben-Shachar D, et al, "Brain iron and dopamine receptor function," *Adv Biochem Psychopharmacol,* 37:309-21; 1982. (Brain iron is concentrated in DA structures (important to attention and learning). Deficiency in rats interferes with brain protein synthesis, and reduces D2 receptor binding sites, downregulating DA activity.)

Youdim MB, Ashkenazi R, et al, "Modulation of dopamine receptor in the striatum by iron: Behavioral and biochemical correlates," *Adv Neurol,* 40:159-70; 1984.

Youdim M, "Nutrient deprivation and brain function: Iron," *Nutrition,* 16(7-8):504-8; 2000.

Copper

Arthur JR, Beckett GJ, "Thyroid function," 55(3):658-668; 11/1999. (Too much or too little iron, zinc, and copper adversely alter thyroid metabolism.)

Balch JF, Balch PA, *Prescription for Nutritional Healing,* Avery, Garden City Park, NY, 1990.

Br Med J, 289:273-6; 8/1984.

Casdorph HR Walker M, *Toxic Metal Syndrome,* Avery, Garden City Park, NY, 1995.

Garrison RH, Somer E, *The Nutrition Desk Reference,* Keats, New Canaan, CN, 1985.

Hoffer Abram, *Orthomolecular Medicine for Physicians,* Keats, New Canaan, CN, 1983.

Ieba A, Kata R, et al, "Serum trace elements in animal models and human depression: Part III. Magnesium. Relationship with copper," *Human Psychopharmacol,* 15(8):631-35; 12/2000. (Serum magnesium was significantly lower than controls in 19 unipolars. Levels relative to copper were significantly correlated with severity.)

Jaffe R, Kruesi OR,"The biochemical immunology window: A molecular view of psychiatric case management," *J App Nutr,* 44(2); 1992.

Lieberman S, Bruning N, *The Real Vitamin & Mineral Book,* Avery, Garden City Park, NY, 1990.

Marlowe M, "Decreased magnesium in the hair of autistic children," *J Orthomol Psychiat,* 13:117-22; 1984.

NutriCircles®, Strickland Computer Consulting, Version 3.25, April 29, 1996.

Page LR, *Healthy Healing,* Healthy Healing, CA, 1992.

Pfeiffer CC, Iliev V, "A study of zinc deficiency and copper excess in the schizophrenias," *Intl Rev Neurobiol;* 1972, p 141. (Manganese can triple copper excretion, or more if used with zinc.)

Pfeiffer CC, *Mental and Elemental Nutrients,* Keats, New Canaan, CN, 1975.

Pfeiffer CC, *Nutrition and Mental Illness,* Healing Arts Press, Rochester, VT, 1987.

Quillin P, *Healing Nutrients,* Contemporary Books, Chicago, 1987.

Siwek M, Wrobel A, et al, [The role of copper and magnesium in the pathogenesis and treatment of affective disorders] *Polish, Psychiatr Pol,* 39(5):911-20; 9-10/2005. (Significantly altered.)

Sohler A, Pfeiffer CC, "Excess copper and lead as factors in the aging process," *J Orthomol Med,* 2(2): 97-105; 1987

Strausak D, Mercer JF, et al, "Copper in disorders with neurological symptoms: Alzheimer's, Menke's, and Wilson's diseases," *Brain Res Bull,* 55(2):175-85; 5/2001.

Walsh, WJ, PhD, "Commentary on nutritional treatment of mental disorders, *International Guide to the World of Alternative Mental Health* at: www.alternativementalhealth.com/articles.walshMP.htm#Py Accessed:10/08/2006.

Lithium *(See also pp 309-10)*

Missiha FS, "Lithium, rubidium, and cesium: Cerebral pharmacokinetics and alcohol interactions," *Pharmacol, Biochem & Behav,* 21: 1, 87-92; 1984.

Whybrow, Peter C, MD, *A Mood Apart, Depression, Mania, and Other Afflictions of the Self,* Basic Books, HarperCollins, NY, 1997.

Boron

McGinnis Woody MD, "Pyroluria: Hidden cause of schizophrenia, bipolar, depression, and anxiety symptoms," Orlando, 5/21/2004. At: alternativementalhealth.com/articles/pyroluria.htm

Nielsen FH, Hunt CD, et al, "Effect of dietary boron on mineral, estrogen and testosterone metabolism in postmenopausal women," *FASEB J,* 1(5):394-7; 11/1987. (Intake by postmenopausal women on low-boron diets prevents calcium and magnesium loss, and increases serum 17-beta-estradiol and testosterone, especially where magnesium starts low.)

Rubidium

Baumel S, *Dealing with Depression Naturally,* Keats, New Canaan, CN, 1995.

Brundusino AO, Cairoli S, [The pharmacological action of rubidium chloride in depression], *Minerva Psichiatr,* 37(1):45-9; 3/1996. (Stimulates dopamine. 15 depressives improved relatively rapidly, without signficant side effects.)

Carolei A, Sonsini U, et al, "Pharmacologic action of rubidium chloride. Antidepressant effects: Comparison with imipramine," *Clin Ter,* 75(5): 469-78; 12/1975.

Fieve RR, *Moodswing,* Bantam Books, 1976.

Malek-Ahmadi P, Williams JA, "Rubidium in Psychiatry: Research Implications," *Pharmacol Biochem Behav,* 21(S1):49-50; 1984.

Missiha FS, "Lithium, rubidium, and cesium: Cerebral pharmacokinetics and alcohol interactions, *Pharmacol Biochem Behav,* 21:1, 87-92; 1984.

Paschalis C, Jenner FA, "Effects of rubidium chloride on the course of manic-depressive illness," *JR Soc Med,* 71(5):343-52; 5/1978. (Can increase manic duration, but may reduce mood extremes. No severe side effects, but a long half-life.)

Placidi G, Lenzi A, et al, "Exploration of the clinical profile of rubidium chloride in depression: A systemic open trial," *J Clin Psychopharmacol,* 8(3):184-8; 6, 1988. (Two-thirds of 31 depressives treated with 180-720 mg improved significantly by week 2. Side effects were generally mild: diarrhea, polyuria, excitement.)

Torta R, Ala G, et al, [Rubidium chloride in the treatment of major depression], *Minerva Psichiatr* 34(2):101-10; 6/1993. (360 or 720 mg led to gradual improvement in depression and anxiety in 20 unipolars, mean age 55 (but was not correlated with serum levels). Benefits were greatest to mood, conservatism, work, and psychomotor slowing. Side effects included diarrhea and skin rash.)

Williams RH, Maturen A, et al, "Pharmacologic role of rubidium in psychiatric research," *Compr Ther,* 13(9):46-54; 9/1987. (Therapeutic in some depressions; relatively nontoxic.)

Germanium

Asai K, *Organic germanium: A Medical Godsend,* Kogakusha, 1977. (Feeling of warmth within 10 minutes, healthy glow, cheerfulness, sound sleep, increased mental acuity. Releases oxygen from water and brings it to body tissue.)

Asai K, *Miracle cure: Organic Germanium,* Japan Publications, 1980.

Asai K, "Ge-132, Outline," *Izumihoncho,* 1-6-4, Koami-Shi, Tokyo, 1984.

Balch JF, Balch PA, *Prescription for Nutritional Healing,* Avery, Garden City Park, NY, 1990.

J Pharmacobio-Dynamics, 6:814-20; 1983.

Levine S, Huntington K, "Organic germanium: Restoring health through increased oxygenation," *Total Health,* 18, 1986a.

Levine SA, Kidd PM, "Oxygen nutrition for super health," *J Orthomol Med,* 11(3);145-8; 1986b.

Lieberman S, Bruning N, *The Real Vitamin & Mineral Book,* Avery, Garden City Park, NY, 1990.

Microbiol Immunology, 29:65-74; 1985.

Tanaka T, Chofu Hospital, "Treatment of depressive psychosis," in Asai, K, *Miracle cure: Organic germanium,* 1980. (Up to 70-100 mg per day, divided doses, improved depression and insomnia.)

Cesium

Ali SA, Peet M, et al, "Blood levels of vanadium, caesium and other elements in depressive patients," *J Affect Dis,* 9:187-91; 1985.

Missiha FS, Krantz J, "Effect of cesium ion on cerebral activity of the mouse," *Am J Pharmacol,* 145:17-21; 1973.

Missiha FS, "Cesium ion: Antagonism to chlorpromazine and levodopa-induced behavioral depression in mice," *J Pharm Pharmacol,* 27:873-74; 1975.

Missiha FS, "Antidepressant action of cesium chloride and its modification of chlorpromazine toxicity in mice," *Br J Pharmacol,* 64:9-12; 1977.

Missiha FS, "Lithium, rubidium, and cesium: Cerebral pharmacokinetics and alcohol interactions, *Pharmacol Biochem Behav,* 21:1, 87-92; 1984.

Rogers S, *Depression, Cured at Last,* SK Publishing, Sarasota FL, 1997.

St. John's wort

Ayd Frank J, Jr, MD, "Evaluating interactions between herbal and psychoactive medications," *Psychiatric Times,* XVII(12); 12/2000. At: http://www.mhsource.cm/pt/p001245.html

Blumental M, Busse WR, et al, "The Complete German Commission E Monographs: Therapeutic Guide to Herbal Medicines," *Am Botanical Council,* Austin TX and *Integrative Medicine Communications,* Boston, 1998; pp 156-7.

Brenner R, Asbel V, et al, "Comparison of an extract of hypericum (LI 160) and sertraline in the treatment of depression: A double-blind, randomized pilot study," *Clin Ther,* 22:411-9; 2000.

Cesarin P, "The experimental and clinical pharmacology of St John's wort (Hypericum perforatum L)," *Mol Psychiat,* 4:333-8; 1999. (Low side effects. Some drug interactions.)

Cott JM, Rosenthal N, et al, "St John's wort and major depression," *JAMA,* 286:42-45; 2001.

Cott JM, Fugh-Berman A, "Is St John's wort (Hypericum perforatum) an effective antidepressant?" *J Nerv Ment Dis,* 186(8):500-1; 8/1998.

Ernst, E, et al, "Complementary therapies for depression: An overview," *Arch Gen Psychiat,* 55: 1026-32; 1998.

www.amoryn.com/formulat.html 12/28/2005

Fava M, et al, "A double-blind randomized trial of St. John's Wort, fluoxetine, and placebo in major depressive disorder," *J Clin Psychopharmacol,* 25(5): 441-47; 10/2005. (Small randomized double blind; 1 wk washout. Significantly more effective than the drug. Trend (probably more significant in a larger study) to superiority over placebo. Safe, well tolerated.

Fetrow, Avila, Committee on Safety of Medicines, *Inst for Natural Products Research,* 1999.

Fugh-Berman A, Cott JM, "Dietary supplements and natural products as psychotherapeutic agents," *Psychosom Med,* 61:712-28; 1999. (Valerian or kava, etc., for insomnia. SAMe, folate, tryptophan, phenylalanine, hypericum, or ginkgo, adjunctively for depression.)

Fugh-Berman A, Miller LG, "Herbal medicinals: Selected clinical considerations, focusing on potential drug-herb interactions," *Arch Intern Med,* 159:1957-9; 1999.

Harrer G, Schmidt U, et al, [Comparison of equivalence between the St John's wort extract, LoHyp-57, and fluoxetine], *Arzneimmittelforschung,* 49:289-96; 1999. (Comparable to SSRIs.)

Kim HL, Streltzer J, et al, "St John's wort for depression: A meta analysis of well defined clinical trials," *J Nerv Ment Dis,* 187:532-8; 1999. (Suggests hypericum is 50% better than placebo, and equivalent to antidepressants.)

Klepser TB, Klepser ME, "Unsafe and potentially safe herbal therapies," *Am J Health-System Pharmacy,* 56(2):125-38; 1999. (Views as unsafe: borage, calamus, coltsfoot, comfrey, chapparel, germander, licorice, life root, ma huang. Potentially safe: feverfew, garlic, ginkgo, Asian ginseng, saw palmetto, St Johnswort, valerian.)

Lantz as cited in Fugh Berman 2000.

Linde K, Ramirez G, et al, "St John's wort for depression — an overview and meta-analysis of randomized clinical trails," *BMJ,* 313(7052):253-8; 8/3/96. (Meta-analysis of 23 randomized trials (15 placebo-controlled; 8, comparisons with drugs) involving 1757 mild to moderate depressives. Effectiveness was comparable to meds, and significantly above placebo. Side effects occured in 20% on hypericum, 52% on antidepressants. Dropouts due to side effects were 0.8% on hypericum; 3.0% on meds.)

Mowrey, Daniel B, PhD, *The Scientific Validation of Herbal Medicine,* Keats, New Canaan, CN, 1986.

Muldner H, Soller M, [Antidepressive effect of a hypericum extract standardized to the active hypericine complex], *Arzneim Forsch,* 34:918-20; 1984. (Improvement in anxiety, depression, insomnia, anorexia in 15 female patients.)

Murray MT, Pizzorno J, *Encyclopedia of Natural Medicine,* Prima, Rocklin, CA, 1998.

Murray, Michael T, ND, *Stress, Anxiety & Insomnia,* Prima, Rocklin, CA, 1995.

Nierenberg AA, Burt T, et al, "Mania associated with St John's wort", *Biol Psychiat,* 46(12):1707-8; 12/15/1999. (2 cases of temporary mania.)

Roby CA, Anderson GD, et al, "St John's Wort: Effect on CYP3A4 activity," *Clin Pharmacol Ther,* 67(5):451-7; 2000.

Ruschitzka, et al, Committee on Safety of Medicines, Inst for Natural Products Research 2000.

Schrader E, "Equivalence of St John's wort extract (Ze 117) and fluoxetine: A randomized controlled study in mild to moderate depression," *Intl Clin Psychopharmacol,* 15:61-68; 2000.

Somner, H, "Improvement of psychovegetative complaints by hypericum," *4th International Congress on Psychotherapy,* Munich, 9/10-3, 1992, abst SL55.

Stoll AL, *The Omega-3 Connection,* Simon & Schuster, NY, 2002.

Suzuki, O, et al, [Inhibition of monamine oxidase by hypericin], *Planta, Medica,* 50:272-74; 1984.

Szegedi A, Kohnen R, et al, "Acute treatment of moderate to severe depression with hypericum extract WS 5570 (St John's wort): Randomized controlled double blind non-inferiority trial versus paroxetine," BMJ, 330:503; 3/2005. (251 moderate-to-severe major depressives from over 21 psychiatric practices. The herb was at least as effective as the drug, and better tolerated.)

Tenney L, *Stress,* Woodland Health Books, 1987.

Woelk, H, "Multicentric practice study analyzing the functional capacity in depressive patients," *4th Intl Congress on Psychotherapy,* Munich, 9/10-13, 1992, abst. SL54.

Ginkgo biloba

Auguet M, De Feudis V, Clostre F, "Effects of ginkgo biloba on arterial smooth muscle responses to vasoactive stimuli," *Gen Pharmac,* 13:169; 1982.

Auget M, et al, [Pharmacological basis for the vascular effects of Ginkgo biloba extract], *Presse Med,* 15(31):1524-8; 1986.

Bolanos-Jimenez, et al, "Stress induced 5HT 1A receptor desensitization: Protective effects on Ginkgo biloba extract (Egb 761)," *Fundam Clin Pharmacol,* 9:169-74; 1995.

Braquet P, Hosford D, "Ethnopharmacology and the development of natural PAF antagonists as therapeutic agents," *J Ethnopharmacol,* 32:135-39; 1991.

Cohen A, "Treatment of antidepressant-induced sexual dysfunction with Ginkgo biloba extract," *New Research Report from the Proceedings of the APA Annual meeting,* Abst #716; 1996.

Cohen AJ, Bartilik BD, "Ginkgo biloba for drug-induced sexual dysfunction," *Proceedings of the APA Annual Meeting,* San Diego, 1997.

Cohen GD, "The magic bullets are blanks. Purported shortcuts to improving the aging mind," *AJGP,* 6(33): 185-95; 1998.

Etienne A, Hecquet F, et al, "Comparison of the effects of an extract of Ginkgo biloba and chloropromazine on the osmotic fragility, in vitro, of rat erythrocytes," *J Pharmacol,* 13(291); 1982.

Gaby AR, "Ginkgo biloba extract: A review," *Alt Med Rev,* 1996.

Gebner, et al, [Study of the long-term action of a Ginkgo biloba extract on vigilence and and mental performance as determined by means of quantitative pharmaco-EEG and psychosomatic measurements], *Arznern-Forsch,* 35:1459-65; 1985.

Hofferberth B, [Effect of Ginkgo biloba extract on neurophysiological and psychometric measurement results in patients with cerebro-organic syndrome. A double-blind study versus placebo], *Arneimittelforsch,* 39:918-22; 1989.

Itil TM, Eralp E, et al, "The pharmacological effects of Ginkgo biloba, a plant extract on the brain of dementia patients in comparison with tacrine," *Psychopharmacol Bull,* 34(3):391-7; 1998. (Comparable with a number of cognitive activators and antidementia drugs.)

Kanowski S, et al, "Proof of efficacy of the Ginkgo biloba special extract EGB 761 in outpatients suffering from mild to moderate primary degenerative dementia of the Alzheimer type of multi-infarct dementia," *Pharmacopsychiat,* 29:47-56; 1996.

Kleijnen J, Knipschild P, "Ginkgo biloba for cerebral insufficiency," *Br J Clin Pharmacol,* 34:352-8; 1992.

Kniegistein et al, "Neuroprotective effects of Ginkgo biloba constituents," *Eur J Pharma Sci;* 1995.

Mowrey, DB, *Next Generation Herbal Medicine,* Keats, New Canaan, CN, 1990.

Murray MT, *The Healing Power of Herbs,* Prima Pub, Rocklin CA, 1995.

Murray MT, Pizzorno J, *Encyclopedia of Natural Medicine,* Prima, Rocklin, CA, 1998.

Peter H, [Vasoactivity of ginkgo bilboa preparation], in B Dumbovith, ed, *4th Conference Jungian Ther Invert Pharmacol, Soc Pharmacol,* Hungary, 1968; pp 177.

Petkov, et al, [Memory effects of standardized extracts of Panax ginseng (G115), Ginkgo biloba (GK501), and their combination (Gincosan R (PHL-00701)], *Planta Med,* 59:106-13; 1993.

Racagni G, et al, [Neurotransmitter changes during cerebral aging. The effect of Ginkgo biloba extract], *Presse Med,* 15(31):1488-90; 1986.

riverhouse.com.au/factsheets/ginkgo.html "Fact sheet: Ginkgo biloba"

Schubert H, Halama P, [Depressive episode primarily unresponsive to therapy in elderly patients: Efficacy of Ginkgo biloba extract (EGB 761) in combination with antidepressants], *Geratr Forsch,* 3:45-53; 1993. (40 older antidepressant-unresponsive patients with mild cognitive dysfunction were randomly assigned to 80 mg gingko, 3x/day, or placebo. The gingko group showed 50% reduction in depression (HAM-D) at 4 wks, 68% at 8 wks. Placebo, under 10%.

Werbach MR, Murray MT, *Botanical Influences on Illness,* Third Line Press, Tarzana, CA, 1994.

Zeng X, Liu M, "Gingko biloba for acute ischaemic stroke," *Cochrane Database of Systematic Reviews,* Issue 4, #CD003691; 2005.

Ginseng

Farnsworth NR, et al, "Siberian ginseng: Current status as an adaptogen," *Econ Med Plant Res,* 1: 156-215; 1985.

Fulder SJ, "Ginseng and the hypothalamic-pituitary control of stress," *Am J Clin Med,* 9(2):112-8; 1981.

Gonzalez-Seiji, et al, 1995, cited in Ayd 12/2000.

Hal S, Yokoyama H, et al, [Stimulation of pituitary-adrenocortical system by ginseng saponins], *Endocrinologica Japonica,* 26(6):661-5; 1979.

Jones BD, Runikis AM, et al, "Interaction of ginseng with phenelzine," *J Clin Psychopharmacol,* 7(3):201-2; 6/1987.

Karman B, *Siberian Ginseng: Latest research on the fabled oriental tonic herb,* Keats, 1988.

Kehara M, Shibata Y, et al, [Effect of ginseng saponins on cholesterol metabolism, III Effect of ginsenoside Rb on cholesterol synthesis in rats fed on high fat diet], *Chem Pharma Bull,* Tokyo, 26(9):2844-54.

Medon PJ, Ferguson PW, et al, "Effects of Eleutherococcus senticosus extracts on hexobarbital metabolism in vivo and in vitro," *J Ethnopharmacol,* 1984. (May interact with barbiturates.)

Pefkov VW, [About the method of operation of Panax ginseng], *Arzneimittel-Forschumg,* 11, 288-95; 1961.

Shader RI, Greenblatt DJ, "Bees, ginseng, and MAOIs revisited," *J Clin Psychopharmacol,* 8(4): 235; 8/1988.

Vogler BK, Pittler MH, et al, "The efficacy of ginseng. A systematic review of randomized clinical trials," *J Clin Pharmacol,* 55:567-75; 1999.

Wong HCG, Miller LG, "Probably false authentication of herbal plants: Ginseng," *Arch Intern Med,* 159:1142-43; 1999.

Gotu kola

Balch JF, Balch PA, *Prescription for Natural Healing,* Avery, Garden City Park, NY, 1990.

Chen Y, Han T, et al, [Effect of total triterpenes from centella asiatica on the depression behavior and concentration of amino acid in forced swimming mice], *Zhong Yao Cai,* 26(12):870-3; 12/2003. (Triterpenes reduce immobility and benefit amino balance, suggesting antidepressant activity.)

Chen Y, Han T, et al, [Effect of total triterpenes of centella asiatica on the corticosterone levels in serum and contents of monoamine in depression rat brain], *Zhong Yao Cai,* 28(6):492-6; 6/2005. (Significantly reduced corticosterone, suggesting benefit to HPA axis; and increased Ser, NE, DA.)

Kloss Jethro, *Back to Eden,* Woodbridge Press, Santa Barbara, CA, 1973.

Mowrey DB, *The Scientific Validation of Herbal Medicine,* Keats, New Canaan, CN, 1986a.

Murray MT, *The Healing Power of Herbs,* Prima Pub, Rocklin CA, 1995; pp 173-83.

Noni la'au

Abbot IA, The geographic origin of the plants most commonly used for medicine by Hawaiians, *J Ethnopharmacol,* 14:213-22; 1985.

American Chemical Society, "Noni plant may yield new drugs to fight tuberculosis," press release, *The 2000 International Chemical Congress of Pacific Basin Societies.*

Atkinson N, "Antibacterial substances from flowering plants. 3. Antibacterial activity of dried Australian plants by a rapid direct plate test," *Austral J Exper Biol,* 34:17-26; 1956.

Bushnell OA, Fukuda M, et al, "The antibacterial properties of some plants found in Hawaii," *Pacific Sci,* 4:167-83; 1950.

Elkins R, *Noni: Prize Herb of the South Pacific,* Woodland Publishing, Pleasant Grove, UT, 1997.

Heinicke RM, "The pharmacologically active ingredient of Noni," *Bull Natl Tropical Bot Garden,* 1985a.

Henicke RM, *Pacific Tropical Botanical Garden Bulletin,* 1985b.

Henicke RM, "The Xeroxine system: A new cellular mechanism that explains the health promoting action of noni and bromelian," *Direct Source Publishing,* 2001.

Hirazumi A, et al, "Anticancer activity of Morinda citrifolia (Noni) on intraperitoneally implanted Lewis lung carcinoma in syngenetic mice," *Proc West Pharmacol Soc,* 37:145-6; 1994.

Hirazumi A, Furusawa E, et al, "Immunomodulation contributes to the anticancer activity of Morinda citrifolia (noni) fruit juice," *Proc West Pharmacol Soc,* 39:7-9; 1996b.

Langford J, Doughty A, et al, "Effects of Morinda citrifolia on auditory function and quality of life in patients with decreased bone mineral density and auditory function," *J Comp Altern Med,* submitted 2002. (Improves depression and mental health.)

Leach AJ, Leach DN, et al, "Antibacterial activity of some medicinal plants of Papua New Guinea," *Sci New Guinea,* 14:1-7; 1988. (Countering *E coli, H pylori.*)

Mueller BA, Scott MK, et al, "Noni juice (Morinda citrifolia): Hidden potential for hyperkalemia?" *Am J Kidney Dis,* 35:310-2; 2000. (High potassium.)

Rai RK, "Screening of indigenous plants for anthelmintic action against human Ascaris Lumbricoides: Part II," *Indian J Physiol Pharmacol,* 19:47-9; 1975. (Insecticide, nematode.)

Saxema AK, Panhotra BR, "Herbal remedies: Renal tragedies," *Swiss Med Wkly,* 2003.

Solomon N, "Nature's amazing healer, Noni," *Woodland Publishing,* Pleasant Grove, UT, 1998.

Solomon N, "The Noni phenomenon." *Direct Source Publishing,* 1999.

Solomon N, "Tahitian noni juice: How much, how often, for what," *Direct Source Publishing,* 2000.

Solomon N, "Tahitian noni juice — The pain fighter," Direct Source, 2001.

Wang MY, Brett JW, et al, "Morinda citrifolia: A literature review and recent advances in Noni research," *Acta Pharmacol Sin,* 23(12):1127-1141; 2002.

Goji

Chan HC, Chang RC, et al, "Neuroprotective effects of Lycium barbarum Lynn on protecting retinal ganglion cells in an ocular hypertension model of glaucoma," *Exp Neurol,* 203(1):269-73; 1/2007.

Cheng CY, Chung WY, et al, "Fasting plasma zeaxanthin response to Fructus barbarum L (wolfberry; Kei Tze) in a food-based human supplementation trial," *Br J Nutr,* 3(1):123-30; 1/2005.

gojibook.com/ BRO9.html Acccessed 3/2008.

He YL, Ying Y, et al, [Effects of Lycium barbarum polysaccharide on tumor microenvironment T-lymphocyte subsets and dendritic cells in H22-bearing mice], *Zhong Xi Yi Jie He Xue Bao,* 3(5): 374-7; 9/2005.

Health Magazine, "Goji, Powerful health benefits from a tiny red berry," 8/2006.

Jia YX, Dong JW, et al, [The effect of lycium barbarum polysaccharide on vascular tension in two-kidney, one clip model of high blood pressure], *Sheng Li Zue Bao,* 50(3):309-14; 6/1998.

Lee DG, Park Y, et al, "Antifungal effects of phenolic amides isolated from the root bark of Lycium chinense," *Biotechnol Lett,* 26(14):1125-30; 7/2004.

Lee DG, Park Y, et al, "Antimicrobial property of (+)-lyoniresinol-3alpha-O-beta-D-glucopyranoside isolated from the root bark of Lycium chinense Miller against human pathogenic microorganisms," *Biotechnol Lett,* 28(9):1031-6; 9/2005. (Protects from some antibiotic-resistant microbes (Staph, Candida.)

Li XM, Ma YL, et al, "Effect of the Lycium barbarum polysaccharides on age-related oxidative stress in aged mice" *J Ethnopharmacol,* 111(3):504-11; 2007.

Mindell E, Handell R, *Goji: The Himalyan Health Secret,* Momentum Media, Dallas, TX, 2005.

Wu H, Guo H, et al, [Effect of Lycium barbarum polysaccharide on the improvement of antioxidant ability and DNA damage in NIDDM rats], *Yakugaku Zasshi,* 126(5):365-71; 2006.

Yu MS, Leung SK, et al, "Neuroprotective effects of anti-aging oriental medicine Lycium barbarum against beta-amyloid peptide neurotoxicity," *Exp Gerontol,* 40(8-9):716-27; 8-9/2005.

Rhodiola

amoryn.com/formula.html 12/28/2005

Brekhman I, Dardymov I, "New substances of plant origin which increase non-specific resistance," *Ann Pharmacol,* 9:419-30; 1969.

Brown R, et al, "Rhodiola rosea: A phytomedical overview," *HerbalGram,* 56:40-52; 2002. (Activates cerebral cortex and limbic system, enhancing cognition, attention, memory and learning.)

Darbinyan V, Kteyan A, et al, "Rhodiola rosea induced fatigue — A double blind cross-over study of a standardized extract SHR-5 with a repeated low-dose regimen on the mental performance of healthy physicians during night duty," *Phytomedicine,* 7(5): 365-71; 2000. (Double blind crossover. 56 physicians. Significant improvement in mental performance.)

Kelly G, "Rhodiola rosea — A possible plant adaptogen," *Altern Med Rev,* 6(3):293-302; 6/2001. (Increases resistance to various biological, physical and chemical stressors. Reputed antidepressant, CNS enhancing effects. Benefits stress-related difficulty with work performance, sleep, appetite, irritability, hypertension, headache, fatigue. Influences monoamine level and activity, and opioid peptides.)

Mamedov Nazim, "Adaptogenic, geriatric, stimulant and antidepressant plants of Russian Far East," *J Cell Molecular Biology,* 4(71-5); 2005. (Traditionally used to restore energy, prolong life.)

Ramazanove Z, *Rhodiola rosea — Adaptogen for mental and physical health,* Ch 3 unpub manu

www.vrp.com/art/1225.asp

Bacopa

Roodenrys S, Booth D, "Chronic effects of brahmi (Bacopa monnieri) on human memory," *Neuropsychopharmacol,* 27(2):279-81; 2002.

Stough C, Lloyd J, "The chronic effects of an extract of Bacopa monniera (Brahmi) on cognitive function in healthy human subjects," *Psychopharmacol (Berl),* 156(4):481-4; 2001. (Improves learning, memory)

www.en.wikipedia.org/wiki/bacopa_monnieri

Suma

Bartram T, *Encyclopedia of Herbal Medicine*

rain-tree.com/suma.htm

Green tea

Cooper R, Morre J, et al, "Medicinal benefits of green tea: Part I. Review of noncancer health benefits," *J Altern Complement Med,* 11(3):521-8; 6/2005.

Dharmananda S, *Biosci, Biotech, Biochem,* 1998, (Rats created 26% more tryptophan; less anxiety.)

Eschenauer G, Sweet BV, "Pharmacology and therapeutic uses of theanine," *Am J Health Syst Pharm,* 63(1):26-30; 2006. (Dose dependent increase in alpha waves 40 minutes post ingestion.)

Hintikka J, Tolmunen T, et al, "Daily tea drinking is associated with a low level of depressive symptoms in the Finnish general population," *Eur J Epid,* 20(4); 4/2005. (Of 2011 subjects, daily tea drinkers showed reduced depression scores and prevalence. With 5+ cups, no depression. Multivariate logistic regression model, adjusted for age, sex, etc.)

Kakuda T, "Inhibiting effect of theanine on caffeine stimulation evaluated by EEG in the rat," *Biosci, Biotech, Biochem,* 64:287-93; 2000.

Kobayahi K, Nagato Y, et al, "Effects of L-theanine on the release of alpha-brain waves in human volunteers," *Nippon Nogei Kagakukaishi,* 72(2):153-7; 1998. (In 8 women with high or low anxiety, 200 mg produced alpha waves in occipital and parietal regions, especially in those with greater anxiety.)

Lekh RJ, et al, "L-theanine — A unique amino acid of green tea and its relaxation effect in humans," *Food Sci Tech,* 10(6-7):199-204; 1999.

Makhtar, H, Wamg Z.Y, et al, "Tea components: Antimutagenic and anticarcinogenic effects," *Prev Med,* 21:351-60; 1992. (Catechins protect the liver from oxidative stress.)

Mason R, "L-theanine boosts alpha waves, promotes alert relaxation," *Alt Complementary Ther,* 7(2):91-95; 4/2001.

Mitcher L, Toews VT, *The Green Tea Book: China's Fountain of Youth.*

Yamada T, Terashima T, et al, "Effects of theanine, r-glutamylethylamide, on neurotransmitter release and its relationship with glutamic acid neurotransmission," *Nutr Neurosci,* 8(4):219-26; 8/2005. (Animal study. Theanine may inhibit excitatory and promote inhibitory messages, especially glycine.)

Cacao

Bruinsman K, Taren DL, "Chocolate: Food or drug?" *J Am Diet Assn,* 99(10):1249-56; 10/1999. (Anandamides, methylxanthines, biogenic amines)

Dallard I, Cathebras P, [Is cocoa a psychotropic drug? Psychopathologic study of a population of subjects self-identified as chocolate addicts], *Encephale,* 27(1):181-6; 3-4 2001.

Jorm AF, Christensen H, et al, "Effectiveness of complementary and self-help treatment for depression," *MJA,* 176(10S):84-95; 2002.

Schuman M, Gitlin MJ, et al, "Sweets, chocolate, and atypical depressive traits," *J Nerv Ment Dis,* 175(8): 491-5; 8/1987. (More common in females.)

IV IM

Balch JF, Balch P, *Prescription for Nutritional Healing,* Avery, Garden City Park, NY, 1990.

Gaby A, "Intravenous vitamin and mineral therapy" Presented at: *Nutritional Therapy in Medical Practice,* conference, Seattle, 1998.

Gaby AR, Intravenous nutrient therapy: "The Myers Cocktail" *Alt Med Rev,* 7(5):389-403; 2002.

Joan M Larson, PhD, interview with author, 6/ 2008

Hugh Riordan, MD interview with author, 10/1995.

Saleeby, JP, MD, "Nutrient Cocktail for Schizophrenia and Bipolar Disorder." At: www.alternativementalhealth.com/articles/cocktail.htm Accessed: 9/6/2005. (Drs. Ian Gaby and Harry Adelson are conducting a pilot study at Naturopathic Med Ctr at UI Bridgeport, and Saleeby, in Savannah.)

Shealy CN, Cady RK, "Magnesium deficiency in depression and chronic pain," *Magnes Trace El,* 9:333; 1997.

Biotype intro

Cooney C, *Methyl Magic,* Andrews McMeel Publishing, Kansas City, 1999; pp 154-66.

Hoffer A, *Adventures in Psychiatry, The Scientific Memoirs of Dr Abram Hoffer,* KOS Pub, Caledon, ON, Canada, 2005.

www.hriptc.org

www.islandnet.com/~hoffer/hofferhp.ht

Jaffe R, Kruesi O, "The biochemical immunology window: A molecular view of psychiatric case management," *J Appl Nutr,* 44(2); 1992.

Larson, Joan Matthews, PhD, interview with author, 7/2008.

Lesser, Michael, MD, interview with author, 8/2008.

Pfeiffer CC, *Nutrition and Mental Illness,* Healing Arts Press, Rochester, VT, 1987.

Pfeiffer CC, *The Schizophrenias Ours to Conquer,* Bio-Communications Press, Wichita, KS, 1988.

Riordan, Hugh, MD, interview with author, 10/1995.

Walsh WJ, "Biochemical treatment of mental illness and behavior disorders," 11/1997 At: www.hriptc.org/BioTreatment.html

Walsh WJ, "Biochemical individuality and nutrition." At: www.hriptc.org/biochemical_individuality.html Accessed: 2000.

Walsh WJ, "A biological basis for neurologic disorders: autism, hyperactivity, attention deficit disorder,depression, obsessive-compulsive disorder, Tourette's syndrome, and violence, An interview with William J Walsh, PhD," *Latitudes,* 5(2):1-8, 2002. At: www.Latitudes.org

Walsh WJ, "Metal metabolism and human function," At: www.hriptc.org/metal_metabolism.html Accessed: 12/2004

Walsh WJ, "Zinc deficiency, metal metabolism, and behavior disorders," At: hriptc.org/zinc_deficiency.html Accessed: 12/2004

Walsh, WJ, "Commentary on nutritional treatment of mental disorders," *International Guide to the World of Alternative Mental Health.* At: www.alternativementalhealth.com/articles.walshMP.htm#Py Accessed:10/08/2006

Walsh, William J, PhD, interview with author, November, 2007, and July 2008.

Pyrrole disorder

Bibus DM, Holman RT, Walsh WJ, "Fatty acid profiles of schizophrenic phenotypes," *Abst, 91ST Annual Mtg, AOCS,* San Diego, 4/25-28/2000.

Bitsas, C, "Nutrients and Depression: Food for your mood." At: hriptc.org Accessed 2002.

Braverman E, Pfeiffer CC, *The Healing Nutrients Within,* Keats, New Canaan, CN, 1987.

diagnose-me.com.cond.C372380.html

Derrien, Benoir, 1929. (High zinc in urine of porphyric patient. Deficiency may cause the psychiatric symptoms.)

Gold MS, *The Good News About Depression,* Villard Books NY, 1987; pp138.

Hoffer A, Osmond H, Malvaria: A new psychiatric disease, Acta Psychiat Scand, 39:335-66; 1963.

Hoffer A, "Behavioral Nutrition," *J Orthomol Psychiat,* 8(3):169-75; 1979.

Hoffer, Abram, MD, PhD, interview with author, April, 1995.

Hoffer A, *Adventures in Psychiatry, The Scientific Memoirs of Dr Abram Hoffer,* KOS Pub, Caledon, ON, Canada, 2005.

Irvine D, Bayne W, and Miyashita H, *Nature,* 224(81); 1969. (Identification of kryptopyrrole in urine and its relation to psychosis.)

Jaffe R, Kruesi OR, "The biochemical-immunology window: A biomolecular view of psychiatric case management," *J App Nutr,* 44(2); 1992.

Kimura, I, Kimura, J, "Preliminary reports on the metabolism of trace elements in neuropsychiatric diseases: Zinc in schizophrenias", *Proc Japan Acad Sci,* 1965; p. 943. (Autopsy found 50% less Zn in frontal, occipital, and hippocampal areas.)

Tom Lane, personal communication, 5-6/1997.

McGinnis W, "Pyroluria: Hidden cause of schizophrenia, bipolar, depression, and anxiety symptoms," Orlando, 5/21/2004. *At:* alternativementalhealth.com/articles/pyroluria.htm

McDermott JF, "Emily Dickinson revisited: a study of periodicity in her work," *Am J Psychiatr,* 158(5): 686-90; 5/2001.

Mc Lardy, T, "Hippocampal zinc in chronic alcoholism and schizophrenia," *IRCS J Med. Sci,* 2:1010; 1973. (Zinc reduced 30% in early onset schizophrenia.)

O'Reilly, Hughes, *Dis Nerv Syst,* 26; 1962. (non-schizophrenics, 42%; schizophrenics, 52%; disturbed children 24%; general population 11%.)

Pfeiffer CC, "Observations on trace and toxic elements in hair and serum," *J Orthomol Psychiat,* 3(4):259-64; 1974.

Pfeiffer CC, Sohler, A, et al, "Treatment of pyroluric schizophrenia (malvaria) with large doses of pyridoxine and a dietary supplement of zinc," *J Orthomol Psychiat,* 3(4):292-3; 1974.

Pfeiffer CC, LaMola, Scott, "Zinc and manganese in the schizophrenias," *J Orthomol Psychiat,* 12: 215-34; 1983.

Pfeiffer CC, *Nutrition and Mental Illness,* Healing Arts Press, Rochester, VT, 1987.

Pfeiffer, CC, *The Schizophrenias Ours to Conquer,* rev ed, Bio-Communications Press, Wichita, KS, 1988.

Pfeiffer CC, Audette L, "Pyroluria, zinc and B6 deficiencies," *Intl Clin Nutr Rev,* 8(3):107-110; 1988.

Pfeiffer CC, "The schizophrenias '76," *Biol Psychiat,* 2:773-5; 1976.

Pfeiffer CC, Bacchi, D, "Copper, zinc, manganese, niacin and pyridoxine in the schizophrenias," *J Appl Nutr,* 27:9-39, 1975.

Pfeiffer CC, Iliev V, "A study of zinc deficiency, copper excess in the schizophrenias," *Intl Rev Neurobiol,* 72:141. (Manganese can triple copper excretion; zinc enhances this effect.)

Ridges P, "Biochemical research into schizophrenia in relation to pink spot excretion," *J Orthomol Psychiat,* 1(1):18-26; 1972.

Ross J, *The Mood Cure,* Viking Penguin, NY, 2002.

Shaw W, "Possible synergistic effects of nonesterified fatty acids and lysolecithins, a toxic methionine metabolite, and ammonia in the production of hepatic encephalopathy and schizophrenia," *J Orthomol Med,* 3(3), 1988.

Sohler A, "A rapid screening test for pyroluria; useful in distinguishing a schizophrenic subpopulation", *J Orthomol Psychiat,* 3(4):273-79, 1974.

Vedantam S, "Did a bipolar trait bring a turn for the verse?" 5/14/2001. At: Washingtonpost.com/ac2/wp-dyn?pagename=article&node=&contentId=A2262

Vonnegut M, *The Eden Express,* Praeger, NY, 1975.

Wallwork J, Sandstead H, "Effect of zinc deficiency on brain catecholamine concentration," *Fed Proc,* 40:939; 1981. (Catecholamines increased.)

Walsh WJ, "Biochemical treatment: Medicines for the next century," *NOHA News,* 16(3); 1991.

Walsh, William J, PhD, interview with author, September, 1995.

Walsh WJ, "Biochemical treatment of mental illness and behavior disorders," 11/17/97. At: www.hriptc.org/BioTreatment.html

Walsh WJ, "Biochemical individuality and nutrition," At: www.hriptc.org/biochemical_individuality.html Accessed: 2000a.

Walsh WJ, "A biological basis for neurologic disorders: autism, hyperactivity, attention deficit disorder,depression, obsessive-compulsive disorder, Tourette's syndrome, and violence, An interview with William J Walsh, PhD," *Latitudes,* 5(2):1-8, 2002. At: www.Latitudes.org

Walsh, WJ, "Commentary on nutritional treatment of mental disorders." At: www.alternativementalhealth.com/articles/walshMP.htm Accessed: 10/2006.

Walsh, William J, PhD, interview with author, November, 2000c, November, 2007, July 2008.

Werbach M, *Nutritional Influences on Mental Illness,* Third Line Press, Tarzana, CA, 1991.

Methylation biotypes & chart

Agnoli A, Andreoli V, "Effects of S-adenosyl-L-methionine upon depression symptoms," *J Psych Res,* 13:434-54; 1976. (Daily IM injection of 45 mg SAM benefited depressed mood, suicidal tendencies, intellectual sluggishness, performance. 80% improved in 4-6 days.)

Bell KM, et al, "S-adenosylmethionine treatment of depression: A controlled clinical trial," *Am J Psychiat,* 145(9):1110-14; 1988. (SAM produced greater improvement than imipramine and less side effects. Benefit was rapid.)

Bell KM, Potkin SG, et al, [S-adenosylmethionine blood levels in major depression: Changes with drug treatment], *Acta Neurol Scand Suppl,* 154: 15-18; 1994. (SAM is necessary for proper catecholamine function. Some depressives are low.)

Berlanga C, et al, "Efficacy of S-adenosyl-L-methionine in speeding the onset of action of imipramine," *Psychiat Res,* 44:257-62; 12/1992.

Bibus DM, Holman RT, Walsh WJ, "Fatty acid profiles of schizophrenic phenotypes," *Abst, 91ST Annual Mtg, AOCS,* San Diego, 4/25-28/2000.

Blandina P, et al, "Stimulation of the histamine H_2 receptor in the rat hypothalamus releases endogenous NE," *J Pharmacol Exp Ther,* 249: 45-51; 1989.

Bottiglieri T, Hyland K, [S-adenosylmethionine levels in psychiatric and neurological disorders: A review], *Acta Neurol Scand,* 154S:19-26; 1994.

Braverman E, *The Healing Nutrients Within,* Keats, New Canaan, CN, 1987.

Bressa GM, [S-adenosyl-L-methionine (SAMe) as antidepressant: Meta-analysis of clinical studies], *Acta Neurol Scand,* 154S, 7-14; 1994. (Comparable to tricyclics. On average, over 6 randomized controlled trials, 70% responded (30%, in placebo). Relatively rapid, few side effects (nausea, restlessness, mild anxiety). Some drug interactions. Can trigger mania, especially IV or with antidepressants.)

Carney MWP, "Rapid antidepressant response with SAMe. A double-blind study," *Ala J Med Sci,* 25(3): 16; 1988.

Conlay LA, et al, "Effects of running the Boston marathon on plasma concentrations of large neutral amino acids," *J Neural Transmission,* 76: 65-71; 1989.

Cooney C, *Methyl Magic,* Andrews McMeel Publishing, Kansas City, 1999; pp 154-66.

Cousens G, *Depression Free for Life,* Quill, HarperCollins, NY, 2001

Crayhon R, *The Carnitine Miracle,* M Evans, 1998.

de Vanna M, Rigamonti R, "Oral S-adenosyl-L-methionine in depression," *Curr Ther Res,* 52: 478-85; 9/1992.

Fieve RR, *Moodswing,* Bantam Books, 1976.

Fredericks C, "Carlton Fredericks' *Nutrition Guide for the Prevention & Cure of Common Ailments & Diseases,* Simon & Schuster, NY, 1982.

Goodnick PJ, Sandoval R, "Psychotropic treatment of chronic fatigue syndrome and related disorders," *J Clin Psychiat,* 54:13-20; 1/1993.

Goodwin RD, Jacobi F, et al, "Mental disorders and asthma in the community," *Arch Gen Psychiat,* 60: 1125-30; 2003.

Green JP, "Histamine and the nervous system," *Fed Proc,* 23:1095-1102; 1964.

Green JP, "Uptake, storage and release of histamine. Uptake and binding of histamine," *Fed Proc,* 26(1): 211-28; 1-2/1967.

Green JP, "Histamine as a neurotransmitter," in Lipton, DeMascio, Killam, eds, *Psychopharmacology: A Generation of Progress,* Raven, NY, 1978a; pp 319-32.

Green JP, Maayani S, Weinstein H, "Defining the histamine H2 receptor in the brain," *NIDA Res Monog,* (22):38-59; 1978b.

Green JP, "Histamine receptors," *Psychopharmacology, The Third Generation of Progress,* HY Meltzer, ed, Raven, NY, 1987; pp 273-79.

Gulat-Marnay, et al, "Modulation of histamine release and synthesis in the brain mediated by alpha1 adrenoreceptors," *J Neurochem,* 53:519-24; 1989.

Hasanah, CI, Khan UA, "Reduced red-cell folate in mania," *J Affect Disord,* 46, 95-99; 1997.

Hill SJ, et al, "Alpha2 adrenoreceptor mediated inhibition of histamine release from rat cerebral cortical slices," *Br J Pharmacol,* 95:1213-19; 1988.

Hitzemann R, Mark C, et al, "Characteristics of phospholipid methylation in human erythrocyte ghosts: Relationship(s) to the psychoses and affective disorders," *Biol Psychiat,* 20:397-407; 1985.

Hoffer A, et al, "Treatment of schizophrenia with nicotinic acid and nicotinamide," *J Clin Exp Psychopath,* 18:131-58, 1957.

Hoffer A, Osmond H, "Treatment of schizophrenia with nicotinic acid: A ten-year follow-up," *Acta Psychiatr Scand,* 40:171-89; 1964.

Hoffer A,"The effect of nicotinic acid on the frequency and duration of rehospitalization of schizophrenic patients; a controlled comparison study," *Int J Neuro Psych,* 2:234-240; 1966.

Hoffer A, "Treatment of schizophrenia with a therapeutic program based upon nicotinic acid as the main variable," in O Wallaas, ed, *Molecular Basis of Some Aspects of Mental Activity,* V3, Academic Press, NY, 1967.

Hoffer A, "Mega vitamin B3 therapy for schizophrenia," *Can Psych Assoc,* 16:499-504; 1971.

Hoffer A, "Mechanism of action of nicotinic acid and nicotinamide in the treatment of schizophrenia," in D Hawkins, L Pauling, eds, *Orthomolecular Psychiatry,* WH Freeman and Co, San Francisco, 1973.

Hoffer A, MD, PhD, "Mega amino acid therapy," *J Orthomol Psychiat,* 9(1):2-5; 1980.

Hoffer A, "Nutrition and behavior," in *Medical Applications of Clinical Nutrition,* J Bland, ed, Keats, New Canaan, CN, 1983.

Hoffer A, *Common Questions on Schizophrenia and their Answers,* Keats, New Canaan, CN, 1987.

Hoffer A, *Adventures in Psychiatry, The Scientific Memoirs of Dr Abram Hoffer,* KOS Pub, Caledon, ON, Canada, 2005.

Horrobin DF, Bennett CN, "Depression and bipolar disorder: Relationships to impaired fatty acid and phospholipid metabolism, and to diabetes, cardiovascular disease, immunological abnormalities, cancer, aging and osteoporosis. Possible candidate genes," *Prostaglandins, Leukot, Essent Fatty Acids,* 60:217-34; 1999.

Hough LB, et al, "Inhibition of brain histamine metabolism by metoprine," *Biochem Pharmacol,* 35:307-10; 1988.

Issidorides MR, Lykouras EP, et al, "Histochemical changes of peripheral blood leukocytes during lithium treatment," *Bibl Psychiatr,* (160):38-44; 1981. (Cytoplasmic basic protein was reduced in blood eosiniophils of 16 bipolars, 2 and 12 mo after starting lithium, suggesting an influence on histamine metabolism.)

Jaffe R, Kruesi OR, "The biochemical-immunology window: A biomolecular view of psychiatric case management," *J App Nutr,* 44(2); 1992.

Kagan B, Sultzer DL, et al, "Oral S-adenosyl-methionine in depression: A randomized, double-blind, placebo-controlled trial," *Am J Psychiat,* 147(5):591-95; 1990. (Randomized double blind. Depression decreased significantly among 18 major depression patients given gradually increasing doses of SAM (perhaps up to 800 mg) 2x/day for 21 days vs placebo. Side effects were mild and short-term, except for one patient who became manic.)

Kruesi, Oscar Rogers, MD, interview with author, February, 1996.

Lipinski JP, Cohen BM, et al, "Open trial of S-adenosylmethionine for treatment of depression," *Am J Psychiat,* 141:448-50; 3/1984.

Low NC, Merikangas KR, "The comorbidity of migraine," *CNS Spectr,* 8:433-4, 437-444; 2003.

Meck W, Church R, "Nutrients that modify the speed of internal clock and memory storage processes," *Behav Neurosci,* 101: 465-75; 1987.

www.methyl.org

Miller CL, Dulay JR, "The high affinity niacin receptor HM74A is decreased in the anterior cingulate cortex of individuals with schizophrenia," *Brain Res Bull,* 77(1):33-41; 9/2008.

Muscettola G, Galzenati, et al, "SAM versus placebo: A double-blind comparison in major depressive disorders," *Lancet,* 7/1984.

Nijinsky R, *Nijinsky,* Simon & Schuster, NY, 1934.

Osmond H, Hoffer A, "Massive niacin treatment in schizophrenia: Review of a nine year study," *Lancet,* 1:316-20; 1962. (Decreased long-term suicide rate.)

Osmond H, Hoffer A, "Naturally occurring endogenous major and minor tranquilizers," *J Orthomol Psychiat,* 9(3):198-205; 1980.

Pfeiffer CC, Iliev V, "A study of zinc deficiency and copper excess in the schizophrenias," *Intl Rev Neurobiol,* 1972; p.141.

Pfeiffer CC, Bacchi D, "Copper, zinc, manganese, niacin and pyridoxine in the schizophrenias," *J App Nutr,* 27(2):9-39; 1975.

Pfeiffer CC, LaMola S, "Zinc and manganese in the schizophrenias," *J Orthomol Psychiat,* 12:215-34; 1983. (Copper may increase 1-3 mo. before falling. This usually can be prevented with Mn, B6 and D-penicillamine. (Avoid penicillamine if possible.)

Pfeiffer CC, *Nutrition and Mental Illness,* Healing Arts Press, Rochester, VT, 1987.

Pfeiffer CC, *The Schizophrenias Ours to Conquer,* rev ed, Bio-Communications Press, Wichita, KS, 1988.

Phillipu, A, et al, "In vivo release by histamine agonists and antagonists of endogenous catecholamines in the cat hypothalamus," *Naunyn-Schmiedeberg's Arch Pharmacol,* 326:116-23, 1984.

Pilc A, Nowak JZ, "Influence of histamine on the serotenergic system of the rat brain, *Eur J Pharmacol,"* 55:269-72; 1979.

Prast, et al, "Modulation by dopamine receptors of histamine release in the rat hypothalamus," *Naunyn-Schmiedeberg's Arch Pharmacol,* 344: 301-5; 1993.

Prast H, et al, "In vivo modulation of histamine release in the hypothalamus by adrenoreceptor agonists and antagonists", *Naunyn-Schmiedeberg's Arch Pharmacol,* 344:183-86; 1991.

Prell GE, et al, "Histamine metabolities in cerebrospinal fluid of patients with chronic schizophrenia: Their relationships to levels of other aminergic transmitters and ratings of symptoms," *Schizophr Res,* 14:93-104; 1995.

Richelson E, "Pharmacology of antidepressants in use in the United States," *Clin Psychiat,* 43:4; 1982. (Tricyclics may act via antihistamine effects.)

Rogers S, *Depression, Cured at Last,* SK Publishing, Sarasota FL, 1997.

Rosenbaum JF, et al, "An open-label pilot study of oral S-adenosyl-L-methionine in major depression: Interim results," *Psychopharmacol Bull,* 24(1):189-94; 1988.

Rosenbaum JF, et al, [The antidepressant potential of oral S-adenosyl-L-methionine], *Acta Psychiatr Scand,* 81:432-36; 5/1990.

Salmaggi, et al, "Double-blind, placebo-controlled study of S-adenosyl-L-methionine in depressed postmenopausal women," *Psychother Psychosom,* 59(1):34-40; 1993.

Sahley BJ, *Healing with Amino Acids,* Pain & Stress Center Pub., TX, 1995.

Schwartz, J, "Histaminergic mechanisms in the brain," *Annu Rev Pharmacol Toxicol,* 17:325-39; 1977. (Stimulates adenosyl cyclase, Zn-heparin-H complex.)

Schwartz JC, et al, "Histaminergic transmission in the mammalian brain," *Physiol Rev,* 71:1-51; 1991.

Smythies JR, "The role of one-carbon cycle in neuropsychiatric disease, *Biol Psychiat,* 19(5):755-58; 5/1984. (Methylation reactions are important in coupling receptors to adenylate cyclase and in neurotransmitter release. Methylation (and the Vmax of MAT) may be increased in some manics, decreased in some depressives and schizophrenics. MAT produces the potent methylatort, SAM.)

Stoll AL, *The Omega-3 Connection,* Simon & Schuster, NY, 2002.

Wada H, et al, "Is the histaminergic nervous system a regulatory center for whole-brain activity?" *Trends Neurosci,* 14:415-18; 1991.

Walker D, "Journey through paranoia and beyond," *J Orthomol Med,* 1(3):158-68; 1986.

Walsh WJ, "Biochemical treatment: Medicines for the next century," *NOHA News,* 16(3); 1991.

Walsh, William J, PhD, interview with author, April, 1995.

Walsh WJ, Rehman F, "Methylation syndromes in mental illness," *Neurosci Soc Abst,* New Orleans, 11/1997a.

Walsh WJ, "Biochemical treatment of mental illness and behavior disorders." At: www.hriptc.org/BioTreatment.html Accessed: 11/1997b.

Walsh WJ, "Biochemical individuality and nutrition," *NOHA News,* XXV(2):6-8; 2000a.

Walsh WJ, "Biochemical individuality and nutrition," at: www.hriptc.org/biochemical_individuality.html Accessed: 2000b.

Walsh, William J, PhD, interview with author, November, 2000c.

Walsh WJ, "Metal-metabolism and human functioning." At: http://www.hriptc.org/mhfres.htm Accessed: 10/31/2000d.

Walsh WJ, "A biological basis for neurologic disorders: Autism, hyperactivity, attention deficit disorder, depression, obsessive-compulsive disorder, Tourette's syndrome, and violence, An interview with William J Walsh, PhD," *Latitudes,* 5(2):1-8, 2002. At: www.Latitudes.org

Walsh WJ, "Metal metabolism and human function," At: www.hriptc.org/metal_metabolism.html Accessed: 12-6-2004a.

Walsh WJ, "Zinc deficiency, metal metabolism, and behavior disorders." At: hriptc.org/zinc_deficiency.html Accessed: 12/6/2004b.

Walsh, WJ, PhD, "Commentary on nutritional treatment of mental disorders," *International Guide to the World of Alternative Mental Health.* At: www.alternativementalhealth.com/articles.walshMP.htm#Py Accessed:10/08/06

Walsh, William J, PhD, interview with author, November 2007, and July 2008.

Wurtman RH, "Effects of dietary amino acids, carboydrates and choline on neurotrnsmitter synthesis," *Mount Sinai J Med,* 55:75-86; 1/1988.

Young SN, "The use of diet and dietary components in the study of factors controlling affect in humans: A review," *J Psychiat Neurosci,* 18(5):235-44; 1993.

Homocysteinuria

Bell IR, Morrow FD, [Low thyroxine levels in female psychiatric inpatients with riboflavin deficiency: Implications for folate-dependent methylation], *Acta Psychiatr Scand,* 85(5):360-3; 1992. (Low B2 may mark thyroxine status in some females. Deficiency may compromise methylation pathways in some.)

Bottiglieri T, Lanundry M, et al, "Homocysteine, folate, methylation, and monoamine metabolism in depression," *J Neurol, Neurosurg, Psychiat,* 2000.

Cooney C, "Methyl Magic and the Mind," *Methyl Magic,* Andrews McMeel Publishing, Kansas City, 1999; pp 154-66.

Cravo ML, Gloria LM, et al, "Hyperhomocysteinemia in chronic alcoholism: Correlation with folate, vitamin B12, and B6 status," *Am J Clin Nutr,* 63: 220-24; 1996.

Duthie SJ, Whalley LJ, et al, "Homocysteine, B vitamin status, and cognitive function in the elderly," *Am J Clin Nutr,* 2002.

Fava M, "Folate, vitamin B12, and homocysteine in major depressive disorder", *Am J Psychiat* At: ajp.psychiatryonline.org Accessed: 1997.

Hultberg, B, Berglund, M, et al, "Elevated plasma homocysteine in alcoholics," *Alcohol Clin Exp Res,* 17:687-89; 1993.

Lipton SA, Kin WK, et al, "Neurotoxicity associated with dual actions of homocysteine at the N-methyl-D-aspartate receptor," *Proc Natl Acad Sci,* 94:5923-28; 1997.

Miller AL, Kelly GS, "Homocysteine metabolism: Nutritional modulation and impact on health and disease," *Alt Med Rev,* 2(4):234-55; 1997.

Morris MS, "Folate, homocysteine, and neurological function," *Nutr Clin Care,* 5(3):124; 2002.

Narath HJ, Joosten E, et al, "Effects of vitamin B6, folate, and B6 supplements in elderly people with normal serum vitamin concentrations," *Lancet,* 346: 85-89; 1995.

Nygard O, Refsum H, et al, "Coffee consumption and plasma total homocysteine: The Hordaland Homocysteine Study," *Am J Clin Nutr,* 65:136-43; 1997.

Papakostas GI, Ptersen T, "Serum folate, vitamin B12, and homocysteine in major depressive disorder, Part I," *J Clin Psychiat,* 2004.

Pfeiffer CC, *The Schizophrenias Ours to Conquer,* Bio-Communications Press, Wichita, KS, 1988.

Regland, B, Johansson, BV, et al, "Homocysteinemia is a common feature of schizophrenia," *J Neural Transm Gen Sect,* 100:165-69; 1995.

Reutens S, Sachdev P, "Homocysteine in neuropsychiatric disorders of the elderly," *Intl J Geriat Psychiat,* 17:859-64; 2002.

Reynolds EH, Carney MW, Toone BK, "Methylation and mood," *Lancet,* 2(8396):19608; 7/1984. (Review. SAM appears as effective as major antidepressants clomipramine and amitriptyline.)

Tolmunen T, Hintikka J, "Association between depressive symptoms and serum concentrations of homocysteine," *Am J Clin Nutr,* 2004.

Tiemeier H, van Tuijl HR, et al, "Vitamin B12, folate and homocysteine in depression: The Rotterdam study," *Am J Psychiat,* 159:2099-2101; 12/2002.

Ubbink JB, van der Merwe, A, et al, "Hyper-homocysteinemia and the response to vitamin supplementation," *Clin Investig,* 71:993-98; 1993.

Neutotoxins

Akil M, Brewer GJ, "Psychiatric and behavioral abnormalities in Wilson's disease," *Adv Neurol,* 65: 171-8; 1995. (Two-thirds presented with psychiatric symptoms, and in half of those Wilson's was not initially diagnosed. In early stages, it's detected in less than 1%. Depression occurs in 20-30% or more.)

Atchison WD, "Effects of neurotoxicants on synaptic transmission: Lessons learned from electrophysiological studies," *Neurotoxicol Teratol,* 10(5):393-416; 1988.

Pfeiffer CC, Bacchi D, "Copper, zinc, manganese, niacin and pyridoxine in the schizophrenias," *J App Nutr,* 27(2); 1975.

Stohs SJ, Bagchi D, "Oxidative mechanisms in the toxicity of metal ions," *Free Radic Biol Med,* 18(2): 321-36; 2/1995.

Copper

Bitas C, "Nutrients and depression: Food for your mood," At: hriptc.com.

Braverman E, Pfeiffer CC, *The Healing Nutrients Within,* Keats, New Canaan, CN, 1987.

Cooney C, "Methyl magic and the mind," *Methyl Magic,* Andrews McMeel Publishing, Kansas City, 1999; pp 154-66.

Cutler A, *Amalgam Illness: Diagnosis and Treatment,"* Andrew Cutler, WA, 1999 & www.noamalgam.com

Cutler A, *Hair Test Interpretation: Finding Hidden Toxicitities,* Andrew Cutler, 2004.

Cutler A, Amalgam illness, at: home.earthlink.net/~moriam/ANDY_INDEX.html & onibasu.com/archives/am/552.html & /am/520.html (2007)

Crayton JW, Walsh WJ, "Elevated serum copper levels, in women with a history of postpartum depression," *J Trace Elements in Medicine & Biology,* 21(1):17-21, 2007. (In over 78 women with a history of postpartum depression, serum copper was significantly elevated, vs. 148 depressives with no such histories, and controls.)

Gold MS, *The Good News About Depression,* Villard Books NY, 1987.

Drevets WC, Videen TO, "Functional anatomical study of unipolar depression," *J Neurosci,* 12: 3628-41; 1992.

Frerreira KT, "The effect of Cu^2 on isolated frog skin," *Biochim Biophys Acta,* 203(3):555-67; 6/1970.

George MS, Ketter TA, et al, "Brain regions involved in recognizing facial emotion or identity: An oxygen-15 PET study," *J Neuropsychiat Clin Neurosci,* 5: 384-94; 1993.

Gold MS, *The Good News About Depression,* Villard Books NY, 1987.

Goldstein L, Pfeiffer CC, "Effects of single oral doses of trace elements on the quantitated EEG of normal subjects and chronic schizophrenia," *Psychopharm Bull,* 14(3):55-7; 7/1978. (EEGs indicate CNS stimulation from 5 mg copper similar to that produced by an equivalent dose of dexedrine.)

Gur RE, Mozley PD, et al, "Resting cerebral glucose metabolism in first-episode and previously treated patients with schizophrenia relates to clinical features," *Arch Gen Psych,* 52(8):8/1995.

Hitier, Yvonne, "Repercussions of ascorbic acid deficiency on tissue ceruloplasmin and copper levels," *Intl J Vitamin Nutr Res,* 46(1):48-57; 1976.

Krauthammer, C, Klerman GL, "Secondary mania: Manic syndromes associated with antecedent physical illness or drugs," *Arch Gen Psychiatr,* 35(11); 11/1978.

Krishnachavi, as quoted in Pfeiffer 1987.

Migliorelli R, Starkstein SE, et al, "SPECT findings in patients with primary mania," *J Neuropsychiat Clin Neurosci,* 5:379-83; 1993.

Nicholson G, et al, "Effect of D-penicillamine on schizophrenic patients," *Lancet, 1:344,* 1966. (Double blind. Copper excretion correlated with improvement.)

Pfeiffer CC, Papaioannou R, Sohler A, "Effect of chronic zinc intoxication on copper levels, blood formation, and polyamines," *J Orthomol Psychiat,* 9(2); 1980.

Pfeiffer CC, Bacchi D, "Copper, zinc, manganese, niacin and pyridoxine in the schizophrenias," *J App Nutr,* 27(2); 1975.

Pfeiffer CC, LaMola S, "Zinc and manganese in the schizophrenias," *J Orthomol Psychiat,* 12: 215-34; 1983.

Pfeiffer CC, *Nutrition and Mental Illness,* Healing Arts Press, Rochester, VT, 1987.

Pfeiffer CC, *The Schizophrenias Ours to Conquer,* Bio-Communications Press, Wichita, KS, 1988.

Robinson RG, "Comparison of mania and depression after brain injury: Causal factors," *Am J Psychiat,* 145:172-8; 1988.

Robinson RG, "Mood disorders following stroke: New findings and future directions," *J Geriatr Psychiatr,* 22(1):1-15; 1989.

Scheuhammer AM, Cherian MG, "Effects of heavy metal cations and sulfhydryl reagents on striatal D2 dopamine receptors," *Biochem Pharmacol,* 34(19): 3405-13; 1985.

Sohler A, Pfeiffer CC, "Oral zinc in normal subjects: Effect on serum copper, iron, calcium and histidine," *J Orthomol Psychiat,* 9(1); 1980.

Starksten SE, Boston JD, et al, "Mechanism of mania after brain injury: 12 case reports and review of the literature," *J Nerv Ment Dis,* 176(2):87-100; 1988.

Starkstein SE, Robinson RG, "Affective disorders and cerebral vascular disease," *Br J Psychiat,* 154: 170-82; 1989.

Starkstein SE, Mayberg HS, et al, "Mania after brain injury: Neuroradiologic and metabolic findings," *Ann Neurol,* 27(6):652-9; 6/1990.

Stohs SJ, Bagchi D, "Oxidative mechanisms in the toxicity of metal ions," *Free Radic Biol Med,* 18(2): 321-36; 2/1995.

US Congress, Office of Technology Assessment, *Neurotoxicity: Identifying and Controlling Poisons of the Nervous System,* U.S. Government Printing Office, publication #OTA-BA-436; 1990; p.46.

Walsh WJ, "Biochemical treatment of mental illness and behavior disorders." At: www.hriptc.org/BioTreatment.html Accessed: 11/17/1997.

Walsh WJ, "Metal-metabolism and human functioning." At: http://www.hriptc.org/mhfres.htm Accessed: 10/31/2000a.

Walsh WJ, "Biochemical individuality and nutrition." At: www.hriptc.org/biochemical_individuality.html Accessed: 2000b.

Walsh, William J, PhD, interview with author, November, 2000c.

Walsh WJ, Usman A, et al,"Disordered Metal Metabolism in a large autism population," APA Annual Meeting, New Orleans, 5/2001.

Walsh WJ, "A biological basis for neurologic disorders: Autism, hyperactivity, attention deficit disorder, depression, obsessive-compulsive disorder, Tourette's syndrome, and violence, An interview with William J Walsh, PhD," *Latitudes,* 5(2):1-8; 2002. At: www.Latitudes.org

Walsh WJ, "Metal metabolism and human function." At: www.hriptc.org/metal_metabolism.html Accessed 12/6/2004.

Walsh WJ, "Zinc deficiency, metal metabolism, and behavior disorders." At: hriptc.org/zinc_deficiency.html Accessed 12/6/2004.

Walsh WJ, "Commentary on nutritional treatment of mental disorders, *International Guide to the World of Alternative Mental Health.* At: www.alternativementalhealth.com/articles.walshMP.htm#Py Accessed:10/08/2006.

Walsh WJ, at: hriptc.org/aggressive_behavior.html Accessed: 2007.

Walsh, William J, PhD, interview with author, December, 2007.

Walsh, William J, PhD, interview with author, July 2008

Other metals

Adachi T, Yasutake A, et al, "Influence of dietary protein and sulfur amino acids on the fate of methyl mercury in mice," *Toxiciology,* 93:225-34; 1994.

Anuradha B, Varalakshmi P, "Protective role of DL-alpha-lipoic acid against mercury-induced neural lipid peroxidation," *Pharmacol Res,* 39(1): 67-80; 1/1999. (Therapeutic for mercury-induced peroxidation and altered antioxidant status in cortex, cerebellum and sciatic nerves.)

Applegarth DA, Ross PM, "Pollution, mercury and the clinical chemist," *Clin Biochem,* 9(4): 179; 8/1976.

Aposhian H, Vasken, "DMSA and DMPS — water soluble antidotes for heavy metal poisoning," *Ann Rev Pharmacol Toxicol,* 23:193-215; 1983. (Chelating mercury, lead, cadmium and arsenic.)

Aposhian HV, Maiorino RM, et al, "Mobilization of heavy metals by newer, therapeutically useful chelating agents," *Toxicol,* 97(1-3):23-38; 3/1995.

Atchison WD, "Effects of neurotoxicants on synaptic transmission: Lessons learned from electrophysiological studies," *Neurotoxicol Teratol,* 10(5):393-416; 1988.

Arch Pediatr Adolesc Med, "Lead in air linked to increase in homicides," 155:5769-82; 5/2001.

Bernard S, McGinnis W, "Autism: A unique form of mercury poisoning." At: www. autism.com/ari/mercurylong.html Accessed: 2000.

Berniew. At: home.earthlink.net/~berniew1/violence.html home.earthlink.net/~berniew1/depress.html Accessed: 2006.

Banks WA, Kastin AJ, "Aluminum increases permeability of the blood brain barrier to labelled DSIP and beta-endorphin: Possible implications for senile and dialysis dementias," *Lancet,* 26:1227-29, 11/1983.

Biesel WR, "Single nutrients and immunity," *Am J Clin Nutr,* 35:417-468.

Biewenga GP, Haenen GR, et al, "The pharmacology of antioxidant lipoic acid," *Gen Pharmacol,* 29(3): 315-31; 9/1997. (Chelates pro-oxidant metals (including iron, copper, cadmium), and scavenges reactive oxygen species, regenerates endogenous antioxidants (E, C, glutathione), and repairs oxidative damage. Also supports NADH activity.)

Bjorksten J, "Possibilities and limitations of chelation as a means for life extension," *J Advancement Med,* 2:77-88; 1989. (Suggests EDTA.)

Bolger PM, Schwetz BA, "Mercury and health," *NEJM,* 347:22, 1735-6; 2002.

Bowdler NC, Beasley DS, "Behavioral effects of aluminum ingestion," *Pharmacol Biochem Behav,* 10:505-12; 1979.

Brockel BJ, Cory-Slechta DA, "Lead, attention, and impulsive behavior," *Pharmacol Biochem Behav,* 60(2):545-52.

Buchet JP, Lauwerys RR, "Influence of 2,3-dimercaptopropane-1-sulfonate [DMPS] and dimercaptosuccinic acid [DMSA] on the mobilization of mercury from tissues of rats pretreated with mercuric chloride, phenylmercury acetate or mercury vapors," *Toxicol,* 54(3):323-33;

3/1989. (DMSA and DMPS only clear extracellular mercury, not what's in the organs. DMPS is initially more effective, but then slows to DMSA levels. Effects of either on brain mercury are minimal.)

Burns JM, Baghurst PA, et al, "Lifetime low-level lead exposure to environmental lead and children's emotional and behavioral development at ages 11-13," *Am J Epid,* 149(8):740-9; 1999.

Bryce-Smith, D, "Behavioral effects of lead and other heavy metal pollutants," *Chem Britain,* 8(6): 240-43; 1972.

Calabrese EJ, *Nutrition and Environmental Health,* V1, John Wiley and Sons, NY, 1980; pp 94-519.

Campbell AMG, Williams ER, et al, "Motor neurone disease and exposure to lead," *J Neurology, Neurosurg, Psychiat,* 33:877-85; 1970.

Casdorph HR, Walker M, *Toxic Metal Syndrome: How Metal Poisoning Can Affect Your Brain,* Avery, Garden City Park, NY, 1995.

Chapman. At: www.ehponline.org/members/2000/suppl-1/29-56/chapman/chapman-full.html

Chapman L, Chan HM, "The influence of nutrition on methyl mercury intoxication," *Environ Health Perspect,* 108 (S1):29-56; 2000.

Chimelnicka J, Konsta-Szumska E, et al, "Effect of interaction between zinc, mercury and selenium in rats (retention, metallothionein, endogenous copper)," *Arch Toxicol,* 53:165-75; 1983.

Chowdhury BA, Chandra RK, "Biological and health implications of toxic heavy metal and essential trace element interactions," *Prog Food Nutr Sci,* 11:55-113; 1987.

Crapper-McLachlan DR, Dalton AJ, "Alterations in short-term retention, conditioned avoidance response acquisition and motivation following aluminum-induced neurofibrillary degeneration," *Physiology and Behavior,* 10:925-933; 1973.

Crapper-McLachlan DR, Tomko GJ, "Neuronal correlates of an encephalopathy associated with aluminum neurofibrillary degeneration," *Brain Res,* 97:253-264; 1975.

Crichton RR, Florence A, et al, "Aluminum and iron in the brain — prospects for chelation," *Coord Chem Rev,* 228(2):365-71; 2002.

Cutler A, *Amalgam Illness: Diagnosis and Treatment,"* Andrew Cutler, WA, 1999 & www.noamalgam.com

Cutler A, *Hair Test Interpretation: Finding Hidden Toxicitities,* Andrew Cutler, 2004.

Cutler A, Amalgam illness, at: home.earthlink.net/~moriam/ANDY_INDEX.html And: onibasu.com/archives/am/552.html & /am/520.html 2007.

Dart RC, Hurlbut KM, et al, "Pharmacokinetics of meso-2, 3-dimercaptosuccinic acid in patients with lead poisoning and in healthy adults," *J Pediatr,* 125(2):309-16; 8/1994.

Dean W, "Research confirms benefits of chelation with EDTA." At: www.yourwholenutrition.com/readon.asp?id=236

Dean W, "Crosslinkage theory of aging — new life for an old theory, PART I, II," *Vitamin Res News,* 16: 1,1,10-12; 2002a & 16:1,2,1-3; 2002b.

Dean W, "Crosslinkage theory of aging — the neurotoxic effects of aluminum, Part III," *Vitamin Res News,* 16:1,3,1,10-12; 2002c.

Dean W, "Crosslinkage theory of aging — AGEs and crosslinkage theory, Part III," *Vitamin Res News,* 16: 1,5,1, 4-7; 2002d.

Djerassi, E, Berova, N, "The possibilities of allergic reactions from silver amalgam restorations," *Int Dent J,* 19(4):481-88; 1969.

Domanska-Janik K, Bourre JM, "Effect of mercury on rabbit myelin CNP-ase in vitro", *Neurotoxicol,* 8(1):23-32; Spring/1987. (Mercury may irreversibly inhibit CNPase; however enough lipoic acid restores activity and removes mercury.)

Dontsov AE, "Phytosorbent prepared from sunflower seed husks prevents mercuric chloride accumulation in kidney and muscle of adult rabbits," *Arch Environ Health,* 1/2000. (Seed husks lowered levels over 25x in kidneys; almost 5x in muscle.)

Doyle JJ, Bernhoft RA, et al, "The effects of low level dietary cadmium on blood pressure, Na, K, and water retention in growing rats," *J Lab Clin Med,* 86(1):57-63; 1975.

Eggleston DW, "Effect of dental amalgam and nickel alloys on T-lymphocytes," *J Prosthetic Dentistry,* 51(5):617-23; 1984.

Ely JT, "Potential breakthrough on mercury problems," summarized in *Mercury Toxicity—New Treatment Possibilities,* Well Mind Assn; 7-8/1994.

Emory E, Pattillo R, et al, "Neurobehavioral effects of low-level lead exposure in human neonates," *Am J Obstet Gynecol,* 181:S2-11; 1999.

Ewan KB, Pamphlett R, "Increased inorganic mercury in spinal motor neurons following chelating agents," *Neurotoxicol,* 17(2):343-9; Summer/1996. (4 wks DMSA or DMPS increased mercury in frozen lumbar spinal cord sections of mice injected with Hg. Authors suggest chelation increases circulating levels, allowing more to enter the nervous system at neuromuscular junctions.)

Fasciana GS, *Are Your Dental Fillings Poisoning You?,* Keats Inc, New Canaan, CN, 1986.

Fleischer, MA, "Mercury: A 21st Century Killer," At: www.yourwholenutrition.com/readon.asp?id=145 (Mercury may promote artherosclerosis, oxidized LDL and blood clots. Hair levels predict carotid atherosclerosis progression. Hg is directly related to risk of heart attack, countering benefits of fish. Cardiovascular disease increases in exposed workers.)

Fox MRS, "Effect of essential minerals on cadmium toxicity: A review," *Food Sci,* 39(2):321-24; 1974.

Godfrey ME, Huggins H, "The pathophysiology of long-term exposure to dental amalgam: A potential hazard for senile dementia," *Clin Pract Altern Med,* 1(2):107-12; 2000.

Gold MS, *The Good News About Depression,* Villard Books, NY, 1987. (Lead syndrome can look like porphyria; can promote hyperactivity, autistic symptoms or mental retardation in children; cognitive and behavioral changes, and depression in adults; at high doses, peripheral nerve disorders, change in personality. Also, headache, metallic taste, abdominal cramps, constipation, nausea. Symptoms may recur during treatment with release from bones.)

Gordon GF, "Insight preventive medicine," *Osteopathic Med,* 3(5):5-9; 1978.

www.GotMercury.org

Goyer RA, "Toxic effects of metals," in CD, Klaassen, MO Amdur, and J Doull, eds, *Casarett and Doull's Toxicology,* Macmillan, NY, 1986.

Gregus Z, Stein AF, et al, "Effect of lipoic acid on biliary excretion of glutathione and metals," *Toxicol Appl Pharmacol,* 114(1):88-96; 5/1992. (Enhances excretion of inorganic mercury 12-37x in rats.)

Grunert, R.R, "The effect of DL-alpha-lipoic acid on heavy-metal intoxication in mice and dogs," *Arch Biochem- Biophys,* 86:190-94; 1960.

Halsey NA, "Limiting infant exposure to thimerosal in vaccines," *JAMA,* 282(18):1763-66; 1999.

Hanson M, *Mercury bibliography, (3rd ed), 285 symptoms of mercury toxicity and 12,000 mercury citations,* Bio-Probe, Inc, Orlando, FL.

Hart RP, "Neuropsychological effects of occupational exposure to cadmium," *J Clin Exp Neuropsychol,* 11(6):933-43; 1989.

Harvey NS, Jarratt J, et al, "Trace elements and the electroencephalogram during long-term lithium treatment," *Br J Psychiat,* 160:654-58; 5/1992. (Irregular cortical activity (EEG) in 12 patients was associated with Br and Va elevation and increased lithium side effects. Bromine may be therapeutic.)

Herbert, V, Colman, N, et al, "Folic acid and vitamin B12," in RS Goodhardt, ME Shils, eds, *Modern Nutrition in Health and Disease,* Lea & Febiger, Philadelphia, 1980.

Hetnarski B, Wisniewski HM, et al, "Central cholinergic activity in aluminum-induced neurofibrillary degeneration," *Annals of Neurology,* 7:489-490; 1980.

Hill CH, Maltrone G, et al, "In vivo interaction of cadmium with copper, zinc, and iron," *J Nutr,* 80(3): 227-35; 1963.

Huggins HA, "Mercury: A factor in mental disease?" *J Orthomol Psychiat,* 11(1):3-16; 1982.

Huggins HA, *It's All in Your Head: The Link Between Mercury Amalgams and Illness,* Avery, Garden City Park, NY, 1993; & www.hugnet.com

Imura N, Naganuma A, "Mode of modifying action of selenite on toxicity and behavior of mercury and other metals," *Nutr Res,* (1S):499-507; 1985.

Jaffe R, Kruesi OR, "The biochemical-immunology window: A molecular view of psychiatric case management," *J App Nutr,* 44(2); 1992.

Jiang HM, Han GA, et al, "Clinical significance of hair cadmium content in the diagnosis of mental retardation in children," *Chin Med J,* 103(4):331-4; 4/1990.

Keith RL, Setiarahardjo I, et al, "Utilization of renal slices to evaluate the efficacy of chelating agents for removing mercury from the kidney," *Toxicol,* 116:67-75; 1997.

Kessel I, O'Connor JT, *Getting the Lead Out,* Plenum, NY, 1997.

Kupsinel R, "Mercury amalgam toxicity," *J Orthomol Psychiat,* 13(4):140-57; 1984.

Kim R, Rotnitsky A, et al, "A longitudinal study of low-level lead exposure and impairment of renal function: The Normative Aging Study," *JAMA,* 275: 1177-81; 1996.

Lai JK, Guest JF, et al, "The effects of cadmium, manganese and aluminum on sodium-potassium-activated and magnesium activated adenosine triphosphatase activity and choline uptake in rat brain synaptosomes," *Biochem Pharmacol,* 29: 141-46; 1980.

Lai JK, Lim L, "Differences in the inhibitory effect of cadmium, manganese and aluminum on the uptake of dopamine by synaptosomes from forebrain and from striatum of the rat," *Biochem Pharmacol,* 30: 3123-25; 1981.

Larson JM, *Alcoholism — The Biochemical Connection,* Villard Books, NY, 1992.

Lawson L, *Staying Well in a Toxic World,* Lynwood Press, Evanston, IL, 1993.

Leskova GE, [Protective effect of lipoic acid amide in experimental mercurialism], *Gig Tr Zabol,* (6): 27-30; 6/1979. (Lipoic reduced brain and organic mercury 50% vs controls.)

Levander O, Cieng L, "Micronutrient interactions, Vitamins minerals and hazardous elements," in *J NY Acad Soc,* 355:1-372; 1980.

Leviton A, Bellinger D, et al, "Pre- and post-natal low-level lead exposure and children's dysfunction in school," *Environ Res,* 60(1):30-43; 1993.

Lin Ja-Liang, Lin-tan, Dan-Tzu, et al, "Environmental lead exposure and progression of chronic renal diseases in patients without diabetes," *NEJM,* 348: 4, 277-86; 2003.

Lob M, [Pollution caused by lead and mercury], *Soz Praventivmed,* 20(2):73-78; 3-4/1975.

Loginov AS, Nilova TV, et al, "Preparations of alpha lipoic acid: The dynamics of their content in the blood and their effect on hemostasis in lesions of the human liver," *Farmakol Toksikol,* 53(2):47-50; 1990.

Lustberg M, Silbergeld E, "Blood lead levels and mortality," *Arch Intern Med,* 162:2443-9; 2002. (John Hopkins analysis of US census and NHANES-III data, estimates 15% of adults (29 million) from 1976-80 had blood lead at least 20mcg/dL. Such levels (vs. 10 mg/DL or less) were associated with a 39% increase in mortality; 46% increase in cardiovascular deaths; 68%, in cancer.)

Magos L, "Overview on the protection given by selenium against mercurials," in T Suzuki, N Imura, TW Clarkson, eds, *Advances in Mercury Toxicology,* Plenum Press, NY, 1991; pp 289-97.

Maji T, Yoshida A, "Therapeutic effect of dietary iron and ascorbic acid on cadmium toxicity of rats," *Nutr Rep Int,* 10(3):139-49; 1974.

Marden PA, "Increased lead burden — cause or consequence of chronic renal insufficiency?" *NEJM,* 4:343-6; 2003.

Marlowe M, Errara J, et al, "Increased lead and mercury levels in emotionally disturbed children," *J Orthomol Psychiatr,* 12:260-7; 1983a.

Marlowe M, Errara J, "Increased lead and cadmium burdens among mentally retarded children and children with borderline intelligence," *Am J Ment Defic,* 87(5):477-83; 1983b.

Marlowe M, Moon C, "Low mercury levels and childhood intelligence," *J Orthomol Med,* 1(1):

43-49; 1986.

Miller EG, Perry WL, et al, "Prevalence of mercury hypersensitivity in dental students," *J Dent Res,* 64:338, Abst.1472, 3/1985. (Age of fillings plays a role.)

Moore LS, Fleischman A, "Subclinical lead toxicity," *J Orthomol Psychiat,* 4(1):61-70; 1975.

Muir M, "Current controversies in the diagnosis and treatment of heavy metal toxicity," *Alt Comp Ther,* 6/1997; pp.170-78.

Nebenfuhrer L, et al, "Mercury allergy in Budapest," *Contact Dermatitis,* 10(2):121-22; 1984.

Needelman HL, Riess JA, "Bone lead levels and delinquent behavior," *JAMA,* 275(5):363-9;1996.

Nevin R, "How lead exposure relates to temporal changes in IQ, violent crime, and unwed pregnancy," *Environ Res,* 83(1):1-22; 2000.

noamalgam.com

North American Contact Dermitiis Group, "Epidemiology of contact dermatitis in North America: 1972," *Arch Dermatol,* 108:537-40; 1973.

Oliver DJ, "Lead and hyperactivity," *J Abnorm Child Psychol,* 5(4):4405-16; 1977.

J Orthomol Psychiat, Editorial, 11(1):2; 1982.

J Orthomol Psychiat, "Psychiatric changes induced by mercury poisoning," 12(3):170-74; 1975.

Packer L, "Alpha-lipoic acid as a biological anti-oxidant," *Free Rad Biol Med,* 19(2):227-50; 1995.

Page LR, *Healthy Healing,* Healthy Healing Pub, CA, 1992.

Papaioannou R, Sohler A, Pfeiffer CC, "Reduction of blood lead levels in battery workers by zinc and vitamin C," *J Orthomol Psychiat,* 7(2):94-106; 1978.

Patterson JE, Weissberg BG, et al, "Mercury in human breath from dental amalgams," *Bull Environ Contam Toxicol,* 34:459-468; 1985.

Peraza MA, Ayalafierro F, et al, "Effects of micronutrients on metal toxicity," *Environ Health Perspect,* 106(S1):203-16; 1998.

Petering HG, Johnson MA, et al, "Studies of zinc metabolism in the rat: I.Dose-response effects of cadmium," *Arch Environ Health,* 28(2):93-101; 1971.

Petit TL, et al, "Early lead exposure and the hippocampus," *Neurotoxicol,* 4(1):74-79; 1983.

Pfeiffer CC, "Blood histamine, basophil counts and trace elements in the schizophrenias," *Rev Can Biol,* 73-6S:31; 1972.

Pfeiffer CC, *Mental and Elemental Nutrients,* Keats, New Canaan CT, 1975.

Pfeiffer CC, *The Schizophrenias Ours to Conquer,* Bio-Communications Press, Wichita, KS, 1988.

Pihl RO, Parkes M, "Hair element content in learning disabled children, *Science,* 1948:204-206; 1977.

Pihl RO, Ervin F, "Lead and cadmium levels in violent criminals," *Psychol Rep,* 66(3.1):839-44; 1990.

Planas-Bohne F, "The influence of chelating agents on the distribution biotransformation of methylmercuric chloride in rats," *J Pharmacol Exp Ther,* 217(2):500-4; 5/1981.

Pleva J, "Mercury poisoning from dental amalgam," *J Orthomol Psychiat,* 12(3):184-93; 1983.

Rifat SL, Eastwood MR, et al, "Effect of exposure of miners to aluminum powder," *Lancet,* 336:1162-65, 11/10/1990.

Ross J, *The Mood Cure,* Viking Penguin, NY, 2002.

Sachs HK, McCaughran DA, et al, "Lead poisoning without encephalopathy," *Am J Diseases of Children,* 133:786-790; 1979.

Salonen JT, Seppanen K, et al, "Intake of mercury from fish, lipid peroxidation, and the risk of myocardial infarction and coronary, cardiovascular, and any death in eastern Finnish men," *Circulation,* 91(3):645-55; 1995.

Saverhoff MW, Michaelson IA, "Hyperactivity and brain catecholamines in lead-exposed developing rats," *Science,* 182:1022-24; 1973.

Schauss AG, "Comparative hair mineral analysis in a randomly selected "normal " population and violence criminal offenders, *Int J Biosocial Res,* 1: 21-41; 1981.

Scheuhammer AM, Cherian MG, "Effects of heavy metal cations and sulfhydryl reagents on striatal D2 dopamine receptors," *Biochem Pharmacol,* 34(19): 3405-13; 1985.

Schiele R, et al, "Studies on the mercury content in brain and kidney related to number and condition of amalgam fillings," *Viewpoints from Medicine and Dental Medicine Symposium,* Institute of Occupational and Social Medicine, U Erlanger-Nurnberg, Cologne, Germany, 3/12/1984.

Silverud RL, "Health effects after dental amalgam removal," *J Orthomol Med,* 5(2):95-106; 1990.

Smith JB, Dwyer SD, et al, "Cadmium evokes inositol polyphosphate formation and calcium mobilization. Evidence for a cell surface receptor that cadmium stimulates and zinc antagonizes," *J Biol Chem,* 264(13):7115-8; 5/1989.

Solomon NW, Viteri FE, "Biological interaction of ascorbic acid and mineral nutrients [iron, selenium, copper, nickel, manganese, zinc, cobalt, cadmium, mercury, vitamin C," *Adv Chem Ser,* 200:551-69; 1982.

Steinwall, O, "Chemotoxic blood-brain barrier damage with special regard to some mercurial effects," in L Roizin, et al, eds, *Neurotoxicology,* Raven Press, NY, 1977.

Stewart-Pinkham SM, "The effect of ambient cadmium air pollution on the hair mineral content of children," *Sci Total Environ,* 78:289-96; 1989.

Stern H, "Lead, lithium and manic-depressive psychosis," *The Chicago Medical School Quarterly,* 28:87-95; 1969.

Stock A, "Nothing new under the sun: Experiences with mercury poisoning," *J Orthomol Psychiat,* 12(3):202-7; 1983. (re: E Jaensch, MD, 1926)

Stohs SJ, Bagchi D, "Oxidative mechanisms in the toxicity of metal ions," *Free Radic Biol Med,* 18(2): 321-36; 2/1995.

Stretesky P, et al, "Homicide rates linked to lead levels," *Arch Pediatr Adolesc Med,* 5/2001.

Sumathi R, Devi VK, et al, "DL alpha-lipoic acid protection against cadmium-induced tissue lipid peroxidation," *Med Sci Res,* 22:23-25; 1994.

Sumathi R, Baskaran G, et al, "Relationship between glutathione and DL alpha-lipoic acid against cadmium-induced hepatotoxicity, *Jpn J Med Sci Biol,* 49(2):39-48; 1996. (Rat study. Pretreatment with lipoic acid decreased liver damage and overall toxicity on cadmium exposure.)

Suzuki S, Taguchi T, et al, "Dietary factors influencing the retention rate of orally administed CdCl3 in mice, with special reference to calcium and protein concentrations in diet," *Ind Health,* 7(3,4):155-62; 1969.

Svare CW, et al, "The effect of removing dental amalgam on mercury blood levels," *J Dent Res,* 60(9):1668-70; 1981.

Taylor J, *The Complete Guide to Mercury Toxicity from Dental Fillings,* Scripps, San Diego, CA, 1988.

Tirosh O, Sen CK, et al, "Neuroprotective effects of alpha-lipoic acid and its positively charged amide analogue," *Free Radic Biol Med,* 26(11-12):1418-26; 6/1999. (Protects from glutamate cytotoxicity, cell peroxidation, and loss of cellular glutathione.)

Thatcher RW, Lester ML, "Effects of low levels of cadmium and lead on cognitive functioning in children," *Arch Environ Health,* 37(3):159-66; 1982.

Townsend Letter for Doctors and Patients, "Psychiatric disturbances and toxic metals," 4/2002.

Trakhtenberg IM, Leskova GE, et al, [Protective action of lipoic acid in poisoning by organic mercury compounds (experimental data)], *Gig Tr Prof Zabol,* (9):25-8; 9/1974. (Lipoic is effective on organic mercury.)

Trakhtenberg IM, Talakin I, et al, [Prophylactic use of pectin in occupational mercurialism], *Gig Tr Prof Zabol,* (7):33-6; 7/1980.

Trakhtenberg IM, Lukovenko VP, [The prophylactic use of pectin in chronic lead exposure in industry] *Gig Tr Prof Zabol,* (1-2):132-6; 1-2/1995.

U.S. Congress, Office of Technology Assessment, *Neurotoxicity: Identifying and Controlling Poisons of the Nervous System,* U.S. Government Printing Office, pub #OTA-BA-436; 1990.

Walsh TJ, Schulz DW, et al, "Acute exposure to triethyl lead enhances the behavioral effects of dopaminergic agonists: Involvement of brain dopamine in organolead neurotoxicity," *Brain Res,* 363(2):222-29; 1/22/1986. (Intensifies cognitive and behavioral effects, motor stimulation, hyperactivity, stereotypy.)

Walsh WJ, Usman A, et al, "Disordered metal metabolism in a large autism population," Presented at the APA annual meeting, New Orleans, 5/2001. At: www.hriptc.org/metal_autism.html

Walsh WJ, "Metal-metabolism and human functioning." At: www.hriptc.org/metal_metabolism.html Accessed: 12/6/2004.

Walsh WJ, "Biochemical individuality and nutrition." At: www.hriptc.org/biochemical_individuality.html

Walsh WJ, "Commentary on nutritional treatment of mental disorders," *International Guide to the World of Alternative Mental Health.* At: www.alternativementalhealth.com/articles.walshMP.htm#Py Accessed: 10/08/06.

Walsh, William J, PhD, interview with author, July 2008.

Weiner R, Ross M, "Occupational health monitoring practices of registered mercury-using workplaces with Gauteng," *S Afr Med J,* 86(8):943-6; 1996.

Weintraub S, *Minding Your Body,* Complementary Medicine Pub. Co, Portland, OR, 1995.

Whanger PD, "Selenium in the treatment of heavy metal poisoning and chemical carcinogenesis," *J Trace Elem Electrol Health Dis,* 6:209-21; 1992.

Woodruff, Croft MH, "Mercury Amalgams," *Country Health,* 13(4):28; 7-8/1995.

Zamm AV, "Removal of dental mercury: Often an effective treatment for the very sensitive patient," *J Orthomol Med,* 5(3):138-42; 1990.

Ziff S, *Silver Dental Fillings: The Toxic Timebomb,* Aurora Press, 1984.

Ziff S, Ziff M, *Infertility & Birth Defects,* Bio-Probe, Orlando, FL, 1987.

Ziff S, Ziff MF, et al, *Dentistry without mercury,* Bio-Probe, Inc, 1997.

Other toxins

U.S. Congress, Office of Technology Assessment, *Neurotoxicity: Identifying and Controlling Poisons of the Nervous System,* US Government Printing Office, publication #OTA-BA-436; 1990; p 46.

Tobacco

Am J Addiction, 2:315-9; 1993.

Boyd W, "Smoking and mental illness", *JAMA,* 11/22/2000. (Harvard Medical School study of 4,411 responders to a National Comorbidity Survey.)

The Brown University Digest of Addiction, "Theory and Application," 6/1994; p 7.

Douglass J, et al, "Effects of raw food diet on hypertension and obesity," *South Med J,* 788(7): 841; 1985. (In hypertensives who smoke or drank, 80% abstained spontaneously when on a diet of 62% uncooked food.)

Greden, J, "Caffeine and tobacco dependence," in *Comprehensive Textbook of Psychiatry,* Wilkins, Baltimore, 1985; pp 1026-33.

Handelman GH, Packer L, et al, "Destruction of tocopherols, carotenoids and retinol in human plasma by cigarette smoke," *Am J Clin Nutr,* 63: 559-65; 1996.

Hoffer A, *Orthomolecular Medicine for Physicians,* Keats, New Canaan, CN, 1983.

Hoffer A, "Nutrition and behavior" in J Bland, ed, *Medical Applications of Clinical Nutrition,* Keats, New, Canaan, CN, 1983.

Hughes JR, Hatsukami DK, et al, "Prevalence of smoking among psychiatric outpatients," *Am J Psychiat,* 143:993-97; 1986.

Humiston K, in Burton Goldberg Group, ed, *Alternative Medicine,* Future Medicine, Puyallup, WA, 1993.

Mowrey DB, *Next Generation Herbal Medicine,* Keats, New Canaan, CN, 1990.

Munro LH, Burton G, et al, "Plasma RRR-alpha-tocopherol concentrations are lower in smokers than in non-smokers after ingestion of a similar oral load of this antioxidant vitamin," *Clin Sci,* 92: 87-93; 1997.

Murray MT, "Lifestyle and dietary factors in depression," *Am J Natural Med,* 2:10-15; 1995.

Ott A, *Lancet,* June 1998. (Over two years, 105/6,870 Netherlanders over 55 developed Alzheimer's; 41, other dementias. Smoking was associated with more than double the risk of Alzheimer's, and an increased risk of vascular dementia.)

Philpott WH, "Maladaptive reactions to frequently used foods and commonly met chemicals as precipitating factors in many chronic physical and chronic emotional illnesses," in R Williams, D Kalita, eds, *A Physician's Handbook on Orthomolecular Medicine,* Keats, New Canaan, CN, 1977.

Philpott W, Kalita D, *Brain Allergies: The Psychonutrient Connection,* Keats, New Canaan, CN, 1980, 87.

Vieweg WV, David JJ, et al, "Correlation of cigarette-induced increase in serum nicotine levels with arginine vasopressin concentrations in the syndrome of self-induced water intoxication and psychosis (SIWIP)," *Can J Psychiat,* 31(2):108-11; 3/1986. (10 SIWIP patients included one bipolar. Smoking can alter diuresis. Limbic-hypothalamic neurotransmitters may induce both SIWIP and inappropriate vasopressin release.)

Walsh WJ, quoted in *Alternative Medicine,* Burton Goldberg Group, ed, Future Medicine, Puyallup, WA, 1993.

Caffeine

Bolton S, Null G, "Caffeine, psychological effects, use and abuse," *J Orthomol Psychiat,* 10(3):202-11; 1981.

Boulenger P, "Panic attack and the caffeine factor," *Psychopharmacol Bull,* 18:53-57. (In 30 panic disorder patients, anxiety and depression correlated with caffeine intake. Subjects showed a heightened sensitivity to caffeine as compared to controls.)

Brody JE, "Bodily interaction found to explain caffeine withdrawal headache," *New York Times,* 4/24/1982.

Bruce M, Lader M, "Caffeine abstention in the management of anxiety disorders," *Psychol Med,* 19:211-4; 1989.

Casdorph HR, Walker M, *Toxic Metal Syndrome: How Metal Poisoning Can Affect Your Brain,* Avery, Garden City Park, NY, 1995.

Christensen, L, "Psychological distress and diet — effects of sucrose and caffeine," *J Appl Nutr,* 40(1):44-50; 1988. (Double blind.)

Christensen L, Burrows R, "Dietary treatment of depression," *Behav Ther,* 21:183-93; 1990. (Depressives assigned to avoid sugar and caffeine showed significantly greater improvement than those avoiding red meat and artificial sweeteners. 3 in the sugar/caffeine group showed caffeine sensitivity.)

Gaby AR, "Preventing and Reversing Osteoporosis," Prima, Rocklin CA, 1994.

Galton, Lawrence, *You May Not Need A Psychiatrist,* Simon & Schuster, NY, 1979.

Greden, John F, et al, U Michigan Med Ctr and Ann Arbor VA Hosp, 1976. (Caffeine was associated with increased anxiety, fatigue, and depression, with little awareness of its role in symptoms.)

Greden, J, "Caffeine and tobacco dependence," in *Comprehensive Textbook of Psychiatry,* Wilkins, Baltimore, 1985; pp 1026-33. (Greater intake of caffeine correlated with more severe depression.)

Heaney RP, "Effects of nitrogen, phosphorus and caffeine on calcium balance in women," *J Lab Clin Med,* 99:46-55; 1982.

Hernandez-Avila M, et al, "Caffeine, moderate alcohol intake, and risk of fractures of the hip and forearm in middle-aged women," *Am J Clin Nutr,* 54:157-63; 1991.

Hoffer, Abram, MD PHD, *Orthomolecular Medicine for Physicians,* Keats, New Canaan, CN, 1983.

Hollingbery PW, et al, "Effect of dietary caffeine and aspirin on urinary calcium and hydroxyproline excretion in pre and postmenopausal women," *Fed Proc,* 44:1149; 1985.

Hughes JR, et al, "Caffeine self-administration, withdrawal and adverse effects among coffee drinkers," *Arch Gen Psychiat,* 48:611-17; 1991. (Double blind.)

Kreitsch, K, et al, "Prevalence, presenting symptoms, and psychological characteristics of individuals experiencing a diet-related mood disturbance," *Behav Ther,* 19:593-614; 1988. (50% reacted to caffeine or sucrose.)

Lee MA, Flegel P, et al, "Anxiogenic effects of caffeine on panic and depressed patients," *Am J Psychiat,* 145:632-35; 1988. (Caffeine can increase anxiety in people prone to panic attacks.)

Levi L, "The effect of coffee on the function of the sympathoadrenomedullary system in man," *Act Med Scand,* 181:431-8, 1967. (Caffeine increases epinephrines.)

McManamy MC, Schube PG, "Caffeine intoxication," *NEJM,* 215(6):16-20.

Mikkelsen E.J, "Caffeine and schizophrenia," *Behavioral Med*; 12/1980. (High intake correlated with anxiety or psychosis. Heavy coffee drinkers on psych wards showed more extreme psychosis. Animal studies suggest caffeine increases NE; and initially, DA, followed by a prolonged decrease.)

Mikkelsen E.J, "Caffeine and schizophrenia," *J Clin Psychiat,* 39(9); 9/1978.

Moore, Daniel T, PhD, "A holistic approach for treating manic depressive disorders," At: familyclinic.simplenet.com/bipolar/bipaper.html 1998.

Murray MT, "Lifestyle and dietary factors in depression," *Am J Natural Med,* 2:10-15; 1995.

Neil JF, Himmelhoch JM, et al, "Caffeinism complicating hypersomnic depressive episodes", *Compr Psychiat,* 19:377-85; 1978.

Partoles M, et al, "Caffeine intake lowers the level of phenylalanine, tyrosine and thyroid hormones in rat plasma," *Ircs Med Sci,* 12:1002-3; 1984.

Robertson D, Freilich JC, et al, "Effects of caffeine on plasma activity, catecholamines, and blood pressure," *NEJM,* 298:181-6; 1978.

Silverman K, Evans SM, et al, "Withdrawal syndrome after the double-blind cessation of caffeine consumption," *NEJM,* 327:1109-14; 1992.

Tondo L, Rudas N, "The course of a seasonal bipolar disorder influenced by caffeine," *J Affect Disord,* 22(4):249-51; 9/1991. (Case report. Stopping heavy caffeine intake may have contributed to sudden remission of a severe seasonal bipolar disorder.

Uhde TW, et al, "Caffeine and behavior. Relation to psychopathology and underlying mechanisms. Caffeine: Relationship to human anxiety, plasma MHPG, and cortisol," *Psychopharm Bull,* 20(3): 4216-30; 1984.

Zander RH, *Saturday Evening Post,* 5-6/1982, pp 50-4.

Alcohol

Ackerson A, Jaques B, "Nutritional support in alcohol dependency: Hepatoprotection and detoxification," *Tyler Research and Information Series,* Gresham, OR, 1997.

Airola P, *How to Get Well,* Health Plus, Phoenix, AZ, 1979.

Baker H, et al, "Inability of chronic alcoholics with liver disease to use food as a source of folates, thiamin and vitamin B6," *Am J Clin Nutr,* 28: 1377-80; 1975.

Baker, "Plasma vitamin B12 titres as indicators of disease severity and mortality of patients with alcoholic hepatitis," *Alcoholism,* 22(1):15; 1987.

Balch JF, Balch P, *Prescription for Nutritional Healing,* Avery, Garden City Park, NY, 1990.

Bertelli A, Cerrati A, et al, "Protective action of L-carnitine and coenzyme Q-10 against hepatic triglyceride infiltration induced by hyperbaric oxygen and ethanol," *Drugs Exp Clin Res,* 1920: 65-68; 1993.

Brady KT, Lydiard RB, "Bipolar affective disorder and substance abuse," *J Clin Psychopharmacol,* 12(1S):17-22S; 2/1992. (NIMH catchment area data indicate that of all axis I disorders, bipolar is most associated with substance abuse or dependence. Alcohol and cocaine abuse are far more common than in the general population. Anticonvulsant, antikindling agents may help.)

Branchey L, et al, "Depression, suicide and aggression in alcoholics and their relationship to plasma amino acids," *Psychiat Res,* 12(3): 219-26; 1984. (Tryptophan is low compared to competing aminos in alcoholics with histories of both aggression and depression, but not necessarily with depression alone.)

Brigham PM, "The Psychopharmacology of Bipolar Disorder." At: http://people.ne.mediaone.net/pmbrig/BP_pharm.html Accessed: 6-11-01 (Some bipolars may stop drinking when depressed.)

Broida, Marian, RN, *New Hope for People with Depression,* Prima (Random House), Roseville CA, 2001.

Brown SA, Schuckit MA, "Changes in depression among abstinent alcoholics," *J Stud Alcohol,* 49:412-7; 1988. (Patients in alcohol treatment programs start with a very high rates of depression, which decline rapidly after abstention.)

Cleary JP, "Niacinamide and addictions," letter, *J Nutr Med,* 1:83-4; 1990. (500-1000 mg/day stopped drug and alcohol craving, which resurfaced when B3 was discontinued.)

Cousens G, *Depression Free for Life,* Quill, HarperCollins, NY, 2001.

Deak G, Muzes G, et al, "Immunomodulator effect of silymarin therapy in chronic alcoholic disease," *Orvosi Hetilap,* 131(24):1291-2, 1295-6; 1990.

Dees SC, "An experimental study of the effects of alcohol and alcoholic beverages on allergic reactions," *Ann Allergy,* 7:185; 1949.

Davidson KM, "Diagnosis of depression in alcohol dependence: Changes in prevalence with drinking status," *Br J Psychiat,* 166:199-204; 1995.

Dunner DL, "A restrospective chart review of 188 bipolars," 1/1992-12/1993." (Demographics, clinical features, and course were different in bipolars with preexisting substance abuse, vs those whose abuse began during the illness, and nonusers.)

Dutta P, Seirafi J, et al, "Acute ethanol exposure alters hepatic glutathione metabolism in riboflavin deficiency," *Alcohol,* 12(1):43-47; 1995.

Feinman JA, Dunner DL, "The effect of alcohol and substance abuse on the course of bipolar affective disorder," *J Affect Disord,* 37(1):43-49; 1996. (Over 60% of bipolar I and almost 50% of bipolar II have a history of substance abuse.)

Gloria L, Cravo M, et al, "Hyperhomocysteinemia in chronic alcoholism: Correlation with folate, vitamin B12 and vitamin B6 status," *Am J Clin Nutr,* 63(2): 220-24; 1996.

Gunther RM, "Role of nutritional therapy in alcoholism treatment," *Intl J Biosocial Res,* 4(1): 5-18; 1983. (Enhanced diet plus multivitamins. 6-month follow-up revealed 81% still sober.)

Hawkins DR, "Diagnosing the schizophrenias," *J Orthomol Psychiat,* 5(1):18-25, 1976.

Hoffer A, "Vitamin B3, niacin and its amide." At: Doctoryourself.com/hoffer_niacin.html Accessed: 4/2007

Ikeda H, "Effects of taurine on alchohol withdrawal," letter, *Lancet,* 2:509; 1977.

Kahan F, Hoffer A, Osmond H, *New Hope for Alcoholics,* University Books, NY, 1966.

Ketter, "Defining the standard of care across the bipolar spectrum: Q & A, April 9,2000; DC, Faculty: Terrence A Ketter MD," Bipolar Disorders Information Center. At: http://www.mhsource.com/bipolar/defketter.html Accessed: 6/11/2001.

Keung WM, "Biochemical studies of a new class of alcohol dehydrogenase inhibitors from Radix Puerpuerariae," *Alcoholism Clin Exp Res,* 17(6): 1254-60; 1993.

Larson JM, *Alcoholism — The Biochemical Connection,* Villard Books, NY, 1992.

Larson, Joan Matthews, PhD, interview with author, June 9, 2008.

Liebber CS, Robins SJ, et al, "Hepatic phosphatidyl ethanolamine methyltransferease activity is decreased by ethanol and increased by phosphatidylcholine," *Alcoholism, Clin Exp Res,* 18(3):592-95; 1994.

Malto JM, Alvarez L, et al, "S-adenosyl-L-methionine

synthetase and methione metabolism deficiencies in cirrhosis," *Adv Exp Med Biol*, 368:113-17; 1994.

Murray MT, Pizzorno JE, *Encyclopedia of Natural Medicine,* Prima, Rocklin CA, 1998.

Murray MT, "Lifestyle and dietary factors in depression," *Am J Natural Med,* 2:10-15; 1995.

Norton VP, "Interrelationships of nutrition and voluntary alcohol consumption in experimental animals," *Br J Addiction;* 72(3):205-12; 1977. (Rats preferred alcohol over water only when low in B.)

Page LR, *Healthy Healing*, Healthy Healing Pub, CA, 1992.

Par A, "Pathogenesis and management of alcoholic liver injury," *Acta Physiologica Hungarica*, 80(1-4): 325-50; 1992.

Pfeiffer CC, *Nutrition and Mental Illness,* Healing Arts Press, Rochester, VT, 1987.

Pfeiffer CC, *The Schizophrenias Ours to Conquer,* Bio-Communications Press, Wichita, KS, 1988.

Rogers LL Pelton RB, et al, "Amino acid supplementation and voluntary alcohol consumption by rats," *J Biol Chem,* 220:321-323; 1956.

Rogers LL, Pelton RB, "Effects of glutamine on IQ scores of mentally deficient children," *Rep Biol Med,* 15:84-90; 1957a.

Rogers LL, Pelton RB, "Glutamine in the treatment of alcoholism," *Quart St,* 18:581-87; 1957b.

Rush AJ, "Toward an understanding of bipolar disorder and its origin," *J Clin Psychiat,* 64:4-8; 2003b.

Sachan DS, Cha YS, "Acetylcarnitine inhibits alcohol dehydrogenase," *Chem Biophys Res Comm,* 203(3):1496-501; 1994.

Schuppan D, Atkinson J, et al, "Alcohol and liver fibrosis — pathochemistry and treatment," *Zeitschrift fur Gastroenterologie,* 33(9):546-50; 1995.

Shelock S, "Nutrition and the alcoholic," *Lancet,* 1: 436-8; 1984. (Difficulty absorbing B1, B6, folic acid, B12, A, E, calcium, EFAs; and storing A, B6, zinc.)

Smith RF, "A five year field trial of massive nicotinic acid therapy of alcoholics in Michigan," *J Orthomol Psychiat,* 3:327-32; 1974.

Smith RF, "Status report concerning the use of megadose nicotinic acid in alcoholics," *J Orthomol Psychiat,* 7:52-5; 1978.

Spencer H, et al, "Alcohol osteoporosis," *Am J Clin Nutr,* 41:847; 1985.

Tanaka, T, Ando, M, et al, "Effects of alanine and glutamine administration on the inhibition of liver regeneation by acute ethanol treatment," *Alcohol and Alcoholism,* 1S:41-45; 1993.

Tanner AR, et al, "Depressed selenium and vitamin E levels in an alcoholic population: Possible relationship to hepatic injury through increased oxidation," *Dig Dis Sci,* 31:1307-12; 1986.

Walsh WJ, PhD, "Commentary on nutritional treatment of mental disorders," *International Guide to the World of Alternative Mental Health.* At: www.alternativementalhealth.com/articles.walshMP.htm#Py Accessed:10/08/2006.

Walsh, William J, PhD, interview with author, November, 2007.

Weinisch S, et al, "Can megadoses of thiamine prevent ethanol-induced damages of rat hippocampal CA1 pyramidal neurons," *Z Ehnahrungswiss,* 35(3):166-272; 1996.

Whybrow PC, *A Mood Apart, Depression, Mania, and Other Afflictions of the Self,* Basic Books, HarperCollins, NY, 1997.

Wilson B, "The vitamin B3 therapy: The first communication to AA's Physicians," 1967; & "A second Communication to AA's Physicians," 1968.

Winokur G, Coryell W, et al, "Alcoholism in manic-depressive (bipolar) illness: familial illness, course of illness, and the primary/secondary distinction," *Am J Psychiat,* 152(3):365-68; 3/1995. (Alcoholism is more likely in bipolars. Family history of alcoholism and affective disorder was similar in alcoholic and nonalcoholic bipolars. Secondary alcoholism was more likely to remit than primary. Primary alcoholics showed significantly fewer affective episodes at followup, suggesting less severe bipolar illness, perhaps triggered by alcoholism.)

Wickramasinghe SN, Hasan R, "In vitro effects of vitamin C, thioctic acid and dihydrolipoic acid on the cytotoxicity of post-ethanol serum," *Biochemical Pharmacology*.

Winokur G, Coryell W, et al, "Familiar alcoholism in manic-depressive (bipolar) disease," *Am J Med Genet,* 67(2):197-201; 4/9/1996. (NIMH. Alcoholism occured more frequently in relatives of bipolar I patients (especially if alcoholic) than in controls.)

Zie CI, Kawamoto A, et al, "Mechanism of antioxidant action of pueraria glycoside (PG)-1 (an isoflavonoid) and mangiferin (a xanthonoid)," *Chem Pharm Bull,* 40(3):721-24; 1992.

Substance abuse. Prescription drugs.

Alao AO, Yolles JC, "Isonazid-induced psychosis," *Ann Pharmacother,* 32(9):889-91; 9/1998. (Psychosis in a 31-year old woman partially resolved after withdrawal. Other case reports note associated mania, OCD, psychosis. Authors suggest checking for B6 deficit via urinary tryptophan metabolites.)

Dr. Manfred Anke, Karl Marx School, Leipzig Germany, as reported in Hoffer, 1983.

Brady KT, Lydiard RB, "Bipolar affective disorder and substance abuse," *J Clin Psychopharmacol,* 12(1S):17-22S; 2/1992.

Braverman E, Pfeiffer CC, *The Healing Nutrients Within,* Keats, New Canaan, CN, 1987.

Brigham PM, "The Psychopharmacology of Bipolar Disorder," At: http://people.ne.mediaone.net/pmbrig/BP_pharm.html Accessed: 6-11-01. (Substance abuse is prevalent and could be a symptom (e.g., judgment impairment), a cause, self-medication, or due to common risk factors.)

Costall B, Naylor R, "Mesolimbic and extrapyramidal sites for the mediation of sterotyped behavior patterns and hyperactivity by amphetamine and apomorphine in the rat," in EH Ellinwood, MM Kilbey, eds, *Cocaine and Other Stimulants, Advances in Behavioral Biology, V21,* Plenum, NY, 1977; pp 47-76.

Cousens G, *Depression Free for Life,* Quill, HarperCollins, NY, 2001.

Dunner DL, "A retrospective chart review of 188 bipolars, 1/1992-12/1993."

Feinman JA, Dunner DL, "The effect of alcohol and substance abuse on the course of bipolar affective disorder," *J Affect Disord,* 37(1):43-49; 1996.

Frye MA, Ketter TA, "Defining the standard of care across the bipolar spectrum: Q & A, April 9,2000; SF, Faculty: Mark A Frye MD, Terrence A Ketter," Bipolar Disorders Information Center. At: http://www.mhsource.com/bipolar/defzarate.html Accessed: 6/11/2001.

Gant C, *End Your Addiction Now,* Warner, 2002.

Gerner RH, Post RM, "A dopaminergic mechanism in mania," *Am J Psychiat,* 133:1177-80; 1976. (Case report. Amphetamines repeatedly induced mania. Lag time, in 2 instances, was 32-34 hrs.)

Gold MS, *The Good News About Depression,* Villard Books, NY, 1987.

Goodwin, Jamison, *Manic Depressive Illness,* Oxford University Press, 1990.

Ketter TA, "Defining the standard of care across the bipolar spectrum: Q & A, April 9,2000, DC, Faculty: Terrence A Ketter MD," Bipolar Disorders Information Center. At: http://www.mhsource.com/bipolar/defketter.html Accessed: 6/11/2001. (If still functional, it's not drug abuse, though kindling may lead to episodes and mixed states, compromise lithium response, and generally worsen the illness.)

Larson, Joan Matthews, PhD, interview with author, June 9, 2008.

Matthews-Larson, Joan, PhD, *7 Weeks to Sobriety,* Fawcett Columbine, 1997.

McLellan AT, Childress AR, et al, "Drug abuse and psychiatric disorders: Role of drug choice," in A Alterman, ed, *Substance abuse and Psychopathology,* Plenum, NY, pp 137-72.

Mendez MF, "Mania self-induced with cough syrup [letter]," *J Clin Psychiat,* 53(5):173-4; 5/1992.

Page LR, *Healthy Healing,* Healthy Healing Pub, CA, 1992.

Pfeiffer CC, *Nutrition and Mental Illness,* Healing Arts Press, Rochester, VT, 1987.

Pfeiffer CC, *The Schizophrenias Ours to Conquer,* Bio-Communications Press, Wichita, KS, 1988.

Regier DA, Farmer ME, et al, "Comorbidity of mental disorders with alcohol and other drug abuse: Results from the Epidemiological Catchment Area (ECA) study," *JAMA,* 264:2511-18; 1990.

Rosenblatt S, *Beyond Valium,* GP Putnam's Sons, NY, 1981.

Rush AJ, "Bipolar disorder: Origin, recognition, and treatment," *J Clin Psychiat,* 64:3 2003a.

Rush AJ, "Toward an understanding of bipolar disorder and its origin," *J Clin Psychiat,* 64:4-8; 2003.

Scheel-Kruger J, Baestrup C, "Cocaine: Discussion of the role of dopamine in the biochemical mechanism of action," in *Cocaine and other Stimulants,* Plenum, NY, 1977.

Snyder, *Biological Aspects of Mental Disorder,* Oxford U Press, NY, 1980.

Steiner W, Laporta M, Chouinard G, "Neuroleptic-induced supersensitivity psychosis in patients with bipolar affective disorder," *Acta Psychiatr Scand,* 81(5): 437-40; 5/1990. (Case reports. 5 bipolars developed mesolimbic supersensitivity psychosis subsequent to neuroleptic treatment.)

Strakowski SM, DelBello MP, "The co-occurrence of bipolar and substance use disorders," *Clin Psychol Rev,* 20(2):191-206; 2000.

Tohen M, Zarate CA, "Bipolar disorder and comorbid substance abuse disorder," in JF Goldberg, M Harrow eds, *Bipolar disorders: Clinical course and outcome,* AP Press, DC, 1999; pp 171-84.

Torrey, EF, *Surviving Schizophrenia: A Family Manual,* rev ed, Harper & Row, NY, 1988.

Trimble MR, "Anticonvulsant-induced psychiatric disorders. The role of forced normalization," *Drug Saf,* 15(3):159-66; 9/1996.

Walsh WJ, "Biochemical treatment: Medicines for the next century," *NOHA NEWS,* 16(3), Summer 1991.

Walsh WJ, "Commentary on nutritional treatment of mental disorders," *International Guide to the World of Alternative Mental Health.* At: www.alternativementalhealth.com/articles.walshMP.htm#Py Accessed:10/08/2006.

Weiss RD, Mirin SN, "Substance abuse as an attempt at self-medication," *Psychiat Med,* 3: 357-67; 1987.

Whybrow PC, *A Mood Apart, Depression, Mania, and Other Afflictions of the Self,* Basic Books, HarperCollins, NY, 1997.

Winokur G, Turvey C, et al, "Alcoholism and drug abuse in three groups — Bipolar I, unipolars, and their acquaintances," *J Affect Disord,* 50:81-89; 1998.

Excitotoxicity

Almeida LMV, Pineiro CC, et al, "Resveratrol increases glutamate uptake, glutathione content, and S100B secretion in cortical astrocyte cultures," *Cell Molec Neurobiol,* 27(5); 2007.

alternativemental health.com/articles/pyroluria.htm

Balch JF, Balch P, *Prescription for Natural Healing,* Avery, Garden City Park, NY, 1990.

Bartholini G, "GABA receptor agonists: Pharmacological spectrum and therapeutic agents," *Med Res Rev,* 5(1):55-75; 1-3/1985. (Review.)

Blaylock R, *Excitotoxins: The Taste that Kills,* Health Press, Santa Fe, NM, 1995.

Bodnar RJ, et al, "Neonatal monosodium glutamate effect upon analgesic responsivity and immonocytochemical ACTH/beta-lipoptropin," *Neuroendocrinology,* 30:280-84; 1980.

Brambilla P, Perez J, et al, "GABAergic dysfunction in mood disorders," *Molec Psychiat,* 8(8):721-3; 2003. (Low GABA in some animal models and affectives. Drugs which increase GABA activity have been helpful. GABA support may help some bipolars.)

Braverman E, Pfeiffer CC, *The Healing Nutrients Within,* Keats, New Canaan, CN, 1987.

Chalecka-Franaszek E, Chuang DM, "Lithium activates the serine kinase Akt-1 and suppresses glutamate-induced inhibition of Akt-1 activity in neurons," *Proc Natl Acad Sci USA,* 96(15):8745-50; 7/20/1999. (The means by which lithium is protective against glutamate-induced excitotoxicity may involve modulation of Akt-1 activity.)

Choi DW, "Glutamate neurotoxicity: A three-stage process," in A Guicotti, ed, *Neurotoxicity of Excitatory Amino Acids,* FIDA Research Foundation Symposium Series, 4: 235-42; 1990.

Coyle JT, et al, "Excitatory amino acid neurotoxins: Selectivity, specificity, and mechanisms of action," *Neurosci Res Prog Bull,* 19:4; 1981.

Dawson R, Simpkins JW, et al, "Age and dose dependent effects of neonatal monosodium glutamate (MSG) administration to female rats," *Neurotox Teratp,* 11:331-337; 1989. (MSG influences DA neuron ontogenesis and migration in the hypothalamus of the neonatal rat.)

Dasgupta B, Milbrandt J, "Resveratrol stimulates AMP kinase activity in neurons," *PNAS,* 2007. (AMPK senses cellular energy. It may decrease over-stimulation by reducing energy output when AMP:ATP is high.)

de Souza CT, Nunes WM, et al, "Insulin secretion in monosodium glutamate (MSG) obese rats submitted to aerobic exercise training," *Physiol Chem Phys Med NMR,* 35(1):43-53; 2003

Eby G, "Magnesium & stress: Rapid recovery from severe, treatment-resistant depression using magnesium," Austin, Texas, 12/9/2001.

Erb J, Erb TM, *The Slow Poisoning of America,* Paladins Press, 2003.

Federation of American Societies for Experimental Biology (FASEB), *Report to FDA,* 1995.

Gold MS, *The Good News About Depression,* Villard Books, NY, 1987.

Greenamyre JT, Young AB, "Excitatory amino acids and Alzheimer's disease," *Neurobiology of Aging,* 10:593-602; 1989.

Itamura CA, Mauri M, et al, "Plasma and platelet excitatory amino acids in psychiatric disorders," *Am J Psychiat,* 150:1731-33; 1993. (Plasma glutamate was significantly elevated in 15 affectives.)

Kendell SF, Krystal JH, et al, "GABA and glutamate systems as therapeutic targets in depression and mood disorders," *Expert Opinon on Therapeutic Targets,* 9(1):153-68; 2/2005.

Klingberg H, Brankack J, "Long-term effects on behavior after postnatal treatment with monosodium-L-glutamate," *Biomed Biochem,* 46:705-11; 1987.

Krystal JH, Sanacora G, et al, "Glutamate and GABA systems as targets for novel antidepressant and mood-stabilizing treatments," *Mol Psychiat,* 7S(1): 71-80; 2002. (Stabilizers and antidepressants may partly work by modulating GABA and glutamate. Stabilization raises GABA and repletes deficits. Glutamate-suppressing drugs can be antimanic. MRS suggests major depression may be associated with low cortex GABA. Clinical work suggests antidepressants suppress NMDA/glutamate receptors.)

Levine J, Panchalingam K, et al, "Increased cerebrospinal fluid glutamine levels in depressed patients," *Biol Psychiat,* 47(7):586-93; 2000.

Maragos WF, Greenamyre JT, et al, "Glutamate dysfunction in Alzheimer's disease: An hypothesis," *TINS,* 10:65-68; 1987.

Martini B, "The connection between Aspartame® (an artificial sweetener) and panic attacks, depression, bipolar disorder, memory problems, and other mental symptoms," *Time Magazine,* 2002. Reprinted at: www.alternativementalhealth.com/articles/aspartame.htm Accessed 9/6/2005

McGinnis W, "Pyroluria: Hidden cause of schizophrenia, bipolar, depression, and anxiety symptoms," Orlando FL, 5/21/2004.

Mebane, AH, "L-glutamine and mania," letter, *Am J Psychiat,* 141(10); 1984.

Michael N, Erfurth A, et al, "Acute mania is accompanied by elevated glutamate/glutamine levels within the left dorsolateral prefrontal cortex," *Psychopharmacol,* 168(3); 7/2003. (Proton MRS of 8 manics found significantly elevated levels.)

www.mpwhi.com

Nairn AC, et al, "Protein kinases in the brain," *Ann Rev Biochem,* 54:931-76; 1985.

Olney JW, et al, "Glutamate induced brain damage in infant primates," *J Neuropath Exp Neur,* 31: 464-487; 1972.

Olney JW, Price MT, "Excitotoxic amino acids as neuroendocrine probes," in EG McGreer, JW Olney, PL McGreer, eds, *Kainic Acid as a Tool in Neurobiology,* Raven Press, New York; 1978.

Olney JW, "Application of neurotoxins in neurobiology," *Neurosci Res Bull,* 14(4):384; 1981.

Olney JW, "Excitotoxic food additives: Functional teratological aspects," *Prog Brain Res,* 18:283-294; 1988. (Typical prepared foods can expose children to 20-fold plasma glutamate elevation.)

Olney JW, "Glutamate, a neurotoxic transmitter," *J Child Neurol,* 4:218-25; 1989.

Page LR, *Healthy Healing,* Healthy Healing Pub, CA, 1992.

Pfeiffer CC, *The Schizophrenias Ours to Conquer,* Bio-Communications Press, Wichita, KS, 1988.

Plaitakis A, "Glutamate dysfunction and selective motor degeneration in amyotrophic lateral sclerosis: An hypothesis," *Ann Neurol,* 28:3-8; 1990.

Roberts H J, *Aspartame disease: An Ignored Epidemic,* Sunshine Sentinel Press, West Palm Beach, FL; 2002. At: susentpress@aol.com

Shimicu K, Mizutari A, et al, "Electron microscopic studies on the hypothalamic lesions in the mouse fetus caused by monosodium glutamate," *Teratology,* 8:105; 1973.

Slagle P, *The Way Up Newsletter,* #28; 4/15/2001.

Spencer PS, Nunn PB, "Guam amyotrophic-lateral-sclerosis-Parkinsonism-dementia linked to plant toxin excitant neurotoxin," *Sci,* 237:517-22; 1987.

Tanaka K, Shimada M, "Hypothalamic lesion induced by injection of monosodium glutamate in suckling period and subsequent development of obesity," *Exp Neurol,* 62(1):191-9; 10/1978

Vaddadi K, "Dyskinesias and their treatment with essential fatty acids: A review," *Prostaglandins Leukot Essent Fatty Acids,* 55(1 & 2):89-94; 7-8/1996. (Fatty acid deficiencies may play a role in excitotoxicity.)

Walton RG, Hudak R, et al, "Adverse reactions to aspartame: Double-blind challenge in patients from a vulnerable population," *Biol Psychiat,* 34(1-2):13-17; 7/1993. (Crossover. Halted at 13 depressives (rather than 40), due to the severe reactions to 30 mg/kg/d over 1 wk. Depressive history significantly increased reactivity.)

Zarate CA, Jing DU, et al, "Regulation of cellular plasticity cascades in the pathophysiology and treatment of mood disorders," *Ann NY Acad Sci,* 1003:273-91; 2003. (NMDA antagonists inhibit glutamate release, and potentiate AMPA, enhancing glutamatergic plasticity.)

Zarate CA, Singh JB, et al, "A randomized trial of N-methyl-D-aspartate antagonist in treatment-resistant major depression," *Arch Gen Psychiat,* 63(8):856-64; 2006. (Injection of an NMDA antagonist led to 71% improved, 29% remission, 35% for at least 1 wk.)

Organic solvents; Pesticides

Anger WK, "Neurobehavioral evaluation of soil and structural fumigators using methyl bromide and sulfuryl fluoride," *Neurotoxicol,* 7(3):137-156; 1986.

Bayer M, "Reversing the effects of pesticide poisoning," *Emergency Med,* 2/29/1992.

Cheremisinoff NP, King J, *Toxic Properties of Pesticides,* Marcel Dekker, NY, 1994.

Gershon S, Shaw FH, "Psychiatric sequelae of chronic exposure to organophosphate insecticides," *Lancet,* (1):1371; 1961.

Gold MS, *The Good News About Depression,* Villard Books, NY, 1987.

Hayes WJ, *Pesticides Studied in Man,* Williams & Wilkins, Baltimore, 1982.

Hayes WJ, Laws ER, *Handbook of Pesticide Toxicology,* Academic Press, NY, 1991.

Mancuso TF, "Carbon disulfide as a cause of suicide, epidemiological study of viscose rayon workers," *J Occupational Med,* 14:595-60; 1972.

Oliver T, *Dangerous Trades,* Murray, London, 1902.

Pfeiffer CC, *The Schizophrenias Ours to Conquer,* Bio-Communications, Wichita, KS, 1988.

Pryor, G.T, "Biomedical studies on the effects of abused inhalant mixtures,"*Annual report #2,* NIDA contract # 271-77-3402, 1978; pp 62-67, 97-104.

www.resveratrolandmooddisorders.wordpress

Robinowitz R, Roberts WR, et al, "Carcinogenicity and tetratogenicity vs psychogenicity: Psychological characteristics associated with self-reported Agent Orange exposure among Viet Nam combat veterans who seek treatment for substance abuse," *J Clin Psychol,* 45:718-28; 1989.

Rowntree DW, Nevin S, Wilson A, "The effects of diisopropylfluorophosphate in schizophrenia and manic depressive psychoses," *J Neurol Neurosurg Psychiat,* 13:47; 1950.

Sarter-M, *Psychopharmacology-Berl,* 114(4):539-50; 5/1994.

Senakayake N, et al, "Neurotoxic effects of organophosphates," *NEJM,* 316:761; 1987.

Spencer PS, et al, "n-hexane, n-methyl and n-butyl ketone," in PS Spencer, HH Schaumberg, eds, *Exp Clin Neurotox,* Williams & Wilkins, Baltimore, 1980; pp 456-75.

Triebig G, et al, "Congress report: International working group on the epidemiology of the chronic neurobehavioral effects of organic solvents," *International Arch Occupat Environ Health,* 61: 423-24; 1989.

US Congress, Office of Technology Assessment, *Neurotoxicity: Identifying and Controlling Poisons of the Nervous System,* US Government Printing Office, pub #OTA-BA-436; 1990.

US Congress, Office of Technology Assessment, *Pesticide Residues in Food,* US Government Printing Office, DC,1988.

Yanez M, Fraiz N, "Inhibitory effects of cis- and trans-resveratol on noradrenaline and 5-hydroxytryptamine uptake and on monoamine oxidase activity," *Biochem Biophys Res Comm,* 344(2); 2006.

Zhang H, Zhou M, "Resveratrol attenuates early pyramidal neuron excitability impairment & death in acute rat hippocampal slices caused by oxygen-glucose deprivation, *Exp Neurol,* 212(1):44-52; 2008.

Health intro

alternativementalhealth.com Newsletter #30.

Bibus DM, Holman RT, Walsh WJ, "Fatty acid profiles of schizophrenic phenotypes," Abst, 91ST Annual Mtg, AOCS, Sand Diego, 4/25-28; 2000.

Brooks JO, III, Hoblyn JC, "Secondary mania in older adults," *Am J Psychiat,* 162:11; 11/2005.

Connor TJ, Leonard BE, "Depression, stress and immunological activation: the role of cytokines in depressive disorders," *Life Sci,* 62:583-606; 1998.

Corsello S, "Stress and its effect on health," in K Greenberg, ed, *Challenging Orthodoxy,* Keats, New Canaan, CN, 1991.

Davidson K, "Schizophrenia-like psychoses associated with organic cerebral disorders: A review," *Psychiatric Developments,* 1:1-34; 1983.

Eastwood MR, Trevelyan MH, "Relationship between physical and psychiatric disorder," *Psychol Med,* 2(4):363-72; 1972.

Engler F, Vetter P, [Affective and schizophrenic syndromes in multiple sclerosis. Review of the literature and case reports], *Schweiz Arch Neurol Psychiatr,* 142(4):367-78; 1991. (Including, neuroborrelioses, syphilis, some viral encephalitis)

Frankel P, Madsen F, *Stop Homocysteine Through the Methylation Process,* Research Corner Pub, 1998.

Gardner ER, Hall, RC, "Physical illness presenting as psychiatric disease—II," *Arch Gen Psychiat,* 1981.

Gardner ER, Hall RCW, "Medical screening of psychiatric patients," *J Orthomol Psychiat,* 9(3): 207-15; 1980.

Gold MS, *The Good News About Depression,* Villard Books, NY, 1987; pp 233-4. (Hope improves lymphocyte function. Helplessness/despair increases digestive problems, cancer; interferes with growth; creates cardiovascular and immune disorders.)

Ikelman J, "The Affective Spectrum," Joyce Ikelman's Info on Bipolar Disorder (Manic Depression). At: frii.com/~parrot/bip.html Accessed: 8/8/1999.

Jaffe R, Kruesi OR, "The biochemical-immunology window: A molecular view of psychiatric case management," *J App Nutr,* 44(2); 1992.

Koran L, *Medical Evaluation Field Manual,* 1988.

Koyranyi EK, "Morbidity and rate of undiagnosed physical illness in a psychiatric clinical population," *Arch Gen Psych,* 36:414-19; 1979.

Krauthammer C, Klerman GL, "Secondary mania: Manic syndromes associated with antecedent physical illness or drugs," *Arch Gen Psychiat,* 35(11):11/1978.

Levine S, [The management of resistant depression], *Acta Psychiatr Beig,* 86(2):141-51; 3-4/1986.

Maes M, "Interleukin-2 and interleukin-6 in schizophrenia and mania: Effects of neuroleptics and mood stabilizers," *J Psychiatr Res,* 29:141-52; 1995.

Maes M, Smith R, et al, "Fatty acid composition in major depression: Decreased omega 3 fractions in cholesteryl esters and increased c20:4 omega 6/c20:5 omega 3 ratio in cholesteryl esters and phospholipids," *J Affect Disord,* 38:35-46; 1996.

Maes M, Smith RS, "Fatty acids, cytokines, and major depression," *Biol Psychiat,* 43:313-4; 1998.

Maes M, Christophe A, et al, "Lowered omega 3 polyunsaturated fatty acids in serum phopholipids and cholesteryl esters of depressed patients," *Psychiat Res,* 85(3):275-91; 1999.

Murray M, Pizzorno J, *Encyclopedia of Natural Medicine,* Prima, Rockland, CA, 1998.

McIntyr, S, Roman J, "Is there a stethoscope in the house (and is it used?)," *Arch Gen Psychiat,* 34: 1147-1151; 1975.

Papez JW, Bateman, JF, "Changes in nervous tissues and study of living organisms in mental disease," *J Nerv Men Dis,* 114:5; 1951.

Papez J, "Living organisms in nerve cells as seen under dark contrast, phase microscope," *Trans Amer Neur Assoc*; 1952.

Papez, JW, "Form of living organisms in psychotic patients," *J Nerv Men Dis,* 116:5; 1952.

Pfeiffer CC, *Nutrition and Mental Illness,* Healing Arts Press, Rochester, VT, 1987.

Pfeiffer CC, *The Schizophrenias Ours to Conquer,* rev ed, Bio-Communications Press, Wichita, KS, 1988.

Philpott WH, "Immunological deficiency in schizophrenia. Schizophrenia as a variant syndrome in the nutritional deficiency addiction-diabetes mellitus-infection disease process," *CSF, 5th Annual Meeting,* Winnipeg, Canada, 6/6/1976.

Rudin DO, et al, *The Omega 3 Phenomenon,* Rawson Assn, NY, 1987.

Schachter M, "The diagnosis and treatment of hypothyroidism," 1996, At healthy.net/scr.article.asp?ID=528

Smith RS, "The macrophage theory of depression," *Med Hypotheses,* 35:298-306; 1991.

Snyder, Solomon, MD, *Madness and the Brain,* McGraw Hill, NY, 1974.

Sterberg EM, Chrousos GP, et al, "The stress response and the regulation of inflammatory disease," *Annals Internal Med,* 1117, 854-866; 1992.

Stoll AL, *The Omega-3 Connection,* Simon & Schuster, NY, 2002.

Torrey EF, *Surviving Schizophrenia,* rev ed, Harper & Row, NY, 1988. (Schizophrenia research especially focuses on lymphocytes and immunoglobulins. Antipsychotics also affect immunity.)

Trowbridge JP, "Update on the yeast syndrome," in K Greenberg, ed, *Challenging Orthodoxy,* Keats, New Canaan, CN, 1991.

Walsh WJ, "Commentary on nutritional treatment of mental disorders," *International Guide to the World of Alternative Mental Health.* At: www.alternativementalhealth.com/articles.walshMP.htm#Py Accessed:10/08/2006.

GI integrity & function

Andrews H, Barczak P, et al, "Psychiatric illness in patients with inflammatory bowel disease," *Gut* 28: 1600-4; 1987 (91 Crohn's patients self reported a 34% prevalence of psychiatric illness.)

Balch JF, Balch P, *Prescription for Natural Healing,* Avery, Garden City Park, NY, 1990.

Bland J, *The 20-Day Rejuvenation Diet Program,* Keats, New Canaan, CN, 1997.

Research by Dr. Ralph Bolton, described in Adams, R, and Murray F, *Megavitamin Therapy,* Larchmont Books, NY, 1973.

Braverman E, *The Healing Nutrients Within,* Keats, New Canaan, CN, 1987.

Canty DJ, Zeisel SH, "Lecithin and choline in human health and disease," *Nutr Rev,* 52(10): 327-393; 10/1994.

Christopher JR, *School of Natural Healing,* Provo, UT, 1976.

Cochia R, "Antidepressive properties of L-glutamine," *Acta Psychiatr Belg,* 76:658-66; 1976.

Cousens G, *Depression Free for Life,* Quill, HarperCollins, NY, 2001.

Darman A, "Natural treatment of manic depression explained," At: geocities.com/allen_dar/index.html Accessed: 3/2008. (Malabsorption, etc.)

Dwivedi C, Heck WJ, et al, "Effect of calcium glucarate on beta-glucuronidase activity and glucarate content of certain vegetables and fruits," *Biochem Med Metab Biol,* 3:83-92; 1990.

Eaton KK, Howard JM, "Abnormal gut fermentation: Laboratory studies reveal deficiency of B vitamins, zinc, and magnesium," *J Nutr Environ Med,* 14(2): 115-20; 5-6/2004. (Abnormal gut fermentation associated with low B, zinc and magnesium.)

Fraga F, de Juana Velasco P, et al, "Metabolic role of gluatmine and its importance in nutritional therapy," *Nutr Hosp,* 11(4):215-25; 7-8/1996. (Supports immunity, structure, function, and metabolism of intestinal mucosa. Stimulates liver glycogen synthesis; provides energy for cell division, and growth of rapidly reproducing GI cells, and immune cells; stimulates protein synthesis and inhibits its degradation; supports carbon and nitrogen transport.)

Gilasson S, et al., *Nutritional Therapies Featuring the Core Program for Diet Revision,* Persona, Winnepeg, Manitoba, Canada, 1991.

Glass CBJ, Slomiany BL, "Derangements of biosynthesis, production and secretion of mucous in gastrointestinal injury and disease," *Adv Exp Med Biol,* 89:311-47; 1976.

Gold M, *The Good News About Depression,* Villard Books, NY, 1987.

Helzer JE, Chammas S, "A study of the association between Crohn's disease and psychiatric illness," *Gastroentero,* 86(2):324-30; 1984. (50 Crohn's patients showed significantly greater depression, and reported significantly greater obsessional or phobic symptoms, vs. 50 with chronic physical illness.

Hidaka H, et al, "Effects of fructooligosaccharides on intestinal flora and human health," *Bifodobacteria Microflora,* 5(1):37-50; 1986.

Jaffe R, Kruesi OR, "The biochemical immunology window: A molecular view of psychiatric case management," *J App Nutr,* 44(2); 1992.

Jain P, Khanna NK, [Evaluation of anti-inflammatory and analgesic properties of L-glutamine], *Agen Act,* 11:243-49; 1981.

Larson JM, *Depression Free, Naturally,* Ballantine Wellspring, NY, 2001.

Levine J, Panchalingam K, et al, "Increased cerebrospinal fluid glutamine levels in depressed patients," *Biol Psychiat,* 47(7):586-93; 2000.

Levine SA, Rheinhardt MS, "Biochemical-pathology initiated by free radicals, oxidant chemicals, and therapeutic drugs in the etiology of chemical hypersensitivity disease," *J Orthomol Psychiat,* 12(3):166-83; 1983.

Manna V, Marucci N, "Effects of short-term administration of cytidine, uridine and L-glutamine, alone or in combination on the cerebral electrical activity of patients with chronic cerebral vascular disease," *Int J Clin Pharm Res,* 8:199-210; 1988.

Mebane AH, "L-glutamine and mania," letter, *Am J Psychiat,* 141(10); 1984. (After 4 gm L-glutamine/day for 2 wks, a patient with no affective history experienced grandiosity, insomnia,hyperactive motor and verbal behavior, ended with 1 wk withdrawal. With 2 gm/day for 1 wk, a dysthymic patient experienced increasing manic symptoms.)

Minakuchi C, et al, [Clinical studies of autonomic instability with abdominal symptoms — effectiveness of gamma-oryzanol]" *Shin-Shin Igaku,* 17(4):12; 1977.

Mitsuoka T, "Bifidobacteria and their role in human health," *J Indust Microbiol,* 6:263-68; 1990.

Murray MT, *Encyclopedia of Nutritional Supplements,* Prima, 1996.

Murray MT, Pizzorno J, *Encyclopedia of Natural Medicine,* Prima, 1998.

Papez JW, "Form of living organisms in psychotic patients," *J Nerv Men Dis,* 116:5; 1952.

Papez, JW, Bateman, JF, "Changes in nervous tissues and study of living organisms in mental disease," *J Nerv Men Dis,* 114:5; 1951.

Paslawski TM, et al, "Effects of the MAO inhibitor phenelzine on glutamine and GABA concentations in rat brain," *Prog Brain Res,* 196:181-86; 1995. (Decreases brain glutamine, increases GABA.)

Pfeiffer CC, *The Schizophrenias Ours to Conquer,* Bio-Communications Press, Wichita, KS, 1988.

Pfeiffer CC, *Nutrition and Mental Illness,* Healing Arts Press, Rochester, VT, 1987.

Philpott W, Kalita D, *Brain Allergies: The Psychonutrient Connection,* Keats, New Canaan, CN, 1987.

Philpott WH, "Immunological deficiency in schizophrenia. Schizophrenia as a variant syndrome in the nutritional deficiency addiction-diabetes mellitus-infection disease process," *CSF, 5th Annual Meeting,* Winnipeg, Canada, 6/6/1976.

Ravel JM, et al, "Reversal of alcohol toxicity by glutamine," *J Biol Chem;* 9/1982.

Rhodes JM, et al, "Altered lectin binding by colonic epithelial glycoconjugates in ulcerative colitis and Crohn's disease," *Dig Dis Sci,* 33(11): 1359-63; 1988.

Riordan, Hugh, MD, interview with the author, October, 1995.

Rogers LL, Pelton RB, et al, "Amino acid supplementation and voluntary alcohol consumption by rats," *J Biol Chem,* 220:321-323; 1956.

Rogers LL, Pelton RB, "Effects of glutamine on IQ scores of mentally deficient children," *Rep Biol Med,* 15:84-90; 1957a.

Rogers LL, Pelton RB, "Glutamine in the treatment of alcoholism," *Quart St,* 18:581-87; 1957b.

Ross H, t al., *Hypoglycemia, The Disease Your Doctor Won't Treat,* Pinnacle Books, 1989.

Slagle P, "Benefits of the amino acid, L-glutamine, *The Way Up Newsletter,* Vol. 28, 4/15/2001.

Slagle P, *The Way Up from Down,* St Martin's Paperbacks, NY, 1992.

Souba WW, et al, "Glutamine metabolism by the gastrointestinal tract," *J Parent Enteral Nutr,* 9: 608-27; 1985.

Souba WW, et al, "The role of glutamine in maintaining a healthy gut and supporting the metabolic response to injury and infection," *J Surgical Res,* 48(4):383-91; 1990.

Tate G, et al, "Suppression of acute and chronic inflammation by dietary gamma linolenic acid," *J Rheumatol,* 16(6):729-34; 1989.

Trowbridge JP, "Update on the yeast syndrome," in K Greenberg, ed, *Challenging Orthodoxy,* Keats, New Canaan, CN, 1991.

Walsh WJ, "Biochemical treatment of mental illness and behavior disorders." At: www.hriptc.org/BioTreament.html Accessed: 11/17/1997.

Walsh WJ, "Biochemical individuality and nutrition," www.hriptc.org/biochemical_individuality.html 2000a.

Walsh WJ, "Biochemical individuality and nutrition," *NOHA News,* XXV(2):6-8; 2000b.

Walsh WJ, "Metal-metabolism and human functioning." At: http://www.hriptc.org/mhfres.htm Accessed: 10/31/2000c.

Walsh WJ, "A biological basis for neurologic disorders: Autism, hyperactivity, attention deficit disorder,depression, obsessive-compulsive disorder, Tourette's syndrome, and violence, An interview with William J Walsh, PhD," *Latitudes,* 5(2):1-8, 2002. At: www.Latitudes.org

Walsh WJ, "Metal metabolism and human function," At: www.hriptc.org/metal_metabolism.html Accessed 12-6-2004a

Walsh WJ, "Zinc deficiency, metal metabolism, and behavior disorders." At: Walsh hriptc.org/zinc_deficiency.html Accessed: 12/6/2004b

Walsh, WJ, "Commentary on nutritional treatment of mental disorders," *International Guide to the World of Alternative Mental Health.* At: www.alternativementalhealth.com/articles.walshMP.htm#Py

Accessed:10/08/2006.
Walsh, William J, PhD, interview with author, November, 2007.
Weintraub S, *Minding Your Body,* Complementary Medicine Pub. Portland, OR, 1995.
Young LS, et al, "Patients receiving glutamine-supplemented intravenous feedings report an improvement in mood," *J Pen,* 17:422-27; 1993.
Young LS, Schelting M, et al, "Can tests of patient well-being be used to evaluate nutritional efficacy? An affirmative answer," *J Pen,* 14:20; 1992.

Candida

Anderson J, Faass N, et al, *Inner Health,* 1997
Balch JF, Balch PA, *Prescription for Nutritional Healing,* Avery, Garden City Park, NY, 1990.
Bellamy W, Wakabayashi H, et al, "Killing of Candida albicans by lactoferricin B, a potent antimicrobial peptide derived the N-terminal region of bovine lactoferrin," *Med Microbiol Immun,* 182(2):97-105; 1993.
Christopher JR, *School of Natural Healing,* Provo, UT, 1976.
Crook, William, MD, *The Yeast Connection,* Vantage Books, NY, 1986.
Donsbach KW, *Candida Albicans & Systemic Candidiasis,* 1987.
Galland L, "Nutrition and Candidiasis," *J Orthomol Psychiat,* 14(1):50-60; 1985.
Hudson T, "Yeast infections and natural medicine," *Evergreen Nutrition,* 6/1997.
Ingram C, *The Cure is in the Cupboard,* Knowledge House, Buffalo Grove, IL, 1997.
Krohn J, *The Whole Way to Allergy Relief & Prevention,* Harley & Marks, Port Roberts, WA, 1991.
Larson JM, *Alcoholism — The Biochemical Connection,* Villard Books, NY, 1992.
Mitsuoka Y, "Intestinal flora and aging," *Nutr Rev,* 50:438-46; 1992.
Murray M, Pizzorno JE, *Encyclopedia of Natural Medicine,* Prima, Rockland, CA, 1998.
Prescatore F, *Allergy and Asthma Cure,* Wiley & Sons, NJ, 2000.
J Reprod Med, 36(8):593-597; 1977. (Boric acid capsules inserted 2x/day for 2 weeks were 98% successful in 100 women nonresponsive to prescription antifungals.)
Rose E, *Lady of Cray, Healing Candida: The Nightmare Chemical Epidemic,* Butterfly Pub, Santa Monica, CA, 1985. (Personal account.)
Ross J, *The Mood Cure,* Viking Penguin, NY, 2002.
B Russell-Manning, ed, *Home Remedies for Candida,* Greensward Press, San Francisco, 1988.
Therapiewoche, 36:3352-58; 1986. (Women using echinacea had a 43% decrease in recurrent yeast infection.)
Trowbridge J, Walker M, *The Yeast Syndrome,* Bantam Books, NY, 1986.
Truss CO, "Tissue injury induced by Candida albicans, mental and neurological manifestations," *J Orthomol Psychiat,* 7(1):17-37; 1978.
Truss CO, "Restoration of immunologic competence to Candida albicans," *J Orthomol Psychiat,* 9(4):287-301; 1980.
Truss CO, "The role of Candida albicans in human illness," *J Orthomol Psychiat,* 10(4):228-38; 1981.
Truss CO, *The Missing Diagnosis,* Orian Truss, Birmingham, Alabama, 1983.
Truss CO, "Metabolic abnormalities in patients with chronic candidiasis: The acetylaldehyde hypothesis," *J Orthomol Psychiat,* 13(2):66-93; 1984.
Vajdani A, Rahimian P, "Immunological cross reactivity between Candida albicans and human tissue," *J Clin Lab Immunol,* 48:1-15; 1996. (On the potential for autoimmune response to Candidiasis.)
Walsh WJ, "A biological basis for neurologic disorders: autism, hyperactivity, attention deficit disorder, depression, obsessive-compulsive disorder, Tourette's syndrome, and violence, An interview with William J Walsh, PhD," *Latitudes,* 5(2):1-8; 2002. At: www.Latitudes.org
Walsh WJ,"Commentary on nutritional treatment of mental disorders," *International Guide to the World of Alternative Mental Health* At: www.alternativementalhealth.com/articles.walshMP.htm#Py Accessed: 10/08/2006.
Zamm AV, "Candida albicans therapy, is there ever an end to it?" *J Orthomol Med,* 1(4):261-66; 1986.

Allergy

Ali M, "Correlation of IgE antibodies with specificity for pollen and mold allergy with changes in electrodermal skin responses following exposure to allergens," *Am J Clin Pathology,* 91(3):357; 1989. (Double blind. EAV response to molds and pollens was 73% correlated with microELISA IgE results.)
Ashkenazi A, et al, "Immunologic reaction of psychotic patients to fractions of gluten," *Am J Psychiat,* 136(10):1306-09; 1979. (Peripheral blood lymphocytes of some psychotics (e.g., celiacs) react to gluten by forming a leukocyte migration inhibition factor. Malabsorption may not be a factor.)
Balch, J, Balch PA, *Prescription for Nutritional Healing,* Avery, Garden City Park, NY, 1990.
Bell I, Miller C, et al, "An olfactory-limbic model of multiple chemical sensitivity — Possible relationships to affective spectrum disorders and to kindling," *Biol Psychiat,* 32:218; 1992.
Ciacci C, Iavarone A, et al, "Depressive symptoms in adult celiac disease, *Scand J Gastroenterol,* 33(3): 247-50; 1998. (Depressive symptoms are a feature of the disease, and respond to nutritients which address celiac disease.)
Coca AF, *The Pulse Test,* Barricade Bks, NY, 1994.
Cott, A, "Fasting: Controlled treatment for schizophrenia," *J Orthomol Psychiat,* 3(4):301-11; 1974.
Davies S, Stewart A, *Nutritional Medicine,* Pan Books, London, 1987; p 403. (A 32-year-old woman with 10 yrs severe mood swings improved markedly in 2 mo on fruit, vegetables, rice, meat, fish. 3 days after eating bread she became severely depressed. It took 8 wks of the above diet to regain benefits.)
Daykin PN, "Stomach acid and hyperactivity," *J Orthomol Psychiat,* 5(3):212-14; 1976.
Dean G, Hanniffy L, et al, "Schizophrenia and coeliac disease," *J Irish Med Assoc,* 68:545-546; 1975.
Dohan FC, et al, "Is schizophrenia rare if grain is rare?" *Biol Psychiat,* 19:385-99; 1984.
Dohan FC, et al, "Relapsed schizophrenics: More rapid improvement on a cereal-free diet," *Br J Psychiat,* 115:595-6; 1969.
Egger J, Stolla A, McEwen LM, "Controlled trial of hyposensitization in children with food-induced hyperkinetic syndrome," *Lancet,* 339:1150-53; 1992.
Faelten, et al, *The Allergy Self-help Book,* Rodale Press, Emmaus, PA, 1983.
Gold MS, *The Good News About Depression,* Villard Books, NY, 1987.
Graham B, "Laboratory testing for schizophrenia and bipolar disorder." At: nutrtional-healing.com.au/content/articles Accessed 3/2008.
Green, "Living with schizophrenia," *J Orthomol Psychiat,* 14(1):39-41; 1985.
Hemmings WA, "Dietary protein reaches the brain," *J Orthomol Psychiat,* 6(4):309-16; 1977.
Hershey, Jane, *Why Can't My Child Behave?* Pear Tree Press, Alexandria, VA, 1996.
Hoffer A, *Common Questions about Schizophrenia and their Answers,* Keats, New Canaan, CN, 1987.
Hoffer, Abram, MD, PhD, interview with author, April, 1995.
Hoffer A, *Orthomolecular Medicine For Physicians,* Keats, New Canaan, CN, 1983.
Horrobin DF, "Prostaglandin deficiency and endorphin excess in schizophrenia," *J Orthomol Psychiat,* 8(1):13-19; 1979.
Humiston KE, et al, "Psychological stress of clearing from food allergies," *J Orthomol Psychiat,* 7(2):124-6; 1979.
Hunter BT, *Gluten Intolerance,* Keats, New Canaan, CN, 1987.
Jaffe R, Kruesi OR, "The biochemical-immunology window: A molecular view of psychiatric case management," *J App Nutr,* 44(2); 1992.
King DS, "Can allergic exposure provoke psychological symptoms? A double blind test," *Biol Psychiatr,* 16(1):3-19, 1981.
Krohn J, *The Whole Way to Allergy Relief and Prevention,* Hartley & Marks, Port Roberts, WA, 1991.
Krop J, Swierczek, J, et al, "Comparison of ecological testing with the Vega test method in identifying sensitivies to chemicals, foods and inhalants," *Am J Acupuncture,* 13(3):253-59; 1985. (Double blind. In 66% of tests, the neutralizing dose indicated by EAV was the same as that suggested by intradermal and sublingual tests.)
Krop J, Lewith GT, "A double blind, randomized, controlled investigation of electrodermal testing in the diagnosis of allergies," *AAEM, 32nd Annual Meeting,* La Jolla, CA, 10/26/1997.
Lamkin, MacPherson P, "Allergies and schizophrenia: Immune system starvation?" *J Orthomol Psychiat,* 10(4):249-62; 1981.
Tom Lane, personal communication, 5-6/1997.
Lawson L, *Staying Well in a Toxic World,* Lynwood Press, Evanston, IL, 1993.
Lemmo W, "Mental health care: Under the microscope" At: www.lemmo.com/mental.html#microscope Accessed: 2003.
Lesser M, *Nutrition and Vitamin Therapy,* Bantam 1985.
Lesser, Michael, MD, personal communication, 2002.
Levin AS, The *Type 1, Type 2 Allergy Relief Program,* Jeremy P Tarcher, Inc, CA, 1983.
Levine SA, Rheinhardt MS, "Biochemical-pathology initiated by free radicals, oxidant chemicals, and therapeutic drugs in the etiology of chemical hypersensitivity disease," *J Orthomol Psychiat,* 12(3):166-83; 1983.
Lewis A, Clowatre Dallas, *Melatonin and the Body Clock,* Keats.
Malzberg B, "A statistical study of mental disease among natives of foreign white parentage in New York State," *Psych Quarterly,* 10:127-42; 1936.
Mandell M, "Cerebral reactions in allergic patients: Illustrative case histories and comments," *2nd International Congress of Social Psychiatry, London,* Keats, New Canaan, CN, 1969.
Mandell M, *Dr Mandell's 5 Day Allergy Relief System,* Thomas Y Crowell, NY, 1979.
Messer M, et al, "Studies on the mechanism of destruction of the toxic action of wheat gluten in coeliac disease by crude papain," *Gut,* 5:295-303; 1964.
Messer M, Baume PE, "Oral papain in gluten intolerance," *Lancet,* 1976; ii, pp 1022.
Mowrey DB, *The Scientific Validation of Herbal Medicine,* Keats, New Canaan, CN, 1986a.
Mowrey DB, *Proven Herbal Blends,* Keats, New Canaan, CN, 1986b.
Murray MT, *Stress, Anxiety & Insomnia,* Prima, Rocklin, CA, 1995.
Murray MT, Pizzorno J, *Encyclopedia of Natural Medicine,* Prima, Rocklin, CA, 1998.
Mycroft FJ, et al, "MIF-like sequences in milk and wheat proteins," letter, *NEJM,* 307(14):895; 1982.
Null G, Feldman M, *Good Food, Good Mood,* St. Martin's, NY, 1988.
Pfeiffer CC, *Nutrition and Mental Illness,* Healing Arts Press, Rochester, VT, 1987.
Pfeiffer CC, *The Schizophrenias Ours to Conquer,* Bio-Communications Press, Wichita, KS, rev ed, 1988.
Philpott WH, at APA/BPA meeting, 1974, reported in Hoffer, 1987.
Philpott WH, "Maladaptive reactions to frequently used foods and commonly met chemicals as precipitating factors in many chronic physical and chronic emotional illnesses," in R Williams, D Kalita, eds, *A Physicians Handbook on Orthomolecular Medicine,* Keats, New Canaan, CN, 1977.
Philpott WH, "Selective substance reactivity in pancreatic insufficiency," *J Orthomol Psychiat,* 7(3):179-89; 1978a.
Philpott WH, "Methods of reversing the stimuli-evoked pancreatic insufficiencies of chronic

degenerative diseases," *J Orthomol Psychiat,* 7(3): 190-201; 1978b.

Philpott WH, et al, "Ecologic-metabolic profile of schizophrenia," *J Orthomol Psychiat,* 8(2):84-105; 1979.

Philpott WH, Philpott K, "Principles of bio-ecologic medicine," *J Orthomol Psychiat,* 11(3): 204-7; 1982.

Philpott WH, Kalita D, *Brain Allergies: The Psychonutrient Connection,* Keats, New Canaan, CN, 1980, 1987.

Quillin P, *Healing Nutrients,* Contemporary Books, Chicago, 1987.

Randolph TG, et al, *An Alternative Approach to Allergies,* Lippincott and Crowell, 1979.

Randolph TG, "Ecologic orientation in medicine: Comprehensive environmental control in diagnosis and therapy," *Annals Allergy,* 23:7-22; 1/1965.

Randolph TG, "Domiciliary chemical air pollution in the etiology of ecologic mental illness," *Intl J Soc Psychiat,* 16(4):70; 1971.

Rapp D, *Is This Your child?* William Morrow, NY, 1991.

Rees E, "Clinical observations on the treatment of schizophrenic and hyperactive children with megavitamins," *J Orthomol Psychiat,* 2(3):93-103; 1973.

Riperre V, "Some varieties of food intolerance in psychiatric patients: An overview," *Nutr Health,* 3(3):125-36; 1984.

Riordan, Hugh, MD, interview with the author, October, 1995.

Rix KJ, et al, "Food antibodies in acute psychoses," *Psychol Med,* 15(2):347-54; 1985. (Possible association of mania with IgE antibodies to wheat or rye.)

Rockwell S, *The Rotation Game: A Diversified Rotation Diet,* and *Allergy Recipies,* Sally J Rockwell, Seattle, WA, 1996.

Rogers S, *Depression: Cured at Last,* SK Pub, Sarasota FL, 1997.

Rudin DO, "The major psychoses and neuroses as omega-3 essential fatty acid deficiency syndrome: Substrate pellagra," *Biol Psychiat,* 16:837-50; 1981.

Rudin, DO, et al, *The Omega 3 Phenomenon,* Rawson Assn, NY, 1987.

Singh MM, et al, "Gluten and schizophrenia," *Lancet,* 2:689; 1976a.

Singh, M.M, Kay S.R, "Wheat gluten as a pathogenic factor in schizophrenia," *Science,* 191:401-2, 1976b. (Double blind. 10/14 responded to milk-and-cereal-free diet, mainly nonparanoid patients with poor previous outcome.)

Steinberg, et al, "Allergic rhinitis can alter mood and cognitive function," Presentation at American Academy of Allergy Asthma and Immunology Meeting, SF, 1997. At: PharmInfo.net (81% of 32 allergic rhinitis patients reported increased irritability, fatigue, inattention, sadness; reduced positive affect and engagement; slow thinking. Memory and learning tests showed deficits. Fatigue, and low activity and motivation were significantly greater vs. controls.)

Thomas AJ, Davis S, et al, "Elevation of cell adhesion molecule immunoreactivity in the anterior cingulate cortex in bipolar disorder," *Biol Psychiat,* 55(6):652-5; 3/15/2004. (Postmortem image analysis suggests bipolars experience immune inflammation in the anterior cingulate cortex.)

Torrey EF, *Schizophrenia and Civilization,* Jason Aaronson, NY, 1980.

Torrey EF, *Surviving Schizophrenia,* rev ed, Harper & Row, NY, 1988.

Tsuei JJ, Lehman CW, et al, "A food allergy study utilizing the EAV acupuncture technique," *Am J Acupuncture,* 12(2):105-116; 1984. (Double blind. EAV results matched patient history 74% of the time; rechallenge tests, 77%; skin testing, 71%; RAST, 69%.)

Walsh D, "Coeliac disease and schizophrenia," *Br Med J,* 2:242; 1973.

Walsh D, "Epidemiological methods applied to an Irish problem," in D Leigh, J Noorbakhsh, eds, *Epidemiological Studies in Psychiatry,* World Psychiatric Association, London, 1974.

Walsh M, *Schizophrenia: Straight Talk for Families and Friends,* William Morrow & Co, NY, 1985.

Walsh, WJ, "Commentary on nutritional treatment of mental disorders," *International Guide to the World of Alternative Mental Health.* At: www.alternativementalhealth.com/articles.walshMP.htm#Py Accessed:10/08/2006

Washburn CF, Reichert RG, "An hypothesis for a mechanism for the pathogenesis of psychomimetic symptoms in gluten/gliadin sensitive individuals," *J Orthomol Med,* 5(3):175-8; 1990.

Weintraub S, *Minding Your Body,* Complementary Medicine Pub Co, Portland, OR, 1995.

Wunderlich R, "Desensitizing allergy injections: A biological and psychological tool to behavioral change," *J Orthomol Psychiat,* 5(2):138-147; 1976.

Young LT, Li PP, et al, "Cerebral cortex Gs-alpha protein levels and forskolin-stimulated cyclic AMP formation are increased in bipolar affective disorder," J Neurochem, 61(3):890-8; Sep 1993. (Gs alpha immunoreactivity significantly elevated in prefrontal, temporal and occipital cortex.)

Zioudrou C, et al, "Opioid peptides derived from food proteins," *J Biol Chem,* 254(7):2446-9; 4/10/1979.

Lancet, 11/14/98; 1582-5. (19/28 celiacs exhibited peripheral neuropathy. MRIs showed cerebellar ataxia in 6 (which may increase over time). Strict avoidance of gluten reversed altered gait and limb movement in some.)

Sugar

Adams R, Murray F, *Megavitamin Therapy,* Larchmont Books, NY, 1973.

Airola P, *How to Get Well,* Health Plus, Phoenix, AZ, 1974.

Allen FM, "Blueberry leaf extract: Physiologic and clinical properties in relation to clinical metabolism," *JAMA,* 89:1577-81; 1927.

Balch JF, Balch PA, *Prescription for Nutritional Healing,* Avery, Garden City Park, NY, 1990.

Bennett JB, "Physiological and biochemical changes in impaired sugar metabolism," *J Orthomol Psychiat,* 3(4):246-53.

Bernstein RK, *Dr Bernstein's Diabetes Solution,* Little, Brown, 2003.

Bever BO, Zahnd GR, "Plants with oral hypoglycemic action," *Quart J Crude Drug Res,* 17:139-96; 1979.

Bolton R, as described in Adams 1973.

Boniface R, Robert AM, "Effect of anthocyanine on connective tissue metabolism in the human," *Klin Monatsbl Augenheikd,* 209:368-72; 1996.

Buckley RE, "Hypoglycemic kindling of limbic system disorder," *J Orthomol Psychiat*; 1978, pp 118-21.

Cavallo MG, Fava D, "Cell-mediated immune response to beta casein in recent-onset insulin-dependent diabetes: Implications for disease pathogenesis," *Lancet,* 348:926-28; 1996.

Cheraskin E, "The prevention of hypovitaminosis C," *JAMA,* 254(20):2894; 11/1985.

Christensen L, "Psychological distress and diet — effects of sucrose and caffeine," *J Appl Nutr,* 40(1):44-50; 1988. (Double blind.)

Christopher JR, *School of Natural Healing,* Provo, UT, 1976.

Cicero AFG, Derosa G, et al, "What do herbalists suggest to diabetic patients in order to improve glycemic control? Evaluation of scientific evidence and potental risks," *Acta Diabetologica,* 41(3); 9/2004. (685 questionaires returned from Italian herbalists. Most recommended: gymnema, psyllium, fenugreek, bilberry, garlic, Chinese ginseng, dandelion, burdock, prickly pear cactus, bitter melon, chromium, B6, zinc, biotin, alpha lipoic acid, fructooligosaccharides, vanadium, C, E, selenium.)

Cott A, "Controlled fasting treatment for schizophrenia," *J Orthomol Psychiat,* 3(4):301-11; 1974.

Cousens G, *Depression Free for Life,* Quill, HarperCollins, NY, 2001.

Currier W, et al, "Hypoglycemia: The end of your sweet life," in R Williams, D Kalita, eds, *A Physician's Handbook on Orthomolecular Medicine,* Keats, New Canaan, CN, 1979.

Dolhofer R, et al, "Increased glycosylation of serum albumin in diabetes mellitus," *Diabetes,* 24: 417-22; 1980.

Droy-Lefaix MT, Vennat JC, et al, "Effect of Ginkgo biloba extract on chloroquine induced retinal alterations," *Lens Eye Toxic Res,* 9:521-528; 1992.

Dufy W, *Sugar Blues,* Warner Books, NY, 1975.

Erasmus U, *Fats that Heal, Fats that Kill,* Alive Books, Burnaby, Canada, rev ed, 1995.

Evans G, *The Picolinates,* Keats, New Canaan, CN, 1989.

Gaby AR, "Preventing and Reversing Osteoporosis," Prima, Rocklin CA, 1994.

Gilasson S, et al, *Nutritional Therapies Featuring the Core Program for Diet Revision,* Persona, Winnepeg, Manitoba, Canada, 1991.

Gold M, et al, *The Good News About Depression,* Villard Books, NY, 1987.

Goodwin, Jamison, *Manic Depressive Illness,* Oxford University Press, 1990.

Hamdorf G, "Experimental clinical endocrinology and diabetes," *J Exp Clin Endocrinology and Metabolism,* 104:126-27; 1995.

Head KA, "Type 1 diabetes: Prevention of the disease and its complications," *Alt Med Rev,* 2(4): 256-81; 1997.

Heninger GR, Mueller PS, "Carbohydrate metabolism in mania before and after lithium carbonate treatment," *Arch Gen Psychiat,* 23:310-9; 1970.

Hoffer A, *Orthomolecular Medicine For Physicians,* Keats, New Canaan, CN, 1983.

Jones T, Borg W, et al, *J Pediatrics,* 1(126):171-7; 1995. (Sucrose can multiply adrenalin tenfold.)

Karjalainen J, Martin J, et al, "A bovine albumin peptide as a possible trigger of insulin-dependent diabetes," *NEJ,* 327:302-7; 1992.

Lagrue G, Robert AM, et al, "Pathology of the microcirculation in diabetes and alterations of the biosynthesis of intracellular matrix molecules," *Front Matrix Biol,* 7:324-35; 1970.

Larson, Joan Matthews, PhD, interview with author, June 2008.

Lemmo W, "Mental health care – Under the microscope," 2003. At: www.lemmo.com/mental.html#Microscope

Lesser M, *Nutrition & Vitamin Therapy,* Bantam Books, NY, 1983.

Lesser, Michael, MD, interview with author, August 2008.

Levy-Marchal C, Karjalainen J, et al, "Antibodies against bovine albumin and other diabetic markers in French children," *Diabetes Care,* 18:1089-94; 1995.

Maiorana A, O'Driscoll G, Green D, "The effect of combined aerobic and resistance exercise training on vascular function in type 2 diabetes," *J Am Coll Cardiol,* 38:860-66; 2001.

Moore DT, "A holistic approach for treating manic depressive disorders," at: familyclinic.simplenet.com/bipolar/bipaper.html 1998. (Clients report sugar and caffeine can start a mild manic episode; likewise, junk, chemicalized food)

Murray MT, *Natural Alternatives to Over-the-counter and Prescription Drugs,* William Morrow & Co, NY, 1994.

Murray MT, *Stress, Anxiety & Insomnia,* Prima, Rocklin CA, 1995a.

Murray MT, "Lifestyle and dietary factors in depression," *Am J Nat Med,* 2:10-15; 1995b.

Murray MT, *Encyclopedia of Natural Medicine,* Prima, Rocklin, CA, 1998.

Page LR, *Healthy Healing,* Healthy Healing Pub, CA, 1992.

Passwater R, *GTF Chromium,* Keats, New Canaan, CN, 1982.

Perez-Bravo F, Carrasco E, et al, "Genetic predisposition and environmental factors leading to the development of insulin-dependent diabetes mellitus in Chilean children," *J Mol Med,* 74:105-9; 1996.

Pfeiffer CC, *Nutrition and Mental Illness,* Healing Arts Press, Rochester, VT, 1987.

Pfeiffer CC, *The Schizophrenias Ours to Conquer,* Bio-Communications Press, Wichita, KS, rev ed, 1988.

Sorenson M, *Mega Health*, National Inst of Fitness, Utah, 1992.

Philpott WH, "Selective substance reactivity in pancreatic insufficiency," *J Orthomol Psychiat*, 7(3):179-89; 1978a.

Philpott WH, "Methods of reversing the stimuli-evoked pancreatic insufficiencies of chronic degenerative diseases," *J Orthomol Psychiat*, 7(3): 190-201; 1978b.

Philpott WH, Kalita D, *Brain Allergies: The Psychonutrient Connection*, Keats, New Canaan, CN, 1987.

Philpott WH, Philpott K, "Principles of bio-ecologic medicine," *J Orthomol Psychiat*, 11(3): 208-15; 1982.

Prange AJ, Whybrow PC, Loosen PT, "Depression and Other Mental Symtoms in Endocrine Disorders: An Overview," in U Halbreich, ed, *Hormones and Depression*, Raven Press, NY, 1987, pp. 313-324.

Quillin P, *Healing Nutrients*, Contemporary Books, Chicago, 1987.

Ribes G, Sauvaire Y, et al, "Antidiabetic effects of subfractions from fenugreek seeds in diabetic dogs," *Proc Soc Exp Biol Med*, 182:159-66; 1986.

Riordan, Hugh, MD, interview with the author, October, 1995.

Rix KJ, et al, "Food antibodies in acute psychoses," *Psychol Med*, 15(2):347-54; 1985. (Possible association of mania with IgE antibodies to wheat or rye.)

Rogers S, *Depression, Cured at Last*, SK Publishing, Sarasota FL, 1997.

Ross H, "Hypoglycemia," *J Orthomol Psychiat*, 3(4): 240-5; 1974.

Ross H, *Hypoglycemia, The Disease Your Doctor Won't Treat*, Pinnacle Books, 1989.

Ross J, *The Mood Cure*, Viking Penguin, NY, 2002.

Saffar JH, "Osteoporotic effect of a high-carbohydrate kiet, in golden hamsters," *Arch Oral Biol*, 26:393-97; 1981.

Sarkar S, Pranava M, et al, "Demonstration of the hypoglycemic action of Momordica charantia in a validated animal model of diabetes," *Pharmacol Res*, 33:1-4; 1996.

Saukkonen T, Savilahti E, et al, "Increased frequency of IgM antibodies to cow's milk proteins in Hungarian children with newly diagnosed insulin-dependent diabetes mellitus," *Eur J Pediatr*, 155:885-89; 1996.

Scharrer A, Oher M, [Anthocyanosides in the treatment of retinopathies]" *Klin Monatsbl Augenheilkd*, 178:386-89; 1981.

Schlauss A, Bolton R, *Ethnology*, 12:227; 7/1973.

Science News, 133(4):62; 1/22/1988.

Shanmugasundarum ER, Rajeswari G, et al, "Use of gymnema sylvestre leaf in the control of blood glucose in insulin-dependent diabetes mellitis, *J Ethnopharmacol*, 30:281094; 1990.

Sharma RD, Raghuram TC, et al, "Effect of fenugreek seeds on blood glucose and serum lipids in type 1 diabetes," *Eur J Clin Nutr*, 44:301-6; 1990.

Shibib BA, Khan LA, et al, "Hypoglycemic activity of Coccinia indica and Momordica charantia in diabetic rats: Depression of the hepatic gluconogenic enzymes glucose-6-phosphatase and fructose-1-6-bisphosphatase and elevation of both liver and red-cell shunt enzyme glucose-6-phosphate dehydrogenase," *Biochem J*, 292:267-70; 1993.

Slagle P, "Artificial sweeteners," *The Way Up Newletter Archives*, #39 At: thewayup.com/newletters/newsarch.htm

Smith T, *Renewal: The antiaging revolution*, Rodale Press, Emmaus, PA, 1998.

Sorenson M, *Mega Health*, National Inst of Fitness, Utah, 1992.

Srivastava Y, Bhatt HV, et al, "Hypoglycemic and life prolonging properies of gymnema sylvestre leaf extract in diabetic rats," *Israeli J Med Sci*, 21:540-42; 1985. (Insulin levels rose, islet and beta cells doubled, pancreatic weight increased 30%.)

Stein D, *The Natural Remedy Book for Women*, The Crossing Press, Freedom, CA, 1992.

Sullivan K, *The miracle of vitamin D*, Wise Traditions in Food, Farming and the Healing Arts, Weston A Price Foundation, Fall 2000.

Tate G, et al, "Suppression of acute and chronic inflammation by dietary gamma linolenic acid," *J Rheumatol*, 16(6):729-34; 1989.

Tenney L, *Stress*, Woodland Health Books, 1987.

Tritschier HJ, et al, "Thioctic (lipoic) acid: A therapeutic metal-chelating antioxidant?" *Biochem Pharmacol*, 1:123-26; 1995.

Vaarala O, Klemetti P, et al, "Cellular immune response to cow's milk beta-lactoglobulin in patients with newly diagnosed IDDM," *Diabetes*, 45:178-82; 1996.

Vahasalo P, Petays T, et al, "Relation between antibodies to islet cell antigens, other autoantigens and cow's milk protein in diabetic children and unaffected siblings at the clinical manifestation of IDDM," *Autoimmunity*, 23:165-74; 1996.

Walsh WJ, "Metal metabolism and human function." At: www.hriptc.org/metal_metabolism.html Accessed 12/6/2004a

Walsh WJ, "Zinc deficiency, metal metabolism, and behavior disorders." At:hriptc.org/zinc_deficiency.html Accessed: 12/6/2004b

Walsh, WJ, "Commentary on nutritional treatment of mental disorders, *International Guide to the World of Alternative Mental Health*. At: www.alternativementalhealth.com/articles.walshMP.htm#Py Accessed: 10/08/2006.

Weidener G, Connor SL, et al, "Improvements in hostility and depression in relation to dietary change and cholesterol lowering. The family heart study," *Ann Intern Med*, 117(10):820-3; 11/15/1992. (Reduced depression, aggressive hostility, and plasma cholesterol with low-fat, high-complex-carbohydrate diet.)

Weintraub S, *Minding Your Body*, Complementary Medicine Pub. Co, Portland, OR, 1995.

Weyerer S, Kupfer B, "Physical exercise and psychological health," *Sports Med*, 17:108-16; 1994.

Wilihinder J, et al, "The insulin-releasing activity of the tropical plant, Momordica charantia," *Acta Biol Med Germ*, 41:1,229-40; 1982.

Williams D, *Nobody Nowhere*, Times Books, 1992.

Wilson, Stephanie, ND, interview with author, December, 1997.

Yudkin J, "Sweet and dangerous," Bantam Books, NY, 1973.

Endocrine/brain interactions

Burch EA, Goldshmidt T, "Neuroendocrine testing in psychiatry: Progress toward a disease model of depression," *Affective Disorders Reassessed*, 1983; pp 151-78.

Burman P, Hetta J, et al, "Growth hormone treatment affects brain neurotransmitters and thyroxine," *Clin Endocrinol (Oxf)*, 44(3):319-24; 3/96. (GH passing into the CSF decreased fT4, increased aspartate, HVA, and T3, suggesting antidepressant benefit.)

Coupland N, Glue P, "Blunting growth hormone release in mania," *Am J Psychiat*, 149(9):1286-7; 9/1992.

Dinan TG, Yatham LN, et al, "Blunting of noradrenergic-stimulated growth hormone release in mania," *Am J Psychiat*, 148(7):936-8; 7/1991.

Fisher G, Pelonero AL, et al, "Mania precipitated by prednisone and bromocriptine [letter]," *Gen Hosp Psychiat*, 13(5):345-6; 9/1991.

Gold MS, *The Good News About Depression*, Villard Books, NY, 1987.

U Halbreich, ed, *Hormones and Depression*, Raven Press, NY, 1987; pp. 313-324.

Lemmo W, "Mental health care: Under the microscope" At: www.lemmo.com/mental.html#microscope Accessed: 2003.

Mason J, "Emotion as reflected in patterns of endocrine integration," in L Levi, ed, *Emotions - Their parameters and measurement*, Raven, NY, 1975; pp 142-81.

Mason JW, Kosten TR, et al, "Multidimensional hormonal discrimination of paranoid schizophrenic from manic patients," *Biol Psychiat*, 29(5):457-66; 3/1/91. (No more than 70% of diagnoses could be distinguished by a single hormone (as mean NE, E, testosterone, and fT4 overlapped); 95%, when three or more were considered together.)

Matussek N, "History and development of the clonidine test," in M Ansseau, R Von Frenckelle, G Franck, eds, *BioMarkers of Depression*, 1992; pp 39-41.

Meltzer HY, "An Overview of Hormones and Monoamine Receptors," in U Halbreich, ed, *Hormones and Depression*, Raven Press, NY, 1987, pp 49-57.

Morgan B, Morgan R, *Hormones*, Price Stern & Sloan, LA, 1989.

Pfeiffer CC, *The Schizophrenias: Ours to Conquer*, Bio-Communications Press, Wichita KS, 1988.

Prange, AJ, Whybrow PC, Loosen PT, "Depression and Other Mental Symtoms in Endocrine Disorders: An Overview," in U Halbreich, ed, *Hormones and Depression*, Raven Press, NY, 1987; pp 313-324.

Sachar EJ, in D Freeman, JE Dyrud, eds, *American Handbook of Psychiatry*, Basic Books, NY, 1975; pp 299-313. (Hypothyroidism is accompanied by depression in over 40% of patients.)

Thyroid

Affelou S, Auriacombe M, et al, [Administration of high dose levothyroxine in treatment of rapid cycling bipolar disorders. Review of the literature and initial therapeutic application apropos of 6 cases], *Encephale*, 23(3):209-17; 5-6/1997. (Open label study. After almost 2 years of T4, 2/6 rapid cyclers completely remitted, 2 showed 67% improvement, and 2 did not respond.)

Aghini-Lombaqrdi F, Antonangeli L, et al, "The spectrum of thyroid disorders in an iodine-deficient community: The Pescopagano survey," *J Clin Endocrinol Metab*, 84(2):561-6; 2/99. (Of 1411 residents of an iodine-deficient Italian village, goiter occured in 16% of children, almost 60% of adults; nodularity, in 0.5% of children, 28.5% of persons aged 56-65. Of adults, 2.9% had current or prior hyperthyroidism (double that in iodine-sufficient regions); 29 had toxic goiter. Overt hypothyroidism was present in 0.2% of adults; subclinical, in 3.8%. Serum thyroglobulin or thyro-peroxidase antibodies were found in 12.6% of the population; diffuse autoimmune thyroiditis in 3.5%. Autoimmune hypothyroid was comparable to that found in iodine-sufficent regions, though serum thyroid antibodies were more common. Goiter, nodularity and functional autonomy increased with age.)

Airola P, *How to Get Well*, Health Plus, Phoenix AZ, 1974.

Alm PO, Klinteberg B, et al, [Criminality and psychopathy as related to thyroid activity in former juvenile delinquents], Acta *Psychiatr Scand*, 94(2): 112-7; 8/1996. (70 people, aged 38-46, with psychopathic personality traits and criminality starting by age 15, vs 35 controls. T3 (but not TSH) was significantly related to criminality, but not psychopathology. It was greater in those persistantly criminal; above-mean T3 was associated with 3.8x more deliquency than if below mean.)

Arem R, *The Thyroid Solution*, Ballantine Books, NY, 114-17; 1999.

Asher Ridha, *Br Med J*, 2:555-562; 1949

Balch JF, Balch P, *Prescription for Nutritional Healing*, Avery, Garden City Park, NY, 1990.

Banki CM, *Eur J Pharmacol*, 41:311-315;1977.

Bargagna S, Canepa G, et al, "Neuropsychological follow-up in early-treated congenital hypothyroidism: A problem-oriented approach," *Thyroid*, 10(3): 243-49; 3/2000. (24 children. Neurological scores were lower and defects greater with more severe hypothyroid. These children were prone to problems with balance, coordination, movement quality, fine motor and head movement. 50% experienced language disorders at ages 3 and 5.)

Barnes BO, Galton L, *Hypothyroidism: The Unsuspected Illness*, Thomas Y Crowell, NY, 1976. www.brodabarnes.org

Bastenie PA, Vanhaelst L, et al, "Preclinical hypothyroidism: A risk factor for coronary-heart disease," *Lancet*, 1:203; 1971.

Basedow CA, cited in Greer 1968.
Bastenie PA, Neve P, et al, "Clinical and pathological significance of asymptomatic atrophic thyroiditis, A condition of latent hypothyroidism," *Lancet,* 1: 915-918; 1967.
Bauer MS, Whybrow PC, Winokur A, "Rapid cycling bipolar affective disorder. I. Association with grade I hypothyroidism," *Arch Gen Psychiat,* 47(5):427-32; 5/1990. (7/30 rapid cyclers were grade I; 8, grade II; 3, grade III hypothyroid. Only 63% were taking lithium or CBZ. Authors suggest hypothyroidism may predispose bipolars to rapid cycling.)
Baumgartner A, Volz HP, et al, "Serum concentrations of thyroid hormones in patients with nonseasonal affective disorders during treatment with bright and dim light," *Biol Psychiat,* 40(9): 899-907; 11/1/1996. (1 wk bright light treatment in 34 non-SAD depressives led to significant but slight improvement, inversely correlated with T4.)
Bell IR, Morrow FD, "Low thyroxine levels in female psychiatric inpatients with riboflavin deficiency: Implications for folate-dependent methylation," *Acta Psychiatr Scand,* 85(5):360-63; 5/1992. (9/52 acute patients were B2-deficient. They also had low T4, and a nonsignificant tendency to depression. B2, via *FAD,* is used in a methylation pathway.)
Bernstein L, "Abrupt cessation of rapid-cycling bipolar disorder with the addition of low-dose L-tetraiodothyronine to lithium (letter)," *J Clin Psychopharmacol,* 12(6):443-4; 12/1992.
Bland J, *The 20-Day Rejuvenation Diet Program,* Keats, New Canaan, CN, 1997.
Boillet D, Szoke A, "Psychiatric manifestations as the only clinical sign of hypothyroidism. Apropos of a case," *Encephale,* 24(1):65-8; 1-2/1998. (A hypothyroid 63-year-old male showed no physical signs, but presented with persecutory delusions, agitation, aggression, and memory impairment. Hormone replacement reversed mental symptoms.)
Bommer M, Naber D, "Subclinical hypothyroidism in recurrent mania," *Biol Psychiat,* 31(7):729-34; 4/1/1992.
Bottlender R, Rudolf D, et al, "Are low basal serum levels of the thyroid stimulation hormone (b-TSH) a risk factor for switches into states of expansive syndromes (known in Germany as "maniform syndromes" in bipolar I depression?" *Pharmacopsychiat,* 33(2):75-77; 3/2000. (15.4% of patients with lower basal TSH (high thyroid) switched, vs. 5.1% with higher TSH.)
Brauchitch HV, *Psychopharmacologia,* 2:1-21; 1961.
Brigham PM, "The psychopharmacology of bipolar disorder." At http://people.ne.mediaone.net/pmbrig/BP_pharm.html Accessed: 6-11-01.
brodabarnes.org
Brownlie BE, Rae AM, et al, "Psychoses associated with thyrotoxicosis — 'Thyrotoxicoxic psychosis.' A report of 18 cases, with statistical analysis of incidence," *Eur J Endocrinol,* 142(5):438-44; 5/2000. (The younger patients had Graves; the older, toxic nodular goitre. Over half showed marked thyroid elevation. In 2, mood swings started when thyroid levels fell with treatment. 7 patients had mania; 7, depression; 2, schizophreniform; 1, paranoid; 1, delirium. In 9, affective psychosis was concurrent with thyrotoxicosis (possibly a trigger).)
Burger HG, Patel YC, in L Martini, GM Besser, eds, *Clinical Neuroendocrinology,* Academic Press, N&Y, 1977; 69-131.
Campbell M, Shapiro T, in RI Shader, ed, *Manual of Psychiatric Therapeutics,* Little Brown and Co, Boston, 1976; pp 137-62.
Capasso G, De Tommaso G, et al, "Effects of thyroid hormones on heart and kidney functions," *Miner Electrolyte Metab,* 25(1-2):56-64; 1-4/99. (Hypothyroidism (if parathyroids are normal) depresses heart contractile and electrical activity, and decreases kidney Na and K activity and fluid reabsorption.)
Centanni M, Canettieri G, et al, "Effect of tryptophan on the early tri-iodothyronine uptake in mouse thymocytes," *Eur J Endocrinol,* 143(1):119-23; 7/2000. (T3 uptake was reduced (and varied with dose) in tissue incubated with tryptophan.)
Cavalca GG, Covezzi E, et al, *Riv Sper Freniat,* 98: 271-300; 1974.
Chang KD, Keck PE Jr, et al, "Differences in thyroid function between bipolar manic and mixed states," *Biol Psychiat,* 43(10):730-3; 5/15/98. (Most rapid cycling studies find increased thyroid axis abnormalities. This study also suggests mixed states (which, similarly, are more common in women, not very responsive to lithium, and tend to poor outcome) show more thyroid axis dysfunction than manics.)
Christopher JR, *School of Natural Healing,* Provo, UT, 1976.
Cleare AJ, McGregor A, et al, "Thyroxine replacement increases central 5-hydroxytryptamine activity and reduces depressive symptoms in hypothyroidism," *Neuroendocrinol,* 64(1):65-69; 7/1996. (T3 replacement in 7 hypothyroids significantly increased 5-HT-mediated cortisol response. TSH correlated with depressive symtoms; cortisol, inversely.)
Clinical Society of London, *Transactions of the Clinical Society of London,* 21S, Longmans, London, 1888.
Cohen KL, Swigar ME, *JAMA,* 242:254-57; 1979.
Cole DP, Thase ME, et al, "Slower treatment response in bipolar depression predicted by lower pretreatment thyroid function," *Am J Psychiat,* 159(1):116-21; Jan, 2002. (Bipolars may be particularly sensitive to normal variations in thyroid parameters. Antidepressant response was significantly slower if low thyroid.)
Coleman R, Hay RJ, "Chronic mucocutaneous Candidasis associated with hypothyroidism: A distinct syndrome," *Br J Dermatol,* 136(1):24-29; 1/1997.
Coppen A, Whybrow PC, et al, *Arch Gen Psychiat,* 26:234-242;1972b.
Cowdry RW, Wehr TA, et al, "Thyroid abnormalities associated with rapid cycling bipolar illness," *Arch Gen Psychiat,* 40:414-20; 1983. (Over 50% of rapid cyclers.)
Crayhon R, *The Carnitine Miracle,* M Evans & Co, 1998.
D'Alecy LG, "Thyroid hormone in neural rescue," *Thyroid,* 7(1):115-24; 2/1997. (In dogs resuscitated 30 sec and 9 min post-cardiac arrest, TT4, TT3, and FT3 were dramatically decreased; rT3, elevated. L-T4 (but not T3) significantly improved nerve function by 24 hrs, perhaps by redressing serum hypothyroid, thus enhancing oxygen uptake and transport.)
Darby, P, "Causes and natural treatments for bipolar disorder." At: www.alternativementalhea lth.com/articles/bipolartreatment.htm Accessed: 2/12/2006.
de Br"atter P, Negretti de Bratter VE, "Influence of high dietary selenium intake on the thyroid hormone level in human serum," *J Trace Elem Med Biol,* 10:163-66; 1996. (Though selenium supports T4-to-T3 conversion, high intake in Se-rich areas of Venezuela was associated with reduced T3 formation.)
de Escobar DM, Obregon MF, del Rey FE, "Is neuropsychological development related to maternal hypothyroidism or to maternal hypothyroxinemia?" *J Clin Endocrin Metab,* 2000; pp 3975-3987.
Delange F, Lecomte P, "Iodine supplementation: Benefits outweigh risks," *Drug Saf,* 22(2):89-95; 2/2000a.
Duntas LH, Panastasiou L, et al, "Incidence of sideropenia and effects of iron repletion treatment in women with subclinical hypothyroidism," *Exp Clin Endocrinol Diabetes,* 107(6):356-60; 1999. (20% of the world population sideropenic, usually due to iron deficit. Of 57 subclinical hypothyroid women, 17 had low iron; 9 also had low ferritin; 8, low hematocrit and hemoglobin. Iron intake nonsignificantly increased T4 and slightly decreased TSH. Authors suggest sideropenia may be common in subclinical hypothyroidism.)
Duval F, Mokrani MC, et al, "Effect of antidepressant medication on morning and evening thyroid function tests during a major depressive episode," *Arch Gen Psychiat,* 53(9):833-40; 9/96. (30 euthyroid depressives were given 1 mo antidepressants. In responders, basal serum fT4 (8 AM & 11 PM) and fT3 (8 AM) decreased; thyrotropin (11 PM) increased.)
Dzurec LC, "Experiences of fatigue and depression before and after low-dose L-thyroxine supplementation in essentially euthyroid individuals," *Res Nurs Health,* 20(5):389-98; 10/1998. (Females (vs males) with normal thyroid labs experienced substantially more disruption of their lives due to fatigue and depression; and benefitted physically and mentally with low-dose T4.)
Earle BV, "Thyroid hormone and antidepressants in resistant depressions," *Am J Psychiat,* 126:143; 1970.
Eidi M, Eidi A, et al, "Effects of Salvia officiinalis L (sage) leaves on memory retention and its interaction with the cholinergic system in rats," *Nutrition,* 22(3): 321-6; 3/2006.
Engstrum G, Svensson TH, et al, "Thyroxine and brain catecholamines: Increased transmitter synthesis and increased receptor sensitivity," *Brain Res,* 77:471; 1974. (Hyperthyroids synthesize more 3H-DA and 3H-NE from 3H-tyrosine. Probenecid increased HVA and slightly increased 5-HIAA.)
Engstrum G, Strumbom TH, et al, "Brain monoamine synthesis and receptor sensitivity after single or repeated administration of thyroxine," *J Neural Transmission,* 37:1; 1975.
Eversole G. At: www.leaflady.org
Extein I, Pottash ALC, Gold MS, et al, "The thyroid stimulating hormone response to thyrotropin-releasing hormone in mania and bipolar depression," *Psychiatr Res,* 2:199-204, 1980.
Extein I, Pottash ALC, Gold MS, *Psychiat Res,* 4: 49-53; 1981.
Fan LF, Huang YR, et al, "Study on quality of sleep and mental health in patients with hyperthyroidism," *Chung Hua Hu Li Tsa Chih,* 32(8):435-9; 8/1997.
Fardella C, Gloger S, "High prevalence of thyroid abnormalities in a Chilean psychiatric outpatient population," *J Endocrinol Invest,* 23(2):102-6; 2/2000.
Feighner JP, King LJ, et al, *Am J Psychiat,* 128: 1230-38; 1972.
Fowler PBS, "Pre-myxoedema: A cause of preventable coronary heart disease," *Proc Roy Soc Med,* 70:297-99; 1977.
Frye MA, Ketter TA, "Defining the standard of care across the bipolar spectrum: Q & A, April 9,2000; SF, Faculty: Mark A Frye MD, Terrence A Ketter MD," *Bipolar Disorders Information Center.* Athttp://www.mhsource.com/bipolar/defzarate.html Accessed: 6/11/01.
Frye MA, Denicoff KD, et al, "Association between lower serum free T4 and greater mood instability and depression in lithium-maintained bipolar patients," *Am J Psychiat,* 156(12):1909-14; 12/1999.
Fukuhara K, Kvetnansky R, et al, "Interrelations between sympathoadrenal system and hypothalamo-pituitary-adrenocortical thyroid systems in rats exposed to cold stress," *J Neuroendocrinol,* 8(7):553-41; 7/1996. (In rats under cold-stress, glucocorticoids restrain catecholamine activity, but when the thyroid is not effective in maintaining body heat, adrenal medulla activity increases to do so.)
Gaby AR, *Preventing and Reversing Osteoporosis,* Prima, Rocklin CA, 1994.
Galton, Lawrence, *You May Not Need A Psychiatrist: How Your Body May Control Your Mind,* Simon & Schuster, NY, 1979.
Gibson JG, "Emotions and the thyroid gland: A critical appraisal," *J Psychosom Res,* 6:93; 1962.
Gjessing H, *Arch Psychiat Nervenkr,* 191:247; 1953.
Gjessing LR, "The switch mechanism in periodic catatonia and manic-depressive disorder, *Chronobiologia,* 2(4):307-16; 10-12/1975. (In both, autonomic and catecholamine metabolism switch suddenly with behavioral changes. Mania and catatonia may be superimposed on depression or schizophrenia respectively, and have reverted with drugs that interfere with catecholamine activity. Catecholamine changes may be due to thyroid, hypothalamus or limbic imbalances. During

catatonia some metabolite may accumulate until it crosses a threshhold, triggering a switch to overt schizophrenia. Thyroid hormone can be helpful.)

Gloger S, Fardella C, et al, "Relevance of thyroid function assessment in psychiatric patients," *Rev Med Chil,* 125(11):1351-6; 11/97. (Retrospective study of 102 psychiatric patients. 40 had thyroid disorders (16, hypothyroid; 7, subclinical hypothyroid; 5, hyperthyroid; 12, goiter or positive antibodies but normal thyroid. Positive antibodies occured in 16 overall.)

Gold PW, Goodwin FK ,et al, "Pituitary thyrotropin response to thyrotropin releasing hormone in affective illness: Relationship to spinal fluid amine metabolites," *Am J Psychiat,* 1(2-3):1028-1031; 1977. (Increased serotinergic activity may inhibit TSH response to stimulation.)

Gold MS, Pottash ALC, et al, "Distinguishing unipolar and bipolar depression by thyrotropin release test," *Lancet,* 2:411-12; 1979.

Gold MS, Pottash ALC, et al, "TRH induced TSH response in unipolar, bipolar and secondary depression: Possible utility in clinical assessment and differential diagnosis," *Psychoneuroendocrinol,* 5:147-155; 1980.

Gold MS, Pottash ALC, Extein I, "Hypothyroidism and depression: Evidence from complete thyroid function evaluation," *JAMA,* 245:1919-1922; 1981.

Gold MS, Pottash ALC, "Thyroid Dysfunction or Depression?" in *Affective Disorders Reassessed;* 1983; pp 179-91.

Gold MS, et al, *The Good News About Depression,* Villard Books, NY, 1987.

Goodwin FK, Prange AJ, Post RM, et al, "Potentiation of antidepressant effects by L-triiodothyronine in tricyclic nonresponders," *Am J Psychiat,* 139: 34-38; 1982.

Gordin A, Saarinen P, et al, "Serum thyrotropin and the response to thyrotropin releasing hormone in symptomless autoimmune thyroiditis and in borderline and overt hypothyroidism," *Acta Endocrinol,* 75:274-85; 1974.

Graves RJ, "Clinical lectures on the practice of medicine," *The New Sydenham Society,* London, 1843.

Great Smokies Diagnostic Laboratory, editor, "Prevalence of Thyroid Imbalance; Thyroid in Pregnancy," *Great Smokies Connection,* 11(12); 2/28/2001. At: http://www.gsdl.com/news/connections/index.html

Great Western Laboratories, "Hyperthyroidism and 'Bipolar Disorder,' When thyroid imbalance 'masquerades' as a mood disorder." At: www.alternativementalhealth.com/articles/hypothyroid.htm Accessed: 2/7/05.

Greer S, Parsons V, "Schizophrenia-like psychosis in thyroid crisis," *Br J Psychiat,* 114:1357-62; 1968.

Gull, *Br Med J,* 2:258-529; 1873.

Gupta RP, Verma PC, et al, "Effect of experimental zinc deficiency on thyroid gland in guinea pigs," *Ann Nutr Metab,* 41(6):376-81; 1997. (Following 30 days zinc deficiency, T3 and T4 were supressed, and the thyroid shrank and paled, showing atrophy and follicle degeneration. Other effects: scaly skin lesions, edema and swelling of back limbs, abnormal posture, hair loss, depression.)

Haggerty JJ Jr, Evans DL, et al, "The presence of anti-thyroid antibodies in patients with affective and nonaffective psychiatric disorders," *Biol Psychiat,* 27(1):51-60; 1/1/1990. (Antithyroid antibodies in 5/65 depressives; 4/31 bipolars; and 7/68 other psychiatric patients.)

Hak AE, Pols HA, et al, "Subclinical hypothyroidism is an independent risk factor for atherosclerosis and myocardial infarction in elderly women: the Rotterdam Study," *Ann Intern Med,* 132(4):270-78; 2/15/2000. (In this study subclinical hypothyroidism was associated with greater age-related aorthic atherosclerosis and myocardial infarction, increasing slightly if autoimmunity was also involved.)

Hall RC, Dunlap PK, "Thyroid disease and abnormal thyroid function tests in women with eating disorders and depression," *J Fla Med Assoc,* 82(3):187-92; 3/1995. (Over age 30, 53% of female depressives with eating disorder had thyroid disease; 17% in those with only depression. At ages 11-29, incidence of thyroid disease was equivalent in the two groups.)

Haskett RF, Rose RM, "Neuroendocrine disorders and psychopathology," *Psychiatr Clin North Am,* 4:239-252; 1981.

Hauser P, McMillin JM, et al, "Resistance to thyroid hormone: Implications for neurodevelopmental research on the effects of thyroid hormone disrupters," *Toxicol Ind Health,* 14(1-2):85-101; 1998. (Perinatal exposure to dioxins, PCBs, etc, has been associated with learning, memory, and attention difficulties, similar to the neurodevelopmental problems found with thyroid dysfunction. Such chemicals may alter the binding of thyroid hormone receptors.)

Hawkins DR, "Diagnosing the schizophrenias," *J Orthomol Psychiat,* 5(1):18-25; 1976.

Hayashi M, Patel AJ, "An interaction between thyroid hormone and nerve growth factor in the regulation of choline acetyltransferase activity in neuronal cultures, derived from the embryonic rat brain, *Brain Res,* 433(1):109-20; 1987.

www.healthychoicenaturals.com/t-Thyroid_Natural_Nutrients.aspx

Heaney RP, "Effects of nitrogen, phosphorus and caffeine on calcium balance in women," *J Lab Clin Med,* 99:46-55; 1982.

Hendrick V, Altshuler L, et al, "Psychoneuroendo crinology of mood disorders. The hypothalamic-pituitary-thyroid axis," *Psychiatr Clin North Am,* 21(2):277-92; 6/98. (Review. Women are more vulnerable to thyroid dysfunction, and more responsive to thyroid.)

Hickie J, Bennett B, et al, "Clinical and subclinical hypothyroidism in patients with chronic and treatment-resistant depression," *Aust N Z J Psychiat,* 30(2):246-52; 4/1992. (Of 93 mood-disordered inpatients, 22% of antidepressant-resistant patients had subclinical or clinical hypothyroidism, vs. 2% of responsive patients. Free thyroxine (fT4) was inverse to depression duration.)

Hernandez-Avila M, et al, "Caffeine, moderate alcohol intake, and risk of fractures of the hip and forearm in middle-aged women," *Am J Clin Nutr,* 54:157-63; 1991.

Hofbauer LC, Spitzweg C, et al, "Selenium-induced thyroid dysfunction," *Postgrad Med J,* 73:103-4; 1997. (In one patient, high doses of IV selenite led to marked hypothyroidism, corrected with iodine.)

Hojo Y, Ikeda U, et al, "Thyroid hormone stimulates Na(+)-Ca2+ exchanger expression in rat cardiac myoctes," *J Cardiovasc Pharmacol,* 29(1):75-80; 1/1997.

Hollingberry PW, et al, "Effect of dietary caffeine and aspirin on urinary calcium and hydroxyproline excretion in pre and postmenopausal women," *Fed Proc,* 44:1149; 1985.

Hollister LE, Davis KL, Davis BM, *Hospital Practice,* 11/1973, pp 103-110.

Howie AF, Walker SW, et al, "Thyroidal extracellular glutathione peroxidase: a potential regulator of thyroid hormone synthesis," *Biochem J,* 308(3): 713-7; 6/1995.

Jackson AS, "Hypothyroidism," *JAMA;* 1957, pp. 121-65.

Jackson IM, "The thyroid axis and depression," Thyroid, 8(10):951-6; 10/1998. (Most depressives show slightly elevated T4, decreased TSH response to TRH, and blunted nocturnal TSH increase, suggesting hyperthyroid. These measures often normalize when depression resolves.)

Jacoby JH, Mueller G, "Thyroid state and brain monoamine metabolism," *Endocrinol,* 97:1332; 1975.

Jain VK, *Psychiatr Clin,* 5:121-130;1972.

Jennings IW, *Vitamins in Endocrine Metabolism,* Charles C. Thomas, Springfield, IL, 1970.

Josephson AM, MacKenzie TB, "Appearance of manic psychosis following rapid normalization of thyroid status," *Am J Psychiat,* 136:846-47; 1979. (A 34-year-old Graves female became hypothyroid, but with 4 days high-dose T4 became manic. She had a history of hypomania.)

Josephson AM, MacKenzie TB, "Thyroid-induced mania in hypothyroid patients," *Br J Psychiat,* 137: 222-28; 1980.

Joyce PR, "The prognostic significance of thyroid function in mania," *J Psychiatr Res,* 25(1-2):1-6; 1991. (Over one-third of 31 manics had elevated thyroid, largely fT4I. This was associated with greater sleep disturbance and with being male. Lower fT4I predicted more 1-yr hospital admissions.)

Kar A, Panda S, et al, "Relative efficacy of three medicinal plant extracts in the alteration of thyroid hormone concentrations in male mice," *Ethnopharmacol,* 81(2):281-5; 7/2002.

Kastin AJ, Ehrensing RH, et al, "Improvement in mental depression with decreased thyrotropin response after administration of thyrotropin-releasing hormone," Lancet, 2:74-82; 1972.

Kato Y, Haraguchi K, et al, "Reduction of thyroid hormone levels by methylsufonyl metabolites of polychlorinated biphenyl cogeners in rats," *Arch Toxicol,* 72(8):541-4; 7-8/1998.

Kennedy DO, Pace S, et al, "Effects of cholinesterase inhibiting sage (Salvia officinalis) on mood, anxiety, and performance on a psychological stressor battery," *Neuropsychopharmacol,* 10/5/2005.

Kent GN, Stuckey BG, et al, Postpartum thyroid dysfunction: Clinical assessment and relationship to psychiatric affective morbidity, *Clin Endocrinol (Oxf),* 51(4):429-38; 10/1999.

Kieley WF, Adrain AD, et al, *Psychosom Med,* 38: 233-241; 1976.

Kilzieh N, Akiskal HS, "Rapid cycling bipolar disorder. An overview of research and clinical experience," *Psychiatr Clin North Am,* 22(3):585-607, 1999. (Rapid cycling is most clearly associated with greater incidence in women, perhaps reflecting a greater tendency to cyclothymia, hypothyroidism, or antidepressant use.)

Kirov G, "Thyroid disorders in lithium-treated patients," *J Affect Disord,* 50(1):33-40; 7/1998. (Retrospective study. Of 209 lithium-treated affectives, 4.9% of females had thyrotoxicosis prior to treatment. 3.4% of males, and 14.9% of females (most rapidly, if over 50) developed hypothyroidism during treatment .)

Klaiber EL, Braverman DM, et al, in TM Itil, G Laudahn, WM Herrman, eds, *Psychotropic Action of Hormones,* Spectrum Pub Co, NY, 1976; pp 135-54.

Klein M, Barb'e F, et al, "Lead poisoning secondary to hyperthyroidism: Report of two cases," *Eur J Endocrinol,* 138(2):185-8; 2/1998. (Hyperthyroidism and hyperparathyroidism increase bone turnover, potentially releasing stored lead.)

K"ohrle J, "Thyroid hormone deiodinases--a selenoenzyme family acting as gate keepers to thyroid hormone action," *Acta Med Austriaca,* 23(1-2):17-30; 1996.

Koutras DA, "Thyroidopathies," *Ann NY Acad Sci,* 900:77-88; 2000.

Krohn J, *The Whole Way to Allergy Relief & Prevention,* Hartley & Marks, Port Roberts, WA, 1991.

Kronfol Z, Grenen JF, et al, "Application of biological markers in depression secondary to thyrotoxicosis," *Am J Psychiat,* 139:1319-22; 1982.

Kusalic M, "Grade II and grade III hypothyroidism in rapid cycling bipolar patients, *Neuropsychobiol,* 25(4):177-81; 1992. (6 /10 rapid cyclers had grade II or III hypothyroidism. T4 with lithium significantly decreased frequency and intensity of episodes.)

Langer, Stephen E, MD, *Solved: The Riddle of Illness,* Keats, New Canaan, CN, 1984.

Larsen PR, "Thyroid-pitutiary interaction," *NEJM,* 306:23-32; 1982.

Lasser RA, Baldessarini RJ, "Thyroid hormones in depressive disorders: A reappraisal of clinical utility," *Harv Rev Psychiat,* 4(6):291-305; 3-4/1997.

Lauberg P, Pedersen KM, et al, "Iodine intake and the pattern of thyroid disorders: A comparative epidemiological study of thyroid abnormalities in the elderly in Ireland and Jutland, Denmark," *J Clin Endocrinol Metab,* 83(3):765-9; 3/1998. (Low iodine correlated with hyperfunction and goiter, high intake with impaired thyroid. Mild deficit may help protect against autoimmune thyroiditis. Thyroid antibodies mark autoimmunity or may be secondary to goiter development.)

Lauberg P, "Forskolin stimulation of thyroid secretion of T4 and T3," *GEBS Lett,* 21:170(2): 273-6; 5/1984.

Lauberg P, B"uolow, Pedersen I, et al, "Low incidence rate of overt hypothyroidism compared with hyperthyroidism in an area with moderately low iodine intake," *Thyroid,* 9(1):33-8; 1/1999. (Iodine intake in Jutland, Denmark is moderately low. Over 569,108 person/years, new hypothyroidism was 13.5/100,000/year; hyperthyroidism was 38.7. 79% of hypothyroids showed spontaneous autoimmune thyroiditis. Only congenital hypothyroids showed more hypothyroidism than hyper.)

Lazarus JH, "The effects of lithium therapy on thyroid and thyrotropin-releasing hormone," *Thyroid,* 8: 909-13; 1998. (Lithium inhibits ATPase, cAMP, and intracellular enzymes. Its effectiveness may, in part, be due to inhibition of inositol phospholipid metabolism.)

Lee S, Chow CC, et al, "Thyroid function and psychiatric morbidity in patients with manic disorder receiving lithium therapy," *J Clin Psychopharmacol,* 20(2):204-9; 4/2000. (Increased TSH stimulation of the thyroid may contribute to the development of a mania. Over 46 manics, baseline FT4 was high normal; FT3 and TSH, normal. In month 1 of lithium treatment, decreases in FT3 and FT4 correlated significantly with improvement in psych symptoms. By month 6, FT3 was not significantly different than baseline, but FT4 was significantly lower. TSH increased steadily over the 6 months.)

Lee S, Privalsky ML, "Heterodimers of retinoic acid receptors and thyroid hormone receptors display unique combinatorial regulatory properties," *Mol Enocrinol,* 19(4):863-78; 4/2005. Epub 1/13/2005.

Li D, Li T, et al, "Functional evidence for retinoid X receptor (RXR) as a nonsilent partner in the thyroid hormone receptor/RXR heterodimer," *Mol Cell Biol,* 22(16):5782-92; 2002.

Linkowski P, Brauman H, et al, "Thyrotropin response to thyrotropin releasing hormone in unipolar and bipolar affective illness," *J Affect Dis,* 3:9-16; 1981.

Linkowski P, Van Wettere JP, et al, *Br J Psych,* 143: 401-05; 1983. (TSH response was virtually absent with history of violent suicidal behavior, normally distributed in those nonviolently suicidal. Suggests blunting may be due to increased thyroid, cortisol, or DA activity.)

Loosen PT, Prange AJ, et al, *Arch Gen Psychiat,* 36: 540-47; 1979.

Loosen PT, Wilson IC, et al, *Am J Psychiat,* 130: 1145-49; 1983.

Loosen PT, Prange AJ, in CB Nemeroff and AJ Dunn, eds, *Peptides, Hormones and Behavior,* Spectrum Pub, NY, 1984; pp 533-577. (Review of brain/thyroid relationships.)

Loosen PT, "Thyroid Hormones and Affective State," in U Halbreich, ed, *Hormones and Depression,* Raven Press, NY, 1987; pp 357-83.

Loosen PT, "Effects of thyroid hormones on central nervous system in aging [see comments]," *Psychoneuroendocrinol,* 17(4):355-74; 8/1992. (Laboratory and clinical studies reveal an interweaving of thyroid and brain function. Animal studies indicate a neuroregulatory role in the brain, influencing behavior. Thyroid is especially important to human brain development and maturation.)

LoPresti JS, "Laboratory tests for thyroid disorders," *Otolaryngol Clin North Am,* 29(4):557-75; 8/1996.

Mackowiak P, Ginalska E, et al, "The influence of hypo- and hyperthyreosis on insulin receptors and metabolism," *Arch Physiol Biochem,* 107(4): 273-79; 10/1999.

Mano T, Sakamoto H, et al, "Effects of thyroid hormone on catecholamine and its metabolite concentrations in rat cardiac muscle and cerebral cortex," *Thyroid,* 8(4):353-8; 1998. (Catecholamine levels varied with thyroid status, and influence CNS and cardiovascular symptoms associated with thyroid dysfunction.)

Marangell LB, George MS, et al, "Carbamazepine increases CSF thyrotropin-releasing hormone in affectively ill patients," *Arch Gen Psychiat,* 51: 625-8; 1994.

Marangell LB, Ketter TA, et al, "Inverse relationship of peripheral thyrotropin-stimulating hormone levels to brain activity in mood disorders," *Am J Psychiat,* 154(2):224-30; 2/1997a. (In medication-free affectives, T3, T4, and FT4 showed no significant relationships to cerebral glucose metabolism and blood flow, while peripheral TSH (a more sensitive measure), was inversely related to both. Results suggest manipulating the thyroid axis may help treat mood disorders.)

Marangell LB, George MS, et al, "Carbamazepine increases CSF thyrotropin-releasing hormone (TRH) in refractory depressed patients," *Arch Gen Psychiat,* 54:214-22; 1997b.

Morgan B, Morgan R, *Hormones,* Price, Stern, Sloan, Los Angeles, CA, 1989.

Morse DC, Wehler EK, et al, "Alterations in rat brain thyroid hormone status following pre- and postnatal exposure to polychlorinated biphenyls (Aroclor 1254)," *Toxicol Appl Pharmacol,* 136(2):269-79; 2/1996. (Suggests PCB accumulation can decrease fetal plasma and brain T4. In late gestational fetuses brain T3 levels may be maintained due to compensation by brain type II thyroxine 5'-deiodinase activity.)

Musselman DL, Nermeroff CB, "Depression and endocrine disorders: Focus on the thyroid and adrenal system," *Br J Psychiat,* (30S):123-8; 6/96.

Nath J, Safar R, "Late-onset bipolar disorder due to hyperthyroidism," *Acta Psychiat Scand,* 104: 72; 2001.

Oomen HA, Schipperijin AJ, Drexhage HA, "The prevalence of affective disorder and in particular of a rapid cycling of bipolar disorder in patients with abnormal thyroid function tests," *Clin Endocrinol (Oxf),* 45(2):215-23; 8/1996. (Cross-sectional admission survey of 3756 psychiatric patients. Highly significant correlation of rapid cycling with early forms of autoimmune thyroid disease, in some cases measurable only by thyroperoxidase antibodies. Affective disorder was weakly associated with subclinical hypothyroidism.

Page LR, *Healthy Healing,* Healthy Healing Pub, CA, 1992.

Panda S, Kar A, "Changes in thyroid hormone concentrations after administration of ashwagandha root extract to adult male mice," *J Pharm Pharmacol,* 50(9):1065-8; 9/1998.

Panda S, Kar A, "Guggulu (Commiphora mukul) induces triiodothyronine production: Possible involvement of lipid peroxidation," *Life Sci,* 65(12): 137-41; 1999a.

Panda S, Kar A, "Withania somnifera and Bauhinia purpurea in the regulation of circulating thyroid hormone concentrations in female mice," *J Ethnopharmacol,* 67(2):233-9; 11/1999b

Panda S, Kar A, "Guggulu (Commiphora mukul) potentially ameliorates hypothyroidism in female mice," *Phytother Res,* 19(1):78-80; 1/2005.

Parry CH, "Collections from the unpublished writings of the late Caleb Hillier Parry," V1, Underwoods, London, 1825.

Pfeiffer CC, *The Schizophrenias Ours to Conquer,* Bio-Communications Press, Wichita, KS, rev ed, 1988.

Pies RW, "The diagnosis and treatment of subclinical hypothyroid states in depressed patients," *Gen Hosp Psychiat,* 19(5):344-54; 9/1997. (Subclinical hypothyroidism may play a role in depression, mood-cycling, and slow response to treatment. Autoimmune thyroiditis, which can lead to hypothyroidism, is also found in depression, especially, postpartum.)

Placidi GP, Boldrini M, "Prevalence of psychiatric disorders in thyroid diseased patients," *Neuropsychobiol,* 38(4):222-5; 11/1998. (Increased panic disorder, phobia, depression, OCD, bipolar disorder, and cyclothymia in 93 thyroid patients.)

Prange AJ, Whybrow PC, Loosen PT, "Depression and other mental symtoms in endocrine disorders: An overview," in U Halbreich, ed, *Hormones and Depression,* Raven Press, NY, 1987; pp. 313-324.

Prange AJ Jr, "Novel uses of thyroid hormones in patients with affective disorders," *Thyroid,* 6(5): 537-43; 10/96. (Thyroid has been used to augment treatment for both mania and depression, even in euthyroids, but perhaps especially in patients with sluggish thyroids. T4 has been used for rapid cycling; T3, because of more rapid onset, for depression. In women, T3 decreases antidepressant lag time. In 2/3 of the approximately 30% who respond poorly to antidepressants, T3 augmentation hastens response. Lithium, which has anti-thyroid activity, converts failures to successes at a similar rate.)

Radovic B, Schmutzler C, et al, "Xanthohumol stimulates iodide uptake in rat thyroid-derived FRTL-5 cells," *Mol Nutr Food Res,* 49(9):832-6; 9/2005.

Rao ML, Ruhrmann S, et al, "Low plasma thyroid indices of depressed patients are attenuated by antidepressant drugs and influence treatment outcome," *Pharmacopsychiat,* 29(5):180-6; 9/96. (Suggests adequate thyroid is needed to compensate for decreases in hormone availability by antidepressants.)

Reed K, Bland RD, *Acta Psychiatr Scand,* 56:421-26; 1977. (Masked myxedematic madness.)

Roca RP, Blackman MR, et al, "Thyroid hormone elevations during acute psychiatric illness: Relationship to severity and distinction from hyperthyroidism," *Endocr Res,* 16(4):415-47; 1990. (Transient hyperthyrosinemia can occur during acute psychiatric illness. In this study, 22/45 acute patients showed significantly elevated thyroid indices. Peak FT4I in depressives was accompanied by increased TSH (which, in acute depression is not suppressed (as it is in hyperthyroids) by abundant thyroid hormone, but may go on to elevate peripheral thyroid levels.)

Rold'an MB, Alonso M, et al, "Thyroid autoimmunity and adolescents with Type 1 diabetes mellitus," *Diabetes Nutr Metab,* 12(1):27-31; 2/1999.

Roodenrys S, Booth D, et al, "Chronic effects of Brahmi (Bacopa monnieri) on human memory," *Neuropsychopharmacol,* 27(2):279-81; 8/2002.

"Rosses' survey," *Thyroid,* 10(9):821-827; 2000.

Ross J, *The Mood Cure,* Viking Penguin, NY, 2002.

Rudas S, Schmitz M, et al, "Treatment of refractory chronic depression and dysthmia with high-dose thyroxine," *Biol Psychiat,* 45(2):229-33; 1/15/1999. (Of 9 treatment-resistant depressives given high-dose T4 antidepressant augmentation over 8 wks, 5 responded completely; 1, partially; 1 failed to respond; 2 dropped out due to side effects.)

Ruz M, Codoceo J, et al, "Single and multiple selenium-zinc-iodine deficiencies affect rat thyroid metabolism and ultrastructure," *J Nutr,* 129(1): 174-80; 1/1999. (Over 6 wks, Zn, Se/Zn, and Se/iodine-deficient rats showed significantly depressed T3. In low-iodine gps, serum and fT4 decreased significantly, while TSH increased (i.e., thyroid was underactive). Se or Se/Zn-deficiency suppressed the thyroid's glutathione peroxidase activity, but not if iodine was low. In Zn and Se/Zn-deficient groups, follicle cells altered or may have been destroyed; less so, if iodine was also low.)

Sachar EJ, in D Freeman and JE Dyrud, eds, *American Handbook of Psychiatry,* Basic Books, NY, 299-313; 1975.

Saffar JH, "Osteoporotic effect of a high-carbohydrate diet, in golden hamsters," *Arch Oral Biol,* 26:393-97; 1981.

Sairam K, Dorababu M, et al, Antidepressant activity of standardized extract of Bacopa monniera in experimental models of depression in rats, *Phytomedicine,* 9(3):207-11; 4/2002.

Saker KE, Fike JH, et al, "Brown seaweed-treated (Tasco) conserved forage enhances antioxidant status and immune function in heat-stressed lambs, *J Anim Physiol Anim Nutr (Berl),* 88(3-4): 122-30; 4/2004.

Salaman M, *Foods that Heal,* Stafford Pub, Menlo Park, CA, 1989.

Schachter M, "The diagnosis and treatment of hypothyroidism," 1996, At healthy.net/scr.article.asp?ID=528

Schmiedebergs *Arch Pharmacol,* 354(6):755-64;

12/1996. (Thyroid may directly affect alpha 1-adrenoceptor-mediated heart activity, rather than through sympathetic mediation.)

Shakir, quoted at: http://people.ne.mediaone.net/pmbrig/BP_pharm.html Accessed: 2001 (A previously stable, hypothyroid bipolar taking T4, developed a TSH over 20 after starting a multi with iron.)

Sher L, Rosenthal NE, Wehr TA, "Free thyroxine-stimulating hormone levels in patients with seasonal affective disorder and matched controls," *J Affect Disord,* 56(2-3):195-9; 12/1999. (Winter fT4 was slightly but significantly lower in SAD patients.)

Shopsin B, "Effects of lithium on thyroid function: A review," *Dis Nerv Syst,* 31:237-44; 1970.

Simpson SG, al-Mufti R, "Bipolar II affective disorder in eating disorder inpatients," *J Nerv Ment Dis,* 180(11):719-22; 11/92.

Skibola CF, Curry JD, et al, "Brown kelp modulates endocrine hormones in female Sprague-Dawley rats and human luteinized granulosa cells," *J Nutr,* 135(2):296-300; 2/2005.

Slagle P, "Low thyroid," *The Way Up Newletter Archives,* #12 At: thewayup.com/newletters/newsarch.htm

Snyder PJ, Utiger RD, "Response to thyrotropin releasing hormone (TRH) in normal man," *J Clin Endocrinol Metab,* 34:380-85; 1972a.

Snyder PJ, Utiger RD, "Thyrotropin responses to thyrotropin releasing hormone in normal females over forty," *J Clin Endocrinol Metab,* 34:1096-98; 1972b. (Normal women (but not men), especially with age, are prone to elevated TSH response.)

Spencer H, et al, "Alcohol osteoporosis," *Am J Clin Nutr,* 41:847; 1985.

Spoov J, Lahdelma L, "Should thyroid augmentation precede lithium augmentation — a pilot study," *J Affect Disord,* 49(3):235-9; 6/98. (In 22 antidepressant-resistant patients, 4 wks T4 followed by 4 wks lithium augmentation was more effective than the reverse.)

St°alenheim EG, von Knorring L, et al, "Serum levels of thyroid hormones as biological markers in a Swedish forensic psychiatric population," *Biol Psychiat,* 43(10):755-61; 5/15/1998. (In a 30 year followup, criminality, antisocial disorder, personality disorder, and psychopathology were associated with elevated T3 and decreased T4.)

Stanbury JB, Ermans AE, et al, "Iodine-induced hyperthyroidism: Occurence and epidemiology," *Thyroid,* 8(1):83-100; 1/1998. (Analysis of reports plus experience in Tasmania, Zaire, Zimbabwe, Brazil. Excess iodine may induce thyrotoxicosis, especially in the elderly with chronic nodular goiter, and in iodine-deficient regions. Cellular mutations may produce autonomous function, and thyrotoxicity, or unexpressed Graves may become active as iodine becomes sufficient. The elderly with heart disease are at particular risk.)

Stancer HC, Persad E, "Treatment of intractable rapid-cycling manic-depressive disorder with levothyroxine. Clinical observations," *Arch Gen Psychiat,* 39:311-2; 1982. (Nonresponders often improve with high-dose thyroid.)

Stockdale T, "A discussion of the relationship between selenium, thyroxine, and indigestion," *Nutr Health,* 12(2):131-4; 98. (Wheat low in seleno-methionine is not as easily digested. Low selenium also depresses deiodinases, fostering hypothyroid.)

Stough C, Lloyd J, et al, The chronic effects of an extract of Bacopa monniera (Brahmi) on cognitive function in healthy human subjects, *Psychopharmacol (Berl),* 156(4):481-4.

Sure B, Easterling L, "The protective action of vitamin B1 against the toxicity of DL-thyroxine," *J Nutr,* 42: 221-5; 1950.

Surks MI, DeFesi CR, "Normal serum free thyroid hormone concentrations in patients treated with phenytoin or carbamazepine. A paradox resolved," *JAMA,* 275(19):1495-8; 5/15/96.

Svensson TH, "Central alpha adrenoceptors and affective symptoms and disorders," in *Depressive Disorders, Symposium,* Rome 5/9-11,1977; FK Schattauer Verlag, NY; pp 248-53.

Temple R, Berman M, et al, "The use of lithium in the treatment of thyrotoxicosis," *J Clin Invest,* 51: 2746-2756; 1972.

thyroidinfo.com

Tidesley NT, Kennedy DO, et al, "Positive modulation of mood and cognitive performance following administration of acute doses of Salvia lavandulae folia essential oil to healthy young volunteers," *Physiol behav,* 83(5):699-709; 1/2005.

Tomasi TE, Hellgren EC, et al, "Thyroid hormone concentrations in black bears (Ursus americanus): Hibernation and pregnancy," *Gen Comp Endocrinol,* 109(2):192-9; 2/1998. (fT3, TT3, fT4 were lower in December. fT3 and fT4 remained low during hibernation.)

Tremont G, Stern RA, "Use of thyroid hormone to diminish the cognitive side effects of psychiatric treatment," *Psychopharmacol Bull,* 33(2):273-80; 1997. (T3 helps protect neurons and support memory. Bipolar cognitive function is significantly linked to thyroid status, rather than lithium.)

Tripathi YB, Malhotra OP, "Thyroid-stimulating action of Z-guggulsterone obtained from Commiphora mukul," *Planta Med,* 50(1):78-80; 2/1984.

Tsang HH, "Natural approaches to suboptimal thyroid," Dr Hing Hau Tsang Newsletter #118. At: http://tsangenterprise.com/news118.htm Accessed 9-21-2007.

Tsimihodimos V, Bairaktari E, et al, "The incidence of thyroid function abnormalities in patients attending an outpatient lipid clinic," *Thyroid,* (4):365-8; 4/99. (Of 248 lipid patients, 7 had asymptomatic biochemical hypothyroidism; 11, subclinical hypothyroidism. In 4 with TSH over 12, small doses of levothyroid significantly improved lipid parameters. In 3, hyperthyroid influenced lipid profile and response to treatment. Authors find thyroid abnormalities common in their patients, and suggest thyroid can significantly alter lipid profile.)

Tsutsui S, Yamazaki Y, *J Int Med Res,* 7:138-46; 1979.

Tunbridge WMG, Brewis M, et al, "Natural history of autoimmune thyroiditis," *Br Med J,* 282:252-62; 1981.

van der Hooft CS, Hoekstra A, et al, "Thyrotoxicosis following the use of ashwagandha," *Ned Tijdschr Geneeskd,* 149(47):2637-8; 11/2005.

van Sande J, Cochaux P, et al, Forskolin stimulates adenylate cyclase and iodine metabolism in thyroid, *GEBS Lett,* 150(1):137-41; 12/1982.

van Wassenaer AG, Kok JH, et al, "Thyroxine administration to infants of less than 30 weeks gestational age decreases plasma tri-iodothyronine concentrations," *Eug J Encocrinol,* 139(5): 508-15; 11/1998. (200 preterm infants were given T4 or placebo for 6 wks. This prevented hypothyroxinemia, but TSH and T3 decreased. Authors suggest adding T3.)

Vitale M, Di Matola T, et al, "Iodide excess induces apoptosis in thyroid cells through a p53-independent mechanism involving oxidative stress," *Endocrinol,* 141(2):598-605; 2/2000. (Toxicity has been observed in some animals fed iodine-rich feed. In vitro, excess can alter cell morphology and inhibit growth. This study suggests iodine oxidation by peroxidases creates free radical damage in the thyroid, killing cells. Toxicity was blocked by inhibiting peroxidase enzymatic activity.)

Wang S, Mason J, et al, "Relationships between thyroid hormones and symptoms in combat-related posttraumatic stress disorder," *Psychosom Med,* 57(4):398-402; 1995. (fT3, T3, T4 correlated with hyperarousal.)

Wang C, Crapo LM, "The epidemiology of thyroid disease and implications for screening," *Endocrinol Metab Clin North Am,* 26(1):189-218; 3/97. (5% of females have overt hypo or hyperthyroidism; 15% of the general population has palpable goiters; 10%, abnormal TSH; up to 50%, microscopic nodules; 3.4%, occult papillary carcinomas.)

Watts DL, "The nutritional relationships of the thyroid," *J Orthomol Med,* 4(3); 1989.

Weinberg AD, Katzell TD, *Lancet,* 1:1104-05; 1977.

Weiss RE, Stein MA, Refetoff S, "Behavioral effects of liothyronine (L-T3) in children with attention deficit hyperactivity disorder in the presence and absence of resistance to thyroid hormone," *Thyroid,* 7(3): 389-93; 6/1997. (Prospective, randomized, double blind, placebo-controlled, cross-over. 50-75% of children resistant to thyroid (RTH) have ADHD. Rapid-acting thyroid (liothyronine) benefitted hyperactivity and impulsivity in such children.

Wenzel KW, Meinhold H, et al, "Classification of hypothyroidism in evaluating patients after radioiodine therapy by serum cholesterol, T4, F4-index, total T3, basal TSH, and TRH test," *Eur J Clin Invest,* 4:141-48; 1974.

West SA, Sax KW, et al, "Differences in thyroid function studies in acutely manic adolescents with and without attention deficity hyperactivity disorder (ADHD)," *Psyc00hopharmacol Bull,* 32(1):63-66; 1996. (T4 concentration in 20 adolescents with ADHD and bipolar disorder was lower than in 10 with bipolar disorder alone.)

Whybrow P, Ferrell R, in AJ Prange, ed, *Thyroid Axis, Drugs and Behavior,* Raven, NY, 1974; pp 5-28.

Whybrow P, Hurwitz R, in *Hormones, Behavior, and Psychopathology,* 38(1):103-113; 1981.

Whybrow PC, "The therapeutic use of triiodothyronine and high dose thyroxin in psychiatric disorder," *Medica Austraca,* 21:47-52; 1994.

Whybrow PC, "Sex differences in thyroid axis function: Treatment implications for affective disorders," *Depression,* 3:33-42; 1995.

Wiessel M, [Administration of thyroid hormones in therapy of psychiatric illnesses], *Acta Med Austriaca,* 26(4):129-31; 1999.

Williams RH, "Metabolism and mentation," *J Clin Endocrinol Metab,* 31(5):461-79; 11/1970.

Wilson IC, Prange AJ, *NEJM,* 282:1063-67; 1970.

Wilson ED, *Wilson's Syndrome: The Miracle of Feeling Well,* Cornerstone Publishing Co, Orlando,1991. wilsonsthyroidsyndrome.com

Wright ML, Pikula A, et al, "Effect of melatonin on the response of the thyroid to thyrotropin stimulation in vitro," *Gen Comp Endocrinol,* 108(2):298-305; 11/1997. (Elevated (but not moderate) melatonin inhibited thyroid response to TSH in amphibians.)

Wright M, Cuthbert KL, et al, "Direct influence of melatonin on the thyroid and comparison with prolactin," *J Exp Zool,* 286(6):625-31; 5/1/2000.

Yildirimkaya M, Ozata M, et al, "Lipoprotein(a) concentration in subclinical hypothyroidism before and after levo-thyroxine therapy," *Endocr J,* 43(6): 73-6; 12/1996. (Elevated total cholesterol, LDL, and apolipoprotein B, improved on T4 therapy.)

Yudkin J, "Sweet and dangerous," Bantam Books, NY, 1973.

Zwaveling J, Batink HD, et al, "Thyroid hormone modulates inotropic responses, alpha adrenoceptor density and catecholamine concentrations in the rat heart," *Naunyn Schmiedebergs Arch Pharmacol,* 354(6):755-64; 12/96. (Thyroid may directly affect alpha 1-adrenoceptor-mediated heart activity, rather than through sympathetic mediation.)

Adrenals

Adler GS, "Cushings Syndrome," At: www.emedicine.com/pnr/topic485.htm Accessed: 12/28/2002.

Ansseau M, "Biological markers of depression," *Proceedings of the International Congress of Biological Markers of Depression: State of the Art,* Liege Belgium, 6/13-15, 1990; in M Ansseau, R Von Frenckell, G Franck, eds, *Excerpta Medica,* Elsevier Sci Pubs, NY, 1991; pp 4-9.

Burch, EA, Goldshmidt TJ, "Neuroendocrine testing in psychiatry: Progress toward a disease model of depression," in *Affective Disorders Reassessed,* 1983; pp 151-78.

Carroll BJ, "Anxiety/depression: Current management and future directions. Biologic markers and treatment response," *J Clin Psychiat,* 44(8):30-40; 9/1983. (DST.)

Carroll BJ, et al., "Neuroendocrine regulation in depression. II. Discrimination of depressed from nondepressed patients," *Arch Gen Psychiat,* 33: 1051-58; 1976.

www.geocities.com/jti026/finalsemcushings4.html

Accessed: 2/3/2005
LJ De Groot, ed, *Endocrinology,* V2, WB Saunders Co, Phil; 1995
Gold MS, MD, *The Good News About Depression,* Villard Books, NY, 1987.
U Halbreich, ed, "Hormones and Depression," Raven Press, NY, 1987; pp 357-83.
Jimerson DC, Insel TR, "Increased plasma MHPG in dexamethasone-resistant depressed patients," 2/1983. (In 15 depressives, nonsuppression, robustly correlated with adrenergic activation, as evidenced by increased MHPG.)
Kathol RG, Delahunt JW, et al, "Transition from bipolar affective disorder to intermittent Cushing's Syndrome: Case report," *J Clin Psychiat,* 46(5): 194-96; 5/1985.
Mathis C, et al, "The neurosteroid pregnenolone sulfate blocks NMDA antagonist-induced deficits in a passive avoidance memory task," *Psychopharmacol (Berl),*10/1994; pp, 201-6. (Pregnenolone is often low in affectives, especially during active depression.)
Meltzer HY, Fang VS, et al, "Effect of dexamethasone on plasma prolactin and cortisol levels in psychiatric patients," *Am J Psychiat,* 139(6):763-68; 6/1982. (DST suppressed both plasma cortisol and prolactin. In some patients, abnormal cortisol may reflect a pituitary rather than limbic issue.)
Mendlewicz J, "Hypothalamic-pituitary-adrenal axis function in chronic schizophrenia: Association with clinical features," *Neuropsychobiol,* 25:1-7; 1992.
Morgan BLG, Morgan R, *Hormones,* Price, Stern, Sloan, Los Angeles, CA, 1989.
Murray MT, *Glandular Extracts,* Keats, New Canaan, CN, 1994.
Musselman DL, Nermcroff CB, "Depression and endocrine disorders: Focus on the thyroid and adrenal system," *Br J Psychiat,* (30S):123-8; 6/1996. (Depression in patients with altered thyroid or adrenal axis is well-documented. Adrenal axis changes can include: enlarged pituitary and adrenals, adrenocorticoid oversecretion, elevated corticotropin-releasing factor.)
Pfeiffer CC, *The Schizophrenias Ours to Conquer,* Bio-Communications Press, Wichita, KS, rev ed, 1988.
Prange AJ, Whybrow PC, Loosen PT, "Depression and other mental symtoms in endocrine disorders: An overview," in U Halbreich, ed, *Hormones and Depression,* Raven Press, NY, 1987; pp. 313-324.
Reus Victor I, MD, "Behavioral implications of HPA dysfunction," in U Halbreich, ed, *Hormones and Depression,* Raven Press, NY, 1987.
Risch SC, Levine RJ, et al, "Limbic-hypothalamic-pituitary-adrenal axis activity and ventricular to brain ratio studies in affective illness and schizophrenia," *Neuropsychopharmacol,* 6(2):95-100; 2/1992. (CSF and CRF cortisol were significantly elevated in the more severely depressed.)
Rogers S, *Depression, Cured at Last,* SK Publishing, Sarasota FL, 1997.
Rose RM, "Endocrine abnormalities in depression and stress — An overview," in U Halbreich, ed, *Hormones and Depression,* Raven Press, NY, 1987, pp 31-48.
Ross J, *The Mood Cure,* Viking Penguin, NY, 2002.
Rubin RT, Young WM, et al, "17-hydroxy-corticosteroid and vanillylmandellic acid excretion in a rapidly cycling manic-depressive," *Psychosom Med,* 30:162-71; 1968.
Sachar EJ, in D Freeman, JE Dyrud, eds, *American Handbook of Psychiatry,* Basic Books, NY, 299-313; 1975.
Schlesser MA, Rush AJ, et al, *Psych Res,* 9:59-67; 1983.
Slagle P, *The Way Up from Down,* St Martin's Paperbacks, NY, 1992.
Smith TJ, *Renewal: The anti-aging revolution,* Rodale Press, Emmaus PA, 1998.
Snyder, Solomon, MD, *Biological Aspects of Mental Disorder,* Oxford U Press, NY, 1980.
Stokes PE, Frazer A, "Unexpected neuroendocrine-transmitter relationships," *Psycho Pharmacol Bull,* 17(1):72-75; 1981.
Stokes PE, Stoll PM, et al, "Pretreatment DST and hypothalamic-pituitary-adrenocortical function in depressed and comparison groups. A multicenter study," *Arch Gen Psychiat,* 4(13):257-67; 1984. (Pretreatment DST was less predictive: positive in 8/77 normals, 35/111 depressed, 8/16 manics. Rate in bipolar and unipolar depressed was similar (about 30%). Age correlated with plasma cortisol.)
Swann AC, Stokes PE, et al, "Hypothalamic-pituitary-adrenocortical function in mixed and pure mania," *Acta Psychiatr Scand,* 85(4):270-4; 4/1992. (In 19 hospitalized manics, cortisol did not correlate with agitation or mania, but increased with depression. 3/9 pure manics were DST nonsuppressors.)
Targum SD, "Neuroendocrine dysfunction in schizophreniform disorder. Correlation with six-month clinical outcome.," *Am J Psychiat,* 140: 309-313; 1983.
Ur E, Turner TH, et al, "Mania in association with hydrocortisone replacement for Addison's disease," *Postgrad Med J,* 68(795):41-3; 1/1992. (A depressed woman with adrenocortical insufficiency experienced acute mania upon hydrocortisone treatment, perhaps due to cerebral oversensitivity due to the prolonged lack. Manic symptoms are also reported in normals on supraphysiological doses.)
Watson S, Gallagher P, et al, "Hypothalamic-pituitary-adrenal axis function in patients with bipolar disorder," *Br J Psychiat,* 184:496-502; 2004.
Whybrow P, Hurwitz R, *Hormones, Behav Psychopathol,* 38(1):103-113; 1981.

Sex hormones

Adams PW, Wynn V, et al, "Vitamin B6, depression, and oral contraception," letter, *Lancet* II, 516-7; 1974.
Adams PW, Wynn V, et al, "Effect of pyridoxine hydrochloride upon depression associated with oral contraception," *Lancet* ii:899-904; 1973. (Double blind. Positive.)
Angst J, "The course of affective disorders: II. Typology of bipolar manic-depressive illness," *Arch Psychiat Nervenkr,* 226:65-73; 1978.
Bermond P, "Therapy of side effects of oral contraceptive agents with vitamin B6," *Acta Vitaminol Enzymol,* 4(1-2):45-54; 1982. (Poor B6 and tryptophan metabolism was associated with OC-related depression, anxiety, glucose intolerance, and low libido. If levels were low, 40 mg B6/day relieved symptoms.)
Brigham PM, "The Psychopharmacology of Bipolar Disorder." At: http://people.ne.mediaone.net/pmbrig/BP_pharm.html Accessed: 6-11-2001.
Brush MG, Perry M, "Pyridoxine and the premenstrual syndrome," *Lancet,* 1399; 5/15/85. (70-80% of 630 with PMS responded.)
Bukreev VI, "Effect of pyridoxine on the psycho-pathology and pathochemistry of involutional depressions," *Zh Nevropatol Psikhiatr,* 78(3):402-08; 1978. (B6 is a cofactor of DOPA decarboxylase, critical to catecholamine synthesis. Intake by 31 involutional melancholics and 17 late-onset manic depressives led to symptomatic improvement, and increased NE excretion.)
Carter CS, Getz L, "Monogamy and the prairie vole," *Sci Am,* 268:100-106; 1993.
Connelly AJ, Mason JI, "Placental steroid hormones," *Clin Endocrin Metab,* 4:249-272; 1990.
Davis S, Jean Hailes Foundation, presentation at World Menopause Day Conference, 10/18/2000.
Dean C, Kendall RE, "The symptomatology of puerperal illnesses," *Br J Psychiat,* 139:128-133; 1981.
http//dir.salon.com/books.feature/2000/06/01/plath2/index.html
Doll H, et al, "Pyridoxine (vitamin B6) and the premenstrual syndrome: A randomized crossover trial," *J Royal Coll Gen Practitioners,* 39:364-368; 9/1989.
Getz L, Carter S, "Prairie vole partnerships," *Am Sci,* 84:56-62; 1996. (3/4 remain mated til one partner dies.)
Glick ID, Quitkin FM, et al, "The influence of estrogens, progestins and oral contraceptives on depression," in U Halbreich, ed, *Hormones and Depression,* Raven Press, NY, 1987; pp 339-55.
Gold MS, *The Good News About Depression,* Villard Books, NY, 1987.
Goodwin FK, Jamison KR, *Manic-Depressive Illness,* Oxford University Press, NY, 1990.
Gunn ADG, "Vitamin B6 and premenstrual syndrome (PMS)," *Int J Vitam Nutr Res,* 27S:213-24. (Review. Benefits PMS depression.)
Hertoghe T, *Hormone solution,* Harmony, 2002. holisticonline.com/remedies/hrt_herbs_summary.htm
Insel TR, "Oxytocin; A neuropeptide for affiliation: Evidence from the behavioral, receptor, autoradiographic, and comparative studies," *Psychoneuroendocrinol,* 17:3-35; 1992.
Insel TR, Shapiro L, "Oxytocin receptor distribution reflects social organization in monogamous and polygamous voles," *Proc Nat Acad Sci,* 89:5981-5985; 1992.
Kendall KE, Schnurr PP, "The effects of vitamin B6 supplementation on premenstrual syndrome," *Ob Gyn,* 70:145-49; 1987.
Kleijnen J, Riet GT, et al, "Vitamin B6 in treatment of the premenstrual syndrome — a review," *Brit J Obstet Gynaecol,* 97:847-52; 1990. (Research inconsistent.)
Kusalic M, Engelsmann F, "Effect of lithium maintenance treatment on hypothalamic pituitary gonadal axis in bipolar men," *J Psychiat Neurosci,* 21(3):181-6; 5/96. (61 stable, lithium-treated euthymic bipolar men showed higher prolactin, luteinizing hormone, and testosterone, which after 2 yrs (5 for testosterone) decreased to normal.)
Lam DH, Jones SH, et al, *Cognitive therapy for bipolar disorder: A therapist's guide to concepts, methods, and practice,* Wiley, Chichester UK, 1999.
Liebenluft E, Fiero PL, Rubinow DR, "Effects of the menstrual cycle on dependent variables in mood disorder research," *Arch Gen Psych,* 51: 761-81; 1994.
Leibenluft E, "Women with bipolar illness: Clinical and research issues," *Am J Psychiat,* 153(2):163-73; 1996. (Rapid cycling and, perhaps depression, more common in women.)
Meltzer ES, Kumar R, "Purperal mental illness, Clinical features and classifications: A study of 142 mother and baby admissions," *Br J Psychiat,* 147: 647-654; 1985. (Virtually all postpartum mania occured within 2 wks of delivery.)
Moses K, *The Real Sylvia Plath,* 2003.
OHara MW, Schlechte JA, et al, "Prospective study of postpartum blues: Biological and psychosocial factors," *Arch Gen Psych,* 48:801-6; 1991. (Family or individual history of depression and extent of estrogen drop were the most significant predictors.)
Pfeiffer CC, *Nutrition and Mental Illness,* Healing Arts Press, Rochester, VT, 1987.
Pfeiffer CC, *The Schizophrenias Ours to Conquer,* Bio-Communications Press, Wichita, KS, rev ed, 1988.
Plath S, *Nick and the Candlestick,* 1963.
Prange AJ, Whybrow PC, Loosen PT, "Depression and Other Mental Symtoms in Endocrine Disorders: An Overview," in U Halbreich, ed, *Hormones and Depression,* Raven Press, NY, 1987, pp. 313-324.
Ross J, *The Mood Cure,* Viking Penguin, NY, 2002.
Shapira B, Oppenheim G, et al, "Lack of efficacy of estrogen supplementation to imipramine in resistant female depressives," *Biol Psychiat,* 20(5): 576-9; 1985.
Sibisi CD, "Sex differences in the age of onset of bipolar affective illness," *Br J Psychiat,* 156:842-5; 6/1990. (UK sample showed middle-aged women had higher inception rates for mania than men. Cumulate admissions were approximately equivalent.)
Slagle P, "Testosterone," *The Way Up Newletter Archives,* #21 At: thewayup.com/newletters/newsarch.htm
Slagle P, "Hormone replacement therapy," *The Way Up Newletter Archives,* #34 At: thewayup.com/newletters/newsarch.htm
Tuttle D, "Report: Jonathan Wright, MD," *LE Magazine;* 4/2005. At: lef.org/magazine/mag2005/apr2005_report_female_02.htm
Venkatarangam SH, Kutcher SP, et al, "Secondary mania with steroid withdrawal," *Can J Psychiat,* 33(7):631-2; 10/1988.

Wehr TA, Sack DA, Rosenthal NE, "Sleep production as a final common pathway in the genesis of mania," *Am J Psychiat,* 144:201-204; 1987.

Wynn V, et al, "Tryptophan, depression and steroidal contraception," *J Steroid Biochem,* 6:965-70; 1975. (Placebo-controlled. Highly effective in severely depressed B6-deficient women on OCs.)

Organic brain disorders

Agnelucci L, et al, "Nerve growth factor bind in aged rat CNS: Effect of acetyl-L-carnitine," *J Neurosci Res,* 20:491; 1988.

Bagley, Christopher, PhD, "Organic brain disorders in the aetiology of schizophrenia," *Schizophrenia,* 3(3-4):150-6; 1971.

Balch JF, Balch PA, *Prescription for Nutritional Healing,* Avery, Garden City Park, NY, 1990.

Baxter LR, Phelps ME, et al, "Cerebral metabolic rates for glucose in mood disorders. Studies with positron emission tomography," *Arch Gen Psychiat,* 1985.

Bella R, et al, "Effect of acetyl-L-carnitine on geriatric patients suffering from dysthymic disorders," *Intl J Clin Pharmacol Res,* 10(6):355-60; 1990.

Bharath S, Hsu M, et al, "Glutathione, iron and Parkinson's disease," *Biochem Pharmacol,* 64(5-6): 9/2002. (GSH supports mitochondrial function, and helps prevent substantia nigra oxidative damage. Iron probably contributes to the oxidative stress.)

Blaylock R, *Excitotoxins: The Taste that Kills,* Health Press, Santa Fe, NM, 1995.

Braverman E, Pfeiffer CC, *The Healing Nutrients Within,* Keats, New Canaan, CN, 1987.

Brooks JO, et al, "Acetyl-L-carnitine shows decline in younger patients with Alzheimer's disease," *Intl J Clin Pharmacol Res,* 10:101; 1990.

Campos L, World Academy of Multidisciplinary Neurotraumatology. At: alternativementalhealth.com/articles/headinjury.htm Accessed: 2005

Casdorph HR, Walker M, *Toxic Metal Syndrome: How Metal Poisoning Can Affect Your Brain,* Avery, Garden City Park, NY, 1995.

Cohen-Cole SA, Stoudemire A, "Major depression and physical illness. Special considerations in diagnosis and biologic treatment," *Psychiat Clin North Am,* 10(1):1-17; 3/1987.

Cole T. At: alternativementalhealth.com/articles/headinjury.htm Accessed: 2005.

Crayhon R, *The Carnitine Miracle,* M Evans & Co, 1998.

Crook TH, "Effects of phosphatidyl-serine in age-associated memory impairment," *Neurology,* 41: 644; 1991.

Cummings JL, "Depression and Parkinson's disease," *Am J Psychiat,* 1992.

Cummings JL, "Behavioral and psychiatric symptoms associated with Huntington's disease," *Adv Neurol,* 65:179-86; 1995.

Cummings JL, 1994, quoted in Nasraddine 1997a

Davidson, K, "Schizophrenia-like psychoses associated with organic cerebral disorders: A review," *Psychiatric Developments,* 1:1-34; 1983.

Engler F, Vetter P, [Affective and schizophrenic syndromes in multiple sclerosis, Review of the literature and case reports], *Schweiz Arch Neurol Psychiatr,* 1991.

Erkfritz G. At:alternativementalhealth.com/articles/headinjury.htm

National Neurotrauma Society. At: www.edc.gsph.pitt.edu/neurotrauma/ncbi.nim.nih.gov/entrezquery.fcgi?cmd+Retrieve&db=PubMed&list_uids+12059045&dopt=Abstract

Folstein SE, *Huntington's Disease: A Disorder of Families,* John Hopkins Press, Baltimore, 1989.

Fry-Welch D, Pfalzer LA, "Effect of bee venom therapy on isometric knee strength in people with multiple sclerosis," *Neurol Report,* 20:4:13-4; 1996.

Filey CM, Kleinschmidt-DeMasters BK, "Neurobehavioral presentations of brain neoplasms," *West J Med,* 1995.

Galton, Lawrence, *You May Not Need A Psychiatrist: How Your Body May Control Your Mind,* Simon & Schuster, NY, 1979.

Gammerman AF, Yourkevitch ID, eds, *Wild Medical Plants,* Bello-Russ Pubs, Acad Sci, Inst Exp Botanics Microbiology, Minsk, Bello-Russia, 1965.

Gelenberg AJ, Gibson CJ, et al, "Neurotransmitter precursors for the treatment of depression," *Psychopharm Bull,* 18(1):7-18; 1982.

Gold MS, *The Good News About Depression,* Villard Books, NY, 1987.

Gross CG, "Neurogenesis in the adult brain: Death of a dogma," *Nature Rev, Neurosci,* 1(2):67-73; 2000.

Hauser RA, "Bee venom therapy for treating multiple sclerosis," *Alt Comp Ther,* 7:1:37-45; 2001.

Hoffer A, *Orthomolecular Medicine for Physicians,* Keats, New Canaan, CN, 1983.

Hoffer A, "Huntington's Disease, A follow-up," *J Orthomol Psychiat,* 13(1):42-44; 1984.

Hoffman D, *The New Holistic Herbal,* Element Books, GB, 1990.

Horrobin DF, Bennett CN, "Depression and bipolar disorder: Relationships to impaired fatty acid and phospholipid metabolism and to diabetes, cardiovascular disease, immunological abnormalities, cancer, and osteoporosis. Possible candidate genes," *Prostaglandins, Leukot, Essent Fatty Acids,* 60:217-34; 1999.

Humphrey K. At: alternativementalhealth.com/articles/headinjury.htm 2005

Irle E, Peper M, et al, "Mood changes after surgery for tumors of the cerebral cortex," *Arch Neurol,* 1994.

Ivy A, in Burton Goldberg Group, ed, *Alternative Medicine,* Future Medicine, Puyallup, WA, 1993.

Jaffe R, Kruesi OR, "The biochemical-immunology window: A molecular view of psychiatric case management," *J App Nutr,* 44(2); 1992.

Jenner P, et al, "Oxidative stress as a cause of nigral cell death in Parkinson's disease and incidental Lewy body disease," *Ann Neurol,* 32:282-87; 1992.

Jorge RE, Robinson RG, Starkstein SE, et al, "Influence of major depression on 1-year outcome in patients with traumatic brain injury," *J Neurosurg,* 1994.

Jorge RE, "Secondary mania following traumatic brain injury," 1993a. At: ajp.psychiatryonline.org.

Jorge RE, Depression and anxiety following traumatic brain injury," 1993b. At: neuro.psychiatryonline.org

Kidd PM, *Phosphatidyl serine, Nature's Brain Booster,* Total Health Comm, St George UT, 2005.

Kloss J, *Back to Eden,* Lifeline Books, Riverside CA 1973.

Krasnoperova MG, et al, "Use of cholinomimetics in the treatment of endogenous autism in children," *Zhurnal Nevrologii I Psikhiatrii,* 6:35; 2004.

Krauthammer C, Klerman GL, "Secondary mania: Manic syndromes associated with antecedent physical illness or drugs," *Arch Gen Psychiatr,* 35(11):11/1978.

Lemmo W. At: alternativementalhealth.com/articles/headinjury.htm Accessed: 2005

Lishman WA, "The psychiatric sequelae of head injury: A review," *Psychol Med,* 3:304-18; 1973.

Mayberg HS, "PET imaging of cortical S2 serotonin receptors after stroke," *Am J Psychiat,* 145:937-43; 1988.

Maggioni M, et al, [Effects of phosphatidylserine therapy in geriatric patients with depressive disorders], *Act Psychiatr Scand,* 81:265; 1990.

Mayberg HS, "Cognitive impairments and depression in Parkinson's disease," *J Neurol,* Neurosurg Psychiat, 1990.

Mayberg HS, "Paralimbic frontal lobe hypometabolism in depression associated with Huntington's disease," *Neurol,* 42(9):1791-7; 1992.

Mayberg HS, Solomon DH, "Depression in Parkinson's disease: A biochemical and organic viewpoint," *Adv Neurol,* 65:49-60; 1995.

McCaldron RJ, "Somato-psychic disorders," *J Orthomol Med,* 4(1); 1989.

McCance-Katz EF, "Serotonergic dysfunction in depression associated with Parkinson's disease," *Neurology,* 42(9):1813-4; 1992.

McKenzie C, At: alternativementalhealth.com/articles/headinjury.htm Accessed: 9-6-2005.

McLoughlin D, "Bipolar disorder and cerebral sarcoidosis," *Br J Psychiat,* 1991.

Mervis RF, Parker KL, et al "Chronic dietary choline and phosphatidylcholine induces dendritic growth in pyramidal cells of aging mouse neocortex," in RJ Wurtman, et al, eds, "Alzheimer's Disease: Advances in Basic Research and Therapies," *Proceedings of the Fourth Meeting of the International Study Group on the Pharmacology of Memory Disorders Associated with Aging,* Zurich, Switzerland, 1987. (PC or choline increased dendritic material 125-166%.)

Meshikovsky M, *Medical Preparations,* Ekarstvennye Sredstva, Medicina Pubs, Moscow, 1967.

Minden SL, Schiffer RB, "Affective disorders in multiple sclersosis. Review and recommendations for clinical research," *Arch Neurol,* 1990.

Mowrey DB, *The Scientific Validation of Herbal Medicine,* Keats, New Canaan, CN, 1986.

Murray MT, Pizzorno JE, *Encyclopedia of Natural Medicine,* Prima, Rockland, CA, 1998.

Nasreddine ZS, Cummings JL, *Depression in neurological diseases,* John Wiley & Sons, 1997a

Nasreddine, et al, "Depression and Cognitive Impairment," *Neuropharmacol,* 53:695-9; 1997b.

National Neurotrauma Society, At: www.edc.gsph.pitt.edu/neurotrauma/ncbi.nim.nih.gov/entrezquery.\fcgi?cmd+Retrieve&db=PubMed&list_uids+12059045&dopt=Abstract

Page LR, *Healthy Healing,* Healthy Healing Pub, CA, 1992.

Perlmutter D, *BrainRecovery.com, Powerfultherapy for Challenging Brain Disorders,* The Perlmutter Health Center, Naples, FL, 2001

Petersen RC, Kokmen E, "Cognitive and psychiatric abnormalities in multiple sclerosis," *May Clin Proc,* 1989.

Pfeiffer CC, *The Schizophrenias Ours to Conquer,* Bio-Communications Press, Wichita, KS, 1988.

Quillin P, *Healing Nutrients,* Contemporary Books, Chicago, 1987.

Randrup A, Munkvad I, *Mania, depression and brain dopamine, Current developments in psychopharmacology,* Spectrum pub, 1975.

Reisch T, Brekenfeld C, et al, "A case of hydrocephalus occlusus presenting as bipolar disorder," *Acta Psychiatr Scand,* 112(2)159-63; 8/2005.

Robinson RG, Starkstein SE, "Mood disorders following stroke: New findings and future directions," *J Geriatr Psychiat,* 1989.

Rother J, et al, "Hypoglycemia presenting as basilar artery thrombosis," *Stroke,* 23:112-13; 1992.

Schiffer RB, Babigian HM, "Behavioral disorder in multiple sclerosis, temporal epilepsy, and amyotrophic lateral sclerosis: An epidemiological study," *Arch Neurol,* 41:1067-9; 1984.

Sechi G, Deledda MG, et al, "Reduced intravenous glutathione in the treatment of early Parkinson's disease," *Prog Neuropsychopharmacol Biol Psychiat,* 20(7):1159-70; 10/1996. (600 mg, IV, 2x/d. for 1 mo. All improved significantly (averaging 42%.)

Shoumitro Deb, Lyons I, et al, "Neurobehavioral symptoms one year after a head injury," *Br J Psychiat,* 174:360-65; 1999a.

Shoumitro D, Lyons I, et al, "Rate of psychiatric illness one year after traumatic brain injury," *Am J Psychiat,* 1999b.

Silver JM, Yudofsky SC, et al, "Depression in traumatic brain injury," *Neuropsychiat Neuropsychol Behav Neurol,* 1991.

Stein D, *The Natural Remedy Book for Women,* The Crossing Press, Freedom, CA, 1992.

Swank RL, "Multiple sclerosis: Twenty years on low fat diet," *Arch Neurol,* 23:260-74; 1970.

Swank RL, *The Multiple Sclerosis Diet Book,* Doubleday, Garden City, NY, 1977.

Tenney L, *Stress,* Woodland Health Books, 1987.

Walsh WJ. At: alternativementalhealth.com/articles/headinjury.htm Accessed: 2005.

Wenstrup D, Ehmann W, "Trace element imbalances in isolated subcellular fractions of Alzheimer's disease brains," *Brain Res,* 533:125-31; 1990.

Werbach MR, *Nutritional Influences on Mental Illness,* Third Line Press, Tarzana, CA, 1991.

Werbach, MR, *Nutritional Influences on Illness,* 2nd ed, Third Line Press, Tarzana, CA, 1993.

Werbach MR, Murray MT, *Botanical Influences on Illness,* Third Line Press, Tarzana, CA, 1994.

Wood M. At: alternativementalhealth.com/articles/headinjury.htm Accessed: 2005.

Wu A, Molteni R, et al, "A saturated-fat diet aggravates the outcome of traumatic brain injury on hippocampal plasticity and cognitive function by reducing brain-derived neurotrophic factor," *Neurosci,* 119:365-75; 2003. (A diet high in sugar and fat decreases brain-derived neurotrophic factor, which is critical to plasticity and recovery from injury.)

Wurtman RJ, "The fate of C14-dihydroxy-phenylalanine (C-14-DOPA) in the whole mouse," *J Pharmacolog Exp Ther,* 174 (3):351-6; 1970.

Wurtman RJ, "Meeting report: Workshop of the international study group (ISG) on the pharmacology of memory disorders associated with aging," *J Neural Transmission,* 47(4); 12/1980.

Walsh, William J, PhD, interview with author, April, 1995.

Immune & autoimmune disorders

Aladjem, H, *The Sun Is My Enemy,* Prentice-Hall, Englewood Cliffs, NJ, 1972. (Personal recovery from lupus with IM niacin.)

Balch JF, Balch PA, *Prescription for Nutritional Healing,* Avery, Garden City Park, NY, 1990.

Bechter K, Herzog S, "MRI in psychiatric patients with serum antibodies against Borna disease virus," *Psychiat Res,* 1989.

Bode L, Ferzt R, et al, "Borna disease virus infection and affective disorders in man," *Arch Virol,* Suppl, 1993.

Christopher JR, *School of Natural Healing,* Provo, UT, 1976.

Connor TJ, Leonard BE, "Depression, stress and immunological activation: The role of cytokines in depressive disorders," *Life Sci,* 62(7):583-606; 1998.

Davidson, K, "Schizophrenia-like psychoses associated with organic cerebral disorders: A review." *Psychiatric Developments,* 1:1-34; 1983.

Erasmus U, *Fats that Heal, Fats that Kill,* Alive Books, Burnaby, Canada, rev ed, 1995.

Fallon BA, Nields JA, et al, "Psychiatric manifestation of Lyme borreliosis," *J Clin Psychiat,* 54(7):263-8; 2/1993.

Fisher CM, "Hypomanic symptoms caused by herpes simplex encephalitis," *Neurol,* 1996.

Fu ZF, Amsterdam JD, et al, "Detection of Borna disease virus-reactive antibodies from patients with affective disorders by western immunoblot technique," *J Affect Disord,* 27(1):61-8; 1993.

Galton L, *You May Not Need A Psychiatrist: How Your Body May Control Your Mind,* Simon & Schuster, NY, 1979.

Gold M, *The Good News About Depression,* Villard Books, NY, 1987.

Gosztonyi G, Ludwig, et al, "Borna disease — neuropathology and pathogenesis," *Curr Top Microbiol Immunol,* 1995.

Hajek T, Pakova B, et al, "Higher prevalence of antibodies to Borrelia burdorferi in psychiatric patients than in healthy subjects," *Am J Psychiat,* 159:297-301; 2/2002.

Hoffer A, *Orthomolecular Medicine for Physicians,* Keats, New Canaan, CT, 1983; pp 41, 180-81.

Kristensson K, Norrby E, "Persistence of RNA viruses in the central nervous system," *Ann Rev Microbiol,* 40:159-84; 10/1986.

Krauthammer C, Klerman GL, "Secondary mania: Manic syndromes associated with antecedent physical illness or drugs," *Arch Gen Psychiatr,* 35(11):11/1978.

Lemmo W, "Mental health care: Under the microscope" At: www.lemmo.com/mental.html#microscope Accessed: 2003.

Lendvai, Saravay SM, et al, "Creutzfeldt-Jakob disease presenting as secondary mania," *Psychosomatics,* 40:6; 11-12; 1999.

Livingston V, "Some cultural, immunological and biochemical properties of progentor cryptocides," *Trans NY, Acad. Sci,* 36(6):569-582; 6/1974.

"Lyme disease research studies — Brain imaging." At: www.lymedisease.about.com Accessed: 1-23-2001.

Maes M, "Evidence for an immune response in major depression: A review and hypothesis," *Prog Neuropsychopharmacol Biol Psychiat,* 19(1): 11-38; 1995.

Maes M, Smith RS, "Fatty acids, cytokines, and major depression," *Biol Psychiat,* 43(5):313-4; 1998.

Major LF, Brown GL, et al, "Carcinoid and psychiatric symptoms," *South Med J,* 1973.

Masterson J, "Lysine, herpes, schizophrenia and MCTD: A confirmation of the viral theory of schizophrenia from a longitudinal study," *J Orthomol Med,* 1(2):97-109; 1986. (Suggests a connection between growth, thymus suppression, herpes (and its lysine/arginine imbalance), and flareups of schizophrenia or lupus.)

Murray MT, Pizzorno JE, *Encyclopedia of Natural Medicine,* Prima, Rockland, CA, 1998.

Page LR, *Healthy Healing,* Healthy Healing Pub, CA, 1992.

Pfeiffer CC, *The Schizophrenias Ours to Conquer,* rev ed, Bio-Communications Press, Wichita, KS, 1988.

Philpott WH, "Immunological deficiency in schizophrenia/ Schizophrenia as a variant syndrome in the nutritional deficiency addiction-diabetes mellitus-infection disease process," *CSF, 5th Annual Meeting,* Winnipeg, Manitoba, Canada, 6/6/1976.

Plutchok JJ, Tikofsky RS, et al, "Tc-99m HMPAO brain SPECT imaging in chronic Lyme disease," *J Spiro Tick Diseases,* 6(3):117-22; 1999. (In one study, brain abnormalities were evident in 74% of 19 Lyme patients.)

Salaman M, *Foods that Heal,* Stafford Pub, Menlo Park, CA, 1989.

Shaw, William D, PhD, "Possible synergistic effects of nonesterified fatty acids and lysolecithins, a toxic methionine metabolite, and ammonia in the production of hepatic encephalopathy and schizophrenia," *J Orthomol Med,* 3(3); 1988.

Smith RS, "The macrophage theory of depression," *Med Hypotheses,* 35(4):298-306; 1991.

Steinberg KD, Hirsch SR, et al, "Influenza infection causing manic psychosis," *Br J Psychiat,* 120(558): 531-5; 5/1972.

Stoll AL, *The Omega-3 Connection,* Simon & Schuster, NY, 2002.

Veach, Harry O, MD, "Reconstructive medication," *J Orthomol Psychiat,* 3(1):20-21; 1974.

Weisman Y, Huminer D, et al, "Borna disease virus antibodies among workers exposed to infected ostriches," *Lancet,* 1994.

Werbach MR, *Nutritional Influences on Mental Illness,* Third Line Press, Tarzana, CA, 1991.

Werbach MR, *Nutritional Influences on Illness,* 2nd ed, Third Line Press, Tarzana, CA, 1993.

Werbach MR, Murray MT, *Botanical Influences on Illness,* Third Line Press, Tarzana, CA, 1994.

Immune support

Balch JF, Balch PA, *Prescription for Nutritional Healing,* Avery, Garden City Park, NY, 1990.

Beyer, RE, "The role of ascorbate in antioxidant protection of biomembranes: Interaction with vitamin E and coenzyme Q," *J Bioenerget,* 26(4): 349-58; 1994.

Bland J, *The 20-Day Rejuvenation Diet Program,* Keats, New Canaan, CN, 1997.

Christopher J, *School of Natural Healing,* Provo, UT, 1976.

Erasmus U, *Fats that Heal, Fats that Kill,* Alive Books, Burnaby, Canada, rev ed, 1995.

Galton L, *You May Not Need A Psychiatrist: How Your Body May Control Your Mind,* Simon & Schuster, NY, 1979.

Gold M, *The Good News About Depression,* 1987.

Hoffer A, *Orthomolecular Medicine for Physicians,* 1983.

Kehrer JP, "Free radicals as mediators of tissue injury and disease," *Crit Rev Toxicol,* 23(1):21-48; 1993.

Ketterer B, Coles B, et al, "The role of glutathione in detoxication," *Environmental Health Perspectives,* 49:59-69; 1983.

Kidd PM, "Glutathione: Systemic protectant against oxidative and free radical damage," *Alt Med Rev,* 2(3):155-76; 1997.

Mowrey DB, *The Scientific Validation of Herbal Medicine,* Keats, New Canaan, CN, 1986a.

Mowrey DB, *Proven Herbal Blends,* Keats, New Canaan, CN, 1986b.

Murray MT, Pizzorno JE, *Encyclopedia of Natural Medicine,* Prima, Rockland, CA, 1998.

Nichols TW, "Alpha-lipoic acid: Biological effects and clinical implications," *Alt Med Rev,* 2(3):177-83; 1997.

Passwater RA, "Lipoic acid: The metabolic anti-oxidant," Keats, New Canaan, CT, 1995; pp 1-47.

Page LR, *Healthy Healing,* Healthy Healing Pub, CA, 1992.

Philpott, William H, "Immunological deficiency in schizophrenia. Schizophrenia as a variant syndrome in the nutritional deficiency addiction-diabetes mellitus-infection disease process," *CSF, 5th Annual Meeting,* Winnipeg, Manitoba, Canada, 6/6/1976.

Smith RS, "The macrophage theory of depression," *Med Hypotheses,* 35:298-306; 1991.

Salaman M, *Foods that Heal,* Stafford Pub, Menlo Park, CA, 1989.

Sullivan K, "The miracle of vitamin D," Wise Traditions in Food, Farming and the Healing Arts, Weston A Price Foundation, Fall, 2000.

Veach HO, "Reconstructive medication," *J Orthomol Psychiat,* 3(1):20-21; 1974.

Werbach MR, *Nutritional Influences on Mental Illness,* Third Line Press, Tarzana, CA, 1991.

Werbach, MR, *Nutritional Influences on Illness,* 2nd ed, Third Line Press, Tarzana, CA, 1993.

Werbach MR, Murray MT, *Botanical Influences on Illness,* Third Line Press, Tarzana, CA, 1994.

Liver Detox

Anderson KE, Kappas A, "Dietary regulation of cytochrome P450," *Annu Rev Nutr,* 11:141-67; 1991.

Beutler E, "Nutritional and metabolic aspects of gluathione," *Ann Rev Nutr,* 9:287-302; 1989.

Bland JS, Bralley JA, "Nutritional upregulation of hepatic detoxification enzymes," *J Applied Nutr,* 44; 1992.

Bland J, *The 20-Day Rejuvenation Diet Program,* Keats, New Canaan, CN, 1997.

Cooper AL, "Biochemistry of sulfur-containing amino acids," *Ann Rev Biochem,* 53:187-222; 1983.

Dickerson JWT, et al, "Activity of drug-metabolizing enzymes in the liver of growing rats fed on diets high in sucrose, glucose, fructose or an equimolar mixture of glucose and fructose," *Proc Nutr Soc,* 30:271-28A; 1971.

Grant DM, "Detoxification pathways in the liver," *J Inher Metab Dis,* 12:421-30; 1991. (Glycine is an antioxidant and detoxifier, and is used in liver conjugation reactions.)

Guengerich FP, "Effects of nutritive factors on metabolic processes involving bioactivation and detoxication chemicals," *Ann Rev Nutr,* 4:207-31; 1984.

Kendler BS, "Taurine: An overview of its role in preventive medicine," *Prev Med,* 18:79-100. (Important in transforming xenobiotics during phase II conjugation.)

Levy G, "Sulfate conjugation in drug metabolism: Role of inorganic sulfate," *Federation Proc,* 45: 2235-2240; 1986. (Sulfation is a rate-limiting step in liver phase II conjugation.)

Makhtar H, Wamg ZY, et al, "Tea components: Antimutagenic and anticarcinogenic effects," *Prev Med,* 21:351-60; 1992 (Catechins, found in green tea, may help defend against hepatic oxidative stress, and may counter environmental toxins by interacting with P450 enzymes.)

Percival, M, "Detoxification," *Nutritional Pearls,* 23; 1/1996.

Queen HS, "Reversing chemical or neurotoxic induced damage to the brain and nervous system," *Health Talk,* 9(2):9-16; 1990.

Tahiliani AG, Beinlich, CJ, "Pantothenic acid in health and disease," *Vitamins and hormones,* 46: 165-227; 1991. (B5 supports acetylation, amino conjugation, CoA synthesis.)

Yim CY, Hibbs JB, et al, "Use of N-acetyl cysteine to increase intracellular glutathione during the induction of antitumor response by IL-2," *J Immunol,* 152:5796-5805; 1994.

Lifestyle; Stress

Agid O, Shapira B, et al, "Environment and vulnerability to major psychiatric illness: A case control study of early parental loss in major depression, bipolar disorder and schizophrenia," *Mol Psychiat,* 4(2):163-172; 3/99. (Early parental loss, especially when due to permanent separation rather than death, was significantly associated with major depression. In 76 bipolars, early parental loss was also common. Controls with such losses had lower income, more divorce and physical illness, and were more likely to live alone and to use tobacco. Future studies should control for psychiatric illness in parents, making them more likely to leave.)

Alhambra MA, Fowler TP, et al, "EEG biofeedback: A new treatment option for ADD/ADHD," *J Neurother,* 1995.

Alloy LB, Reilly-Harrington NA, et al, "Cognitive styles and life events in subsyndromal unipolar and bipolar disorders: Stability and prospective prediction of depressive and hypomanic mood swings," *J Cognitive Psychother,* 13:21-40; 1999. (Negative cognitive style was more prevalent in patients with abnormally negative mood, even with occasional mania/hypomania.)

Ambelas A, "Psychologically stressful events in the precipitation of manic episodes," *Br J Psychiat,* 135: 15-21; 1979.

Aston-Jones G, Foote SL, Bloom FE, "Anatomy and physiology of locus ceruleus neurons: functional implications," in MG Zeitler, CR Lake, *Norepinephrine,* Williams and Wilkins, Baltimore; pp 92-116.

Bauer MS, Whybrow PC, "Thyroid hormones and the central nervous system in affective illness: Interactions which may have clinical signifcance," *Integrative Psychiat,* 6:75-100; 1988.

Bowers WA, "Treatment of depressed inpatients. Cognitive therapy plus medication, relaxation plus medication, and medication alone," *Br J Psychiat,* 156:73-78; 1990. (Augments antidepressants.)

Broota A, Dhir R, "Efficacy of two relaxation techniques in depression," *J Pers Clin Stud,* 6: 83-90; 1990.

Burrows GD, "Affective Disorders and Hypnosis," in RO Stanley, GD Burrows, PB Bloom, eds, *International Handbook of Clinical Hypnosis,* 2001.

Cavanaugh JT, van Beck M, et al, "Case-control study of neurocognitive function in euthymic patients with bipolar disorder: An association with mania," *Br J Psychiat,* 180:320-6; 2002.

Chadwick P, Lowe C, "A cognitive approach to modifying delusions," *Behavior Res Ther,* 32:355-67; 1994.

Coe CL, Mendoza SP, et al, "Mother-infant attachment in the squirrel monkey: Adrenal response to separation," *Behavior Biol,* 22:256-263; 1978.

Connor TJ, Leonard BE, "Depression, stress and immunological activation: The role of cytokines in depressive disorders," *Life Sci,* 62:583-606; 1998.

Corrigan FM, "Mindfulness, dissociation, EMDR, and the anterior cingulate cortex: A hypothesis," *Contemporary Hypnosis,* 19(1):8-17; 2002.

Dennerstein, eds, *Handbook of Hypnosis and Psychosomatic Medicine,* 1980; pp 149-70.

Depue RA, Luciana M, et al, "Dopamine and the structure of personality: Relation of agonist-induced dopamine activity to positive emotionality," *J Personality Soc Psychol,* 67:485-98; 1994.

Depue RA, Colins PF, et al, *A Model of Neurobiology: Environmental Interaction in Developmental Psychopathology,* Oxford Press, NY, 1996.

Depue RA, Collins PF, "Neurobiology of the structure of personality: Dopamine, facilitation of incentive motivation, and extraversion," *Behav Brain Sci,* 22: 491-569; 1998.

Devilly GJ, Spence, SH, "The relative efficacy and treatment distress of EMDR and a cognitive behavior trauma treatment in the amelioration of posttraumatic stress disorder," *J Anxiety Disord,* 13(1-2):131-57; 1999.

Dryden SC, "Hypnosis in the treatment of depression," *Psycholog Reports,* 58(3):923-9; 1986.

Ellicott A, Hammen C, et al, "Life events and the course of bipolar disorder," *Am J Psychiatr,* 147(9): 1194-98; 1990. (Survival analysis, controlling for medication levels. Over 2 yrs, in 61 bipolar outpatients, stressful life events were significantly associated with relapse.)

Field T, Grizzle N, et al, "Massage and relaxation therapies: Effects on depressed adolescent mothers," *Adolescence,* 31:903-11; 1996.

Field T, Morrow C, et al, "Massage reduces anxiety in child and adolescent psychiatric patients," *J Am Acad Child Adolesc Psychiat,* 31:125-31; 1992.

Field T, "Massage therapy effects," *Am Psychol,* 53:1270-81; 1998. (Increases vagal activation and improves facial expression and vocalizations. May counter depression by shifting right frontal to balanced or left frontal activation.)

Gold PW, Goodwin FK, "Clinical and biochemical manifestations of depression. Relation to the neurobiology of stress," *NEJM,* 319 (7):413-20; 8/1988.

Gray JA, "Brain systems that mediate both emotion and cognition," *Cognit Emot,* 4:269-88; 1990.

Gray JA, "Neural systems, emotions, and personality," in J Madden IV, ed, *Neurobiology of Learning, Emotion, and Affect,* Hillsdale Press, NY, 1991; pp 273-306.

Han JS, "Electroacupuncture: An alternative to antidepressants for treating affective diseases?" *Int J Neurosci,* 29:79-92; 1986. (Double blind. As effective as tricyclics.)

Hosboer F, "Neuroendocrinology of mood disorders," in FE Bloom, DJ Kupfer, eds, *Psychopharmacology: The Fourth Generation of Progress,* Raven, NY, 1995; pp 957-69.

Hunt N, Bruce-Jones W, et al, "Life events and bipolar affective disorder," *J Affect Disord,* 25:13-20; 1992. (Adverse events were several times more likely within 1 mo. before an episode.)

Jacobson L, Sapolsky R, "The role of the hippocampus in feedback regulation of the hypothalamic-pituitary-adrenocortical axis," *Endocrine Rev,* 12: 118-34; 1991.

James T, "The use of NLP and time line therapy TM techniques in treating depression," 2003 At: www.tltinfo.com.au/depres.html

Johnson SL, Sandrow D, et al, "Life events involving goal-attainment and increases in manic symptoms," presented at the Annual Conference of the Association for the Advancement of Behavior Therapy, Toronto, CAN; 11/1999a.

Johnson SL, Winett C, et al, "Social support and the course of bipolar disorder," *J Abnorm Psychol,* 108: 558-566; 1999b.

Johnson SL, Meyer B, et al, "Social support and self-esteem predict changes in bipolar depression but not mania," *J Affect Disord,* 58:79-86; 2000.

Jorm AF, Christensen H, et al, "Effectiveness of complementary and self-help treatment for depression," *Med J Australia,* 176(10S):84-95; 2002.

Kahn JS, Kehle TJ, et al, "Comparison of cognitive-behavioral relaxation training, and self-modeling interventions for depression among middle school students," *School Psychol Rev,* 19:196-211; 1990.

Kennedy S, Thompson R, et al, "Life events precipitating mania," *Br J Psychiat,* 142:398-403; 1983.

Kingdon DG, Turkington D, "Cognitive-behavioral therapy of schizophrenia," Guilford Press, NY; 1994.

Koob GF, "Behavioral actions of corticotrophin releasing factor in the central nervous system," *J Cell Biochem,* Suppl 12D:299-309; 1988.

Koob, "Behavioral responses to stress," in MR Brown, GF Koob, C Rivier, *Stress, Neurobiology & Neuroendocrinology,* Marcel Bekker, NY, 1991; pp 255-271.

Kuehner C, Weber I, "Responses to depression in unipolar depressed patients: An investigation of Nolen-Hoeksema's response styles theory," *Psychol Med,* 29(6):1323-33; 11/1999. (Depression may be associated with rumination, supporting Hocksema's response style theory that distraction is helpful.)

Ladd CO, Owens MJ, et al, "Persistent changes in corticotrophin-releasing factor neuronal systems induced by maternal deprivation," *Endocrinol,* 137:1212-18; 1996.

Laidlaw L, Naito A, "Mood changes after self-hypnosis and Johrei prior to exams," *Contemporary Hypnosis,* 20(1):25-39; 2003.

Lam DH, Wong G, "Prodromes, coping strategies, insight and social functioning in bipolar affective disorders," *Psychol Med,* 27:1091-1100; 1997. (Social function is better if patients can recognize mania.)

Lam DH, Jones SH, et al, "Cognitive therapy for bipolar disorder: A therapist's guide to concepts, methods and practice," Wiley, Chichester UK, 1999.

Lemmo W, "Mental health care: Under the microscope" At: www.lemmo.com/mental.html#microscope Accessed: 2003.

Lesser, Michael, MD, interview with author, August 2008.

Levine S, "Psychobiologic consequences of disruption in mother-infant relationships," in NA Krasnoger, EM Blass, MA Hoffer, WP Smotherman, eds, Academic Press, Orlando, 1987; pp 359-376.

Lozano BE, Johnson SL, "Personality traits as predictors of mania and depression," Annual Conference of the Association for the Advancement of Behavior Therapy, Toronto, 11/1999.

Luo H, Meng F, et al, "Clinical research on the therapeutic effect of the electroacupuncture treatment in patients with depression," *Psychiat Clin Neurosci,* 52:S338-40; 1998.

Miklowitz DJ, Goldstein MJ, *Bipolar disorder: A family-focused treatment approach,* Guilford Press, NY,1997.

Malkoff-Schwartz S, Frank E, et al, "Stressful life events and social rhythm disruption in the onset of manic and depressive episodes: A preliminary investigation," *Arch Gen Psychiat,* 55(8):702-7; 1998. (As compared to euthymic periods, at least one severe event in the 8 wks pre-onset was common, in 20 manics, 29 bipolar depressed.)

Matheson, G, "Modification of depressive symptoms through posthypnotic suggestion," *Am J Clin Hypnosis,* 22(1):61-64; 1979.

Martin M, "On the induction of mood," *Clin Psychol Rev,* 10:669-97; 1990.

Miklowitz DJ, Goldstein MJ, et al, "Family factors and the course of bipolar affective disorder," *Arch Gen Psychiatr,* 45:2225-30; 1988.

Miklowitz DJ, Goldstein MJ, *Bipolar disorder: A family-focused treatment approach,* Guilford Press, NY, 1997.

Moore DT, "A Holistic Approach for Treating Manic Depressive Disorders." At: familyclinic.simplenet.com/bipolar/bipaper.html Accessed: 1998. (Hypnosis, meditation, accelerated conditioning, relaxation, etc., mainly help at the outset of a mood swing, and often change body parameters comparably to meds. Self-hypnosis can prevent a mania, reduce depression.)

Murphy GE, Carney RM, et al, "Cognitive behavior therapy, relaxation training, and tricyclic antidepressant medication in the treatment of depression," *Psychol Rep,* 77:403-20; 1995.

Newman CF, Leahy RL, et al, *Bipolar Disorder: A Cognitive Therapy Approach,* Am Psychological Assn, DC, 2002.

O'Connell RA, Mayo JA, et al, "Social support and long term lithium outcome," *Br J Psychiat,* 147:272-75; 1985. (Social support (resources, relationships, other buffers against negative life events) correlated most with good outcome on global assessment, social adjustment and affective episode scales.)

Otto MW, Reilly-Harrington N, et al, "Psycho-educational and cognitive-behavioral strategies in the management of bipolar disorder," *J Affect Disord,* 73:171-81; 2003.

Post RM, Rubinow DR, et al, "Conditioning and sensitization in the longitudinal course of affective illness," *Br J Psychiat,* 149:191-201; 1986.

Priebe S, Wildgrube C, et al, "Lithium prophylaxis and expressed emotion," *Br J Psychiatr,* 154:396-

99; 1989.

Reilly-Harrington NA, Alloy LB, et al, "Cognitive styles and life events interact to predict bipolar and unipolar symptomatology," *J Abnorm Psychol*, 198: 567-78; 1999.

Reynolds WM, Coats KI, "A comparison of cognitive-behavioral therapy and relaxation training for the treatment of depression in adolescents," *J Consult Clin Psychol*, 54:653-60; 1986.

Rosenfeld P, "EEG biofeedback of frontal alpha asymmetry in affective disorders," *Biofeedback*, 1997.

Rosenfeld JP, "An EEG biofeedback protocol for affective disorders," *Clin Electroencephalogr*, 2000. At: ncbi.nim.nih.gov

Rush AJ, "Toward an understanding of bipolar disorder and its origin," *J Clin Psychiat*, 64:4-8; 2003. (Poor social support can worsen depression and delay recovery.)

Sachar E, "Corticosteroid response to the psychotherapy of depressions: Evaluation during confrontation of loss," *Arch Gen Psychiat*, 16: 461-70; 1967.

Sachar E, "Disrupted cortisol secretion in psychotic depression," *Arch Gen Psychiat*, 28:19-24; 1973.

Sahley BJ, *Healing with Amino Acids*, Pain & Stress Center Pub, TX, 1995.

Selye H, *The Stress of Life*, McGraw-Hill, NY, 1978.

Spitz R, "Anaclitic depression: An inquiry into the genesis of psychiatric conditions in early childhood," *Psychoanalytic Study of the Child*, 2: 313-347; 1942.

Stoll AL, *The Omega-3 Connection*, Simon & Schuster, NY, 2002.

Suomi S, "Early stress and adult emotional reactivity in rhesus monkeys," *The Childhood Environment & Adult Disease, Ciba Foundation Symposium*, 156: 171-188; 1991a.

Suomi S, "Uptight and laid-back monkeys: Individual differences in response to social challenges," in S Branch, W Hall, E Dooling eds, *Plasticity of Development*, MIT Press, Cambridge, Mass, 1991b; pp 27-55.

Suomi SJ, Harlow HF, et al, "Effect of repetitive infant-infant separation of young monkeys," *J Abnorm Psychol*, 76:161-172; 1970.

Sutherland C, "Neurosomatic treatment for depression: A preliminary report on a group treatment program," *Frontier Perspectives*, 10(2); 2001. At: lifeworks-group.com.au

Vellucci SV, "Primate social behavior — anxiety or depression?" *Pharmacol Ther*, 47:167-180; 1990.

Walsh J, Connelly PR, "Supportive behaviors in natural support networks of people with serious mental illness," *Health Soc Work*, 21(4):296-303; 11/1996.

Walsh WJ, "Commentary on nutritional treatment of mental disorders," *International Guide to the World of Alternative Mental Health*. At: www.alternativementalhealth.com/articles.walshMP.htm#Py Accessed: 10/08/2006.

Weissman MM, Bland RC, et al, "Cross-national epidemiology of major depression and bipolar disorder," *JAMA*, 276:293-99; 1996.

Whybrow PC, "Sex differences in thyroid axis function: Treatment implications for affective disorders," *Depress*, 3:33-42; 1995.

Winters KC, Neale JM, "Mania and low self-esteem," *J Abnorm Psychol*, 94:282-90; 1985.

Optimizing diet

Airola P, *How to Get Well*, Health Plus, Phoenix, AZ, 1974.

Anderson KE, Kappas, A, "Dietary regulation of cytochrome P450," *Ann Rev Nutr*, 11:141-67; 1991.

Balch JF, Balch PA, *Prescription for Nutritional Healing*, Avery, Garden City Park, NY, 1990.

Beutler E, "Nutritional and metabolic aspects of gluathione," *Ann Rev Nutr*, 9:287-302; 1989.

Bland JS, Bralley JA, "Nutritional upregulation of hepatic detoxification enzymes," *J Applied Nutr*, 44; 1992.

Bland J, *The 20-Day Rejuvenation Diet Program*, Keats, New Canaan, CN, 1997.

Blauer S, *The Juicing Book*, Avery, Garden City Park, NY, 1989.

Calbom C, Keane M, *Juicing for Life*, Avery, Garden City Park, NY, 1992.

Cooper AL, "Biochemistry of sulfur-containing amino acids," *Ann Rev Biochem*, 53:187-222; 1983.

Cott A, *Fasting: The Ultimate Diet*, Bantam, 1975.

Cott A, "Fasting, controlled treatment for schizophrenia," *J Orthomol Psychiat*, 3(4):301-11; 1974.

Cousens G, *Depression Free for Life*, Quill, HarperCollins, NY, 2001.

Davis B, *Rapid Healing Foods*, Parker, NY, 1980.

DesMaisons K, *Potatoes not Prozac*, Radiant Recovery, Alburquerque NM.

Dickerson JWT, et al, "Activity of drug-metabolizing enzymes in the liver of growing rats fed on diets high in sucrose, glucose, fructose or an equimolar mixture of glucose and fructose," *Proc Nutr Soc*, 30:271-28A; 1971.

Grant DM, "Detoxification pathways in the liver," *J Inher Metab Dis*, 12:421-30; 1991. (Glycine is used in liver conjugation reactions.)

Guengerich FP, "Effects of nutritive factors on metabolic processes involving bioactivation and detoxication chemicals," *Ann Rev Nutr*, 4:207-31; 1984.

Gursche S, *Healing with Herbal Juices*, Alive Books, Vancouver, 1993.

HealthComm, Intl, "Modified elimination diet," and "Diet Summary," Form 29, 2/7/1995.

Hoffer A, "Nutrition and behavior," in J Bland, ed, *Medical Applications of Clinical Nutrition*, Keats, New Canaan, CN, 1983.

Hoffer A, *Orthomolecular Medicine For Physicians*, Keats, New Canaan, CN, 1983.

Hoffer A, *Common Questions on Schizophrenia and their Answers*, Keats, New Canaan, CN, 1987.

Kendler BS, "Taurine: An overview of its role in preventive medicine," *Prev Med*, 18:79-100. (Important in transforming xenobiotics during phase II conjugation.)

Lee W, *The Book of Raw Fruit and Vegetable Juices and Drinks*, Keats, New Canaan, CN, 1982.

Lesser M, *Nutrition & Vitamin Therapy*, Bantam Books, NY, 1983.

Levy G, "Sulfate conjugation in drug metabolism: Role of inorganic sulfate," *Federation Proc*, 45: 2235-2240; 1986. (Sodium sulfate, supplies sulfur for sulfation reactions. Sulfation is a rate-limiting step in liver phase II conjugation.)

Makhtar H, Wamg ZY, et al, "Tea components: Antimutagenic and anticarcinogenic effects," *Prev Med*, 21:351-60; 1992.

Miller CL, Dulay JR, "The high affinity niacin receptor HM74A is decreased in the anterior cingulate cortex of individuals with schizophrenia," *Brain Res Bull*, 77(1):33-41; 9/2008.

Murray, MT, *Encyclopedia of Natural Medicine*, Prima, Rocklin, CA, 1998.

Page LR, *Healthy Healing*, Healthy Healing Pub, CA, 1992.

Percival, M, "Detoxification," *Nutritional Pearls*, 23; 1/1996.

Pfeiffer CC, *Nutrition and Mental Illness*, Healing Arts Press, Rochester, VT, 1987.

Pfeiffer CC, *The Schizophrenias Ours to Conquer*, rev ed, Bio-Communications Press, Wichita, KS, 1988.

Pritchard P, *Healing with Whole Foods*, North Atlantic Books, Berkeley CA, 1993.

Queen HS, "Reversing chemical or neurotoxic induced damage to the brain and nervous system," *Health Talk*, 9(2):9-16; 1990.

Sachs J, *Nature's Prozac*, Prentice Hall, Paramus NJ, 1997.

Salaman M, *Foods that Heal*, Stafford Pub, Menlo Park, CA, 1989.

Shelton HM, *Fasting Can Save Your Life*, Natural Hygiene, 1981.

Tahiliani AG, Beinlich CJ, "Pantothenic acid in health and disease," *Vitamins and Hormones*, 46: 165-227; 1991.

Walker N, *Fresh Vegetable and Fruit Juices*, Norwalk Press, Prescott, AZ, 1970.

Walsh WJ, "Commentary on nutritional treatment of mental disorders," *International Guide to the World of Alternative Mental Health*. At: www.alternativementalhealth.com/articles.walshMP.htm#Py Accessed: 10/08/2006.

Walsh, William J, PhD, interview with author, November, 2007.

Werbach MR, *Nutritional Influences on Mental Illness*, Third Line Press, Tarzana, CA, 1991.

Werbach MR, *Nutritional Influences on Illness*, 2nd ed, Third Line Press, Tarzana, CA, 1993.

Werbach MR, Murray MT, *Botanical Influences on Illness*, Third Line Press, Tarzana, CA, 1994.

Yim CY, Hibbs JB, et al, "Use of N-acetyl cysteine to increase intracellular glutathione during the induction of antitumor response by IL-2," *J Immunol*, 152:5796-5805; 1994.

Young SN, "The use of diet and dietary components in the study of factors controlling affect in humans: A review," *J Psychiat Neurosci*, 18(5):235-44; 1993.

Exercise, Oygen

Babyak MA, Blumenthal JA, et al, "Exercise treatment for major depression: Maintenance of therpeutic benefit at 10 months," *Psychosom Med*, 62:633-8; 2000. (Less relapse than with antidepressants.)

Blumenthal JA, Babyak MA, et al, "Effects of training on older patients with major depression," *Arch Intl Med*, 159:19-26; 1999.

Doyne EJ, Ossip-Klein DJ, et al, "Running versus weight lifting in the treatment of depression," *J Consult Clin Psychol*, 55:748-54; 1987. (Randomized, controlled. Both were beneficial.)

Hoffer A, *Orthomolecular Medicine for Physicians*, Keats, New Canaan, CN, 1983.

Janakiramaiah N, Gangadhar BN, et al, "Anti-depressant efficacy of Sudarshan Kriya Yoga (SKY) in melancholia: A randomized comparison with electroconvulsive therapy (ECT) and imipramine," *J Affect Disord*, 57:255-7; 2000. (The benefit of breathwork was equivalent to that of imipramine.)

Jorm AF, Christensen H, et al, "Effectiveness of complementary and self-help treatment for depression," *Med J Australia*, 176(10S):84-95; 2002.

Khumar SS, Kaur S, "Effectiveness of shavasana on depression among university students," *Indian J Clin Psychol*, 20:82-7; 1993. (30 days, 20 min/day, improved multiple depressive symptoms vs controls.)

LemmoW, "Mental health care: Under the microscope" At: www.lemmo.com/mental.html#microscope Accessed: 2003.

McCann L, Holmes DS, "Influence of aerobic exercise on depression," *J Pers Soc Psychol*, 46:1142-7; 1984. (More effective than relaxation therapy.)

McNeil JK, Le Blanc E, et al, "The effect of exercise on depressive symptoms in the moderately depressed elderly," *Psychol Aging*, 6:487-8; 1991. (Comparable to social contact.)

Murray MT, "Lifestyle and dietary factors in depression," *Am J Natural Med*, 2:10-15; 1995.

Ott J, "The Eyes Dual Function," *The Eye Ear Nose and Throat Monthly*, V. 53; 7/1974.

Pfeiffer CC, *Nutrition and Mental Illness*, Healing Arts Press, Rochester, VT, 1987.

Pfeiffer CC, *The Schizophrenias Ours to Conquer*, rev ed, Bio-Communications Press, Wichita, KS, 1988.

Pinchasov BB, Shurgaja AM, et al, "Mood and energy regulation in seasonal and non-seasonal depression before and after midday treatment with physical exercise or bright light," *Psychiat Res*, 92: 29-42; 2000. (Exercise was superior to placebo and more effective than light in non-SAD individuals.)

Quillin P, *Healing Nutrients*, Contemporary Books, Chicago, 1987.

Singh NA, Clements KM, et al, "The efficacy of exercise as a long-term antidepressant in elderly subjects: A randomized controlled trial," *J Gerontol A Biol Sci Med Sci*, 56A:M497-504; 2001. (Improvement persists over time.)

Riordan, Hugh, MD, in *Alternative Medicine*, Burton Goldberg Group, ed, Future Medicine, Puyallup, WA, 1993.

Stewart NJ, McMullin LM, et al, "Movement therapy

with depressed inpatients: A randomized multiple single case design," *Arch Psychiatr Nurs,* 8:22-9; 1994. (Some improved on treatment days.)

Weyerer S, Kupfer B, "Physical exercise and psychological health," *Sports Med,* 17:108-16; 1994.

Whitman W, "Song of Myself, poem X."

Weil A, *Breathing: The Master Key to Self Healing,* Sounds True, 1999.

Williams R, *Biochemical Individuality,* John Wiley & Sons, Texas, 1956.

Rhythms

Ambelas A, "Psychologically stressful events in the precipitation of manic episodes," *Br J Psychiat,* 135: 15-21; 1979.

Ansseau, Marc, "Biological markers of depression," M Ansseau, R Von Frenckell, G Franck, eds, *Proceedings, International Congress of Biological Markers of Depression: State of the Art,* Liege Belgium, 6/13-15, 1990, Elsevier Sci Pubs, Excerpta Medica, NY, 1991; pp 4-9.

Arendt J, "The pineal hormone melatonin in seasonal and circadian rhythms," in PH Redfern, IC Campbell, JA Davies, et al, eds, *Circadian Rhythms in the Central Nervous System,* Macmillan, London, 1985; pp 15-24.

Aschoff J, "Circadian rhythms in man," *Science,* 148: 1427-32; 1965.

Avery DH, Wildschiodtz G, Rafaelsen O, "REM latency and temperature in affective disorder before and after treatment," *Biol Psychiat,* 17: 463-470; 1982.

Avery D, Dahl K, "Bright light therapy and circadian neuroendocrine functions in seasonal affective disorder," in J Schulkin, ed, *Hormonally Induced Changes in Mind and Brain,* Academic Press, San Diego, 1993; chapter 11.

Avery DH, Eder DN, et al, "Dawn simulation and bright light in the treatment of SAD: A controlled study," *Biol Psychiat,* 50:205-16; 2001.

Bauer MS, Donner DL, "Validity of seasonal pattern as a modifier for recurrent mood disorders for DSM-IV," *Comp Psychiat,* 34:159-70; 1993.

Bauer M, Gyulai L, et al, "Testing definitions of dysphoric mania and hypomania: Prevalence, clinical characteristics, and inter-episode stability," *J Affect Dis,* 32:201-11;1994.

Beck-Friis J, Kjellman BF, et al, "Serum melatonin in relation to clinical variables in patients with major depressive disorder and a hypothesis of a low melatonin syndrome," *Acta Psychiatr Scand,* 71: 319-30; 1985a. (Low in major depression.)

Beck-Friis J, Kjellman BF, et al, "The pineal gland and melatonin in affective disorders," in GM Brown, SD Wainwright, eds, *The Pineal Gland: Endocrine Aspects* (Advances in the Biosciences, V53) Pergamon, Oxford, 1985b.

Bersani G, Garavini A, "Melatonin add-on in manic patients with treatment resistant insomnia," *Prog Neuropsychopharmaol, Biol Psychiat,* 24(2): 185-91; 2/2000.

Birdsall TC, "The biological effects and clinical uses of the pineal hormone melatonin," *Alt Med Rev,* 1(2):94-102; 1996.

Delito JA, Moline M, et al, "Effects of phototherapy on non-seasonal unipolar and bipolar depressive spectrum disorders," *J Affect Disord,* 23(4):231-7; 12/1991.

Bittman EL, Demsey RJ, et al, "Pineal melatonin secretion drives the reproductive response to daylength in the ewe," *Endocrinol,* 113:2276-83; 1983.

Boyce PM, "6-Sulphatoxymelatonin in melancholia," *Am J Psychiat,* 142:125-127; 1985.

Branchey L, Weinberg U, et al, "Simultaneous study of 24-hour patterns of melatonin and cortisol secretion in depressed patients," *Neuropsychobiol,* 8:225-232; 1982.

Brigham PM At: mediaone.net/pmbrig/BP_pharm.htm Accessed: 2001

Broadway J, Arendt JH, et al, "Bright light phase shifts the human melatonin rhythm during the Antarctic winter," *Neurosci Letters,* 79:185-189; 1987.

Brown R, Kocsis JH, et al, "Differences in nocturnal melatonin secretion between melancholic depressed patients and control subjects," *Am J Psychiat,* 142: 811-816; 1985.

Bubenik GA, Smith PS, Schams D, "The effect of orally administered melatonin on the seasonality of deer pelage exchange, antler development, LH, FSH, prolactin, testosterone, T3, T4, cortisol, and alkaline phosphatase," *J Pineal Res,* 3:331-49; 1986.

Bunney WE, Murphy DL, et al, "The 'switch process' in manic-depressive illness," *Arch Gen Psychiat,* 27: 295-302; 1972.

Bunney WE, Wehr TR, "The switch process in manic-depressive psychosis," *Ann Intern Med,* 1977.

Buysse DJ, Tu XM, et al, "Pretreatment REM sleep and subjective sleep quality distinguish depressed psychotherapy remitters and nonremitters," *Biol Psychiat,* 45(2):205-13; 1/15/1999. (Midlife recurrently depressed females unresponsive to psychotherapy had elevated phasic REM and significantly worse sleep quality (perhaps reflecting limbic and brain stem arousal.)

Christopher JR, *School of Natural Healing,* Provo, UT, 1976.

Clark DM, Teasdale JD, "Diurnal variation in clinical depression and accessibility of memories of positive and negative experience," *J Abnorm Psychol,* 91: 87-95; 1982.

Claustrat B, Chazot G, et al, "A chronological study of melatonin and cortisol secretion in depressed subjects: Plasma melatonin, a biochemical marker in major depression," *Biol Psychiat,* 19:1215-28; 1984.

Corfman E, "Depression, manic depressive illness, and biological rhythms," US Dept HEW, Public Health Serv; Alcohol, Drug, & Mental Health Administration, Maryland.

Cousens G, *Depression Free for Life,* Quill, HarperCollins, NY, 2001.

Cowgill, "Season of birth in man," *Ecology,* 47: 614-623; 1966.

Dahlitz M, Alvarez B, et al, "Delayed sleep phase syndrome response to melatonin," *Lancet,* 1:1121-24; 1991.

Delito JA, Moline M, et al, "Effects of phototherapy on non-seasonal unipolar and bipolar depressive spectrum disorders," *J Affect Disord,* 23(4):231-7; 12/1991.

D'Mello DA, McNeil JA, et al, "Seasons and bipolar disorder," *Ann Clin Psychiat,* 7(1):11-18; 3/1995. (Michigan male bipolar admissions peaked in spring; females, in spring and fall. Aggressive behavior in both peaked in spring.)

Dunne A, "Some effect of the quality of light on health," *J Orthomol Med,* 4(4):229-32; 1989.

Ehlers CL, Frank E, et al, "Social zeitgebers and biological rhythms: A unified approach to understanding the etiology of depression," *Arch Gen Psychiatr,* 45:948-52; 1988.

Ehlers CL, Kupfer DJ, et al, "Biological rhythms and depression, The role of zeitgebers and zeitstorers," *Depression,* I: 285-93; 1993.

Eiber R, Escande M, [Sleep electroencephalography in depression and mental disorders with depressive comorbidity], *Encephale,* 15(5):381-90; 9-10/1999.

Faedda GL, Tondo L, et al, "Seasonal mood disorders. Patterns of seasonal recurrence in mania and depression," *Arch Gen Psychiat,* 50(1); 1/1993. (Fall-winter depression, spring-summer mania. Suicide rate is highest in spring and fall, May and Oct, when sun/dark ratio changes most rapidly.)

Frank E, Kupfer DJ, et al, "Interpersonal and social rhythm therapy for bipolar disorder: Integrating interpersonal and behavioral approaches," *Behav Ther,* 17:143-149; 1994.

Gaby A, *Townsend Letter for Doctors and Patients,* 50-54, 126-31, 8-9/2000.

Garrison RH, Somer E, *The Nutrition Desk Reference,* Keats, New Canaan, CN, 1985.

Glickman G, Byrne B, "Light therapy for seasonal affective disorders with blue narrow-band ligh-emitting diocides (LEDs)," *Biol Psychiatr,* 59(6): 502-7; 2006.

Gloth FM III, Alam W, Hollis B, "Vitamin D vs broad spectrum phototherapy in the treatment of seasonal affective disorder," *Nutr Health Aging,* 3(1):5-7; 1999. (Small single blind, randomized controlled. One-time oral dose of 100,000 IU improved depression better than light therapy in SAD patients. Improvement significantly correlated with 25(OH)D. No added benefit when used with light therapy.)

Gold MS, *The Good News About Depression,* Villard Books, NY, 1987.

Goodwin, Jamison, *Manic Depressive Illness,* Oxford University Press, 1990.

Halaris A, ed, *Chronobiology and psychiatric disorders,* Elsevier, NY, 1987.

Hartman E, "Longitudinal studies of sleep and dream patterns in manic-depressive patients," *Arch Gen Psychiat,* 19:312-29; 1968.

Hartmann E, Spinweber CL, "Sleep induced by L-typtophan. Effect of dosages within normal dietary intake," *J Nerv Ment Dis,* 167(8):497-9; 1979.

Hartmann E, Cravens J, et al, "Hypnotic effects of L-tryptophan," *Arch Gen Psychiat,* 31(3):394-7; 9/1974.

Hartmann E, "L-tryptophan: A rational hypnotic with clinical potential," *Am J Psychiat,* 134:366-70; 1977. (Review of 9 studies. Unlike hypnotics, it doesn't distort sleep physiology.)

Hauri P, Chernik D, Hawkins D, "Sleep of depressed patients in remission," *Arch Gen Psychiat,* 31:386-91; 1974. (Stage 4, probably Ser-dependent, slow-wave sleep disturbance remained after remission.)

Healy D, "Rhythm and blues: Neurochemical, neuropharmacological and neuropsychological implications of a hypothesis of circadian rhythm dysfunction in the affective disorders," *Psychopharmacol,* 93:271-85; 1987.

Hobson JA, *The Dreaming Brain,* Basic Books, NY, 1988.

Huether G, et al, "Effects of tryptophan administration on circulating melatonin levels in chicks and rats: Evidence for stimulation of melatonin synthesis and release in the gastrointestinal tract," *Life Sci,* 51:945-53; 1992.

Hyman JW, *The Light Book,* Jerry M Tarcher Inc, LA, 1990.

Iguchi HM, Kato K, Ibayashi H, "Age-dependent reductions in serum melatonin concentrations in healthy human subjects," *J Clin Endocrinol,* 55: 27-29; 1982.

Jain S, Kaliaperumal VG, et al, "Climate and admissions for mania in the tropics," *J Affect Disord,* 26(4):247-50; 12/1992. (No seasonal trends for manic admissions, over 9 yrs, in a tropical hospital, where climate was relatively constant.)

Jan JE, Connolly MB, et al, "Melatonin treatment of non-epileptic myoclonus in children," *Dev Med Child Neurol,* 41:255-59; 1999.

Jouvet M, "Biogenic amines and the states of sleep," *Sci,* 163:32-41; 1969.

Kamo J, Shinichiro T, et al, "Season and mania," *Japan J Psychiatr Neurol,* 47(2):473-74; 1993.

Kasper S, Wehr TA, "The role of sleep and wakefulness in the genesis of depression and mania," *Encephale,* 18S(1):45-50; 1/1992. (Sleep deprivation augmenting antidepressants can produce sustained improvement, but may trigger mania, especially in rapid cyclers.)

Kennedy S, Thompson R, et al, "Life events precipitating mania," *Br J Psychiat,* 142:398-403; 1983.

Ketter RA, "Defining the standard of care across the bipolar spectrum: Q & A, April 9, 2000; DC, Faculty: Terrence A Ketter MD," Bipolar Disorders Information Center. At: http://www.mhsource.com/bipolar/defketter.html

Klein DC, "Melatonin and puberty," *Sci,* 224:6; 1984.

Kloss J, *Back to Eden,* Lifeline Books, Riverside CA 1973.

Iguchi HM, Kato K, Ibayashi H, "Age-dependent reductions in serum melatonin concentrations in healthy human subjects," *J Clin Endocrinol Mrysn,* 55:27-29; 1982.

Krieger Dorothy T, "Abnormalities in circadian periodicity in depression," in DJ Kupfer, TH Monk,

JD Barchas, eds, *BioRhythms & Mental Disorders,* Guilford Press, 1988.

Kripke DF, Mullaney DJ, et al, "Circadian rhythm disorders in manic-depressives," *Biol Psychiat,* 13: 335-50; 1978. (Episodes may be caused by a beat phenomena as rhythms go in and out of phase.)

Kripke DF, "Light treatment for nonseasonal depression: Speed, efficacy and combined treatment," *J Affect Disord,* 49:109-17; 1998.

Krohn J, *The Whole Way to Allergy Relief & Prevention,* Hartley & Marks, Point Roberts, WA, 1991.

Kuhs H, Farber D, et al, "Serum prolactin, growth hormone, total corticoids, thyroid hormones and thyrotropin during serial therapeutic sleep deprivation," *Biol Psychiat,* 39(10):857-64; 5/15/1996. (13 antidepressant-treated depressives were given 4 wks of 6 partial-late-night sleep deprivation. On day 1, T3 and TSH were consistently elevated, T4 less so. After a full night's sleep, TSH reverted to baseline, but T3 elevation continued.)

DJ Kupfer, TH Monk, JD Barchas, eds, *BioRhythms and Mental Disorders,* Guilford Press, 1988.

Lagoguey M, Reinbery A, *J Physiol,* 257:19-20; 1976.

Lam RW, Levitan Rd, et al, "L-tryptophan augmentation of light therapy in patients with seasonal affective disorder," *Can J Psychiat,* 42: 303-6; 1997.

Lambert GW, Reid C, et al, "Effect of sunlight and season on serotonin turnover in the brain," *Lancet,* 360(9348):1840-2, 2002 (Summer sun increases serotonin twice as much as winter.)

Lansdowne AT, Provost SC, "Vitamin D3 enhances mood in healthy subjects during winter," *Psychopharmacol, Berl,* 135(4):319-23; 1998. (Randomized double blind. Among 44 subjects, 400 or 800 IU, vs placebo, significantly enhanced positive affect over 5 days in late winter.)

Larson JM, *Alcoholism — The Biochemical Connection,* Villard Books, NY, 1992.

Lee TMC, Chan CCH, "Dose-response relationship of phototherapy for seasonal affective disorder: A meta analysis," *Acta Psychiatr Scand,* 99:3151-23; 1999. (Response improves with brighter light.)

Lerner AB, Nordlund JJ, "Melatonin: Clinical pharmacology," *J Neural Transm,* 13S:339-347; 1978.

Lesser M, *Nutrition & Vitamin Therapy,* Bantam Books, NY, 1983.

Lemmo W, "Mental health care: Under the microscope" At: www.lemmo.com/mental.html#microscope Accessed: 2003.

Lewy AJ, Markey SP, "Analysis of melatonin in human plasma by gas chromatography negative chemical ionization mass spectrometry," *Science,* 201:741-43; 1978.

Lewy AJ, Wehr TA, Gold PW, et al, "Plasma melatonin in manic-depressive illness," in E Usdin, IJ Kopin, J Barchas, eds, *Catecholamines: Basic and Clinical Frontiers,* V2, Pergamon, NY, 1979.

Lewy A, Wehr T, et al, "Light suppresses melatonin secretion in humans," *Science,* 210:1267-69; 1980.

Lewy AJ, Wehr T, Goodwin P, et al, "Manic depressive patients may be supersensitive to light," *Lancet,* 383-4; 1981.

Lewy A, Kern H, Rosenthal N, Wehr T, "Bright artifical light treatment in manic depressive patients with a seasonal mood cycle," *Am J Psychiatr,* 139: 1496-1498; 1982.

Lewy AJ, "Biochemistry and regulation of mammalian melatonin production," in R Relkin, ed, *The Pineal Gland,* Elsevier, NY, 1983; pp 77-128.

Lewy AJ, "Human melatonin secretion (II): A marker for the circadian system and the effects of light," in RN Post, JC Ballenger, eds, *Neurobiology of Mood Disorder,* Williams & Wilkins, Baltimore, 1984; pp 215-26.

Lewy A, Nurnberger J, et al, "Supersensitivity to light: Possible trait marker for manic depressive illness," *Am J Psychiatr,* 142:725-27; 1985.

Lieberman PB, Strauss JS, "The recurrence of mania: Environmental factors and medical treatment," *Am J Psychiat,* 141:77-80; 1984.

Lieberman S, Bruning N, *The Real Vitamin & Mineral Book,* Avery, Garden City Park, NY, 1990.

Lockley SW, Brainard SW, et al, "High sensitivity of the human circadian melatonin rhythm to resetting by short wavelength light," *J Clin Endocrinol Metab,* 88:4502-5; 6/2003.

Lockely SW, et al, "Short-wavelength sensitivity for the direct effects of light on alertness, vigilance and the waking electroencephalogram in humans," *Sleep,* 29:161-8; 2006.

Loew D, [L tryptophan. An essential amino acid for structural and functional metabolism], *Fortschr Med,* 115:40-42; 1997.

Marczynski TJ, Yamaguchi N, Ling GM, et al, "Sleep induced by the administration of melatonin (5-methoxy-N-acetyltryptamine) to the hypothalamus in unrestrained cats," *Experientia,* 20:435-37; 1964.

Maurizi CP, "The mystery of Alzheimer's disease and its prevention by melatonin," *Med Hypotheses,* 45(4):339-40; 10/1995. (Melatonin is frequently deficient in Alzheimer's. Damage to brain mitochondria may be due to hydroxyl radicals, for which melatonin is a scavenger.)

Mayeda, Aimee, Nurnberger JR, "Melatonin and circadian rhythms in bipolar mood disorder," in M Del Shafii, S Lea Shaffii, eds, *Bio Rhythms, Mood Disorders, Light Therapy, and the Pineal Gland,* Am Psych Press, DC, 1990.

Mendlewicz J, Linkowski P, et al, "Abnormal 24 hour pattern of melatonin secretion in depression," *Lancet,* 2:1362; 1979.

Moore RY, Klein DC, "Visual pathways and the central neural control of a circadian rhythm in pineal serotonin N-acetltransferase activity," *Brain Res,* 71:17-33; 1974.

Mowrey DB, *The Scientific Validation of Herbal Medicine,* Keats, New Canaan, CN, 1986.

Mueller PS, et al, "Diagnosis and treatment of severe light-sensitive seasonal energy syndrome (SES) and its relationship to melatonin anabolism," *Fair Oaks Hospital Library Letter,* 2:9; 9/1984.

Mulder RT, Cosgriff JP, et al, "Seasonality of mania in New Zealand," *Aust N Z J Psychiat,* 24(2): 187-90; 6/1990. (Over 5 yrs, manic admissions peaked in spring and summer, but not consistently each year and not in older females, or young first admissions.)

Murakami N, Hayafuji C, Sasaki Y, et al, "Melatonin accelerates the reentrainment of the circadian adrenocortical rhythm in inverted illumination cycle," *Neuroendocrinol,* 36:385-91; 1983.

Myers DH, Davies P, "The seasonal incidence of mania and its relationship to climactic variables," *Psychol Med,* 8(3):433-40; 8/1978. (In Britain, it's concentrated in summer, low in winter.)

Nair NPV, Hariharasubramanian N, et al, "Circadian rhythm of plasma melatonin in endogenous depression," *Prog Neuropsychopharmacol Biol Psychiat,* 8:715-18; 1984.

Neumeister A, Prascgaj-Rieder N, et al, "Effects of tryptophan depletion in fully remitted patients with seasonal affective disorder during summer," *Psychol Med,* 2(28); 1998.

Nurnberger J, Berretinin W, et al, "Supersensitivity to melatonin suppression by light in young people at high risk for affective disorder. A preliminary report," *Neuropsychopharmacol,* I:217-23; 1989.

Osher Y, Yaroslavsky Y, et al, "Predominant polarity of bipolar patients in Israel," *World J Biol Psychiat,* 1(4):187-9; 10/2000. (Mania predominant in S Israel.)

Ott J, "The Eyes Dual Function," *The Eye Ear Nose and Throat Monthly,* V. 53; 7/1974.

Ott J, *Health and Light,* Simon and Schuster, NY, 1973.

Page LR, *Healthy Healing,* Healthy Healing Pub, CA, 1992.

Parekh PI, Ketter TA, et al, "Relationships between thyroid hormone and antidepressant responses to total sleep deprivation in mood disorder patients," *Biol Psychiat,* 43(5):392-4; 3/1998. (Sleep deprivation is temporarily antidepressant in 50%. Here, deprivation in 34 medication-free affectives significantly increased 8AM TSH, T3, T4, and fT4. Increased TSH correlated with antidepressant benefit.)

Peck DF, "Climactic variables and admissions for mania: A reanalysis," *J Affect Disord,* 20(4):149-50; 1990. (Strong relation of sun to manic admissions one month later.)

Pfeiffer CC, *Nutrition and Mental Illness,* Healing Arts Press, Rochester, VT, 1987.

Pfeiffer CC, *The Schizophrenias Ours to Conquer,* Bio-Communications Press, Wichita, KS, 1988.

Pflug B, "The effect of sleep deprivation on depressed patients," *Acta Psychiatr Scand,* 53: 148-58; 1976.

Quillin P, *Healing Nutrients,* Contemporary Books, Chicago, 1987.

Redman J, Armstrong S, et al, "Free-running activity rhythms in the rat: Entrainment by melatonin," *Science,* 219:1089-91; 1983.

Robertson LM, Takahashi JS, "Circadian clock in cell culture, I: Oscillation of melatonin release from dissociated chick pineal cells in flow through microcarrier culture; II: In vitro photic entrainment of melatonin oscillation from dissociated chick pineal cells, *J Neurosci,* 8:12-21; 8:22-30; 1988ab.

Rosen L, Targum S, et al, "Prevalence of seasonal affective disorder at four latitutes," *Psychiat Res,* 31: 131-144; 1990.

Rosenthal NE, Sack DA, et al, "Seasonal affective disorder: A description of the syndrome and preliminary findings with light therapy," *Arch Gen Psychiatr,* 41:72-80; 1984.

Rusack B, Zucker I, "Neural regulation of circadian rhythms," *Physiol Rev,* 59:449-526; 1979.

Sack DA, Nurnberger JI, Rosenthal NE, et al, "Potentiation of antidepressant medications by phase advance of the sleep-wake cycle," *Am J Psychiat,* 142:606-8; 1985. (Selective REM deprivation can also be antidepressant and can promote mania.)

Sack DA, Rosenthal NE, et al, "Biological rhythms in psychiatry," in HY Meltzer, ed, *Psychopharma cology, The Third Generation of Progress,* Raven, NY, 1987.

Sadun AA, Schaechter JD, et al, "A retino-hypothalamic pathway in man: Light mediation of circadian rhythms," *Brain Res,* 301:371-77; 1984.

Sandyk R, Pardeshi R, "The relationship between ECT nonresponsiveness and calcification of the pineal gland in bipolar patients," *Int J Neurosci,* 54(3-4):301-6; 10/1990.

Sayer HK, Marshall S, et al, "Mania and seasonality in the southern hemisphere," *J Affect Disord,* 23(3): 151-6; 11/1991. (Admissions peak spring/summer.)

Schilgen B, Tolle R, "Partial sleep deprivation as therapy for depression," *Arch Gen Psychiat,* 37: 267-71; 1980.

Schneider-Helmet, D, et al, "Evaluation of L-tryptophan for treatment of insomnia: A review," *Psychopharmacol,* 89(1):1-7; 1986. (Doesn't distort sleep physiology.)

Shibata S, "Biological rhythms and drugs," *Nihon Shinkei Seishin Yakurigaku Zasshi,* 19(1):11-20; 2/1999.

Shillab G, "Orthomolecular Frontiers," *Nutr Ment Health,* Winter/2007; p 2.

Sitarem N, Gillin JC, Bunney WE, "The switch process in manic-depressive illness," *Arch Psychiatr Scand,* 58:267-78; 1978.

Slagle P, "Low moods/ Light therapy/ L-tyrosine," *The Way Up Newletter Archives,* #3 At: thewayup.com/newletters/newsarch.htm

Slagle P, "Melatonin," *The Way Up Newletter Archives* #7 At: thewayup.com/newletters/newsarch.htm

Smeraldi E, Benedetti F, et al, "Sustained antidepressant effect of sleep deprivation combined with pindolol in bipolar depression. A placebo controlled trial," *Neuropsychopharmacol,* 20(4): 380-85; 4/1999. (15/20 responded to 3 cycles of total sleep deprivation plus pindolol (which blocks the 5HT1A receptor). With lithium also, response lasted 6 mo in 65%. Results suggest Ser contributes to, and helps sustain, sleep deprivation benefits.)

Stein D, *The Natural Remedy Book for Women,* Crossing Press, Freedom, CA, 1992.

Strakowski SM, Hudson JI, et al, "Four cases of obstructive sleep apnea associated with treatment-resistant mania," *J Clin Psychiat,* 52(4):156-8; 4/91.

Suhail K, "Social Psychiatry and Psychiatric Epidemiology," *Cochrane,* 33(5); 4/1998. (Depression was highest in winter. Mania clustered around the summer in women only.)

Sullivan K, *The miracle of vitamin D,* Wise Traditions in Food, Farming and the Healing Arts, Weston A Price Foundation, Fall 2000.

SunlightD.org

Terman M, Terman J, et al, "Light therapy for seasonal affective disorder. A review of efficacy," *Neuropsychopharmacol,* 2:1-22; 1989

Terman M, Terman JS, "Treatment of seasonal affective disorder with high-output negative ionizer," *J Altern Complement Med,* 1:87-92; 1995. (May increase serotonin. High density ionization better than low.)

Terman M, Terman JS, et al, "A controlled trial of timed bright light and negative air ionization for treatment of winter depression," *Arch Gen Psychiat,* 55:875-82; 1998.

Ursin R, "The effect of 5-hydroxytryptophan and L-tryptophan on wakefulness and sleep patterns in the cat," *Brain Res,* 106:106-15; 1976.

Vieth R, Kimball S, et al, "Randomized comparison of the effects of the vitamin D3 adequate intake versus 100 mcg (4000 IU) per day on biochemical responses and the wellbeing of patients," *Nutr J,* 3(8); 7/2004. (130 adults with normal D (24 ng/mL in summer, about 16 in winter). Those most likely to develop depression were given 600 or 4000 IU summer through winter. Both achieved at least 40 ng/mL. Mood improved with increasing D, even in the winter, most so in those taking 4000 IU.)

Waldhauser F, Dietzel M, "Daily and annual rhythms in human melatonin secretion: Role in puberty control," *Ann NY Acad Sci,* 453:205-14; 1985.

Waldhauser F, Weiszenbacher G, et al, "Alterations in nocturnal serum melatonin levels in humans with growth and aging," *J Clin Endocrinol Metab,* 66:648-52; 1988.

Walsh, William J, PhD, interview with author, April, 1995.

Wehr TA, Wirz-Justice A, Goodwin FK, et al, "Phase advance of the circadian sleep-wake cycle as an antidepressant," *Science,* 206:710-13; 1979.

Wehr TA, Goodwin FK, "Desynchronization of circadian rhythms as a possible source of manic-depressive cycles," *Psychopharmacol Bull,* 16: 19-20; 1980.

Wehr T, Goodwin F, et al, "Forty-eight-hour sleep-wake cycles in manic depressive illness: Naturalistic observation and sleep deprivation experiments," *Arch Gen Psychiatr,* 39:559-65; 1982.

Wehr TA, Sack D, Rosenthal N, et al, "Circadian rhythm disturbances in manic-depressive illness," *Fed Proc,* 42:2809-13; 1983.

Wehr TA, Sack D, Rosenthal N, "Sleep reduction as a final common pathway in the genesis of mania," *Am J Psychiat,* 144:2; 2/1987a.

Wehr TA, Sack DA, et al, "Seasonal affective disorder with summer depression and winter hypomania," *Am J Psychiatr,* 144(12):1602-03; 1987b.

Wehr, Thomas A, "Sleep and biological rhythms in affective illness," in DJ Kupfer, TH Monk, JD Barchas, eds, *Biorhythms and Mental Disorders,* Guilford Press, 1988.

Wehr TA, Sack DA, et al, "Rapid cycling affective disorder: Contributing factors and treatment responses in 51 patients," *Am J Psychiatr,* 145: 179-84; 1988.

Wehr TA, "Sleep-loss as a possible mediator of diverse causes of mania," *Br J Psychiat,* 159:576-8; 10/1991.

Wehr TA, Turner EH, et al, "Treatment of a rapidly cycling bipolar patient by extended bed rest and darkness to stabilize the timing and duration of sleep," *Biol Psychiatr,* 43:822-28; 1998.

Werbach M, Murray MT, *Botanical Influences on Illness* Third Line Press, Tarzana, CA, 1994.

Wettenberg L, "The relationship between the pineal gland and the pituitary adreanl axis in health, endocrine and psychiatric conditions," *Psychoneuroendocrinol,* 8:75-80; 1983.

Wever RA, "Use of light to treat jet lag: Differential effects of normal and bright artificial light on human circadian rhythms," *NY Acad Sci,* 453: 282-304; 1985.

Wever RA, *The Circadian System of Man: Results of Experiments Under Temporal Isolation,* Springer-Verlag, NY, 1979.

Wever, Rutger A , "Order and disorder in human circadian rhythmicity: Possible relationship to mental disorder," in David J Kupfer MD, Timothy H Monk, PhD, Jack D Barchas MD, eds, *BioRhythms and Mental Disorders,* Guilford Press, 1988.

Whybrow PC, Bahr R, "A study of seasonal behavior, in animals and humans," *The Hibernation Response,* Arbor House, NY, 1988.

Wileman SM, Eagles JM, et al, "Light therapy for seasonal affective disorder: Randomized controlled trial," *Br J Psychiat,* 178:311-6; 2001.

Wirz-Justice A, Arendt J, "Diurnal, menstrual cycle and seasonal indole rhythms in man and their modification in affective disorders," in J Obiols, C Ballus, E Gonzalez, et al, eds, *Biological Psychiatry Today,* Elsvier, Amsterdam, 1979.

Wirz-Justice A, Graw P, et al, "Natural light treatment of seasonal affective disorder," *J Affect Disord,* 37:109-20; 1996.

Wirz-Justice A, "Beginning to see the light," *Arch Gen Psychiat,* 55:861-2; 1998.

Zatz M, Brownstein MJ, "Intraventricular carbachol mimics the effect of light on the circadian rhythm in the rat pineal gland," *Science,* 203:358-61, 1979.

Zatz M, Brownstein MJ, "Injection of alpha-bungarotoxin near the suprachiasmatic nucleus blocks the effects of light on nocturnal pineal enzyme activity," *Brain Res,* 213:438-42; 1981.

Zhdanova IV, Wartman RJ, "Sleep inducing effects of low doses of melatonin ingested in the evening," *Clin Pharmacol Thera,* 57:552-58; 1995.

Anxiety, OCD, eating disorders, PTSD, borderline, etc.

Abbey LC, "Agorophobia," *J Orthomol Psychiat,* 11:243-59; 1982. (B1, B3, B6, folic acid, or B12, correcting specific deficiencies, created dramatic improvement in 19/23, completely stopped panic attacks in 11.)

Alberti KG, Nattrass M, "Lactic acidosis," *Lancet* ii: 25-9; 1977.

Alvarez WC, "Puzzling 'nervous storms' due to food allergy," *Gastroenterol,* 7:241-2; 1946.

Amadeo S, Abbar M, et al, "Clinical study of 5 families with bipolar disorder," *Encephale,* 18 S (1):78-82; 1/1992. (In each pedigree, at least one bipolar suffered an additional disorder (borderline, panic, retardation, anorexia, bulimia, etc.)

Bauer MS, Whybrow PC, "Validity of rapid cycling as a modifier for bipolar disorder I, DSM-IV," *Depress,* 1:11019; 1993.

Bauer M, "Rapid cycling," in R Joffe, J Calabrese, eds, *Anticonvulsants in Psychiatry,* Marcel Dekker, NY, 1994a; pp 1-26.

Bauer MS, Calabrese J, et al, "Multi site data reanalysis: Rapid cycling as a modifier for bipolar disorder in DSM IV," *Am J Psychiatr;* 1994b.

Bell C, Abrams J, "Tryptophan depletion and its implications for psychiatry," *Br J Psychiatr,* 178:399-405; 2001. (Important in maintaining antidepressant response in panic patients. Also benefits OCD.)

Bell IR, Wyatt JK, et al, "Effect of dairy-containing diets on cognitive processing and plasma b-endorphins," *J Am Coll Nutr,* 13(5):530; 1994.

Benton D, Cook R, "The impact of selenium supplementation on mood," *Biol Psychiat,* 29(11): 1092-8; 1991. (Double blind crossover. Especially if depleted, improved anxiety, depression, fatigue.)

Brady KT, Lydiard RB, "Bipolar affective disorder and substance abuse," *J Clin Psychopharmacol,* 12(1S):17-22S; 2/1992.

Brewerton TD, Murphy DL, et al, "Test meal responses following m-chlophenylpiperazine in bulimics and controls," *Neuropsychopharmacol,* 11(1):63-71; 1994.

Brigham PM, "The Psychopharmacology of Bipolar Disorder," At: http://people.ne.mediaone.net/pmbrig/BP_pharm.html Accessed: 6-11-01.

Bruce M, Lader M, "Caffeine abstention in the management of anxiety disorders," *Psychol Med,* 19:211-4; 1989.

Buist RA, "Anxiety neurosis: The lactate connection," *Int Clin Nutr Rev,* 5:1-4; 1986.

Challem JJ, Lewin R, "Obsessive-compulsive behavior. There are nutritional answers," *Lets Live,* 6/1982. (Tryptophan helps anxious obsessions more than pleasurable ones.)

Colodny L, Hoffman, Ronald L, "Inositol: Clinical Applications for exogenous use," *Alt Med Rev,* 3(6):4323-447.

Dalvit-McPhillips S, "A dietary approach to bulimia treatment," *Physiol Behav,* 33(5):769-75; 1984.

Drewnowski A, Krahn DD, et al, "Nalaxone, an opiate blocker, reduces the consumption of sweet, high-fat foods in obese and lean female binge eaters," *Am J Clin Nutr,* 61(6):1206-12; 1995.

Duke P, Hochman G, *A Brilliant Madness, Living with Manic-Depressive Illness,* Bantam Books, NY 1992.

Durlach J, Durlach V, et al, "Magnesium and therapeutics," *Magnes Res,* 7(3-4):313-28; 1994. (Review. Chronic deficiency was associated with anxiety, insomnia, fatigue, labile emotions.)

Fux M, Levine J, et al, "Inositol treatment of obsessive-compulsive disorder," *Am J Psychiat,* 153(9):1219-21; 1996.

Gaby AR, "Vitamin B3, Part 2: Powerful tool in nutritional medicine," *Nutrition and Healing,* 12/1995. (Especially if anxiety is due to reactive hypoglycemia.)

Heseker H, Kubler W, et al, "Psychological disorders as early symptoms of a mild-to-moderate vitamin deficiency," *Ann NY Acad Sci,* 660:352-7; 1992. (Low B1, B6 B12, C, or E associated with anxiety.)

Himmelhoch J, Mulla D et al, "Incidence and significance of mixed affective states in a bipolar population," *Arch Gen Psychiatr,* 33:1062-66; 1976a.

Hoes MJ, et al, "Hyperventilation syndrome, treatment with L-tryptophan and pyridoxine; Predictive value of xanthurenic acid excretion," *J Orthomol Psychiat,* 10(1):7-15; 1981. (9/13 recovered.)

Hoes MJ, "Monoamines in psychiatry: The role of serotonin in depression, anxiety and stress," *Acta Psychiatr Belg,* 82(3):287-309, 1982.

Howat PM, Varner LM, et al, "The effect of bulimia upon diet, body fat, bone density and blood components," *J Am Diet Assoc,* 89(7):929-34; 1989.

Hoyse SE, "Experiences with L-tryptophan in a child and family psychiatric department," *J Int Med Res,* 10(3):157-9; 1982. (12 children. Good results.)

Hudson J, Pope H, of McLean in Massachusetts quoted in, "The Affective Spectrum, Joyce Ikelman's Info on Bipolar Disorder (Manic Depression)." At: frii.com/~parrot/bip.html Accessed: 8/1999.

Hughes JR, et al, "Caffeine self-administration, withdrawal and adverse effects among coffee drinkers," *Arch Gen Psychiat,* 48:611-17; 1991.

Humphries L, Vivian B, et al, "Zinc deficiency and eating disorders," *J Clin Psychiat,* 50(12):456-9; 1989.

Huwig-Poppe C, Voderholzer U, et al, "The tryptophan depletion test. Impact on sleep in healthy subjects and patients with obsessive compulsive disorder," *Adv Exp Med Biol,* 467:35-42; 1999. (Important for sleep in OCD.)

Joborn C, et al, "Psychiatric symptomology in patients with primary hyperparathyroidism," *Ups J Med Sci,* 91(1):77-87; 1986. (Hyperparathyroidism increases calcium and commonly produces anxiety. In some, low calcium is associated with anxiety.)

Kahn RS, Westenberg HG, et al, "Effect of a serotonin precursor and uptake inhibitor in anxiety disorders; a double-blind comparison of 5-hydroxytryptophan, clomipramine and placebo," *Int Clin Psychopharmacol,* 2(1):33-45; 1987. (5HTP improved anxiety, as did the SSRI. Ser may be particularly important in agorophobia and panic.)

Kennedy B, et al, "Similarity between the action of nicotinamide and diazepam on neurotransmitter metabolism in the rat," *Biochem Soc Trans,* 8(1): 59; 1980.

Ketter TA, "Defining the standard of care across the bipolar spectrum: Q & A, April 9, 2000; DC, Faculty: Terrence A Ketter MD," Bipolar Disorders Information Center. At: http://www.mhsource.com/bipolar/defketter.html Accessed: 6/11/2001.

King DS, "Can allergic exposure provoke psychological symptoms? A double-blind test," *Biol Psychiat,* 16(1):3-19, 1981. (Also exhaust, chlorine.)

Kinzler E, Kromer J, et al, "Clinical efficacy of a kava extract in patients with anxiety syndrome: Double-blind placebo-controlled study over 4 weeks," *Arzneim Forsch,* 41:584-8; 1991.

Levi L, [The effect of coffee on the function of the sympathoadrenomedullary system in man], *Acta Med Scand,* 181:431-8, 1967.

Levin P, Lazrove S, et al, "What psychological testing and neuroimaging tell us about the treatment of post-traumatic stress disorder by Eye Movement Desensitization and Reprocessing," *J Anxiety Disord,* 13(1-2):159-72; 1-4/1999. (With successful EMDR, recall of the threat elicited increased anterior cingulate gyrus and left frontal lobe activity in 4/6, enhancing discernment of real vs. imagined threat, but not necessarily reducing limbic arousal.)

Levine J, Fux M, et al, "Double-blind placebo-controlled, crossover trial of inositol treatment for panic disorder," *Am J Psychiat,* 152(7)/l1084-6; 1995. (Significant decline in number of panic attacks and severity of agorophobia.)

Lindenberg D, Pitule-Schodel H, "DL-kavain in comparison with oxazepam in anxiety disorders: A double-blind study of clinical effectiveness," *Forsche Med,* 108:49-50, 53-4; 1990.

Mc Cleane GJ, Watters CH, "Pre-operative anxiety and serum potassium," *Anaesthesia,* 45(7):583-5; 1990. (The most anxious showed less potassium.)

McClain CJ, Stuart MA, et al, "Zinc, appetite regulation and eating disorders," *Prog Clin Biol Res,* 380:47-64; 1993.

McClain CJ, Stuart MA, et al, "Zinc status before and after zinc supplementation of eating disorder patients, *J Am Coll Nutr,* 11(6):694-700; 1992.

McElroy S, Keck P, et al, "Clinical and research implications of the diagnosis of dysphoric or mixed mania or hypomania," *Am J Psychiat,* 149: 1633-44; 1992.

Mills DE, Ward RP, "Effects of eicopentaenoic acid (20:5 omega 3) on stress reactivity in rats," *Proc Soc Exp Biol Med,* 182(1):127-31; 1986.

Mills DE, Prkachin KM, et al, "Dietary fatty acid supplementation alters stress reactivity and performance in man," *J Hum Hypertens,* 3:111-6; 1989. (Double blind. GLA may be particularly effective for stress.)

Mizuno TI, Yukari YM, [Prophylactic effect of L-5HTP on self mutilation in the Lesch Nyhan syndrome], *Neuropadiatrie,* 6:13-23; 1975.

Mohler H, et al, "Nicotinamide is a brain constituent with benzodiazepam-like action," *Nature,* 278:563-5; 1979.

Monteiro MG, et al, "Subjective feelings of anxiety in young men after ethanol and diazepam infusions," *J Clin Psychiat,* 51(1):12-16; 1990.

Murphy D, et al, "Obsessive compulsive disorder as a 5-HT subsystem-related behavioral disorder," *Br J Psychiat,* 155:15-24; 1989.

Nusbaum M, "Food for thought: The problem of anorexia nervosa and bulimia," *J Orthomol Med,* 1(44):242-8; 1986.

Kaye WH, Welzin TE, "Neurochemistry of bulimia nervosa," *J Clin Psychiatr,* 52:221-8; 1991.

http://www.metamodels.com/maps/hpp.html

O'Connell RA, Mayo JA, et al, "PDQ-R personality disorders in bipolar patients," *J Affect Disord,* 23(4)-217-21; 12/91. (Ratings indicated personality disorders in 58% of 50 bipolars. Borderline was most common; histrionic disorder was also frequent.)

Patrick L, "Eating disorders, A review of the literature with emphasis on medical complications and clinical nutrition," *Altern Med Rev,* 7(3):184-202; 6/2002. (Inositol, zinc.)

Peselow E, Sanfilipo M, et al, "Relationship between hypomania and personality disorders before and after successful treatment," *Am J Psychiat,* 152: 232-238; 1995. (Cluster B: Erratic & Dramatic (borderline, etc.), and Cluster C: Anxious & Fearful (avoidant, etc.) are each twice as common as Cluster A: Odd & Eccentric (schizoid, etc.).)

Pfeiffer CC, *Nutrition and Mental Illness,* Healing Arts Press, Rochester, VT, 1987.

Pfeiffer CC, *The Schizophrenias Ours to Conquer,* Bio-Communications Press, Wichita, KS, 1988.

Pijl H, Cohen AF, et al, "Plasma amino acid ratios related to brain serotonin synthesis in response to food intake in bulimia nervosa," *Biol Psychiat,* 38(10):659-68; 1995.

Rainey JM, Jr, et al, "Specificity of lactate infusion as a model of anxiety," *Psychopharmacol Bull,* 20(1):45-9; 1984. (Glucose infusion can produce panic attacks.)

Ramussen SA, "Lithium and tryptophan augmentation in clomipramine-resistant obsessive compulsive disorder," *Am J Psychiat,* 141(10): 1283-5; 1984.

Regier DA, Farmer ME, et al, "Comorbidity of mental disorders with alcohol and other drug abuse: Results from the Epidemiological Catchment Area (ECA) study," *JAMA,* 264:2511-18; 1990.

Replogie WH, Eicke FJ, "Megavitamin therapy in the reduction of anxiety and depression among alcoholics," *J Orthomol Med,* 4(4):221-4; 1989. (Niacin-B6-C-E created significant improvement as compared to placebo.)

Robertson D, Freilich JC, et al, "Effects of caffeine on plasma activity, catecholamines, and blood pressure," *NEJM,* 298:181-6; 1978.

Rudin DO, "The major psychoses and neuroses as omega-3 essential fatty acid deficiency syndrome: Substrate pellagra," *Biol Psychiat,* 16:837-50; 1981.

Salzer HM, "Relative hypoglycemia as a cause of neuropsychiatric illness," *J Natl Med Assoc,* 58(1): 12-17; 1966. (85% of hypoglycemics with anxiety responded to a high-protein, low-carbohydrate, caffeine-free diet, frequent meals, and calcium glycerophosphate injections.)

Seelig MS, Berger AR, et al, "Latent tetany and anxiety, marginal Mg deficit and normocalcemia," *Cis Ner Syst,* 36:461-5; 1975. (Mild magnesium deficiency often produces anxiety.)

Silverman K, Evans SM, et al, "Withdrawal syndrome after the double-blind cessation of caffeine consumption," *NEJM,* 327:1109-14; 1992.

Singh T, "Kava: An overview," *J Ethnopharmacol,* 37:13-45; 1992.

Slagle P, "Mood & stress control/ Essential fatty acids," *The Way Up Newletter Archives,* #9 At: thewayup.com/newletters/newsarch.htm

Slagle P, "Anxiety & Taurine," *The Way Up Newletter Archives,* #16 At: thewayup.com/newletters/newsarch.htm

Strakowski SM, Tohen M, Stoll AL, et al, "Comorbidity in mania at first hospitalization," *Am J Psychiatr,* 149:554-56; 1992.

Tohen M, Zarate CA, "Bipolar disorder and comorbid substance abuse disorder," in JF Goldberg, M Harrow, eds, *Bipolar disorders: Clinical course and outcome,* APA Press, DC, 1999; pp 171-84.

Uhde TW, et al, "Caffeine and behavior. Relation to psychopathology and underlying mechanisms. Caffeine: Relationship to human anxiety, plasma MHPG, and cortisol," *Psychopharm Bull,* 20(3): 4216-30; 1984.

Volpi E, et al, "Nicotinamide counteracts alcohol-induced impairment of hepatic protein metabolism in humans," *J Nutr,* 127:2199-204; 1997.

Walsh, WJ, "Commentary on nutritional treatment of mental disorders," *International Guide to the World of Alternative Mental Health.* At: www.alternativementalhealth.com/articles.walshMP.htm#Py Accessed:10/08/2006

Wang S, Mason J, et al, "Relationships between thyroid hormones and symptoms in combat-related post-traumatic stress disorder," *Psychosom Med,* 57(4):398-402; 1995. (fT3, T3, T4 correlated with hyperarousal.)

Werbach MR, *Nutritional Influences on Mental Illness,* Third Line Press, Tarzana, CA, 1991.

Weltzin TE, "Serotonin activity in anorexia and bulimia nervosa: Relationship to the modulation of feeding and mood," *J Clin Psychiat,* 52:12S: 41-8; 1991.

Wendel OW, Beebe WE, "Glycolytic activity in schizophrenia," in D Hawkins, L Pauling, eds, *Orthomolecular Psychiatry: Treatment of Schizophrenia,* WH Freeman, SF, 1973. (Glucose can elevate lactate and decrease pyruvate.)

Weston PG, et al, "Magnesium sulphate as a sedative," *Am J Med Sci,* 165:431-3; 1923.

Williams RD, Mason HL, et al, "Induced thiamine (vitamin B1) deficiency in man; relation of depletion of thiamine to development of biochemical defect and of polyneuropathy," *Arch Intern Med,* 71: 38-53; 1943. (Prolonged B1 restriction associated with fear, agitation, emotional instability. Reversed with intake.)

Yaryurah Tobias JA,Bhagavan HN," L-tryptophan in obsessive-compulsive disorders," *Am J Psychiat,* 134(11):1298-9; 1977. (Tryptophan, B3, B6.)

Yaryurah Tobias JA, *Presentation to the Third Congress of Biological Psychiatry,* Stockholm, reported in *Clinical Psychiat News;* 9/1981.

Zang DX [A double-blind clinical study of L-tryptophan and placebo in treated neurosis], *Chung Hua Shen Ching Ching Shen Ko Tso Chih,* 24(2):77-80; 1991. (3gm/day tryptophan was effective in 91% of 79, creating marked improvement in 58%.)

Behavior & conduct disorders, delinquency, violence

B´en´ezech M, Bourgeois M, *Encephale,* 18 Spec (1):89-90; 1/1992.

home.earthlink.net/~berniew1/violence.html
home.earthlink.net/~berniew1/depress.html
home.earthlink.net/~berniew1/tmlbn.html

Braverman E, "In patients who commit violent crimes, are bitemporal abnormalities a characteristic?" *J Orthomol Med,* 8(3):54-6; 1993.

Buckley RE, "Hypoglycemia, temporal lobe disturbance and aggressive behavior," *J Orthomol Psychiat,* 8(3):188-92; 1979.

Cromwell PF, Arabide BR, et al, "Hair mineral analysis: Biochemical imbalances and violent criminal behavior," *Psycholog Rep,* 64:259-66; 1989.

Goldstein M, "Brain research and violent behavior. A summary and evaluation of the status of biomedical research on brain and aggressive violent behavior," *Arch Neurol,* 30(1):1-35; 1/1974.

Walsh WJ, at: hriptc.org/aggressive_behavior.html

Hibbeln JR, Umhau JC, et al, "Do plasma polyunsaturates predict hostility and depression," *World Rev Nutr Diet,* 82:175-86; 1997. (Low omega 3 strongly associated with depression.)

Mawson AT, "Corn consumption, tryptophan, and cross-national homicide rate," *J Orthomol Psychiat,* 7:227-30; 1978. (Nations with greater corn consumption, and presumably lower tryptophan, showed significantly higher homicide rates.)

Moyer KE, "Allergy and aggression," *Psychology Today,* 7/1975; pp 77-79.

J Orthomol Med, "Nutritional influences on aggressive behavior," 7(1): 45-51, 1992.

Pfeiffer CC, *The Schizophrenias Ours to Conquer,* Bio-Communications Press, Wichita, KS, 1988.

Pihl RO, Ervin F, "Lead and cadmium levels in violent criminals," *Psychol Rep,* 66(3):839-44; 1990. (Greater in violent vs nonviolent male criminals.)

Raleigh MJ, "Differential behavioral effects of tryptophan and 5-hydroxytryptophan on vervet monkeys: Influence of catecholamine systems," *Psychopharmacology* (Berlin), 93(1):44-50; 1987. (5HTP, in some cases, may increase aggression, perhaps due to its influence on catecholamines.)

Rapp D, *Is This Your child?* William Morrow, NY, 1991.

Reed B, *Food, Teens & Behavior,* Natural Press, Manitowoc, WI, 1983.

Schauss AG, Simonsen CE, "A critical analysis of the diets of chronic juvenile offenders," *J Orthomol Psychiat,* 8(3):149-57, 8(4):222-6; 1979. (Significant correlation with milk intake.)

Schauss AG, *Diet, Crime and Delinquency,* Parker

House, Berkeley, CA, rev ed, 1981a.
Schauss AG, "Comparative hair mineral analysis in a randomly selected "normal" population and violent criminal offenders," *Int J Biosocial Res,* 1: 21-41; 1981b.
Schauss, A.G, "Nutrition and antisocial behavior," *Int Clin Nutr Rev,* 4(4):172-77; 1984. (Decreased milk associated with reduced antisocial behavior in inmates at several Michigan detention centers.)
Schmidt K, et al, "Clinical ecology treatment approach for juvenile offenders," *J Behav Ecology Biosocial,* 2(1); 1981. (Elevated hair aluminum in 22 delinquents.)
Schoenthaler SJ, "The Los Angeles probation department diet-behavior program: An empirical evaluation of six institutional settings," *Int J Biosocial Res,* 5(2):88-98; 1983. (Decreased dietary refined sugar was correlated with significantly less violence among male criminals and delinquents.)
Volavka, J, et al, "Tryptophan treatment of aggressive psychiatric inpatients," *Biol Psychiat,* 28(8):728-32; 1990. (Double blind. Tryptophan reduced the need for sedatives to control violent behavior.)
Walsh W, *Science News,* 124:122-5; 1983. (In the violent member of each of 24 sibling pairs, aged 8-18, and in 96 violent males vs controls, violence was generally associated with high Cd, Ca, Fe, Pb, and low Co, Li, Zn; episodic violence, with high Cu, K, Na; antisocial personality with low Cu, high K.)
Walsh W, "Biochemical treatment: Medicines for the next century," *NOHA NEWS,* 15(3); 1991.
Walsh W, Isaacson HR, et al, "Elevated blood copper/zinc ratios in assaultive young males," *Neuroscience Annual Meeting, Abstract of papers,* Miami Beach, 1994.
Walsh W, "Zinc deficiency, metal metabolism, and behavior disorders," *A Report of the Health Research Institute,* Naperville, IL; 3/1996.
Walsh W, Isaacson HR, et al, "Elevated blood copper/zinc ratios in assaultive young males," *Physiol Behav,* 62(2):327-9; 8/1997. (Mean ratio 1.4 in 135 assaultive males vs. 1.02 in 18 controls.)
Walsh WJ, Glab LB, et al, "Reduced violent behavior following biochemical therapy," *Physiol Behav,* 2004.

Suicide

Beck AT, Brown GK, et al, "Suicide ideation at its worst point: A predictor of eventual suicide in psychiatric outpatients," *Suicide Life Threat Behav,* 29(1):109; 1999.
B´en´ezech M, Bourgeois M," *Encephale,* 18S(1): 89-90; 1/1992. (Forensic studies generally link depression to suicide and homicide; mania to relatively benign penal infractions. 15-28% of killers are depressed.)
Bowden CL, "Comparison of open versus blinded studies in bipolar disorder," in JF Goldberg, M Harrow, eds, *Bipolar disorders: Clinical course and outcome,* Am Psychiatric Press, DC, 1999; pp 149-70.
Branchey L, et al, "Depression, suicide and aggression in alcoholics and their relationship to plasma amino acids," *Psychiat Res,* 12(3):219-26; 1984.
Ellis TE, Newman CF, *Choosing to live: How to defeat suicide through cognitive therapy,* New Harbinger, Oakland; 1996.
Erasmus U, *Fats that Heal, Fats that Kill,* Alive Books, Burnaby, Canada, rev ed, 1995.
Gold MS, *The Good News About Depression,* Villard Books, NY, 1987.
Hoffer A, Osmond H, "Schizophrenia and suicide," *Schizophrenia,* 1(1); 1967.
Hoffer A, et al, "Postscript, Aug 1977 [to Hoffer, 1967]," *J Orthomol Psychiat,* 7(1):57-67; 1978.
Kitahara, "Insufficient ascorbic acid uptake from the diet and the tendency for suicide," *J Orthomol Med,* 2(4); 1987.
Lam DH, Jones SH, et al, *Cognitive therapy for bipolar disorder: A therapist's guide to concepts, methods, and practice,* Wiley, Chichester UK, 1999.
Lester D, PhD, "Fat consumption and suicide," *J Orthomol Med,* 5(1):20-221; 1990.
Marano, HE, "Managing bipolar disorder: A major advancement in treatment helps those who suffer," *Psychology Today,* 6/30/2005.
Miles CP, "Conditions predisposing to suicide: A review," *J Nerv Ment Disease,* 164:231-46; 1977.
Pfeiffer CC, *Nutrition and Mental Illness,* Healing Arts Press, Rochester, VT, 1987.
Simpson SG, Jamison KR, "The risk of suicide in patients with bipolar disorders," *J Clin Psychiatr,* 60(S2):53-56;1999. (15%.)
Tsuange MT, Woolson RF, "Mortality in patients with schizophrenia, mania, depression, and surgical conditions," *Brit J Psychiat,* 1301, 162-6, 1977.
Webb WL, Gehi M, "Electrolyte and fluid imbalance: Neuropsychiatric manifestation," *Psychosomatics,* 22(3):199-203; 1981. (Low potassium was associated with weakness, fatigue, depression, organic brain syndrome, suicides. Excess can also be detrimental.)
Winokur G, Tsuang M, "The Iowa 500: Suicide in mania, depression and schizophrenia," *Am J Psychiat,* 132:650; 1975.

Bipolar delusions & psychosis

Brigham Peter M, MD, "The Psychopharmacology of Bipolar Disorder." At: http://people.ne.mediaone.net/pmbrig/BP_pharm.html Accessed: 6-11-01
Edelman E, *Natural Healing for Schizophrenia,* Borage Books, Eugene, OR, 2001.
Hoffer A, *Common Questions about Schizophrenia and their Answers,* Keats, New Canaan, CN, 1987.
Hoffer A, "Bipolar disorder and antioxidants," *Townsend Letter,* 2008, submitted.
Horrobin DF, Bennett CN, "New gene targets related to schizophrenia and other psychiatric disorders: Enzymes, binding proteins and transport proteins involved in phospholipid and fatty acid metabolism," *Prostaglandins Leukot Essent Fatty Acids,* 60:141-67; 1999.
Kidd, PM, "Bipolar disorder as cell membrane dysfunction. Progress toward integrative management," *Alt Med Rev,* 9(2):107-35; 2004.
Kytle E, *The Voices of Robby Wilde,* Seven Locks Press.
Lesser, Michael, MD, interview with author, 8/2008.
Miller CL, Dulay JR, "The high affinity niacin receptor HM74A is decreased in the anterior cingulate cortex of individuals with schizophrenia," *Brain Res Bull,* 77(1):33-41; 9/2008. (The postmortem anterior cingulate cortex of 12 schizophrenics vs 14 bipolars and 14 normals, showed decreased activation of high affinity niacin receptors. Ketones (produced by a high protein, low carbohydrate diet) might help stimulate such receptors.)
Moller HJ, "Bipolar disorder and schizophrenia: Distinct illnesses or a continuum?" *J Clin Psychiatr,* 64:23-27; 2003.
Pfeiffer CC, *Nutrition and Mental Illness,* Healing Arts Press, Rochester, VT, 1987.
Pfeiffer CC, *The Schizophrenias Ours to Conquer,* Bio-Communications Press, Wichita, KS, 1988.
Rush AJ, "Bipolar disorder: Origin, recognition, and treatment," *J Clin Psychiat,* 64:3, 2003.

Childhood concerns

Baker, Sidney M, MD, "Food allergies and autism spectrum problems in children," *Autism Res Rev Intl,* 10(4):3; 1996.
Blaylock R, *Excitotoxins: The Taste that Kills,* Health Press, Santa Fe, NM, 1995.
Bodnar RJ, et al, "Neonatal monosodium glutamate effect upon analgesic responsivity and immonocytochemical ACTH/beta-lipoptropin," *Neuroendocrinol,* 30:280-84; 1980.
Bowden CL, "Toward an integrated biological model of bipolar disorder," in R Joffe, LT Young, eds, *Bipolar Disorder: Biological models and their Clinical Applications,* Marcel Dekker, NY, 1997.
Bowden CL, Calabrese, et al, "Who enters therapeutic trials? Illness characteristics of patients in clinical drug studies of mania," *Psychopharmacol Bull,* 31:103-9; 1995.
Bowden CL, "Strategies to reduce misdiagnosis of bipolar depression," *Psychiatr Serv, APA,* 52: 51-55; 1/2001.
www.bpkids.org Accessed: 2002b
Brigham PM, "The Psychopharmacology of Bipolar Disorder." At: http://people.ne.mediaone.net/pmbrig/BP_pharm.html Accessed: 6-11-01.
Carlson GA, Kashani JH, *J Affect Disord,* 15(3): 219-26; 11-12/1988a. (Teens with manic symptoms showed greater ADD, conduct, anxiety, psychotic, dysphoric, compulsive, and labile symptoms.)
Chabrinski, Ted, "The other half," *Rising up Crazy,* NY; Summer, 1973.
Child and Adolescent Bipolar Foundation (CABF), "About early-onset bipolar disorder," at: www.bpkids.org Accessed: 2002.
Clarke TW, "The relation of allergy to character problems in children: A survey," *Allergy,* 3-4/1950; pp 175-87.
Cott A, "Treatment of learning disabilities," *J Orthomol Psychiat,* 3(4):343-55, 1974.
Cott A, "Treating schizophrenic children," *Schizophrenia,* 1(1):44-59; 1969.
Duke P, Hochman G, *A Brilliant Madness, Living with Manic-Depressive Illness,* Bantam Books, NY; 1992.
Edwards HE, Dortok D, et al, "Prenatal stress alters seizure thresholds and the development of kindled seizures in infant and adult rats," *Horm Behav,* 42: 437-47; 2002.
Fredericks C, *Psycho-Nutrition,* Grosset & Dunlap, NY, 1976.
Frye MA, Ketter TA, "Defining the standard of care across the bipolar spectrum: Q & A, April 9,2000; SF, Faculty: Mark A Frye MD, Terrence A Ketter MD," Bipolar Disorders Information Center. At: http://www.mhsource.com/bipolar/defzarate.html Accessed: 6/11/2001. ("The means by which episodes are prevented influences the course of the illness.")
Gelenberg AJ, Hopkins HS, "Report on efficacy of treatments for bipolar disorder," *Psychopharmacol Bull,* 29(4):447-56; 1993.
Geller B, Luby J, "Child and adolescent bipolar disorder: A review of the past 10 years," *J Am Acad Child Adolesc Psychiat,* 36:1168-76; 1997.
Geller B, Sun K, et al, "Complex and rapid-cycling in bipolar children and adolescents: A preliminary study," *J Affect Disord,* 34(4):259-68; 1995.
Gold MS, *The Good News About Depression,* Villard Books, NY, 1987.
Goldstein S, "Developmental Medicine and Child Neurology," in *Handbook of Neurodevelopmental and Genetic Disorders in Adults,* Guilford Press, 2005.
Green RG, "Subclinical pellagra: Its diagnosis and treatment," *Schizophrenia,* 2(2 & 3):70-79; 1970.
Gross CG, "Neurogenesis in the adult brain: Death of a dogma," *Nature Rev Neurosci,* 1(2): 67-73; 2000.
Hoffer A, in J Bland, ed, *Medical Applications of Clinical Nutrition,* Keats, New Canaan, CN, 1983.
Ivy, Andrew, MD, quoted in *Alternative Medicine,* Burton Goldberg Group, ed, Future Medicine, Puyallup, WA, 1993.
Kidd PM, "Bipolar disorder as cell membrane dysfunction. Progress toward integrative management," *Alt Med Rev,* 9(2):107-35; 2004. (Neurodegenerative disorders often show impaired mitochondrial citric acid cycle and oxidative phosphorylation enzymes, and low energy and reserves; electron leakage creates free radicals, damaging mitochondria and neurons. Support may include: minerals, B, E, K; antioxidant and energetic cofactors (alpha lipoic acid, CoQ10, NADH, etc.); trophic nutrients (ALCAR, GPC and PS, which support mitochondria, conserve growth factor receptors, and improve cognition); and DHA (which combines with GPC and PS to form membrane phospholipids).)
Klingberg, H, Brankack J, et al, "Long-term effects on behavior after postnatal treatment with monosodium-L-glutamate," *Biomed Biochem Acta,* 46:705-11; 1987.
Kluger J, Song S, "Young and bipolar," *Time,* 160: 38-46, 51; 2002.
Kracke K, "Biochemical bases for behavioral disorders in children," *J Orthomol Psychiat,* 11(4): 289-96; 1982.
Krasnoperova MG, et al, [Use of cholinomimetics

in the treatment of endogenous autism in children], *Zhurnal nevrologii i psikhiatrii,* 6:35; 2004.

Krohn J, et al, *The Whole Way to Allergy Relief & Prevention,* Harley & Marks, Port Roberts, WA, 1991.

Kun, Lee Dae, Pusan Research Center on Child Problems, Korea. Communication with Bernard Rimland, 1989, reported in Rimland 1990. (80% of 39 autistics improved on DMG.)

Larson JM, *Alcoholism — The Biochemical Connection,* Villard Books, NY, 1992.

Larson JM, *Depression Free, Naturally,* Ballantine Wellspring, NY, 2001.

Last U, Mandel B, et al, "In search of psychological markers of bipolar manic-depressive illness. Commonalities in psychological functioning between adult euthymic BMDI patients and offspring of BMDI-affected parents," *Isr J Psychiat Relat Sci,* 26(1-2):775-84; 1989.

Lish J, Dime-Meenan S, et al, *J Affect Disord,* 31: 281-94; 1994.

Marano, HE, "Managing bipolar disorder: A major advancement in treatment helps those who suffer," *Psychology Today,* 6/30/05. (Incidence in the young is rising. Average onset is now 19. Omega 6 may play a role. Hyperactivity meds can trigger the first mania.)

Osher Y, Mandel B, et al, "Rorschach markers in offspring of manic-depressive patients," *J Affect Disord,* 59(3):231-6; 9/2000. (Relatively severe thought disorder, unconventional perceptions, and reduced cognitive mediation of affect.)

Pfeiffer CC, *Nutrition and Mental Illness,* Healing Arts Press, Rochester, VT, 1987.

Pfeiffer CC, *The Schizophrenias Ours to Conquer,* Bio-Communications Press, Wichita, KS, rev ed, 1988.

Philpott WH, "Professional dyslexia about dyslexia," *J Orthomol Psychiat,* 6(1):27-32; 1977.

Post RM, Leverich GS, et al, "Developmental vulnerabilities to the onset and course of bipolar disorder," *Dev Psychopathol,* 13:581-98; 2001.

Rapp D, *Is This Your child?* William Morrow, NY, 1991.

Reninger JE, "The multi-disciplinary treatment of hyperactive learning-disabled children," *J Orthomol Psychiat,* 9(3):171-82; 1980.

Rimland B, "An orthomolecular study of psychotic children," *J Orthomol Psychiat,* 3(4):371-7; 1974.

Rimland B, "Dimethylglycine for autism," Autism Research Institute, Pub 110; 8/1996. (Suggests starting children at half a 125 mg tab DMG, and gradually increasing to 1-4 tabs/day; 2-8 for adults. If hyperactivity increases, folate may help.)

Rimland, B, "Dimethylglycine (DMG), a nontoxic metabolite, and autism," *Autism Res Rev International,* 4(2):3; 1990.

Rush AJ, "Bipolar disorder: Origin, recognition, and treatment," *J Clin Psychiat,* 64:3, 2003a

Rush AJ, "Toward an understanding of bipolar disorder and its origin," *J Clin Psychiat,* 64:4-8; 2003b.

Stoll AL, Severus WE, et al, "Omega 3 fatty acids in bipolar disorder: A preliminary double-blind, placebo-controlled trial," *Arch Gen Psychiat,* 56(5): 407-12; 5/1999. (Over 4 mo, the fish oil group did significantly better, with considerable symptomatic improvement and longer remissions. Literature suggests comparability to lithium or VPA.)

Tohen M, Waternaux CM, Tsuang MT, "Outcome in mania. A 4-year prospective follow-up of 75 patients utilizing survival analysis," *Arch Gen Psychiat,* 47(12):1106-11; 12/1990.

van Os J, Jones P, et al, "Developmental precursors of affective illness in a general population birth cohort," *Arch Gen Psychiat,* 54:625-31; 1997.

von Hildheimer G, *Allergy, Toxins, and the Learning-Disabled Child,* Academic Therapy Pubs, San Rafael, CA, 1974.

Walsh, WJ, "Commentary on nutritional treatment of mental disorders," *International Guide to the World of Alternative Mental Health.* At: www.alternativementalhealth.com/articles.walshMP.htm#Py Accessed:10/08/2006.

Weintraub S, *Minding Your Body,* Complementary Medicine Pub. Co, Portland, OR, 1995.

West SA, Strakowski SM, "Phenomenology and comorbidity of adolescents hospitalized for the treatment of acute mania," *Biol Psychiat,* 1996.

Winokur G, Clayton PJ, et al, *Manic Depressive Illness,* Mosby, St Louis, MO; 1969.

Wozniak J, Cawford MH, et al, "Antecedents and complications of trauma in boys with ADHD: Findings from a longitudinal study," *J Am Acad Child Adolesc Psychiat,* 38:48-55; 1999.

Learning disorders

Birdsall TC, "The biological effects and clinical uses of the pineal hormone melatonin," *Alt Med Rev,* 1(2):94-102; 1996.

Birdsall TC, "5-hydroxytryptophan: A clinical/ effective serotonin precursor," *Alt Med Rev,* 1998.

Brigham PM, "The Psychopharmacology of Bipolar Disorder." At: http://people.ne.mediaone.net/pmbrig/BP_pharm.html Accessed: 6-11-01.

Bruinsman K, Taren DL, "Chocolate: Food or drug?" *J Am Diet Assoc,* 99(10):1249-56; 10/1999. (Contains anandamides, methylxanthines, biogenic amines.)

Burgess JR, Stevens L, et al, "Long chain poly-unsaturated fatty acids in children with attention-deficient hyperactivity disorder," *Am J Clin Nutr,* 71(1):3327-30; 2000

Cott A, "Treatment of learning disabilities," *J Orthomol Psychiat,* 3(4):343-55, 1974.

Crook, William, M.D, *Solving the Puzzle of Your Hard to Raise Child?.*

Dallard I, Cathebras P, [Is cocoa a psychotropic drug? Psychopathologic study of a population of subjects self-identified as chocolate addicts], *Encephale,* 27(1):181-6; 3-4 2001.

Divan H, Kheifets L, et al, "Prenatal and postnatal exposure to cell phone use and behavioral problems in children," *Epidemiology,* 19(4):523-9; 7/2008.

Egger J, Carter CM, et al, "Controlled trial of oligoantigenic treatment in the hyperkinetic syndrome," *Lancet,* 1:540-45; 1985.

Feingold BF, *Why Your Child is Hyperactive,* Random House, NY, 1975.

Frye MA, Ketter TA, "Defining the standard of care across the bipolar spectrum: Q & A, April 9,2000; SF, Faculty: Mark A Frye MD, Terrence A Ketter," Bipolar Disorders Information Center. At: http://www.mhsource.com/bipolar/defzarate.html Accessed: 6/11/2001.

Gaby AM, *Townsend Letter for Doctors & Patients,* 50-54, 126-31, 8-9/2000.

Hardell L, Carlberg M, et al, "Long-term use of cellular phones and brain tumors: Increased risk associated with use for more than or equal to 10 years," *Occupational Environ Med,* 64(9):626-32; 9/2007.

Hours M, Bernard M, et al, "Cell phones and risk of brain and acoustic nerve tumors: The French Interphone Case-Control Study," *Rev Epidemiol Sante Publique,* 55(5):321-32; 10/2007.

Hershey J, *Why Can't My Child Behave?* Pear Tree Press, Alexandria, VA, 1996.

Ketter, Frye, "Defining the standard of care across the bipolar spectrum: Q & A, April 9,2000; SF, Faculty: Mark A Frye MD, Terrence A Ketter MD," Bipolar Disorders Information Center. At: http://www.mhsource.com/bipolar/defzarate.html Accessed: 6/11/2001.

Marlowe M, Moon C, "Low mercury levels and childhood intelligence," *J Orthomol Med,* 1(1): 43-49; 1986.

National Academy of Science, *Toxicity Testing: Strategies to Determine Needs and Priorities,* NAS Press, DC, 1989.

Ott J, *Health and Light,* Simon and Schuster, NY, 1973.

Pfeiffer CC, *Nutrition and Mental Illness,* Healing Arts Press, Rochester, VT, 1987.

Pfeiffer CC, *The Schizophrenias Ours to Conquer,* rev ed, Bio-Communications Press, Wichita, KS, 1988.

Rapp D, *Is This Your child?* William Morrow, NY, 1991.

Sevilla I, Aguirre N, "Study on the effects of super blue green algae on the nutritional status and school performance of first, second and third grade children attending the Monsenor Velez School in Naindaime, Nicaragua," *Universidad Centroamericana, Falcultad de Ciencias Agropecuarias,* 1995.

Thompson GO, et al, "Blood levels and children's behavior: Results from the Edinburgh lead study," *J Child Psychol Psychiat,* 30(4):515-28; 1989.

tsangenterprise.com/news90.htm 2007

Wever RA, "Order and disorder in human circadian rhythmicity: Possible relationship to mental disorder," in DJ Kupfer, TH Monk, JD Barchas, eds, *Biorhythms and Mental Disorders,* Guilford Press, 1988.

Wozniak J, Biederman J, "Diagnostic and therapeutic dilemnia in the management of pediatric-onset bipolar disorder," *J Clin Psychiat,* 62S(14):10-5; 2001.

Wozniak J, Spencer T, et al, "The clinical characteristics of unipolar vs bipolar major depression in AHDH youth," *J Affect Disord,* 82(1S):59-69; 2004. (Bipolars are more prone to severe depression, suicidality, anhedonia, conduct disorder, severe oppositional defiant disorder, agoraphobia, OCD, alcohol abuse, hospitalizations, psych disorders in close relatives.)

Wozniak J, Biederman J, "Childhood mania: Insights into diagnostic and treatment issues," *J Assoc Acad Minor Phys,* 8(4):78-84.1997. (Often associated with ADHD, irritability, mixed states.)

Autism

Autism Research Institute, "Parent ratings of behavioral effects of drugs and nutrients," ARI Pub#34E; 7/1994. (In 2050 autistics, B6 and magnesium were reported helpful in 46%; detrimental, in 5%.)

Baker SM, Pangborn J, *Defeat Autism Now! Clinical Options Manual for Physicians,* 1997.

Baker SM, "Food allergies and autism spectrum problems in children," *Autism Research Review International,* 10(4):3; 1996.

Barthelemy C, Garreau B, "Behavioral and biological effects of oral magnesium, vitamin B6, and combined magnesium-B6 administration in autistic children," *Magnesium Bulletin,* 3:150-53; 1981. (Double blind. Highly significant benefit.)

Belmonte MK, Cook EH, et al "Autism as a disorder of neural information processing: Directions for research and targets for therapy," *Mol Psychiatry,* 9(7):646-63; 2004.

Baranek GT, "Efficacy of sensory and motor interventions for children with autism," *J Autism Developmental Disord,* 32(5); 2002.

Blaylock R, *Excitotoxins: The Taste that Kills,* Health Press, Santa Fe, NM, 1995.

Bodnar RJ, et al, "Neonatal monosodium glutamate effect upon analgesic responsivity and immonocytochemical ACTH/beta-lipoptropin," *Neuroendocrinol,* 30:280-84; 1980.

Cott A, "Treatment of learning disabilities," *J Orthomol Psychiat,* 3(4):343-55, 1974.

Courchesne E, "Brainstem, cerebellar and limbic neuroanatomical abnormalities in autism," *Curr Opin Neurobiol,* 7(2):269-78; 1997.

Duker PC, Seys D, "Long-term use of electrical aversion treatment with self-injurious behavior," *Res Devel Disab,* 17(4):293-301; 1996.

Ellman G, "Pyridoxine effectiveness on autistic patients at Sonoma State Hospital," *Res Conf Autism,* San Diego, CA, 11/1/1981. (Double blind.)

Fudenberg H, "Typical course of an autistic patient," *NeuroImmuno Ther Res,* 2001. At: nitrf.org/autistic.html

Gerlach EK, *Autism Treatment Guide,* Four Leaf Press, Eugene, 1993.

Grandin T, "My experiences as an autistic child and review of selected literature," *J Orthomol Psychiat,* 13(3); 1984.

Harris, et al, *J Autism & Devel Disab,* 21(3):261-290; 1991. (Intensive early intervention highly effective in mild to moderate autism.)

Heeley AG, Roberts GE, "A study of tryptophan metabolism in psychotic children," *Develop Med Child Neurol,* 3:708-718; 1966.

Hoffer A, in J Bland, ed, *Medical Applications of Clinical Nutrition,* Keats, New Canaan, CN, 1983.

Israngkun PP, Newman HA, et al, "Potential biochemical markers for infantile autism," *Neurochem Pathol,* 5(1):51-70; 1986.

Jonas C, Etienne T, et al, "Clinical and biochemical indications of the use of vitamin B6 and magnesium in the treatment of residual autism in the adult," *Therapie*, 39:661-69; 1984. (Double blind. B6 and magnesium were helpful.)

Kane P, "Reversing autism with nutrition," *Altern Med Dig*, 19:36-45.

Kaplin M, Carmody DP, "Postural orientation modifications in autism in response to ambient lenses," *Child Psychiat and Hum Devel*, 27(2):81-91; 1996. (Corrective prism lenses improved head tilt, ball catching, tense facial expressions.)

Klerman GL, Weisman MM, "Increasing rates of depression," *JAMA*, 261:2229-35; 1989.

Klingberg, H, Brankack, J, et al, "Long-term effects on behavior after postnatal treatment with monosodium-L-glutamate," *Biomed Biochem Acta*, 46:705-11; 1987.

Knivsberg AM, et al, *Brain Dysf*, 3:315; 1991.

Kun LD, Pusan Research Center on Child Problems, Korea. Communication with Bernard Rimland, 1989, reported in Rimland, 1990. (80% of 39 autistic children improved on DMG.)

LeLord G, Muh JP, et al, "Effects of pyridoxine and magnesium on autistic symptoms: initial observations," *J Autism Devel Disord*, 111(2):219-30; 1981. (Double blind. Behavioral improvement.)

Lovaas I, et al, *J Consult Clin Psychol*, 65(1):3-9; 1987. (9/19 low-functioning autistics given intensive early intervention were able to be mainstreamed vs. 1/40 with less intensive training.)

McDouble CJ, Naylor ST, et al, "Effects of tryptophan depletion in drug-free adults with autistic disorder," *Arch Gen Psychiat*, 53:993-1000; 1996. (Depletion significantly affected self-mutilation, rocking, pacing, anxiety, general well-being.)

McEachin, Smith, et al, *Am J Mental Retardation*, 4:359-91; 1993.

Megson MN, "Is autism a G-alpha protein defect reversible with natural vitamin A," *Med Hypotheses*, 54(6):979-83; 6/2000.

Olney JW, Price MT, "Excitotoxic amino acids as neuroendocrine probes," in EG McGreer, JW Olney, PL McGreer, eds, *Kainic Acid as a Tool in Neurobiology*, Raven Press, New York; 1978.

Olney JW, "Glutamate, a neurotoxic transmitter," *J Child Neurology*, 4:218-25; 1989.

Pfeiffer CC, *The Schizophrenias Ours to Conquer*, Bio-Communications Press, Wichita, KS, rev ed, 1988.

Reichelt KL, Hole K, et al, "Biologically active peptide-containing fractions in schizophrenia and childhood autism," *Adv Biochem Psychopharmac*, 28:627-43; 1981.

Reichelt KL, Ekrem J, et al, "Gluten, milk proteins and autism: Dietary intervention effects on behavior and peptide secretion," *J Appl Nutr*, 42(1); 1990.

Reichelt KL, Knivsberg AM, et al, "Probable etiology and possible treatment of childhood autism," *Brain Dysf*, 4(66):308-19; 1991.

Rimland B, "An orthomolecular study of psychotic children," *J Orthomol Psychiat*, 3(4):371-7; 1974.

Rimland B, Callaway E, "The effects of high doses of vitamin B6 on autistic children: A double-blind crossover study," *Am J Psychiatr*, 135:472-75; 1978. (Double blind. 11/15 improved.)

Rimland B, "Controversies in the treatment of autistic children: Vitamin and drug therapy," *J Child Neurol*, S68-S72; 1988.

Rimland B, "Dimethylglycine, a nontoxic metabolite, and autism," *Autism Res Rev Intl*, 4(2):3; 1990.

Rimland B, "Form letter regarding high dosage vitamin B6 and magnesium therapy for autism and related disorders," *ARI Pub #39F*, 4/1996. (Averages 8 mg B6 and 3 mg Mg/lb body weight. Support with Ca, B, C, Zn, etc. DMG may support speech.)

Rimland B, "ARI Recommendations on treatments for autistic and other mentally and neurologically handicapped children," ARI Pub #49; 5/1996a. (B6, Mg, DMG, etc, *as relevant;* avoid junk food; treat allergies (dairy, wheat, chocolate, etc), Candida, etc. Early intensive behavior intervention, emphasizing positive reinforcement with only mild adverse stimuli; structured, well-planned teaching; Sensory and Auditory Integration Training.)

Rimland B, "Dimethylglycine for autism," ARI Pub #110; 8/1996b. (Suggests starting at 62.5 mg/day, gradually going to 125-500; double for adults. Increased hyperactivity may indicate need for folate.)

Shattock P, Kennedy A, et al, "Role of neuropeptides in autism and their relationships with classical neurotransmitters," *Brain Dysf*, 3(5-6):328-45; 1990.

Shimicu K, Mizutari A, et al, "Electron microscopic studies on the hypothalamic lesions in the mouse fetus caused by monosodium glutamate," *Teratology*, 8:105; 1973.

Shulman R, "Optometry's role in the treatment of autism," *J Optomet Vision Develop*, V. 25; Winter/1994. (With corrective lenses, 45% showed good progress, 30% fair, 25% slow.)

Walsh WJ, "Disordered metal metabolism in autism spectrum disorder," *DAN! conference*, 2001a.

Walsh WJ, Usman A, et al, "Disordered metal metabolism in a large autism population," Presented at the *APA Annual Meeting*, May, 2001b, New Orleans. At: www.hriptc.org/metal_autism.html

Walsh WJ, "Metal metabolism and human function," At: www.hriptc.org/metal_metabolism.html Accessed: 12/2004a

Walsh WJ, "Zinc deficiency, metal metabolism, and behavior disorders," At: hriptc.org/zinc_deficiency.html Accessed: 12/2004b

Walsh, William J, PhD, interview with author, July 2008.

Williams D, *Nobody, Nowhere*, Avon Books, NY, 1992.

Williams D, *Somebody Somewhere*, Times Books, NY, 1992.

Yao Y, Walsh WJ, "Altered vascular phenotype in autism," *Arch Neurol*, 64:1161-4; 2006. (Platelet and vascular endothelium activation, oxidative stress contribute to onset and symptoms of autism.)

Elderly concerns

Donaldson S, *By force of Will, The Art and Life of Ernest Hemingway*, Viking, 1977, 2001.

Fieve RR, *Moodswing*, Bantam Books, 1976.

Gold MS, *The Good News About Depression*, 1987.

Hemingway GH, *Papa, A personal memoir*, Houghton Mifflin, Boston, 1976.

Hemingway L, *My brother, Ernest Hemingway*, Fawcett, Greenwich, CN, 1961.

Kidd PM, Bipolar disorder as cell membrane dysfunction, Progress toward integrative management," *Alt Med Rev*, 9(2):107-35; 2004.

McLerndon J, *Papa*, Popular Library, NY, 1972.

Shullman KI, "Neurologic comorbidity and mania in old age," *Clin Neurosci*, 4(1):37-40; 1997a.

Shullman KI, "Disinhibition syndromes, secondary mania and bipolar disorder in old age," *J Affect Disord*, 46(3):175-82; 12/1997b.

Yalom I, Yalom M, "Ernest Hemingway: A psychiatric view," *Arch Gen Psychiatr*, 24, 6/1971.

Appendix I: Neural communication

Alpha Diagnostic International, "Vesicular monoamine transporters," At: www.4adi.com/flr/vmat.html Accessed 2000.

Avissar S, Nechamkin Y, et al, "Differential G protein measures in mononuclear leukocytes of patients with bipolar mood disorder are state dependent," *J Affect Disord*, 43(2):85-94; 4/1989. (G proteins activate second messengers, setting switches on the membrane and nucleus. WBC G-proteins are highly elevated in mania, reduced in depression.)

Barton PG, Gunstone FD, "Hydrocarbon chain packing and molecular motion in phospholipid bilayers formed from unsaturated lecithins. Synthesis and properties of sixteen positional isomers of 1, 2-dioctadecenolyl-sn-glycero-3-phosphorylcholine," *J Biol Chem*, 250(12):4470-76; 1975. (Omega 3 alters membrane properties and may make them resistant to hydrolysis by phospholipases, thereby producing less DAG, IP3, and thus less PKC and Ca release.)

Brown AS, Mallinger AG, et al, "Elevated platelet membrane phosphatidyl inositol-4,5-bisphosphate in bipolar mania," *Am J Psychiat*, 150:1252-4; 1993.

Changeaux, JP, *Neuronal Man*, Pantheon, 1985.

Chen G, Manji HK, et al, "Chronic sodium valproate selectively decreases protein kinase C alpha and epsilon in vitro," *J Neurochem*, 63:2361-4; 1994.

Dubovsky SL, Christiano J, et al, "Increased platelet-intracellular calcium concentration in patients with bipolar affective disorders," *Arch Gen Psychiat*, 46: 632-8; 1989.

Dubovsky SL, Murphy J, et al, "The calcium second messenger system in bipolar disorders: Data supporting new research directions," *J Neuropsychiat Clin Neurosci*, 4:3-14; 1992.

Fields A, Li PP, et al, "Increased cyclic AMP-dependent protein kinase activity in postmortem brain from patients with bipolar affective disorder," *J Neurochem*, 73:1704-10; 1999.

Friedman E, Wang HY, "Receptor-mediated activation of G proteins is increased in postmortem brains of bipolar affective disorder subjects," *J Neurochem*, 67(3):1145-52; 9/1996. (G protein / receptor binding and trimeric status were enhanced in bipolars, perhaps underlying excessive signaling and affective changes.)

Friedman E, Hoau-Yan Want, et al, "Altered platelet protein kinase C activitiy in bipolar affective disorder, manic episode," *Biol Psychiat*, 33:520-5; 1993.

www.genome.jp/kegg/pathway/map/map00380.html

Horrobin DF, Bennett CN, "Depression and bipolar disorder: Relationships to impaired fatty acid and phospholipid metabolism and to diabetes, cardiovascular disease, immunological abnormalities, cancer, aging and osteoporosis. Possible candidate genes," *Prostaglandins, Leukot, Essent Fatty Acids*, 60:217-34; 1990.

Knable MB, "Schizophrenia and bipolar disorder: Findings from studies of the Stanley Foundation Brain Collection," *Schizophr Res*, 39(2):149-52, 163; 9/29/1999. (Frontal cortical interneuron abnormalities, in different neural populations in schizophrenic vs bipolar brains. In familial bipolar and major depression, altered cingulate glial density.)

Lenox RH, Hahn CG, "Overview of the mechanisms of action of lithium in the brain: Fifty year update," *J Clin Psychiat*, 61S(9):5-15; 2000. (Lithium's effects on GSK-3 beta and PKC may help regulate membrane phosphorylation, stabilizing mood. Modification of transcription factors may stabilize expression of genes overseeing signaling.)

Manji HK, Bebchuk JM, et al, "Modulation of CNS signal transduction pathways and gene expression by mood-stabilizing agents: Therapeutic implications," *J Clin Psychiat*, 60S(2):27-39, 40-41, 113-6; 1999a. (PKC regulates neurotransmitter release and neuron excitability. Tamoxifen, like lithium and valproate, inhibits PKC and moderates mania. Downstream such meds may alter AP-1 transcription factors (perhaps via kinases and GSK-3 beta).

Manji HK, McNamara R, et al, "Signalling pathways in the brain: Cellular transduction of mood stabilization in the treatment of manic-depressive illness," *Aust NZJ Psychiat*, 33S:65-83; 12/1999b. (Treatment appears to regulate signaling and gene expression, influencing amplification and integration of signalling cascades. Studies especially pinpoint lithium's supression of PKC alpha and epsilon, and their major substrate, MARCKS. Research also finds effects on GSK-3 beta and on neuroprotective/neurotrophic proteins.)

Manji HK, Lenox RH, "Protein kinase C signaling in the brain: molecular transduction of mood stabilization in the treatment of manic-depressive illness," *Biol Psychiat*, 46(10):1328-51; 11/15/1999c. (Research suggests lithium and valproate target PKC alpha and epsilon, and MARCKS. Possibly, GSK-3 beta and the AP-1 transcription factors.)

Medini L, Colli S, "Diets rich in n-9, n-6 and n-3 fatty acids differentially affect the generation of inositol phosphates and of thromboxane by stimulated platelets in the rabbit," *Biochem Pharmacol*, 39(1): 129-33; 1990.

Modica-Napolitano JS, Renshaw PF, "Ethanolamine and phosphoethanolamine inhibit mitochondrial function in vivo: Implications for mitochondrial dysfunction hypothesis in depression and bipolar disorder," *Biol Psychiat*, 55:273-77; 2004.

Moyer D, *Too good to be true? Nutrients Quiet the Unquiet Mind*, Nu-Tone Press, Penn Valley,

CA, 2003.
Perez J, Tardito D, et al, "Abnormalities of cyclic adenosine monophosphate signaling in platelets from untreated patients with bipolar disorder," *Arch Gen Psychiat,* 56(3):248-53; 3/1999. (Platelets of 112 drug free bipolars. cAMP-dependent PKA was elevated in 29 depressed and 31 manic bipolars as compared to euthymics and controls. Rap1, a PKA substrate, was high in all bipolars.)
Perez J, Tardito D, et al, "Altered Rap1 endogenous phosphorylation and levels of Rap1 in platelets from patients with bipolar disorder," *J Psychiatr Res,* 34(2): 99-104; 3-4/2000. (Increased cAMP-dependent phosphorylation, perhaps due to elevated Rap 1, may contribute to symptoms.)
Reiach JS, Li PP, et al, "Reduced adenyl cyclase immunolabeling and activity in postmortem temporal cortex of depressed suicide victims", *J Affect Disord,* 56(2-3):141-51; 12/1999. (Perhaps contributing to cAMP signaling cascade disturbances.)
Schreiber G, Avissar S, "Lithium sensitive hyperfunction: A dynamic model for the pathogenesis of bipolar affective disorder," *Med Hypotheses,* 35(3):237-43; 7/91a. (Lithium may inhibit G protein function, thereby affecting phophatidylinositol and cAMP, which influence PKA and PKC, and, in turn, phosphorylation, perhaps thereby destabilizing mood.)
Schreiber G, Avissar S, et al, "Hyperfunctional G proteins in mononuclear leukocytes of patients with mania," *Biol Psychiat,* 29(3):273-80; 1991b. (G proteins were hyperactive in untreated manics, vs. lithium-treated euthymics and normals.)
Schreiber G, Avissar S, "G proteins as biochemical tools for diagnosis and monitoring treatments of mental disorders," *Isr Med Assoc J,* 2 S:86-91; 7/2000. (Distinctive patterns of function and immunoreactivity in depression and mania in G alpha-s, -alpha-i, -beta subunit proteins coupled to beta adrenergic, muscarinic or DA receptors are normalized with affective treatment.)
Soares JC, Mallinger AG, Abnormal phosphatidyl-inositol (PI) signalling in bipolar disorder," *Biol Psychiat,* 39:461-4; 1996.
Soares JC, Mallinger AG, et al, "Effects of lithium on platelet membrane phosphoinositides in bipolar disorder patients: A pilot study," *Psychopharmacol (BERL),* 149:12-6; 2000.
Soares JC, Dippold CS, et al, "Increased platelet membrane phosphatidylinositol-4,5-bisphosphate in drug-free depressed bipolar patients," *Neurosci Lett,* 299:150-2; 2001.
Sperling RI, Benincaso AI, et al, "Dietary omega-3 polyunsaturated fatty acids inhibit phosphoinositide formation chemotaxis in neutrophils," *J Clin Invest,* 91(2):651-60; 1999.
Spleiss O, van Calker D, et al, "Abnormal G protein alpha(s) - and alpha(i2)-subunit mRNA expression in bipolar affective disorder," *Mol Psychiat,* 3(6):512-20; 11/98. (Major disturbances in cAMP signalling. G proteins are usually at the beginning of signalling pathways. Messenger RNA of G protein alpha(s) was markedly elevated in bipolars, treated with lithium or not. Messenger RNA of G alpha(i2) was increased in lithium-treated (but not untreated) bipolars and not particularly responsive to cAMP.)
Stoll AL, Severus WE, "Mood stabilizers: Shared mechanisms of action at postsynaptic signal-transduction and kindling processes," *Harv Rev Psychiat,* 4(2):77-89; 1996. (Literature review.)
Stoll AL, Marangell LB, "In reply," *Arch Gen Psychiat,* 56(5):415-6; 1999a.
Stoll AL, Locke CA, et al, "Omega-3 fatty acids and bipolar disorder: A review," *Prostaglandins Leukot Essent Fatty Acids,* 60:329-37; 1999b.
Vawter MP, Freed WJ, et al, "Neuropathology of bipolar disorder," *Biol Psychiat,* 48:486-504; 2000.
Wang HY, Friedman E, "Lithium inhibition of protein kinase C activation-induced serotonin release," *Psychopharmacology (Berl),* 99:213-8; 1989.
Wang HY, Friedman E, "Enhanced protein kinase C activity and translocation in bipolar affective disorder brains," *Biol Psychiat,* 40:568-75; 1996.
Wang HY, Markowitz P, et al, "Increased membrane-associated protein kinase C activity and translocation in blood platelets from bipolar affective disorder patients," *J Psychiatr Res,* 33(2):171-79; 3-4/1999. (PKC signal transduction was increased among 44 manics, vs 25 depressives and 43 schizophrenics.)
Young LT, Li PP, et al, "Postmortem cerebral cortex Gs alpha-subunit levels are elevated in bipolar affective disorder, *Brain Res,* 553(2):323-6; 7/12/1991. (Gs alpha immunoreactivity was significantly increased in the occipital (80%) & frontal cortex; nonsignificantly in the cerebellum of 7 postportem bipolars vs controls, perhaps due to increased responsiveness & disturbed signal transduction.)
Young LT, Bezchlibnyk et al, "Amygdala cyclic adenosine monophosphate response element binding protein phosphorylation in patients with mood disorders: Effects of diagnosis, suicide, and drug treatment," *Biol Psychiat,* 55(6):570-7; 3/2004.
Zubieta Joh-Kar, "Excessive monoaminergic synaptic terminals associated with bipolar disorder," *Am J Psychiat,* 157:1619-28; 2000.

Appendix II: Brain structures

Adler CM, Holland SK, et al, "Abnormal white matter tracts in bipolar disorder: A diffusion tensor imaging study," *Bipolar Disord,* 6(3):197-203; 6/2004.
Adler CM, Levine AD, Strakowski SM, "Changes in gray matter volume in patients with bipolar disorder," *Biol Psychiat,* 58(2):151-7; 2005.
Adolphs R, Tranel D, et al, "Impaired recognition of emotion in facial expressions following bilateral damage to the human amygdala," *Nature,* 371: 669-72; 1994.
Aggleton JP, Passingham RE, "Syndrome produced by lesions of the amygdala in monkeys," *J Compar Physiol Psychol,* 95:961-977; 1981.
Altshuler LL, Bartzokis G, et al, "An MRI study of temporal lobe structures in men with bipolar disorder or schizophrenia," *Biol Psychiat,* 48(2): 147-62; 7/14/2000.
American Academy of Family Physicians. At: http://www.aafp.org/afp/990501ap/quantum.html (Ice water treatment.) At: alternativementalhealth.com/articles/ice.htm Accessed: 9/6/2005.
Amsterdam JD, Mozley DP, "Temporal lobe asymmetry with Iofetamine (IMP) SPECT imaging in patients with major depression," *J Affect Disorders,* 24:43-53; 1991.
Anand A, Shekhar A, "Brain imaging studies in mood and anxiety disorders: Special emphasis on the amygdala," *Ann NY Acad Sci,* 985:370-88; 4/2003.
Baxter LR, Phelps ME, et al, "Cerebral metabolic rates for glucose in mood disorders: Studies with positron emission tomography and gluorodeoxyglucose F 18," *Arch Gen Psychiatr,* 42:441-47; 1985.
Bearden CE, Hoffman KM, et al, "The neuro-psychology and neuro-anatomy of bipolar affective disorder, A critical review," *Bipolar Disord,* 3:106-50; 2001.
Benes FM, Vincent SL, et al, "The density of pyramidal and nonpyramidal neurons in anterior cingulate cortex of schizophrenic and bipolar subjects," *Biol Psychiat,* 50(6):395-406; 9/15/2001. (Stimulation, e.g., by mesocortical DA projections altered by stress, or the amygdala, may damage the GABA system or otherwise disturb cell migration in early development.)
Blumberg HP, Charney DS, et al, "Frontotemporal neural systems in bipolar disorder," *Semin Clin Neuropsychiat,* 7(4):243-54; 10/2002. (Ventral and medial prefrontal, and amygdala changes.)
Blumberg HP, Martin A, et al, "Frontostriatal abnormalities in adolescents with bipolar disorder: Preliminary observations from functional MRI," *Am J Psychiat,* 160(7):1345-7; 7/2003.
Blumberg HP, Kaufman J, et al, "Significance of adolescent neurodevelopment for the neural circuitry of bipolar disorder," *Ann NY Acad Sci,* 10213:76-83; 6/2004.
Botteron KN, Figiel GS, et al., "MRI abnormalities in adolescent bipolar affective disorder," *J Am Acad Child Adolesc Psychiat,* 31(2):258-61; 3/1992. (Recent MRIs find focal signal hyperintensities in the deep white matter in some bipolars. Case report of such findings in an adolescent in her first mania.)
Brambilla P, Harenski K, et al, "MRI investigation of temporal lobe structures in bipolar patients," *J Psychiatr Res,* 37(4):287-95; 7-8/2003. (May be enlarged in adult bipolars.)
Bruder GE, Stewart JW, et al, "Abnormal cerebral laterality in bipolar depression: Convergence of behavioral and brain event-related potential findings," *Biol Psychiat,* 32(1):33-47; 7/1/92. (Bipolars (vs. unipolars and normals) performed less well on visuospatial tasks for the left visual field, and on brain event-related potentials in audiospatial and temporal discrimination tasks, suggesting right dysfunction of the arousal/attention system of the temporoparietal and perhaps frontal brain.)
Bruno SD, Barker GJ, "A study of bipolar disorder using magnetization transfer imaging and voxel-based morpholometry," *Brain,* 127:2433-40; 11/2004.
Buchsbaum MS, Wu J, et al, "Frontal cortex and basal ganglia metabolic rates assessed by positron emission tomography with [^{18}F]2-deoxyglucose in affective illness," *J Affect Dis,* 10:137-52; 1986.
Chang K, Adleman NE, et al, "Anomalous prefrontal-subcortical activation in familial pediatric bipolar disorder: A functional magnetic resonance imaging investigation," *Arch Gen Psychiat,* 61(8):781-92; 8/2004. (Especially anterior cingulate cortex, left dorsolateral prefrontal cortex, left putamen, left thalamus, and right inferior frontal gyrus.)
Chang K, Adleman N, et al, "Decreased N-acetylaspartate in children with familial bipolar disorder," *Biol Psychiat,* 53(11):1059-65; 6/2003.
Chang K, "The neuroscience of early-onset bipolar disorder." At: http://www.invisiblechild.org/2005_handouts/ChangHandout.htm
Clark L, Iversen SD, et al, "A neuropsychological investigation of prefrontal cortex involvement in acute mania," *Am J Psychiat,* 158(10):1605-11; 10/2001. (Enhances verbal memory, focus, performance.)
Coffman JA, Bornstein RA, et al., "Cognitive impairment and cerebral structure by MRI in bipolar disorder," *Biol Psychiat,* 27(11):1188-96; 6/1990.
Curtis VA, Dixon TA, et al, "Differential frontal activation in schizophrenia and bipolar illness during verbal fluency," *J Affect Disord,* 66(2-3): 111-21; 10/2001.
Dasari M, Friedman L, et al, "A magnetic resonance imaging study of thalamic area in adolescent patients with either schizophrenia or bipolar disorder as compared to healthy controls," *Psychiat Res,* 91(3): 155-62; 10/11/1999.
Davidson RJ, Abercrombie H, et al, "Regional brain function, emotion, and disorders of emotion," *Curr Opin Neurobiol,* 9(2):228-34; 4/1999. (Neuroimaging indicates prefrontal and parietal cortex, anterior cingulate, and amygdala dysfunction may be critical in depression and anxiety.)
DelBello MP, Zimmerman ME, et al, "Magnetic resonance imaging analysis of amygdala and other subcortical brain regions in adolescents with bipolar disorder," *Bipolar Disord,* 6(1):43-52; 2/2004.
Drevets WJ, *Neuroscience,* 12:3628-3641; 1992. (In recurrent depressives, PFC circulation was increased, especially in the left hemisphere (which stores emotional meaning and codes feelings from the amygdala and hippocampus), and the cingulate gyrus (which contains the amygdala and part of the thalamus), perhaps fostering rumination. Blood flow was decreased in the posterior brain, where vision is located, perhaps contributing to withdrawal.)
Drevets WC, Price JL, et al, "Subgenual prefrontal cortex abnormalities in mood disorders," *Nature,* 386:824-7; 1997.
Drevets WC, Ongur D, et al, "Neuroimaging abnormalities in the subgenual prefrontal cortex: implications for the pathophysiology of familial mood disorders," *Mol Psychiat,* 3(3):220-6 190-1; 5/1998.
Drevets WC, *Ann Rev Med,* 49:331-61; 1998. (In recovered depressives, left amygdala circulation is abnormal. Perhaps also with distrubed sleep or Ser.)
Drevets WC, "Prefrontal cortical-amygdalar metabolism in major depression," *Ann NY Acad Sci,* 877:614-37; 6/29/1999. (Resting blood flow and glucose metabolism is abnormal in the amygdala and associated PFC regions. Depressive severity and plasma cortisol correlate with amygdala metabolism. Hypermetabolism during remission increases risk of

relapse. Perhaps to counter this hypermetabolism and emotional response, orbital PFC metabolism decreases. This may eventually lower grey matter volume and glia in both regions (MRIs shows reductions in the posterior orbital and anterior cingulate cortex (which contains the amygdala).)

Drevets WC, Price JL, et al, "Glucose metabolism in the amygdala in depression: Relationship to diagnostic subtype and plasma cortisol levels," *Pharmacol Biochem Behav,* 71(3):431-47; 3/2002.

Dupont RM, Jerniga TL, et al, "Subcortical abnormalities detected in bipolar affective disorder using magnetic resonance imaging. Clinical and neuropsychological significance," *Arch Gen Psychiat,* 47(1):55-59; 1/1990. (MRI revealed subcortical signal hyperintensities in 9/19 bipolars. These 9 tended toward decreased fluency and recall, and more hospitalizations.)

Fossati P, Harvey PO, et al, "Verbal memory performance of patients with a first depressive episode and patients with unipolar and bipolar recurrent depression," *J Psychiatr Res,* 38(2):137-44; 3-4/2004. (Prefrontal verbal memory deteriorates with acute depression.)

Frey BN, Folgierini M, et al, "A proton magnetic resonance spectroscopy investigation of the dorsolateral prefrontal cortex in acute mania," *Hum Psychopharmacol,* 20(2):133-39; 1/12/2005.

Frey BN, Fonseca MM, et al, [Neuropathological and neurochemical abnormalities in bipolar disorder], *Rev Bras Psiquiatr,* 26(3):180-8; 9/2004.

George MS, Ketter TA, et al, "Brain activity during transient sadness and happiness in healthy women," *Am J Psychiat,* 152:341-51; 1993.

Goodwin, Jamison, *Manic Depressive Illness,* Oxford University Press, 1990.

Gross CG, "Neurogenesis in the adult brain: Death of a dogma," *Nature Rev Neurosci,* 1(2):67-73; 2000. (Adults can grow new neurons (hippocampus)).

Gur, *Science,* 267:528-331; 1995.

Gur, *Psychiat Res,* 52:215-36; 1994.

Gyulai L, Alavi A, et al, "Iofetamine (IMP) single photon computed emission tomography in rapid cycling bipolar disorder — A clinical study," *Biol Psychiat,* 2001.

Haldane M, Frangou S, "New insights help define the pathophysiology of bipolar affective disorder: Neuroimaging and neuropathology findings," *Prog Neuropsychopharmacol Biol Psychiat,* 28(6):943-60; 9/2004.

Hamner MB, Lorberbaum JP, et al, "Potential role of the anterior cingulate cortex in PTSD: Review and hypothesis," *Depress Anxiety,* 9(1):1-14; 1999. (NE is chronically activated. NE projections from the locus coeruleus may decrease anterior cingulate gating, exaggerating response.)

Harrison PJ, "The neuropathology of primary mood disorder," *Brain,* 125:1428-49; 2002. (MRIs showed reduced volume.)

Hirayasu Y, Shenton ME, et al, "Subgenual cingulate cortex volume in first-episode psychosis," *Am J Psychiat,* 156(7):1091-93; 7/1999. (Previous work finds reduced gray matter volume and glucose use in the left subgenual cingulate of familial bipolar and unipolar depressed. This study of 41 first episode patients finds the left subgenual cingulate smaller in familial affective disorder, than in nonfamilial, schizophrenics, and controls.)

Hirsh S, study, cited in Horrobin 2000.

Horrobin DF, "The role of essential fatty acids in schizophrenia," *ISOM, Nutritional Medicine Today Conf,* Vancouver, BC, 4/2000.

Hurd YL, "Subjects with major depression or bipolar disorder show reduction of prodynorphin mRNA expression in discrete nuclei of the amygdaloid complex," *Mol Psychiat,* 7(1):75-81; 2002.

Jested DV, Lohr JB, Goodwin, FK, "Neuroanatomical studies of major affective disorders. A review and suggestions for further research," *Br J Psychiat,* 53: 444-459; 1988. (Post injury depression is generally associated with injury to the left (language) hemisphere, especially temporal and frontal-limbic regions. Indifferent euphoria, similar to mania, is less common, but tends to follow injury to the right, (spacial) hemisphere or basal ganglia.)

Jurjus GJ, Nasrallah HA, et al, "Developmental brain anomalies in schizophrenia and bipolar disorder: A controlled MRI study," *J Neuropsychiatr Clin Neurosci,* 5:375-78; 1993a.

Jurjus GJ, Nasrallah HA, et al, "Cavum septum pellucidum in schizophrenia, affective disorders, and healthy controls: A magnetic resonance imaging study," *Psychological Med,* 23:319-22; 1993b.

Kennedy SH, Javanmard M, et al, "A review of functional neuroimaging in mood disorders: positron emission tomography and depression," *Can J Psychiat,* 42(5):467-75; 6/1997. (With manipulation of affect, cognition, activity, meds, etc., PET suggests PFC and limbic abnormalities, including anterior cingulate, and amygdala changes).

Ketter TA, Kimbrell TA, et al, "Effects of mood and subtype on cerebral glucose metabolism in treatment-resistant bipolar disorder," *Biol Psychiat,* 49(2):97-109; 1/15/2001.

Ketter RA, Drevets WC, "Neuroimaging studies of bipolar depression: Functional neuropathology, treatment effects, and pedictors of clinical response," *Clin Neurosci Res,* 2:182-92; 2002.

Ketter, Frye, "Defining the standard of care across the bipolar spectrum: Q & A, April 9, 2000, SF, Faculty: Mark A Frye MD, Terrence A Ketter MD," Bipolar Disorders Information Center. At: http://www.mhsource.com/bipolar/defzarate.html Accessed: 6/11/2001.

Kidd PM, "Bipolar disorder as cell membrane dysfunction, Progress toward integrative management," *Alt Med Rev,* 9(2):107-35; 2004.

Lawrence NS, Williams AM, et al, "Subcortical and ventral prefrontal cortical neural responses to facial expressions distinguish patients with bipolar disorder and major depression," *Biol Psychiat,* 55(6):578-87; 1/15/2004. (Ventral PFC response to emotional expressions is enhanced in bipolars.)

Ladue J, in JP Aggleton, ed, *The Amygdala: Neurobiological Aspects of Emotion, Memory and Mental Dysfunction,* William Wiley-Liss, NY, 1992; pp 339-51.

Lauterbach EC, "Bipolar disorders, dystonia, and compulsion after dysfunction of the cerebellum, dentatorubrothalamic tract, and substantia nigra," *Biol Psychiat,* 40(8):726-30; 10/15/1996. (3/15 subjects developed bipolar disorder following focal cerebellar lesions, 2 with rapid cycling and dystonia. Authors suggest nigra pars reticulata dysfunction, and reduced cerebellar output to limbic, thalamic, basal ganglia, etc, may create the neural oscillation found in rapid-cyclers and dystonia.)

Lopez-Larson MP, DelBello MP, et al, "Regional prefrontal gray and white matter abnormalities in bipolar disorder," *Biol Psychiat,* 52(2):93-100; 7/2002.

Malhi GS, Lagopoulos J, et al, "Cognitive generation of affect in hypomania, an fMRI study," *Bipolar Disord,* 6(4):271-85; 8/2004a.

Malhi GS, Ivanovski B, et al, "Bipolar Disorder: It's all in your mind? The neuropsychological profile of a biological disorder," *Can J Psychiat,* 49(12): 813-819; 12/2004b.

Manji HK, Lenox RH, "Signalling: Cellular insights into the pathophysiology of bipolar disorder," *Biol Psychiat,* 48(6):518-30; 9/15/2000. (Anterior cingulate, amygdala, PFC, laterality.)

Matsuo K, Watanabe A, et al, "Prefrontal hemodynamic response to verbal-fluency task and hyperventilation in bipolar disorder measured by multi-channel near-infared spectroscopy," *J Affect Disord,* 82(1):85-92; 10/2004. (Vascular hypofrontality.)

Mayberg HS, Brannan SK, et al, "Cingulate function in depression: A potential predictor of treatment response," *Neuroreport,* 8(4):1057-61; 3/1997a.

Mayberg HS, "Limbic-cortical dysregulation: A proposed model of depression," *J Neuropsychiat Clin Neurosci,* 9:471-81; 1997b.

Mayberg HS, Liotti M, et al, "Reciprocal limbic-cortical function and negative mood: Converging PET findings in depression and normal sadness," *Am J Psychiat,* 156(5):675-82; 5/1999. (Mood inverse to attention. Sadness increased limbic-paralimbic (subgenual cingulate, anterior insula) blood flow; decreased neocortex (right dorsolateral, prefrontal, inferior parietal) flow; reversed on recovery.)

McDonald C, Zanelli J, et al, "Meta-analysis of magnetic resonance imaging brain morphometry studies in bipolar disorder," *Biol Psychiat,* 56(6): 411-17; 9/15/2004. (Left subgenual PFC, amygdala, thalamus, anterior limbic, other cortical regions, visual areas, right lateral and 3rd ventricle, etc.)

Michael N, Erfurth A, et al, "Acute mania is accompanied by elevated glutamate/glutamine levels with the left dorsolateral prefrontal cortex," *Psychopharmacology,* (Berl), 4/9/2003 [Epub ahead of print].

Migliorelli R, Starkstein SE, et al, "SPECT findings in patients with primary mania," *J Neuropsychiat Clin Neurosci,* 5:359-83; 1993. (Patients who developed mania post-stroke or brain injury tended to reduced circulation in right limbic/PFC/temporal/thalamic structures.)

Monkul ES, Yildiz A, Soares J [Magnetic resonance spectroscopy (MRS) applications in bipolar disorder], *Turk Psikiyatri Derg,* 15(2):138-47; 2004.

Morice R, "Cognitive inflexibility and prefrontal dysfunction in schizophrenia and mania," *Br J Psychiat,* 157:50-4; 7/1990. (Schizophrenics and manics performed poorly on the Wisconsin Card Sorting Test, suggesting cognitive inflexibility and/or PFC dysfunction.)

Nasrallah H, Coffman J, et al, "Structural brain imaging findings in affective disorders: An overview," *J Neuropsychiat Clin Neurosci,* 1:21-26; 1989.

Ongur D, Drevets WC, et al, "Glial reduction in the subgenual prefrontal cortex in mood disorders," *PNAS,* 95:13290-95; 1998. (PFC glia loss may alter stress-related autonomic and endocrine response, and limbic DA reward-related function.)

Pang A, Lewis SW, "Bipolar affective disorder minus left prefrontal cortex equals schizophrenia," *Br J Psychiat,* 168(5):647-50; 5/1996.

Pardo JV, Pardo PJ, et al, "Neural correlates of self-induced dysphoria," *Am J Psychiat,* 150:713-719; 1993.

Post R, DeLisi L, et al, "Glucose utilization in the temporal cortex of affectively ill patients: Positron emission tomography," *Biol Psychiatr,* 22:545-553; 1987.

Price JL, "Prefrontal cortical networks related to visceral function and mood," *Ann NY Acad Sci,* 877: 383-96; 6/29/1999. (Functional imaging indicates abnormal medial and orbital PFC activity in bipolar and major depression. Volume may be reduced, as may glia density. Ventromedial PFC lesions have been associated with sociopathic behavior.)

Rajkowska G, "Postmortem studies in mood disorders indicate altered numbers of neurons and glial cells," *Biol Psychiat,* 48(8):766-77; 10/15/2000. (Stress tends to compromise function of the hippocampus (which stores emotion-laden memory).)

Rajkowska G, Halaris A, et al, "Reductions in neuronal and glial density characterize the dorsolateral prefrontal cortex in bipolar disorder," *Biol Psychiat,* 49(9):741-52; 5/1/2001.

Robinson RG, Boston JD, et al, "Comparison of mania and depression after brain injury: Causal factors," *Am J Psychiat,* 145(2):172-78; 2/1988. (In patients who developed secondary mania, injury tended to concentrate in right limbic-connected regions, and family history showed significantly more affective disorder. Injury in poststroke depressives focused on left PFC and basal ganglia.)

Rossi A , Stratta P, et al., "Temporal lobe structure by magnetic resonance in bipolar affective disorders and schizophrenia," *J Affect Disord,* 21(1):19-22; 1/91. (In both, when lateral differences occurred, the left temporal lobe was smaller.)

Rubinstein M, Cepeda C, et al, "Dopamine D4 receptor-deficient mice display cortical hyperexcitability," *J Neurosci,* 21(11):3756-3763; 6/2001.

Rosoklija G, Toomayan G, et al, "Structural abnormalities of subicular dendrites in subjects with schizophrenia and mood disorders: Preliminary findings," *Arch Gen Psychiat,* 57:349-

56; 2000. (Perhaps minor synaptic and dendritic abnormalities.)

Rubinstein JS, Fletcher PC, et al, "Decision-making in mania: a PET study," *Brain,* 124(12):2550-63; 12/2001.

Scherk H, Reith W, et al, [Changes in brain structure in bipolar affective disorders], *Nervenarzt,* 75(9): 861-72; 9/2004.

Shastry BS, "Bipolar disorder: an update," *Neurochem Int,* 46(4):273-9; 3/2005. (Ser and NE)

Soares JC, Mann JJ, "The functional neuroanatomy of mood disorders," *J Psychiatr Res,* 31(4):393-432; 7-8/1997. (Neuroimaging most consistently shows decreased PFC metabolism and blood flow, correlating with severity, perhaps especially in older depressives. Bipolars show temporal, and perhaps other limbic abnormalities. Depressed affectives may have reduced basal ganglia metabolism and blood flow. Frontal and cerebellar abnormalities may be associated with cognitive impairment. Antidepressants, but not ECT, may reverse some of these changes.)

Stoll AL, Renshaw PF, et al, "Neuroimaging in bipolar disorder: What have we learned," *Biol Psychiat,* 48(6):505-17; 2000. (Structural imaging suggests increased hyperintensities. Lesions may reflect the illness or cardiovascular risks, which are common. Cerebellar shrinkage and anomalies can occur; less so, increased sulcal prominence.)

Starkstein SE, Boston JD, et al, "Mechanisms of mania after brain injury: 12 case reports and review of the literature," *J Nerv Ment Dis,* 176:87-100;1988.

Starksten SE, Robinson RG, "Affective disorders and cerebral vascular disease," *Br J Psychiat,* 154: 170-182; 2/1989. (30-50% of post-stroke patients develop depressions which can last a year or more. Lesions of the left frontal or basal ganglia, or prior subcortical atrophy were common. Ser and NE systems might also be involved. Social support, history, demographics and severity of impairment were only weakly associated. Mania was rare, and strongly associated with limbic-connected right hemisphere lesions, plus some predisposing factor (e.g., seizure disorder, subcortical atrophy, genetic susceptibity, perhaps, frontal dysfunction.)

Starkstein SE, Mayberg HS, et al, "Mania after brain injury: Neuroradiological and metabolic findings," *Ann Neurol,* 27(6):652-9; 6/2990. (8 patient series suggests a role for the basal right temporal lobe in secondary mania.)

Strakowski SM, Wilson DR, et al, "Stuctural brain abnormalities in first-episode mania," *Biol Psychiat,* 33:602-09; 1993a.

Strakowski SM, Woods BT, et al, "MRI subcortical signal hyperintensities in mania at first hospitalization," *Biol Psychiat,* 33(3):204-06; 1993b.

Strakowski SM, DelBello MP, et al, "Brain magnetic resonance imaging of structural abnormalities in bipolar disorder," *Arch Gen Psychiat,* 56(3): 254-60; 3/1999. (In 24 manics, structural volumes along mood-modulating pathways were altered (e.g., amygdala enlargement), though not particularly associated with state or degree of illness.)

Strakowski SM, DelBello MP, "Neuroimaging in bipolar disorder," *Bipolar Disord,* 2(3):148-64; 2000.

Strakowski SM, Adler CM, et al, "Volumetric MRI studies of mood disorders: Do they distinguish unipolar and bipolar disorder?" *Bipolar Disord,* 4(2):80-88; 4/2002.

Strakowski SM, Adler CM, et al "A preliminary FMRI study of sustained attention in euthymic, unmedicated bipolar disorder," *Neuropsychopharmacol,* 29(9): 1734-40; Sep 2004.

Strakowski SM, DelBellow MP, Adler CM, "The functional neuroanatomy of bipolar disorder: A review of neuroimaging findings," *Molec Psychiat,* 2005.

Swayze VW, Andreasen NC, et al, "Structural brain abnormalities in bipolar affective disorder. Ventricular enlargement and focal signal hyperintensities," *Arch Gen Psychiat,* 47(11): 1054-59; 11/1990. (Hyperintensities were most common in bipolars, who then trended toward larger ventricles. Enlargement was most prominent in schizophrenic males.)

Talan J, "Loss of key brain cells linked to mental illness," *Newsday,* printed in *Denver Post,* 10/22/ 1997. (Manics, impulsiveness, without regard for consequence, may be due to anterior cingulate dysfunction, dissociating emotion from anticipation of reward.)

Thomas AJ, Davis S, et al, "Elevation of cell adhesion molecule immunoreactivity in the anterior cingulate cortex in bipolar disorder," *Biol Psychiat,* 55(6):652-5; 3/15/2004.

Torrey EF, Barci BM, et al, "Neurochemical markers for schizophrenia, bipolar disorder, and major depression in postmortem brains," *Biol Psychiat,* 57(3):252-60; 2/1/2005.

Vawter MP, Freed WJ, et al, "Neuropathology of bipolar disorder," *Biol Psychiat,* 48(6):486-504; 9/15/2000.

Winsberg ME, Sachs N, et al, "Decreased dorsolateral prefrontal N-acetyl aspartate in bipolar disorder," *Biol Psychiat,* 47(6):475-81; 3/15/2000.

Yurgelun-Todd DA, Gruber SA, et al, "fMRI during affect discrimination in bipolar affective disorder," *Bipolar Disord,* 2(3 Pt 2):237-48; Sept 2000.

Appendix III: Side effects of psychiatric medications

Abramson J, *Overdosed America,* Harper Collins, 2004.

Adams, JD, Klaidman LK, et al, "Alzheimer's and Parkinson's disease: Brain levels of gluathione, glutathione disulfide, and vitamin E," *Mol Clin Neuropathol,* 14:213-226; 1991.

Adler I, Peslow E, et al, "Vitamin E in tardive dyskinesia: Effects of longer term treatment," *Am Coll Neuropsychopharmacol Abs*; 1992; p 213. (25 patients improved up though 36 wks.)

Antman EM, Stone PH, et al, "Calcium blocking agents in the treatment of cardiovascular disorders," *Ann Intern Med,* 93:873-85; 1980.

APA, "Tardive dyskinesia," *APA Task Force Report,* 1980. (Reviews reports of 40-60% incidence.)

Baldessarini RJ, "Risks of discontinuing maintenance treatments," (abstract), *Paper presented at the 149th annual meeting of the American Psychiatric Association,* NY, 5/1996. (Poor response on resuming lithium and increased need for neuroleptics.)

Borg and Cotzias, quoted in Davies 1972.

Baumel S, *Dealing with Depression Naturally,* Keats, New Canaan, CN, 1995.

Bowden CL, Rhodes LJ, "Mania in children and adolescents: Recognition and treatment," *Psychiatric Annals,* 26(7S):430-434; 1996.

Bowden CL, "Comparison of open versus blinded studies in bipolar disorder," in JF Goldberg, M Harrow, eds, *Bipolar disorders: Clinical course and outcome,* Am Psychiatric Press, DC, 1999; pp 149-70.

Braverman E, *Path Wellness Manual,* Pub for Achieving Total Health, NJ, 1994.

Breggin, PR, *Electro-Shock, Its Brain Disabling Effects,* Springer, NY, 1979.

Breggin PR, *Psychiatric Drugs: Hazards to the Brain,* Springer, NY, 1983.

Breggin PR, *Toxic Psychiatry,* St Martin's Press, NY, 1991.

Brigham PM, "The Psychopharmacology of Bipolar Disorder, Peter M Brigham, MD, updated 5-9-01." At: http://people.ne.mediaone.net/pmbrig/BP_pharm.html Accessed: 6-11-2001.

Broida, Marian, RN, *New Hope for People with Depression,* Prima, Roseville CA, 2001.

Cadet, JL, et al, "Possible involvement of free radicals in neuroleptic induced movement disorders. Evidence from treatment of tardive dyskinesia with vitamin E," *Ann NY Acad Sci,* 570:176-85, 1989.

Chakos MH, Lieberman JA, et al, "Increase in caudate nuclei volumes of first-episode schizophrenic patients taking antipsychotic drugs," *Am J Psychiat,* 151(10):1430-6, 1994.

Chouinard, as reported in *Clin Psychiat News*; 6/ 1990. (Patients on neuroleptics 15 years or more, had an almost certain risk of developing TD.)

Cohen D, Cailloux-Cohen S, l'AGIDD-SMQ, *Guide Critique des Medicaments de l'Ame,* Les Editions de l'Homme, Quebec, 1995. (TD affects 10-15% of acute, 35-40% of chronic, and 50-70% of elderly North American psychiatric patients.)

Cohen, G, "Oxy-radical toxicity in catecholamine neurons," *Neurotoxicology,* 5:77-82; 1984.

Colodny L, Hoffman, Ronald L, "Inositol: Clinical Applications for exogenous use," *Alt Med Rev,* 3(6):4323-447.

Coryell W, Solomon D, et al, "Lithium discontinuation and subsequent effectiveness," *Am J Psychiat,* 155:895-98; 1998. (Study does not confirm discontinuation refractoriness, though finds lithium benefits occured in the first 32 weeks, but semi-annual follow-ups over 5 yrs showed no advantage, with patients nonsignificantly worse than those not using lithium.)

Cousens G, *Depression Free for Life,* Quill, HarperCollins, NY, 2001.

Davies, *The Clinical Significance of the Essential Biological Metals,* Charles C Thomas, Springfield, IL, 1972.

Dawson E, in *Diseases of the Nerv Sys;* 1970.

Denicoff KD, Smith-Jackson EE, et al, "Comparative prophylactic efficacy of lithium, carbamazepine, and the combination in bipolar disorder," *J Clin Psychiat,* 58:470-78; 1997.

Deveaugh-Geiss, J, Manion L, "High dose pyridoxine in tardive dyskinesia," *J Clin Psych,* 39: 573-5, 1978. (Reduced frequency and severity of involuntary movements.)

Diler RS, Avci A, "SSRI-induced mania in obsessive-compulsive disorder," *J Am Acad Child Adolesc Psychiat,* 38(1):6-7; 1/1999.

Dilsaver SC, Greden JF, "Antidepressant with-drawal-induced activation (hypomania and mania): Mechanism and theoretical significance," *Brain Res,* 319(1):29-48; 3/1984. (Antidepressant withdrawal overactivates the cholinergic system. Eventually catecholamine activity may increase to counter this, then cholinergics, etc. Cycling may thus accelerate, and homeostatic mechanisms, deteriorate. Lithium down-regulates cholinergic receptors, and otherwise supports monoaminergic/cholinergic homeostasis.)

Dubvosky SL, Franks RD, "Intracellular calcium ions in affective disorders: A review and an hypothesis," *Biol Psychiat,* 18:781-97; 1983.

Elkashef AM, Ruskin PE, et al. At: http: //www.ncbi.nlm.nih.gov/entrez/query.fcgi?cmd=Retrieve&db=pubmed&dopt=Abstract&list_uids=1987837

Elkashef AM, et al, "Vitamin E in the treatment of tardive dyskinesia," *Am J Psychiat,* 147(4):505-6, 1990. (Suggests abundant antioxidants, plus 200 mg phosphatidyl serine, 1000 mg purified lecithin, 2000 mg flax oil, 2000 mg omega 3 fish oil, all 2x/day.)

Erasmus U, *Fats that Heal, Fats that Kill,* Alive Books, Burnaby, Canada, rev ed, 1995.

Fann WE, et al, "Deanol in tardive dyskinesia: A preliminary report," *Psychopharmacol,* 42(2); 1/ 1975. (Increases striatum Ach which is antagonistic to DA. Provides relief within 1-2 wks.)

Fieve RR, *Moodswing,* Bantam Books, 1976.

Freeman MP, Freeman SA, et al, "The comorbidity of bipolar and anxiety disorders: Prevalence, psychobiology, and treatment issues," *J Affect Disord,* 68:1-23; 2002.

Frye, Ketter, "Defining the Standard of Care Across the Bipolar Spectrum: Q & A, April 9, 2000; SF, Faculty: Mark A Frye MD, Terrence A Ketter MD," Bipolar Disorders Information Center, At: http: //www.mhsource.com/bipolar/defzarate.html Accessed: 6/11/2001.

Gant, Charles, *End Your Addiction Now,* Warner Books, 2002

Gelenberg Alan J, et al, "Choline and lecithin in the treatments of tardive dyskinesia: Preliminary results from a pilot study,"*Am J Psychiat,* 136(6): 772-6; 1979. (All 5 males improved.)

Gelenberg AJ, Kane JM, et al, "Comparison of standard and low serum levels of lithium for maintenance treatment of bipolar disorder," *NEJM,* 321:1489-93; 1989.

Gelenberg AJ, et al, "A crossover study of lecithin treatment of tardive dyskinesia," *J Clin Psychiat,* 51(4):149-53, 1990. (Double blind crossover. Minimal, but definite effect of lecithin.)

Gernaat HB, Van de Woude J, et al, "Fluoxetine and Parkinsonism in patients taking carbamazepine," *Am J Psychiat,* 148:1604-5; 1991. (Associated with moderate to severe Parkinsonian symptoms.)

Gillberg IC, Heligren L, Gillberg C, "Psychotic disorders diagnosed in adolescence: Outcome at age 30 years," *J Child Psychol Psychiat,* 34:1173-85; 1993.

Gitlin MJ, Swendsen J, et al, "Relapse and impairment in bipolar disorder," *Am J Psychiat,* 152:1635-40; 1995.

Glaser William, MD, TD Clinic, New Haven, CN. (68% developed some degree of TD after 25 years of maintenance neuroleptics.)

Gold MS, *The Good News About Depression,* Villard Books, NY, 1987

Graham DG, "Oxidative pathways for catecholamines in the genesis of neuromelanin and cytotoxic quinones," *Mol Pharmacol,* 14: 633-43; 1978.

Gross CG, "Neurogenesis in the adult brain: Death of a dogma," *Nature Rev Neurosci,* 1(2):67-73; 2000.

Gur RE, Cowell P, et al, "A follow up magnetic resonance imaging study of schizophrenia," *Arch Gen Psychiat,* 55(145):152; 1998a. (In first episode schizophrenia, larger medication doses were associated with greater reductions in frontal and temporal volume, and more neurobehavioral deterioration.)

Gur, RE, Maany V, et al, "Subcortical MRI volumes in neuroleptic-naive and treated patients with schizophrenia," *Am J Psychiat,* 155(12):177-1717; 1998b.

Gutton, Michael, et al, *J Psychiat,* 4/1989.

Hawkins D, "Treatment of Schizophrenia," in D Hawkins, L Pauling, eds, *Orthomolecular Psychiatry,* WH Freeman and Co, SF, 1973.

Hawkins D, "Prevention of tardive dyskinesia with high vitamin doses: A study of 58,000," *J Orthomol Med,* 1(1):24-6; 1986.

Hawkins D, "Successful prevention of tardive dyskinesia," *J Orthomol Med,* 4(1):35-36; 1989.

Healy D, Medicines and Healthcare Products Regulatory Authority, Department of Psychological Medicine, North Wales, 2003. At: http://www.drugawareness,org/Archives/3rd Qtr_2004/record0003.html and record0012.html (FDA found in 2-3% of cases, antidepressants raised risk of suicidal thoughts or actions. Even healthy volunteers became aggressive, hostile.)

Hoffer A, "A tardive dyskinesia treated with manganese," letter, *Can Med Assn J,* 117(8):859, 1977. (Nursing home in Vancouver, using Mn, etc, where tardive dyskinesia is no longer problem.)

Hoffer A, *Orthomolecular Medicine for Physicians,* Keats, New Canaan, CN, 1983a.

Hoffer A, "Nutrition and behavior," in J Bland, ed, *Medical Applications of Clinical Nutrition,* Keats, New Canaan, CN, 1983b.

Hoffer A, "Editorial, Toxic: vitamins," International bulletin board for orthomolecular medicine (IBBOM) At: www.orthoeurope.com/IBBOM/index.php Accessed: 1/22/2004.

Jackson IV, et al, "Treatment of tardive dyskinesia with lecithin," *Am J Psychiat,* 136(11):1458-60, 1979. (Double blind crossover. 6 patients, all improved.)

Jackson IV, et al "Lecithin administration in tardive dyskinesia: Clinical and medical correlates," *Biol Psychiat,* 16:85, 1981. (Double blind crossover.)

Jenner, P, "Oxidative damage in neurodegenerative disease," *Lancet,* 9/17/1994; pp 796-98.

Joffe RT, Post RM, et al, "Hematological effects of carbamazepine in patients with affective illness," *Am J Psychiat,* 142(10):1196-99; 10/1985.

Kaufman KR, Gerner R, "Lamotrigine toxicity secondary to sertraline," *Seizure,* 7:163-5; 1998.

Ketter TA, Kimbrell TA, et al, "Effects of mood and subtype on cerebral glucose metabolism in treatment-resistant bipolar disorder," *Biol Psychiat,* 49(2):97-109; 1/15/2001.

Ketter TA, Bipolar Disorders Information Center, http://www.mhsource.com/bipolar/defketter.html Accessed: 6/11/2001.

Kidd, PM, "Bipolar disorder as cell membrane dysfunction. Progress toward integrative management," *Alt Med Rev,* 9(2):107-35; 2004.

Koczerginski D, Kennedy SH, et al, "Clonazepam and lithium — A toxic combination in the treatment of mania?" *Intl Clin Psychopharmacol,* 4:195-9; 1989.

Kruesi, Oscar Rogers, MD, interview with author, February, 1996.

Kukopulos A, Reginaldi D, et al, "The long term prophylaxis of affective disorders," *Adv Biochem Psychopharmacol,* 49:127-47; 1995. (11/129 may have developed tolerance, or discontinuation refractoriness.)

Kunin RA, "Manganese and niacin in the treatment of drug induced dyskinesias," *J Orthomolecular Psych,* 5(1): 4-27, 1976. (14/15 pts. responded to Mn alone or Mn plus niacin, often with striking improvement.)

Lancet "Neuroleptics in progressive structural brain abnormalities in psychiatric illness," (Research letters), 352(9130)784; 1998. (Computerized tomography before initial neuroleptic treatment and five years later suggests risk of atrophy increases 4-6% for each 10 gm neuroleptics. Frontal atrophy was unrelated to diagnosis.)

Larson, JM, *Depression Free, Naturally,* Fawcett Columbine, 1997.

Larson, Joan Matthews, PhD, interview with author, June 9, 2008.

LemmoW, "Mental health care: Under the microscope" At: www.lemmo.com/mental.html#microscope Accessed: 2003.

Lerner V, Miodownik C, "Vitamin B6 treatment for tardive dyskinesia: A randomized, double-blind, placebo-controlled, crossover study, *J Clin Psychiat,* 68(11):1648-54; 2007. (50 schizoaffectives or schizophrenics received 1200 mg B6/day, or placebo. The B6 group showed statistically significant improvements in all measures, vs. controls.)

Lesser M, *Nutrition & Vitamin Therapy,* Bantam Books, NY, 1983.

Leverich GS, Post M, Frye MA, unpub data, 1998, cited in Post 1999. (Efficacy lost after an average of 2.8 years in 45% of severely ill patients)

Lohr, JB, et al, "Alpha tocopherol in tardive dyskinesia," letter, *Lancet,* 1:913-4; 1987. (15 patients, mean 43% improvement.)

Lohr JB, Cadet, JL, et al, "Vit E in treatment of tardive dyskinesia: The possible involvement of free radical mechanisms," *Schiz Bull,* 14:291-6, 1988. (Double blind crossover. 13/15 patients with moderate TD were started on 400 IU, increased to 1200 IU after 4 wks. Symptoms reduced almost 50%.)

Lohr, JB, Browning, JA, "Free radical involvement in neuropsychiatric illnesses," *Psychopharmacol Bull,* 31:159-65; 1995.

Maj M, Piozzi R, Kemali D, "Long term outcome of lithium prophylaxis in patients initially classified as complete responders," *Psychopharmacol (Berl.),* 98: 535-38; 1989. (Breakthrough episodes after 2 yrs in a substantial number of initially lithium-responsive and remitted patients. Similarly for another 5 yrs.)

Millett K, *The Loony Bin Trip,* Simon & Schuster, NY, 1990.

Moller HJ, Nasrallah HA, "Treatment of bipolar disorder," *J Clin Psychiat,* 64:9-17; 2003.

Moore NC, Lerer B, et al, "Three cases of carbamazepine toxicity," *Am J Psychiat,* 142(8): 974-75; 8/1985. (Hepatitis, fatal aplastic anemia, severe skin reaction.)

Moore DT, "A holistic approach for treating manic depressive disorders," 1998. At: familyclinic.simplenet.com/bipolar/bipaper.html (The same dose rarely maintains effectiveness. Multiple adjustments are required.)

Nair N, "Drug therapy of schizophrenias in the community," *J Orthomol Psychiat,* 6(4):348-53; 1977.

Nasrallah HA, Kuo I, "Side effects in the treatment of bipolar affective disorder," *Medscape Psychiat Ment Health,* 8/29/2003.

Nasrallah HA, et al, "Variable clinical response to choline in tardive dyskinesia," *Psychol Med,* 1493: 697-700; 1984. (Double blind crossover. 7/11 partial or minimal improvement, 2 worse.)

Nilddon, S, Hottonin, D.F, et al, "Essential fatty acids and abnormal involuntary movements in the general male population: A study of men born in 1933," *Prostaglandins Leukot Essent Fatty Acids,* 55(1 & 2): 83-87; 7-8/1996. (Neuroleptics and cigarettes (and perhaps, impaired LA to AA metabolism) associated with dyskinesia, free radical formation, and lipid peroxidation.)

Nielsen EB, Lyon M, "Evidence for cell loss in corpus striatum after long-term treatment with a neuroleptic drug (flupenthixol) in rats," *Psychopharmacol,* 59 85-89; 1978. (10% cell loss. Chronic intake may cause irreversible anatomical changes.")

O'Connell RA, Mayo JA, et al, "Outcome of bipolar disorder on long-term treatment with lithium ," *Br J Psychiat,* 159:123-29; 1991.

Page Linda Rector, ND, PhD, interview with author, October, 1994.

Paulsen JS, Heaton RK, et al, "Neuropsychological impairment in tardive dyskinesia," *Neuropsychol,* 8(2):227-41; 1994. (Review. The worse the TD, the more the neuropsychological impairment, with both perhaps due to brain alterations.)

Pfeiffer CC, *Nutrition and Mental Illness,* Healing Arts Press, Rochester, VT, 1987.

Pfeiffer CC, *The Schizophrenias Ours to Conquer,* rev ed, Bio-Communications Press, Wichita, KS, 1988.

Post RM, Leverich GS, et al, "Carbamazepine prophylaxis in refractory affective disorders: A focus on long-term follow-up, *J Clin Psychopharmacol,* 10:318-27; 1990.

Post RM, "Transduction of psychosocial stress into the neurobiology of recurrent affective disorder," *Am J Psychiat,* 149:999-1010; 1992.

Post RM, Ketter TA, et al, "Assessment of anticonvulsant drugs in patients with bipolar affective illness," in I Hindmarch, PD Stonier, eds, *Human Psychopharmacology Methods and Measures,* vol 4, Wiley, Chichester, England, 1993a; pp 71-84.

Post RM, Leverich GS, et al, " Lithium tolerance and discontinuation as pathways to refractoriness," in NJ Birch, C Padgham, MS Hughes, eds, *Lithium in Medicine and Biology,* Marius Press, Lancashire, England, UK, 1993b; pp 72-84. (34.8% of 66 patients developed tolerance over long term prophylaxis.)

Post RM, Weiss SRB, "The neurobiology of treatment-resistant mood disorders," in FE Bloom, DJ Kupger, eds, *Psychopharmacology: The Fourth Generation of Progress,* Raven Press, NY, 1995; pp 1155-1170.

Post 1996 unpub data cited in Post 1999. (*40.7%* of 27 responders developed tolerance to carbamazepine after an average of 3.6 years.)

Post RM, Denicoff KD, et al, "Long-term outcome of anticonvulsants in affective disorders," in JE Goldberg, M Harrow eds, *Bipolar Disorders: Clinical Course and Outcome,* Am Psychiatric Press, Inc, DC, 1999.

Post RM, Leverich GS, "A re-evaluation of the role of antidepressants in the treatment of bipolar depression: Data from the Stanley Foundation bipolar Network," *Bipolar Disorders,* 5(6):396; 12/2003. (Antidepressant augmentation created modest response. About 18% switched to hypomania or mania. Of the 15-20% who remained well on antidepressants for over 2 mo, depression recurred in about 35% by 1 yr.)

Pozo P, Alcantara AG, "Mania-like syndrome in a patient with chronic schizophrenia during olanzapine treatment," *J Psychiat Neurosci,* 23(5): 309-10; 11/1998.

Plyushch L, Press conference reported in *US News & World Report,* 2/16/1976.

Psychiat News, "Lithium and memory loss," 12/5/1986.

Reeves RR, McBride WA, "Olanzapine-induced mania," *J Am Osteopath Assoc,* 98(10):549-50; 10/1998.

Richman DL, *Dr. Caligari's Psychiatric Drugs,* Network Against Psychiatric Assault, Berkeley, 3rd ed. with add, 1987; 1992 update.

Rudra P, "A review of hemiologic side effects of

lithium," *Hosp Community Psychiat,* 36:127-8; 1985.

Sachdev P, Hume F, et al, [Negative symptoms, cognitive dysfunction, tardive akathisia and tardive dyskinesia], *Acta Psychiatr Scand,* 93(6):451-59; 1996. (Review. Many studies, including this one, relate TD to cognitive deficits. None exclude it. This study found a stronger link with tardive akathisia. Cognitive deficits can also occur with other movement disorders.)

Sachs G, Printz DJ, et al, "Expert Consensus Guideline Series: Medication, Treatment of Bipolar Disorder, 2000," At: www.psychguides.com

Salama AA, Shafey M, "A case of severe lithium toxicity induced by combined fluoxetine and lithium carbonate," *Am J Psychiat,* 146:278; 1989.

Saltz BL, Werner MG, "Prospective study of tardive dyskinesia incidence in the elderly," *JAMA,* 226: 2402-6; 1991.

Sarantidis D, Waters B, "Predictors of lithium prophylaxis effectiveness," *Prog Neuropsychopharmacol,* 5:507-10; 1981.

Schatzberg A, Cole J, *Manual of Clinical Psychopharmacol,* Am Psych Press, 1986. (3-4% increased likelihood per year of use. Occurs in 50-60% of chronic institutionalized patients.)

Sovner R, Davis JM, "A potential drug interaction between fluoxetine and valproic acid," *J Clin Psychopharmacol,* 11:389; 1991.

Sovner, Robert, pamphlet for Sandoz, 1986. (Up to 56% of chronic patients.)

Swann AC, Bowden CL, et al, "Mania: Clinical and biological predictors of outcome," *ACNP Scientific Abstracts,* 1997, p252. (The greater the illness and prior episodes, the more likely the patient will be nonresponsive to lithium.)

Steiner W, Laporta M, Chouinard G, "Neuroleptic-induced supersenstivity psychosis in patients with bipolar affective disorder," *Acta Psychiatr Scand,* 81(5): 437-40; 5/1990. (5 case reports.)

Sterling P, "U.S. neuroscience: Psychiatry's drug addiction," *New Republic,* 12/9/1979, p 17.

Stoll AL, Severus WE, "Mood stabilizers: Shared mechanisms of action at postsynaptic signal-transduction and kindling processes," *Harv Rev Psychiat,* 4(2):77-89; 1996. (Literature review.)

Stoll AL, Locke CA, et al, "Omega-3 fatty acids and bipolar disorder: A review," *Prostaglandins Leukot Essent Fatty Acids,* 60:329-37; 1999b.

Stoll AL, *The Omega-3 Connection,* Simon & Schuster, NY, 2002.

Teicher M, McLean Hospital, MA, 1990. (6 patients developed "intense, violent, suicidal thoughts" after taking fluoxetine.)

Tkacz C, "A preventive measure for tardive dyskinesia," *J Intl Acad Preventive Med,* 8(5):5-8, 1984. (Not one case in 10,000 outpatients and 1,000 inpatients receiving nutrient-based treatments.)

Trimble MR, "Anticonvulsant-induced psychiatric disorders. The role of forced normalization," *Drug Saf,* 15(3):159-66; 9/1996.

Vaddadi, K.S, et al, "A double blind trial of essential fatty acid supplementation in patients with tardive dyskinesia," *Psychiat Res,* 27(3):313-23, 1989. (Membrane omega 3 correlated inversely with the severity of the dyskinesia.)

Vaddadi, K, "Dyskinesias and their treatment with essential fatty acids: A review," *Prostaglandins Leukot Essent Fatty Acids,* 55(1-2):89-94; 7-8/1996.

Waddington JL, Youssef HA, "Cognitive dysfunction in chronic schizophrenia followed prospectively over 10 years and its longitudinal relationship to the emergence of tardive dyskinesia," *Psychol Med,* 26:681-688; 1996. (Onset of orofacial dyskinesia was associated with cognitive deterioration.)

Walsh, WJ, "Commentary on nutritional treatment of mental disorders," *International Guide to the World of Alternative Mental Health.* At: www.alternativementalhealth.com/articles.walshMP.htm#Py Accessed:10/08/2006.

Walsh, William J, PhD, interview with author, November, 2007.

Watkins, Lana, OPHD, Psychosomatic Society, Denver 3/4/2006. (Antidepressants increased risk of cardiovascular fatality 55%.)

Werbach MR, *Nutritional Influences on Mental Illness,* Third Line Press, Tarzana, CA, 1991. (Uncontrolled trials show improvement with niacin, B6, E, Mn, tryptophan. Small double blind crossovers support use of phosphatidyl choline.)

Weiss SRB, Clark M, et al, "Contingent tolerance to the anticonvulsant effects of carbamazepine: Relationship to loss of endogenous adaptive mechanisms," *Brain Res Rev,* 20:305-325; 1995. (Tolerance in animals was associated with failure of seizure-related adaptions, such as increased TRH and GABA receptors.)

Werry JS, McClellan JM, et al, "Childhood and adolescent schizophrenic, bipolar, and schizoaffective disorders: A clinical and outcome study," *J Am Acad Child Adolesc Psychiat,* 30: 457-65; 1991.

Whybrow PC, *A Mood Apart, Depression, Mania, and Other Afflictions of the Self,* Basic Books, HarperCollins, NY, 1997.

Yahr MD, et al, "Reversal of L-dopa effects in Parkinsonism," *Trans Am Neurol Assoc,* 95:81-5, 1969.

Zaslove M, Silverio T, et al, "Severe riboflavin deficiency: A previously undescribed side effect of phenothiazines," *J Orthomol Psychiat,* 12(2): 111-112; 1983.

Appendix IV: Biochemical tests

Bland J, *The 20-Day Rejuvenation Diet Program,* Keats, New Canaan, CN, 1997.

Braverman E, Path Wellness Manual, Publications for Achieving Total Health, Princeton, NJ, 1994.

Carl C. Pfeiffer Institute, tests given at the Princeton Bio Center Laboratory, Princeton, NJ.

Cutler A, "Amalgam Illness: Diagnosis and Treatment of Mercury Poisoning." At: home.earthlink.net/~moriam/ANDY_INDEX.html And: onibasu.com/archives/am/552.html & am/520.html Accessed: 2007

Gardner ER, Hall RCW, "Medical screening of psychiatric patients," *J Orthomol Psychiat;* 9(3): 207-15; 1981.

Gilasson S, *Nutritional Therapies Featuring the Core Program for Diet Revision,* Persona, Winnepeg, Manitoba, Canada, 1991.

Gold MS, *The Good News About Depression,* Villard Books NY, 1987.

Graham B, "Laboratory testing for schizophrenia and bipolar disorder," At: nutritional-healing.com.au/content/articles Accessed 3/2008. (Allergies, GI microbes, red cell fatty acids, hair minerals, serum copper and ceruloplasmin, urinary pyrroles.)

Jaffe R, Kruesi OR, "The biochemical-immunology window: A molecular view of psychiatric case management," *J App Nutr,* 44(2); 1992.

Larson JM, *Depression Free, Naturally,* Ballantine Wellspring, NY, 2001.

Lesser, Michael, MD, interview with author, August 2008.

Murray MT, Pizzorno J, *The Encyclopedia of Natural Medicine,* Prima, Rocklin, CA, 1998.

Pfeiffer CC, "Psychiatric hospital vs. Brain Bio Center in diagnosis of biochemical imbalances," *J Orthomol Psychiat,* 5(1); 1976.

Pfeiffer CC, *The Schizophrenias Ours to Conquer,* Bio-Communications Press, Wichita, KS, 1988.

Taylor RL, *Mind or Body: Distinguishing Psychological from Organic Disorders,* McGraw-Hill, NY, 1982.

Walsh WJ, "A biological basis for neurologic disorders: autism, hyperactivity, attention deficit disorder,depression, obsessive-compulsive disorder, Tourette's syndrome, and violence, An interview with William J Walsh, PhD," *Latitudes,* 5(2):1-8, 2002. At: www.Latitudes.org

Walsh WJ, "Metal metabolism and human function," At: www.hriptc.org/metal_metabolism.html Accessed: 12/2004

Walsh WJ, "Zinc deficiency, metal metabolism, and behavior disorders," At: hriptc.org/zinc_deficiency.html Accessed: 12/2004.

Walsh, WJ, "Commentary on nutritional treatment of mental disorders," *International Guide to the World of Alternative Mental Health.* At: www.alternativementalhealth.com/articles.walshMP.htm#Py Accessed:10/08/2006.

Walsh, William J, PhD, interview with author, November, 2007.

Watts D, "Trace elements and neuropsychological problems as reflected in tissue mineral analysis (TMA) patterns," *J Orthomol Med,* 5(3):159-66; 1990.

Werbach, MR, *Nutritional Influences on Illness,* 2nd ed, Third Line Press, Tarzana, CA, 1993.

To order

Natural Healing *for* Bipolar Disorder: Send $39^{95} plus $5^{00} shipping

Natural Healing *for* Schizophrenia: Send $29^{95} plus $4^{00} shipping

Check or money order only. Inquire for discounts on multiple copies.
For out-of-country orders, write checks in US dollars, drawn on a US bank.

To: **Borage Books, 3003 West 11th Ave, #144, Eugene, OR 97402**
Or call: **(541) 683-8720**
Or email: **msgs@boragebooks.com**

Call for our most recent contact info. Or visit our website at: **www.boragebooks.com**

The author is available for educational workshops, seminars, interviews, & media presentations.
She welcomes any comments, questions, experiences, additions, criticisms, etc.
sent c/o Borage Books at the above addresses.

Natural Healing *for* Schizophrenia & Other Common Mental Disorders

"Edelman has provided a superb, detailed account of orthomolecular treatment... the best treatment of schizophrenia which is available today."

Abram Hoffer MD, PhD,
Father of orthomolecular medicine

"An invaluable resource for every family afflicted by not only schizophrenia, but any mental illness...This book enlightens us all in the medical professional, and will give great hope and comfort to families."

Oscar Rogers Kruesi, MD, FACP
New Health Initiatives, Morristown Memorial Hospital

"A magnificent and needed contribution to the field of mental health... Both a scholarly text and a practical guidebook. Well-organized, clearly written, and comprehensive in scope, it will without doubt change the lives of suffers and familities with mental illness... a superb work, a beacon of hope."

Ralph Golan, MD
Author, *Optimal Wellness*

"Could qualify as a textbook which should be required reading for every mental health professional."

Hugh D Riordan MD
Center for Improvement of Human Functioning, International

"A much-needed, immensely readable guide to nutitional... treatment of schizophrenia."

Roberta Foss Morgan, DO
Carl C Pfeiffer Institute, Princeton, NJ

Index